Essentials of Cemented Knee Arthroplasty

Erik Hansen • Klaus-Dieter Kühn
Editors

Essentials of Cemented Knee Arthroplasty

With forewords from Michael D. Ries (University of California, San Francisco) and Patrick Sadoghi (Medical University of Graz, Austria)

Springer

Editors
Erik Hansen
Department of Orthopaedic Surgery
University of California San Francisco UCSF
San Francisco, CA
USA

Klaus-Dieter Kühn
Department of Orthopedic Surgery
Medical University of Graz
Graz, Austria

ISBN 978-3-662-63112-6 ISBN 978-3-662-63113-3 (eBook)
https://doi.org/10.1007/978-3-662-63113-3

Cover illustration © Left figure: Hansen E., Kühn K.D. Essentials of cemented Knee Arthroplasty (2022). Chapter 28 Zaid M.B., Vail T.P. Posterior Stabilized Total Knee Arthroplasty. Fig. 28.2 left / Right figure © Heraeus Medical GmbH.

This Springer imprint is published by the registered company Springer-Verlag GmbH, DE part of Springer Nature.
The registered company address is: Heidelberger Platz 3, 14197 Berlin, Germany

Foreword

The final surgical treatment of end-stage osteoarthritis (OA) of the knee joint is total knee arthroplasty (TKA), with over 1 million cases performed annually worldwide, including over 15.000 cases per year in Austria, and more than 350 of these implanted by the Division of Knee Surgery at the Department of Orthopaedics and Trauma at the Medical University of Graz.

Contemporary TKA has substantially evolved over the past 130 years, since the first prosthesis was implanted early in 1890 by Themistocles Gluck in a 17-year-old female suffering from a tuberculous knee joint. The prosthesis was made of ivory in a hinged design as Gluck was the first surgeon who additionally experimented with bone cement including copper amalgam, plaster of Paris, and stone putty, which hardened rapidly after mixing. Whilst many of Gluck´s devices ultimately failed because of chronic infection, we have to admit that today, 130 years later, we still face the same obstacles, namely the best materials producing the lowest wear, the ideal alignment and biomechanics, the cementation technique (Gluck favoured osseointegration although his implants could be well fixed with "cement" alone), and the treatment of early or late infection after TKA.

130 years later, we still face equal challenges such as revision surgery after failed TKA (Gluck´s ivory prosthesis had to be removed), the adequate management of postoperative complications (some of his cases ended in fistula formation), selection of the ideal patient for surgery (Gluck already recognized outcome of surgeries after previous infections) and improvement of rehabilitation or even fast-track approaches. All these aspects are still in the focus of research worldwide, and various projects are currently performed at our department in Graz, Austria.

In addition, various new technologies emerged over the past decades, such as robotics, patient-specific instrumentation, preoperative planning and computer-assisted surgery, which had significant impact with respect to accuracy and reproducibility of our results as knee surgeons. However, various level II studies performed at our own institution did not reveal significant clinical benefits for our patients operated on by high-volume surgeons and have, therefore, not been implemented in our daily practice.

In 2020, our approach in Graz consisted of systematic preoperative and postoperative patients´ assessment (including 100% of the assessed patients in level IV studies and approx. 75% of the assessed patients in level II studies); a totally cemented, fixed TKA design using a cobalt-chromium-molybdenum (CoCrMo) alloy with or without titanium-nitride coating; surgical helmet systems; an extension gap first technique with conventional (mechanical) or kinematic alignment; and patient-specific instrumentation in case of intramedullary pathologies.

We can be excited regarding the future of TKA and I sincerely hope that this book feeds your interest on this ongoing scientific field.

Patrick Sadoghi
Medical University of Graz
Graz, Austria

Foreword

It is with great pleasure that I write the foreword to *Essentials of Cemented Knee Arthroplasty*, edited by Erik Hansen and Klaus-Dieter Kühn. The US and European editors have done a remarkable job of assembling international experts in the field to contribute timely and well-written chapters on a topic which is considered the "gold standard" for total knee arthroplasty, but has evolved and developed over the past 50 years.

Cemented total knee arthroplasty remains one of the most clinically successful, cost-effective treatments for degenerative or inflammatory arthritis of the knee. It is anticipated that the volume of procedures performed in the coming decades will grow significantly. However, even a small proportion of replacements which do not meet expectations suggest that there is still room for improvement in the outcome of this procedure for a substantial number of patients.

Essentials of Cemented Knee Arthroplasty is a very comprehensive "one-stop-shop" book. It includes separate parts dedicated to surgical indications, surgical techniques, clinical outcomes, partial and total knee implant options, implant design, and PMMA. It goes further to discuss complications and management of failed total knee arthroplasty. Other topics covering healthcare economics and new technology which may influence the future role of total knee arthroplasty have been included. In short, there are few texts which are as all-encompassing and written by such a collection of international experts.

There is a strong focus on the subject of polymethylmethacrylate (PMMA) with many chapters highlighting tips and tricks of using bone cement during surgery. There are also numerous chapters dedicated to related topics, including the pros and cons of antibiotic-loaded bone cement (ALBC), antibiotic cement spacers for treatment of periprosthetic joint infection, and use of bone cement in revision total knee arthroplasty.

While there are many textbooks focused on knee arthroplasty, what makes this textbook really standout is the compilation of international authors and perspectives on the subject matter of knee arthroplasty. A quick preview of the Table of Contents reveals novel contributions from international experts from all the major continents. These varied perspectives add depth to the subject matter and makes the messages all the more "universal".

Michael D. Ries
University of California, San Francisco
San Francisco, CA, USA

Preface

Who would've or could've imagined how different the world would be when we first embarked on this project over a year ago? Upon reflection, a couple of things truly stand out to me. For one, the COVID pandemic has reinforced that *we are truly an interconnected global community*, whether it be in relation to the spread of the virus or, more importantly, the concerted international effort to develop effective treatment strategies including vaccines. Parallels can be drawn with the scope of this textbook. We set out to draw together the world experts in the field of knee arthroplasty, both because we saw value in including the varied perspectives of individual authors from all the major continents, but we also wanted a text that was relevant to the practice of knee replacement surgery throughout the globe.

Additionally, the last several months have only reinforced the importance of *reliance on sound science and an evidence-based approach rather than personal opinion*. Each of the chapters included in this textbook is heavily referenced with the most relevant, recent literature to ensure that the readers are provided accurate up-to-date information. As with the development of any novel therapeutics to prevent or treat the Corona virus, there will undoubtedly be varied approaches and strategies. Similarly, in the field of knee arthroplasty, there are numerous philosophical differences in surgical techniques and optimal implant design, and we wanted to be inclusive of these important differences. We included a part on healthcare economics to recognize that the practice of medicine cannot be divorced from the larger issues of access, geographical differences, and increasingly constrained healthcare resources. There is also a novel part on databases to highlight both national and international trends in the utilization of knee arthroplasty, as well as provide macro-level data to complement other more commonly used research methodologies. We also believed that incorporating a part on the use of technology in the field of arthroplasty was timely and relevant, as it is clear that the field is heading towards greater adoption of innovative technological solutions for many current unsolved problems.

In closing, I want to express my deepest gratitude to my co-editor Professor Kühn, Barbara Krampitz (the heart and soul of the book), as well as all of the individual authors who graciously contributed to this textbook. Despite COVID-19's disruption to family life, our clinical practices, and social norms in general, you all demonstrated remarkable resilience and an unwavering commitment to furthering knowledge in the field of arthroplasty when you were being simultaneously pulled in numerous disparate directions. I have been heartened by this international collaborative effort and am hopeful that the same spirit will get us through this current pandemic.

Humbly and respectfully,
Erik Hansen, MD
University of California, San Francisco

Erik Hansen
San Francisco, CA, USA

Acknowledgment

First of all, I wish to extend my very special thanks to Dr. Barbara Krampitz for the arduous work associated with the making of this book, especially for all organizing steps with Erik, contributors, Springer, colleagues, computer specialists, and translators.

Naturally, my special thanks go to all contributors worldwide for providing their exceptional expertise and knowledge.

I also owe great thanks to Doctor E. Hansen (University of San Francisco (UCFS); California USA) for his reliable and exceptional cooperation. Erik has supervised most authors from the USA with greatest professionalism, and our constructive exchange has been decisive for the success of this book.

Furthermore, I would like to extend my thanks to all who provided scientific help and fruitful discussions, in particular Christof Berberich, who contributed two chapters (ALBC – discussing fear of resistance; infection risk-adjusted antibiotic prophylaxis strategies in arthroplasty – low-dose single vs. high-dose dual ALBC) and provided thoughts on the initial table of contents which gave momentum to the book design. I would also like to thank Lothar Kiontke who provided loads of inspiration as well.

The motivated willingness of Dr. E. Lieb to support this extensive book in every phase of its creation and flexibility besides writing her doctoral thesis was amazing. She deserves extraordinary thanks. In addition, she has contributed significantly to the article Collaboration with Professor Dr. Morlock, University of Hamburg.

Since the book includes various contributions from many different countries, it was often necessary to contact the authors directly. This would not have been possible without B. Webb (USA), Dr. E. Lieb (F), A. Peyer (SA), M. Zaijer (B, NL), R. Gossens (B), S. Tye (AUS), Dr. C. Berberich (S), L. Kiontke (USA), S. Chua (SG), T. Furokawa, C. Hirai, and Y. Sasaki (J), Dr. B. Krampitz (ETH), and I. Martinez Kardeskog (S). A book of such scope requires the critical review of impartial experts. The main participants we would like to thank are: S. Ubong, P. Vidal, B. Webb, N. Pezic, C. Abt, D. Kratzmeier, A. Mensendieck, Dr. A. Holl, and O. Vornkahl.

For the correspondence and translation from Japanese, we thank V. Aue (► www.alealibris.de) (independent translator Japanese–English/Japanese–German) and Dr. H. Dürr (LahnPharma) (translation from German to English).

Furthermore, I would like to thank M. Zimni for the creation of the book cover and other graphics, and A. Lenzen, D. Kraplow, and Y. Bell of Springer for managing the publication of the book.

As a freelance editor, Karin Dembowsky has devotedly edited the book, checked it for conclusiveness, and put the finishing touches on it.

The support of the IT department was invaluable. J. Matuliauskas was always on hand to manage the valuable articles, illustrations, and tables.

Last but not least, I would like to thank Professor Patrick Sadoghi (Medical University of Graz) for writing a foreword. He emphasizes the relevance of such a book from the current research approaches of the Medical University Hospital of Graz, Austria. I also would like to thank Professor Andreas Leithner (Medical University of Graz, Head and Chair of the Department of Orthopedic Surgery) for the opportunity and freedom to create the present book.

Klaus-Dieter Kühn
Medical University of Graz
Graz, Austria

Contents

IV Treatment

V Clinical Care Pathways

VI Implant Design

IX Cementing Technique

X Complications

XI Management – Revision

Contributors

Matthew P. Abdel Department of Orthopaedic Surgery, Mayo Clinic, Rochester, MN, USA
abdel.matthew@mayo.edu

Abdullah Aftab Department of Orthopedics, Hospital for Special Surgery, New York, NY, USA
AftabA@hss.edu

Vignesh K. Alamanda, MD OrthoVirginia, Reston, VA, USA

Sachin Allahabadi San Francisco Department of Orthopaedic Surgery, University of California, San Francisco, CA, USA
Sachin.Allahabadi@ucsf.edu

Derek F. Amanatullah Department of Orthopaedic Surgery, Stanford Medicine, Redwood City, CA, USA
dfa@stanford.edu

Kenoma Anighoro Department of Surgery and Perioperative Care, Dell Medical School at The University of Texas at Austin, Austin, TX, USA
kenoma.anighoro@austin.utexas.edu

Jean-Noël Argenson Service de Chirurgie Orthopedique, Aix-Marseille University, Hospital Sainte-Marguerite, Marseille, France
jean-noel.argenson@ap-hm.fr

Jaymeson R. Arthur Department of Orthopedic Surgery, Mayo Clinic Arizona, Phoenix, AZ, USA
arthur.jay@mayo.edu

Michael P. Ast Hospital for Special Surgery, Department of Orthopaedic Surgery, New York, NY, USA
astm@hss.edu

Matthew S. Austin The Rothman Institute, Thomas Jefferson University Hospital, Philadelphia, PA, USA
matt.austin@rothmanortho.com

Samik Banerjee Department of Orthopaedic Surgery, Rothman Institute/Thomas Jefferson University Hospital, Philadelphia, PA, USA
samik.banerjee@rothmanortho.com

Ankit Bansal Orthopedic Centers of Colorado, Denver, CO, USA

Jeffrey Barry Department of Orthopaedic Surgery, University of California, San Francisco, CA, USA
jeff.barry@ucsf.edu

Christof Berberich Medical Training, Heraeus Medical GmbH, Wehrheim, Germany
christof.berberich@heraeus.com

Keith R. Berend JIS Orthopedics, New Albany, OH, USA
BerendKR@jisortho.com

Christie Bergerson Exponent, Inc., Philadelphia, PA, USA
cbergerson@exponent.com

Stefano A. Bini Department of Orthopaedic Surgery, University of California, San Francisco, San Francisco, CA, USA
stefano.bini@ucsf.edu

Michael P. Bolognesi Hospital South, Orange Zone, Duke University Medical Center, Durham, NC, USA
michael.bolognesi@duke.edu

Krit Boontanapibul Chulabhorn International College of Medicine, Department of Orthopaedics, Thammasat University, Pathum Thani, Thailand

Kevin J. Bozic Department of Surgery and Perioperative Care, Dell Medical School at The University of Texas at Austin, Austin, TX, USA
kevin.bozic@austin.utexas.edu

Daniel N. Bracey Colorado Joint Replacement, Denver, CO, USA

James A. Browne Department of Orthopaedic Surgery, University of Virginia, Charlottesville, VA, USA
Jab8hd@hscmail.mcc.Virginia.edu

Scot Brown Department of Orthopaedic Surgery, Rothman Institute/Thomas Jefferson University Hospital, Philadelphia, PA, USA
scot.brown@rothmanortho.com

Brian P. Chalmers Department of Orthopedic Surgery, Adult Reconstruction and Joint Replacement, Hospital for Special Surgery, New York, NY, USA
chalmersb@hss.edu

J. Parker Chapman Department of Orthopedic Surgery, University of Florida College of Medicine, Gainesville, FL, USA
chapmjp@ortho.ufl.edu

Antonia F. Chen Department of Orthopedic Surgery, Brigham and Women's Hospital, Boston, MA, USA
afchen@bwh.harvard.edu

Darwin Chen Department of Orthopedic Surgery, The Mount Sinai Hospital, New York, NY, USA
darwin.chen@mountsinai.org

Jimmy Chow Orthopedic Institute of the West, Department of Orthopaedic Surgery, Phoenix, AZ, USA
jimmy@ChowHipandKnee.com

Zachary K. Christopher Department of Orthopedic Surgery, Mayo Clinic Arizona, Phoenix, AZ, USA
christopher.zachary@mayo.edu

Kyle H. Cichos Department of Orthopaedic Surgery, University of Alabama at Birmingham, Birmingham, AL, USA
kcichos@uab.edu

Samuel J. Clarkson Rothman Orthopaedic Institute, Thomas Jefferson University, Philadelphia, PA, USA
samuel.clarkson@rothmanortho.com

H. John Cooper Department of Orthopedic Surgery, Columbia University Irving Medical Center, New York, NY, USA
hjc2008@cumc.columbia.edu

P. Maxwell Courtney Department of Orthopaedic Surgery, Rothman Institute/Thomas Jefferson University Hospital, Philadelphia, PA, USA
paul.courtney@rothmaninstitute.com

Jonathan Dattilo Anderson Orthopaedic Research Institute, Department of Orthopaedic Surgery, Alexandria, VA, USA

Douglas A. Dennis Colorado Joint Replacement, Denver, CO, USA
ddennis@colaradojoint.com

Steven D. Donohoe Department of Orthopedics, Southern California Permanente Group, Panorama City, CA, USA

Sarah Fischer Institute of Biomechanics, TUHH Hamburg University of Technology, Hamburg, Germany
Sarah.Fischer.1@TUHH.de

Simon Garceau Department of Orthopaedic Surgery, NYU Langone Health, NYU Langone Orthopedic Hospital, New York, NY, USA

Elie S. Ghanem Department of Orthopaedic Surgery, University of Alabama at Birmingham, Birmingham, AL, USA
eghanem@uab.edu

Emmanuel Gibon Department of Orthopedic Surgery, University of Florida College of Medicine, Gainesville, FL, USA
gibonef@ortho.ufl.edu

Jeremy Gililland Department of Orthopedics, University of Utah, Salt Lake City, UT, USA
jeremy.gililland@hsc.utah.edu

Ioannis Gkiatas Hospital for Special Surgery, New York, NY, USA
Gkiatasi@hss.edu

Stuart B. Goodman Department of Orthopaedic Surgery, Stanford Medicine, Redwood City, CA, USA
goodbone@stanford.edu

Hugh Gorman Department of Orthopedic Surgery, Brigham and Women's Hospital, Boston, MA, USA
hgorman1@bwh.harvard.edu

Karan Goswami Rothman Orthopaedic Institute, Thomas Jefferson University, Philadelphia, PA, USA

Chancellor F. Gray Department of Orthopedic Surgery, University of Florida College of Medicine, Gainesville, FL, USA
graycf@ortho.ufl.edu

Robert Greenhow Orthopedic Centers of Colorado, Denver, CO, USA

Joshua A. Greenspoon Department of Orthopaedic Surgery, Rush University Medical Center, Chicago, IL, USA

Steve B. Haas Department of Orthopedic Surgery, Adult Reconstruction and Joint Replacement, Hospital for Special Surgery, New York, NY, USA
haas@hss.edu

Fares Haddad The Princess Grace Hospital and The Wellington Hospital, University College London Hospitals, London, UK
fares.haddad@nhs.net

David P. Hagan Department of Orthopedic Surgery, University of Florida College of Medicine, Gainesville, FL, USA
hagandp@ortho.ufl.edu

Nils P. Hailer Department of Surgical Sciences/Orthopaedics, Uppsala University Hospital, Uppsala, Sweden
Nils.Hailer@surgsci.uu.se

William Hamilton Anderson Orthopaedic Research Institute, Department of Orthopaedic Surgery, Alexandria, VA, USA

Charles P. Hannon Department of Orthopaedic Surgery, Rush University Medical Center, Chicago, IL, USA

Erik Hansen Department of Orthopaedic Surgery, University of California San Francisco UCSF, San Francisco, CA, USA
erik.hansen@ucsf.edu

Matthew A. Harb Department of Orthopaedic Surgery, University of Virginia, Charlottesville, VA, USA
MAH4XR@hscmail.mcc.virginia.edu

Carl L. Herndon Department of Orthopedic Surgery, Columbia University Irving Medical Center, New York, NY, USA
ch3181@cumc.columbia.edu

Carlos A. Higuera Cleveland Clinic Florida, Levitetz Department of Orthopaedic Surgery, Cleveland Clinic Blvd, Weston, FL, USA
higuerc@ccf.org

Craig A. Hogan School of Medicine, Department of Orthopedics, Aurora, CO, USA
craig.hogan@ucdenver.edu

Sherina Holland Department of Orthopaedic Surgery, North Shore Hospital, Auckland, New Zealand
Sherina.holland@waitematadhb.govt.nz

Derek Holyoak Exponent, Inc., Philadelphia, PA, USA
dholyoak@exponent.com

Paul Hoogervorst Department of Orthopedic Surgery, University of Minnesota, Minneapolis, MN, USA
hooge034@umn.edu

Patrick K. Horst Department of Orthopedic Surgery, University of Minnesota, Minneapolis, MN, USA
phorst@umn.edu

Shayan Hosseinzadeh Department of Orthopedic Surgery, Brigham and Women's Hospital, Boston, MA, USA
Shayan.Hosseinzadeh@childrens.harvard.edu

James I. Huddleston Department of Orthopedic Surgery, Stanford Medicine, Redwood City, CA, USA
jamesh3@stanford.edu

Christophe Jacquet Service de Chirurgie Orthopedique, Aix-Marseille University, Hospital Sainte-Marguerite, Marseille, France

Jean-Yves Jenny Pôle Locomax, University Hospital Strasbourg, Strasbourg, France
jean-yves.jenny@chru-strasbourg.fr

Daniel O. Johansen David Geffen School of Medicine, University of California Los Angeles, Santa Monica, CA, USA
DJohansen@mednet.ucla.edu

Cynthia A. Kahlenberg Hospital for Special Surgery, Department of Orthopaedic Surgery, New York, NY, USA
kahlenbergc@hss.edu

Eli Kamara Department of Orthopaedic Surgery, Albert Einstein College of Medicine, Bronx, NY, USA
Albert Einstein College of Medicine, Montefiore Medical Center, Bronx, NY, USA
Ekamara@montefiore.org

Atul F. Kamath Orthopaedic and Rheumatologic Institute, Cleveland Clinic, Cleveland, OH, USA
kamatha@ccf.org

Asim Khan NHS Foundation Trust, University College London Hospitals, Bloomsbury, UK
muhammad.khan93@nhs.net

Bradley A. King Mercy Health Orthopaedic Surgery, Cincinnati, OH, USA

Takao Kodama Department of Orthopedic Surgery, JCHO Saitama Medical Center, Saitama, Japan
kodamat@t.toshima.ne.jp

Bryan T. H. Koh Department of Orthopaedic Surgery, National University Health Systems, Singapore, Singapore

Chad A. Krueger Rothman Institute, Department of Orthopaedic Surgery, Sidney Kimmel Medical College at Thomas Jefferson University, Philadelphia, PA, USA
Chad.Krueger@rothmanortho.com

Klaus-Dieter Kühn Department of Orthopedic Surgery, Medical University of Graz, Graz, Austria
Klaus.kuehn@medunigraz.at

Kevin A. Lawson Department of Orthopedic Surgery, Stanford Medicine, Redwood City, CA, USA

Tsun-Yee Law Holy Cross Hospital, Inc., Department of Orthopaedic Surgery, Fort Lauderdale, FL, USA

Gwo-Chin Lee Department of Orthopaedic Surgery, University of Pennsylvania, Philadelphia, PA, USA
gwo-chin.lee@uphs.upenn.edu

Jessica Lee CU Hip Clinic, Champion Center, Department of Orthopaedic Surgery, Boulder, CO, USA
jessica.lee@cuanschutz.edu

Alex Lencioni School of Medicine, Department of Orthopedics, University of Colorado, Aurora, CO, USA
Alex.Lencioni@Cuanschutz.edu

Benjamin J. Levens Department of Orthopaedic Surgery, Albert Einstein College of Medicine, Bronx, NY, USA
Belevens@montefiore.org

Gladius Lewis Department of Mechanical Engineering, The University of Memphis, Memphis, TN, USA
glewis@memphis.edu

Elke Lieb Department of Market Access, Europe, Heraeus Medical GmbH, Wehrheim, Germany
Elke.lieb@heraeus.com

Adolph V. Lombardi Jr JIS Orthopedics, New Albany, OH, USA
LombardiAV@jisortho.com

William J. Long Department of Orthopedic Surgery, Adult Reconstruction and Joint Replacement, Hospital for Special Surgery, New York, NY, USA

Jess H. Lonner Rothman Institute, Department of Orthopaedic Surgery, Sidney Kimmel Medical College at Thomas Jefferson University, Philadelphia, PA, USA
Jess.Lonner@rothmanortho.com

David Craig Loucks Orthopedic Centers of Colorado, Englewood, CO, USA

Zia Maharaj Charlotte Maxeke Johannesburg Academic Hospital, Arthroplasty Unit, Department of Orthopaedic Surgery, Johannesburg, South Africa

Arthur L. Malkani Department of Orthopaedics, University of Louisville, Louisville, KY, USA
arthur.malkani@louisville.edu

Kevin K. Mathew Northwell Health Orthopedics, Lenox Hill Hospital, New York, NY, USA

Ruben A. Mazzucchelli Division of Orthopaedics and Traumatology, Kantonsspital Winterthur, Winterthur, Switzerland

Spencer J. Montgomery Department of Orthopedic Surgery, Stanford Medicine, Redwood City, CA, USA

Michael A. Mont Northwell Health Orthopedics, Lenox Hill Hospital, New York, NY, USA
mmont@northwell.edu

Vikaesh Moorthy Yong Loo Lin School of Medicine, National University of Singapore, Singapore, Singapore

Michael Morlock Institute of Biomechanics, TUHH Hamburg University of Technology, Hamburg, Germany
morlock@tuhh.de
biomechanik@tuhh.de

Denis Nam Department of Orthopaedic Surgery, Rush University Medical Center, Chicago, IL, USA
denis.nam@rushortho.com

Nader A. Nassif Hoag Orthopedic Institute, Irvine, CA, USA

Newport Orthopedic Institute, Newport Beach, CA, USA
Nnassif@newportortho.com

Brandon H. Naylor Northwell Health Orthopedics, Lenox Hill Hospital, New York, NY, USA

Daniel A. Oakes Department of Orthopaedic Surgery, Keck School of Medicine of USC, Los Angeles, CA, USA
daniel.oakes@med.usc.edu

Matthieu Ollivier Service de Chirurgie Orthopedique, Aix-Marseille University, Hospital Sainte-Marguerite, Marseille, France

Kevin Ong Exponent, Inc., Philadelphia, PA, USA
kong@exponent.com

Matan Ozery Cleveland Clinic Florida, Levitetz Department of Orthopaedic Surgery, Cleveland Clinic Blvd, Weston, FL, USA
mozer003@med.fiu.edu

Tejbir S. Pannu Cleveland Clinic Florida, Levitetz Department of Orthopaedic Surgery, Cleveland Clinic Blvd, Weston, FL, USA
pannut@ccf.org

Javad Parvizi Rothman Orthopaedic Institute, Thomas Jefferson University, Philadelphia, PA, USA

Department of Orthopaedic Surgery, Rothman Institute and Jefferson, Philadelphia, PA, USA

Neel R. Patel JIS Orthopedics, New Albany, OH, USA

Colin T. Penrose Hospital South, Orange Zone, Duke University Medical Center, Durham, NC, USA
Colin.penrose@duke.edu

Jurek Rafal Tomasz Pietrzak Charlotte Maxeke Johannesburg Academic Hospital, Arthroplasty Unit, Department of Orthopaedic Surgery, Johannesburg, South Africa

Robert Pivec The Rothman Institute, Thomas Jefferson University Hospital, Philadelphia, PA, USA
robert.pivec@rothmanortho.com

Hernan A. Prieto Department of Orthopedic Surgery, University of Florida College of Medicine, Gainesville, FL, USA
prieth@ortho.ufl.edu

Amar S. Ranawat Department of Orthopedics, Hospital for Special Surgery, New York, NY, USA
ranawatamar@hss.edu

Michael D. Ries Reno Orthopaedic Clinic, Reno, NV, USA
riesm@orthosurg.ucsf.edu

Martin Roche Hospital for Special Surgery Florida, Department of Orthopaedic Surgery, West Palm Beach, FL, USA
martin@mroche.com

Robert P. Runner Department of Orthopaedic Surgery, Rancho Los Amigos National Rehabilitation Center, Downey, CA, USA
rrunner@dhs.lacounty.gov

Anas Saleh Department of Orthopaedic Surgery, Cleveland Clinic Indian River Hospital, Vero Beach, FL, USA
saleha3@ccf.org

Hytham S. Salem Northwell Health Orthopedics, Lenox Hill Hospital, New York, NY, USA

Giulio Santi School of Orthopaedic Surgery, Università degli Studi di Milano, Milano, Italy
giulio.santi@unimi.it

Pablo Sanz-Ruiz Orthopedic and Trauma Service, Marañon on General University Hospital, Complutense University, Madrid, Spain

Nana O. Sarpong Department of Orthopedic Surgery, Columbia University Irving Medical Center, New York, NY, USA
no2282@cumc.columbia.edu

Adam A. Sassoon David Geffen School of Medicine, University of California Los Angeles, Santa Monica, CA, USA
Asassoon@mednet.ucla.edu

Axel Schmidt Service de Chirurgie Orthopedique, Aix-Marseille University, Hospital Sainte-Marguerite, Marseille, France

Isaac Schultz Cleveland Clinic Florida, Levitetz Department of Orthopaedic Surgery, Cleveland Clinic Blvd, Weston, FL, USA

Ran Schwarzkopf Department of Orthopaedic Surgery, NYU Langone Health, NYU Langone Orthopedic Hospital, New York, NY, USA
ran.schwarzkopf@nyulangone.org

Travis Scudday Hoag Orthopedic Institute, Irvine, CA, USA
Orthopedic Specialty Institute, Irvine, CA, USA
tscudday@osiortho.com

Peter K. Sculco Hospital for Special Surgery, New York, NY, USA
SculcoP@hss.edu

Thomas P. Sculco Hospital for Special Surgery, New York, NY, USA
SculcoT@hss.edu

Ahmed Siddiqi Orthopedic Institute of Central Jersey, Manasquan, NJ, USA

Mark J. Spangehl Department of Orthopedic Surgery, Mayo Clinic Arizona, Phoenix, AZ, USA
spangehl.mark@mayo.edu

Bryan D. Springer, MD OrthoCarolina Hip & Knee Center, Charlotte, NC, USA
bryan.springer@orthocarolina.com

Matthew W. Squire Rush Copley Center for Joint Preservation and Replacement, Rush Copley Medical Center, Aurora, IL, USA
orthosquire1@gmail.com

Thomas M. Steck Department of Orthopaedic Surgery, Keck School of Medicine of USC, Los Angeles, CA, USA
thomas.steck@med.usc.edu

Russell Presley Swann Orthopedic Centers of Colorado, Denver, CO, USA

Atsushi Takahashi Joint Surgery, Sports Clinic Ishinomaki, Ishinomaki, Japan
a-takahashi@jss-clinic.com

John P. Taliaferro Department of Orthopaedic Surgery, University of Virginia, Charlottesville, VA, USA
JPT2SH@hscmail.mcc.virginia.edu

Timothy L. Tan Department of Orthopaedic Surgery, Rothman Institute and Jefferson, Philadelphia, PA, USA
timothy.tan@rothmanortho.com

Thomas P. Vail Department of Orthopaedic Surgery, University of California, San Francisco, San Francisco, CA, USA
thomas.vail@ucsf.edu

Craig Della Valle Department of Orthopaedic Surgery, Rush University Medical Center, Chicago, IL, USA
craig.dellavalle@rushortho.com

Dries Van Doninck Department of Orthopedic Surgery, University Hospitals Leuven, Leuven, Belgium

Frank Verheyden Department of Orthopedic Surgery, H. Hart Hospital, Lier, Belgium
frank.verheyden@hhzhlier.be

Maarten Verheyden Department of Orthopedic Surgery, University Hospitals Leuven, Leuven, Belgium

Jesus M. Villa Cleveland Clinic Florida, Levitetz Department of Orthopaedic Surgery, Cleveland Clinic Blvd, Weston, FL, USA
villaj2@ccf.org

Wilson Wang Department of Orthopaedic Surgery, Yong Loo Lin School of Medicine, National University of Singapore, Singapore, Singapore
wilson_wang@nuhs.edu.sg

Derek Ward San Francisco Department of Orthopaedic Surgery, University of California, San Francisco, CA, USA
derek.ward@ucsf.edu

Annette W-Dahl Department of Clinical Sciences Lund/Orthopedics, Lund University, Lund, Sweden
annette.w-dahl@med.lu.se

Benjamin M. Wooster Department of Orthopaedic Surgery, OrthoCarolina, Charlotte, NC, USA
benjamin.wooster@orthocarolina.com

Seid Mohammed Yasin Department of Orthopedic Surgery, Yekatit 12 Hospital Medical College, Addis Ababa, Ethiopia

Piers J. Yates Orthopaedics WA, Murdoch and The Mount Private Hospitals, Orthopaedic Research Foundation WA, Fiona Stanley and Fremantle Hospitals Group, University of Western Australia, Perth, WA, Australia

Simon W. Young Department of Orthopaedic Surgery, North Shore Hospital, Auckland, New Zealand
Simon.young@auckland.ac.nz

Musa B. Zaid Department of Orthopaedic Surgery, University of California, San Francisco, San Francisco, CA, USA
Musa.Zaid@ucsf.edu

Yoav S. Zvi Department of Orthopedic Surgery, Montefiore Medical Center, Bronx, NY, USA
yzvi@montefiore.org

History

Contents

The History of Total Knee Arthroplasty

Ioannis Gkiatas, Thomas P. Sculco, and Peter K. Sculco

Contents

E. Hansen, K.-D. Kühn (eds.), *Essentials of Cemented Knee Arthroplasty*,
https://doi.org/10.1007/978-3-662-63113-3_1

1.1 Introduction

Total knee arthroplasty (TKA) is one of the most commonly performed surgical procedures with the number of TKAs nearly tripling in a 13-year period (Kurtz 2005). In 2020, approximately 1,065,000 TKAs will be performed in the United States, and this number will likely increase over time (Singh et al. 2019). The success of TKA is based on excellent implant survivorship and the alleviation of joint pain and improvement of function in the majority of patients.

The biomechanical principles and component materials that are used today were initially conceptualized and developed in the early 1970s. While TKA in 2020 can be performed in a multitude of ways—either manually or robotically, with resection or retention of the ACL and PCL, utilizing various (i.e., symmetric, asymmetric, medial congruent, and ultracongruent) insert designs, and adhering to mechanical or kinematic alignment priniciples—all of these modern practices can be traced back to the engineers and orthopedic surgeons in the 1970s and 1980s. The purpose of this chapter is to highlight the key developments in the history of TKA design in order to shed light on more recent developments.

> The success and failures of the early period in TKA design may also provide more information on the risks and benefits of more recently released designs and support the adage "those who do not know history are doomed to repeat it!"

Many international surgeons and engineers were involved in this effort and today there has been a consensus on the condylar design of knee replacement in most centers.

1.2 First Attempts

During the nineteenth century, the idea of treating knee arthritis with replacement materials was spawned and initially took form as a soft tissue interposition between the joint surfaces with or without bone resection of distal femur and proximal tibia (Amendola et al. 2012). The first attempts are reported in 1860 when Verneuil (Verneuil 1860) proposed the interposition of soft tissues in order to reconstruct the articular surface of the knee joint. One year later, Ferguson (Ferguson 1861) attempted to eradicate the arthritic joint by resecting the entire knee joint. The concept of prosthetic material interposed in the arthritic knee joint was further evolved in 1880. Implants made from ivory were described by Thermestocles Gluck who proposed their stabilization to bone using cement made from colophony, pumice, and plaster of Paris (Amendola et al. 2012). Despite the great innovation of Gluck, the first results were not promising so other ideas and concepts continued to be pursued such as the interposition of other tissues within the knee joint (Heaton and Dorr 2003).

In 1886, Ollier described a procedure similar to Verneuil's with the use of muscle instead of joint capsule (Murray 1991), and in 1894 Helferich presented successful results in transforming an ankylosed knee to a functional one using a resection arthroplasty and the use of muscle as interposed tissue (Helferich 1894). The use of subcutaneous fat, fascia lata, and patellar fat pad by Murphy in 1913 (Murphy 1913), Putti in 1920 (Putti 1921), and Albee in 1928 (Albee 1928), respectively, did not prove to be ideal materials nor the prepatellar bursa proposed by Cambel in 1921 (Campbell 1921). The other proposed alternatives such as chromized pig bladder, cellophane, sheets of nylon, and skin also did not prove effective (Baer 1918; Samson 1949; Kuhns 1964; Brown et al. 1958).

1.3 Early Attempts Using Metallic Prostheses to Treat Knee Arthritis

The first metallic implants for knee replacement were designed in 1937 and 2 years later a vitallium interposition mold was placed over the femur in patients (Campbell 1940). Some years later Smith-Petersen, who had experience from hip arthroplasty, introduced a distal femur prosthesis for the knee made from vitallium (Riley 1976). Lacheretz in 1952 (Lacheretz 1953) as well as Kraft and Levinthal in 1954 (Kraft and Levinthal 1954) implanted an acrylic distal femur prosthesis. At Massachusetts General Hospital, orthopedic surgeons reported a series of 78 cases using a modification of Smith-Petersen arthroplasty but with poor results (Jones et al. 1967). This prosthesis was a distal femoral implant fixed with an intramedullary femoral stem which tended to erode the articulating cartilage and often created a depression in the tibial plateau (Murray 1991).

- **MacIntosh & McKeever Tibial Plateau Design**

MacIntosh in the late 1960s (MacIntosh 1958) introduced the idea of acrylic tibial plateau hemiarthroplasty which was originally described by Jansen for the treatment of proximal tibia deformities (Murray 1991). Another similar implant to the MacIntosh implant was designed by McKeever (1960). Both of these implants resulted in good early outcomes. These "hemiarthroplasties" were employed frequently in patients with rheumatoid arthritis and were semilunar in shape, came in multiple sizes, were made of cobalt chrome, and were placed over the medial and lateral tibial plateau (Fig. 1.1).

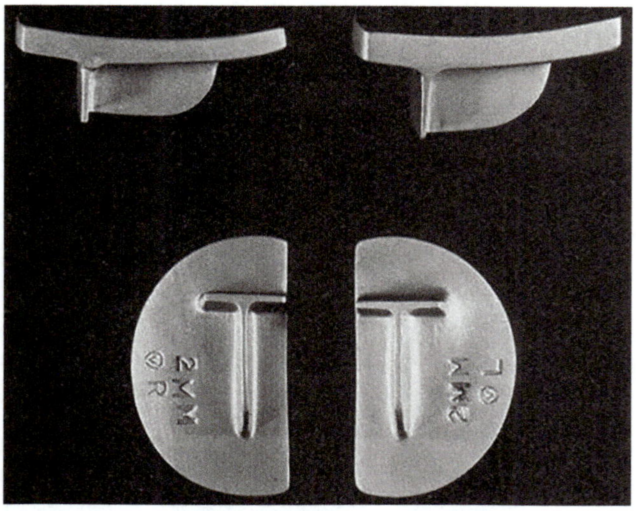

■ **Fig. 1.1** The MacIntosh & McKeever tibial plateau design. (Orthobullets—free learning and collaboration community for physicians, ▸ www.orthobullets.com)

Hinged Total Knee Implants

Hinge prosthetic devices were popularized first in Europe. An experimental hinged total knee implant was initially proposed by Judet et al. (1947), and the early results at 2 years with this prosthesis were first reported in 1949 by Magnoni and d' Intignano (Magnoni and d'Intignano 1949). The hinged acrylic prostheses were modified and fabricated into metal implants by Walldius (1953). This implant was a fixed axis hinge, had several sizes, was somewhat bulky (Shiers 1954; YOUNG 1963), and became widely accepted in Europe and particularly in Scandinavia.

Guepar Hinged Prosthesis

Using the experience with the Walldius prosthesis, another fixed-axis hinge, the Guepar hinged prosthesis, was developed in the 1970s by a consortium of designers primarily from France (Ranawat and Sculco 1985). This implant was also used in the United States in cases of severe deformity with marked ligamentous insufficiency. The early results with the Guepar were excellent, but failures eventually occurred primarily with implant loosening and migration due to the fixed axis nature of the implant and the severe torsion loads at the intramedullary bone–cement interface (Hoikka et al. 1989) (■ Fig. 1.2).

Freeman–Swanson TKA Design

One of the first successful collaborations of a bioengineer and orthopedic surgeon occurred in London in the late 1960s. Alfred Swanson of the Imperial College, a brilliant engineer, and Michael Freeman, a master innovative hip and knee surgeon, designed a unique knee implant known as the ICLH (Imperial College London Hospital) knee arthroplasty (■ Fig. 1.3). This knee had a "roller and trough" design and the cruciate ligaments could be sacrificed. The contact area for the components was quite extensive in an attempt to reduce focal loading and wear. The concept of soft tissue balancing was also derived from this collaboration where ligament asymmetry was dealt with by releasing the tight ligament on the concave side of the deformity and this was balanced with the lax ligament on the convex side of the deformity.

> This concept was pivotal to subsequent knee design and success and is still utilized today.

The publication by Todd, Freeman, and Sculco documented this technique for the first time and it was presented at the AAOS in 1974 (Freeman et al. 1973, 1977). As knee replacement design evolved, all components at this time consisted of a polyethylene component on the tibial side mated with a metal femoral component. All components were fixed with methylmethacrylate cement popularized by John Charnley in hip arthroplasty. Tibial fixation of the polyethylene was enhanced by fins, grooves, slots, or other shallow irregularities on the undersurface of the prosthesis.

1.4 The Concept of Modern TKA

During the early evolution of total knee replacement design, there existed a strong debate about whether the femoral and tibial components should be monoblock or unicondylar (and individually resurface each femoral condyle and each tibial plateau surface with an implant).

The Polycentric Knee

Gunston who had visited Charnley and discussed knee replacement design with him was a strong proponent of individual components, and this evolved into the Polycentric knee (Gunston 2006) (■ Fig. 1.4). The Polycentric knee had four individual components which were quite narrow and fit into grooves on the femoral and tibial surfaces. The technique was difficult and there was little stability inherent in this device leading to component subsidence, dislocation of the individual components, and eventual failure.

The Duocondylar Prosthesis

Developed in 1971, the Duocondylar prosthesis from the Hospital for Special Surgery had a bridged monoblock condylar design with two thin femoral condylar surfaces (■ Fig. 1.5). This Duocondylar design consisted of a flat, high-density polyethylene tibial plateau, which was in two parts, whereas the femoral component

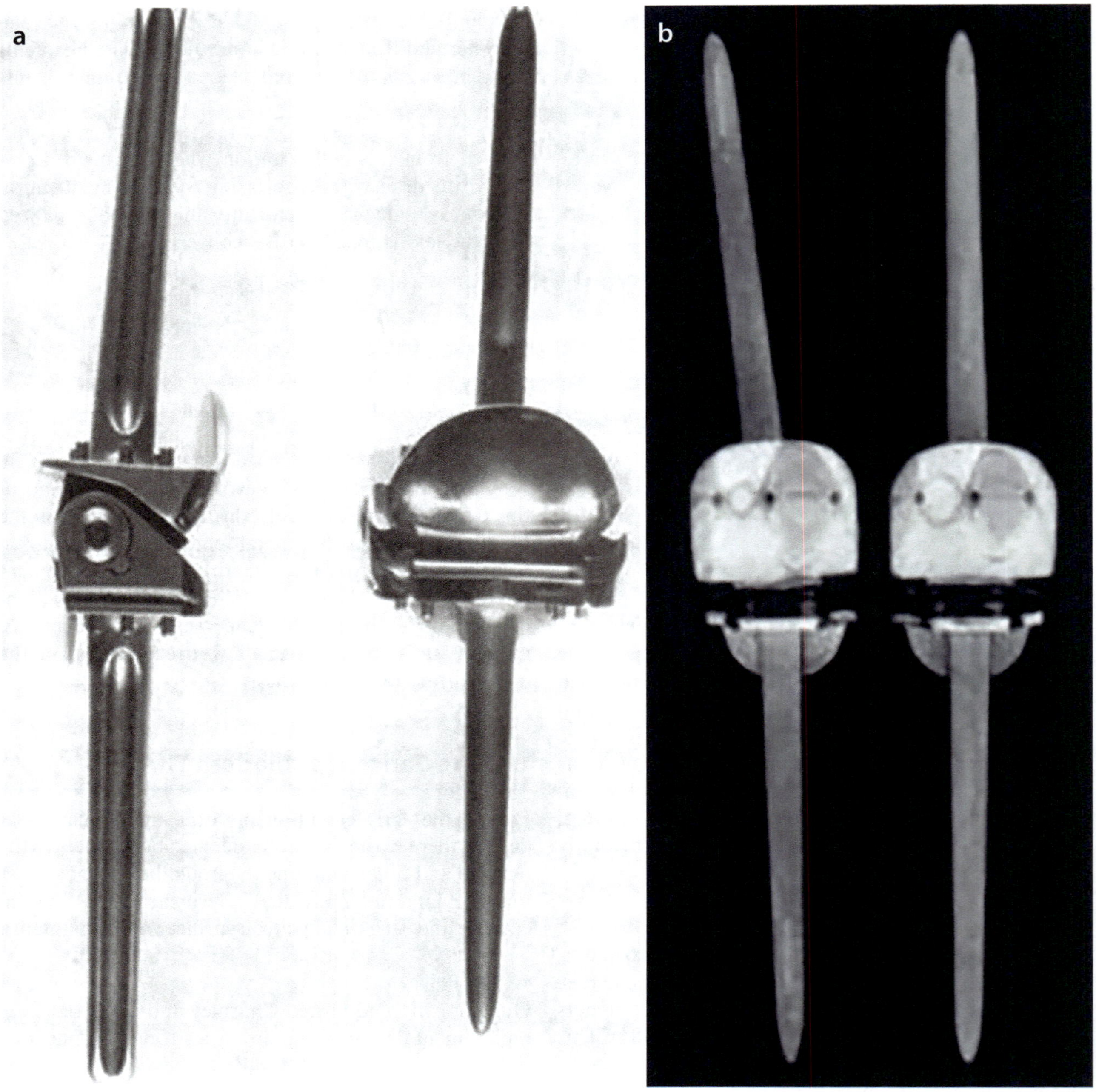

Fig. 1.2 **a** The Walldius prosthesis (Orthobullets—free learning and collaboration community for physicians, ▶ www.orthobullets.com). **b** The Guepar prosthesis. (From leNobel and Patterson 1981. © The British Editorial Society of Bone and Joint Surgery, with permission)

had a metal bridge connecting the two thin metallic condyles. The patellofemoral joint remained unresurfaced (Ranawat and Sculco 1985). This implant was one of the first to be introduced with instrumentation for improved alignment although very rudimentary (Heaton and Dorr 2003). Both cruciate ligaments had to be preserved with the Duocondylar knee and this increased its failure rate especially in knees with severe deformity and inflammatory arthritis with ligamentous damage. The design of this implant was later modified in order to include a polyethylene patellar replacement which was named the Duopatellar prosthesis (Ranawat and Ranawat 2012).

The Total Condylar Prosthesis

A major breakthrough in implant design occurred when the total condylar (TC) prosthesis was introduced in 1974 and this was adopted quickly worldwide and became the design platform for future knee implant development (Fig. 1.6). It was again a collaboration between a biomechanical engineer, Peter Walker, an

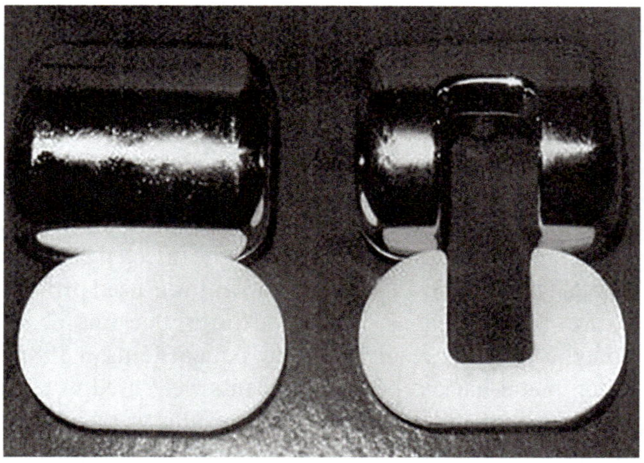

Fig. 1.3 The Freeman–Swanson TKA design. (Reprinted from (Insall and Scott 2018), © 2018, with permission from Elsevier)

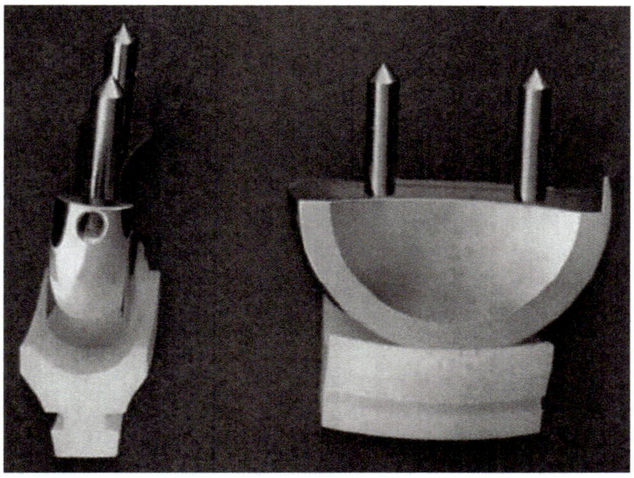

Fig. 1.4 The Polycentric knee designed by Gunston. (From Gunston 2006, by courtesy of Wolters Kluwer Health, Inc.)

innovative designer, and Drs. John Insall and Chitranjan Ranawat, surgeons at the Hospital for Special Surgery (HSS) in New York City. The fundamental concept was the replacement of all three components of the knee with a single tibial all-polyethylene component. Both cruciate ligaments were sacrificed and knee stability was achieved with the deep dish design of the polyethylene tibial component and increased congruence with the femoral component. A dome-shaped, single-lugged, polyethylene component was generally also used with this component.

The Insall–Burstein TKA Prosthesis

In 1978, Dr. John Insall in collaboration with the bioengineer Albert Burstein designed the posterior stabilized (PS) TKA at HSS which was called the Insall–Burstein knee (IB). The IB design included a cam-post mechanism and an all-polyethylene tibia and later a metal tibial tray to more evenly distribute tibial load. The IB II implant was developed several years later and offered modularity with a tibial component that engaged the metal tray and a locking clip. This allowed changing the

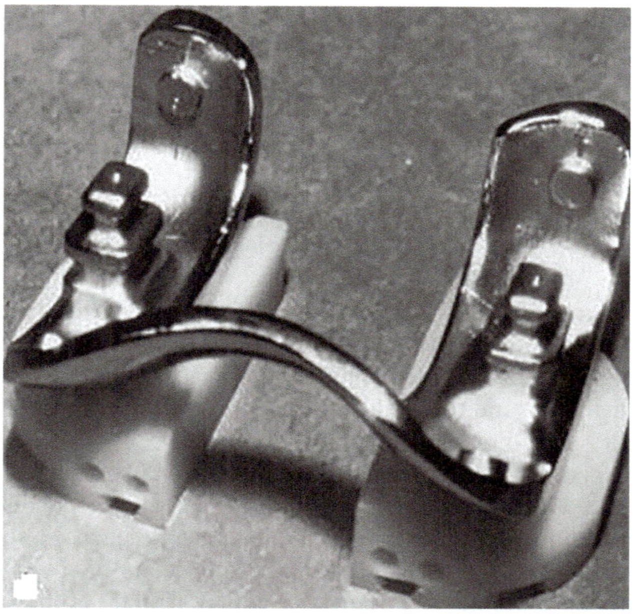

Fig. 1.5 The Duocondylar prosthesis. (Reprinted from Insall and Scott 2018, © 2018, with permission from Elsevier)

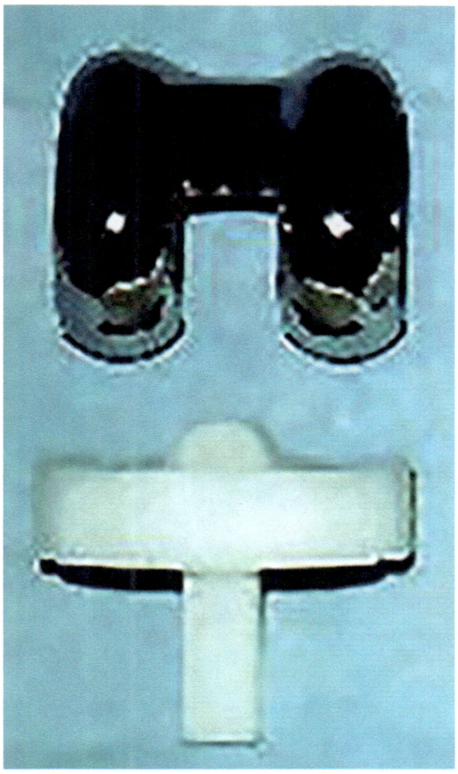

Fig. 1.6 The total condylar prosthesis. (Parcells and Tria 2016, courtesy of the U.S. National Library of Medicine)

polyethylene if needed rather than having to remove the entire tibial component. This implant was extremely successful and formed the basis for subsequent posterior stabilized designs (▣ Fig. 1.7). A patellar polyethylene component was generally used in all cases in the IB systems.

▪ Press-Fit Condylar Prosthesis and Porous-Coated Anatomic Prosthesis

A group of Boston surgeons led by Drs. Richard Scott and Thomas Thornhill used the same concepts but believed in the preservation of the posterior cruciate ligament, and this philosophy led to the development of the press-fit condylar (PFC) design (Depuy Synthes, Warsaw, Indiana). In the early 1980s, David Hungerford and Kenneth Krackow developed the porous-coated anatomic (PCA) cruciate-retaining knee which was also a condylar design. They popularized the concept of anatomic placement of the tibial component in approximately 3° varus which has seen a resurgence of interest by surgeons interested in the kinematic philosophy of knee replacement. These surgeons are often credited for the development of modern surgical instrumentation to make implantation more reproducible (▣ Fig. 1.8).

> In 1976, the first constrained condylar TKA, the TC III, was designed with an elevated and widened tibial eminence for improved joint stability in knees with severe deformity and marked ligamentous laxity and for the growing demand for revision total knee replacement (Ranawat and Ranawat 2012).

1.5 Patella

Patellectomy was commonly performed in the early treatment for severe patellofemoral arthritis (Murray 1991). In 1955, McKeever designed a patellar implant which was a metallic prosthesis fitted to the patella with a screw (McKeever 1955) (▣ Fig. 1.9). In 1989, Insall designed a metal button that was cemented into the resected arthritic patella (Insall et al. 1980). This implant was used primarily for isolated patellofemoral arthritis but was abandoned after poor results in many patients (Insall 1982). Later, metal-backed patellar implants were used in total knee replacement, however, their results were inferior mainly due to the reduced thickness of the polyethylene, which resulted in polyethylene wear through, fracture of the polyethylene, and separation of the polyethylene from the metal backing (Andersen et al. 1991). As a result of these failures, most current patellar implants are all polyethylene designs, although more recently, good early outcomes have been observed with uncemented patella buttons with highly cross-linked polyethylene.

▪ Concept of Posterior Cruciate Ligament Preservation

> In the early 1970s, Yamamoto and Kodoma reported the first implantation of a uncemented condylar cruciate-sparing prosthesis (Kodama–Yamamoto prosthesis) (Yamamoto 1979).

Other surgeons such as Scott, Thornhill, Hungerford, and Krackow also supported the concept of trying to

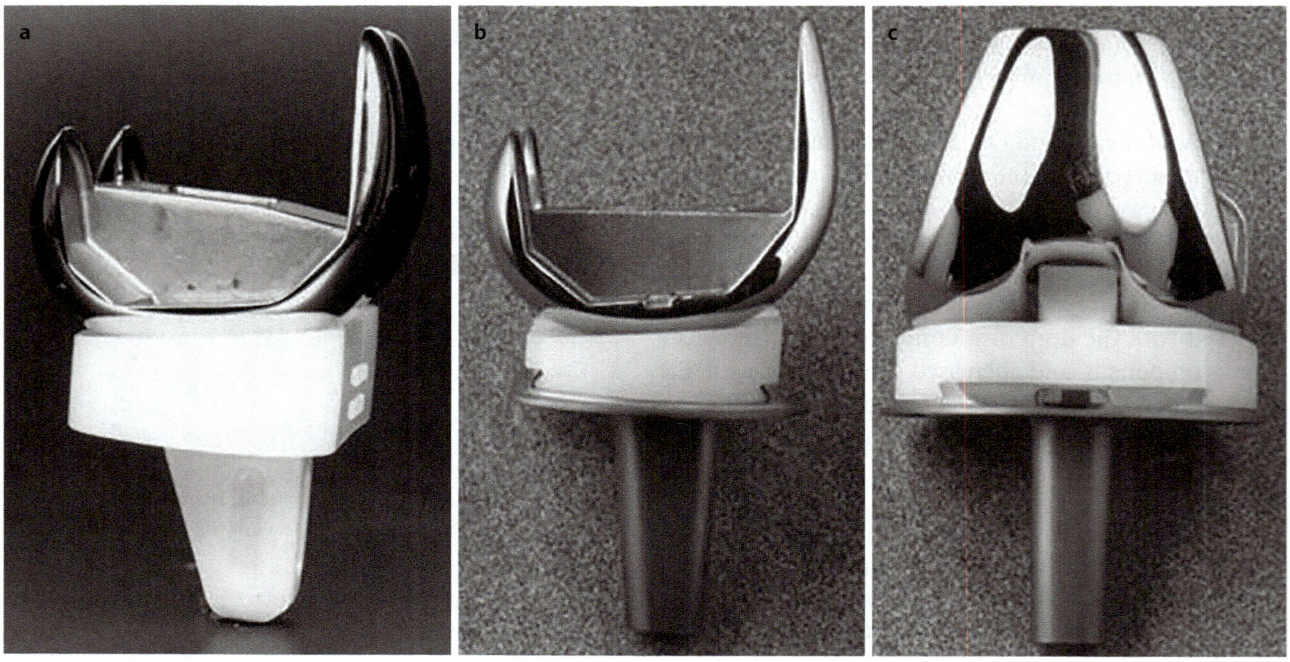

▣ **Fig. 1.7** **a** The Insall–Burstein TKA prosthesis. **b**, **c** The Insall–Burstein II TKA prosthesis. (Reprinted from Insall and Scott 2018, © 2018, with permission from Elsevier)

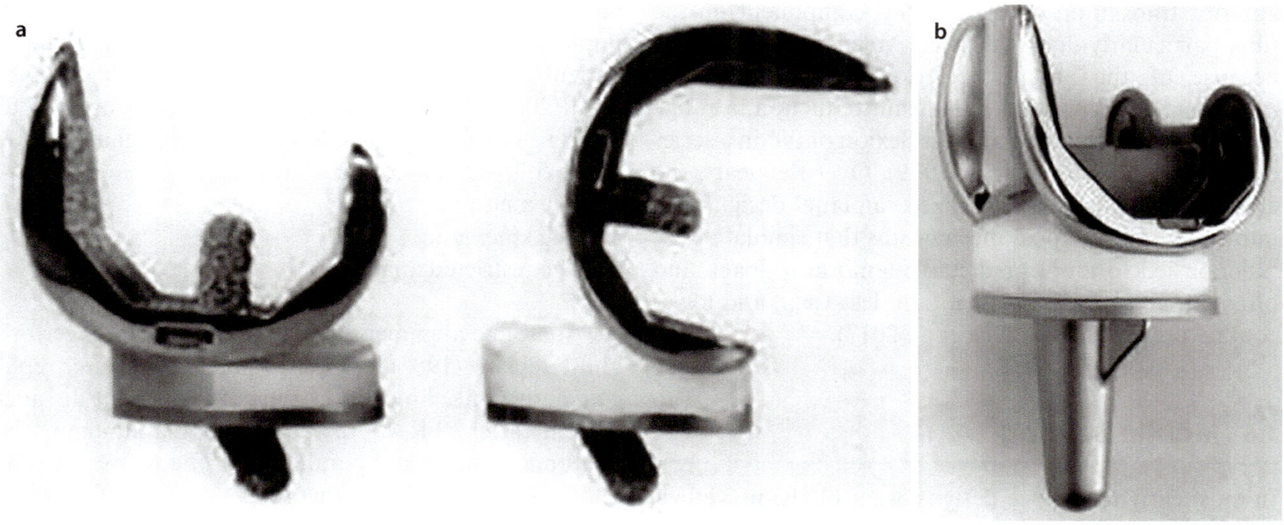

Fig. 1.8 **a** Porous-coated anatomic prosthesis. **b** Press-fit condylar prosthesis. (From Heaton and Dorr 2003, by courtesy of Wolters Kluwer Health, Inc.)

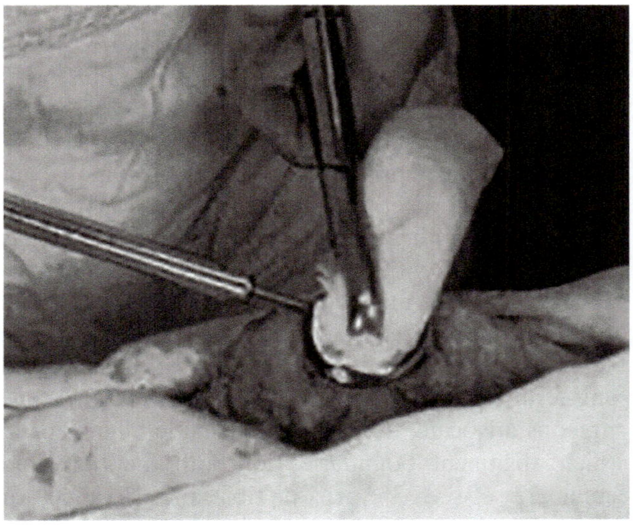

Fig. 1.9 The insertion of the cemented metallic patellar implant with a screw. (McKeever 1955)

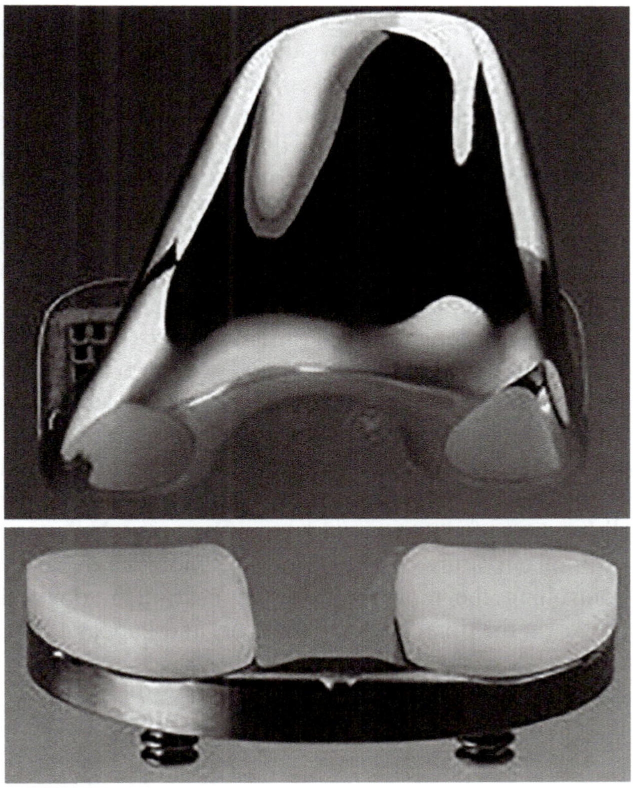

Fig. 1.10 Prosthesis which allows the preservation of both cruciate ligaments. (From Cloutier et al. 1999, by courtesy of Wolters Kluwer Health, Inc.)

preserve the posterior cruciate ligament (Waugh et al. 1973; Townley and Hill 1974). The posterior cruciate retraining implants generally had a horseshoe tibial component to allow preservation of ligament insertion.

Cloutier from Canada advocated preserving both cruciate ligaments and the polyethylene component had to be modular or have a larger central opening to preserve both ligaments (Amendola et al. 2012) (Fig. 1.10).

The difficulty with posterior cruciate preservation (and ACL if also preserved) has always been the proper balancing of this ligament to prevent posterior tethering of the joint by a tight cruciate and thereby increased posterior polyethylene wear and potentially reduced knee flexion. Additionally, if the cruciate is too tight, the kinematics of the knee will be altered and femoral rollback may be less predictable than in a posterior cruciate substituting design where it is controlled via the cam-post mechanism.

The rationale for posterior cruciate preservation was that despite the wide success of the TC, PCL sacrificing prosthesis, there remained a concern of "paradoxical" anterior translation of the femoral component on the tibia particularly during flexion (Amendola et al. 2012) because of the absent posterior cruciate ligament. Additionally, there was a significant reduction in range of motion with reported average flexion of 90° in a series of 220 patients (Insall et al. 1979). Over the years, the evolution of posterior stabilized implants design with improved cam and post mechanisms that simulate PCL function led to more predictable femoral rollback and offered a greater range of motion, less wear, and lower contact pressures (Dall'Oca et al. 2017).

1.6 Mobile Bearing

In most early total knee designs, wear of the polyethylene was a major concern that could compromise the longevity and function of the replacement.

■ **Oxford Knee and LCS Knee Replacement System**

The concept of mobile-bearing components was first introduced by Goodfellow and O'Connor in 1976 in order to decrease focal polyethylene loading and hopefully reduce polyethylene wear. They designed a bicondylar knee prosthesis known as the Oxford knee in which the polyethylene bearing freely moved on the metal tibial tray (Goodfellow and O'Connor 1978). This mobile polyethylene insert was called a "mensical bearing" design and the congruency of the insert with the femoral component imitated the medial compartment and associated mensical congruency in the native knee (Heaton and Dorr 2003). The Oxford knee was used primarily in Europe whereas in the United States, a new design, the New Jersey Low-Contact-Stress (LCS) Knee Replacement System (Depuy Synthes), was developed by Buechel and Pappas in 1977. This implant was designed to resist the dislocation of the meniscal bearing by using decreasing radii of curvature on the posterior femoral side and by controlling the movement of the bearing in dovetail tracks on the tibial platform (Buechel and Pappas 1986).

> Mobile bearing designs are less popular than fixed bearing knees as polyethylene wear has been less of a problem in newer designs and the mobile bearing knee tended to be somewhat less stable and harder to balance.

1.7 The Evolution of Alignment Parameters: Anatomic Versus Kinematic Versus Restricted Kinematic

As knee replacement design progressed, alternative alignment techniques have been proposed in order to improve the functional outcomes (Rivière et al. 2017). It has been reported that despite outstanding long-term implant survivorship with mechanical alignment, patient dissatisfaction may be as high as 20% (Baker et al. 2007; Bourne et al. 2010). Technical options to improve satisfaction include variation in alignment such as the following:

- The anatomic
- The kinematic
- The restricted anatomic

Anatomic alignment was introduced by Hungerford and Krackow (1985) in order to potentially better replicate native knee kinematics and reduce patient dissatisfaction after TKA. In addition, maintaining the anatomic oblique and parallel joint line between femur and tibial articulations theoretically allows for better load distribution on the tibial component and provides better patella biomechanics as it reduced lateral retinacular ligament stretching during knee flexes (Klatt et al. 2008; Ghosh et al. 2009). This alignment was popular early after its introduction. Errors in alignment, particularly of the tibial component with excessive varus, led to increased polyethylene wear and implant failure and ultimately led to its falling out of favor as a mechanical alignment target (Oussedik et al. 2020).

Contemporary principles behind kinematic alignment can be characterized as an evolution of anatomical alignment as both are based on restoring a patient's native alignment with the placement of tibial and femoral components to match the pre-arthritic state (Howell et al. 2013). The debate continues whether kinematic alignment negatively impacts knee biomechanics and long-term implant survivorship. For this reason, some surgeons advocate "restricted" kinematic alignment in which alignment boundaries for both the tibia and femur are set (i.e., 3° varus or tibia and 3° valgus for femur). The long-term survivorship and functional outcomes compared to mechanical alignment (as advocated by Insall) continue to be debated (Oussedik et al. 2020; Howell et al. 2013).

1.8 The Evolution of Femoral Component Design

The development of the condylar-resurfacing TKA design arose from two different concepts, allowing the prosthesis to determine the knee kinematics (posterior stabilized) concept or to preserve posterior cruciate ligament and allow the retained soft tissue to influence knee kinematics. Each philosophy continues to have its proponents and critics. The early condylar designs were PCL sacrificing but not did adequately substitute PCL function which led to unreliable femoral rollback on the tibia and often allowed anterior translation as the knee flexed (Dall'Oca et al. 2017). Resultant increased polyethylene wear may have also resulted in these early TC designs (Robinson 2005). In addition, the absence of "rollback" resulted in impingement of the posterior femoral metaphysis against the tibial articular surface at approximately 95° of flexion. This along with other design issues (such as limited sizing) likely led to the restriction of motion in the early condylar designs.

> To correct these issues, the posterior cruciate-substituting design was developed in 1978 by adding a central cam mechanism to the articular surface geometry of the total condylar prosthesis.

The cam on the femoral component engaged a central post on the tibial articular surface at approximately 70° of flexion and caused the contact point of the femorotibial articulation to be posteriorly displaced, effecting femoral rollback and allowing further flexion (Causero et al. 2014).

1.9 The Evolution of Tibial Component Design

The initial tibial component had a metaphyseal stem in order to resist varus–valgus forces of the prosthesis during asymmetrical loading. It was all-polyethylene and later metal backing was added. This alteration allowed more uniform stress transfer to the underlying cancellous metaphyseal bone and additionally protected the polyethylene from deformation (Causero et al. 2014). Separate tibial plateau components were abandoned for one piece units early in knee replacement development (Causero et al. 2014). However, while the metal backing improved load distribution in the tibial metaphysis, modularity introduced another interface, the concept of backside wear. The PFC design (DePuy Synthes, Warsaw IN) and other similar locking mechanism designs demonstrated increased backside wear, polyethylene particles that led to large amounts on osteolysis in some cases. Despite inferior loading characteristics, several studies have demonstrated excellent long-term survivorship with all-polyethylene tibias and they continue to be used today.

> In reference to tibial component shape, both symmetric and asymmetric designs continue to be used today with excellent long-term outcomes.

1.10 The Evolution of Polyethylene—The Growth of Mid-Level Constraint

Over the years there have been several design adaptions of the polyethylene liners in order to both improve the stability of the joint and better replicate natural knee kinematics. The PS design was a modification of the earlier total condylar design which was lax mainly in flexion.

> The liner in a PS prosthesis, where both cruciate ligaments are sacrificed, has a post, which engages the femoral cam at approximately 40–90° of flexion. In contrast to PS liners, CR polyethylene liners, where the PCL should be retained, do not have the central post and are typically flat.

They are also required to guide the knee through the range of motion and provide appropriate stability in all planes. The newer ultracongruent designs aim to prevent the paradoxical anterior translation of the femur that takes place in some CR designs. The PCL can be retained or sacrificed but typically is sacrificed.

> In the 1990s, medial pivot liners were designed and developed to simulate knee kinematics. The medial compartment is deeper and keeps the medial femoral condyle relatively stable as a "pivot point," and the lateral compartment is flatter allowing for some natural translation via the "screw home" mechanism (Macheras et al. 2017).

The evolution of polyethylene constraint has progressed through several iterations. The original TC knee had a dishing of the plateau surface to improve congruency and provide some stability in a knee that sacrificed both cruciate ligaments. The posterior cruciate ligament-retaining knees tend to be flat on their surfaces to allow posterior rollback with an intact posterior cruciate ligament controlling the knee kinematics. Asymmetric posterior loading tended to be increased in the flat designs and, therefore, increased congruency and dishing are favored today. It is important to emphasize that the posterior stabilized designs do not provide coronal or sagittal stability. A constrained condylar polyethylene design has an elevated and widened polyethylene eminence which does provide AP, medial lateral, and rotational stability although it cannot substitute for an absent collateral ligament.

> Newer mid-level constraint (MLC) bearings somewhat limit rotation and varus/valgus liftoff but have less constraint than the constrained condylar knee (CCK) insert.

The MLC compared to the PS design has an increased height and width of the polyethylene insert post, leading to a higher level of articulation with the femoral box and increased congruity. It is often used to correct valgus deformity resulting from the lateral bone loss on the femur and deficiency of the medial soft-tissue envelope. In this case, the contact between tibial eminence and femoral box can act to reduce a hyperextension moment (Peters et al. 2001; Dubin and Westrich 2020).

1.11 The Evolution of Fixation in TKA

> The use of cemented implants remains the gold standard as cemented fixation continues to provide durable long-term results in several large-scale registry studies and randomized clinical trials (Papas et al. 2019; Nivbrant et al. 2020).

However, despite early failures with uncemented designs (PCA), uncemented designs are increasingly used and have demonstrated excellent mid-term survivorship in some more recent studies (Fricka et al. 2019). The improvement in highly porous 3D printed titanium coating and enhancements in peg and keel fixation have led to greater adoption. While the material properties have evolved significantly over the years, the initial concepts and usage of uncemented total knee replacements date back to over 40 years.

In 1977, the cementless condylar knee design was introduced. These prostheses were as follows:

- The Kodama–Yamamoto
- The Imperial College London Hospital (ICLH) (Freeman et al. 1983)
- The "Ring" prosthesis (Ring 1980)
- One year later, the Low Contact Stress (LCS) (Buechel and Pappas 1989) (Depuy, Warsaw, IN)

In 1978 as well, Dr. David Hungerford, Robert Kenna, and Dr. Kenneth Krackow designed the first porous-coated uncemented total knee replacement (Hungerford et al. 1982). This initial design was groundbreaking in several aspects. Insertion of the implants followed a press-fit technique. This was the first knee design with a sintered porous-coated surface on the backside of the femoral and tibial implant. The porous-coated anatomical (PCA) total knee, which was a posterior stabilized knee, was manufactured by Howmedica (Rutherford, NJ). Ortholoc I followed in 1982 (Whiteside) (Whiteside 1989), The Tricon-M in 1983 (Smith and Nephew, TN) (Laskin 1988), the Miller Galante (MG-1) (Landon et al. 1986) in 1984, the Anatomic Graduated Component (AGC) in 1984 (Ritter et al. 1992) (Biomet, Warsaw, IN), the Press-Fit Condylar (PFC) in 1985 (Scott and Thornhill 1994) (Depuy, Warsaw, IN), the Natural-Knee in 1985 (Hofmann et al. 1991) (Zimmer, Warsaw IN), and the Genesis I in 1988 (Smith and Nephew, Memphis, TN).

Since instability has proved to be the reason for approximately 19% of revision TKA operations (Siddiqi et al. 2020), appropriate soft tissue balancing is of high importance for a successful TKA. The traditional balancing techniques were mainly subjective and relied on surgeon's experience. Classically, there are two techniques that are used in order to achieve the balance of soft tissues in TKA: measured resection (MR) and gap balancing (GB) (D'Lima et al. 2007). The first one uses fixed osseous landmarks to plan bony cuts and then performs soft tissue releases in order to achieve symmetric flexion and extension gaps (Hungerford et al. 1982), whereas the second one uses the tension of collateral ligament via soft-tissue releases as a guide to balance flexion and extension gaps and set component rotation prior to osseous resection (Freeman et al. 1986).

1.12 Conclusion

The evolution of TKA implant design and surgical technique over the last two centuries is impressive. Orthopedic surgeons have long recognized that the definitive treatment of progressive, symptomatic arthritis is replacement of the articular surfaces with biocompatible, kinematically friendly prostheses. While initial efforts focused more on optimizing the design features of joint replacement implants, the importance of soft tissue balancing was recognized to be an equally important element of successful outcomes. As a result of the complexity of knee joint kinematics, it is now known that both accurate preoperative planning for bone resection and ligament balancing are required for a successful postoperative result. The development of technology, improved instrumentation, and evolution of biomaterials have improved TKA designs over the last several decades. In addition, technology has been integrated into every aspect of TKA and has become an important assistant not only in the preoperative but also in the intraoperative execution of TKA. We owe a great deal of gratitude to those innovative surgeons and engineers who dedicated themselves to the constant improvement of knee implant design and technique and who continue to enable us to provide the reproducible outcomes of improving pain and function in patients with knee arthritis.

Take-Home Messages

- Initial attempts for joint replacement started during the nineteenth century.
- First metallic implants designed were based on the concept of hemiarthroplasty.
- The concept of modern TKA was introduced in the early 1970s with the Duocondylar prosthesis.
- The total condylar prosthesis introduced the idea of all three compartments replacement.
- In the late 1970s, the Insall–Burstein prosthesis was developed.
- There is ongoing research regarding implants design and joint alignment in order to improve knee kinematics.
- Cemented TKA is still the gold standard.

References

Albee F (1928) Original features in arthroplasty of the knee with improved prognosis. Surg Gynecol Obstet 47:312
Amendola L, Tigani D, Fosco M, Dallari D (2012) History of condylar total knee arthroplasty. In: Recent advances in hip and knee arthroplasty. InTech Rijeka, Croatia, p 189
Andersen HN, Ernst C, Frandsen PA (1991) Polyethylene failure of metal—backed patellar components: 111 AGC total knees followedfor 7-22 months. Acta Orthop Scand 62(1):1–3
Baer WS (1918) Arthroplasty with the aid of animal membrane. JBJS s2–16(3):171
Baker PN, van der Meulen JH, Lewsey J, Gregg PJ, National Joint Registry for England and Wales (2007) The role of pain and function in determining patient satisfaction after total knee replacement. Data from the National Joint Registry for England and Wales. J Bone Joint Surg Br 89(7):893–900
Bourne RB, Chesworth BM, Davis AM, Mahomed NN, Charron KDJ (2010) Patient satisfaction after total knee arthroplasty: who is satisfied and who is not? Clin Orthop Relat Res 468(1):57–63
Brown JE, Mcgaw WH, Shaw DT (1958) Use of cutis as an interposing membrane in arthroplasty of the knee. JBJS 40(5):1003
Buechel FF, Pappas MJ (1986) The New Jersey low-contact-stress knee replacement system: biomechanical rationale and review of the first 123 cemented cases. Arch Orth Traumatol Surg 105(4):197–204
Buechel FF, Pappas MJ (1989) New Jersey low contact stress knee replacement system. Ten-year evaluation of meniscal bearings. Orthop Clin North Am 20(2):147–177
Campbell WC (1921) Arthroplasty of the knee—report of cases. JBJS 3(9):430
Campbell WC (1940) Interposition of vit allium plates in arthroplasties of the knee: preliminary report. Am J Surg 47(3):639–641
Causero A, Di Benedetto P, Beltrame A, Gisonni R, Cainero V, Pagano M (2014) Design evolution in total knee replacement: which is the future? Acta Biomed 85 Suppl 2:5–19
Cloutier JM, Sabouret P, Deghrar A (1999) Total knee arthroplasty with retention of both cruciate ligaments. A nine to eleven-year follow-up study. J Bone Joint Surg Am 81(5):697–702. https://www.jbjs.org/
D'Lima DD, Patil S, Steklov N, Colwell CW (2007) An ABJS best paper: dynamic intraoperative ligament balancing for total knee arthroplasty. Clin Orthop Relat Res 463:208–212
Dall'Oca C, Ricci M, Vecchini E, Giannini N, Lamberti D, Tromponi C et al (2017) Evolution of TKA design. Acta Bio-medica: Atenei Parmensis 88(Suppl 2):17
Dubin JA, Westrich GH (2020) Mid-level constraint may correct coronal plane imbalance without compromising patient function in patients with severe osteoarthritis. J Orthop 21:84–87
Ferguson W (1861) Excision of the knee joint: recovery with a false joint and a useful limb. Med Times Gaz 1:601
Freeman MAR, Swanson SAV, Todd RC (1973) Total replacement of the knee using the Freeman-Swanson knee prosthesis. Clin Orthop Relat Res 94:153–170
Freeman MA, Sculco T, Todd RC (1977) Replacement of the severely damaged arthritic knee by the ICLH (Freeman-Swanson) arthroplasty. J Bone Joint Surg Br 59(1):64–71
Freeman MA, McLeod HC, Levai JP (1983) Cementless fixation of prosthetic components in total arthroplasty of the knee and hip. Clin Orthop Relat Res 176:88–94
Freeman MA, Samuelson KM, Levack B, de Alencar PG (1986) Knee arthroplasty at the London Hospital. 1975–1984. Clin Orthop Relat Res 205:12–20
Fricka KB, McAsey CJ, Sritulanondha S (2019) To cement or not? Five-year results of a prospective, randomized study comparing cemented vs cementless Total knee arthroplasty. J Arthroplast 34(7S):S183–S187
Ghosh KM, Merican AM, Iranpour-Boroujeni F, Deehan DJ, Amis AA (2009) Length change patterns of the extensor retinaculum and the effect of total knee replacement. J Orthop Res 27(7):865–870
Goodfellow J, O'Connor J (1978) The mechanics of the knee and prosthesis design. J Bone Joint Surg 60(3):358–369
Gunston FH (2006) Polycentric knee arthroplasty: prosthetic simulation of normal knee movement. 1971. Clin Orthop Relat Res 446:11–12. https://journals.lww.com/clinorthop/pages/default.aspx
Heaton KT, Dorr LD (2003) History of total knee arthroplasty. In: Callaghan JJ, Rosenberg AG, Rubash HE, Simonian PT, Wickiewicz TL (eds) The adult knee. Lippincott Williams and Wilkins, Philadelphia, Baltimore, New York, London, Buenos Aires, Hong Kong, Sydney, Tokyo, pp 15–24
Helferich H (1894) Ein neues Operationsverfahren zur Heilung der knöchernen Kiefergelenksankylose. Arch Klin Chir 48:864–870
Hofmann AA, Wyatt RW, Beck SW, Alpert J (1991) Cementless total knee arthroplasty in patients over 65 years old. Clin Orthop Relat Res 271:28–34
Hoikka V, Vankka E, Eskola A, Lindholm TS (1989) Results and complications after arthroplasty with a totally constrained total knee prosthesis (GUEPAR). Ann Chir Gynaecol 78(2):94–96
Howell SM, Howell SJ, Kuznik KT, Cohen J, Hull ML (2013) Does a kinematically aligned total knee arthroplasty restore function without failure regardless of alignment category? Clin Orthop Relat Res 471(3):1000–1007
Hungerford DS, Krackow KA (1985) Total joint arthroplasty of the knee. Clin Orthop Relat Res 192:23–33
Hungerford DS, Kenna RV, Krackow KA (1982) The porous-coated anatomic total knee. Orthop Clin North Am 13(1):103–122
Insall J (1982) Current concepts review. Patellar pain. J Bone Joint Surg Am 64(4):633

Insall J, Scott WN (2018) Historic development, classification, and characteristics of knee prostheses. In: Insall, Clarke (eds) Surgery of the knee, 6th edn. Elsevier, Amsterdam, pp 1375–1404
Insall J, Scott WN, Ranawat CS (1979) The total condylar knee prosthesis. A report of two hundred and twenty cases. J Bone Joint Surg Am 61(2):173–180
Insall J, Tria AJ, Aglietti P (1980) Resurfacing of the patella. J Bone Joint Surg Am 62(6):933–936
Jones WN, Aufranc OE, Kermond WL (1967) Mold arthroplasty of knee. In: Journal Of Bone And Joint Surgery-American Volume. Journal Bone Joint Surgery Inc 20 Pickering St, Needham, MA, p 1022
Judet J, Judet R, Crepin G, Rigault A (1947) Essais de prothèse ostéo-articulaire. Vol. 55. MASSON EDITEUR 21 STREET CAMILLE DESMOULINS, ISSY, 92789 MOULINEAUX CEDEX 9 …; 302–302 p
Klatt BA, Goyal N, Austin MS, Hozack WJ (2008) Custom-fit total knee arthroplasty (OtisKnee) results in malalignment. J Arthroplast 23(1):26–29
Kraft GL, Levinthal DH (1954) Acrylic prosthesis replacing lower end of the femur for benign giant-cell tumor. JBJS 36(2):368–374
Kuhns JG (1964) Nylon membrane arthroplasty of the knee in chronic arthritis. JBJS 46(2):448
Kurtz S (2005) Prevalence of primary and revision Total hip and knee arthroplasty in the United States from 1990 through 2002. J Bone Joint Surg Am 87(7):1487
Lacheretz M (1953) Traitement des ankyloses. Rev Chir Orthop Par 39:495
Landon GC, Galante JO, Maley MM (1986) Noncemented total knee arthroplasty. Clin Orthop Relat Res 205:49–57
Laskin RS (1988) Tricon-M uncemented total knee arthroplasty. J Arthroplast 3(1):27–38
Macheras GA, Galanakos SP, Lepetsos P, Anastasopoulos PP, Papadakis SA (2017) A long term clinical outcome of the medial pivot knee arthroplasty system. Knee 24(2):447–453
MacIntosh DL (1958) Hemiarthroplasty of the knee using space occupying prosthesis for painful varus and valgus deformities. J Bone Joint Surg 40:1431
Magnoni V, d'Intignano JM (1949) Genou en resine acrylique. Rev Orthop 35:556
McKeever DC (1955) Patellar prosthesis. JBJS 37(5):1074–1084
McKeever DC (1960) Tibial plateau prosthesis. Clin Orthop Relat Res 18:86–95
Murphy JB (1913) I. Arthroplasty. Ann Surg 57(5):593
Murray DG (1991) History of total knee replacement. In: Total knee replacement. Springer, pp 3–15
Nivbrant NO, Khan RJK, Fick DP, Haebich S, Smith E (2020) Cementless versus cemented tibial fixation in posterior stabilized total knee replacement: a randomized trial. J Bone Joint Surg [Internet]. [cited 2020 Jul 1];Publish Ahead of Print. Available from: https://journals.lww.com/10.2106/JBJS.19.01010
Oussedik S, Abdel MP, Victor J, Pagnano MW, Haddad FS (2020) Alignment in total knee arthroplasty. Bone Joint J 102-B(3):276–279
Papas PV, Congiusta D, Cushner FD (2019) Cementless versus cemented fixation in total knee arthroplasty. J Knee Surg 32(07):596–599
Parcells BW, Tria AJ (2016) The cruciate ligaments in total knee arthroplasty. Am J Orthop 45(4):E153–E160
Peters CL, Mohr RA, Bachus KN (2001) Primary total knee arthroplasty in the valgus knee. J Arthroplast 16(6):721–729
Putti V (1921) Arthroplasty. JBJS 3(9):421–430
Ranawat AS, Ranawat CS (2012) The history of total knee arthroplasty. In: The knee joint. Springer, pp 699–707
Ranawat CS, Sculco TP (1985) History of the development of total knee prosthesis at the Hospital for Special Surgery. In: Total-condylar knee arthroplasty. Springer, pp 3–6
Riley JL (1976) The evolution of total knee arthroplasty. Clin Orthop Relat Res 120:7–10
Ring PA (1980) Uncemented surface replacement of the knee joint. Clin Orthop Relat Res 148:106–111
Ritter MA, Keating EM, Faris PM (1992) Design features and clinical results of the anatomic graduated components (AGC) total knee replacement. Contemp Orthop 19:641–641
Rivière C, Iranpour F, Auvinet E, Howell S, Vendittoli P-A, Cobb J et al (2017) Alignment options for total knee arthroplasty: a systematic review. Orthop Traumatol Surg Res 103(7):1047–1056
Robinson RP (2005) The early innovators of today's resurfacing condylar knees. J Arthroplast 20:2–26
Samson JE (1949) Arthroplasty of the knee joint; late results. J Bone Joint Surg Br 31B(1):50–52
Scott RD, Thornhill TS (1994) Posterior cruciate supplementing total knee replacement using conforming inserts and cruciate recession. Effect on range of motion and radiolucent lines. Clin Orthop Relat Res 309:146–149
Shiers LGP (1954) Arthroplasty of the knee: preliminary report of a new method. J Bone Joint Surg 36(4):553–560
Siddiqi A, Smith T, McPhilemy JJ, Ranawat AS, Sculco PK, Chen AF (2020) Soft-tissue balancing technology for total knee arthroplasty. JBJS Rev 8(1):e0050
Singh JA, Yu S, Chen L, Cleveland JD (2019) Rates of Total joint replacement in the United States: future projections to 2020–2040 using the National Inpatient Sample. J Rheumatol 46(9):1134–1140
Townley C, Hill L (1974) Total knee replacement. LWW
Verneuil A (1860) De la création d'une fausse articulation par section ou résection partielle de l'os maxillaire inférieur, comme moyen de rémedier a l'ankylose vraie ou fausse de la machoire inférieure, Rignoux
Walldius B (1953) Arthroplasty of the knee joint employing an acrylic prosthesis. Acta Orthop Scand 23(2):121–131
Waugh TR, Smith RC, Orofino CF, Anzel SM (1973) Total knee replacement: operative technic and preliminary results. Clin Orthop Relat Res (1976–2007) 94:196–201
Whiteside LA (1989) Clinical results of Whiteside Ortholoc total knee replacement. Orthop Clin North Am 20(1):113–124
Yamamoto S (1979) Total knee replacement with the Kodama-Yamamoto knee prosthesis. Clin Orthop Relat Res 145:60–67
YOUNG HH (1963) Use of a hinged vitallium prosthesis for arthroplasty of the knee: a preliminary report. JBJS 45(8):1627–1642

Indications

Contents

Osteoarthritis

Benjamin J. Levens, Eli Kamara, and Erik Hansen

Contents

E. Hansen, K.-D. Kühn (eds.), *Essentials of Cemented Knee Arthroplasty*,
https://doi.org/10.1007/978-3-662-63113-3_2

2.1 Introduction

According to the World Health Organization, musculoskeletal conditions are the leading cause of disability worldwide (Musculoskeletal Conditions 2019). Among these conditions, osteoarthritis (OA) is one of the most common, affecting more than 25% of the adult population (Chen et al. 2017). This number will continue to rise as our population ages and the obesity rate increases. As of 2012, the number of adults with OA in the United States was 27 million. By 2030, that number is projected to reach 67 million (Van Manen et al. 2012). With the prevalence of OA increasing in the population, it is important to understand the pathophysiology, diagnostic features, and treatment options for this disease.

> Osteoarthritis is the degeneration of joint cartilage and underlying bone. One of the most common sites of OA is the knee.

The burden caused by OA is a major reason for medical visits and healthcare costs. Fifty percent of people who are 50 years and older report to have knee pain during the course of a year (Blagojevic et al. 2010). A quarter of them have severe or disabling knee pain, a number that continues to rise. When reviewing the National Health and Nutrition Examination Survey and Framingham Osteoarthritis Studies, Nguyen et al. found the prevalence of knee pain and symptomatic OA roughly doubled in women and tripled in men after adjusting for age and body mass index over a 20-year period (Blagojevic et al. 2010; Nguyen et al. 2011).

2.2 Risk Factors

Knee joint OA results in pain, swelling, stiffness, and limited mobility. The cause of OA is multifactorial. Several patient-specific risk factors have been associated with the development of knee OA including the following:

- Family history
- Increased body mass index (BMI)
- Prior knee injury
- Female gender
- Older age

Other factors are intensive physical activity including certain occupational activities such as kneeling and squatting (Blagojevic et al. 2010). In addition, several genetic factors have been implicated in the cause of OA. Growth factors such as transforming growth factor-β (TGF-β), Wnt3a, and Indian hedgehog, signaling molecules Smad3, β-catenin, and HIF-2α, and transcription factor Runx2 are involved in OA development (Chen et al. 2017). Although several different risk factors have been indicated in the disease, the pathogenesis remains fairly constant.

2.3 Pathophysiology

> On a cellular level, osteoarthritis is the failure to regenerate damaged cartilage.

Chondrocytes are the single cellular component of adult hyaline cartilage and maintain the cartilage matrix under normal conditions. Articular cartilage is composed of type II collagen, which is named hyaline for its glass-like, translucent appearance. Due to lack of vascularity in cartilage, chondrocytes have limited supply of nutrients and oxygen, which normally aid in cellular repair. Early in the process of OA, chondrocytes attempt to repair damaged areas by exhibiting a transient proliferative response increasing the synthesis of cartilage matrix, catabolic cytokines, and matrix-degrading enzymes.

As mentioned previously, Runx2 is a key factor regulating the transcription of genes encoding matrix degradation enzymes in articular cartilage. Upregulation of Runx2 causes increased production of degrading enzymes such as metalloproteinases (MMPs), which break down the extracellular matrix of cartilage and cause apoptotic death of chondrocytes. The resulting cartilage is unable to withstand mechanical stress, leading to a repetitive cycle of further breakdown.

Due to the lack of pain receptors in the cartilage, these findings typically do not present clinically until later in the process. As cartilage debris and catabolic mediators break off from the cartilage and enter the synovial cavity, macrophages from the synovial fluid take up these products and further amplify the inflammatory response by releasing their own proinflammatory markers. Although previously thought of as a noninflammatory disease, recent studies have shown synovial inflammation to be a cause of joint swelling and pain (Chen et al. 2017; Bijlsma et al. 2011; Goldring 2000; Sellam and Berenbaum 2010).

As OA progresses on a molecular level, the resulting process on a macroscopic scale leads to joint space narrowing, subchondral bone sclerosis, osteophyte formation, and cystic changes. These findings can be visualized on plain radiograph and are useful in the diagnosis of OA (Fig. 2.1). More than 50% of patients older than 65 have these radiographic changes, however, many of these patients remain asymptomatic (Brown 2013). For this reason, history and physical are crucial in proper diagnosis and treatment of OA.

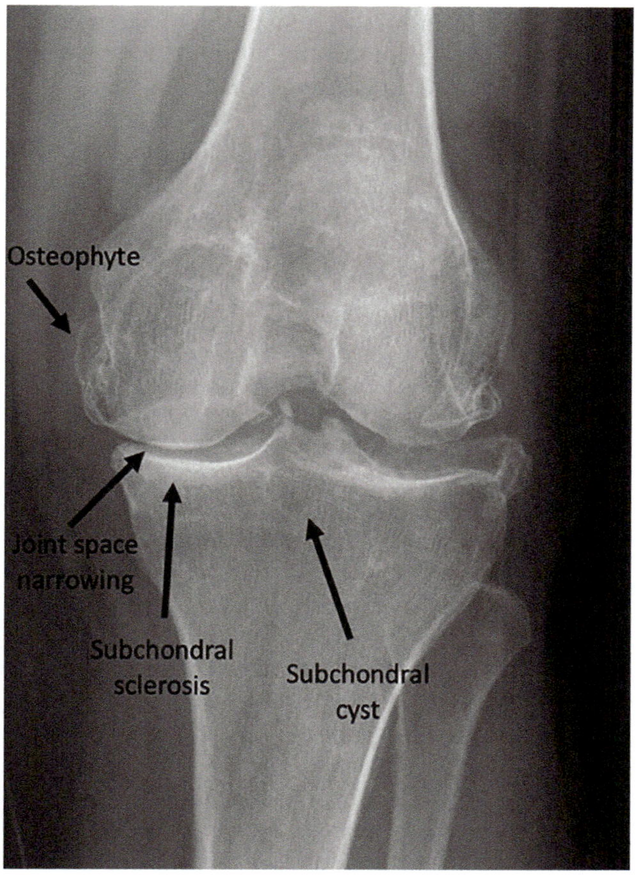

Fig. 2.1 AP weight-bearing radiograph of a knee with significant arthritic changes

2.4 Diagnostic Features

Among the symptoms of OA, pain is the most common initial symptom that patients report to their primary care physician. The pain is typically described as intermittent, worse both during and after weight-bearing activities. In addition to pain, patients also complain of stiffness.

Stiffness associated with OA is most commonly felt in the morning and resolves within a few minutes of getting up. Stiffness can help differentiate OA from Rheumatoid Arthritis (RA). Morning stiffness associated with RA is defined as stiffness that resolves more than 30 minutes after getting up from sleep. Other common symptoms are loss of movement and function, limiting activities of daily living such as climbing stairs, prolonged walking, and doing household chores. The limitations caused by OA can diminish the quality of life resulting in mood changes, anhedonia, and depression (Bijlsma et al. 2011).

2.5 Treatment Options

After diagnosis, proper treatment is important.

The Osteoarthritis Research Society International (OARSI) recommends at least 6 months of nonoperative treatment. If conservative, nonoperative management fails to improve symptoms after 6 months, surgical intervention may be indicated (Van Manen et al. 2012).

2.5.1 Nonoperative Management

There are many different nonoperative treatment modalities available for OA. The OARSI and American Academy of Orthopaedic Surgeons (AAOS) each have recommendations for treatment based on both clinical research and expert opinion.

Weight loss is strongly recommended by both the AAOS and OARSI.

Generally, weight loss is recommended for patients with symptomatic OA of the knee and a BMI ≥25 (Brown 2013). The Framingham Knee Osteoarthritis study showed a greater than 50% reduction in symptoms related to primary knee OA with a decrease in BMI of two or more (Felson et al. 1987). The AAOS and OARSI recommend weight loss by participating in self-managed strengthening and low-impact aerobic exercises, as well as engaging in physical activities focusing on muscle strengthening and range of motion (Scuderi and Insall 1992; Zhang et al. 2008).

In addition to exercise, patients with symptomatic OA also benefit from referral to a physical therapist for evaluation and instruction regarding appropriate exercises. These exercises should focus on pain reduction and improvement of functional capacity. With the assistance of physical therapists, patients can also be evaluated for the need for walking aids such as a cane or walker, which have been shown to reduce pain. In patients with unilateral symptomatic OA, a cane or crutch is recommended on the contralateral side. For bilateral symptomatic OA, a framed or wheeled walker is preferred (Zhang et al. 2008).

Usage of a valgus knee brace compared to neoprene sleeve has been shown to improve Western Ontario McMaster Universities Osteoarthritis Index (WOMAC) scores, although there is only moderate strength of recommendation for this treatment by the OARSI. Similarly, lateral wedged insoles for medial tibiofemoral compartment OA have been shown to reduce pain and improve ambulation. The research on this, however, is conflicting. Several observational studies show symptomatic relief and decrease in lateral thrust of the knee with lateral wedged insoles. However, in several RCTs, there was no improvement in pain scores or functional outcomes at 6 months or 2 years follow-up (Maillefert et al. 2001; Pham et al. 2004). Other therapeutic options such as thermal modalities, transcutaneous electrical nerve stimulation (TENS), and acupuncture are all weakly recommended by the OARSI and lack strong consensus among the existing guidelines. Unlike the OARSI, the AAOS recommends strongly against acupuncture therapy (Scuderi and Insall 1992; Zhang et al. 2008).

The OARSI recommends a multimodal approach of both pharmacological and non-pharmacological options in treating OA. Pharmacologically, the OARSI recommends the use of acetaminophen or paracetamol for the treatment of mild to moderate pain in OA. The previously recommended dose of up to 4 g/day has more recently come into question. The risk of gastrointestinal (GI) and renal toxicity with long-term use of acetaminophen 4 g/day has been equivocal (Garcia Roderiguez and Hernandez-Diaz 2001). For this reason, short-term use is preferred.

> Analogously, non-steroidal anti-inflammatory drugs (NSAIDs) are also strongly recommended by both the OARSI and AAOS, but only for short-term use due to the risk of GI discomfort. Opioids are strongly recommended only for the management of severe pain in exceptional circumstances (Scuderi and Insall 1992; Zhang et al. 2008).

Oral supplementation is another modality that can be used in the treatment of osteoarthritis, albeit with variable results and limited recommendations. The most common supplements are glucosamine and chondroitin, which are components of cartilage. Proponents of these compounds as supplements purport that they stimulate synovial fluid production and improve cartilage healing (Lim et al. 2019). When reviewed in 2005 by Cochrane, pooled analysis of multiple RCTs found improvement in pain and function, however, there was considerable heterogeneity among the studies resulting in questionable outcomes. For this reason, the OARSI only weakly recommends the use of glucosamine and/or chondroitin for symptomatic treatment of knee OA. The AAOS strongly recommends against glucosamine based on lack of effectiveness (Scuderi and Insall 1992; Zhang et al. 2008).

Corticosteroid intra-articular injections are a commonly used noninvasive treatment modality in most orthopedic surgery practices. First tested in a clinical trial by Miller in 1958, corticosteroids have been used for knee OA for over 50 years (Miller et al. 1958). Corticosteroids have a strong anti-inflammatory effect. As mentioned previously, damaged cartilage produces an inflammatory response in the knee joint via the release of cytokines. These cytokines (interleukin-1B, interleukin-6, and tumor necrosis factor alpha) bind to cellular receptors activating intracellular signaling pathways such as mitogen-activated protein kinase (MAPK), nuclear factor kappa-B (NF-kB), and Janus kinase-signal transducer and activator of transcription (JAK STAT). The activation of these pathways triggers the production of arachidonic acid via phospholipase A2. Arachidonic acid is further broken down by cyclo-oxygenase (COX) enzymes into signaling molecules prostaglandin, leukotriene, and thromboxane, which are responsible for the transmission of pain. Corticosteroids bind to glucocorticoid receptors in the cell-inhibiting activation of intracellular signaling cascade. By repressing NF-kB, MAPK, and JAK STAT, further propagation of inflammatory response is prevented. Corticosteroids also inhibit phospholipase A2 which results in decreased production of signaling molecules prostaglandin, leukotriene, and thromboxane. Therefore, through repression of inflammatory cascade, corticosteroids, in theory, reduce pain (Lawrence 2009; Chen et al. 2018). OARSI recommends the use of corticosteroid injections with moderate strength of recommendation. Due to inconclusive research, the AAOS cannot recommend for or against the use of corticosteroid injections. Based on a 2015 Cochrane review, corticosteroid injections were shown to provide a moderate short-term improvement in pain and only small improvement in function. These results, however, were inconclusive due to small effect size and large degree of heterogeneity among studies (Jüni et al. 2015).

Viscosupplementation is another type of intra-articular injection which attempts to restore natural elements to a depleted arthritic knee. The most common viscosupplement is hyaluronic acid (HA), a glycosaminoglycan. Hyaluronic acid is the main component of synovial fluid and acts as a lubricant and shock absorber in the joint providing a chondroprotective effect. Despite the theoretical utility, research on viscosupplementation has been largely inconclusive. In a recent meta-analysis by Jevsevar et al. of only double-blinded RCTs with over 60 patients, there was no clinically significant difference between HA and placebo. However, when all literature in the analysis was included, the HA treatment group was slightly higher than placebo (Jevsevar et al. 2015). The OARSI found that although HA has a delayed onset when compared with corticosteroids, it may have a prolonged duration. The strength of this recommendation, however, is weak. Unlike the OARSI, the AAOS strongly recommends against the use of viscosupplementation for the conservative treatment of OA (Scuderi and Insall 1992; Zhang et al. 2008).

2.5.2 Surgical Intervention: Cemented Total Knee Arthroplasty

When conservative treatment has failed and the patient continues to have pain, stiffness, limited mobility, and/or decreased quality of life, surgical management should be considered. Several surgical options are available for the management of OA with varying degrees of success. For the purpose of this chapter, we will only be discussing cemented total knee arthroplasty (TKA) as a treatment for OA of the knee.

Total knee replacement is the most commonly performed operation amongst orthopedic surgeons. More than 600,000 knee replacements are performed each year in the United States. Primary TKA is projected to increase by 637% by 2030 in the United States (*OKU Hip and Knee 5* 2017). The primary indication for TKA is OA, which accounts for more than 94% of total procedures (Van Manen et al. 2012).

> In terms of TKA technique, cemented arthroplasty remains the gold standard.

Scuderi and Insall describe the technique of fixation of the cement, methylmethacrylate, to the bone surface. Fixation is achieved by the irregular configuration of the bony surface and cement penetration into the microstructure of the cancellous bone. Prior to cementation, pulsatile lavage assists in the removal of debris from the bony indices allowing for adequate penetration of cement (Scuderi and Insall 1992).

More recently, cementless TKA has emerged as another surgical option, but further research is required to comment on long-term durability. Cemented TKA provides the surgeon with optimal outcomes without relying on anatomic cuts and supplemental fixation, which is required to achieve adequate bony ingrowth in cementless fixation (Callaghan and Liu 2010). The immediate fixation from cement allows for immediate, unrestricted weight-bearing and the ability to start rehabilitation more rapidly. Although cementless TKA was initially developed to benefit younger patients, when compared to cemented TKA in patients 60 years and less, both groups were found to have similar functional outcomes and survival rates (Franceschetti et al. 2017; Behery et al. 2017). Cemented TKA has consistently demonstrated long-term success in multiple different survivorship studies. Scuderi and Insall found their 15-year success rate to be around 91% in 1992. More recent studies have shown the survivorship to be 97% at 10 and 12 years (Falatyn et al. 1995; Ranawat et al. 1993). These long-term studies further emphasize the success of cemented TKA as an ideal surgical treatment of OA.

2.6 Conclusion

Osteoarthritis affects millions of patients with a multifactorial genesis. Nonoperative treatment includes weight loss, physical therapy, NSAIDs, and intra-articular injections. When nonoperative treatment is no longer effective, surgical management with cemented TKA is a viable treatment option with proven long-term results.

Take-Home Messages

- Osteoarthritis is a common source of knee pain and can cause a great degree of disability.
- The pathophysiology of osteoarthritis involves cyclical cartilage damage predominantly due to catabolic enzymes secreted by chondrocytes and synovial macrophages.
- The radiographic signs of osteoarthritis include joint space narrowing, subchondral bone sclerosis, osteophyte formation, and cystic changes. Although present in many elderly patients, these findings may be asymptomatic.
- The clinical signs of osteoarthritis are knee pain with weight-bearing activities, morning stiffness lasting less than 30 minutes, decreased range of motion, and crepitus.
- Conservative treatment is recommended for at least 6 months prior to surgical intervention for osteoarthritis. The best conservative therapy involves a combination of pharmacologic and non-pharmacologic modalities.
- Weight loss, low impact exercise, physical therapy, and walking aids are all strongly recommended by either the AAOS and/or OARSI. NSAIDs, acetaminophen, and tramadol are also strongly recommended pharmacologically.
- Although frequently used in practice, the research behind intra-articular injections such as corticosteroids and HA is equivocal and therefore based on only weak to moderate recommendation.
- When conservative treatment measures have been exhausted, total knee arthroplasty is an ideal surgical treatment for symptomatic relief.
- Cemented TKA remains the gold standard for treatment with excellent long-term survivorship.

References

Behery OA, Kearns SM, Rabinowitz JM, Levine BR (2017) Cementless vs cemented Tibial fixation in primary total knee arthroplasty. J Arthroplast 32(5):1510–1515

Bijlsma JW, Berenbaum F, Lafeber FP (2011) Osteoarthritis: an update with relevance for clinical practice. Lancet 377(9783):2115–2126

Blagojevic M, Jinks C, Jeffery A, Jordan KP (2010) Risk factors for onset of osteoarthritis of the knee in older adults: a systematic review and meta-analysis. Osteoarthr Cartil 18(1):24–33

Brown GA (2013) AAOS clinical practice guideline: treatment of osteoarthritis of the knee: evidence-based guideline, 2nd edition. J Am Acad Orthop Surg 21(9):577–579

Callaghan JJ, Liu SS (2010) Cementless tibial fixation in TKA: not a second coming. Orthopedics 33(9):655

Chen D, Shen J, Zhao W et al (2017) Osteoarthritis: toward a comprehensive understanding of pathological mechanism. Bone Res 5:16044

Chen L, Deng H, Cui H et al (2018) Inflammatory responses and inflammation-associated diseases in organs. Oncotarget 9(6):7204–7218

Falatyn S, Lachiewicz PF, Wilson FC (1995) Survivorship analysis of cemented total condylar knee arthroplasty. Clin Orthop Relat Res 317:178–184

Felson DT, Naimark A, Anderson J, Kazis L, Castelli W, Meenan RF (1987) The prevalence of knee osteoarthritis in the elderly: the Framingham Osteoarthritis Study. Arthritis Rheum 30(8):914–918

Franceschetti E, Torre G, Palumbo A et al (2017) No difference between cemented and cementless total knee arthroplasty in young patients: a review of the evidence. Knee Surg Sports Traumatol Arthrosc 25(6):1749–1756

Garcia Roderiguez LA, Hernandez-Diaz S (2001) Risk of upper gastrointestinal complications among users of acetaminophen and non-steroidalantiinflammatory drugs. Epidemiology 12:570e6

Goldring MB (2000) The role of the chondrocyte in osteoarthritis. Arthritis Rheum 43(9):1916–1926

Jevsevar D, Donnelly P, Brown GA, Cummins DS (2015) Viscosupplementation for osteoarthritis of the knee: a systematic review of the evidence. J Bone Joint Surg Am 97(24):2047–2060

Jüni P et al (2015) Intra-articular corticosteroid for knee osteoarthritis. Cochrane Database Syst Rev. https://doi.org/10.1002/14651858. cd005328.pub3

Lawrence T (2009) The nuclear factor NF-kappaB pathway in inflammation. Cold Spring Harb Perspect Biol 1(6):a001651

Lim YZ et al (2019) Nutrients and dietary supplements for osteoarthritis. In: Bioactive food as dietary interventions for arthritis and related inflammatory diseases, 2nd edn. Academic Press. https://www.sciencedirect.com/science/article/pii/B9780128138205000064

Maillefert JF, Hudry C, Baron G, Kieffert P, Bourgeois P, Lechevalier D et al (2001) Laterally elevated wedged insoles in the treatment of medial knee osteoarthritis: a prospective randomized controlled study. Osteoarthr Cartil 9:738e45

Miller JH, White J, Norton TH (1958) The value of intra-articular injections in osteoarthritis of the knee. J Bone Joint Surg Br Vol 40-B(4):636–643

Musculoskeletal Conditions (2019) World Health Organization, World Health Organization. https://www.who.int/news-room/factsheets/detail/musculoskeletal-conditions

Nguyen UA, Zhang Y, Zhu Y, Niu J, Zhang B, Felson DT (2011) Increasing prevalence of knee pain and symptomatic knee osteoarthritis: survey and cohort data. Ann Intern Med 155(11):725–732

Old AB, Long WJ, Scott WN (2017) Chapter 11: Special Considerations in Primary Total Knee Arthroplasty. OKU Hip & Knee 5

Pham T, Maillefert JF, Hudry C, Kieffert P, Bourgeois P, Lechevalier D et al (2004) Laterally elevated wedged insoles in the treatment of medial knee osteoarthritis. A two-year prospective randomized controlled study. Osteoarthr Cartil 12:46e55

Ranawat CS, Flynn WF, Saddler S, Hansraj KK, Maynard MJ (1993) Long-term results of the total condylar knee arthroplasty. A 15-year survivorship study. Clin Orthop Relat Res 286:94–102

Scuderi GR, Insall JN (1992) Total knee arthroplasty. Current clinical perspectives. Clin Orthop Relat Res 276:26–32

Sellam J, Berenbaum F (2010) The role of synovitis in osteoarthritis. Nat Rev Rheumatol 6:625–635

Van Manen MD, Nace J, Mont MA (2012) Management of primary knee osteoarthritis and indications for total knee arthroplasty for general practitioners. J Am Osteopath Assoc 112(11):709–715

Zhang W, Moskowitz RW, Nuki G et al (2008) OARSI recommendations for the management of hip and knee osteoarthritis, Part II: OARSI evidence-based, expert consensus guidelines. Osteoarthr Cartil 16(2):137–162

Osteoarthritis and Other Indications for Total Knee Arthroplasty: An East African Perspective

Seid Mohammed Yasin

Contents

E. Hansen, K.-D. Kühn (eds.), *Essentials of Cemented Knee Arthroplasty*,
https://doi.org/10.1007/978-3-662-63113-3_3

3

3.1 Osteoarthritis

3.1.1 Introduction

> Osteoarthritis (OA) is a disease characterized by degeneration of cartilage and its underlying bone within a joint. It has traditionally been subdivided into either primary (idiopathic) or secondary forms considering its etiology.

Primary osteoarthritis is the most common type of arthritis and one of the commonest reasons for disability worldwide (Kim et al. 2011). It has been estimated that ~7.5% of people over 55 years of age have some knee pain and disability and that ~2% have severe problems. Radiographic evidence of OA occurs in the majority of people of 65 years of age and in about 80% of those aged over 75 years (Arden and Nevitt 2006). About 13% of women and 10% of men aged 60 years and older have symptomatic knee OA (Zhang and Jordan 2010).

> OA of the knee is more prevalent and more severe in women, especially after the age of 55 years, as compared to males.

The prevalence of OA in Africa has not been investigated much. One such study showed that in rural Nigeria, for instance, 1 out of every 5 adults aged ≥40 have symptomatic knee OA (Akinpelu et al. 2011), indicating that the condition is quite rampant in the region.

OA of the knee is particularly important not only for its high prevalence rate compared with other types of OA but also for its presentation at an earlier age and its ongoing increase in incidence in line with the prevalence of aging and obesity.

Total knee arthroplasty (TKA), when indicated, is a very effective way of managing advanced OA as it improves quality of life through improving function and alleviation of pain (Katchy et al. 2018).

3.1.2 Risk Factors

OA is multifactorial and develops through a complex interplay of constitutional and mechanical factors.

Risk Factors for OA of the Knee with Different Degrees of Contributions

- Genetic predisposition
- Old age
- Female sex
- Overweight and obesity
- Knee injury
- Repetitive stress on a joint (e.g., frequent kneeling and prolonged squatting)
- Decreased bone density
- Knee malalignment
- Muscle weakness
- *Meniscal injuries*
- *Other arthritic conditions*
- Joint laxity

Genetic predisposition has been blamed to contribute to the development of primary knee OA. In both genders, knee OA within parents, brothers, or sisters was a significant predictor for symptomatic knee OA in the investigated person (Klussmann et al. 2010).

Aging is known to be an established risk factor for OA. The strong association between age and osteoarthritis may best be explained by age-related changes in the matrix composition and a decrease in chondrocyte function as well as increased responsiveness to stimuli. These changes can interfere with continued internal remodeling, maintenance of the tissue, and loss of cartilage (Hinton et al. 2002).

Obesity, on the other hand, is generally taken as a major risk factor for the occurrence of symptomatic knee OA. This correlation has been supported by numerous publications.

- It has been shown that every 5 kg of weight gain results in a 36% increase in the risk of knee OA.
- On the other hand, another study has reported that 5.1 kg weight reduction over a 10-year period decreased the likelihood of women developing symptomatic knee OA by 50%, revealing the presence of a strong correlation between obesity and OA (Bliddal et al. 2014).

> The pathogenetic role of obesity has been identified to be beyond just a mechanical load on prone joints, in that excess adipose tissue produces humoral factors, altering articular cartilage metabolism. The leptin system has also been postulated to be the link between OA and obesity. These premises may explain the observed prevalence of OA in non-weight-bearing joints such as hand joints of obese subjects (Heidari 2011).

Niu et al. (2009) examined the effect of obesity on knee OA and came up with the following conclusion: Obesity increases the incidence of OA but its contribution to the progression of an already established knee OA may not be as significant. However, this conclusion has so far been an area of debate in the literature.

Occupations that involve knee-straining work activities such as *excessive kneeling and squatting* or *lifting and carrying loads* were found to be associated with symptomatic knee osteoarthritis (Klussmann et al. 2010).

> Other important risk factors include asymmetric mechanical loading, infectious and noninfectious arthritic conditions as well as presence of meniscal injuries.

Regarding sports activities, there are conflicting conclusions among different literatures, some of them regarding sports as risk factors, some others considering them protective against OA, while the rest regarding them as having no effect. In general, evidence show that heavy and repetitive sports could pose some risk of OA whereas *moderate exercises* are *chondroprotective*.

The lifetime risk of developing symptomatic knee OA (i.e., developing the condition by age 85 years) is estimated to be 44.7%, irrespective of sex, race, and level of education. The risk increased in the presence of history of trauma and raised BMI/ obesity (Murphy et al. 2008).

3.1.3 Pathology

> The central pathologic features of OA are the loss of hyaline articular cartilage and changes in the subchondral bone.

The pathogenesis is directly linked to an increase in water content of the articular cartilage with a decrease in proteoglycan content. Collagenase levels increase, thereby disrupting maintained collagen. Proteolytic enzymes and inflammatory cytokines, on the other hand, will increase and end up in an arthritic, painful joint (Martin et al. 2011).

Pathophysiology of the arthritic knee is also known to be related to changes in the autonomic nervous system, blood and lymph flow, fascial tension, limitations in range of motion, and relationships of the length and tension of the muscles around the knee (Van Manen et al. 2012).

3.1.4 Clinical Features

Common symptoms and signs of knee OA include persistent pain, reduced function, crepitus, and swelling. The swelling could result from effusion or could even be secondary to bony enlargement in late presentations.

According to Peat et al. (2007), together with expected demographic features such as age, sex, and body mass index, absence of whole leg pain, difficulty in descending stairs, palpable effusion, fixed-flexion deformity, restricted-flexion range of motion, and crepitus predicted knee OA at sensitivity of 94% and specificity of 93%.

3.1.5 Laboratory Findings

> Complete blood count (CBC), erythrocyte sedimentation rate (ESR), and C-reactive protein (CRP) levels in OA are usually normal.

Synovial fluid is of noninflammatory type. In suspected cases of knee OA, synovial fluid level of anti-CCP can be used for the differentiation of OA from RA (Heidari et al. 2010).

3.1.6 Radiologic Features

Radiologic appearance of an osteoarthritic knee exhibits its attestations for progressive destruction of the articular cartilage like joint space narrowing and reparative processes such as osteophyte formation and subchondral sclerosis.

Subchondral cysts, though taken as one of the cardinal radiological features of OA, are absent in most patients with established OA. Audrey et al. (2014) have documented that subchondral cysts were only present in 30.6% of their study population while narrowed joint space, osteophytes, and subchondral sclerosis were found to be present in 99.5%, 98.1%, and 88.3% of all radiographs in their series, respectively.

Radiologic features are also used for the classification of OA in an attempt to give an idea of severity of the arthritic process and joint degeneration. Kellgren and Lawrence in 1957 came up with a radiologic classification of OA, which has later been endorsed by the WHO and continued to be one of the most accepted radiologic classifications of OA to date (Table 3.1; Figs. 3.1, 3.2, and 3.3).

3.1.7 Management

In obese patients with primary OA of the knee, *weight loss* is the most important strategy to relieve symptoms, including pain, and to check disease progression through *breaking the vicious cycle of events*: reduced activity (because of pain and heavyweight), further weight gain, and decreased muscle strength, leading to further articular damage.

A study on overweight and obese older adults with knee OA estimated that every pound of lost weight

3

Table 3.1 Radiologic grading of OA (adapted from Kellgren and Lawrence 1957)

Grade	Radiologic findings
0	No radiological findings of osteoarthritis
I	Doubtful joint space narrowing and possible osteophytic lipping
II	Definite osteophytes and possible joint space narrowing
III	Moderate multiple osteophytes, definite narrowing of joint space, small pseudocystic areas with sclerotic walls, and possible deformity of bone contour
IV	Large osteophytes, marked joint space narrowing, severe sclerosis, and definite deformity of bone contour

resulted in a fourfold reduction in the load exerted on the knee per step during daily activities, which appears to be clinically meaningful (Bliddal et al. 2014).

The AAOS recommends self-management, exercise, and integrated healthcare programs for patients with knee OA.

> Professionally guided weight loss programs should be incorporated including diet modification and specific exercise programs which do not cause further stress on the knee and its overlying cartilage.

The Framingham knee osteoarthritis study showed a greater than 50% reduction in primary knee OA with a decrease in body mass index of 2 or more (Felson et al. 1987).

Aquatic exercise, gait aids, cognitive behavioral therapy with an exercise component, and self-management programs were the recommended non-pharmacologic options. Moreover, for the first time, mind–body exercises (Tai Chi and Yoga) have recently been recommended as core treatment options for individuals with knee OA.

Topical non-steroidal anti-inflammatory drugs (NSAIDs) were strongly recommended for use in knee OA patients with no comorbidities. High-quality evidence involving a large number of patients showed modest benefits over the course of 12 weeks (Bannuru et al. 2019).

As an initial drug treatment plan, a trial of acetaminophen with other non-pharmaceutical treatments has been recommended before adding NSAIDs, considering the overall cost of NSAIDs and their side effects (Wegman et al. 2004). However, AAOS does not recommend acetaminophen anymore claiming to have found no benefits for it compared to placebo.

Intra-articular corticosteroid injections, on the other hand, reduce knee pain for at least 1 week. They are taken as short-term management options for chronic osteoarthritic conditions (Hepper et al. 2009).

> Hyaluronic acid (HA) injections have a longer term effect in pain control compared with corticosteroids (Bellamy et al. 2006).

The use of glucosamine and chondroitin sulfate for symptomatic knee OA has not been supported by most publications despite the ongoing controversy regarding their patient-reported benefits. All meta-analyses showed that the overall effect of these agents compared to placebo was not statistically significant.

3.1.8 Indications for Total Knee Arthroplasty

> Common diseases that cause knee damage requiring arthroplasty are osteoarthritis, chronic rheumatoid arthritis, and osteonecrosis, while contraindications for knee arthroplasty include purulent arthritis and tuberculosis (Tateishi 2001).

Osteoarthritis, as an indication for surgery, is responsible for majority of TKAs done worldwide. In the USA, one population-based study identified OA to have accounted for 94%–97% of TKA operations (Singh et al. 2010). A search for a similar study in East African countries resulted in almost no data to be mentioned. The only paper identified was from Kenya, by Kigera and Kimpiatu (2015), which showed that *osteoarthritis was the indication for surgery in 96% of TKAs* in their series. Other African countries like Nigeria and Malawi have studies that reported that OA accounted for 100% and 99% of the indications for TKA, respectively (Davies et al. 2019; Katchy et al. 2018).

Knee deformities can be taken both as predisposing conditions for OA and consequences of OA marking severity of the condition and hence necessitating TKA. Analysis of 68 consecutive TKAs performed in Nigeria showed that 26.47% of replaced knees had valgus before surgery, with a mean angle of 22.07° ± 5.73°, whereas 17.65% had varus knees with a mean angle of 14.69° ± 2.84°, and 11.77% knees were found to have flexion deformities with a mean angle of 10.2° ± 1.32°. The rest of 44.11% knees had no deformities (Katchy et al. 2018).

In the presence of radiologic evidence for end-stage degenerative knee joint disease, Osteoarthritis Research Society International (OARSI) recommends TKA for OA when there is a continued pain despite an attempt of

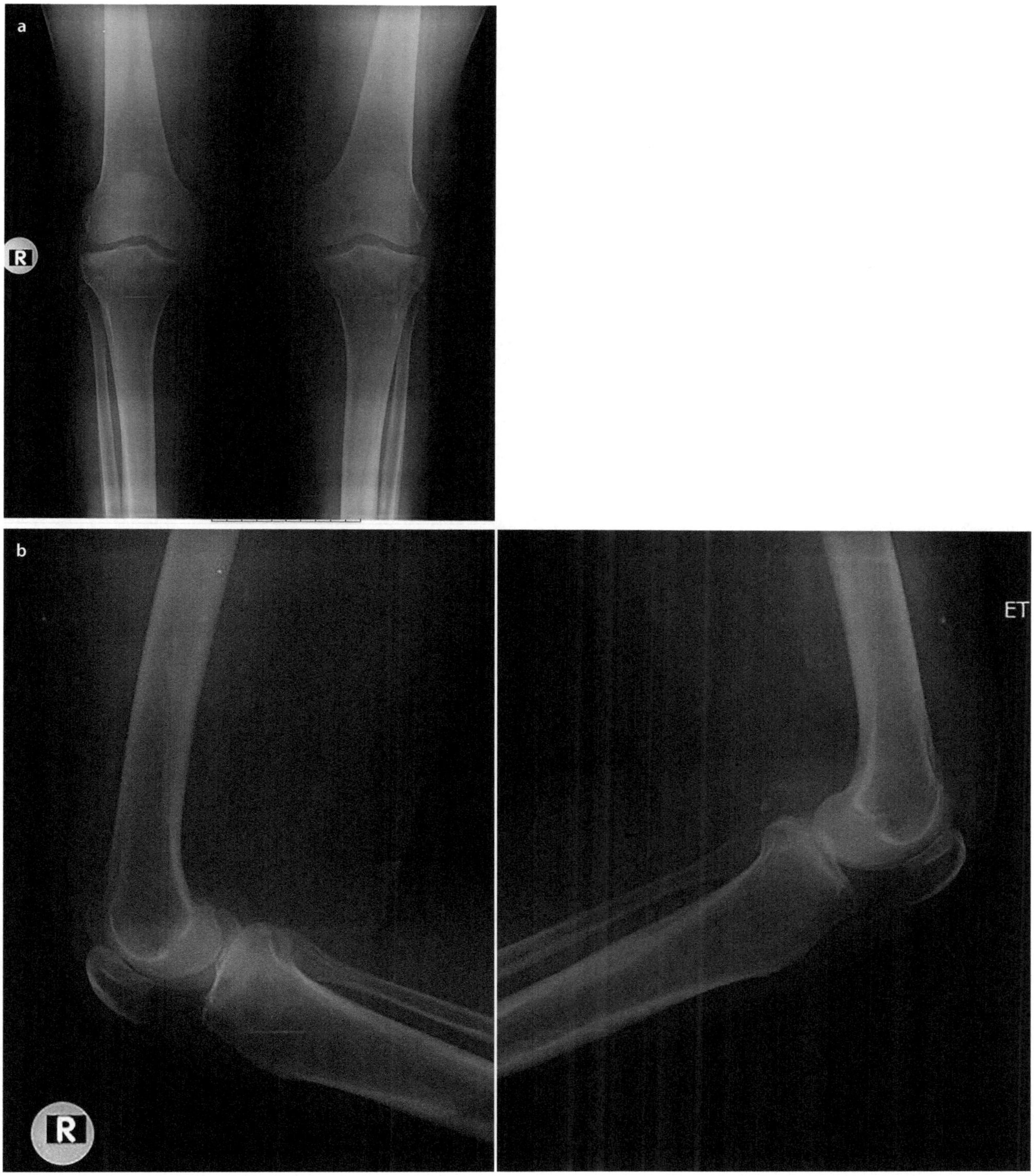

Fig. 3.1 **a**, **b** Mild OA in a 62-year-old Ethiopian woman (Kellgren stage I)

a 6-month course of nonoperative treatment (Zhang et al. 2008). Besides, the decision to pursue TKA should *put the age and body habitus of the patient into consideration*, since the outcome has been variable when TKA was performed for younger and obese individuals in different literatures. This guideline is also applicable for other degenerative joint diseases.

According to Hardorn and Holmes (1997), follow-up of indications for TKA surgeries shows that patients below the age of 60 are less likely to be considered for a TKA and most surgeons want their obese patients to lose weight before surgery.

An additional factor identified to be among determinants of considering candidates for surgery, as several

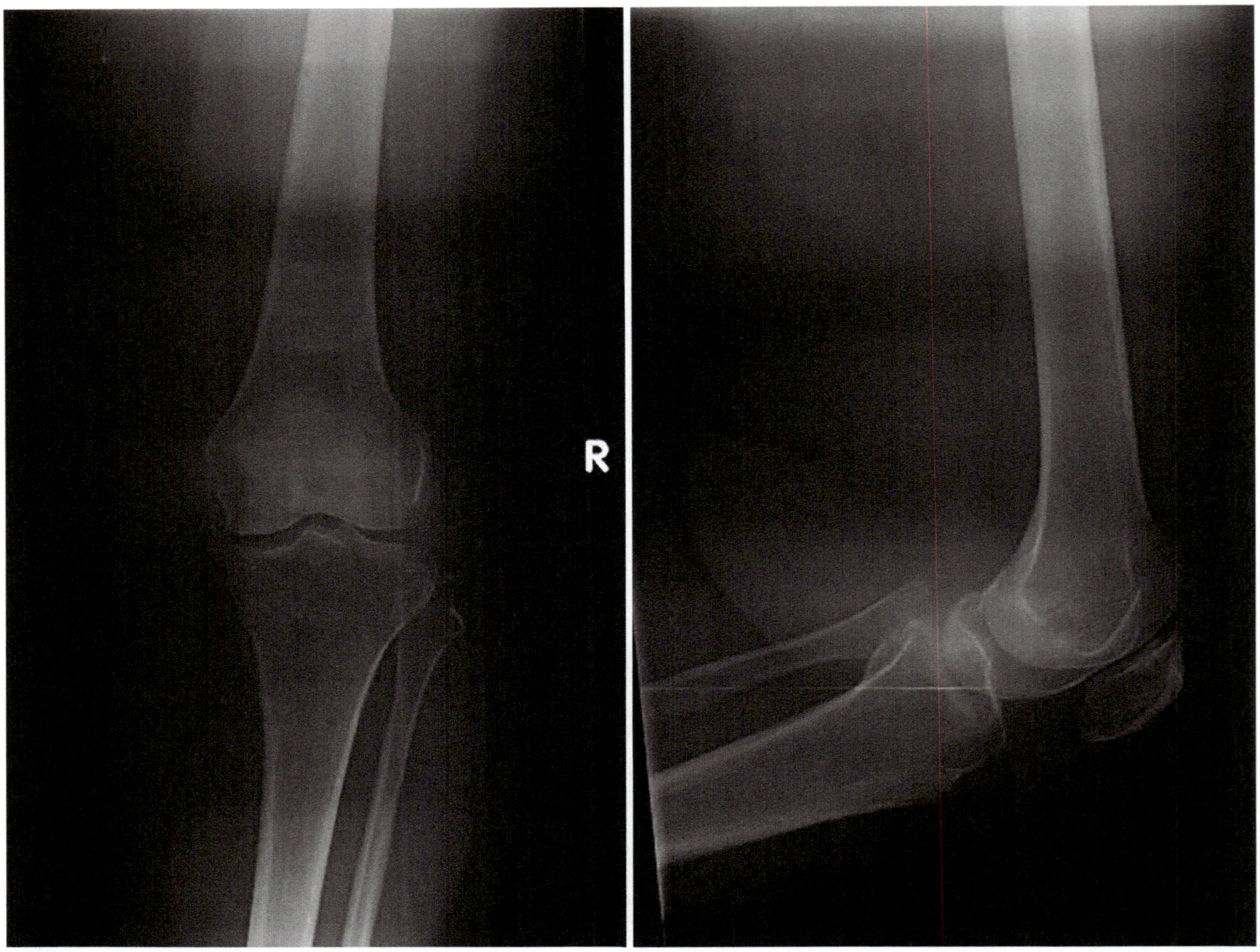

Fig. 3.2 Moderately advanced OA in a 67-year-old Ethiopian man (Kellgren stage II)

studies (summarized by O'Connor and Hooten 2011) have documented, is the presence of an unconscious bias on provider recommendations of TKA for male patients with moderate OA as compared to females with similar conditions.

Despite the numerous researches on the subject and several trials to come up with specific indications for TKA in patients with advanced knee OA, yet there is no consensus on when exactly to do TKA in the disease progress.

However, in the literature review performed by Dieppe et al. (1999), it was concluded that despite the lack of evidence-based indications for TKA in knee OA, daily pain and an attendant X-ray evidence of loss of joint space are taken as key indications for TKA in a consensus-style approach. A high patient motivation was also cited as a common factor contributing to the decision to go ahead with surgery, whereas co-morbidities and technical difficulties were common factors against it.

X-ray features can assist decision-making when both operative and nonoperative options are on the table for a particular patient. But it is wise to note that radiographic appearance of the diseased knee may not always correlate with the degree of pain and disability the patient complains of. It is not uncommon to see patients with comparably affected bilateral knee X-rays, while symptoms are asymmetrical.

McAlindon et al. (1993) have been able to show that radiographic score does not make significant independent contribution to prediction of disability. Quadriceps weakness has rather been found to be the most important factor, signaling the need for a thorough patient evaluation and exhaustion of nonoperative options before coming to a conclusion that TKA is the solution.

The Knee Osteoarthritis Grading System (KOGS) is a radiological grading system of degenerative arthritis of the knee. It is relatively easier to use and has the ability to evaluate all three compartments of the knee to aid the surgeon's decision on the type and timing of knee arthroplasty. Oosthuizen et al. (2018) have regarded KOGS as the first and valid tri-compartmental grading system that can help in decision-making regarding the type and timing of knee arthroplasties based on the preoperative OA status.

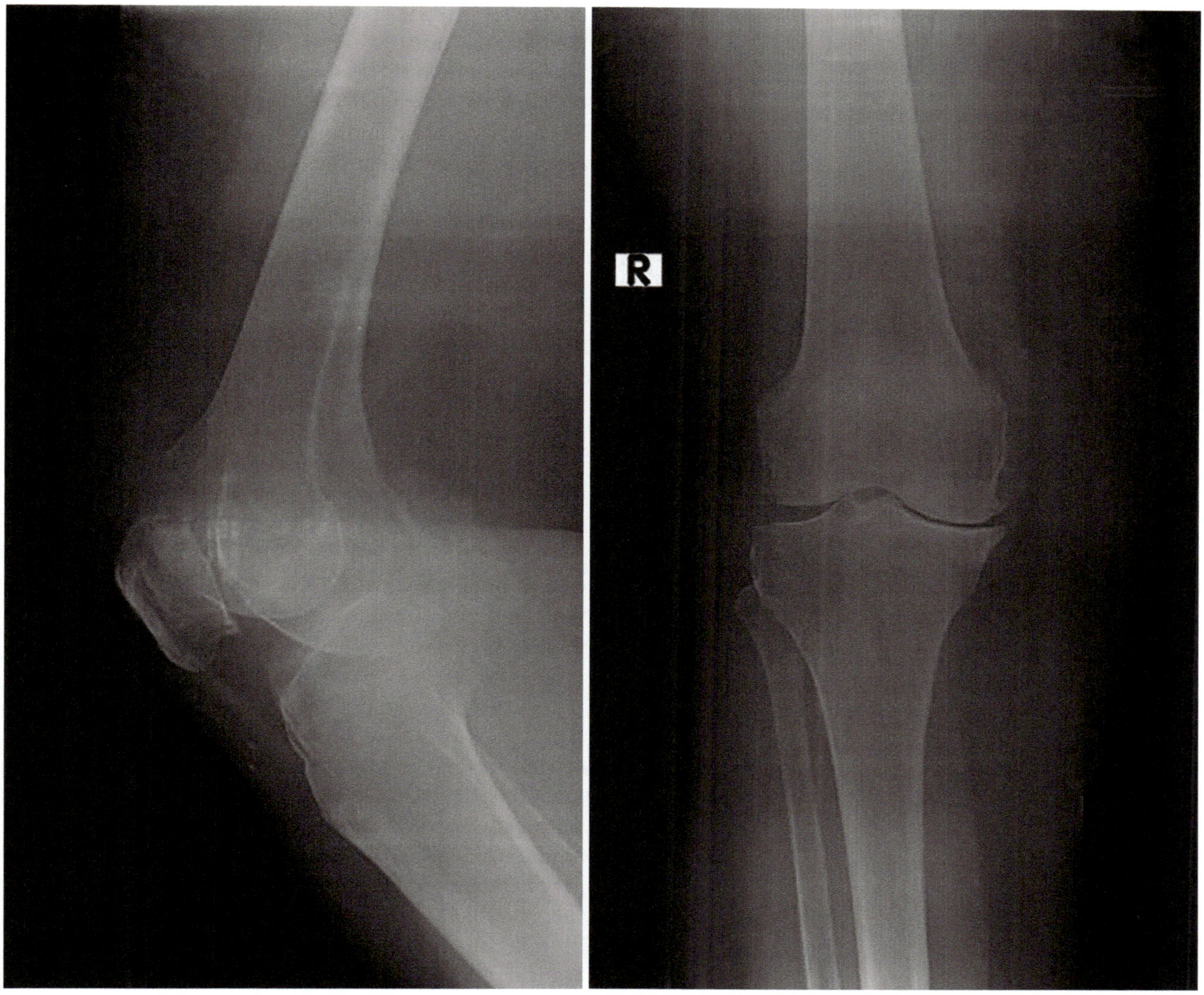

Fig. 3.3 Advanced OA in a 72-year-old Ethiopian woman (Kellgren stage III)

The Delphi consensus technique used by Hardorn and Holmes (1997), trying to derive surgical priorities in knee and hip replacement surgeries using clinical parameters can also be taken as an assistive guide while making decisions (Table 3.2).

Even though this technique, also referred to as "New Zealand priority criteria," has been in use for several years in different institutions, its ability to accurately determine those patients who are most in need of joint replacement surgery has been questioned by Coleman et al. (2005) after comparing it with other scoring systems for disability from musculoskeletal diseases such as the Western Ontario and McMasters Universities Arthritis Index (WOMAC) and the Musculoskeletal Function Assessment (MFA). Its use, hence, should be assisted with other radiologic parameters like KOGS to minimize subjectivity in decision-making.

Table 3.2 Summary of New Zealand priority criteria for major joint replacement[a]

Pain (40%)	Pain severity scored 0–20
	Pain occurrence scored 0–20
Functional activity (20%)	Walking difficulty 0–10
	Other functional impairment 0–10
Movement and deformity (20%)	Pain on active/passive motion 0–10
	Other abnormalities including loss of movement and radiographic change 0–10
Other factors (20%)	Other joints affected 0–10
	Ability to work, act as a caregiver, and live independently 0–10

[a]Patients are scored from 0 to 100 on a scale that describes different levels of severity in four domains: pain, function, joint damage and other factors

3

3.2 Total Knee Arthroplasty in East (and Sub-Saharan) Africa

Given the prevalence of advanced OA requiring TKA in different communities in the world, TKA is taken as an underutilized procedure. This being true even in most civilized countries where access to health care is not a big issue, it would be reasonable to expect a considerable mismatch between the demand and availability of TKA surgeries in less privileged parts of the world such as East Africa.

In most high-income countries healthcare insurance is available to those who can afford it and a state-run safety net program covers the treatment costs for those who cannot afford.

> In contrast, most sub-Saharan African countries (to which East Africa belongs) either do not have health insurers at all or they are yet in the process of developing such a system.

This makes costly procedures such as TKA unaffordable to the majority, not to mention sociocultural barriers, which further diminish the number of candidates.

Therefore, in contrast to the developed countries like Canada, for instance, where willingness to consider total joint arthroplasty is the strongest predictor of the time to such a surgery and income is insignificant as a predictive factor (Hawker et al. 2006).

> In countries like Ethiopia and the rest of East Africa, income is known to be a crucial factor.

In general, in the East African region, TKA surgery is in its infancy for several reasons. Most patients with indications for TKA either do not come to hospitals as from the outset they believe that their condition is an expected stage of their aging process to which one should get used to, or due of a lack of adequate numbers of properly trained knee arthroplasty surgeons and implants the problem is referred to overseas.

Taking a look at the Ethiopian experience, e.g., among cases that were referred abroad for advanced treatments from BLH, the largest hospital in Ethiopia, in 2008, TKA was found to be the third most common indication, being preceded only by total hip replacement and ACL reconstruction (Bezabih and Wamisho 2013).

Over the past several years, knee arthroplasty has been performed in Ethiopia only by visiting surgeons from developed countries in the form of campaigns once in a while. The rest of the patients are referred abroad or obliged to choose living with their ailments because of financial constraints. It is only recently that TKA has started to be performed on a regular basis, though still in very few private hospitals and at costs unaffordable to the huge majority.

Even though there is no published data on the scale of the actual demand for knee arthroplasty or prevalence of the main indications in Ethiopia so far, our experience shows that the number of people with clear indications for TKA is rising from time to time.

In some government hospitals there is a trend of putting the names and contact addresses of patients who are candidates for TKA on a waiting list, relying on links with certain institutions/individual volunteer arthroplasty surgeons who unpredictably visit them for free-of-charge surgeries, in order to help those who cannot afford to travel abroad or cover their own costs in private hospitals. Even though such campaigns have mostly been conducted for total hip arthroplasties (THAs), few campaigns were also conducted addressing those who are in need of TKAs.

Since February 2019, a hospital in the southern part of Ethiopia has started TKA surgeries, probably as the first center in Ethiopia's history to perform TKAs on a regular basis. So far, there are 300 patients on the hospital's waiting list and on average 3–4 are added weekly.

As another example, the largest hospital in the country (BLH), located in the capital city, Addis Ababa, has started to register needy patients with clear indications for TKA. By the end of December 2019, 77 patients were put on the waiting list although there was no announcement of the registration process, no such surgery had been performed in that hospital previously, and there was no known or predicted time when TKA could be done in the future, except for optimistic promises awaiting voluntary surgeons and donors.

> The most probable explanation for the observed rise in the demand for TKAs could be the increase of the aging population and apparent lifestyle changes in the country.

Over the past decade, there are several indicators that more and more people get used to sedentary life and "Western" food items such as fast food alongside increasing urbanization and economic growth. These conditions have increased the prevalence of obesity, one of the main risk factors for OA and progressive knee arthropathy.

While trying to explain the reasons for the observed recent increment in the prevalence of obesity among the Ethiopian community, Dagne et al. (2019) identified new habits like snacking and alcohol drinking as well as an ongoing improvement of the economic status in the society to be the main contributory factors. Compared to previous reports, they also reported that overweight and obesity are on the rise.

Therefore, lifestyle changes, together with the improving trust in modern medicine and the raising awareness (especially in rural areas) regarding the presence of a "medical solution" for the problem mostly conceived as a natural process of aging which the patients are destined to live with for the rest of their lives, are believed to have increased the number of people demanding TKA.

Data on the trend of TKA in the rest of East African countries are not available, probably due to limited experience and short-lived practice of TKA in the region.

Take-Home Messages

- OA of the knee is one of the most prevalent types and has an ongoing increase in incidence in line with prevalence of aging and obesity.
- Family history of the condition, aging, obesity, occupation/type of activity, trauma, other arthritic conditions, and mechanical factors predispose an individual to OA.
- In obese patients, weight loss is an important strategy to check the progression of OA. Exercise programs that do not cause further stress on the knee and its overlying cartilage along with diet modifications should be incorporated into the prevention as well as management strategies of OA.
- There is no internationally agreed protocol for when to pursue TKA in an individual patient with OA or other degenerative joint diseases. But in general, in the presence of radiologic evidence for end-stage degenerative knee joint disease, TKA is recommended when there is a continued pain despite an attempt of a 6-month course of nonoperative treatment.
- The scanty studies done in East Africa showed that by far the vast majority of TKA is done, in the region, for patients with OA.
- Lack of healthcare insurance (i.e., affordability of the surgery) and sociocultural barriers are crucial factors determining the decision to consider TKA in East Africa, besides the clinical decisions.
- The number of patients requiring TKAs is increasing in East Africa, probably because of the increasing incidence of obesity and the society's improving awareness on the availability as well as effectiveness of TKA as a treatment option.

References

Akinpelu AO, Maduagwu SM, Odole AC, Alonge TO (2011) Prevalence and pattern of knee osteoarthritis in a North Eastern Nigerian rural community. East African Orthop J 5:48–54

Arden N, Nevitt MC (2006) Osteoarthritis: epidemiology. Best Pract Res Clin Rheumatol 20(1):3–25

Audrey HX, Abd Razak HR, Andrew TH (2014) The truth behind subchondral cysts in osteoarthritis of the knee. Open Orthop J 8:7–10

Bannuru RR, Bierma-Zeinstra SMA, Blanco FJ et al (2019) OARSI guidelines for the non-surgical management of knee, hip, and polyarticular osteoarthritis. Osteoarthr Cartil 27:1578e1589

Bellamy N, Campbell J, Robinson V et al (2006) Viscosupplementation for the treatment of osteoarthritis of the knee. Cochrane Database Syst Rev 19(2):CD005321

Bezabih B, Wamisho BL (2013) Referrals of Ethiopian orthopedic patients for treatment abroad. COSECSA/ASEA Publication – East Central Afr J Surg 18(1)

Bliddal H, Leeds AR, Christensen R (2014) Osteoarthritis, obesity and weight loss: evidence, hypotheses and horizons – a scoping review. Obes Rev 15:578–586

Coleman B, McChesney S, Twaddle B (2005) Does the priority scoring system for joint replacement really identify those in most need? N Z Med J 118(1215):U1463

Dagne S, Gelaw YA, Abebe Z, Wassie MM (2019) Factors associated with overweight and obesity among adults in Northeast Ethiopia: a cross-sectional study. Diabetes Metab Syndr Obes 12:391–399

Davies PSE, Graham SM, Maqungo S, Harrison WJ (2019) Total joint replacement in sub-Saharan Africa: a systematic review. Trop Dr 49(2):120–128

Dieppe P, Basler HD, Chard J et al (1999) Knee replacement surgery for osteoarthritis: effectiveness, practice variations, indications and possible determinants of utilization. Rheumatology 38:73–83

Felson DT, Naimark A, Anderson J et al (1987) The prevalence of knee osteoarthritis in the elderly: the Framingham Osteoarthritis Study. Arthritis Rheum 30(8):914–918

Hardorn DC, Holmes AC (1997) The New Zealand priority criteria project. Part 1: overview. Br Med J 314:131–314

Hawker GA, Guan J, Croxford R et al (2006) A prospective population-based study of the predictors of undergoing total joint arthroplasty. Arthritis Rheum 54(10):3212–3220

Heidari B (2011) Knee osteoarthritis prevalence, risk factors, pathogenesis and features: part I. Caspian J Intern Med 2(2):205–212

Heidari B, Abedi H, Firouzjahi A, Heidari P (2010) Diagnostic value of synovial fluid anti-cyclic citrullinated peptide antibody for rheumatoid arthritis. Rheumatol Int 30:1465–1470

Hepper CT, Halvorson JJ, Duncan ST et al (2009) The efficacy and duration of intra-articular corticosteroid injection for knee osteoarthritis: a systematic review of level I studies. J Am Acad Orthop Surg 17(10):638–646

Hinton R, Moody RL, Alan W, Thomas SF (2002) Osteoarthritis: diagnosis and therapeutic considerations. Am Fam Physician 65(5):841–848

Katchy AU, Katchy SC, Ekwedigwe HC, Ezeobi I (2018) Total knee replacement in Nigeria: an assessment of early functional outcome of 68 consecutive knees. Niger J Clin Pract 21:1202–1208

Kellgren JH, Lawrence JS (1957) Radiological assessment of osteoarthrosis. Ann Rheum Dis 16:494e502
Kigera JWM, Kimpiatu P (2015) Incidence of early post operative infection after primary total knee arthroplasty at an East African centre. Ann Afr Surg 12:70–72
Kim RH, Springer BD, Douglas DA (2011) Knee reconstruction and replacement. In: Flynn F (ed) Orthopaedic knowledge update. American Academy of Orthopaedic Surgeons, Rosemont, IL, pp 469–475
Klussmann A, Gebhardt H, Nübling M et al (2010) Individual and occupational risk factors for knee osteoarthritis: results of a case-control study in Germany. Arthritis Res Ther 12:R88
Martin JA, Ramakrishnan PA, Lim T et al (2011) Articular cartilage and intervertebral disk. In: Flynn JM (ed) Orthopaedic knowledge update, 10th edn. American Academy of Orthopaedic Surgeons, Rosemont, IL, pp 23–26
McAlindon TE, Cooper C, Kirwan JR, Dieppe PA (1993) Determinants of disability in osteoarthritis of the knee. Ann Rheum Dis 52:258–262
Murphy L, Schwartz TA, Helmick CG et al (2008) Lifetime risk of symptomatic knee osteoarthritis. Arthritis Rheum 59(9):1207–1213
Niu J, Zhang YQ, Torner J et al (2009) Is obesity a risk factor for progressive radiographic knee osteoarthritis? Arthritis Rheum 61:329–335
O'Connor MI, Hooten EG (2011) Breakout session: gender disparities in knee osteoarthritis and TKA. Clin Orthop Relat Res 469:1883–1885
Oosthuizen CR, Takahashi T, Snyckers CH et al (2018) The knee osteoarthritis grading system for arthroplasty. J Arthroplast 34:450e455
Peat G, Thomas E, Duncan R et al (2007) Estimating the probability of radiographic osteoarthritis in the older patient with knee pain. Arthritis Rheum 57(5):794–802
Singh JA, Vessely MB, Harmsen WS et al (2010) A population-based study of trends in the use of total hip and total knee arthoplasty, 1969–2008. Mayo Clin Proc 85(10):898–904
Tateishi H (2001) Indications for total knee arthroplasty and choice of prosthesis. JMAJ 44:153–158
Van Manen MD, Nace J, Mont MA (2012) Management of primary knee osteoarthritis and indications for total knee arthroplasty for general practitioners. J Am Osteopath Assoc 112:709–715
Wegman A, van der Windt D, van Tulder M et al (2004) Nonsteroidal antiinflammatory drugs or acetaminophen for osteoarthritis of the hip or knee? A systematic review of the evidence and guidelines. J Rheumatol 31(2):344–354
Zhang Y, Jordan JM (2010) Epidemiology of osteoarthritis. Clin Geriatr Med 26:355–369
Zhang W, Moskowitz RW, Nuki G et al (2008) OARSI recommendations for the management of hip and knee osteoarthritis: part II. OARSI evidence-based, expert consensus guidelines. Osteoarthr Cartil 16(2):137–162

Inflammatory Arthritis

Zachary K. Christopher, Jaymeson R. Arthur, and Mark J. Spangehl

Contents

E. Hansen, K.-D. Kühn (eds.), *Essentials of Cemented Knee Arthroplasty*,
https://doi.org/10.1007/978-3-662-63113-3_4

4

4.1 Introduction

Patients with inflammatory arthritis planning to undergo total knee arthroplasty (TKA) present several unique challenges for orthopedic surgeons. In this chapter, we will briefly review how to approach the patient with inflammatory arthritis and outline critical preoperative, intraoperative, and postoperative considerations to aid in a successful cemented TKA in this patient population.

Inflammatory arthropathies encompass numerous diseases, all causing systemic inflammation, often with multiple joint involvement. These diseases include the following:

- Rheumatoid arthritis (RA).
- Psoriatic arthritis.
- Ankylosing spondylitis.
- Juvenile idiopathic arthritis (JIA).
- Systemic lupus erythematosus (SLE).

> Rheumatoid arthritis is the most common form of inflammatory arthritis in the United States and the majority of literature on TKA in inflammatory arthritis focuses on this patient population (Schrama et al. 2010; Bongartz et al. 2008; Cancienne et al. 2016).

While each disease entity may have several specific factors that should be considered, it is critical to understand that a common thread among all inflammatory arthropathies is the combination of both local and systemic effects produced by the disease and, therefore, both local and systemic factors must be considered for optimizing outcomes.

> Local effects of inflammatory arthritis include generalized osteopenia, bony erosions and deformity, and soft tissue derangement.

Studies using magnetic resonance imaging (MRI) and ultrasonography (US) have been pivotal in our understanding of the pathogenesis of the inflammatory process at a joint-specific level (Boutry et al. 2007; Sudoł-Szopińska et al. 2017; Henchie et al. 2019). Common findings include synovitis, tenosynovitis, bursitis, and subchondral bone marrow edema and erosions. Studies have shown that it is the subchondral bone that is most significantly affected (Lereim and Goldie 1975; Lereim et al. 1974; Yang et al. 1997). This finding is of particular importance to the arthroplasty surgeon as this is where prosthetic fixation is achieved and where the bone–cement interface is most robustly fixated.

> For this reason, uncemented TKA in this patient population is strongly discouraged.

Further, patients can often exhibit significant cystic changes and focal bone loss.

The surgeon should carefully scrutinize preoperative X-rays to be aware of and prepared to address these bony defects as bone grafting or augmentation is often required.

> Bony deformity as well as ligament incompetence may also be present in these patients.

The surgeon should be prepared with implants that impart a higher level of constraint if necessary. However, as previously noted, the quality of the subchondral bone is often deficient in these patients and increasing constraint imparts more mechanical shear on the bone–cement interface. Hence, each case should be carefully planned when deciding implant options as additional fixation may be required when managing bony deficiency or using an increased level of constraint.

> Systemic effects of inflammatory arthritis include immunosuppression, respiratory and cardiac comorbidities, wound healing issues, cervical spine pathology, dermatologic manifestations, and malnutrition.

Furthermore, long-term corticosteroid use and immunosuppressive medications often render these patients immunocompromised. Therefore, in addition to surgical considerations, it is important to ensure medical optimization prior to the procedure. Consulting with the patient's rheumatologist preoperatively, or consulting one if a patient is presenting with a new diagnosis, is recommended. Assessment by a rheumatologist can aid in optimizing the patient's medication management, which has become the mainstay for treatment for the majority of these conditions.

4.2 Case Example

A 33-year-old female presented to the clinic with several years of bilateral knee pain and a history of rheumatoid arthritis diagnosed 10 years prior. She was being managed by a rheumatologist and had been treated with several medications including prednisone 8 mg daily, hydroxychloroquine 200 mg twice daily, and sulfasalazine 1000 mg twice daily. In addition, she used rituximab twice annually, most recently 3 months prior to presentation. She was dependent on a walker or wheelchair and could only ambulate for very short distances unassisted. She had tried over-the-counter medications including acetaminophen and NSAIDs without significant relief. On examination, she had marked varus malalignment bilaterally and a lateral thrust. Her varus was correctable to nearly neutral. She had good range of motion from 3° to 125° on the left and 0° to 130° on the right. Neurovascular exam was normal. Plain radiographs demonstrated severe bilateral knee deformities with significant tricompartmental arthritis with joint space narrowing, sclerosis, and varus malalignment (◘ Fig. 4.1).

The patient ultimately underwent bilateral-staged TKAs approximately 6 weeks apart. Prior to her surgeries, her prednisone was weaned down to 6 mg/day. This medication was continued in the perioperative period along with sulfasalazine. Preoperative cervical spine films revealed 3 mm anterolisthesis of C1 on C2 (◘ Fig. 4.2). For both knee arthroplasties, varus/valgus-stabilized cemented implants were utilized with 50 mm stem extensions. On the left side, a medial tibial augment was used because of severe medial bone deficiency. On the right, a smaller defect was filled with cement. Prophylactic tobramycin was used in the cement. At most recent follow-up of 3 years postoperative, the patient was doing well with no pain and had returned to activities like 6-mile elliptical exercises. Her knees were stable to varus and valgus stress without laxity, and both knees had excellent range of motion from 0° to 135°. Radiographs demonstrated well-fixed, well-positioned implants without any concerns of loosening (◘ Fig. 4.3).

4.3 Preoperative Considerations

Prior to elective surgery, patients with inflammatory arthritis must undergo a thorough multidisciplinary preoperative evaluation. In addition to the orthopedic evaluation, particular attention should be paid to the cardiovascular system and the cervical spine. Further, preoperative and perioperative medication management in patients with inflammatory arthritis has been a subject of much debate and research and, as such, a significant portion of this chapter will focus on the management of these various medications.

4.3.1 General Medical Evaluation

> As part of the multidisciplinary workup, a thorough cardiac evaluation should be performed.

Studies have shown that patients with inflammatory arthritis such as rheumatoid arthritis are at an increased risk of cardiovascular-related death compared to the general population (Meune et al. 2009; Ogdie et al. 2015; Avina-Zubieta et al. 2012). Lindharden et al. evaluated over four million patients in their cohort study and found that the risk of myocardial infarction in patients with RA was similar to that of patients with diabetes and to that of non-rheumatoid patients who were 10 years older (Lindhardsen et al. 2011). Further, Ogdie et al. showed that psoriatic arthritis may be an independent risk factor for major cardiac events in the perioperative period, particularly in those patients not on disease-modifying antirheumatic drugs (DMARDs) (Ogdie et al. 2015). Based on a patient's cardiac conditions, the primary care/medicine team can determine if further cardiac testing is warranted outside of the standard electrocardiogram and physical examination. Close collaboration with these teams to ensure proper perioperative risk evaluation and medical optimization will help safeguard the best overall outcomes.

> Cervical spine disease is common in patients with inflammatory arthritis, especially in patients with RA (Kwek et al. 1998; Lopez-Olivo et al. 2012; Krause and Matteson 2014).

Abnormalities include atlantoaxial subluxation, atlantoaxial impaction, and subaxial subluxation. Although no clinical practice guidelines have been established for preoperative imaging in patients with inflammatory arthritis, the anesthesiology team should always be made aware of this condition, as intraoperative positioning and method of intubation may be affected based on the presence or absence of cervical spine disease. The anesthesiology team typically requires cervical spine X-ray including flexion–extension views (Lopez-Olivo et al. 2012). Further, based on anesthesia's assessment, the use of regional blocks or flexible fiber optic bronchoscopy has been increasingly utilized in this patient population in order to mitigate potential adverse events related to preexisting cervical spine disease (Kwek et al. 1998).

4.3.2 Medications

There are numerous medications used to treat inflammatory diseases. It is important to understand each class and how to manage these medications pre- and postoperatively. In general, many patients with systemic inflammatory arthritis are generally immunocompromised. The American College of Rheumatology and the American Association of Hip and Knee Surgeons (ACR-AAHKS) published a series of evidence-based guidelines on perioperative medication management that can be used to guide decision-making (◘ Table 4.1; ▶ https://www.rheumatology.org/Portals/0/Files/ACR-AAHKS-Perioperative-Management-Guideline.pdf).

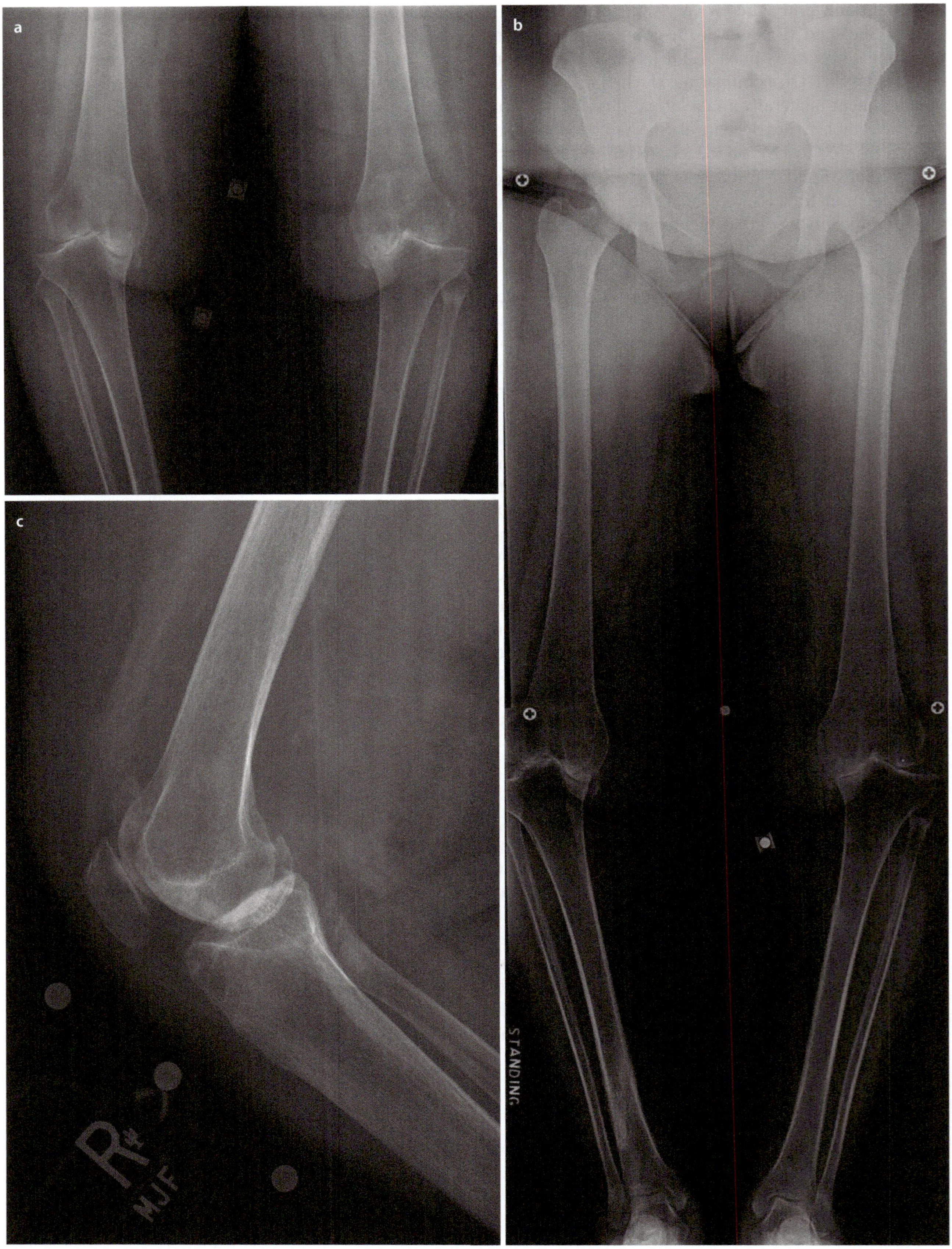

Fig. 4.1 **a–e** Preoperative bilateral knee radiographs

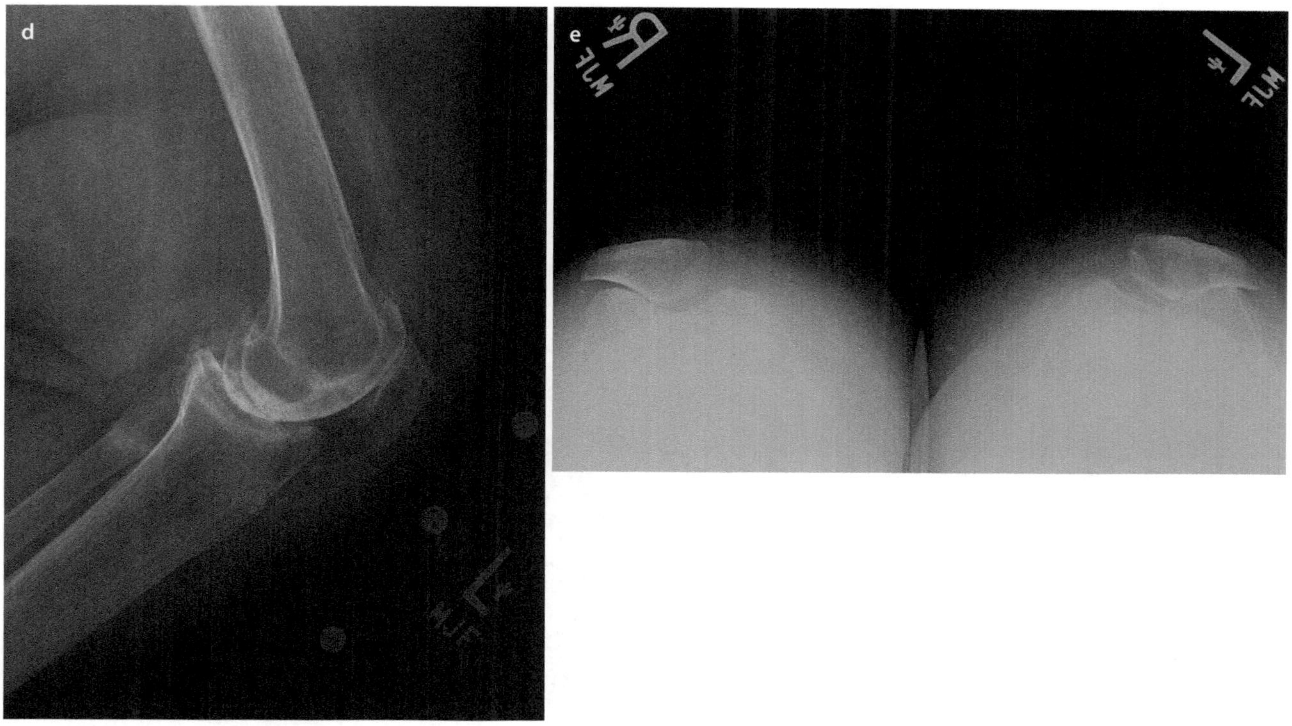

Fig. 4.1 (continued)

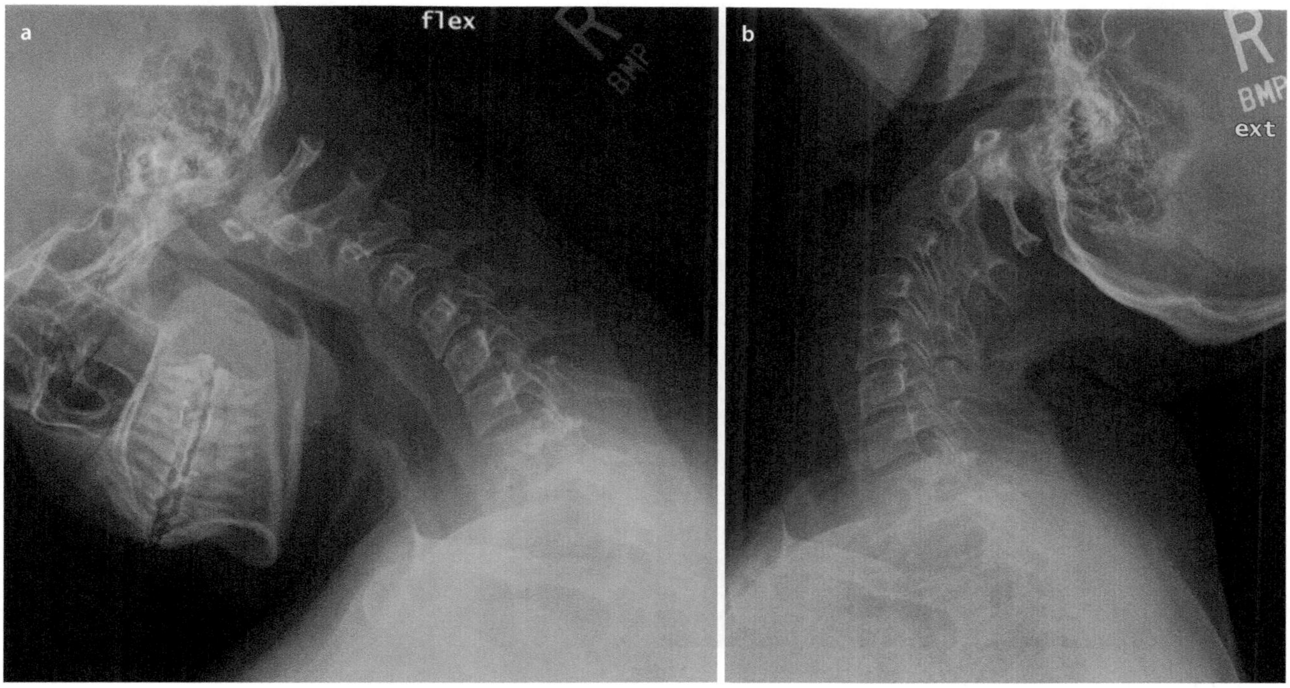

Fig. 4.2 **a**, **b** Preoperative flexion–extension cervical spine radiographs

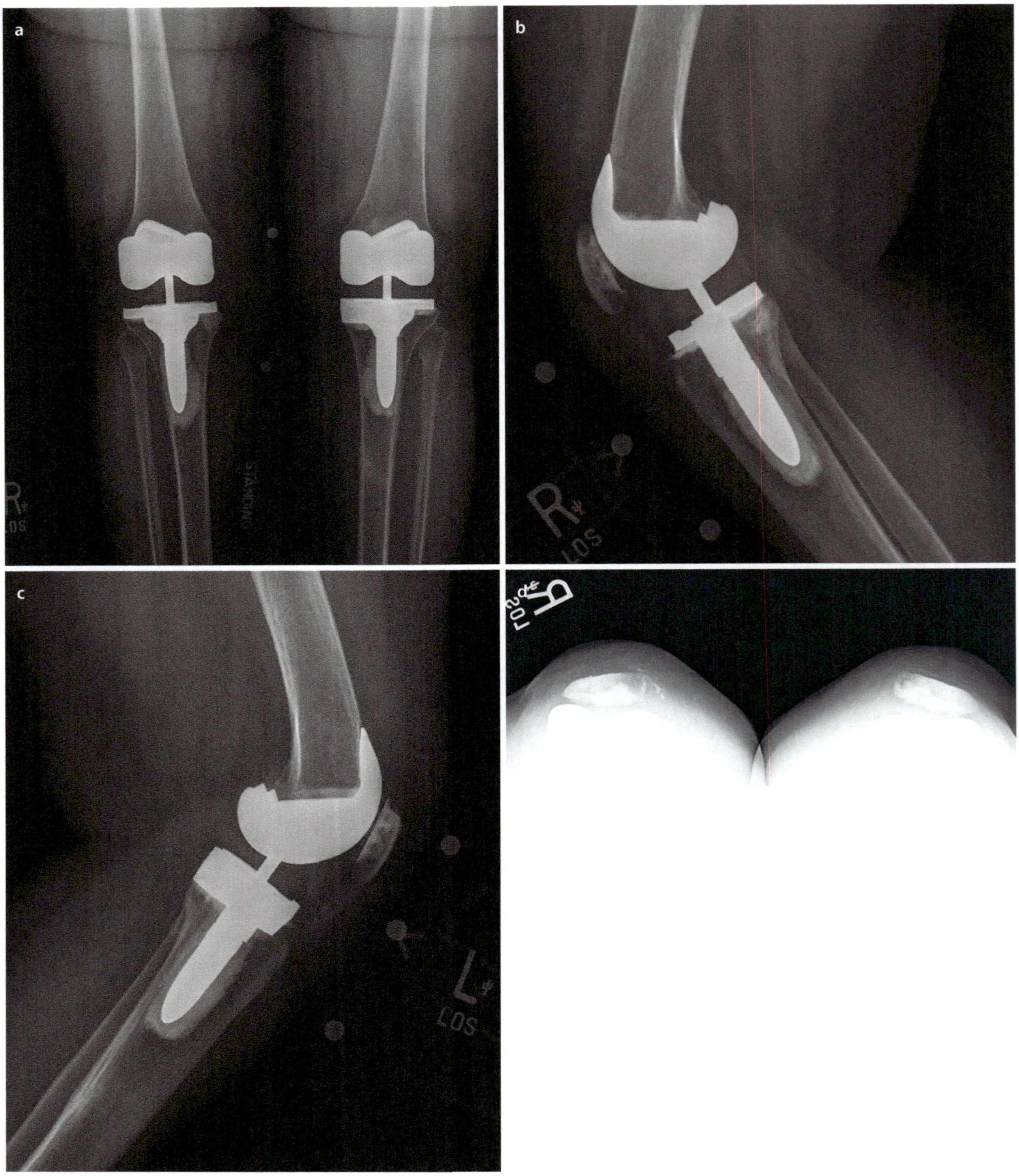

Fig. 4.3 **a–d** Postoperative bilateral knee radiographs

Table 4.1 Perioperative medication management in patients with inflammatory diseases

DMARDs: *Continue* these medications through surgery	**Dosing interval**	**Continue/withhold**
Methotrexate	Weekly	Continue
Sulfasalazine	Once or twice daily	Continue
Hydroxychloroquine	Once or twice daily	Continue
Leflunomide (Arava)	Daily	Continue
Doxycycline	Daily	Continue
Biologic Agents: Stop **these medications prior to surgery at the end of the dosing cycle. *Resume* medications at minimum 14 days after surgery in the absence of wound healing problems, surgical site infection, or systemic infection**	**Dosing interval**	**Schedule surgery (relative to last biologic agent dose administered) during**
Adalimumab (Humira)	Weekly or every 2 weeks	Week 2 or 3
Etanercept (Enbrel)	Weekly or twice weekly	Week 2
Golimumab (Simponi)	Every 4 weeks (SQ) or Every 8 weeks (IV)	Week 5 Week 9
Infliximab (Remicade)	Every 4, 6, or 8 weeks	Week 5, 7, or 9
Abatacept (Orenica)	Monthly (IV) or Weekly (SQ)	Week 5 Week 2
Certolizumab (Cimzia)	Every 2 or 4 weeks	Week 3 or 5
Rituximab (Rituxan)	2 doses 2 weeks apart every 4–6 months	Month 7
Tocilizumab (Actemra)	Every week (SQ) or Every 4 weeks (IV)	Week 5 Week 2
Anakinra (Kineret)	Daily	Day 2
Secukinumab (Cosentyx)	Every 4 weeks	Week 5
Ustekinumab (Stelara)	Every 12 weeks	Week 13
Belimumab (Benlysta)	Every 4 weeks	Week 5
Tofacitinib (Xeljanz): *Stop* this medication 7 days prior to surgery	Daily or twice daily	7 days after last dose
Severe Sle-specific Medications: Continue **these medications in the perioperative period**	**Dosing interval**	**Continue/withhold**
Mycophenolate mofetil	Twice daily	Continue
Azathioprine	Daily or twice daily	Continue
Cyclosporine	Twice daily	Continue
Tacrolimus	Twice daily (IV and PO)	Continue
Not-severe Sle: Discontinue **these medications 1 week prior to surgery**	**Dosing interval**	**Continue/withhold**
Mycophenolate mofetil	Twice daily	Continue
Azathioprine	Daily or twice daily	Continue
Cyclosporine	Twice daily	Continue
Tacrolimus	Twice daily (IV and PO)	Continue

Courtesy of the 2017 American College of Rheumatology/American Association of Hip and Knee Surgeons Guideline for the Perioperative Management of Antirheumatic Medication in Patients With Rheumatic Diseases Undergoing Elective Total Hip or Total Knee Arthroplasty(Goodman et al. 2017)

4

4.3.2.1 Glucocorticoids

Glucocorticoids are often used in treating the following:

- RA.
- Ankylosing spondylitis.
- SLE.
- Psoriatic arthritis.

> The ACR-AAHKS current recommendations are to continue the current daily dose of glucocorticoids in adults with inflammatory arthridities who are undergoing TKA or THA (Goodman et al. 2017). Supratherapeutic "stress-dosing" is not recommended in most patients.

Jain et al. published evidence suggesting that continuation of steroids does not affect postoperative infection rates, and in fact, stopping them can lead to flares which can delay rehabilitation (Jain et al. 2002). However, it does distinguish that doses over 15 mg/day have been reported to increase postoperative infection rates in patients with RA (Somayaji et al. 2013). It is important to note that the current guidelines recommend continuing glucocorticoids at doses <20 mg/day when possible. At higher doses, consultation with the patient's rheumatologist should be considered prior to surgery, as this may indicate inadequate disease control (ACR-AAHKS Guidelines).

4.3.2.2 DMARDs

> The current consensus is that disease-modifying antirheumatic drugs (DMARDs) are safe to continue through the perioperative period.

One of the most significant studies by Grennan et al. evaluated methotrexate and early postoperative complications in patients with RA undergoing elective TJA. They found that continuation of methotrexate did not increase the risk of infections compared to those patients who had the medication discontinued, and in fact continuation of methotrexate may decrease the risk of flares (Grennan et al. 2001). These authors performed a 10-year follow-up study and ultimately adhered to their original conclusions that in the absence of renal failure or sepsis, methotrexate therapy should be continued (Sreekumar et al. 2011). Similar results have been demonstrated in hand and wrist surgery (Jain et al. 2002).

4.3.2.3 Biologics

Biologic agents are those medications that use genetically engineered proteins to target specific immune cells or other cellular proteins to ultimately alter downstream immune responses. Management of biologics in the perioperative period is often more nuanced than the other medication classes. The details of the current recommendations can be found in ◘ Table 4.1 from the ACR-AAHKS. Biologics should be stopped prior to surgery.

> Elective surgery should be scheduled at the end of the dosing cycle with discontinuation of the medications.

The literature demonstrates that the use of biologics increases the risk of infection as well as serious adverse events with odds ratios around 1.5 for both endpoints (Goodman and Figgie 2013). Furthermore, Goodman et al. performed a systematic review and meta-analysis evaluating the use of TNF-α inhibitors in total joint arthroplasty. Their findings confirmed that the use of TNF-α inhibitors resulted in an increased risk of developing a surgical site infection with an odds ratio of 2.47 (95% CI 1.66, 3.68); $P < 0.0001$) (Goodman et al. 2016).

4.3.2.4 SLE-Specific Considerations

Medications including mycophenolate mofetil, azathioprine, cyclosporine, and tacrolimus have SLE-specific indications. The specific dosing intervals in the perioperative period are again found in ◘ Table 4.1. The key difference is whether the medication is being used to treat severe or non-severe SLE. In patients with severe SLE, it is recommended to continue these medications, whereas in non-severe SLE they can be withheld 1 week prior to surgery. Severe SLE is defined as those currently being treated for severe organ involvement including lupus nephritis, myocarditis, hemolytic anemia, and central nervous system lupus, among many others.

4.3.3 Orthopedic Evaluation

Orthopedic evaluation starts with a thorough history focusing on the disease process such as duration of disease, medications, and other joint involvement. A thorough physical exam should be conducted with special attention toward the degree of deformity of the knee, including fixed versus correctible deformities in the coronal and sagittal planes. Further, there is often attenuation of the ligaments in or around the knee; hence determination of ligamentous stability is critical to evaluate as this influences implant choice.

> Preoperative knee radiographs including full-length standing alignment films are recommended. It is also important to discuss patient expectations following TKA in patients with inflammatory arthritis.

Outcomes will be discussed further below, but literature has shown that patients undergoing TKA with inflammatory diseases are on average 10 years younger than those with osteoarthritis (OA) (Lee et al. 2017). Of patients younger than 45 undergoing TKA, a majority had either RA or juvenile RA as the primary diagnosis (Dalury et al. 1995). Fortunately, patient-reported outcome measures in young patients with both OA and inflammatory arthritis are comparable to those in older age groups (Gill et al. 1997). However, it is critical to discuss that the risk of requiring revision surgery for any reason is higher in younger patients. A study published in 2017 demonstrated that the lifetime risk of revision increases up to 35% for those in the age of 50–54 undergoing TKA compared with only 5% in patients older than 70 (Schreurs and Hannink 2017).

4.4 Intraoperative Considerations

With proper preparation, including careful scrutiny of preoperative imaging and detailed physical examination, the arthroplasty surgeon should be aware of the bony defects, soft tissue destruction, and ligament stability. Further, the surgeon should be prepared with a combination of augments, cones, or sleeves, and increasing implant-specific level of constraint to address each patient's specific needs. Because of the overall osteopenia and specifically the effect of the inflammatory process on the subchondral bone, where implant fixation is most critical, cementation is almost exclusively recommended in this patient population.

The posterior cruciate ligament (PCL) provides the main resistance to posterior translation of the tibia on the femur and is critical for femoral rollback during knee flexion. Perhaps one of the most debated topics in patients with inflammatory disease undergoing TKA is the use of posterior stabilized (PS) versus cruciate-retaining (CR) implants. Several studies have been published citing good results for either, and mixed results have been published comparing the two groups (◘ Table 4.2). No meta-analyses have been performed comparing PS and CR TKAs. Some surgeons favor the use of PS citing a higher risk of complications and increased revision rate due to eventual PCL incompetence. Laskin et al. compared patients with RA undergoing TKA with CR and PS implants for a minimum of 6-year follow-up. The group with PCL retention (i.e., CR knees) was noted to have increased recurvatum and posterior instability. Similarly, in the revision setting, patients had a higher incidence of PCL absence (Laskin and O'Flynn 1997).

In contrast, some surgeons favor the use of CR implants when the PCL is present and functioning well. Archibeck et al. demonstrated satisfactory results with posterior cruciate-retaining implants with a 93% survival rate at 10 years. Nine of 72 patients required revision, but 6 of these were related to the metal-backed patella. Only one patient had radiographic or clinical evidence of posterior instability (Archibeck et al. 2001). Similarly, Miller et al. demonstrated a 93% implant survival rate at 20 years in patients with CR implants using posterior instability as the endpoint (Miller et al. 2011). Ashraf et al. performed a review of the literature and found "excellent" long-term survivorship and functional outcomes with up to 25 years of follow-up (Ashraf et al. 2017). Notably, this review was not a meta-analysis. In another study, Hanyu noted good results when selectively using both PS and CR implants in RA patients, citing a 93% survivorship rate at 10 years after adjustment for mortality (Hanyu et al. 1997). These authors used a CR design in 57 knees and PS in the remaining 31 when the PCL was incompetent. There is a need for a systematic review with meta-analysis comparing CR and PS implants to strengthen any recommendations.

> However, if the PCL is found to be deficient or absent intraoperatively, a PS implant is indicated.

Patellar resurfacing in patients with inflammatory arthritis, specifically RA, has been investigated. In 1989 Shoji performed a study of 35 patients with bilateral TKA, one with and one without patellar resurfacing and found no difference in pain, functional improvement, muscle strength, or range of motion (Shoji et al. 1989). About a decade later, Kajino et al. performed a study of simultaneous bilateral TKA with patellar resurfacing unilaterally. They noted similar outcomes, however, they found pain on standing and ascending and descending stairs was noted only in those without patellar resurfacing (Kajino et al. 1997). A more recent study by Bhan et al. concluded that TKA without patellar resurfacing yielded satisfactory results in patients with RA (Bhan et al. 2006).

> There is no consensus on patellar resurfacing in inflammatory arthritis, but surgeons should consider that these conditions affect the entire joint and the patellofemoral joint may be frequently involved.

It would stand to reason that in patients with adequate bone stock, patellar resurfacing is an option. However, if the patella is naturally thin (<20 mm thick), osteopenic, or has significant bone loss secondary to erosions or wear, then patellar resurfacing is not advised.

There is limited literature on the use of antibiotic bone cement in primary total knee arthroplasty in patients with inflammatory arthritis.

4

Table 4.2 Selected studies evaluating PS and CR implants in patients with inflammatory arthritis

Year published	Authors	Prosthesis	Findings	Conclusion (PS vs. CR)
1995	Aglietti et al. (1995)	PS	Cumulative success rate of 96.2% at 13 years	PS implants have excellent results in patients with RA
1997	Laskin and O'Flynn (1997))	PS vs. CR (in both RA and OA)	CR implants in RA: Increased recurvatum and posterior instability, 81% survival rate at 10 years	PS recommended due to posterior instability
1997	Hanyu et al. (1997)	PS vs. CR	93% implant survival at 10 years for all comers, but 31/61 patients died during the study period	Both can have excellent results
2001	Gill and Joshi 2001	CR	90.7% survivorship of implant at 19 years	Good long-term results with CR implants in RA
2001	Archibeck et al. (2001)	CR	95% good to excellent PROMs, 93% survivorship at 10 years, no aseptic loosening	Excellent results with CR when PCL was intact and functioning at the time of surgery
2011	Miller et al. (2011)	CR	At 20 years: 69% survival with revision as the endpoint, 93% survival with posterior instability as the endpoint	PCL insufficiency with instability was rarely the cause of failure following CR TKA in patients with RA
2012	Yamanaka et al. (2012)	CR	No loosening, 96.9% survivorship at 12 years	CR prosthesis is very effective in RA patients at 5 to 12 years postoperative
2015	Lee et al. (2015)	CR	All-cause revision rates: 98.7% at 10 years and 83.6% at 17 years	Possibility of increased loosening rates after 10 years in CR knees
2019	Luo et al. (2019)	PS (multi- vs. single-radius)	97.5% implant survival for the SR at 10 years and 98.3% for the MR group at 10 years	Single- and multi-radius PS prostheses yield satisfactory results at 10 years

A 2003 study by Liu reviewed 60 patients with RA who underwent primary TKA with cefuroxime-loaded bone cement in addition to parenteral antibiotic prophylaxis, and demonstrated no deep infections (Liu et al. 2003).

Studies evaluating high-risk patients suggest that there may be benefits in using low-dose antibiotic-loaded bone cement (ALBC). Chiu et al. randomized 340 patients undergoing primary TKA to cefuroxime-impregnated cement versus a control and showed no deep infection in the ALBC group versus five infections in the control group. It is important to note that all five infections occurred in a higher risk group with diabetes (Chiu et al. 2002).

In a 2006 current concepts review, Jiranek et al. recommended the use of low-dose ALBC in high-risk patients (Fig. 4.4) (Jiranek et al. 2006). Two large retrospective registry studies demonstrated a statistically significant decrease in rates of revision (HR 0.85) (Jameson et al. 2019) and odds for early postoperative infection (OR 0.89) (Chan et al. 2019).

Extrapolating these data, we recommend consideration of either manual or commercially mixed ALBC in patients with inflammatory diseases who are inherently at higher risk for infection.

4.5 Postoperative Considerations

4.5.1 Medications

As discussed previously, medication management is the mainstay of treatment for these systemic diseases. Restarting any medications that were discontinued prior to surgery is important to minimize symptoms, maintain control of the condition, and prevent flare of the disease. The risk and benefits of disease control versus complications must be carefully balanced and it is important to work closely with the patient's rheumatol-

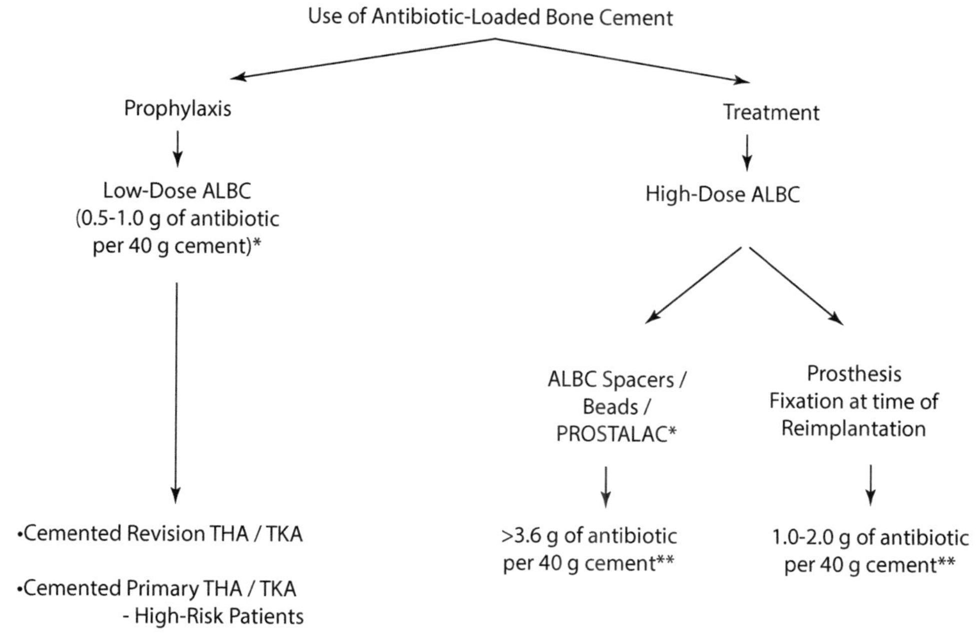

■ **Fig. 4.4** Use of antibiotic-loaded bone cement. (Jiranek et al. 2006)

ogist in decision-making. The recommendations from the ACR-AAHKS publication can be found in ■ Table 4.1 and should serve as a guide to therapy.

4.5.2 Complications

Patients with inflammatory arthropathies are well known to have higher complication rates, particularly infection, compared to those with OA. This is likely due to a combination of chronic inflammation, immune dysfunction, and long-term use of immune-suppressing medications. By the time these patients present for evaluation by an arthroplasty surgeon, they have usually been taking immune-modulating medications including DMARDs, steroids, or biologics for an extended time period. Although historical studies reported infection rates after joint replacement to be as high as 17%(Stern et al. 1989) in patients with inflammatory conditions, more recent data suggest that the rate of infection in patients with inflammatory arthritis following TKA is approximately 2%, which is nearly double that of the general population (Cancienne et al. 2016). Despite several studies evaluating the timing of medication management in the perioperative period, infection risk still remains high in this patient population (Schrama et al. 2010; Bongartz et al. 2008; Ravi et al. 2012).

» Bongartz et al. showed that RA patients had a threefold increased infection rate at 5 years compared to patients with OA. They recommended that surgeons should strongly consider the use of antibiotic-impregnated cement in this patient population (Bongartz et al. 2008).

Similarly, we agree that it is reasonable to use ALBC in this context, however, there is no evidence that it prevents indolent inoculum or late hematogenous infection.

Although many of the common medications used in managing inflammatory arthritis have dramatically improved the quality of life in patients afflicted with these disorders, these medications can also have detrimental effects in the immediate postoperative period. As the primary effect of many of these drugs is to decrease inflammation and the local immune response, this has direct implication on wound healing.

In their review article, Busti et al. thoroughly outline the normal process of wound healing and how therapeutic medications can disrupt this healing (Busti et al. 2005). They outline that during the acute phase of wound healing, often termed the inflammatory phase, growth factors such as platelet-derived growth factor (PDGF) and eicosanoids (e.g., prostaglandins, leukotrienes, and thromboxanes) stimulate chemotaxis, cell permeability, and proliferation of the various cells responsible for wound healing, including macrophages, monocytes, and neutrophils. Further, in both the inflammatory and proliferative phases of wound healing, fibroblasts and smooth muscle cells are drawn to the wound bed to continue to supplement wound healing. In the final phase of wound healing (maturation or remodeling phase), deposition of fibronectin, hyaluronic acid, proteoglycans, and collagen takes place over weeks to months to provide the ultimate strength and integrity of the wound.

Each medication used to treat inflammatory arthridities can affect this pathway in some way. For example, NSAIDs disrupt the synthesis of prostaglandins and leukotrienes thereby blunting the inflammatory phase and limiting cell permeability/chemotaxis (Karukonda et al. 2000). Corticosteroids have been shown to inhibit fibroblast proliferation, vascular proliferation, and wound contraction (Busti et al. 2005; Pollack 1982). DMARDs have numerous mechanisms of action but in general all function to decrease inflammation (Busti et al. 2005). Although each of these medications has theoretical disadvantages with respect to local wound healing, they simultaneously play a role in mitigating the deleterious systemic effects of the inflammatory process. For this reason, extensive clinical studies have been performed to determine which medications should be withheld and the optimal timing. As outlined earlier in the chapter, the American College of Rheumatology and the American Association of Hip and Knee Surgeons in 2017 extensively reviewed available and pertinent literature (Goodman et al. 2017).

> In general, they recommend continuing current doses of glucocorticoids, continuing DMARDs, and holding biologics in the perioperative period. The importance of involving the rheumatologist, especially in patients with multiple medications and/or higher dosing regimens, cannot be understated.

Please see Table 4.1 for more extensive breakdown of each medication recommendation.

Most of the research surrounding inflammatory arthritis and joint replacement have been performed on RA, however recent publications have shed light on other conditions. Cancienne et al. reviewed over 1.7 million patients who underwent primary TKA including 153,531 with RA, 7918 with psoriatic arthritis, and 4575 with ankylosing spondylitis. Infection, revision at all time points, and readmission rates were all significantly higher in these patients compared to those with OA (Cancienne et al. 2016). Schasner et al. showed that patients with juvenile rheumatoid arthritis also have a higher risk of wound dehiscence (Schnaser et al. 2015). In the same study, they demonstrated an increased risk of perioperative periprosthetic fracture in patients with inflammatory arthridities. With the exception of psoriatic arthritis, they demonstrated that all inflammatory conditions had significantly more medical as well as orthopedic complications (Schnaser et al. 2015).

As inflammatory arthritis is a risk factor for delayed wound healing,(Doran et al. 2002; Bernatsky et al. 2007) the issue of prolonged or increased wound drainage may be more commonly encountered in this population. Saleh et al. showed that prolonged wound drainage is a significant risk factor for surgical site infection (Saleh et al. 2002). Further, Johnson et al. demonstrated wound edge hypoxia with excessive knee flexion immediately postoperatively (Johnson et al. 1991). For these reasons, in our clinical practice, if significant drainage is noted or there is concern preoperatively that a patient may suffer from prolonged healing and/or increased drainage, we recommend a brief period of immobilization following surgery until we are satisfied that the wound is sealed with no drainage.

4.5.3 Implant Survivorship

> Results of TKA in patients with inflammatory conditions have been shown to be satisfactory, but slightly inferior to patients undergoing TKA for OA.

Ravi et al. performed a systematic review and meta-analysis comparing complications and outcomes of total joint arthroplasty for RA and OA (Ravi et al. 2012). They report a slightly higher odds ratio of revision at less than 5 years (OR 1.24, 95% CI: 1.10–1.40). At 6–10 years and > 10 years, there were no differences in revision rates in cemented TKA. Similarly, Hernigou compared matched groups of patients with RA and OA undergoing revision TKA and found no difference in re-revision rates at 10-year follow-up. All implants in this study were posterior stabilized and cemented (Hernigou et al. 2017). The patients with RA had lower pre-revision functional scores, but similar postoperative scores, hence a greater change in functional scores compared to the OA revision group.

4.6 Conclusion

Inflammatory arthridities are systemic conditions that often symmetrically affect knees and can lead to severe impairment in daily function. Patients undergoing cemented TKA for inflammatory arthridities can expect good long-term survivorship with excellent improvement in outcome scores. Surgeons should work closely with the patient's rheumatologist especially with regard to perioperative medication management. The decision for PS versus CR implants remains controversial, but when the PCL is deficient or absent, PS components should be utilized. Arthroplasty surgeons should counsel their patients on the increased perioperative risks during and after TKA, with particular emphasis on infection. Cemented TKA is an appropriate procedure for patients with inflammatory disorders who have end-stage knee arthritis. The arthroplasty surgeon should be well versed in the surgical and nonsurgical considerations of the disease in order to provide excellent outcomes for these patients.

Take-Home Messages

- Inflammatory arthritis has complicated local and systemic disease manifestations. Attention to detail of both is critical for successful outcomes.
- These patients require a multidisciplinary team to achieve optimal outcomes.
- High-quality cementation technique is important, secondary to poorer quality of the subchondral bone.
- The addition of prophylactic antibiotics to the cement is recommended in this patient population.
- Manual (e.g., cefuroxime) or commercially (e.g., gentamicin/tobramycin) mixed antibiotics may be used.
- If the PCL is intact, the surgeon can consider using CR implants with good reported results.
- Patellar resurfacing may result in activity-related pain reduction, though resurfacing should be reserved for patients with adequate bone stock.
- Not all rheumatological medications require discontinuation prior to surgery. Guidelines have been established to aid in decision-making for perioperative medication management.

References

Aglietti P, Buzzi R, Segoni F, Zaccherotti G (1995) Insall-Burstein posterior-stabilized knee prosthesis in rheumatoid arthritis. J Arthroplast 10(2):217–225. https://doi.org/10.1016/S0883-5403(05)80131-7

Archibeck M, Berger R, Barden R et al (2001) Posterior cruciate ligament-retaining total knee arthroplasty in patients with rheumatoid arthritis. J Bone Joint Surg Am Vol 83(8):1231–1236

Ashraf M, Sharma OP, Priyavadhana S, Sambandam SN, Mounasamy V (2017) Rationale of cruciate retaining design in rheumatoid arthritis: a review of clinical analysis and its role in rheumatoid arthritis. Open Orthop J 11:1023–1027. https://doi.org/10.2174/1874325001711011023

Avina-Zubieta JA, Thomas J, Sadatsafavi M, Lehman AJ, Lacaille D (2012) Risk of incident cardiovascular events in patients with rheumatoid arthritis: a meta-analysis of observational studies. Ann Rheum Dis 71(9):1524–1529. https://doi.org/10.1136/annrheumdis-2011-200726

Bernatsky S, Hudson M, Suissa S (2007) Anti-rheumatic drug use and risk of serious infections in rheumatoid arthritis. Rheumatology (Oxford) 46(7):1157–1160. https://doi.org/10.1093/rheumatology/kem076

Bhan S, Malhotra R, Eachempati KK (2006) Total knee arthroplasty without patellar resurfacing in patients with rheumatoid arthritis. Publ Assoc Bone Joint Surg® | CORR® 450:157–163. https://doi.org/10.1097/01.blo.0000229277.74194.bf

Bongartz T, Halligan CS, Osmon DR et al (2008) Incidence and risk factors of prosthetic joint infection after total hip or knee replacement in patients with rheumatoid arthritis. Arthritis Rheum 59(12):1713–1720. https://doi.org/10.1002/art.24060

Boutry N, Morel M, Flipo R-M, Demondion X, Cotten A (2007) Early rheumatoid arthritis: a review of MRI and sonographic findings. Am J Roentgenol 189(6):1502–1509. https://doi.org/10.2214/AJR.07.2548

Busti AJ, Hooper JS, Amaya CJ, Kazi S (2005) Effects of perioperative antiinflammatory and immunomodulating therapy on surgical wound healing. Pharmacotherapy 25(11):1566–1591. https://doi.org/10.1592/phco.2005.25.11.1566

Cancienne JM, Werner BC, Browne JA (2016) Complications of primary total knee arthroplasty among patients with rheumatoid arthritis, psoriatic arthritis, ankylosing spondylitis, and osteoarthritis. J Am Acad Orthop Surg 24(8):567–574. https://doi.org/10.5435/JAAOS-D-15-00501

Chan JJ, Robinson J, Poeran J, Huang H-H, Moucha CS, Chen DD (2019) Antibiotic-loaded bone cement in primary total knee arthroplasty: utilization patterns and impact on complications using a national database. J Arthroplasty 34(7S):S188–S194.e1. https://doi.org/10.1016/j.arth.2019.03.006

Chiu F-Y, Chen C-M, Lin C-FJ, Lo W-H (2002) Cefuroxime-impregnated cement in primary total knee arthroplasty: a prospective, randomized study of three hundred and forty knees. J Bone Joint Surg Am 84(5):759–762

Dalury DF, Ewald FC, Christie MJ, Scott RD (1995) Total knee arthroplasty in a group of patients less than 45 years of age. J Arthroplast 10(5):598–602. https://doi.org/10.1016/S0883-5403(05)80202-5

Doran MF, Crowson CS, Pond GR, O'Fallon WM, Gabriel SE (2002) Frequency of infection in patients with rheumatoid arthritis compared with controls: a population-based study. Arthritis Rheum 46(9):2287–2293. https://doi.org/10.1002/art.10524

Gill GS, Joshi AB (2001) Long-term results of Kinematic Condylar knee replacement. J Bone Joint Surg 83(3):4

Gill GS, Chan KC, Mills DM (1997) 5- to 18-year follow-up study of cemented total knee arthroplasty for patients 55 years old or younger. J Arthroplast 12(1):49–54. https://doi.org/10.1016/S0883-5403(97)90046-2

Goodman SM, Figgie M (2013) Lower extremity arthroplasty in patients with inflammatory arthritis: preoperative and perioperative management. J Am Acad Orthop Surg 21(6):355–363. https://doi.org/10.5435/JAAOS-21-06-355

Goodman SM, Menon I, Christos PJ, Smethurst R, Bykerk VP (2016) Management of perioperative tumour necrosis factor α inhibitors in rheumatoid arthritis patients undergoing arthroplasty: a systematic review and meta-analysis. Rheumatology (Oxford) 55(3):573–582. https://doi.org/10.1093/rheumatology/kev364

Goodman SM, Springer B, Guyatt G et al (2017) 2017 American College of Rheumatology/American Association of Hip and Knee Surgeons Guideline for the Perioperative Management of Antirheumatic Medication in Patients With Rheumatic Diseases Undergoing Elective Total Hip or Total Knee Arthroplasty. J Arthroplast 32(9):2628–2638. https://doi.org/10.1016/j.arth.2017.05.001

Grennan DM, Gray J, Loudon J, Fear S (2001) Methotrexate and early postoperative complications in patients with rheumatoid

arthritis undergoing elective orthopaedic surgery. Ann Rheum Dis 60(3):214–217. https://doi.org/10.1136/ard.60.3.214
Hanyu T, Murasawa A, Tojo T (1997) Survivorship analysis of total knee arthroplasty with the kinematic prosthesis in patients who have rheumatoid arthritis. J Arthroplast 12(8):913–919. https://doi.org/10.1016/S0883-5403(97)90161-3
Henchie TF, Gravallese EM, Bredbenner TL, Troy KL (2019) An image-based method to measure joint deformity in inflammatory arthritis: development and pilot study. Comput Methods Biomech Biomed Engin 22(10):942–952. https://doi.org/10.1080/10255842.2019.1607315
Hernigou P, Dubory A, Potage D, Roubineau F, Flouzat-Lachaniette CH (2017) Outcome of knee revisions for osteoarthritis and inflammatory arthritis with postero-stabilized arthroplasties: a mean ten-year follow-up with 90 knee revisions. Int Orthop 41(4):757–763. https://doi.org/10.1007/s00264-016-3319-8
Jain A, Witbreuk M, Ball C, Nanchahal J (2002) Influence of steroids and methotrexate on wound complications after elective rheumatoid hand and wrist surgery. J Hand Surg Am 27(3):449–455. https://doi.org/10.1053/jhsu.2002.32958
Jameson SS, Asaad A, Diament M et al (2019) Antibiotic-loaded bone cement is associated with a lower risk of revision following primary cemented total knee arthroplasty: an analysis of 731,214 cases using National Joint Registry data. Bone Joint J 101-B(11):1331–1347. https://doi.org/10.1302/0301-620X.101B11.BJJ-2019-0196.R1
Jiranek WA, Hanssen AD, Greenwald AS (2006) Antibiotic-loaded bone cement for infection prophylaxis in total joint replacement. JBJS 88(11):2487–2500. https://doi.org/10.2106/JBJS.E.01126
Johnson DP, Eastwood DM, Bader DL (1991) Biomechanical factors in wound healing following knee arthroplasty. J Med Eng Technol 15(1):8–14. https://doi.org/10.3109/03091909109015442
Kajino A, Yoshino S, Kameyama S, Kohda M, Nagashima S (1997) Comparison of the results of bilateral total knee arthroplasty with and without patellar replacement for rheumatoid arthritis. A follow-up note*. JBJS 79(4):570–574
Karukonda SR, Flynn TC, Boh EE, McBurney EI, Russo GG, Millikan LE (2000) The effects of drugs on wound healing–part II. Specific classes of drugs and their effect on healing wounds. Int J Dermatol 39(5):321–333. https://doi.org/10.1046/j.1365-4362.2000.00949.x
Krause ML, Matteson EL (2014) Perioperative management of the patient with rheumatoid arthritis. World J Orthop 5(3):283–291. https://doi.org/10.5312/wjo.v5.i3.283
Kwek TK, Lew TWK, Thoo FL (1998) The role of preoperative cervical spine X-rays in rheumatoid arthritis. Anaesth Intensive Care 26(6):636–641. https://doi.org/10.1177/0310057X9802600604
Laskin RS, O'Flynn HM (1997) The Insall Award. Total knee replacement with posterior cruciate ligament retention in rheumatoid arthritis Problems and complications. Clin Orthop Relat Res 345:24–28
Lee JK, Kee YM, Chung HK, Choi CH (2015) Long-term results of cruciate-retaining total knee replacement in patients with rheumatoid arthritis: a minimum 15-year review. Can J Surg 58(3):193–197. https://doi.org/10.1503/cjs.012014
Lee D-K, Kim H-J, Cho I-Y, Lee D-H (2017) Infection and revision rates following primary total knee arthroplasty in patients with rheumatoid arthritis versus osteoarthritis: a meta-analysis. Knee Surg Sports Traumatol Arthrosc 25(12):3800–3807. https://doi.org/10.1007/s00167-016-4306-8
Lereim P, Goldie IF (1975) Relationship between morphologic features and hardness of the subchondral bone of the medial tibial condyle in the normal state and in osteoarthritis and rheumatoid arthritis. Arch Orthop Unfallchir 81(1):1–11. https://doi.org/10.1007/BF00417022
Lereim P, Goldie I, Dahlberg E (1974) Hardness of the subchondral bone of the tibial condyles in the normal state and in osteoarthritis and rheumatoid arthritis. Acta Orthop Scand 45(1–4):614–627. https://doi.org/10.3109/17453677408989184
Lindhardsen J, Ahlehoff O, Gislason GH et al (2011) The risk of myocardial infarction in rheumatoid arthritis and diabetes mellitus: a Danish nationwide cohort study. Ann Rheum Dis 70(6):929–934. https://doi.org/10.1136/ard.2010.143396
Liu H-T, Chiu F-Y, Chen C-M, Chen T-H (2003) The combination of systemic antibiotics and antibiotics impregnated cement in primary total knee arthroplasty in patients of rheumatoid arthritis--evaluation of 60 knees. J Chin Med Assoc 66(9):533–536
Lopez-Olivo MA, Andrabi TR, Palla SL, Suarez-Almazor ME (2012) Cervical spine radiographs in patients with rheumatoid arthritis undergoing anesthesia. J Clin Rheumatol 18(2):61–66. https://doi.org/10.1097/RHU.0b013e318247bb0d
Luo Z, Zhou Z, Pei F (2019) Long-term results of total knee arthroplasty with single-radius versus multi- radius posterior-stabilized prosthesis in rheumatoid arthritis. Orthopaedic Proceedings 101-B(SUPP_4):47. https://doi.org/10.1302/1358-992X.2019.4.047
Meune C, Touze E, Trinquart L, Allanore Y (2009) Trends in cardiovascular mortality in patients with rheumatoid arthritis over 50 years: a systematic review and meta-analysis of cohort studies. Rheumatology 48(10):1309–1313. https://doi.org/10.1093/rheumatology/kep252
Miller MD, Brown NM, Della Valle CJ, Rosenberg AG, Galante JO (2011) Posterior cruciate ligament-retaining total knee arthroplasty in patients with rheumatoid arthritis: a concise follow-up of a previous report: *. JBJS 93(22):e130. https://doi.org/10.2106/JBJS.J.01695
Ogdie A, Yu Y, Haynes K et al (2015) Risk of major cardiovascular events in patients with psoriatic arthritis, psoriasis and rheumatoid arthritis: a population-based cohort study. Ann Rheum Dis 74(2):326–332. https://doi.org/10.1136/annrheumdis-2014-205675
Pollack SV (1982) Systemic medications and wound healing. Int J Dermatol 21(9):489–496. https://doi.org/10.1111/j.1365-4362.1982.tb01189.x
Ravi B, Escott B, Shah PS et al (2012) A systematic review and meta-analysis comparing complications following total joint arthroplasty for rheumatoid arthritis versus for osteoarthritis. Arthritis Rheum 64(12):3839–3849. https://doi.org/10.1002/art.37690
Saleh K, Olson M, Resig S et al (2002) Predictors of wound infection in hip and knee joint replacement: results from a 20 year surveillance program. J Orthop Res 20(3):506–515. https://doi.org/10.1016/S0736-0266(01)00153-X
Schnaser EA, Browne JA, Padgett DE, Figgie MP, D'Apuzzo MR (2015) Perioperative complications in patients with inflammatory arthropathy undergoing total knee arthroplasty. J Arthroplast 30(9 Suppl):76–80. https://doi.org/10.1016/j.arth.2014.12.040
Schrama JC, Espehaug B, Hallan G et al (2010) Risk of revision for infection in primary total hip and knee arthroplasty in patients with rheumatoid arthritis compared with osteoarthritis: a prospective, population-based study on 108,786 hip and knee joint arthroplasties from the Norwegian Arthroplasty Register. Arthritis Care Res 62(4):473–479. https://doi.org/10.1002/acr.20036
Schreurs BW, Hannink G (2017) Total joint arthroplasty in younger patients: heading for trouble? Lancet 389(10077):1374–1375. https://doi.org/10.1016/S0140-6736(17)30190-3

4

Shoji H, Yoshino S, Kajino A (1989) Patellar replacement in bilateral total knee arthroplasty. A study of patients who had rheumatoid arthritis and no gross deformity of the patella. J Bone Joint Surg Am 71(6):853–856
Somayaji R, Barnabe C, Martin L (2013) Risk factors for infection following total joint arthroplasty in rheumatoid arthritis. Open Rheumatol J 7:119–124. https://doi.org/10.2174/1874312920131210005
Sreekumar R, Gray J, Kay P, Grennan DM (2011) Methotrexate and post operative complications in patients with rheumatoid arthritis undergoing elective orthopaedic surgery–a ten year follow-up. Acta Orthop Belg 77(6):823–826
Stern SH, Insall JN, Windsor RE, Inglis AE, Dines DM (1989) Total knee arthroplasty in patients with psoriasis. Clin Orthop Relat Res 248:108–110; discussion 111. https://doi.org/10.1097/00003086-198911000-00018
Sudoł-Szopińska I, Jans L, Teh J (2017) Rheumatoid arthritis: what do MRI and ultrasound show. J Ultrason 17(68):5–16. https://doi.org/10.15557/JoU.2017.0001
Yamanaka H, Goto K, Suzuki M (2012) Clinical results of Hi-tech Knee II total knee arthroplasty in patients with rheumatoid athritis: 5- to 12-year follow-up. J Orthop Surg Res 7(1):9. https://doi.org/10.1186/1749-799X-7-9
Yang J-P, Bogoch ER, Woodside TD, Hearn TC (1997) Stiffness of trabecular bone of the tibial plateau in patients with rheumatoid arthritis of the knee. J Arthroplast 12(7):798–803. https://doi.org/10.1016/S0883-5403(97)90011-5

Osteonecrosis

Hytham S. Salem, Brandon H. Naylor, Kevin K. Mathew, and Michael A. Mont

Contents

E. Hansen, K.-D. Kühn (eds.), *Essentials of Cemented Knee Arthroplasty*,
https://doi.org/10.1007/978-3-662-63113-3_5

5.1 Introduction

Total knee arthroplasty (TKA) is primarily indicated in the elderly population with end-stage arthritis. However, a subset of patients who undergo TKA has an underlying diagnosis of osteonecrosis.

> The knee is the second most common site for osteonecrosis to develop.

It is generally categorized into three distinct types:
- Secondary
- Spontaneous
- Post-arthroscopic (Jones and Mont 2019)

Due to the propensity for some forms of knee osteonecrosis to manifest at a younger age than osteoarthritis, maximizing the survivorship of TKA implants is increasingly important.

Secondary osteonecrosis of the knee is more likely to present earlier in life, typically affecting patients younger than 45 years (Mont et al. 2000). Secondary osteonecrosis is associated with multiple factors including the following:
- Corticosteroid use
- Excessive alcohol intake
- Sickle-cell disease
- Gaucher's disease
- Myeloproliferative disorders

> The two most common risk factors are corticosteroid use and alcohol abuse (Mont et al. 2000).

Both corticosteroid use and alcohol abuse have been shown to increase bone marrow adipogenesis leading to increased intraosseous pressure, and consequently, hypoperfusion of bone (Wang et al. 2003; Yin et al. 2006). Secondary knee osteonecrosis involves both femoral condyles in greater than 80% of cases and can involve the epiphyseal, metaphyseal, and diaphyseal regions of the distal femur, while proximal tibia involvement is seen in 22% to 36% of patients (Mears et al. 2009; Mont et al. 2000). Patients who have secondary knee osteonecrosis typically describe an insidious onset of knee pain and may also complain of additional joint pain due to the propensity for multiple joint involvement in up to 90% of patients (Mears et al. 2009).

Conversely, spontaneous osteonecrosis of the knee (SPONK) is more commonly diagnosed in the elderly population. Its prevalence has been estimated to be 3.4% in patients older than 50 years and 9.4% in those greater than 65 years of age (Pape et al. 2002). SPONK is most likely to occur as a focal epiphyseal lesion in the medial femoral condyle (Mears et al. 2009). In fact, it has been shown that 94% of SPONK lesions are located in medial condyle (al-Rowaih et al. 1993). Some authors have postulated that this is due to relatively limited intraosseous blood supply of the medial versus lateral condyle (Reddy and Frederick 1998). Conversely, other authors argue that unlike other forms of osteonecrosis, ischemia is not the primary factor that leads to SPONK (Yamamoto and Bullough 2000). Rather, it has been found that subchondral insufficiency fracture with extravasation of fluid into the bone may represent the inciting pathogenic mechanism (Yamamoto and Bullough 2000).

> This hypothesis is supported by evidence that SPONK is most commonly seen in female patients older than 60 years, and that low bone mineral density is a risk factor in these patients (Akamatsu et al. 2012).

Patients who have SPONK typically present with acute onset medial knee pain with tenderness over the medial femoral condyle (Lotke et al. 1982).

A rare form of knee osteonecrosis occurs following arthroscopic knee surgery. Studies have shown that post-arthroscopic knee osteonecrosis occurs after meniscectomy or chondroplasty in 0.2–4% of patients who undergo these procedures (Cetik et al. 2009; Di Caprio et al. 2017; Pruès-Latour et al. 1998). While some theories for the etiology of post-arthroscopic osteonecrosis have been proposed, its exact pathogenic mechanism remains poorly understood. The use of radiofrequency for chondral debridement has been posited as a risk factor, however, recent studies have refuted this theory (Cetik et al. 2009; Turker et al. 2015). Post-arthroscopic knee osteonecrosis most commonly affects the medial femoral condyle and tends to correspond with the location of preexisting knee pathology (Pape et al. 2007). The time between arthroscopic surgery and the onset of symptoms is typically 6 to 8 weeks (Karim et al. 2015). Similar to SPONK lesions, those associated with an arthroscopic surgery present with a sudden onset of pain over the affected region.

Regardless of etiology, TKA may be the only treatment option for patients who have post-collapse knee osteonecrosis and have failed conservative treatment measures. Among the three forms of this condition, TKA for steroid-induced knee osteonecrosis tends to be the most problematic due to two main distinctive factors. As previously mentioned, it is more common in younger patients. Secondly, a more diffuse pattern of necrosis is typically observed when compared to other etiologies (Seldes et al. 1999). For this reason, patients who undergo TKA for steroid-induced knee osteonecrosis may have diminished bone stock potentially compromising component fixation. For example, cases where large areas of necrotic bone remain following bone cuts may have a negative impact on component fixation.

Polymethylmethacrylate (PMMA), or bone cement, is often used for fixation of joint prostheses. Unlike cementless methods which achieve fixation through bony ingrowth around the implant, cemented knee arthroplasties utilize PMMA to fill the space between the implant and the porous trabecular bone. While cementless knee arthroplasties are gaining popularity, they are usually considered in younger patients who typically have adequate bone stock and high metabolic activity (Matassi et al. 2013). Osteonecrosis of the distal femur is characterized by reduced bone quality.

> As a result, cemented TKA has been historically considered as the gold standard in the treatment of end-stage osteonecrosis of the distal femur. However, outcomes for both cemented and cementless TKA in recent literature have been largely successful.

Thus, there are no special considerations regarding fixation methods for TKA in patients who have knee osteonecrosis. In some cases, extensive necrotic bone, particularly in the metaphyseal region, may necessitate a stemmed femoral or tibial component. Quite often, the bone is found to be amenable to cementless fixation. This is the senior author's preferred method as it leads to a less complicated revision surgery, if needed.

5.2 Case Examples

5.2.1 Case Report #1

A 64-year-old female with no history of previous trauma, arthroscopic procedures, steroid use, or alcohol abuse presented with a complaint of a 3-month history of left knee pain without injury. She reported pain on the medial aspect of the knee characterized by intermittent sharp and dull pain, swelling, clicking, and diminished range of motion. Due to the pain, the patient relies on a cane when walking for extended distances. Acetaminophen and ibuprofen have provided minimal relief.

Physical examination showed mild effusion of the left knee with medial joint line and medial femoral condyle tenderness to palpation. Active range of motion was 5–135°. All ligaments appeared stable with negative ligamentous maneuvers. A negative Steinman test but positive McMurray's test with click was identified.

Standing anteroposterior, lateral, merchant, and 45° posteroanterior standing X-rays revealed mild medial joint space narrowing with an osteoarthritic classification of Kellgren and Lawrence Grade II/III. An irregularity of the medial femoral condyle was also identified which may be due to osteochondral defect or osteonecrosis (Fig. 5.1).

The patient was advised that symptoms appear to be secondary to a combination of degenerative arthritis, possible degenerative tear of the medial meniscus, and an osteochondral defect of the medial femoral condyle. An MRI was recommended followed by conservative management with physical therapy and Naproxen 500 mg twice daily for the interim.

MRI findings revealed a complex tear and extrusion of the medial meniscus with a multiloculated parameniscal cyst anterior to the anterior root of the medial meniscus measuring 1.2 × 0.7 cm. A 3.1 × 1.3 cm area of crescentic subchondral low signal was noted in the weight-bearing aspect of the medial femoral condyle with moderate surrounding marrow edema. In concordance with original X-rays, the hypodense signal most likely represented SPONK.

After discussion of findings with the patient, she preferred to follow conservative treatment due to mild improvement with physical therapy and hesitancy toward surgical intervention. The patient returned 2 months later with increasing pain and difficulty carrying out activities of daily living. Repeated radiographs of the left knee revealed collapse of the subchondral bone at the medial femoral condyle reflective of Ficat Stage IV osteonecrosis. Due to the progressive nature of the disease, TKA was recommended for which the patient agreed.

Intraoperatively, degenerative changes and depression of the cartilage were noted at the medial femoral condyle. Subchondral bone softening was also identified. Complete excision of the lesion was obtained during resection of the distal femur during femoral implant preparation. After determining that the femoral bone stock was adequate, cementless prosthetic implants were used. The patient has significantly improved knee pain and is able to carry out activities of daily living with minimal to no assistance at 1-year follow-up.

5.2.2 Case Report #2

A 63-year-old female with past medical history significant for systemic lupus erythematosus, obesity, primary hyperparathyroidism, chronic obstructive pulmonary disease, right knee arthroscopy for Grade III cartilage degeneration 3 years prior, and daily corticosteroid use presented with worsening right knee pain. Physical exam findings show mild joint effusion of the right knee. There is also right knee pain and crepitus with passive range of motion. Tenderness was also elicited over the anterior aspect of the knee upon palpation. Radiographic imaging of the right knee demonstrated mild tricompartmental degeneration with an osteoarthritic classification of Kellgren–Lawrence Grade II/III. There was minor narrowing of the joint spaces with no fracture or insufficiency noted. The patient's symptoms were indica-

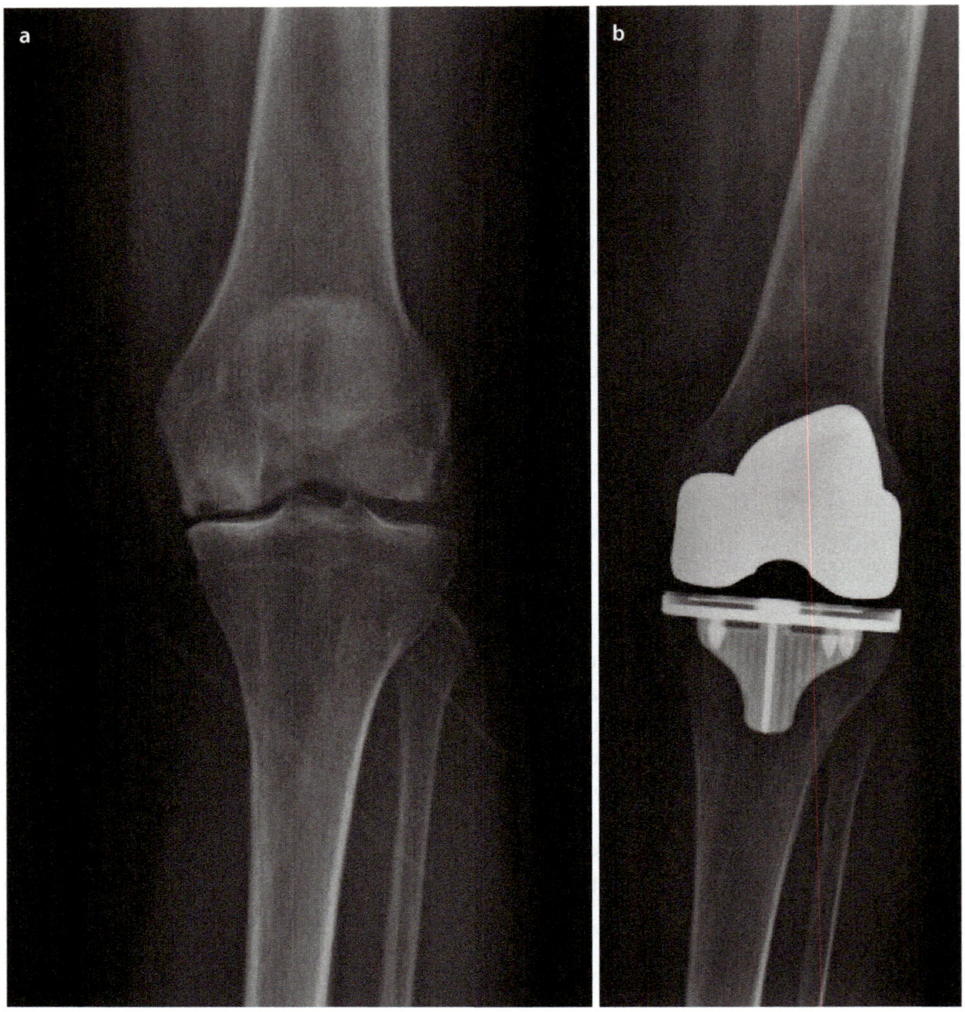

Fig. 5.1 **a** Standing anteroposterior radiograph of the left knee with evidence of an osteonecrotic lesion in the medial femoral condyle (*white arrow*). **b** Anteroposterior radiograph of the left knee after cementless TKA

tive of osteoarthritis. She then received a cortisone injection and conservative strategies including weight loss, physical therapy, and over-the-counter non-steroidal anti-inflammatory drugs were discussed and recommended.

The patient presented again 6 months after the initial visit with progressively worsening right knee pain and difficulty carrying out activities of daily living without assistance. Radiographic imaging demonstrated the evidence of patchy mineralization in the right femur and tibia that was thought to be due to osteonecrosis (Fig. 5.2). An MRI was performed which revealed extensive osteonecrosis involving the distal femur bone marrow extending into the majority of the medial femoral condyle. There is also an irregular contour of the subchondral bone plate which may be indicative of multiple areas of subchondral collapse. Osteonecrosis was also identified in medial tibial plateau without evidence of subchondral insufficiency. Due to a combination of extensive physical and radiographic findings, a TKA was performed. Intraoperative assessment revealed diminished bone quality with large areas of necrotic bone remaining following the bone cuts, prompting cemented fixation of the tibial and femoral components.

5.3 Published Outcome Data

Chalmers et al. (2019) reviewed 167 TKAs in 156 patients who had primary (66%) and secondary (34%) knee osteonecrosis. Outcomes were assessed using Knee Society scores and radiographs after a mean follow-up of 6 years (range, 2 to 12 years) and mean patient age of 61 years (range, 14 to 93 years). All TKAs were fixed with antibiotic cement. Stemmed tibial and femoral components were used in 9% and 7% of cases, respectively. At 10-year follow-up, implant survivorship free from aseptic loosening and any reoperation including revision surgery was 97%. Two TKAs (1%) underwent revision surgery for aseptic loosening of the tibial component. No unrevised TKAs demonstrated radiologic evidence of loosening. The knee component of the KSS

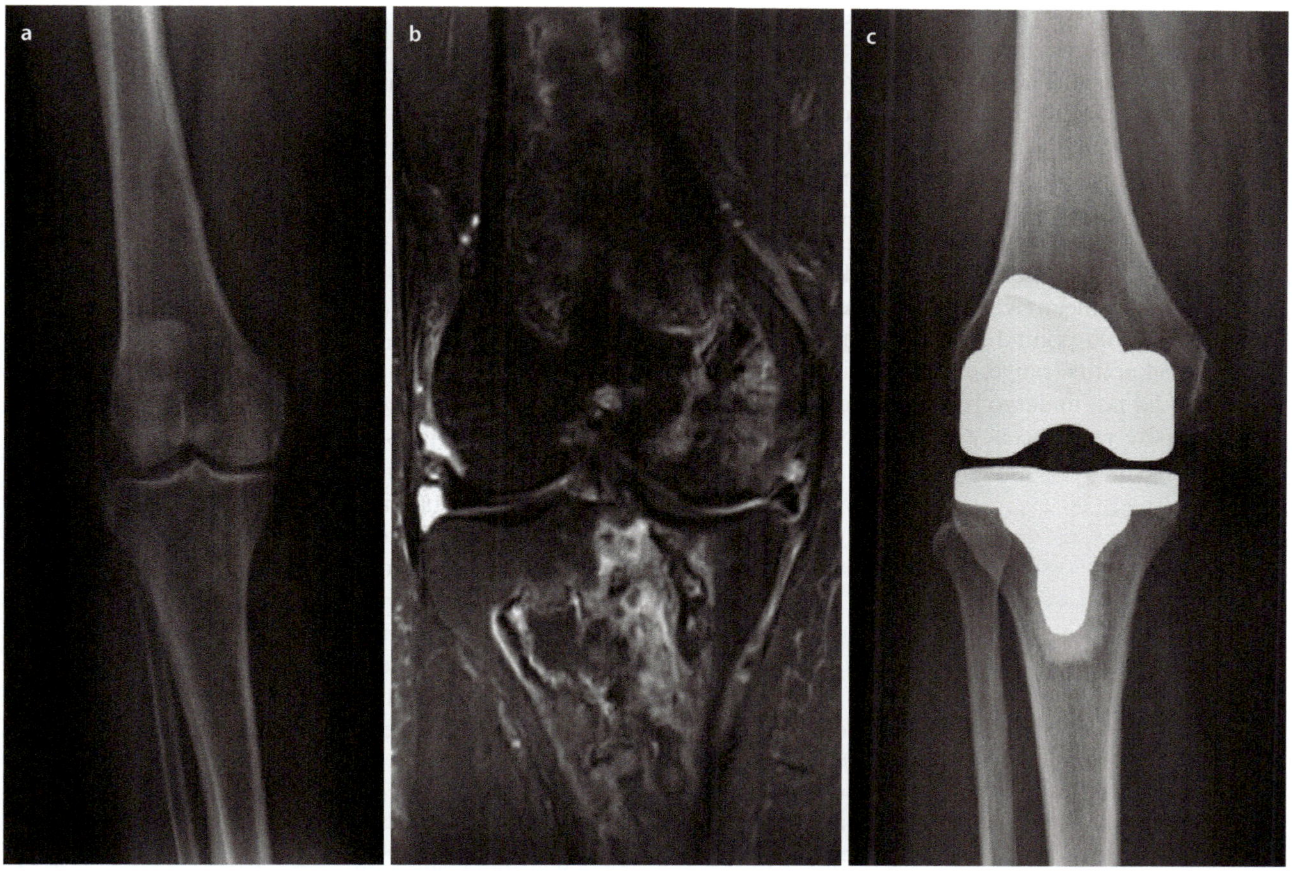

Fig. 5.2 a Standing anteroposterior radiograph of the right knee revealing patchy mineralization of the femur and tibia. b Coronal T2 MRI of the right knee demonstrating extensive necrosis of the proximal tibia and distal femur extending into a majority of the medial femoral condyle. c Anteroposterior radiograph of the left knee after TKA with cemented fixation

improved from 57 points (range, 32 to 87 points) preoperatively to 91 points (range, 49 to 100 points) at final follow-up. The authors concluded that cemented TKA with selective stem utilization resulted in durable survivorship and reliable improvement in patient-reported outcomes for patients who have knee osteonecrosis.

In another study evaluating the outcomes of cemented TKA for osteonecrosis, 32 knees in 30 patients were evaluated after a mean follow-up period of 108 months (range, 49 to 144 months) (Mont et al. 2002). Due to sufficient bone loss or osteonecrotic bone involving the metaphysis, a stemmed femoral component was used in 6 knees and a stemmed tibial component was used in 2 knees. The mean age at the time of arthroplasty was 54 years (range, 31 to 77 years). Twenty-two patients had corticosteroid-associated osteonecrosis and the remaining 8 had SPONK. At final follow-up, 31 of the 32 knees (97%) demonstrated successful clinical outcomes with a mean KSS of 95 points, improving from a preoperative mean of 54 points. There was no radiologic evidence of progressive radiolucency in any cases. Only one unsuccessful clinical outcome was reported at 9-year follow-up in a patient who was undergoing corticosteroid therapy for systemic lupus erythematosus.

> The authors of this study concluded that cement fixation should be used for TKA in patients who have osteonecrosis, and that femoral and/or tibial stems should be utilized when warranted.

Mont et al. (1997) reviewed 31 cementless TKAs in 21 patients under the age of 50 who had a diagnosis of corticosteroid-associated osteonecrosis of the knee. Clinical and radiologic outcomes were reported after a mean 8.2-year follow-up (range, 2 to 16 years). The revision rate for aseptic loosening was 37% (11 knees) and 3 additional knees were revised for periprosthetic joint infection (PJI). Of note, all 6 knees in patients who did not have systemic lupus erythematosus (SLE) had excellent clinical results, while only 11 of 25 knees (44%) were clinically successful in patients who had SLE. While the results of this study are not encouraging for the use of cementless TKA for patients who have knee osteonecrosis, it is important to consider that the technology used for the manufacturing of cementless arthroplasty implants has improved considerably since this study was published in 1997. While limited, there is evidence of improved outcomes in patients who had osteonecrosis and underwent TKA with newer generation cementless implants.

Sultan et al. (2018) evaluated 49 knees in 46 patients who had osteonecrosis and underwent primary cementless TKA. The main outcomes of interest were implant survivorship, clinical outcomes, complications, and radiographic findings after a mean follow-up of 44 months (range, 36 to 96 months). Implant survivorship free from aseptic loosening was 97.9% and all-cause implant survivorship was 95.9%. In total, one knee was revised for aseptic loosening and one knee was revised for a PJI. The mean KSS pain score was 93 points (range, 85 to 100 points) and the mean KSS function score was 84 points (range, 70 to 90 points). Among the cases that did not undergo revision surgery, no evidence of progressive radiolucency, subsidence, or changes in postoperative implant alignment were noted at final follow-up.

> The results of this study indicate that excellent survivorship and clinical outcomes can be achieved with newer generation cementless fixation of TKA in patients who have osteonecrosis.

Seldes et al. (1999) reviewed 31 TKAs in 24 patients who had steroid-induced osteonecrosis of the knee. KSS was used to evaluate clinical outcomes and radiographs were evaluated for alignment and evidence of subsidence or loosening after a mean follow-up time of 64 months (range, 24 to 145 months). The mean patient age was 46 years (range, 27 to 79 years). Cemented implants were used in 22 of 31 cases (71%), while cementless and hybrid fixation was carried out in 8 (26%) and 1 (3%) knees, respectively. In 6 knees (19%), autologous bone grafting was deemed necessary to augment large areas of necrotic bone. In addition, 4 knees required a stemmed tibial component and 1 knee required a stemmed femoral component. The functional component of the KSS improved from 37 points (range, 0 to 80 points) preoperatively to 64 points (range, 20 to 100 points) at final follow-up. The knee component of the KSS improved from 47 points (range, 19 to 70 points) preoperatively to 87 points (range, 51 to 99 points) at final follow-up. In total, 5 knees (16%) required a revision procedure including 3 cemented (13.6%) and 2 cementless (25%) knees. Three of these 5 failures were due to aseptic loosening after 113 months, 61 months, and 144 months. Two of the aseptic revisions were cemented TKAs (9.1%) while 1 was cementless (12.5%). Based on the data presented in this study, it was not possible to assess the optimal fixation technique. However, it appears that cemented and cementless techniques led to adequate outcomes.

5.4 Conclusion

TKA is the treatment of choice for patients who have osteonecrosis of the knee with femoral condyle collapse and failure of conservative treatment. While earlier studies advise against the use of cementless fixation for TKA in the setting of osteonecrosis (Mont et al. 1997), it is important to note the advancements in technology with newer generation cementless implants may have led to better outcomes (Sultan et al. 2018). Several factors must be taken into account when selecting the optimal fixation method for TKA in patients who have osteonecrosis. The overall quality of the distal femoral and proximal tibial bone should be assessed intraoperatively. Gross examination of bone quality should be evaluated and stability of the cementless fixation be ensured. If these factors are not determined to be optimal, cemented fixation should be utilized. The use of stemmed implants or bone grafts should be used judiciously for patients in whom large areas of necrosis may compromise fixation. Overall, the current literature has demonstrated acceptable outcomes of cemented and cementless fixation in appropriately selected patients.

Take-Home Messages

- Patients undergoing total knee arthroplasty for osteonecrosis may be younger in age than those who have osteoarthritis, and thus long-lasting fixation is imperative.
- The overall quality of the distal femoral and proximal tibial bone should be assessed intraoperatively to aid in the selection of cemented versus cementless fixation.
- Corticosteroid-associated knee osteonecrosis is typically found in younger aged patients, is more diffuse in nature compared to spontaneous lesions, and may decrease bone density. All of these factors are important to consider when selecting a fixation method.
- Earlier studies have advocated the use of cemented fixation for osteonecrosis patients undergoing TKA. However, improved biologic fixation may be achieved with newer generation cementless implants compared to older designs.
- Selective use of stemmed implants or bone grafts should be used for patients in whom large areas of necrosis may compromise fixation.

References

Akamatsu Y, Mitsugi N, Hayashi T, Kobayashi H, Saito T (2012) Low bone mineral density is associated with the onset of spontaneous osteonecrosis of the knee. Acta Orthop 83(3):249–255. PMID: 22537352

al-Rowaih A, Bjorkengren A, Egund N, Lindstrand A, Wingstrand H, Thorngren KG (1993) Size of osteonecrosis of the knee. Clin Orthop Relat Res (287):68–75. PMID: 8448962

Cetik O, Cift H, Comert B, Cirpar M (2009) Risk of osteonecrosis of the femoral condyle after arthroscopic chondroplasty using radiofrequency: a prospective clinical series. Knee Surg Sports Traumatol Arthrosc 17(1):24–29. PMID: 18758748

Chalmers BP, Mehrotra KG, Sierra RJ, Pagnano MW, Taunton MJ, Abdel MP (2019) Reliable outcomes and survivorship of primary total knee arthroplasty for osteonecrosis of the knee. Bone Joint J 101-b(11):1356–1361. PMID: 31674235

Di Caprio F, Meringolo R, Navarra MA, Mosca M, Ponziani L (2017) Postarthroscopy osteonecrosis of the knee: current concepts. Joints 5(4):229–236. PMID: 29270561

Jones LC, Mont MA (2019) UpToDate. Wolters Kluwer. Available at: https://www.uptodate.com/contents/osteonecrosis-avascular-necrosis-of-bone#H13728325. Accessed 9 Jan 2020

Karim AR, Cherian JJ, Jauregui JJ, Pierce T, Mont MA (2015) Osteonecrosis of the knee: review. Ann Transl Med 3(1):6. PMID: 25705638

Lotke PA, Abend JA, Ecker ML (1982) The treatment of osteonecrosis of the medial femoral condyle. Clin Orthop Relat Res 171:109–116. PMID: 7140057

Matassi F, Carulli C, Civinini R, Innocenti M (2013) Cemented versus cementless fixation in total knee arthroplasty. Joints 1(3):121–125. PMID: 25606521

Mears SC, McCarthy EF, Jones LC, Hungerford DS, Mont MA (2009) Characterization and pathological characteristics of spontaneous osteonecrosis of the knee. Iowa Orthop J 29:38–42. PMID: 19742083

Mont MA, Myers TH, Krackow KA, Hungerford DS (1997) Total knee arthroplasty for corticosteroid associated avascular necrosis of the knee. Clin Orthop Relat Res 338:124–130. PMID: 9170373

Mont MA, Baumgarten KM, Rifai A, Bluemke DA, Jones LC, Hungerford DS (2000) Atraumatic osteonecrosis of the knee. J Bone Joint Surg Am 82(9):1279–1290. PMID: 11005519

Mont MA, Rifai A, Baumgarten KM, Sheldon M, Hungerford DS (2002) Total knee arthroplasty for osteonecrosis. J Bone Joint Surg Am 84(4):599–603. PMID: 11940621

Pape D, Seil R, Fritsch E, Rupp S, Kohn D (2002) Prevalence of spontaneous osteonecrosis of the medial femoral condyle in elderly patients. Knee Surg Sports Traumatol Arthrosc 10(4):233–240. PMID: 12172718

Pape D, Seil R, Anagnostakos K, Kohn D (2007) Postarthroscopic osteonecrosis of the knee. Arthroscopy 23(4):428–438. PMID: 17418337

Pruès-Latour V, Bonvin JC, Fritschy D (1998) Nine cases of osteonecrosis in elderly patients following arthroscopic meniscectomy. Knee Surg Sports Traumatol Arthrosc 6(3):142–147. PMID: 9704320

Reddy AS, Frederick RW (1998) Evaluation of the intraosseous and extraosseous blood supply to the distal femoral condyles. Am J Sports Med 26(3):415–419. PMID: 9617405

Seldes RM, Tan V, Duffy G, Rand JA, Lotke PA (1999) Total knee arthroplasty for steroid-induced osteonecrosis. J Arthroplast 14(5):533–537. PMID: 10475550

Sultan AA, Khlopas A, Sodhi N et al (2018) Cementless total knee arthroplasty in knee osteonecrosis demonstrated excellent survivorship and outcomes at three-year minimum follow-up. J Arthroplast 33(3):761–765. PMID: 29128233

Turker M, Cetik O, Cirpar M, Durusoy S, Comert B (2015) Postarthroscopy osteonecrosis of the knee. Knee Surg Sports Traumatol Arthrosc 23(1):246–250. PMID: 23443330

Wang Y, Li Y, Mao K, Li J, Cui Q, Wang GJ (2003) Alcohol-induced adipogenesis in bone and marrow: a possible mechanism for osteonecrosis. Clin Orthop Relat Res 410:213–224. PMID: 12771833

Yamamoto T, Bullough PG (2000) Spontaneous osteonecrosis of the knee: the result of subchondral insufficiency fracture. J Bone Joint Surg Am 82(6):858–866. PMID: 10859106

Yin L, Li YB, Wang YS (2006) Dexamethasone-induced adipogenesis in primary marrow stromal cell cultures: mechanism of steroid-induced osteonecrosis. Chin Med J 119(7):581–588. PMID: 16620700

Post-Traumatic Arthritis

Colin T. Penrose and Michael P. Bolognesi

Contents

E. Hansen, K.-D. Kühn (eds.), *Essentials of Cemented Knee Arthroplasty*,
https://doi.org/10.1007/978-3-662-63113-3_6

6.1 Introduction

An injury causing any combination of fractures of the tibia, femur, or patella, as well as periarticular soft tissue injuries involving tendons, muscles, cartilage, and ligaments can eventually lead to a painful and debilitating condition known as post-traumatic arthritis (PTA). Total knee arthroplasty (TKA) is the treatment of choice and should be considered when all conservative measures have failed and after an appropriate evaluation for other etiologies.

Multiple factors can make the TKA more challenging than a routine primary TKA including the following:

- Deformity.
- Hardware present.
- Bone defects.
- Scars from prior incisions or lacerations.
- Ligamentous stability.

For these reasons, it is especially important to have a surgical plan that may include techniques like the following:

- Hardware removal (possibly staged).
- Technological adjuncts.
- Increased constraint.
- The use of cones, sleeves, or augments.
- Extensile approaches for challenging exposure.
- Osteotomies.

The outcomes after TKA in PTA patients when compared to patients with osteoarthritis involve higher complication rates including infection, deep vein thrombosis, and revision, as well as increased cost and lower patient function.

> However, TKA is still a very beneficial operation in this patient population when patients are appropriately indicated for surgery and the operation is performed using good surgical technique.

6.2 Case Examples

6.2.1 Case 1: Femoral Nail

A 61-year-old female presented with bilateral (left worse than right) knee pain with a history of left distal femur fracture after falling down on icy steps which was treated with a retrograde femoral nail (▫ Fig. 6.1). In addition to the retrograde femoral nail, her medical history included pulmonary fibrosis and diabetes and her prior surgical history included a left ankle fracture ORIF, lumbar spine fusion, and a hysterectomy. She was unable to go up- or downstairs and used a walker or crutches inside and required a wheelchair for longer distances. The knee range of motion was 15–90° with no extensor lag. Ligamentous examination demonstrated no significant coronal or sagittal instability. She was initially managed with knee joint corticosteroid injections which provided short-term relief. After thorough discussion of risks and benefits and involvement of the pulmonary and endocrine teams for optimization of her comorbidities, the decision was made to proceed with left total knee arthroplasty. Her prior well-healed midline incision was extended proximally and distally, and computer navigation was used to optimize the cutting block location without the need for an intramedullary guide. Because of her flexion contracture, an additional 2 mm of distal femur was resected, which allowed full extension to be achieved without having to remove the femoral nail. A range of motion from 0° to 110° was achieved intraoperatively with appropriate medial and lateral soft tissue tension using a 13 mm ultracongruent polyethylene liner (▫ Fig. 6.2). At early follow-up, she did well, but unfortunately she died from complications related to her pulmonary condition prior to long-term follow-up.

6.2.2 Case 2: Tibial Plateau Plate

A 63-year-old female, with a history of left bicondylar tibial plateau fracture, treated initially with a knee-spanning external fixator and fasciotomies for compartment syndrome followed by ORIF with dual plating, presented with left knee pain (▫ Fig. 6.3). Her knee range of motion was 5–115° with no extensor lag. Ligamentous examination demonstrated no significant ligamentous laxity. Neurovascular examination was without abnormalities. Fasciotomy incisions were well healed medially and laterally and there was a lateral tibial plateau incision. Inflammatory markers including ESR and CRP were not elevated. After discussion of the risks and benefits and alternative options, the patient requested to proceed with total knee arthroplasty. Prior anterolateral incision was used and then extended proximally in a more medial direction to allow for a medial parapatellar approach. Intraoperatively, she was noted to have advanced tricompartmental arthritic changes with a slight lateral tibial plateau step-off. No gross evidence of infection was present and frozen sections demonstrated no acute inflammation on pathology analysis. Limited hardware removal of the proximal subchondral screws and the proximal portion of the plate using a metal cutting burr and ultrasound gel facilitated the removal of metal shavings. Computer navigation was utilized for accuracy of cuts and component positioning. Knee range of motion and stability were both found to be excellent

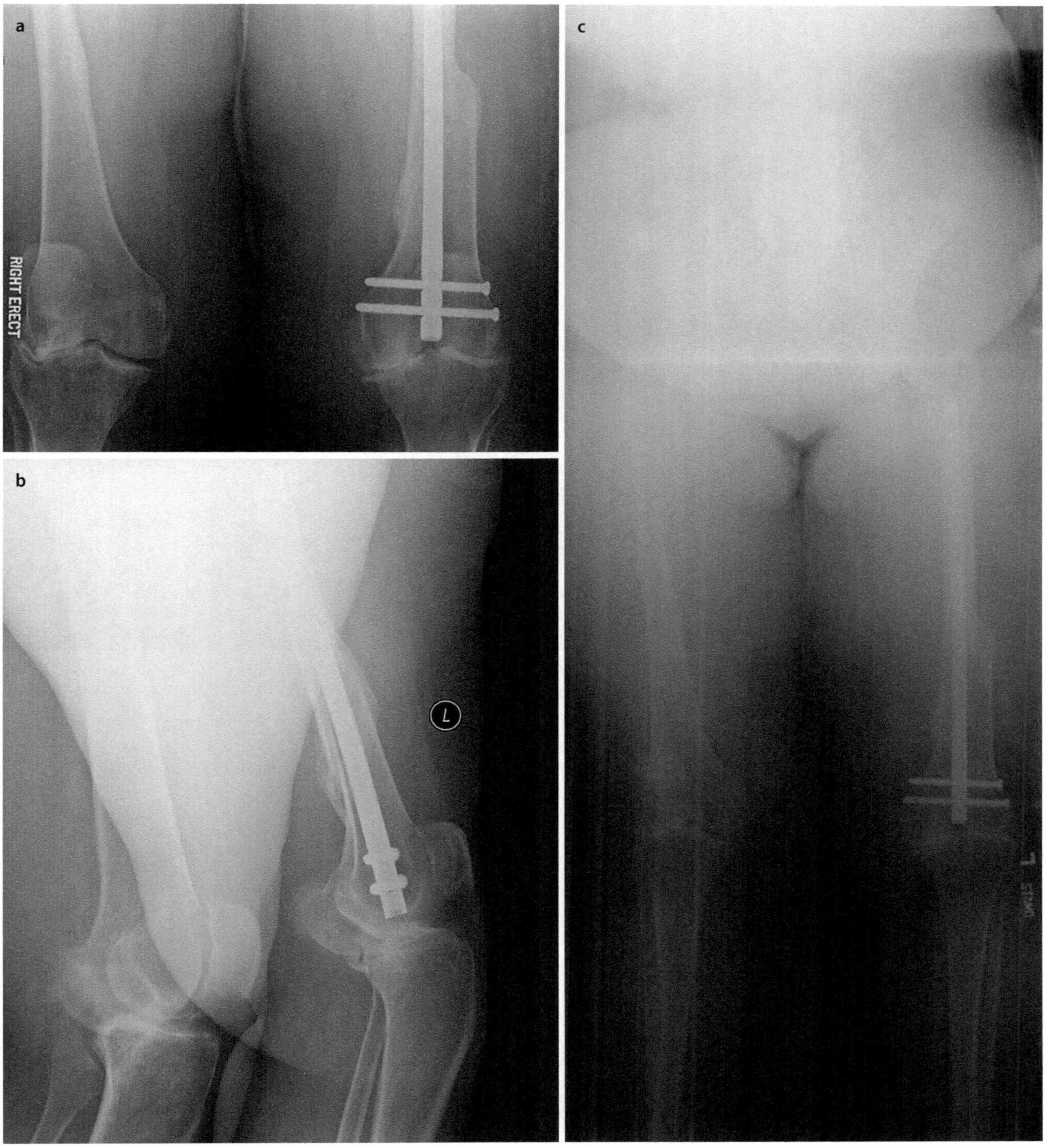

■ **Fig. 6.1** **a–c** Anteroposterior (AP), lateral, and long-standing radiographs of a 61-year-old female with PTA after prior left distal femur fracture treated with retrograde IMN

with primary components and final tibial, femoral, and patellar components were cemented in place (■ Fig. 6.4). At 14-year follow-up, the patient is doing very well with no left knee pain and an excellent range of motion from 0° to 120°. She does have some contralateral knee pain and is considering operative intervention on that side.

6.3 Preoperative Evaluation

Evaluation for post-traumatic painful knees should begin with a thorough patient history with attention to the prior trauma, subsequent treatments, and the time course of symptoms. TKA patients undergoing conversion from a prior surgery are more likely to be younger.

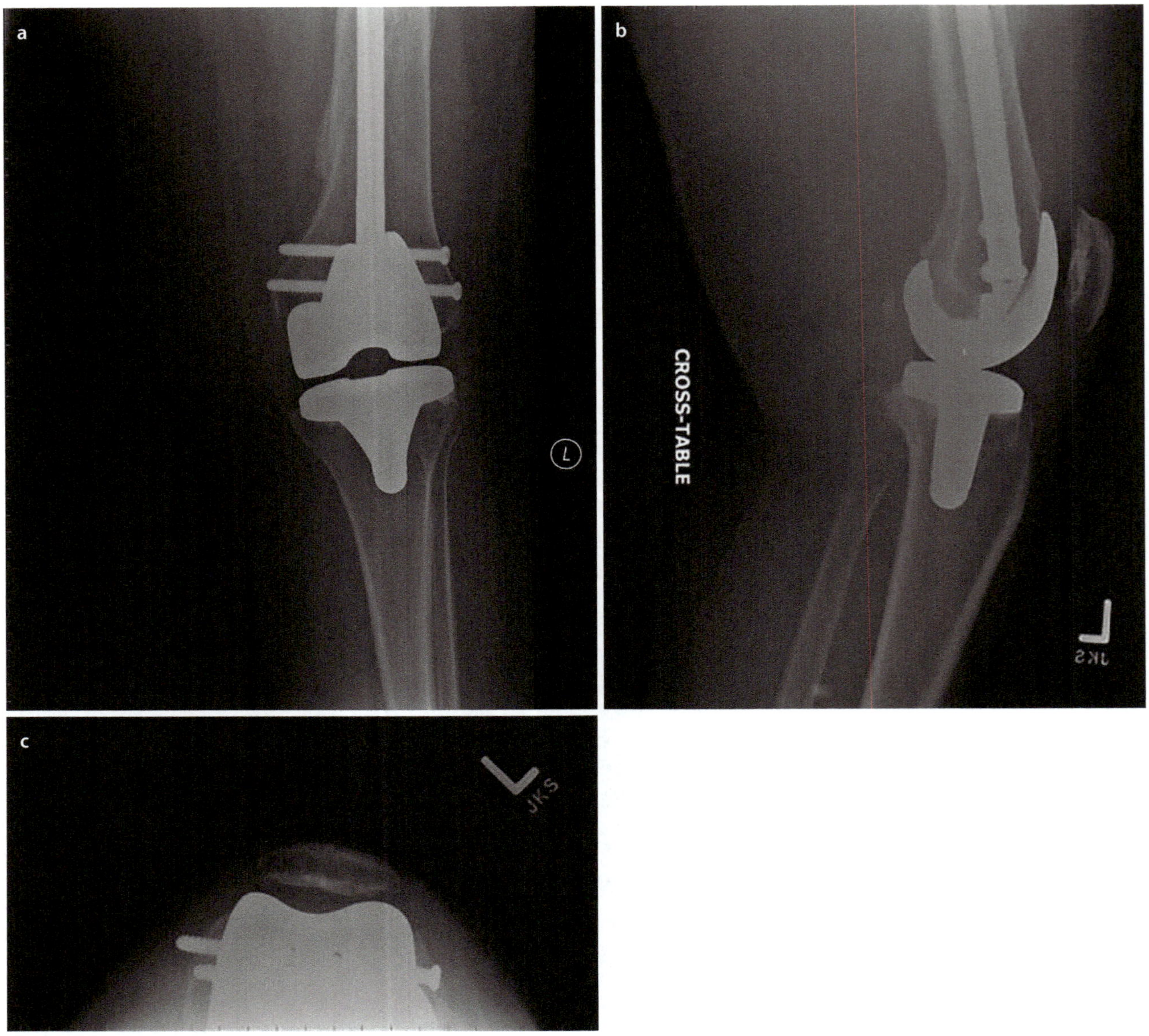

Fig. 6.2 a–c Postoperative radiographs (AP, lateral, and Merchant view) after TKA with hardware retention

Several studies have shown a different comorbidity profile than other TKA patients including higher rates of substance abuse and liver disease, but perhaps a healthier condition overall (Brophy et al. 2014; Brockman et al. 2020; Bala et al. 2015; Dexel et al. 2016; Kester et al. 2016). A physical examination should be performed with attention to ligamentous stability, range of motion, neurovascular function, and skin integrity.

> Radiographic evaluation should include the joint above and below, ideally with a long-standing view to assess alignment and deformity as well as orthogonal views. It is critical to distinguish whether deformity present is intra- or extra-articular or both (Benazzo et al. 2016).

An intra-articular correction can generally be performed with arthroplasty until the point where it leads to ligamentous laxity, compromises ligamentous attachments, or causes excessive bone loss (Sculco et al. 2019). General guidelines have suggested that extra-articular deformity less than 20° on the femur, 30° on the tibia, or 20° in the sagittal plane can be corrected with intra-articular techniques (Sculco et al. 2019). Staged osteotomy followed by knee arthroplasty is recommended for severe deformity cases and those with a significant leg length discrepancy that must be addressed. Peroneal nerve injury is one potential complication when performing acute lengthening, flexion contracture correction, and/or addressing valgus deformity and especially when the magnitude of deformity is large. This can be mitigated through gradual correction such as with

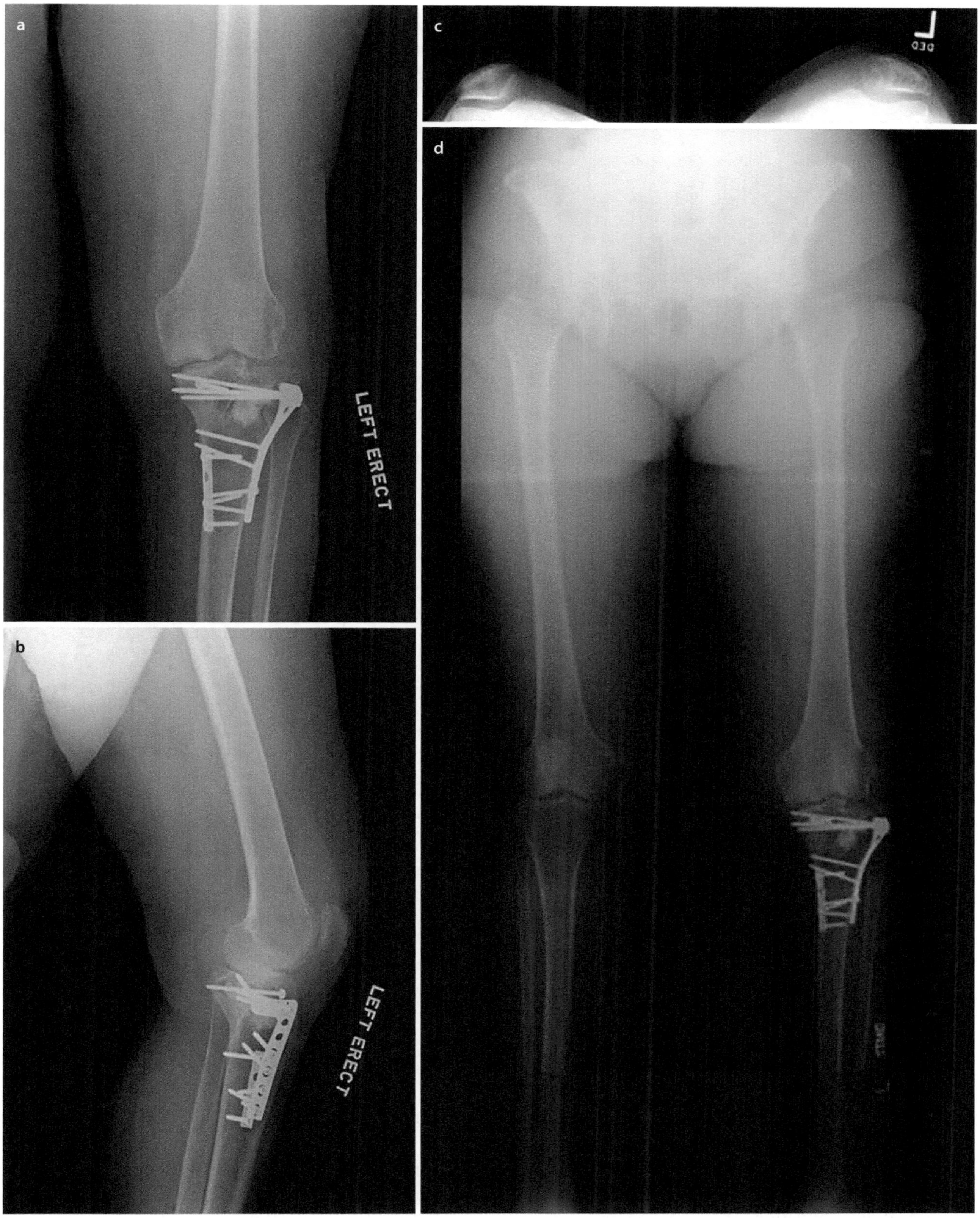

■ **Fig. 6.3** **a–d** AP, lateral, Merchant, and long-standing radiographs of a 63-year-old female, with PTA after left bicondylar tibial plateau fracture initially treated with a knee-spanning external fixator, followed by ORIF

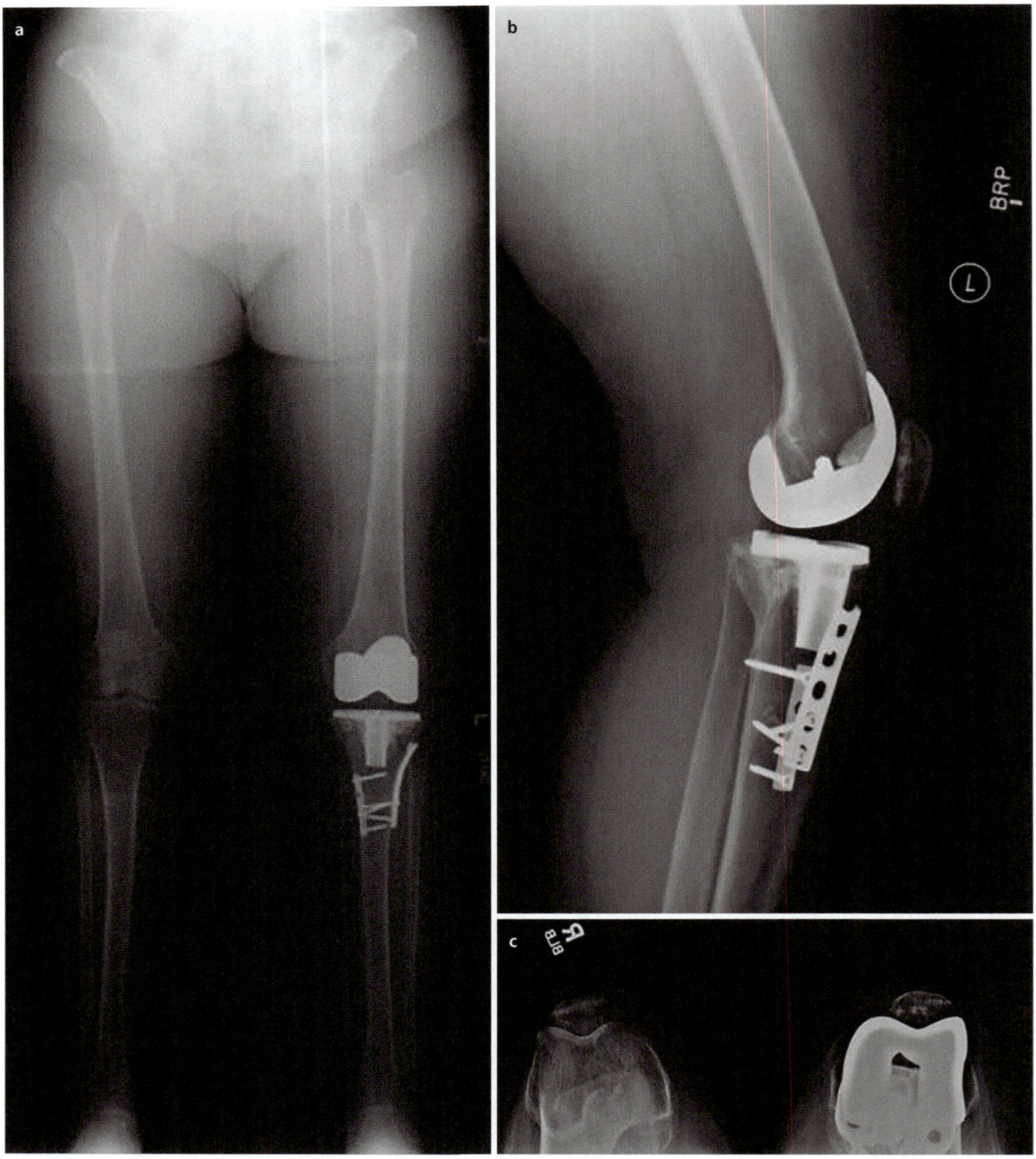

Fig. 6.4 **a–c** Postoperative radiographs after limited hardware removal and TKA using computer navigation

a spatial frame or magnetic growing rod application after osteotomy followed by knee arthroplasty in a staged manner after completion of correction in all planes, removal of fixation, likely with a time interval to allow for pin tract healing. Fixation of osteotomies can also involve intramedullary nails, external fixation, and plates and screws on the femoral, tibial, or both sides of the knee joint (Sculco et al. 2019).

Preoperative templating, intraoperative navigation applications, patient-specific instrumentation (PSI), and/or robotic platforms may provide utility in determining which deformities are correctable through the joint and which require osteotomy (Catani et al. 2012; Denjean et al. 2017). It is important to consider deformities of the tibia and femur separately when both exist, and authors have described a successful correction with osteotomy performed either staged or in the same setting as the arthroplasty (Catonné et al. 2019a; Catonné et al. 2019b; Demir et al. 2018).

> Doing deformity correction and arthroplasty in the same setting has the obvious benefit of only a single surgery. It is a technically challenging procedure with risks of complications related to increased blood loss and cement integration into an osteotomy site which could interfere with healing (Sculco et al. 2019).

Location and integrity of hardware on radiographs should include the number and trajectory of screws and plates, whether or not hardware is broken and if there are any bone defects. Review of prior imaging may be helpful as well as operative reports.

> It can be helpful to know what hardware is present in case it needs to be removed either in part or in full and to be informed about prior surgical approaches, especially if a lateral parapatellar arthrotomy was performed to prevent further devascularization of the patella.

Performing a medial approach after an extensive lateral parapatellar arthrotomy compromises additional geniculate arteries and could lead to osteonecrosis of the patella. The condition of the soft tissues needs to be carefully evaluated including the location of prior scars.

> It is generally recommended that the most lateral incision be used, and if existing incisions are not compatible with surgical exposure then connecting at 90° or greater angles is recommended.

Preoperative consultation with a plastic surgeon is sometimes advisable when skin quality or integrity is in question and local tissue flaps including medial gastrocnemius or even free flaps may be necessary for coverage. The condition of the extensor mechanism should be evaluated with the patient's ability to perform a straight leg raise. Patella alta and baja and extensor lag should be noted. Chronic patellar subluxations or dislocations and patella fractures can be encountered in the PTA patient, thus the subvastus approach and lateral retinacular release may need to be considered (Hudson et al. 2003; In et al. 2009; Houdek et al. 2015). The workhorse medial parapatellar approach to the knee may not always be the best option in the post-traumatic arthritic patient and surgeons should have familiarity with other options including subvastus, quadriceps snip, tibial tubercle osteotomy, banana peel of the patellar tendon, and lateral parapatellar arthrotomy, which can each play a useful role in providing adequate exposure in certain cases (In et al. 2009; Lahav and DiMaio 2007; Lizaur-Utrilla et al. 2015; Lonner et al. 1999; Lahav and Hofmann 2007). Range of motion should also be carefully assessed and documented, as patient expectations and surgical goals should be tailored to a patient's preoperative range of motion.

6.4 Intraoperative Considerations

Planning ahead and having all equipment available including burrs, hardware removal sets with necessary screwdrivers can eliminate intraoperative delays and reduce operative time. The diagnosis of PTA has been linked to both longer operative time and higher infection rates and costs (Dexel et al. 2016; Kester et al. 2016; Ge et al. 2018).

> Preoperative workup for occult infection is important especially in instances of prior infection, open fractures or traumatic arthrotomies, history of wound healing issues postoperative, and radiographic findings concerning osteomyelitis.

Baseline erythrocyte sedimentation rate (ESR) and C-reactive protein (CRP) should be obtained in any post-traumatic patient with any concern for infection, and if either is high, aspiration can yield additional information. In some cases, it may be prudent to remove the hardware in a staged fashion and to obtain intraoperative cultures to exclude infection, prior to proceeding with TKA (Lizaur-Utrilla et al. 2015; Pinter et al. 2020). This approach may be advisable when extensive hardware removal is required, prominent hardware may be contributing to symptoms, or when infection is suspected or has been confirmed. TKA in the PTA patient can be more technically demanding and may require additional resources including techniques, equipment, and implants that many arthroplasty surgeons may not routinely use for uncomplicated primary knee arthroplasty (Dexel et al. 2016; Weiss et al. 2003a). Implants more typically associated with revision knee arthroplasty including cones, sleeves, augments, stems, and higher levels of constraints should be available and used when deemed necessary. Small bone defects can be filled with cement technique, sometimes including a screw used as rebar.

> In general, the lowest level of constraint and hardware that allows for a stable construct and joint

should be used on a case-by-case basis to achieve excellent long-term functional outcomes for the patient (Weiss et al. 2003a; Martin-Hernandez et al. 2018; Pancio et al. 2017).

Similar to knee arthroplasty for other indications, cementless designs can be considered in PTA patients and may be an attractive option for younger patients but must be used judiciously and only for patients with adequate bone quality with careful attention to precision of bone cuts (Buechel 2002).

> Cemented arthroplasty is generally the preferred technique for achieving early fixation with aseptic loosening being a relatively uncommon cause of failure in this patient population (Brockman et al. 2020; Bala et al. 2015).

Unicompartmental arthroplasty, including medial, lateral, or patellofemoral, can be useful in the post-traumatic patient setting when only part of the knee joint is affected, but evaluation of the ligaments and cartilage surfaces in the other compartments is necessary before proceeding in order to reduce the risk of subsequent conversion to TKA (Buechel 2002; Konan and Haddad 2016; Lustig et al. 2012).

> Technological adjuncts including GPS-based, computer navigation, patient-specific instrumentation, or robotics may have helpful applications, particularly in settings where intramedullary guidance is not possible or more difficult due to existing hardware or deformity (Kuo et al. 2011; Manzotti et al. 2012; Manzotti et al. 2014).

These adjuncts may obviate the need for extensive hardware removal, although the modalities that are based on preoperative imaging may encounter difficulties due to metal artifacts. A surgeon should be familiar with these techniques and using them for the first time in a more challenging case is not advised.

6.5 Outcomes

> Outcomes after total knee arthroplasty (TKA) performed for post-traumatic arthritis (PTA) are inferior compared to those for primary osteoarthritis with regard to infection, deep vein thrombosis, implant survival (revision), patient function (including stiffness), and quality of life (Brockman et al. 2020; Bala et al. 2015; Lunebourg et al. 2015; Houdek et al. 2016).

It has been proposed that this should impact reimbursement in a bundled payment model (Kester et al. 2016). Significant improvements in pain control, range of motion, and functional outcome occur after knee arthroplasty in PTA patients, and thus, despite higher risks, it remains the optimal treatment for end-stage degenerative changes in these patients (Bedi and Haidukewych 2009; Saleh et al. 2016; Weiss et al. 2003b). Knee stiffness is more common and manipulation under anesthesia is more frequently required postoperatively for arthrofibrosis in this patient population (Lunebourg et al. 2015; Weiss et al. 2003b; Saini and Trikha 2016). In one large institutional series, the rate of revision for PTA patients was 25% at 15-year follow-up (Houdek et al. 2016). There are some instances with certain fractures in certain patients where TKA may be appropriate acutely after the time of injury (Benazzo et al. 2014; Parratte et al. 2011); however, the focus of this chapter is on TKA in the PTA patient who generally develops degenerative disease years after an injury and has often had surgical treatment shortly after the time of injury.

6.6 Conclusion

While many patients with soft tissue injuries around the knee and fractures of the distal femur, proximal tibia, and patella will eventually develop post-traumatic arthritis if given enough time, not all will require TKA (Scott et al. 2015; Wasserstein et al. 2014). The rate of PTA undoubtedly varies by numerous factors including type and severity of injury, age, genetics, and treatment-related variables. For patients who develop significant pain and negative impact on their quality of life as a result of end-stage degenerative changes associated with PTA, TKA is the optimal treatment for reducing pain and restoring function. Thorough preoperative workup is especially important to evaluate candidacy for arthroplasty and differentiating effects of PTA from other etiologies like infection, nonunion, pathology in the hip or spine. For those patients likely to benefit from TKA, a surgical plan should be created, with backup plans, which can range from resembling a routine primary total or partial knee arthroplasty to complex-staged reconstruction involving revision components and other less frequently used techniques. Outcomes after TKA performed for PTA are well established to be inferior compared to those for primary osteoarthritis; however, significant improvements for these patients do occur after knee arthroplasty, and thus despite higher risks, it remains the optimal treatment for many PTA patients. Surgeons and patients should both be aware of and have a discussion regarding the risks/benefit profile of arthroplasty in the PTA patient population, customized as much as possible to the patient's individual circumstances and goals.

Take-Home Messages

- Evaluation of post-traumatic arthritis begins with a thorough history, physical examination, and radiographs and may include an investigation for occult infection in selected patients.
- Other etiologies of pain must be considered (spine, hip, infection, nonunion).
- Technical considerations may include working around or removing hardware, utilizing technological adjuncts such as navigation, as well as having revision-type implants to address either bone and/or ligamentous deficiencies (e.g., metaphyseal fixation, semi-constrained liners).
- Complications including infection, stiffness/arthrofibrosis, and revision may be higher, but benefits still often outweigh the risks, and shared decision-making with the patient to proceed with surgery when indicated is imperative.

References

Bala A, Penrose CT, Seyler TM, Mather RC 3rd, Wellman SS, Bolognesi MP (2015) Outcomes after total knee arthroplasty for post-traumatic arthritis. Knee 22(6):630–639

Bedi A, Haidukewych GJ (2009) Management of the posttraumatic arthritic knee. J Am Acad Orthop Surg 17(2):88–101

Benazzo F, Rossi SM, Ghiara M, Zanardi A, Perticarini L, Combi A (2014) Total knee replacement in acute and chronic traumatic events. Injury 45(Suppl 6):S98–s104

Benazzo F, Rossi SMP, Combi A, Meena S, Ghiara M (2016) Knee replacement in chronic post-traumatic cases. EFORT Open Rev 1(5):211–218

Brockman BS, Maupin JJ, Thompson SF, Hollabaugh KM, Thakral R (2020) Complication rates in total knee arthroplasty performed for osteoarthritis and post-traumatic arthritis: a comparison study. J Arthroplast 35(2):371–374

Brophy RH, Gray BL, Nunley RM, Barrack RL, Clohisy JC (2014) Total knee arthroplasty after previous knee surgery: expected interval and the effect on patient age. J Bone Joint Surg Am 96(10):801–805

Buechel FF (2002) Knee arthroplasty in post-traumatic arthritis. J Arthroplast 17(4 Suppl 1):63–68

Catani F, Digennaro V, Ensini A, Leardini A, Giannini S (2012) Navigation-assisted total knee arthroplasty in knees with osteoarthritis due to extra-articular deformity. Knee Surg Sports Traumatol Arthrosc 20(3):546–551

Catonné Y, Khiami F, Sariali E, Ettori MA, Delattre O, Tillie B (2019a) Same-stage total knee arthroplasty and osteotomy for osteoarthritis with extra-articular deformity. Part II: femoral osteotomy, prospective study of 6 cases. Orthop Traumatol Surg Res 105(6):1055–1060

Catonné Y, Sariali E, Khiami F, Rouvillain JL, Wajsfisz A, Pascal-Moussellard H (2019b) Same-stage total knee arthroplasty and osteotomy for osteoarthritis with extra-articular deformity. Part I: Tibial osteotomy, prospective study of 26 cases. Orthop Traumatol Surg Res 105(6):1047–1054

Demir B, Özkul B, Saygılı MS, Çetinkaya E, Akbulut D (2018) Deformity correction with total knee arthroplasty for severe knee osteoarthritis accompanying extra-articular femoral deformity: the results are promising. Knee Surg Sports Traumatol Arthrosc 26(11):3444–3451

Denjean S, Chatain F, Tayot O (2017) One-stage computer-assisted total knee arthroplasty and tibial osteotomy. Orthop Traumatol Surg Res 103(3):381–386

Dexel J, Beyer F, Lutzner C, Kleber C, Lutzner J (2016) TKA for posttraumatic osteoarthritis is more complex and needs more surgical resources. Orthopedics 39(3 Suppl):S36–S40

Ge DH, Anoushiravani AA, Kester BS, Vigdorchik JM, Schwarzkopf R (2018) Preoperative diagnosis can predict conversion total knee arthroplasty outcomes. J Arthroplast 33(1):124–129.e121

Houdek MT, Shannon SF, Watts CD, Wagner ER, Sems SA, Sierra RJ (2015) Patella fractures prior to total knee arthroplasty: worse outcomes but equivalent survivorship. J Arthroplast 30(12):2167–2169

Houdek MT, Watts CD, Shannon SF, Wagner ER, Sems SA, Sierra RJ (2016) Posttraumatic total knee arthroplasty continues to have worse outcome than total knee arthroplasty for osteoarthritis. J Arthroplast 31(1):118–123

Hudson J, Reddy VR, Krikler SJ (2003) Total knee arthroplasty for neglected permanent post-traumatic patellar dislocation–case report. Knee 10(2):207–212

In Y, Kong CG, Sur YJ, Choi SS (2009) TKA using the subvastus approach and lateral retinacular release in patients with permanent post-traumatic patellar dislocation: a report of two cases. Knee Surg Sports Traumatol Arthrosc 17(3): 254–259

Kester BS, Minhas SV, Vigdorchik JM, Schwarzkopf R (2016) Total knee arthroplasty for posttraumatic osteoarthritis: is it time for a new classification? J Arthroplasty 31(8):1649–1653.e1641

Konan S, Haddad FS (2016) Midterm outcome of avon patellofemoral arthroplasty for posttraumatic unicompartmental osteoarthritis. J Arthroplast 31(12):2657–2659

Kuo CC, Bosque J, Meehan JP, Jamali AA (2011) Computer-assisted navigation of total knee arthroplasty for osteoarthritis in a patient with severe posttraumatic femoral deformity. J Arthroplast 26(6):976.e917–976.e920

Lahav A, DiMaio FR (2007) Concurrent opening wedge osteotomy and total knee replacement in a patient with posttraumatic arthritis and a varus tibial malunion. Am J Orthop (Belle Mead, NJ) 36(8):E121–E123

Lahav A, Hofmann AA (2007) The "banana peel" exposure method in revision total knee arthroplasty. Am J Orthop (Belle Mead, NJ) 36(10):526–529; discussion 529

Lizaur-Utrilla A, Collados-Maestre I, Miralles-Munoz FA, Lopez-Prats FA (2015) Total knee arthroplasty for osteoarthritis secondary to fracture of the tibial plateau. A prospective matched cohort study. J Arthroplast 30(8):1328–1332

Lonner JH, Pedlow FX, Siliski JM (1999) Total knee arthroplasty for post-traumatic arthrosis. J Arthroplast 14(8):969–975

Lunebourg A, Parratte S, Gay A, Ollivier M, Garcia-Parra K, Argenson JN (2015) Lower function, quality of life, and survival rate after total knee arthroplasty for posttraumatic arthritis than for primary arthritis. Acta Orthop 86(2):189–194

Lustig S, Parratte S, Magnussen RA, Argenson JN, Neyret P (2012) Lateral unicompartmental knee arthroplasty relieves pain and

improves function in posttraumatic osteoarthritis. Clin Orthop Relat Res 470(1):69–76
Manzotti A, Chemello C, Pullen C, Cerveri P, Confalonieri N (2012) Computer-assisted total knee arthroplasty after prior femoral fracture without hardware removal. Orthopedics 35(10 Suppl):34–39
Manzotti A, Pullen C, Cerveri P, Chemello C, Confalonieri N (2014) Post traumatic knee arthritis: navigated total knee replacement without hardware removal. Knee 21(1):290–294
Martin-Hernandez C, Floria-Arnal LJ, Gomez-Blasco A et al (2018) Metaphyseal sleeves as the primary implant for the management of bone defects in total knee arthroplasty after post-traumatic knee arthritis. Knee 25(4):669–675
Pancio SI, Sousa PL, Krych AJ et al (2017) Increased risk of revision, reoperation, and implant constraint in TKA after multiligament knee surgery. Clin Orthop Relat Res 475(6):1618–1626
Parratte S, Bonnevialle P, Pietu G, Saragaglia D, Cherrier B, Lafosse JM (2011) Primary total knee arthroplasty in the management of epiphyseal fracture around the knee. Orthop Traumatol Surg Res 97(6 Suppl):S87–S94
Pinter Z, Jha AJ, McGee A et al (2020) Outcomes of knee replacement in patients with posttraumatic arthritis due to previous tibial plateau fracture. Eur J Orthop Surg Traumatol 30(2):323–328
Saini P, Trikha V (2016) Manipulation under anesthesia for post traumatic stiff knee-pearls, pitfalls and risk factors for failure. Injury 47(10):2315–2319
Saleh H, Yu S, Vigdorchik J, Schwarzkopf R (2016) Total knee arthroplasty for treatment of post-traumatic arthritis: systematic review. World J Orthop 7(9):584–591
Scott CE, Davidson E, MacDonald DJ, White TO, Keating JF (2015) Total knee arthroplasty following tibial plateau fracture: a matched cohort study. Bone Joint J 97-b(4):532–538
Sculco PK, Kahlenberg CA, Fragomen AT, Rozbruch SR (2019) Management of extra-articular deformity in the setting of Total knee arthroplasty. J Am Acad Orthop Surg 27(18):e819–e830
Wasserstein D, Henry P, Paterson JM, Kreder HJ, Jenkinson R (2014) Risk of total knee arthroplasty after operatively treated tibial plateau fracture: a matched-population-based cohort study. J Bone Joint Surg Am 96(2):144–150
Weiss NG, Parvizi J, Hanssen AD, Trousdale RT, Lewallen DG (2003a) Total knee arthroplasty in post-traumatic arthrosis of the knee. J Arthroplast 18(3 Suppl 1):23–26
Weiss NG, Parvizi J, Trousdale RT, Bryce RD, Lewallen DG (2003b) Total knee arthroplasty in patients with a prior fracture of the tibial plateau. J Bone Joint Surg Am 85(2):218–221

Post-Septic Arthritis

Matan Ozery, Isaac Schultz, Tejbir S. Pannu, Jesus M. Villa, and Carlos A. Higuera

Contents

E. Hansen, K.-D. Kühn (eds.), *Essentials of Cemented Knee Arthroplasty*,
https://doi.org/10.1007/978-3-662-63113-3_7

7.1 Introduction

Septic arthritis is a major cause of morbidity and mortality in the adult patient population. The incidence of septic bacterial arthritis is estimated to be around 0.7% of all hospital admissions (Donatto 1998), of which 40–50% are infections of the knee (Kelly 1975). The mortality rates in patients who develop a septic joint range from 5% to 25% (Ferrand et al. 2016; Kaandorp et al. 1997), and there is a strong association between septic arthritis and poor functional clinical outcomes (Kaandorp et al. 1997). Recently, a significantly higher mortality rate has been reported in septic arthritis patients in the setting of infective endocarditis (Anis et al. 2020). Patients who have an underlying joint disease, or have undergone joint arthroplasty are 5–10 times more likely to develop an infection in their joint (Favero et al. 2008; Smith et al. 2006). The two most common ways that a knee becomes infected are through hematogenous spread or direct inoculation.

Hematogenous spread (septicemia/bacteremia) is the more common cause, and may be difficult to recognize in a patient who does not have an obvious underlying joint pathology (Kaandorp et al. 1997). Other risk factors for joint infection include, among others, the following:

- Either advanced or very young age
- Diabetes mellitus
- Skin infection
- Endocarditis
- Rheumatoid arthritis (Kaandorp et al. 1995)

The inflammatory processes triggered by infection often lead to extensive articular tissue damage of the knee, damage which must be addressed through emergent treatment of the infection.

Treatment of the septic knee always includes an antibiotic regimen, which is selected for the bacteria cultured from the joint or the most likely pathogen for the site (Mathews et al. 2010). The most common pathogen is *Staphylococcus aureus*, which may also be penicillin-resistant (Kaandorp et al. 1997). Depending on the type of infection (acute or chronic), the antibiotic regimen is mostly combined with a technique to remove the pathogenic tissue from the joint, whether through needle aspiration, irrigation, and debridement (I & D), or arthroscopy (Mathews et al. 2010). I & D can be done in one of the two ways: either arthroscopically or through open management via arthrotomy.

In cases in which the knee infection is unresolved for a prolonged period of time, joint degeneration ensues. Total knee arthroplasty (TKA) has emerged as the treatment of choice in these patients with end-stage degenerative joint disease after septic arthritis. As compared to the traditional arthrodesis, TKA can result in the following:

- Increased range of motion (ROM)
- Improved pain
- Better quality of life and function

> In a clinical setting, post-septic knee arthritis can present either as an acute, quiescent, or evolutive infection.

It is imperative to choose the appropriate treatment option, and set goals with tailored treatment depending on these different scenarios, highlighting the importance of surgical decision-making based on the details of each individual case. In the current chapter, our objective is to review the literature on the management of septic knee with variable presentations and its associated clinical outcomes and the utility, efficacy, and safety of TKA in patients with native septic joint disease. We also briefly discuss the development of periprosthetic joint infection in TKA after native septic arthritis treatment.

7.2 Definition and Diagnosis of Post-Septic Arthritis

Post-septic arthritis is defined as the arthritis which develops secondary to hematogenous seeding of a joint during a transient or persistent bacteremia (Goldenberg 1998). When bacteria enter the joint space, an acute inflammatory synovitis is triggered and the synovial membrane reacts with a proliferative lining-cell hyperplasia (Goldenberg 1998). The lack of a basement membrane in synovial tissue allows for a rapid spread of microorganisms throughout the joint (Margaretten et al. 2007). An influx of acute and chronic inflammatory cells leads to the release of inflammatory factors which degrade the joint cartilage, and if untreated, within several days, irreversible subchondral bone loss can occur (Goldenberg 1998).

> Any microbial pathogen can cause septic arthritis; however, *Staphylococcus* and *Streptococcus* are the most common infecting organisms (Klippel et al. 2001).

Most cases of septic arthritis are mono-articular and occur in large peripheral joints such as the knee, which accounts for 50% of cases (Goldenberg 1998; Klippel et al. 2001). Septic arthritis can be diagnosed through a positive synovial fluid gram stain or culture, or by a presumptive diagnosis through analysis of purulent synovial fluid with a leukocyte count (Klippel et al. 2001; Miller et al. 2018).

> A synovial fluid aspiration with a leukocyte count >50,000 cells/mL is considered to be diagnostic of a septic joint, however, lower counts do not exclude the diagnosis (Miller et al. 2018).

Serum inflammatory markers such as C-reactive protein and erythrocyte sedimentation rate (ESR) might be useful to detect infection as well. The diagnosis of septic knee requires a strong clinical suspicion depending on the patient presentation, and physical examination, further supported by the results of synovial fluid assay. Differential diagnosis includes gout exacerbation or pseudogout flares that can be differentiated using synovial fluid crystal analysis of uric acid or calcium pyrophosphate presence, respectively. Additionally, some inflammatory arthropathies including rheumatoid arthritis can mimic a septic arthritis, however, in this condition the aspiration of synovial fluid is generally aseptic.

7.3 Approach to Septic Arthritis Depending on the Stage of the Joint Disease

In general, septic arthritis can present in three clinical settings as discussed below.

7.3.1 Acute Septic Arthritis on a Native Knee and Without Degenerative Disease

This scenario describes an acute infection of the joint, with no other preexisting pathology. The initial management often includes both joint irrigation and debridement and a course of postoperative antibiotics. However, in case of gonococcal arthritis, an appropriate antibiotic therapy suffices for majority of the cases. Initial hospitalization is recommended until 1–2 days after resolution of symptoms. Follow-up synovial aspiration to confirm infection eradication is the key in management of gonococcal arthritis (Shirtliff and Mader 2002). If the patient does not respond to the initial treatment, further invasive management is indicated.

> I & D is a relatively efficacious initial surgical treatment in these patients with acute infection of a native knee (Abram et al. 2020). I & D can either be performed arthroscopically or via open arthrotomy.

When comparing the short-term outcomes (e.g., bleeding, adverse events), arthroscopic I & D has shown favorable outcomes compared to open techniques. The literature is divided over infection recurrence and restoration of functional outcomes. While some authors have found no significant difference between the two techniques, others have presented arthroscopic I & D to have more favorable outcomes than an open approach in these areas (Aïm et al. 2015; Faour et al. 2019; Johns et al. 2017). I & D is used as an ideally curative, less functionally limiting treatment for a native septic joint, however, if it does not successfully eradicate the infection or if the joint damage progresses, then TKA, or in worst cases, arthrodesis or amputation may be necessary (Abram et al. 2020). Historically, I & D of the septic joint has demonstrated favorable outcomes with less soft tissue damage and invasiveness than the alternative treatments (Abram et al. 2020; Faour et al. 2019; Shukla et al. 2014), however, more recently it has been suggested that the failure rate of I & D is higher than previously realized.

7.3.2 Quiescent/Cured Septic Arthritis

This type of septic arthritis involves previous septic knee whose resolution is uncertain after a long asymptomatic period (Bauer et al. 2010). A history of septic knee arthritis often leads to long-term consequences which limit functional use of the joint, requiring further corrective treatment.

> Permanent joint damage occurs in 50% of cases of septic arthritis of which the majority occurs in the knee (Goldenberg 1998; Kelly 1975).

Thus, the range of motion and function of the knee may progressively deteriorate. Also, the infective microorganism may still reside in quiescence in these cases (Bauer et al. 2010; Sultan et al. 2019). In both circumstances, total knee arthroplasty may be indicated.

In case of quiescent infection, one-stage total knee arthroplasty with extensive synovectomy has been most commonly performed, as suggested by the literature (Bauer et al. 2010). Preoperative joint biopsy is mandatory to screen for any quiescent infections, however, the false-negative rate for this procedure is high (Bauer et al. 2010). To confirm the presence of infection, intraoperative synovial fluid, tissue, and bone samples are recommended. (Bauer et al. 2010). The antibiotic therapy should then be adapted depending on these culture results (Bauer et al. 2010). These steps are key to preventing prosthetic failure of the TKA in these post-septic cases where the infective status of the knee is unclear.

One-stage TKA begins with removal of all infected tissue and copious lavage of the remaining tissue, and often involves bone cuts. The wound is then packaged with sterile swabs and bandaged, as well as released from the tourniquet. The surgical team then re-scrubs, re-drapes, and gets a new set of instruments, and begins the second part of the procedure. The tourniquet is re-inflated and the joint is prepared and the prosthesis is then implanted in the knee, completing the procedure (Bauer et al. 2010).

> In one-stage TKA, it is important that the infective organism is identified through aspiration prior to surgery, and organism-specific antibiotics are administered perioperatively and loaded in the cement of the prosthesis (Parkinson et al. 2011).

The amount of antibiotic mixed in the cement should not compromise its mechanical properties (Hinarejos et al. 2015).

7.3.3 Evolutive Septic Arthritis with End Degenerative Disease

This type of arthritis results in severe damage to cartilage and bone, eventually leading to functional deterioration of the knee (Bauer et al. 2010). A recent investigation defined this arthritis as the presence of one or more of the following criteria:

- Clinical signs of infection (local erythema, tenderness, effusion, limited range of motion, or presence of a sinus)
- Loss of articular space on radiographic studies
- Femoral heads or articular cartilage damage
- Inflammatory markers (C-reactive protein [CRP] > 10 mg/dL, erythrocyte sedimentation rate [ESR] > 30 mm/h)
- Intraoperative purulence
- Positive synovial fluid or tissue cultures at the time of first stage of antibiotic spacer placement, if applicable (Xu et al. 2019)

> In the setting of evolutive septic knee, two-stage total knee arthroplasty has been the procedure of choice (Bauer et al. 2010; Xu et al. 2019).

The first stage comprises total synovectomy with knee joint resection. The debridement of infected and necrotic tissue is performed. Synovial fluid, deep tissue, and bone samples are obtained for cultures. Joint irrigation is done with 5–9 L of an antiseptic solution. After this, an antibiotic-loaded articulating cement spacer is then inserted. Depending on the culture sensitivity results, antibiotics should be selected and administered at least for 6 weeks after the first stage. For patients with negative cultures, empiric, broad-spectrum antibiotic therapy should be considered.

The appropriate time for implantation is determined based on confirmation of the infection eradication. This is supported by the absence of clinical signs of infection, and gradually decreasing inflammatory markers like ESR and CRP values. Before second stage, some advocate at least a 2-week antibiotic holiday. The second stage includes repeated synovectomy and removal of the previously inserted antibiotic-loaded cement spacer (Bauer et al. 2010). Reconfirmation of the infection resolution is done intraoperatively. Tissue samples are obtained and sent for frozen sections to measure acute inflammation evidenced by more than 5 neutrophils per high-powered field in 5 power fields (Kwiecien et al. 2017). In the next step, the new prostheses are implanted and re-debridement and irrigation are performed.

While TKA (one-stage or two-stage) is indicated in both quiescent and evolutive septic arthritis, the question has always risen about the safe timeline of performing TKA after septic arthritis.

> Recent data suggest that while there is no ideal optimal time point after treatment for septic arthritis for TKA to be performed, it has been demonstrated that waiting at least 1 year is relatively safe (Sultan et al. 2019; Tan et al. 2019).

7.4 Importance of Antibiotic-Loaded Cement for TKA in Post-Septic Arthritis

In both the one-stage and two-stage approaches to post-septic TKA, when implanting the prosthesis, antibiotic-loaded bone cement (ALBC) is commonly used. In ALBC, the antibiotic elutes through pores in the cement to eradicate intra-articular organisms and prevent prosthetic infection (Hinarejos et al. 2015). Commonly, aminoglycosides and vancomycin are used to treat gram-negative and gram-positive species, respectively (Hinarejos et al. 2015). Although high-dose formulation ALBC has been used for a long time for infection prophylaxis, there are many shortcomings, especially with cemented TKA:

- First, there is an inverse relationship between the amount of antibiotic infused with the cement and the compressive and tensile strength of it (Hinarejos et al. 2015). For the antibiotic to elute the cement, a certain degree of porosity is required, and this increase in porosity weakens the mechanical strength

of the cement, ultimately decreasing the longevity of the joint fixation (Hinarejos et al. 2015).
- Second, the antibiotic can leave the joint and can be detected systemically, leading to side effects of the specific antibiotic, hypersensitivity reactions, and antibiotic resistance development because of the slow release, exposing the infecting organism to initially insufficient levels of antibiotic (Hinarejos et al. 2015)

> In general, considering the high-risk profile of post-septic arthritis cases, the use of ALBC in TKA is recommended in all cases.

There are multiple commercial premixed ALBCs available (Jiranek et al. 2006). The majority of them are composed of aminoglycosides in combination with either tobramycin or gentamicin. The major limitation of these commercial ALBCs is the inability to tailor antibiotics for specific organisms. Thus, surgeons still continue to hand-mix antibiotics to the cement in order to target a particular infecting organism. There is no evidence comparing commercially premixed and hand-mixed cement as such in the setting of post-septic arthritis. However, some evidence on this subject comes from the management of periprosthetic joint infection. Chang et al. (2013) tested the following two premixed ALBCs against hand-mixed ALBCs:

- Palacos R + G: 1 g gentamicin in 40 g polymethylmethacrylate (PMMA)
- Simplex P: 1 g tobramycin in 40 g PMMA

While gentamicin-loaded premixed ALBC showed an equal or longer duration of antibacterial action against different bacteria, tobramycin-loaded premixed ABLC did not show any advantage over hand-mixed ABLC (Chang et al. 2013).

7.5 TKA in Post-Septic Arthritis

7.5.1 Clinical Outcomes: One-Stage and Two-Stage

7.5.1.1 One-Stage TKA

Multiple previous reports have shown benefits of one-stage TKA in septic arthritis patients with previous history of sepsis which was considered resolved (Bauer et al. 2010; Lee et al. 2002). Bauer et al. demonstrated the eradication of joint infection in 95% of quiescent septic arthritis patients who underwent one-stage arthroplasty. These favorable outcomes were also reflected in the mean postoperative International Knee Score (IKS) of 91/100 and the mean postoperative IKS functional score of 80/100 (Bauer et al. 2010). On treating 18 out of 20 patients with previous sepsis around the knee with one-stage TKA, Lee et al. showed an improvement in the mean Knee Society scores for pain from 39 points preoperatively to 91 points postoperatively (Lee et al. 2002).

> While these reports show favorable outcomes with the one-stage approach in quiescent septic arthritis, a high rate of PJI after arthroplasty was found in a recent investigation of 62 native knees with quiescent infection which were managed using this approach (Seo et al. 2014).

At a mean follow-up of 6.1 years, as much as 9.7% (6/62) of these cases developed infection. Interestingly, organisms similar to those cultured previously regrew at the time of re-infection (Seo et al. 2014). Thus, more recent studies have considered two-stage arthroplasty in these patients as a rewarding alternative (Anagnostakos et al. 2016; Fleck et al. 2011; Xu et al. 2019).

7.5.1.2 Two-Stage TKA

> Two-stage arthroplasty has been a preferred procedure in the setting of evolutive septic arthritis in old investigations (Bauer et al. 2010). However, as mentioned before, this approach is also now considered as a substitute for quiescent septic arthritis.

In terms of clinical outcomes, the Knee Society (KS) score (Jenny and Diesinger 2011) has been used in the literature as an indicator of clinical function. Nazarian et al. (2003) studied 14 knees with recurrent septic arthritis or chronic periarticular osteomyelitis in which a two-stage approach was used (Nazarian et al. 2003). With this approach, average Knee Society scores markedly improved from the preoperative (46) to the postoperative period (89). In the same cohort, the postoperative average knee functional score was determined to be 78 (Nazarian et al. 2003). Alike results were reported by Bauer et al. (2010) using a two-stage TKA to treat septic arthritis (Knee Society Pain scores and Knee Society Function scores: both 80 out of 100) (Bauer et al. 2010).

Depending on the stage of organism growth cycle, quiescent infections have been shown to achieve better clinical outcomes, as compared to evolutive infections (Bauer et al. 2010). Two-stage approaches using articulating cement spacers molded intraoperatively for infected knees have been associated with favorable postoperative clinical outcomes. The mean Knee Society Pain and mean Knee Society Function scores exhibited an improvement from preoperative 41 and 43 to postoperative 85 and 83, respectively, at the latest follow-up (Shaikh et al. 2014). Clinical outcomes for TKA using impregnated cement spacers in post-septic arthritis have been shown to be comparable to aseptic TKA in terms of range of motion, knee scores, patient satisfaction, and function scores (Lee et al. 2017).

Of note, recent evidence has shown that TKA performed after an episode of septic arthritis is associated with an increased risk of periprosthetic joint infection (Sultan et al. 2019). Factors such as smoking and poor glycemic control (uncontrolled diabetes mellitus) are associated with a higher risk of periprosthetic joint infection after TKA for a native septic joint arthritis. This may be due to poor management of medical comorbidities such as diabetes, smoking, or immunosuppression, which could have caused the initial septic arthritis. Nonetheless, with good management of comorbidities, aggressive physical therapy, and patient education, good clinical outcomes can be achieved (Bauer et al. 2010). Additionally, better clinical outcomes may be achieved by waiting at least 1 year, and preferably 2 years after the initial infection has cleared, before attempting a TKA (Kim et al. 2003; Sultan et al. 2019; Tan et al. 2019).

7.5.2 Complication and Revision Rates of TKA

Complications that arise from the use of TKA to treat septic arthritis are essentially the same as those that arise from any joint arthroplasty. The two categories of complications are broadly classified into:

- Aseptic complications
- Septic complications

When considering septic complications, the most common pathogen remains *Staphylococcus aureus*, which may be treated empirically or through bacterial culture. Common causes of aseptic complications include periprosthetic fracture, aseptic loosening, and polyethylene wear, among others (Lee et al. 2017).

Revision rates after TKA in post-septic arthritis patients have been demonstrated to be much higher than that of TKA patient population, in general.

> In fact, the most common reason for revision in a patient who has had septic arthritis is joint infection (Yu et al. 2018).

It is noteworthy that revision rates for periprosthetic joint infection (PJI) for patients after TKA range from 0.8% to 1.9% in the general population (Ratto et al. 2017), whereas revision rates for PJI are much higher (12%) in patients who received TKA for septic arthritis (Jenny and Diesinger 2011).

In a recent investigation, in patients with history of previously treated native septic arthritis of the same joint, as high as 8% rate of periprosthetic joint infections (5 out of 62 patients) was determined (Sultan et al. 2019).

7.6 Special Considerations for TKA in Post-Septic Arthritis

While TKA is a relatively safe choice for treating degenerative changes after septic arthritis, there are some contraindications to be aware of. Patients with an ongoing infection of the knee or who have a condition that might preclude them from non-emergent surgery (such as a cardiovascular event or systemic immunosuppression) should not undergo a TKA (Schmitt et al. 2017). Other situations in which TKA is contraindicated are neurological disease of the lower extremity (such as a nonfunctional extensor mechanism) and ischemic or thrombotic leg disease (Promish et al. 2018; Thornhill and Lee (n.d.), available at ▶ https://jomi.com/article/13/total-knee-arthroplasty).

One should also take into account the medical profile and lifestyle of the patient. If the patient is unlikely to follow up with physical rehabilitation or cannot lose weight, then TKA is not as likely to be successful. In these instances, alternative methods should be discussed. Finally, in cases where there is significant destruction of the joint and there is severe bone loss or ligamentous incompetence, a constrained implant (Moussa et al. 2017) or on occasions a hinge prosthesis should be considered (Rodríguez-Merchán 2019).

Conclusion

Post-septic arthritis can present either as an acute, quiescent, or evolutive infection. In persistent progressive cases, it can result in degenerative joint disease. Based on the stage of the disease, patients should be treated with aspiration, irrigation, and debridement, or total knee arthroplasty, in combination with a tailored antibiotic protocol depending on the infecting organism, if known. While arthroscopic irrigation and debridement seem to produce better clinical outcomes in the acute setting, total knee arthroplasty appears to be safe at least 1 year after septic arthritis and has been shown to ensure adequate infection control and functional joint outcomes. It is important to counsel patients about the elevated risk of periprosthetic joint infection in these cases. Strong evidence on the choice of surgical approach (one-stage vs. two-stage) in post-septic arthritis is still lacking. Overall, studies investigating total knee arthroplasty in setting of post-septic arthritis are scarce. Further research on this topic is warranted.

Take-Home Messages

- For an appropriate treatment, categorization of post-septic arthritis into acute, quiescent, or evolutive is imperative.
- Both one-stage and two-stage TKAs result in favorable clinical outcomes, but seem to be associated with high rates of postoperative PJI.
- Old investigations suggest the choice of one-stage TKA for quiescent, and two-stage TKA for evolutive septic arthritis.
- Even today, strong evidence is still lacking on the choice of one-stage versus two-stage TKA.
- More studies focusing on the use of TKA for the treatment of post-septic arthritis are warranted.

References

Abram SGF, Alvand A, Judge A et al (2020) Mortality and adverse joint outcomes following septic arthritis of the native knee: a longitudinal cohort study of patients receiving arthroscopic washout. Lancet Infect Dis 20(3):341–349. https://doi.org/10.1016/S1473-3099(19)30419-0

Aïm F, Delambre J, Bauer T, Hardy P (2015) Efficacy of arthroscopic treatment for resolving infection in septic arthritis of native joints. Orthop Traumatol Surg Res 101(1):61–64. https://doi.org/10.1016/j.otsr.2014.11.010

Anagnostakos K, Duchow L, Koch K (2016) Two-stage protocol and spacer implantation in the treatment of destructive septic arthritis of the hip joint. Arch Orthop Trauma Surg 136(7):899–906. https://doi.org/10.1007/s00402-016-2455-3

Anis HK, Miller EM, George J et al (2020) Incidence and characteristics of osteoarticular infections in patients with infective endocarditis. Orthopedics 43(1):24–29. https://doi.org/10.3928/01477447-20191031-02

Bauer T, Lacoste S, Lhotellier L et al (2010) Arthroplasty following a septic arthritis history: a 53 cases series. Orthop Traumatol Surg Res 96(8):840–843. https://doi.org/10.1016/j.otsr.2010.06.009

Chang Y, Tai CL, Hsieh PH, Ueng SW (2013) Gentamicin in bone cement: a potentially more effective prophylactic measure of infection in joint arthroplasty. Bone Joint Res 2(10):220–226. https://doi.org/10.1302/2046-3758.210.2000188

Donatto KC (1998) Orthopedic management of septic arthritis. Rheum Dis Clin N Am 24(2):275–286. https://doi.org/10.1016/s0889-857x(05)70009-0

Faour M, Sultan AA, George J et al (2019) Arthroscopic irrigation and debridement is associated with favourable short-term outcomes vs. open management: an ACS-NSQIP database analysis. Knee Surg Sports Traumatol Arthrosc 27(10):3304–3310. https://doi.org/10.1007/s00167-018-5328-1

Favero M, Schiavon F, Riato L et al (2008) Rheumatoid arthritis is the major risk factor for septic arthritis in rheumatological settings. Autoimmun Rev 8(1):59–61. https://doi.org/10.1016/j.autrev.2008.07.018

Ferrand J, El Samad Y, Brunschweiler B et al (2016) Morbimortality in adult patients with septic arthritis: a three-year hospital-based study. BMC Infect Dis 16:239. https://doi.org/10.1186/s12879-016-1540-0

Fleck EE, Spangehl MJ, Rapuri VR, Beauchamp CP (2011) An articulating antibiotic spacer controls infection and improves pain and function in a degenerative septic hip. Clin Orthop Relat Res 469(11):3055–3064. https://doi.org/10.1007/s11999-011-1903-1

Goldenberg DL (1998) Septic arthritis. Lancet 351(9097):197–202. https://doi.org/10.1016/S0140-6736(97)09522-6

Hinarejos P, Guirro P, Puig-Verdie L et al (2015) Use of antibiotic-loaded cement in total knee arthroplasty. World J Orthop 6(11):877–885. https://doi.org/10.5312/wjo.v6.i11.877

Jenny JY, Diesinger Y (2011) Validation of a French version of the Oxford knee questionnaire. Orthop Traumatol Surg Res 97(3):267–271. https://doi.org/10.1016/j.otsr.2010.07.009

Jiranek WA, Hanssen AD, Greenwald AS (2006) Antibiotic-loaded bone cement for infection prophylaxis in total joint replacement. J Bone Joint Surg Am 88(11):2487–2500. https://doi.org/10.2106/JBJS.E.01126

Johns BP, Loewenthal MR, Dewar DC (2017) Open compared with arthroscopic treatment of acute septic arthritis of the native knee. J Bone Joint Surg Am 99(6):499–505. https://doi.org/10.2106/JBJS.16.00110

Kaandorp CJ, Van Schaardenburg D, Krijnen P et al (1995) Risk factors for septic arthritis in patients with joint disease. A prospective study. Arthritis Rheum 38(12):1819–1825. https://doi.org/10.1002/art.1780381215

Kaandorp CJ, Dinant HJ, van de Laar MA et al (1997) Incidence and sources of native and prosthetic joint infection: a community based prospective survey. Ann Rheum Dis 56(8):470–475. https://doi.org/10.1136/ard.56.8.470

Kelly PJ (1975) Bacterial arthritis in the adult. Orthop Clin North Am 6(4):973–981

Kim YH, Oh SH, Kim JS (2003) Total hip arthroplasty in adult patients who had childhood infection of the hip. J Bone Joint Surg Am 85(2):198–204. https://doi.org/10.2106/00004623-200302000-00003

Klippel JH, Weyand CM, Crofford LJ, Stone JH (2001) Arthritis foundation: primer on the rheumatic diseases, 12th edn. Arthritis Foundation, Atlanta

Kwiecien G, George J, Klika A et al (2017) Intraoperative frozen section histology: matched for Musculoskeletal Infection Society Criteria. J Arthroplast 32(1):223–227. https://doi.org/10.1016/j.arth.2016.06.019

Lee GC, Pagnano MW, Hanssen AD (2002) Total knee arthroplasty after prior bone or joint sepsis about the knee. Clin Orthop Relat Res 404:226–231. https://doi.org/10.1097/00003086-200211000-00036

Lee DH, Lee SH, Song EK et al (2017) Causes and clinical outcomes of revision total knee arthroplasty. Knee Surg Relat Res 29(2):104–109. https://doi.org/10.5792/ksrr.16.035

Margaretten ME, Kohlwes J, Moore D, Bent S (2007) Does this adult patient have septic arthritis? JAMA 297(13):1478–1488. https://doi.org/10.1001/jama.297.13.1478

Mathews CJ, Weston VC, Jones A et al (2010) Bacterial septic arthritis in adults. Lancet 375(9717):846–855. https://doi.org/10.1016/S0140-6736(09)61595-6

Miller JM, Binnicker MJ, Campbell S et al (2018) A guide to utilization of the microbiology laboratory for diagnosis of infectious diseases: 2018 update by the Infectious Diseases Society of America and the American Society for Microbiology. Clin Infect Dis 67(6):e1–e94. https://doi.org/10.1093/cid/ciy381

Moussa ME, Lee YY, Patel AR, Westrich GH (2017) Clinical outcomes following the use of constrained condylar knees in primary total knee arthroplasty. J Arthroplast 32(6):1869–1873. https://doi.org/10.1016/j.arth.2017.01.001

Nazarian DG, de Jesus D, McGuigan F, Booth RE Jr (2003) A two-stage approach to primary knee arthroplasty in the infected arthritic knee. J Arthroplast 18(7, Suppl 1):16–21. https://doi.org/10.1016/s0883-5403(03)00343-7

Parkinson RW, Kay PR, Rawal A (2011) A case for one-stage revision in infected total knee arthroplasty? Knee 18(1):1–4. https://doi.org/10.1016/j.knee.2010.04.008
Promish M, Wang C, Guo YD (2018) Impact of coronal alignment in total knee arthroplasty and functional outcome. Open J Orthop 8:11–23. https://doi.org/10.4236/ojo.2018.81002
Ratto N, Arrigoni C, Rosso F et al (2017) Total knee arthroplasty and infection: how surgeons can reduce the risks. EFORT Open Rev 1(9):339–344. https://doi.org/10.1302/2058-5241.1.000032
Rodríguez-Merchán EC (2019) Total knee arthroplasty using hinge joints: indications and results. EFORT Open Rev 4(4):121–132. https://doi.org/10.1302/2058-5241.4.180056
Schmitt J, Lange T, Günther KP et al (2017) Indication criteria for total knee arthroplasty in patients with osteoarthritis – a multi-perspective consensus study (Indikationskriterien für den endoprothetischen Gelenkersatz bei Gonarthrose – eine multiperspektivische Konsensstudie). Z Orthop Unfall 155(5):539–548. https://doi.org/10.1055/s-0043-115120
Seo JG, Moon YW, Park SH et al (2014) Primary total knee arthroplasty in infection sequelae about the native knee. J Arthroplast 29(12):2271–2275. https://doi.org/10.1016/j.arth.2014.01.013
Shaikh AA, Ha CW, Park YG, Park YB (2014) Two-stage approach to primary TKA in infected arthritic knees using intraoperatively molded articulating cement spacers. Clin Orthop Relat Res 472(7):2201–2207. https://doi.org/10.1007/s11999-014-3545-6
Shirtliff ME, Mader JT (2002) Acute septic arthritis. Clin Microbiol Rev 15(4):527–544. https://doi.org/10.1128/cmr.15.4.527-544.2002
Shukla A, Beniwal SK, Sinha S (2014) Outcome of arthroscopic drainage and debridement with continuous suction irrigation technique in acute septic arthritis. J Clin Orthop Trauma 5(1):1–5. https://doi.org/10.1016/j.jcot.2014.01.004
Smith JW, Chalupa P, Shabaz Hasan M (2006) Infectious arthritis: clinical features, laboratory findings and treatment. Clin Microbiol Infect 12(4):309–314. https://doi.org/10.1111/j.1469--0691.2006.01366.x
Sultan AA, Mahmood B, Samuel LT et al (2019) Patients with a history of treated septic arthritis are at high risk of periprosthetic joint infection after total joint arthroplasty. Clin Orthop Relat Res 477(7):1605–1612. https://doi.org/10.1097/CORR.0000000000000688
Tan TL et al (2019) Total joint arthroplasty after septic arthritis: when can this be safely performed? Presented at: Musculoskeletal Infection Society Annual Open Scientific Meeting, Aug. 2–3, 2019, New York
Thornhill T, Lee D (n.d.) Total knee arthroplasty, JOMI. https://jomi.com/article/13/total-knee-arthroplasty I https://doi.org/10.24296/jomi/13
Xu C, Kuo FC, Kheir M et al (2019) Outcomes and predictors of treatment failure following two-stage total joint arthroplasty with articulating spacers for evolutive septic arthritis. BMC Musculoskelet Disord 20(1):272. https://doi.org/10.1186/s12891-019-2652-7
Yu S, Bolz N, Buza J et al (2018) Orthopaedic Proceedings Vol 99-B, No SUPP 6 Re-revision total knee arthroplasty: Epidemiology and factors associated with outcomes. Published Online: 21 Feb 2018 (boneandjoint.org.uk)

Influence of Lifestyle and Risk Factors on the Development of Knee Arthritis and Outcomes Following Cemented Total Knee Arthroplasty: A US Perspective

Jonathan Dattilo and William Hamilton

Contents

E. Hansen, K.-D. Kühn (eds.), *Essentials of Cemented Knee Arthroplasty*,
https://doi.org/10.1007/978-3-662-63113-3_8

8.1 Introduction

Osteoarthritis (OA) is the most common form of arthritis, affecting over 27 million people in the United States and over 250 million people worldwide (O'Neill et al. 2018; Vos et al. 2012). Among patients aged 63 to 94 years, 33% were found to have radiographic presence of OA (Felson et al. 1987). Additionally, it has been estimated that 45% of adults will develop symptomatic knee OA between the ages of 45 and 85 (Murphy et al. 2008). The risk factors for progression of OA are not well understood. However, knee OA represents a substantial burden to society. The cost of treating OA in developed countries is between 1% and 2.5% of the gross domestic product (GDP) (Hiligsmann et al. 2013; March and Bachmeier 1997). Total knee arthroplasty (TKA) is an extremely successful and cost-effective treatment for advanced knee OA but is not without complications (Price et al. 2018). While there are many additional etiologies of arthritis, including post-traumatic arthritis, osteonecrosis, infectious, and inflammatory arthritis, this chapter will focus on primary osteoarthritis. In the first section, we will examine patient and lifestyle factors that may contribute to the development of knee OA. In the second section, we will review the most common reasons for failure of cemented TKA and the correlation of individual patient variables.

8.2 Patient and Lifestyle Risk Factors Associated with the Development of Knee Osteoarthritis

8.2.1 Patient Factors

8.2.1.1 Genetics

Genetic studies offer a partial explanation for the development of knee OA. Multiple genome-wide association studies (GWAS) have been conducted in the hopes of identifying the molecular pathogenesis of knee OA. Over 30 genetic loci have been associated with OA (Gonzalez and Valdes 2018; Kerkhof et al. 2010; Panoutsopoulou and Zeggini 2013; Zengini et al. 2018), but these have been found to explain only about 25% of heritability (Gonzalez and Valdes 2018), often as a result of differential genetic expression (Zengini et al. 2018). Other genetic efforts have focused on studies of identical twins to quantify the contribution of genetics. When controlling environmental confounders, one study estimated that up to 65% of the variance in knee OA could be attributable to genetic factors (Spector et al. 1996). A second twin study, however, found that twins with OA of the knee were up to five kilograms (kg) heavier than their co-twin without the disease, supporting more of an influence of weight than genetics (Cicuttini et al. 1996). Thus, while there is likely a component of genetic contribution to the development of knee OA, much remains to be investigated prior to clinical application.

8.2.1.2 Gender Differences

> There do seem to be clear gender differences between the burden of knee OA in men and women.

The Framingham study found that there was a slightly greater preponderance of radiographic knee OA in women (34%) than men (31%) (Felson et al. 1987). Additionally, in this study, the presence of symptomatic knee OA was greater in women than men (11.4% vs. 6.8%). There also appear to be differences in presentation between genders. Women demonstrate lower preoperative functional scores before undergoing TKA compared to men (O'Connor 1846), including reduced quadriceps strength, 6-min walk test, and stair-climbing times (Petterson et al. 2007). Additionally, women have lower preoperative Western Ontario and McMaster Universities Arthritis Index (WOMAC) scores (Lingard et al. 2004; MacDonald et al. 2008).

Gender differences among knee OA have lead many researchers to investigate the role of sex hormones in OA development. Menarche at younger age (Leung et al. 2019) and childbirth (Leung et al. 2019; Wise et al. 2013) have been associated with increased knee OA. In fact, in the Million Women study, each additional birth was associated with an 8% increase in relative risk of knee replacement (Liu et al. 2009). Interestingly, age at menopause does not appear to alter the risk of knee replacement (Hussain et al. 2018; Liu et al. 2009), suggesting a temporal effect of estrogen exposure at a younger age on the risk of OA development in women. If this is true, then one may expect exogenous sex hormone supplementation to also influence knee OA. While estrogen-containing oral contraceptives (OCPs) have been reported to reduce the risk of ACL injuries (Herzberg et al. 2017), studies accessing OCP use and risk of TKA compared to nonusers have demonstrated conflicting results (Hussain et al. 2018; Leung et al. 2019; Liu et al. 2009). Similarly conflicting findings have been reported with hormone replacement therapy (HRT) for postmenopausal women. In the Million Women study, patients treated with HRT had significantly increased incidence of knee replacement (Liu et al. 2009), but other studies have reported a reduced risk of OA at the knee after HRT treatment (Spector et al. 1997). Therefore, the currently available evidence does not support a role for HRT in the primary prevention of OA.

In the male population, there is a paucity of evidence on testosterone levels and the development of OA. Testosterone levels have been associated with other known OA risk factors including muscle weakness and BMI, and testosterone levels are known to decrease with age (Harman et al. 2001), but at present the role of testosterone in the etiology of OA warrants further investigation prior to clinical application.

8.2.1.3 Malalignment

Lower extremity malalignment has demonstrated a significant influence on the development of knee OA. In fact, patient self-reported varus or valgus knee malalignment during young adulthood was associated with subsequent development of knee OA later in life (McWilliams et al. 2010). The Multicenter Osteoarthritis Study (Sharma et al. 2010) reported an odds ratio of 3.59 for the development of medial knee OA in patients with varus alignment and an odds ratio of 4.85 for lateral OA in patients with valgus alignment. Subsequent studies have reaffirmed the potent influence of malalignment, with particular risk of varus alignment on the development of medial knee OA (Felson et al. 2005).

8.2.1.4 Obesity

> Obesity is one of the most influential risk factors for the development of knee OA.

The World Health Organization (WHO) defines obesity as a body mass index (BMI) > 30 kg/m^2 (James et al. 2001) (Table 8.1). In the WHO definition, obesity is further stratified into classes 1–3, or sometimes referred to as "moderate," "severe," or "very severe." More commonly, authors have used "obesity" to describe patients with a BMI 30–39.9, "morbid obesity" for patients with BMI 40–49.9, and a new term of "super obesity" for patients with BMI greater than 50 (Sturm 2003) (Table 8.2). For the purposes of this chapter, we will utilize these latter terms to provide consistency with the cited studies.

Among US adults in 2014, 35% of men and 40% of women were obese (Flegal et al. 2016), and predictions estimate will be 65 million more obese adults in the United States by 2030 (Wang et al. 2011). A 2010 report estimated the total annual cost of obesity to the US economy exceeded $215 billion, and that this was probably twice the cost spent on adults of healthy weight (Hammond and Levine 2010). In fact, care for obese patients may account for as much as 21% of all US medical costs (Cawley and Meyerhoefer 2012).

Table 8.1 World Health Organization's classification of obesity (James et al. 2001)

Classification	BMI (kg/m^2)
Underweight	<18.5
Normal range	18.5–24.9
Overweight	≥25
Obese class 1	30–34.9
Obese class 2	35–39.9
Obese class 3	≥40

Table 8.2 Descriptive classification of obesity (Sturm 2003)

Description	BMI (kg/m^2)
Obesity	30–39.9
Morbid obesity	40–49.9
Super obesity	≥50

The risk of knee OA in the obese population has been repeatedly demonstrated (Grotle et al. 2008; Mork et al. 2012; Sturmer et al. 2000). This risk is increased by 3.87 in obese women and 4.78 in obese men (Anderson and Felson 1988). Furthermore, increasing levels of obesity appear to confer additional risks. Patients with a BMI ≥ 35 kg/m^2 required arthroplasty 7 years earlier compared to patients with BMI ≤ 25 mg/kg^2 (Gandhi et al. 2010).

The pathogenesis of OA in the obese patient is multifactorial. Mechanically, two to five times body weight is transmitted across the knee joint during daily activities (Maquet and Pelzer 1977). Reactive forces across the patellofemoral joint are four times the body weight when ascending or descending stairs, and eight times when squatting (Reilly and Martens 1972). Thus these forces are compounded in the obese patient and can precipitate early cartilage wear and the development of knee OA. On a molecular level, adipose tissue may produce abnormal levels of certain hormones and growth factors which can affect cartilage and the underlying bone, possibly leading to degeneration. Adipose tissue releases adipokine, a protein that has been implicated in cartilage inflammation and degradation (Pottie et al. 2006). Furthermore, modest associations between elevated levels of insulin-like growth factor-1 (IGF-1) in the knee have been observed in patients with knee OA (Lloyd et al. 1996), although other studies have not supported this association (Denko et al. 1990). A multitude of additional proinflammatory cytokines is the subject of intense investigation (Courties et al. 2019). While a full discussion is beyond the scope of this chapter, this research is invaluable in elucidating the molecular pathophysiology of adiposity and its influence on OA development.

If obesity is correlated with an increased risk of knee OA, then it follows that weight loss should decrease OA risk, or at the very least symptoms of OA. Indeed, the Framingham study reported that reduction in 2 or more BMI units significantly decreased the odds of developing OA (Felson et al. 1992). Messier conducted a prospective, randomized trial, concluding that modest dietary weight loss in combination with moderate exercise leads to significant improvement in self-reported measures of knee pain, function, and mobility (Messier et al. 2004). In this study, a 5% weight loss over an 18-month period resulted in an 18% improvement in function, and when diet was combined with exercise, this functional improvement increased to 24%. There was no difference in radiographic joint space as a product of weight loss, however. Surgically assisted weight loss offers promising results for the obese suffering from knee pain. In a prospective trial of vertical-banded gastroplasty, 1 year postoperatively patients lost on average 97 pounds, and 87% reported complete relief of pain in one or more joints (McGoey et al. 1990). Specifically regarding the knee, in this study, 57% of patients reported pain prior to gastroplasty, which decreased to 14% at 1-year follow-up. Interestingly, the authors found no difference in patients who lost a moderate amount (< 60 pounds) of weight compared to those who lost a greater amount (>99 pounds), suggesting a possible threshold effect on weight loss. A second bariatric surgery report found that in patients who self-reported knee pain but did not have a formal diagnosis of OA, weight loss was associated with a rapid and dependable means of reversing the early radiologic changes associated with OA (Abu-Abeid et al. 2005).

8.2.2 Lifestyle Factors

8.2.2.1 Nutrition and Dietary Patterns

> Nutritional supplementation among patients suffering from musculoskeletal conditions is common, yet its efficacy is debatable.

One study reported that nearly 18% of patients used some form of dietary supplements (Ficke et al. 2018). Natural vitamin supplementation has been extensively studied, but has not shown promising results. General supplementation with Vitamin D demonstrates conflicting evidence. Felson and colleagues found that Vitamin D status was unrelated to risk of joint space or cartilage loss in knee OA (Felson et al. 2007a), while McAlindon demonstrated that low intake and low serum levels of Vitamin D each appear to be associated with increased risk for progression of knee OA (McAlindon et al. 1996). The same study found relatively poor evidence that Vitamin C may reduce the risk of cartilage loss and disease progression, but had no effect on incident OA. Vitamin K deficiency has been associated with an increased risk of developing radiographic knee OA (Misra et al. 2013) and other authors have suggested some association between lack of Vitamin K-dependent proteins and progression of knee OA (Shea et al. 2015). Unfortunately, while multiple replacement trials have been conducted, no trial has demonstrated significant beneficial evidence in those with established knee OA. Specifically, trials examining replacement of Vitamin A (Canter et al. 2007), Vitamin C (Canter et al. 2007), Vitamin D (Diao et al. 2017), Vitamin E (Wluka et al. 2002), and selenium (Canter et al. 2007), all reported disappointing results. Therefore, the current available evidence does not support making specific recommendations regarding dietary supplementation to prevent or treat established knee OA. Turmeric is a top-selling herbal supplement (Ficke et al. 2018), the principal component of which is curcumin (*Curcuma longa*). Turmeric has historically been used to treat inflammation through a proposed mechanism of limiting pro-inflammatory enzymes in the cyclooxygenase and lipoxygenase families and inflammatory transcription factor nuclear factor kappa beta (Aggarwal and Sung 2009; Jurenka 2009). A prospective trial of turmeric administration in knee OA patients demonstrated decreased biochemical markers of inflammation as well as improvement in patient-reported joint function, supporting its role as an effective herbal anti-inflammatory (Belcaro et al. 2010).

There is limited, poor-quality evidence that any specific diet influences the rate of knee OA. Animal studies have shown that olive oil may lower articular cartilage degradation (Musumeci et al. 2013). A follow-up study suggested that patients who follow a Mediterranean diet, of which olive oil is often a principle component, is associated with lower prevalence of knee OA (Veronese et al. 2017). High intakes of total fat and saturated fatty acids have been correlated with increased structural knee OA progression, while monounsaturated and polyunsaturated fatty acids have been suggested to reduce progression (Lu et al. 2017). At present, however, specific influences of dietary patterns are of very poor and limited evidence.

8.2.2.2 Smoking and Alcohol

Smoking appears to be associated with a reduction in the risk of developing knee OA, though these findings must be interpreted with some caution. A meta-analysis reported the relative risk of developing knee OA for smokers was 0.80, with a more marked effect in men than women (Kong et al. 2017). Hui and colleagues similarly reported that smokers had a lower odds of developing OA at any joint, and suggested one potential mechanism could be that smokers tended to have a lower BMI than nonsmokers (Hui et al. 2011). Leung similarly demonstrated a strong dose-dependent association between increased duration and dosage of smoking with a decreasing risk of total knee arthroplasty (Leung et al. 2014). The authors suggested that nicotine promotes proliferation and collagen synthesis in chondrocytes. However, these results should be interpreted with extreme caution, as the primary outcome measure was patient selection for total knee replacement, which may have been biased if surgeons did not want to operate on smokers due to fear of pulmonary complications or wound healing problems.

Limited evidence exists on the effects of alcohol and knee OA. One study reported that beer consumption appears to increase the risk of developing hip and knee OA, but wine consumption was associated with a reduced risk (Muthuri et al. 2015).

8.2.2.3 Exercise and Muscle Strength

Exercise and its influence on the risk of knee OA is a complicated issue. Anecdotally, many patients and physicians surmise that long-term, high-impact exercise may risk the development of OA. While this may seem plausible, the evidence for this is not wholly convincing. In fact, multiple studies of both the general population as well as recreational runners found no increased risk of knee OA in those who reported undertaking regular, "moderate" physical activity (Felson et al. 2007b; Hannan et al. 1993; Lane et al. 1993; McAlindon et al. 1999; Panush et al. 1995). However, other more intense activities, particularly those that involve deep knee flexion, have shown significant associations with knee OA. In the Framingham study, self-reported "heavy" physical activity with a threshold of greater than 4 h per day had increased odds of knee OA (McAlindon et al. 1999). A second study identified patients who engaged in cycling and prolonged squatting as higher risk for knee OA (Dahaghin et al. 2009).

> Thus, historical assumptions of activity level on knee OA may not be accurate, and warrant further investigation to determine objective threshold measurements by which practitioners can guide patients.

Muscle strength also appears to play a role in the progression of knee OA. Patients with symptomatic knee OA have demonstrated reduced muscle strength, particularly of the quadriceps (Leyland et al. 2012; Murphy et al. 2008). Historically, this has been thought to be secondary to osteoarthritis-related joint symptoms, resulting in reduced activity levels and consequent muscle atrophy. However, more recent studies suggest that muscle weakness predates the onset of knee OA (Oiestad et al. 2010; Segal et al. 2010; Slemenda et al. 1998). Specifically, weakness of the knee extensor mechanism was shown to significantly increase the odds of developing symptomatic OA (Oiestad et al. 2015).

> Therefore, muscle weakness may represent an important modifiable risk factor to help slow the progression of knee OA.

A systematic review of the literature provided an international consensus statement on daily activities and structured exercise related to knee OA (Vignon et al. 2006) (Table 8.3). The authors concluded that activities of daily living (ADL) were a risk factor for knee OA, and that risk increases with intensity and duration of these activities. However, the strength of the supporting data was graded as moderate, and no threshold activity level was able to be defined, limiting clinical utility in patient education.

Table 8.3 International consensus on activity level in knee osteoarthritis patients (Vignon et al. 2006)

Parameter (Level of evidence)	Consensus statement	Recommendation
ADL (Moderate)	ADL is a risk factor for knee OA, which increases with intensity and duration, but no threshold could be defined	Healthy subjects can pursue a high level of physical activity, providing the activity is not painful and does not predispose to trauma
Structured exercise (High)	Strengthening exercises have a favorable effect on pain and function in the sedentary knee OA patient, but it was not possible to identify a specific exercise modality that produces superior results on pain and function	Structured exercises are recommended for the sedentary patient with knee OA
Sport and recreational activities (High)	Sport is a risk factor for knee OA, and this risk correlates with intensity and duration of level of exposure. However, risk of OA associated with sport was lesser than that associated with trauma or obesity	OA patients can continue to engage regularly in recreational sports as long as the activity does not cause pain

ADL activities of daily living, *OA* osteoarthritis

8.2.2.4 Occupation

> Occupation also appears to have a significant effect on the risk of knee OA.

Kwon and colleagues examined men over the age of 50 stratified by occupation type (Kwon et al. 2019). They classified occupations as follows:

- White collar (WC) including managers, professionals, and office workers
- Pink collar (PC) including service and salespersons
- Blue collar (BC) including technicians and device/machine operators
- Agribusiness and low-level (AL) including skilled workers in agriculture and fishery and low-level laborers

8

They observed that the risk for knee OA was highest in AL and BC workers compared to WC. The risk for severe radiographic knee OA was highest in AL followed by BC occupations. WC occupations appeared to be least affected by knee OA and chronic knee pain. These conclusions support that knee OA risk was correlated with the degree of physical labor associated with an occupation. Another occupational study found that jobs requiring repetitive kneeling and squatting, including mining and carpentry, were at increased odds of knee OA (Maetzel et al. 1997). Professional athletes have also been shown to have increased risk of developing knee OA, particularly soccer players and weight lifters (Kujala et al. 1995). However, there may be confounding factors as soccer players may be more prone to knee injuries which could predispose them to post-traumatic arthritis, and weight lifters may be more prone to knee OA secondary to a higher BMI that may be more common in this population.

Additionally, in Vignon and colleagues' systematic international review of activity level in knee OA patients, the authors also concluded that there was a relationship between occupational activity (Vignon et al. 2006). This study found that physically demanding work was associated with knee OA with a high level of evidence. However, the authors were not clearly able to characterize the biomechanical stresses leading to OA, which limits the generalizability of the findings to specific work-related activities. Rather, they simply concluded that work-related activities that produce or maintain pain should be avoided.

8.3 Patient Risk Factors for Adverse Outcome Following Cemented TKA

> Cemented TKA is a successful operation to treat end-stage arthritis of the knee, with reported survivorship of 82% at 25 years across a range of prosthetic designs (Evans et al. 2019).

In a landmark study of outcomes following TKA, Sharkey and colleagues identify the predominant etiologies of failure for modern TKA prostheses at 10-year follow-up (Sharkey et al. 2014).

> In the first 2 years, infection was the most common reason for early revision.

Beyond 2 years, aseptic, or noninfectious, loosening was the predominant mode of failure, accounting for 39.9% of revisions. Additional etiologies for late failure included infection (27.4%), periprosthetic fracture (4.7%), and arthrofibrosis (4.5%). Similar results have also been reported by other authors (Schroer et al. 2013). While infection is undoubtedly an important etiology of TKA failure, it is beyond the scope of this chapter and is covered elsewhere in the text. In this section, we will focus on specific variables which are thought to contribute to aseptic failure of cemented TKA prostheses, and conclude with a brief discussion on factors that may contribute to functional outcomes and patient satisfaction.

8.3.1 Aseptic Loosening

Aseptic loosening is thought to be due to the development of excess wear particles that induce a proinflammatory state, which in turn leads to osteoclast differentiation and macrophage production, ultimately leading to local osteolysis and consequent loosening of the prosthesis (Jiang et al. 2013). Aseptic loosening is an end result, and its etiology can and often may be multifactorial. Causes may include preoperative factors such as obesity, intraoperative malalignment, or postoperative activity level.

8.3.1.1 Obesity

The contribution of obesity to aseptic loosening has been extensively studied, with conflicting results. Multiple studies have supported a positive association between obesity and aseptic loosening (Foran et al. 2004a; Ritter et al. 2011; Schiffner et al. 2019). Several other studies, meanwhile, have refuted these findings (Chaudhry et al. 2019; Si et al. 2015).

> Part of this discrepancy may be due to the fact that loosening is likely multifactorial, and is at least partially influenced by surgeon technique when cementing the prosthesis.

This intuitively may be more difficult in the obese patient for whom exposure may be more challenging, yet this confounding variable may be difficult to objectively measure even in well-designed studies. Similarly, while aseptic loosening has been shown to be the predominant reason for revision at 10 years (Sharkey et al. 2014), other studies with shorter follow-up may not adequately capture this mode of failure. Some authors advocate for prophylactic tibial stem extension when performing cemented TKA in the obese population to help mitigate the risk of aseptic loosening, but this has not been shown to significantly affect early failures at an average of nearly 3-year follow-up (Steere et al. 2018).

We have previously discussed the role of weight loss in reducing the incidence and symptoms associated with knee OA, and is worth discussing the role of weight loss before and after total joint arthroplasty. Many obese patients cite their knee pain as a barrier to exercise and the consequent barrier to weight loss, which presents a challenge for the surgeon. It is a commonly held belief among the medical community that patients will lose weight after undergoing knee arthroplasty, but a meta-analysis reporting 1-year follow-up presented strong evidence that this does not in fact occur within this time period (Inacio et al. 2013). Furthermore, one study demonstrated that at 12-month follow-up, while 12.5% of obese patients had achieved a clinically significant weight loss of 5% after arthroplasty, 21% had actually gained weight. However, a longer term study looking beyond 2-year follow-up did support a statistically significant decrease in weight after TKA, suggesting that TKA may facilitate weight loss, but that these effects may not be appreciable until outside of the follow-up period utilized in prior studies (Duchman et al. 2014).

Additionally, many surgeons refer obese patients for bariatric surgery prior to elective total joint arthroplasty. Springer reported on the fate of these patients, noting that only 23% of referred patients actually attended their bariatric appointment and only 7% underwent bariatric surgery prior to arthroplasty. The authors of this study make an interesting point that some surgeons argue that obese patients cannot lose weight due to their musculoskeletal limitations and, therefore, we should operate on them regardless of BMI. However, the authors state that we would not consent to operate in other forms of uncontrolled disease, such as diabetes or open wounds, and that one might consider a similar stance for obesity. Parvizi et al. reported on the outcomes of patients who underwent bariatric surgery prior to TKA (Parvizi et al. 2000). The mean reduction in BMI was from 49 to 29, and mean time from bariatric surgery to joint replacement was 23 months. In this study, Knee Society scores (KSS) improved significantly postoperatively and no patient required revision at mean follow-up of 3.7 years.

> The authors conclude that morbidly obese patients with severe osteoarthritis who are deemed unsuitable for joint replacement because of weight should be considered for bariatric surgery.

8.3.1.2 Malalignment

Malalignment after TKA has been shown to be a significant reason for revision surgery (Evans et al. 2019). Severe malalignment may predispose to early failure due to abnormal joint biomechanics, while less pronounced malalignment could predispose to implant loosening secondary to abnormal joint forces across the implant–cement or cement–bone interfaces. Preoperative alignment is predictive of postoperative failure, with increased risk associated with greater than 8° of varus or greater than 11° of valgus (Ritter et al. 2013). In patients undergoing TKA with traditional instrumentation, preoperative limb alignment and BMI were significant predictive factors in postoperative limb alignment (Estes et al. 2013). Obesity has been shown in several studies to be a risk factor for postoperative malalignment, including risk in technical errors of component malpositioning (Gaillard et al. 2017; Jarvenpaa et al. 2010), and a higher risk for varus limb malalignment with increased BMI (Gaillard et al. 2017). One study has refuted these findings, showing no difference in malalignment after TKA (Ojard et al. 2018). A study of computer navigation in TKA showed no differences in postoperative limb alignment in the obese compared to non-obese, suggesting a potential benefit of computer navigation to help mitigate the reported risks of malalignment in this population (Shetty et al. 2014).

8.3.1.3 Activity Level

As activity level has historically and perhaps erroneously been associated with increased knee osteoarthritis, similarly we have assumed that increased activity would lead to earlier failure of cemented TKA. In a meta-analysis of aseptic loosening after total hip arthroplasty (THA) and TKA, Chierian and colleagues found that high activity levels were a risk factor for loosening in THA, but this was not replicated in TKA (Cherian et al. 2015). In fact, using the University of California, Los Angeles Activity Scale, Crawford et al. reported that after controlling for confounding variables, highly active patients actually demonstrated increased survivorship at 5-year minimum follow-up compared with lower activity patients (Crawford et al. 2020). While these findings attempt to refute historical dogma, further study is warranted to ascertain if these trends persist with longer follow-up.

8.3.2 Function and Patient Satisfaction

8.3.2.1 Functional Outcomes

While patient functional outcomes are not an objective etiology of TKA failure and may not constitute an isolated reason for revision surgery, these parameters remain crucial in evaluating outcomes of TKA.

> Function after TKA may be influenced by a variety of preoperative and postoperative factors.

Gender studies have demonstrated that women have consistently lower preoperative functional scores at the time of TKA than men, including reduced quadriceps strength, 6-min walk test, stair-climbing times, and preoperative WOMAC scores (Lingard et al. 2004; MacDonald et al. 2008; O'Connor 1846; Petterson et al. 2007). Women also report worse pain than men both before and after arthroplasty (Lingard et al. 2004; MacDonald et al. 2008; Ritter et al. 2008) and do not appear to reach the same final functional levels as men (Dalury et al. 2009; MacDonald et al. 2008; Ritter et al. 2008).

8

Similar to other obesity-related factors and outcomes, the functional outcomes of TKA in the obese population have yielded conflicting results. Boyce et al. reported that among morbidly obese patients, the Knee Society Objective score (KSOS) and Knee Society Functional score (KSFS) were poorer in morbidly obese patients both preoperatively and postoperatively (Boyce et al. 2019). However, the mean improvement in KSOS in this study was the same for obese compared to non-obese patients. Obese patients have also been shown to have lower WOMAC scores, Short Form-36 (SF-36), and Hospital for Special Surgery (HSS) questionnaires (Smith et al. 1992; Stickles et al. 2001). Knee Society scores (KSS) have perhaps been the most widely used outcome metric, but demonstrate substantially conflicting results. Foran and colleagues showed that only 80% of obese patients achieved a KSS greater than 80 points postoperatively compared to 99% of non-obese patients at 80-month follow-up (Foran et al. 2004a). These findings have been replicated in multiple other studies (Collins et al. 2012; Foran et al. 2004a, b; Griffin et al. 1998; Jarvenpaa et al. 2012). However, a nearly equal number of studies have reported no significant differences in scores between obese and non-obese patients (Amin et al. 2006; Benjamin et al. 2001; Bin Abd Razak et al. 2013; Deshmukh et al. 2002; Dewan et al. 2009; Hamoui et al. 2006; Issa et al. 2013), making it impossible to draw definitive conclusions.

8.3.2.2 Patient Satisfaction

> Patient dissatisfaction following TKA has been reported as high as 20% in some studies (Husain and Lee 2015) and has remained relatively stable over the past several decades despite multiple changes in implant design, surgical technique, and perioperative pain protocols.

Outcomes have been shown to be influenced by medical comorbidities, mental health status, socioeconomic status, and ethnicity (Husain and Lee 2015). Regarding socioeconomic status, patients earning annual income less than $25,000 were less likely to be satisfied with TKA outcomes and more likely to have functional limitations after TKA than patients of higher income (Barrack et al. 2014). While we have previously discussed the increased risk of radiographic and symptomatic knee OA in women, it does not appear that there are significant gender differences in patient satisfaction following TKA in women compared to men (O'Connor 1846). Perhaps most interestingly, while obese patients have been shown numerous times to be at risk for a multitude of complications, poorer functional outcomes, and the need for revision surgery following TKA, multiple studies have demonstrated comparable satisfaction scores between the obese and non-obese (Deshmukh et al. 2002; Ersozlu et al. 2008; Yeung et al. 2011).

- **Conclusion**

Knee OA is an extremely common condition affecting millions of individuals annually. However, as this chapter exemplifies, there are a myriad of patient and lifestyle factors that can influence the development of OA. While some factors, notably obesity, may play a more prominent role than others, the true pathogenesis in the individual patient is likely multifactorial and at present time incompletely understood. Similarly, TKA is a very successful operation to treat end-stage OA, yet the longevity of the implant, functional outcome, and satisfaction may all be influenced by a multitude of patient factors. It is our hope that this brief overview of many of these confounding variables provides a resource for the practitioner to counsel patients and, where gaps exist in our current fund of knowledge, a challenge for future research endeavors.

Take-Home Messages

- Women appear to be more susceptible and more adversely affected by knee OA than men, possibly due to hormonal exposure. The therapeutic implications for hormonal treatment, however, remain unclear.
- Obesity is a clear risk factor for knee OA, and obese patients are at risk for multiple perioperative complications, aseptic loosening, and poorer postoperative functional outcomes. Bariatric surgery offers promising results for the obese patient suffering from symptomatic knee OA.
- There is limited, poor-quality evidence on diet and nutritional supplementation in preventing or treating knee OA.
- Exercise and sport participation have demonstrated conflicting results in their influence on the development of knee OA. The greatest risk appears to be associated with activities that induce repetitive microtrauma to the joint.
- Occupation appears to be associated with knee OA, with more labor-intense occupations at greater risk.
- Activity level following TKA has not been clearly shown to be a risk factor for aseptic loosening.
- Satisfaction rates following TKA appear to be associated with socioeconomic status, but these have not demonstrated clear correlations with other risk factors. Specifically, despite higher risk and lower functional scores preoperatively, neither gender nor obesity has clearly demonstrated poorer satisfaction postoperatively.
- Cemented TKA is a successful operation to treat end-stage arthritis of the knee. In the first 2 years, infection was the most common reason for early revision.

References

Abu-Abeid S, Wishnitzer N, Szold A, Liebergall M, Manor O (2005) The influence of surgically-induced weight loss on the knee joint. Obes Surg 15(10):1437

Aggarwal BB, Sung B (2009) Pharmacological basis for the role of curcumin in chronic diseases: an age-old spice with modern targets. Trends Pharmacol Sci 30(2):85

Amin AK, Patton JT, Cook RE, Brenkel IJ (2006) Does obesity influence the clinical outcome at five years following total knee replacement for osteoarthritis? J Bone Joint Surg 88(3):335

Anderson JJ, Felson DT (1988) Factors associated with osteoarthritis of the knee in the first national Health and Nutrition Examination Survey (HANES I). Evidence for an association with overweight, race, and physical demands of work. Am J Epidemiol 128(1):179

Barrack RL, Ruh EL, Chen J, Lombardi AV Jr, Berend KR, Parvizi J, Della Valle CJ, Hamilton WG, Nunley RM (2014) Impact of socioeconomic factors on outcome of total knee arthroplasty. Clin Orthop Relat Res 472(1):86

Belcaro G, Cesarone MR, Dugall M, Pellegrini L, Ledda A, Grossi MG, Togni S, Appendino G (2010) Efficacy and safety of Meriva(R), a curcumin-phosphatidylcholine complex, during extended administration in osteoarthritis patients. Altern Med Rev 15(4):337

Benjamin J, Tucker T, Ballesteros P (2001) Is obesity a contraindication to bilateral total knee arthroplasties under one anesthetic? Clin Orthop Relat Res (392):190

Bin Abd Razak HR, Chong HC, Tan AH (2013) Obesity does not imply poor outcomes in Asians after total knee arthroplasty. Clin Orthop Relat Res 471(6):1957

Boyce L, Prasad A, Barrett M, Dawson-Bowling S, Millington S, Hanna SA, Achan P (2019) The outcomes of total knee arthroplasty in morbidly obese patients: a systematic review of the literature. Arch Orthop Trauma Surg 139(4):553

Canter PH, Wider B, Ernst E (2007) The antioxidant vitamins A, C, E and selenium in the treatment of arthritis: a systematic review of randomized clinical trials. Rheumatology (Oxford) 46(8):1223

Cawley J, Meyerhoefer C (2012) The medical care costs of obesity: an instrumental variables approach. J Health Econ 31(1):219

Chaudhry H, Ponnusamy K, Somerville L, McCalden RW, Marsh J, Vasarhelyi EM (2019) Revision rates and functional outcomes among severely, morbidly, and super-obese patients following primary total knee arthroplasty: a systematic review and meta-analysis. JBJS Rev 7(7):e9

Cherian JJ, Jauregui JJ, Banerjee S, Pierce T, Mont MA (2015) What host factors affect aseptic loosening after THA and TKA? Clin Orthop Relat Res 473(8):2700

Cicuttini FM, Baker JR, Spector TD (1996) The association of obesity with osteoarthritis of the hand and knee in women: a twin study. J Rheumatol 23(7):1221

Collins RA, Walmsley PJ, Amin AK, Brenkel IJ, Clayton RA (2012) Does obesity influence clinical outcome at nine years following total knee replacement? J Bone Joint Surg 94(10):1351

Courties A, Berenbaum F, Sellam J (2019) The phenotypic approach to osteoarthritis: a look at metabolic syndrome-associated osteoarthritis. Joint Bone Spine 86(6):725

Crawford DA, Adams JB, Hobbs GR, Berend KR, Lombardi AV Jr (2020) Higher activity level following total knee arthroplasty is not deleterious to mid-term implant survivorship. J Arthroplast 35(1):116

Dahaghin S, Tehrani-Banihashemi SA, Faezi ST, Jamshidi AR, Davatchi F (2009) Squatting, sitting on the floor, or cycling: are life-long daily activities risk factors for clinical knee osteoarthritis? Stage III results of a community-based study. Arthritis Rheum 61(10):1337

Dalury DF, Mason JB, Murphy JA, Adams MJ (2009) Analysis of the outcome in male and female patients using a unisex total knee replacement system. J Bone Joint Surg 91(3):357

Denko CW, Boja B, Moskowitz RW (1990) Growth promoting peptides in osteoarthritis: insulin, insulin-like growth factor-1, growth hormone. J Rheumatol 17(9):1217

Deshmukh RG, Hayes JH, Pinder IM (2002) Does body weight influence outcome after total knee arthroplasty? A 1-year analysis. J Arthroplast 17(3):315

Dewan A, Bertolusso R, Karastinos A, Conditt M, Noble PC, Parsley BS (2009) Implant durability and knee function after total knee arthroplasty in the morbidly obese patient. J Arthroplast 24(6 Suppl):89

Diao N, Yang B, Yu F (2017) Effect of vitamin D supplementation on knee osteoarthritis: a systematic review and meta-analysis of randomized clinical trials. Clin Biochem 50(18):1312

Duchman KR, Gao Y, Phisitkul P (2014) Effects of total knee and hip arthroplasty on body weight. Orthopedics 37(3):e278
Ersozlu S, Akkaya T, Ozgur AF, Sahin O, Senturk I, Tandogan R (2008) Bilateral staged total knee arthroplasty in obese patients. Arch Orthop Trauma Surg 128(2):143
Estes CS, Schmidt KJ, McLemore R, Spangehl MJ, Clarke HD (2013) Effect of body mass index on limb alignment after total knee arthroplasty. J Arthroplast 28(8 Suppl):101
Evans JT, Walker RW, Evans JP, Blom AW, Sayers A, Whitehouse MR (2019) How long does a knee replacement last? A systematic review and meta-analysis of case series and national registry reports with more than 15 years of follow-up. Lancet 393(10172):655
Felson DT, Naimark A, Anderson J, Kazis L, Castelli W, Meenan RF (1987) The prevalence of knee osteoarthritis in the elderly. The Framingham Osteoarthritis Study. Arthritis Rheum 30(8):914
Felson DT, Zhang Y, Anthony JM, Naimark A, Anderson JJ (1992) Weight loss reduces the risk for symptomatic knee osteoarthritis in women. The Framingham Study. Ann Intern Med 116(7):535
Felson DT, Gale DR, Elon Gale M, Niu J, Hunter DJ, Goggins J, Lavalley MP (2005) Osteophytes and progression of knee osteoarthritis. Rheumatology (Oxford) 44(1):100
Felson DT, Niu J, Clancy M, Aliabadi P, Sack B, Guermazi A, Hunter DJ, Amin S, Rogers G, Booth SL (2007a) Low levels of vitamin D and worsening of knee osteoarthritis: results of two longitudinal studies. Arthritis Rheum 56(1):129
Felson DT, Niu J, Clancy M, Sack B, Aliabadi P, Zhang Y (2007b) Effect of recreational physical activities on the development of knee osteoarthritis in older adults of different weights: the Framingham Study. Arthritis Rheum 57(1):6
Ficke JR, Moroski NM, Ross SD, Gupta R (2018) Integrative medicine as an adjunct to orthopaedic surgery. J Am Acad Orthop Surg 26(2):58
Flegal KM, Kruszon-Moran D, Carroll MD, Fryar CD, Ogden CL (2016) Trends in obesity among adults in the United States, 2005 to 2014. JAMA 315(21):2284
Foran JR, Mont MA, Etienne G, Jones LC, Hungerford DS (2004a) The outcome of total knee arthroplasty in obese patients. J Bone Joint Surg Am 86(8):1609
Foran JR, Mont MA, Rajadhyaksha AD, Jones LC, Etienne G, Hungerford DS (2004b) Total knee arthroplasty in obese patients: a comparison with a matched control group. J Arthroplast 19(7):817
Gaillard R, Cerciello S, Lustig S, Servien E, Neyret P (2017) Risk factors for tibial implant malpositioning in total knee arthrosplasty-consecutive series of one thousand, four hundred and seventeen cases. Int Orthop 41(4):749
Gandhi R, Wasserstein D, Razak F, Davey JR, Mahomed NN (2010) BMI independently predicts younger age at hip and knee replacement. Obesity 18(12):2362
Gonzalez A, Valdes AM (2018) Big data boost for osteoarthritis genetics. Nat Rev Rheumatol 14(7):387
Griffin FM, Scuderi GR, Insall JN, Colizza W (1998) Total knee arthroplasty in patients who were obese with 10 years followup. Clin Orthop Relat Res (356):28
Grotle M, Hagen KB, Natvig B, Dahl FA, Kvien TK (2008) Obesity and osteoarthritis in knee, hip and/or hand: an epidemiological study in the general population with 10 years follow-up. BMC Musculoskelet Disord 9:132
Hammond RA, Levine R (2010) The economic impact of obesity in the United States. Diabetes Metab Syndr Obes 3:285
Hamoui N, Kantor S, Vince K, Crookes PF (2006) Long-term outcome of total knee replacement: does obesity matter? Obes Surg 16(1):35
Hannan MT, Felson DT, Anderson JJ, Naimark A (1993) Habitual physical activity is not associated with knee osteoarthritis: the Framingham Study. J Rheumatol 20(4):704
Harman SM, Metter EJ, Tobin JD, Pearson J, Blackman MR (2001) Longitudinal effects of aging on serum total and free testosterone levels in healthy men. Baltimore Longitudinal Study of Aging. J Clin Endocrinol Metab 86(2):724
Herzberg SD, Motu'apuaka ML, Lambert W, Fu R, Brady J, Guise JM (2017) The effect of menstrual cycle and contraceptives on ACL injuries and laxity: a systematic review and meta-analysis. Orthop J Sports Med 5(7). https://doi.org/10.1177/2325967117718781
Hiligsmann M, Cooper C, Arden N, Boers M, Branco JC, Luisa Brandi M, Bruyere O, Guillemin F, Hochberg MC, Hunter DJ, Kanis JA, Kvien TK, Laslop A, Pelletier JP, Pinto D, Reiter-Niesert S, Rizzoli R, Rovati LC, Severens JL, Silverman S, Tsouderos Y, Tugwell P, Reginster JY (2013) Health economics in the field of osteoarthritis: an expert's consensus paper from the European Society for Clinical and Economic Aspects of Osteoporosis and Osteoarthritis (ESCEO). Semin Arthritis Rheum 43(3):303
Hui M, Doherty M, Zhang W (2011) Does smoking protect against osteoarthritis? Meta-analysis of observational studies. Ann Rheum Dis 70(7):1231
Husain A, Lee GC (2015) Establishing realistic patient expectations following total knee arthroplasty. J Am Acad Orthop Surg 23(12):707
Hussain SM, Wang Y, Giles GG, Graves S, Wluka AE, Cicuttini FM (2018) Female reproductive and hormonal factors and incidence of primary total knee arthroplasty due to osteoarthritis. Arthritis Rheumatol 70(7):1022
Inacio MC, Kritz-Silverstein D, Paxton EW, Fithian DC (2013) Do patients lose weight after joint arthroplasty surgery? A systematic review. Clin Orthop Relat Res 471(1):291
Issa K, Pivec R, Kapadia BH, Shah T, Harwin SF, Delanois RE, Mont MA (2013) Does obesity affect the outcomes of primary total knee arthroplasty? J Knee Surg 26(2):89
James PT, Leach R, Kalamara E, Shayeghi M (2001) The worldwide obesity epidemic. Obes Res 9(Suppl 4):228s
Jarvenpaa J, Kettunen J, Kroger H, Miettinen H (2010) Obesity may impair the early outcome of total knee arthroplasty. Scand J Surg 99(1):45
Jarvenpaa J, Kettunen J, Soininvaara T, Miettinen H, Kroger H (2012) Obesity has a negative impact on clinical outcome after total knee arthroplasty. Scand J Surg 101(3):198
Jiang Y, Jia T, Wooley PH, Yang SY (2013) Current research in the pathogenesis of aseptic implant loosening associated with particulate wear debris. Acta Orthop Belg 79(1):1
Jurenka JS (2009) Anti-inflammatory properties of curcumin, a major constituent of Curcuma longa: a review of preclinical and clinical research. Altern Med Rev 14(2):141
Kerkhof HJ, Lories RJ, Meulenbelt I, Jonsdottir I, Valdes AM, Arp P, Ingvarsson T, Jhamai M, Jonsson H, Stolk L, Thorleifsson G, Zhai G, Zhang F, Zhu Y, van der Breggen R, Carr A, Doherty M, Doherty S, Felson DT, Gonzalez A, Halldorsson BV, Hart DJ, Hauksson VB, Hofman A, Ioannidis JP, Kloppenburg M, Lane NE, Loughlin J, Luyten FP, Nevitt MC, Parimi N, Pols HA, Rivadeneira F, Slagboom EP, Styrkarsdottir U, Tsezou A, van de Putte T, Zmuda J, Spector TD, Stefansson K, Uitterlinden AG, van Meurs JB (2010) A genome-wide association study identifies an osteoarthritis susceptibility locus on chromosome 7q22. Arthritis Rheum 62(2):499
Kong L, Wang L, Meng F, Cao J, Shen Y (2017) Association between smoking and risk of knee osteoarthritis: a systematic review and meta-analysis. Osteoarthr Cartil 25(6):809

Kujala UM, Kettunen J, Paananen H, Aalto T, Battie MC, Impivaara O, Videman T, Sarna S (1995) Knee osteoarthritis in former runners, soccer players, weight lifters, and shooters. Arthritis Rheum 38(4):539

Kwon S, Kim W, Yang S, Choi KH (2019) Influence of the type of occupation on osteoarthritis of the knee in men: the Korean National Health and Nutrition Examination Survey 2010–2012. J Occup Health 61(1):54

Lane NE, Michel B, Bjorkengren A, Oehlert J, Shi H, Bloch DA, Fries JF (1993) The risk of osteoarthritis with running and aging: a 5-year longitudinal study. J Rheumatol 20(3):461

Leung YY, Ang LW, Thumboo J, Wang R, Yuan JM, Koh WP (2014) Cigarette smoking and risk of total knee replacement for severe osteoarthritis among Chinese in Singapore--the Singapore Chinese health study. Osteoarthr Cartil 22(6):764

Leung YY, Talaei M, Ang LW, Yuan JM, Koh WP (2019) Reproductive factors and risk of total knee replacement due to severe knee osteoarthritis in women, the Singapore Chinese Health Study. Osteoarthr Cartil 27(8):1129

Leyland KM, Hart DJ, Javaid MK, Judge A, Kiran A, Soni A, Goulston LM, Cooper C, Spector TD, Arden NK (2012) The natural history of radiographic knee osteoarthritis: a fourteen-year population-based cohort study. Arthritis Rheum 64(7):2243

Lingard EA, Katz JN, Wright EA, Sledge CB (2004) Predicting the outcome of total knee arthroplasty. J Bone Joint Surg Am 86(10):2179

Liu B, Balkwill A, Cooper C, Roddam A, Brown A, Beral V (2009) Reproductive history, hormonal factors and the incidence of hip and knee replacement for osteoarthritis in middle-aged women. Ann Rheum Dis 68(7):1165

Lloyd ME, Hart DJ, Nandra D, McAlindon TE, Wheeler M, Doyle DV, Spector TD (1996) Relation between insulin-like growth factor-I concentrations, osteoarthritis, bone density, and fractures in the general population: the Chingford study. Ann Rheum Dis 55(12):870

Lu B, Driban JB, Xu C, Lapane KL, McAlindon TE, Eaton CB (2017) Dietary fat intake and radiographic progression of knee osteoarthritis: data from the osteoarthritis initiative. Arthritis Care Res 69(3):368

MacDonald SJ, Charron KD, Bourne RB, Naudie DD, McCalden RW, Rorabeck CH (2008) The John Insall Award: gender-specific total knee replacement: prospectively collected clinical outcomes. Clin Orthop Relat Res 466(11):2612

Maetzel A, Makela M, Hawker G, Bombardier C (1997) Osteoarthritis of the hip and knee and mechanical occupational exposure–a systematic overview of the evidence. J Rheumatol 24(8):1599

Maquet PG, Pelzer GA (1977) Evolution of the maximum stress in osteo-arthritis of the knee. J Biomech 10(2):107

March LM, Bachmeier CJ (1997) Economics of osteoarthritis: a global perspective. Baillieres Clin Rheumatol 11(4):817

McAlindon TE, Felson DT, Zhang Y, Hannan MT, Aliabadi P, Weissman B, Rush D, Wilson PW, Jacques P (1996) Relation of dietary intake and serum levels of vitamin D to progression of osteoarthritis of the knee among participants in the Framingham Study. Ann Intern Med 125(5):353

McAlindon TE, Wilson PW, Aliabadi P, Weissman B, Felson DT (1999) Level of physical activity and the risk of radiographic and symptomatic knee osteoarthritis in the elderly: the Framingham study. Am J Med 106(2):151

McGoey BV, Deitel M, Saplys RJ, Kliman ME (1990) Effect of weight loss on musculoskeletal pain in the morbidly obese. J Bone Joint Surg 72(2):322

McWilliams DF, Doherty S, Maciewicz RA, Muir KR, Zhang W, Doherty M (2010) Self-reported knee and foot alignments in early adult life and risk of osteoarthritis. Arthritis Care Res 62(4):489

Messier SP, Loeser RF, Miller GD, Morgan TM, Rejeski WJ, Sevick MA, Ettinger WH Jr, Pahor M, Williamson JD (2004) Exercise and dietary weight loss in overweight and obese older adults with knee osteoarthritis: the Arthritis, Diet, and Activity Promotion Trial. Arthritis Rheum 50(5):1501

Misra D, Booth SL, Tolstykh I, Felson DT, Nevitt MC, Lewis CE, Torner J, Neogi T (2013) Vitamin K deficiency is associated with incident knee osteoarthritis. Am J Med 126(3):243

Mork PJ, Holtermann A, Nilsen TI (2012) Effect of body mass index and physical exercise on risk of knee and hip osteoarthritis: longitudinal data from the Norwegian HUNT Study. J Epidemiol Community Health 66(8):678

Murphy L, Schwartz TA, Helmick CG, Renner JB, Tudor G, Koch G, Dragomir A, Kalsbeek WD, Luta G, Jordan JM (2008) Lifetime risk of symptomatic knee osteoarthritis. Arthritis Rheum 59(9):1207

Musumeci G, Trovato FM, Pichler K, Weinberg AM, Loreto C, Castrogiovanni P (2013) Extra-virgin olive oil diet and mild physical activity prevent cartilage degeneration in an osteoarthritis model: an in vivo and in vitro study on lubricin expression. J Nutr Biochem 24(12):2064

Muthuri SG, Zhang W, Maciewicz RA, Muir K, Doherty M (2015) Beer and wine consumption and risk of knee or hip osteoarthritis: a case control study. Arthritis Res Ther 17:23

O'Connor MI (2011) Implant survival, knee function, and pain relief after TKA: are there differences between men and women? Clin Orthop Relat Res 469(7):1846

O'Neill TW, McCabe PS, McBeth J (2018) Update on the epidemiology, risk factors and disease outcomes of osteoarthritis. Best Pract Res Clin Rheumatol 32(2):312

Oiestad BE, Holm I, Gunderson R, Myklebust G, Risberg MA (2010) Quadriceps muscle weakness after anterior cruciate ligament reconstruction: a risk factor for knee osteoarthritis? Arthritis Care Res 62(12):1706

Oiestad BE, Juhl CB, Eitzen I, Thorlund JB (2015) Knee extensor muscle weakness is a risk factor for development of knee osteoarthritis. A systematic review and meta-analysis. Osteoarthr Cartil 23(2):171

Ojard C, Habashy A, Meyer M, Chimento G, Ochsner JL (2018) Effect of obesity on component alignment in total knee arthroplasty. Ochsner J 18(3):226

Panoutsopoulou K, Zeggini E (2013) Advances in osteoarthritis genetics. J Med Genet 50(11):715

Panush RS, Hanson CS, Caldwell JR, Longley S, Stork J, Thoburn R (1995) Is running associated with osteoarthritis? An eight-year follow-up study. J Clin Rheumatol 1(1):35

Parvizi J, Trousdale RT, Sarr MG (2000) Total joint arthroplasty in patients surgically treated for morbid obesity. J Arthroplast 15(8):1003

Petterson SC, Raisis L, Bodenstab A, Snyder-Mackler L (2007) Disease-specific gender differences among total knee arthroplasty candidates. J Bone Joint Surg Am 89(11):2327

Pottie P, Presle N, Terlain B, Netter P, Mainard D, Berenbaum F (2006) Obesity and osteoarthritis: more complex than predicted! Ann Rheum Dis 65(11):1403

Price AJ, Alvand A, Troelsen A, Katz JN, Hooper G, Gray A, Carr A, Beard D (2018) Knee replacement. Lancet 392(10158):1672

Reilly DT, Martens M (1972) Experimental analysis of the quadriceps muscle force and patello-femoral joint reaction force for various activities. Acta Orthop Scand 43(2):126

Ritter MA, Wing JT, Berend ME, Davis KE, Meding JB (2008) The clinical effect of gender on outcome of total knee arthroplasty. J Arthroplast 23(3):331

Ritter MA, Davis KE, Meding JB, Pierson JL, Berend ME, Malinzak RA (2011) The effect of alignment and BMI on failure of total knee replacement. J Bone Joint Surg Am 93(17):1588

Ritter MA, Davis KE, Davis P, Farris A, Malinzak RA, Berend ME, Meding JB (2013) Preoperative malalignment increases risk of failure after total knee arthroplasty. J Bone Joint Surg Am 95(2):126

Schiffner E, Latz D, Thelen S, Grassmann JP, Karbowski A, Windolf J, Jungbluth P, Schneppendahl J (2019) Aseptic loosening after THA and TKA – do gender, tobacco use and BMI have an impact on implant survival time? J Orthop 16(3):269

Schroer WC, Berend KR, Lombardi AV, Barnes CL, Bolognesi MP, Berend ME, Ritter MA, Nunley RM (2013) Why are total knees failing today? Etiology of total knee revision in 2010 and 2011. J Arthroplast 28(8 Suppl):116

Segal NA, Glass NA, Felson DT, Hurley M, Yang M, Nevitt M, Lewis CE, Torner JC (2010) Effect of quadriceps strength and proprioception on risk for knee osteoarthritis. Med Sci Sports Exerc 42(11):2081

Sharkey PF, Lichstein PM, Shen C, Tokarski AT, Parvizi J (2014) Why are total knee arthroplasties failing today--has anything changed after 10 years? J Arthroplast 29(9):1774

Sharma L, Song J, Dunlop D, Felson D, Lewis CE, Segal N, Torner J, Cooke TD, Hietpas J, Lynch J, Nevitt M (2010) Varus and valgus alignment and incident and progressive knee osteoarthritis. Ann Rheum Dis 69(11):1940

Shea MK, Kritchevsky SB, Hsu FC, Nevitt M, Booth SL, Kwoh CK, McAlindon TE, Vermeer C, Drummen N, Harris TB, Womack C, Loeser RF (2015) The association between vitamin K status and knee osteoarthritis features in older adults: the health. Aging and Body Composition Study. Osteoarthr Cartil 23(3):370

Shetty GM, Mullaji AB, Bhayde S, Lingaraju AP (2014) No effect of obesity on limb and component alignment after computer-assisted total knee arthroplasty. Knee 21(4):862

Si HB, Zeng Y, Shen B, Yang J, Zhou ZK, Kang PD, Pei FX (2015) The influence of body mass index on the outcomes of primary total knee arthroplasty. Knee Surg Sports Traumatol Arthrosc 23(6):1824

Slemenda C, Heilman DK, Brandt KD, Katz BP, Mazzuca SA, Braunstein EM, Byrd D (1998) Reduced quadriceps strength relative to body weight: a risk factor for knee osteoarthritis in women? Arthritis Rheum 41(11):1951

Smith BE, Askew MJ, Gradisar IA Jr, Gradisar JS, Lew MM (1992) The effect of patient weight on the functional outcome of total knee arthroplasty. Clin Orthop Relat Res (276):237–244

Spector TD, Cicuttini F, Baker J, Loughlin J, Hart D (1996) Genetic influences on osteoarthritis in women: a twin study. BMJ 312(7036):940

Spector TD, Nandra D, Hart DJ, Doyle DV (1997) Is hormone replacement therapy protective for hand and knee osteoarthritis in women? The Chingford Study. Ann Rheum Dis 56(7):432

Steere JT, Sobieraj MC, DeFrancesco CJ, Israelite CL, Nelson CL, Kamath AF (2018) Prophylactic tibial stem fixation in the obese: comparative early results in primary total knee arthroplasty. Knee Surg Relat Res 30(3):227

Stickles B, Phillips L, Brox WT, Owens B, Lanzer WL (2001) Defining the relationship between obesity and total joint arthroplasty. Obes Res 9(3):219

Sturm R (2003) Increases in clinically severe obesity in the United States, 1986–2000. Arch Intern Med 163(18):2146

Sturmer T, Gunther KP, Brenner H (2000) Obesity, overweight and patterns of osteoarthritis: the Ulm Osteoarthritis Study. J Clin Epidemiol 53(3):307

Veronese N, Stubbs B, Noale M, Solmi M, Luchini C, Smith TO, Cooper C, Guglielmi G, Reginster JY, Rizzoli R, Maggi S (2017) Adherence to a Mediterranean diet is associated with lower prevalence of osteoarthritis: data from the osteoarthritis initiative. Clin Nutr 36(6):1609

Vignon E, Valat JP, Rossignol M, Avouac B, Rozenberg S, Thoumie P, Avouac J, Nordin M, Hilliquin P (2006) Osteoarthritis of the knee and hip and activity: a systematic international review and synthesis (OASIS). Joint Bone Spine 73(4):442

Vos T, Flaxman AD, Naghavi M, Lozano R, Michaud C, Ezzati M, Shibuya K, Salomon JA, Abdalla S, Aboyans V, Abraham J, Ackerman I, Aggarwal R, Ahn SY, Ali MK, Alvarado M, Anderson HR, Anderson LM, Andrews KG, Atkinson C, Baddour LM, Bahalim AN, Barker-Collo S, Barrero LH, Bartels DH, Basanez MG, Baxter A, Bell ML, Benjamin EJ, Bennett D, Bernabe E, Bhalla K, Bhandari B, Bikbov B, Bin Abdulhak A, Birbeck G, Black JA, Blencowe H, Blore JD, Blyth F, Bolliger I, Bonaventure A, Boufous S, Bourne R, Boussinesq M, Braithwaite T, Brayne C, Bridgett L, Brooker S, Brooks P, Brugha TS, Bryan-Hancock C, Bucello C, Buchbinder R, Buckle G, Budke CM, Burch M, Burney P, Burstein R, Calabria B, Campbell B, Canter CE, Carabin H, Carapetis J, Carmona L, Cella C, Charlson F, Chen H, Cheng AT, Chou D, Chugh SS, Coffeng LE, Colan SD, Colquhoun S, Colson KE, Condon J, Connor MD, Cooper LT, Corriere M, Cortinovis M, de Vaccaro KC, Couser W, Cowie BC, Criqui MH, Cross M, Dabhadkar KC, Dahiya M, Dahodwala N, Damsere-Derry J, Danaei G, Davis A, De Leo D, Degenhardt L, Dellavalle R, Delossantos A, Denenberg J, Derrett S, Des Jarlais DC, Dharmaratne SD, Dherani M, Diaz-Torne C, Dolk H, Dorsey ER, Driscoll T, Duber H, Ebel B, Edmond K, Elbaz A, Ali SE, Erskine H, Erwin PJ, Espindola P, Ewoigbokhan SE, Farzadfar F, Feigin V, Felson DT, Ferrari A, Ferri CP, Fevre EM, Finucane MM, Flaxman S, Flood L, Foreman K, Forouzanfar MH, Fowkes FG, Franklin R, Fransen M, Freeman MK, Gabbe BJ, Gabriel SE, Gakidou E, Ganatra HA, Garcia B, Gaspari F, Gillum RF, Gmel G, Gosselin R, Grainger R, Groeger J, Guillemin F, Gunnell D, Gupta R, Haagsma J, Hagan H, Halasa YA, Hall W, Haring D, Haro JM, Harrison JE, Havmoeller R, Hay RJ, Higashi H, Hill C, Hoen B, Hoffman H, Hotez PJ, Hoy D, Huang JJ, Ibeanusi SE, Jacobsen KH, James SL, Jarvis D, Jasrasaria R, Jayaraman S, Johns N, Jonas JB, Karthikeyan G, Kassebaum N, Kawakami N, Keren A, Khoo JP, King CH, Knowlton LM, Kobusingye O, Koranteng A, Krishnamurthi R, Lalloo R, Laslett LL, Lathlean T, Leasher JL, Lee YY, Leigh J, Lim SS, Limb E, Lin JK, Lipnick M, Lipshultz SE, Liu W, Loane M, Ohno SL, Lyons R, Ma J, Mabweijano J, MacIntyre MF, Malekzadeh R, Mallinger L, Manivannan S, Marcenes W, March L, Margolis DJ, Marks GB, Marks R, Matsumori A, Matzopoulos R, Mayosi BM, McAnulty JH, McDermott MM, McGill N, McGrath J, Medina-Mora ME, Meltzer M, Mensah GA, Merriman TR, Meyer AC, Miglioli V, Miller M, Miller TR, Mitchell PB, Mocumbi AO, Moffitt TE, Mokdad AA, Monasta L, Montico M, Moradi-Lakeh M, Moran A, Morawska L, Mori R, Murdoch ME, Mwaniki MK, Naidoo K, Nair MN, Naldi L, Narayan KM, Nelson PK, Nelson RG, Nevitt MC, Newton CR, Nolte S, Norman P, Norman R, O'Donnell M, O'Hanlon S, Olives C, Omer SB, Ortblad K, Osborne R, Ozgediz D, Page A, Pahari B, Pandian JD, Rivero AP, Patten SB, Pearce N, Padilla RP, Perez-Ruiz F, Perico N, Pesudovs K, Phillips D, Phillips MR, Pierce K, Pion S, Polanczyk GV, Polinder S, Pope CA, Popova S, Porrini E, Pourmalek F, Prince M, Pullan RL, Ramaiah KD, Ranganathan D, Razavi H, Regan M, Rehm JT, Rein DB, Remuzzi G, Richardson K, Rivara FP, Roberts T, Robinson C, De Leon FR, Ronfani L, Room R, Rosenfeld LC, Rushton L, Sacco RL, Saha S, Sampson U, Sanchez-Riera L, Sanman E, Schwebel DC, Scott JG, Segui-Gomez M, Shahraz S, Shepard DS, Shin H, Shivakoti R, Singh D, Singh GM, Singh JA, Singleton J, Sleet DA, Sliwa K, Smith E, Smith JL, Stapelberg

NJ, Steer A, Steiner T, Stolk WA, Stovner LJ, Sudfeld C, Syed S, Tamburlini G, Tavakkoli M, Taylor HR, Taylor JA, Taylor WJ, Thomas B, Thomson WM, Thurston GD, Tleyjeh IM, Tonelli M, Towbin JA, Truelsen T, Tsilimbaris MK, Ubeda C, Undurraga EA, van der Werf MJ, van Os J, Vavilala MS, Venketasubramanian N, Wang M, Wang W, Watt K, Weatherall DJ, Weinstock MA, Weintraub R, Weisskopf MG, Weissman MM, White RA, Whiteford H, Wiersma ST, Wilkinson JD, Williams HC, Williams SR, Witt E, Wolfe F, Woolf AD, Wulf S, Yeh PH, Zaidi AK, Zheng ZJ, Zonies D, Lopez AD, Murray CJ, AlMazroa MA, Memish ZA (2012) Years lived with disability (YLDs) for 1160 sequelae of 289 diseases and injuries 1990-2010: a systematic analysis for the Global Burden of Disease Study 2010. Lancet 380(9859):2163

Wang YC, McPherson K, Marsh T, Gortmaker SL, Brown M (2011) Health and economic burden of the projected obesity trends in the USA and the UK. Lancet 378(9793):815

Wise BL, Niu J, Zhang Y, Felson DT, Bradley LA, Segal N, Keysor J, Nevitt M, Lane NE (2013) The association of parity with osteoarthritis and knee replacement in the multicenter osteoarthritis study. Osteoarthr Cartil 21(12):1849

Wluka AE, Stuckey S, Brand C, Cicuttini FM (2002) Supplementary vitamin E does not affect the loss of cartilage volume in knee osteoarthritis: a 2 year double blind randomized placebo controlled study. J Rheumatol 29(12):2585

Yeung E, Jackson M, Sexton S, Walter W, Zicat B, Walter W (2011) The effect of obesity on the outcome of hip and knee arthroplasty. Int Orthop 35(6):929

Zengini E, Hatzikotoulas K, Tachmazidou I, Steinberg J, Hartwig FP, Southam L, Hackinger S, Boer CG, Styrkarsdottir U, Gilly A, Suveges D, Killian B, Ingvarsson T, Jonsson H, Babis GC, McCaskie A, Uitterlinden AG, van Meurs JBJ, Thorsteinsdottir U, Stefansson K, Davey Smith G, Wilkinson JM, Zeggini E (2018) Genome-wide analyses using UK Biobank data provide insights into the genetic architecture of osteoarthritis. Nat Genet 50(4):549

Lifestyle and Risk Factors for Knee Arthroplasty: A South African Perspective

Zia Maharaj and Jurek Rafal Tomasz Pietrzak

Contents

E. Hansen, K.-D. Kühn (eds.), *Essentials of Cemented Knee Arthroplasty*,
https://doi.org/10.1007/978-3-662-63113-3_9

9.1 Introduction

Total knee arthroplasty (TKA) is the most commonly performed joint replacement procedure worldwide. Approximately 100,000 TKAs in the UK and 155,000 TKAs in the USA were performed in 2018 alone (National Joint Registry 16th Annual Report 2019; American Academy of Orthopaedic Surgeons, American Joint Replacement Registry (AJRR) 2018). The demand for TKA is rising and has been projected to increase by a rate of 85% to reach 1.26 million procedures annually by 2030 in the USA alone (Sloan et al. 2018).

> There is a changing demographic of a younger population presenting for TKA as shown by a disproportionately increased demand in individuals less than 60 years of age (Jain et al. 2005)

9

In 2008, an estimated 7733 revision TKAs were performed in the UK and 17,921 in the USA, respectively. The most common cause for early revision TKA worldwide is periprosthetic joint infection (PJI). In fact, for 63.2% of patients in the USA, PJI is the reason to present for revision surgery within 3 months after the index procedure (National Joint Registry 16th Annual Report 2019; American Academy of Orthopaedic Surgeons, American Joint Replacement Registry (AJRR) 2018).

There are several lifestyle-related risk factors that have been implicated in negatively impacting outcomes including the following:

- Age at index surgery
- Smoking
- Nutritional status

> Younger patient cohorts have shown the highest incidence of need for early revisions (National Joint Registry 16th Annual Report 2019; American Academy of Orthopaedic Surgeons, American Joint Replacement Registry (AJRR) 2018)

In the USA, patients under 50 years of age have the highest incidence of early revision after TKA when compared to older patient cohorts ($p < 0.0001$) (American Academy of Orthopaedic Surgeons, American Joint Replacement Registry (AJRR) 2018). Similar findings have been reported in the UK, demonstrating that young, male patients have the highest risk for revision within 1 year after primary TKA (National Joint Registry 16th Annual Report 2019). Furthermore, an association exists between an increased age at primary TKA and a decreased risk for early revision (Fig. 9.1). Smoking has been associated with a 1.3-fold risk for revision TKA when compared to patients who have never smoked (American Academy of Orthopaedic Surgeons, American Joint Replacement Registry (AJRR) 2018). Malnutrition is implicated in a 2–4.5 times higher risk of readmissions and revisions compared with patients with normal nutritional status (Carli et al. 2019; Kamath et al. 2016).

Revisions after TKA due to postoperative complications place a significant burden on both patients and the healthcare system.

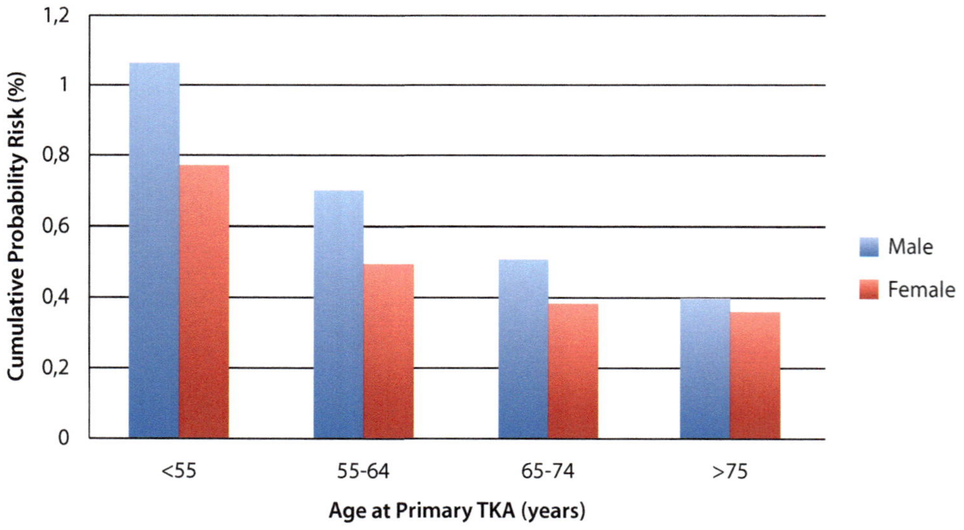

*Total sample results based on 1,193,830 primary Total Knee Arthroplasty (TKA) procedures and 33 292 first revisions between 2003 and 2018. (1)

Fig. 9.1 Risk of revision within 1 year after primary total knee arthroplasty (TKA). Total sample results based on 1,193,830 primary TKA procedures and 33,292 first revisions between 2003 and 2018 (National Joint Registry 16th Annual Report 2019)

> Patients with malnutrition consume three times more hospital resources. This results in annual costs of $11 billion in the USA only (Carli et al. 2019; Tappenden et al. 2013)

In comparison to healthy matched control patients, postoperative complications due to undernutrition can be translated into an additional expense of $3875 per patient (Bala et al. 2020). In obese patients for TKA, an additional cost of $250–$300 exists for every 5-unit increase in Body Mass Index (BMI) beyond 30 kg/m^2 (Martin et al. 2017; Werner et al. 2015a). These inflated costs are even more exaggerated in obese patients undergoing revision TKA with a corresponding additional cost of $600–$650 per 5-unit increase in BMI. Increased costs are due to expenses related to treating increased associated medical co-morbidities, greater analgesic requirements, increased incidence of all-cause hospitalization and total overall healthcare expenditures (Johnston et al. 2020).

> Therefore, it is imperative to identify and optimize lifestyle and modifiable risk factors prior to elective surgery to ensure positive outcomes and mitigate the risk of adverse events.

9.2 Return to Work and Return to Sports

A younger patient demographic has greater potential needs for improved postoperative function and need to return to work (RTW). Additionally, patients who participate in recreational physical activity over their lifetime are prone to develop osteoarthritis (OA) and present for TKA at a younger age.

> Former athletes and physically active individuals have high expectations to return to sports (RTS) after TKA and that has been strongly correlated with patient satisfaction.

RTW is a common goal for patients undergoing TKA with postoperative success rates reported to range between 68% and 85% (van Zaanen et al. 2019). The time of RTW has been shown to vary between 8 and 12 weeks after TKA (Tilbury et al. 2014). Studies have reported a wide variation of return to sports (RTS) after TKA (34–100%) across a spectrum of demographics and including sports ranging across various levels of activity (Barber-Westin and Noyes 2016).

Younger active patients aim to maintain a healthy lifestyle and it is important for the clinician to facilitate these goals. The American Heart Association and the American College of Sports Medicine published guidelines on the levels of physical activity that have been associated with a decreased risk profile for cardiovascular health and premature mortality. The guidelines include both aerobic activity and muscle-strengthening exercises with resistance training. Some studies have associated increased activity after TKA with a higher risk for implant wear and aseptic loosening (Garber et al. 2011; Gerhard et al. 2013; Golant et al. 2010; Granan et al. 2009; Harding et al. 2014) whereas others have reported equivocal outcomes when compared to a sedentary control cohort (Haskell et al. 2007; Healy et al. 2008; Hopper and Leach 2008). The intensity of activity recommended after TKA remains controversial, in particular with regard to moderate- and high-impact forms of exercise.

While there are *no consensus guidelines concerning the recommended level of activity after TKA*, there are two primary approaches to consider namely individualization of postoperative sports participation or didactic instruction of permitted and non-permitted sports activities:

- A popular approach is to consider the premorbid level of activity participation and *individualize postoperative exercise recommendations according to baseline function.*
- An alternative approach is to *discourage participation in moderate- to high-intensity activities for all patients postoperatively.*

The rationale behind the latter approach is that increased intensity of activity could have predisposed the patient to requiring TKA and, furthermore, cause postoperative complications such as implant wear. Vielgut et al. (2016) reported a long-term follow-up study assessing both pre- and postoperative activity levels in patients undergoing TKA (Vielgut et al. 2016). After a mean follow-up of 14.9 years, a significant improvement in pain and function was observed with some patients being able to safely continue high-impact activities (Vielgut et al. 2016). The 1999 Knee Society Survey conveyed a predominant opinion that minimal impact activities such as swimming, cycling, and power walking should be recommended as safe after TKA (Barber-Westin and Noyes 2016; Healy et al. 2008). The benefits of exercise for overall health are undeniable and the current perspective is that surgeons should consider each case individually with the primary aim of meeting patient expectations.

Preoperative Optimization

Preoperative expectations have a significant impact on outcomes and must be addressed in detail for each patient. The current level of activity must be thoroughly questioned and preoperative function should be examined and documented. Advice from healthcare practitioners can be inconsistent and not individualized to patient needs, leading to uncertainty and suboptimal postoperative outcomes (Bardgett et al. 2016). Psychological factors, including self-motivation and an optimistic attitude, have a positive effect on improving patients' outcomes (McGonagle et al. 2019).

> Extensive personalized counseling is necessary to ensure positive and realistic expectations (van Zaanen et al. 2019).

It is imperative to identify factors that enable patients and optimize lifestyle-related barriers which may prevent patients to meet their postoperative goals, respectively.

Preoperative workup must also include patient expectations to RTW and details of the physical level of activity required for work-related physical tasks. Work-related activities that require knee-demanding movements, such as kneeling, squatting, or crouching, remain difficult to perform even after surgery (Kievit et al. 2014). However, operating foot pedals, standing, and other physical activities that are less strenuous on the knee joint can improve after TKA (Kievit et al. 2014). A discussion with the employer may need to be facilitated in order to ensure a successful RTW.

> Job flexibility with employer-facilitated adaptations such as better working area requirements, lighter intensity of duties, and variable hours have shown to have a positive impact on RTW (McGonagle et al. 2019).

Furthermore, physically demanding duties without the supported implementation of alterations in working condition have been associated with a *negative experience of RTW and impeded patient outcomes* (Bardgett et al. 2016).

There are several *nonmodifiable barriers to successful RTS* that have been implicated including the following:

- Age
- Educational status
- Complex factors such as income and domicile

Age over 65 years is a limiting factor regarding both pre- and postoperative activity levels. Elderly patients are unlikely to increase activity levels after TKA despite the reduction in pain (Vielgut et al. 2016). Other modifiable factors include personal beliefs and motivation, social support system, and self-efficacy. The physical effects of surgery such as pain and fatigue have been implicated as the primary barrier preventing RTW (Kievit et al. 2014).

If the current level of function is poor or suboptimal, there may be a role for preoperative rehabilitation. Patients who underwent rehabilitation before TKA have demonstrated a significant decrease in length of hospital stay (Sharma et al. 2019). Recommendations should only be made after a full assessment to formulate a directed goal-based rehabilitation program and ensure patient satisfaction.

9.3 Malnutrition

Patients for TKA with a poor nutritional status are at risk for increased complications, greater morbidity, and high mortality rates postoperatively. (Sayeed et al. 2019) Optimizing the nutritional status of patients undergoing elective TKA preoperatively may reduce the incidence of these complications (Jones et al. 2013; Sayeed et al. 2019).

> The World Health Organization (WHO) has described the global status as a double burden of malnutrition with the coexistence of undernutrition along with overweight and obesity (World Health Organisation (WHO) 2018).

According to the latest WHO estimates approximately 462 million adults are underweight and 1.9 billion adults are overweight, respectively, with over 600 million of these categorically obese (BMI > 30 kg/m^2) (World Health Organisation (WHO) 2018). Malnutrition affects all geographic regions and spans socioeconomic population groups (World Health Organisation (WHO) 2018). Malnutrition, including both undernutrition and overnutrition, can be defined according to biochemical and anthropometric measurements (■ Table 9.1).

9.4 Undernutrition

A systematic review of 20 total joint arthroplasty (TJA) population studies in the USA reported an incidence of undernutrition of 40–60%. However, the difficulty of identifying poor nutrition was highlighted in a review of 105 academic institutions in the USA, which reported that *undernutrition may be missed in as many as 80% of cases.*

Undernutrition has been associated with male gender and revision surgery but not with age. Despite the prevalence and consequences of undernutrition, there are no standardized guidelines for screening, risk stratification, or management protocols for patients undergoing TKA. Anthropometric measurements are less accurate than biochemical markers at identifying undernutri-

Table 9.1 Summary of parameters defining malnutrition (World Health Organisation (WHO) 2018; Springer et al. 2017)

Undernutrition		Overnutrition	
Serum marker	Measurement	Classification	BMI (kg/m^2)
Albumin (g/dL)	<3.5	Overweight	25–29.9
Total lymphocyte count ($cells/mm^3$)	<1500	Obesity	30–39.9
Transferrin (μg/dL)	<200	Morbid obesity	40–49.9
Anthropometry	Measurement	Super obesity	>50
BMI (kg/m^2)	<18.5		

BMI Body Mass Index

tion. However, triceps skinfold and arm muscle circumference have been found to correlate with serum albumin.

> The use of either low serum albumin or low serum transferrin increases the sensitivity and specificity of defining malnutrition, especially as both have been shown to directly predict increased complications (Carli et al. 2019; Huang et al. 2013; Tobert et al. 2018).

Markers of nutritional status include blood sample measurements of the following:

- Zinc
- Vitamin D
- Transferrin
- Albumin
- Total lymphocyte count

Low preoperative serum albumin is the most accurate predictor of postoperative infective complications.

> Greene et al. (2020) reported that a serum albumin of <3.5 g/dL or a total lymphocyte count of <1500 cells/mm^3 inferred a seven- and fivefold increased risk of major wound complications after TJA (Greene et al. 1991).

The infective consequences of undernutrition are physiologically due to an impaired immune system with a decreased number of lymphocytes. Wound healing is impaired due to the inhibition of collagen synthesis and fibroblast proliferation. Additionally, increased tissue edema and suboptimal oxygen tension compromise tissue tensile strength and contribute to poor healing with postoperative wound problems and potential wound dehiscence (Blevins et al. 2018; Carli et al. 2019; Greene et al. 1991; Ryan et al. 2018; Tsantes et al. 2019).

PJI is the most common reason for revision in patients undergoing TKA with undernutrition.

> The risk of superficial skin infections (SSI) is 2–3 times higher in undernourished patients, while the likelihood of deep PJI rises by 2.3–3.6 times, respectively.

The likelihood of an early revision within 30 days of primary TKA as a result of SSI is tenfold higher in undernourished patients (Carli et al. 2019; Huang et al. 2013; Schroer et al. 2018). In comparison with other modifiable risk factors including anemia, uncontrolled diabetes, narcotic and tobacco use, Schroer et al. (2018) showed that undernutrition was associated with the highest rate of 90-day readmissions (Schroer et al. 2018). In addition to PJI, undernutrition is an independent risk factor for renal and neurovascular adverse events and hematoma or seroma formation. Bala et al. (2020) reported significantly more major complications in protein-malnourished patients when compared with a control cohort undergoing TJA (Bala et al. 2020). The increase in postoperative complications included more pulmonary embolisms, acute myocardial infarctions, occlusive strokes, and respiratory and heart failures (Courtney et al. 2016).

Preoperative Optimization

The benefit of preoperative optimization of the nutritional status remains controversial and still a paucity of literature exists. In a randomized prospective study investigating the effect of a multimodal approach to preoperative nutritional supplementation, Alito and de Aguilar-Nascimento (2016) demonstrated significantly reduced hospital stay and decreased C-reactive protein (CRP) levels in blood on day 2 postoperatively (Alito and de Aguilar-Nascimento 2016). Nishizaki et al. (2015) demonstrated that preoperative supplementation of β-hydroxy-β-methylbutyrate, L-arginine, and L-glutamine (HMB/Arg/Gln) was protective of quadriceps strength at 2 weeks postoperatively in 23 randomized patients undergoing TKA (Nishizaki et al. 2015). Cao et al. (2017) reported a decreased length of hospital stays and lower rates of wound ooze in patients who had received carbohydrate and protein nutritional supplementation preoperatively (Cao et al. 2017). Various studies have been conducted on nutritional supplementation; however, neither a standardized management protocol nor parameters indicative of effective treatment are yet to be established.

9.5 Overnutrition

In 2017, obesity affected approximately 58% of adults worldwide, with regional estimates exceeding 70% for the USA, Chile, and Mexico, respectively (Organisation for Economic Co-operation and Development (OECD) 2019). In many countries in Africa, a similar development is emerging. Obesity is classified according to BMI with recent additions of subclassifications for severe obesity including morbid obesity and super obesity (Table 9.1). The incidence of morbidly obese patients is rising with an increase of 70% between 2000 and 2010 and now accounts for approximately 7% of people in the USA (Springer et al. 2017; Sturm 2007; Sturm and Hattori 2013). A direct correlation exists between obesity and the development of osteoarthritis (OA) of the knee. Obese patients are 3–5 times more likely to suffer from knee OA than normal or overweight patients (Odum et al. 2013; Werner et al. 2015a). It has been shown that a 4% increase in the incidence of OA exists with each unit increase in age-adjusted BMI. (Bagsby et al. 2016; Sahyoun et al. 1999)

9

> Subsequently, approximately, 80–95% of patients for TKA are overweight or obese (Changulani et al. 2008; Pellegrini et al. 2017).

In addition, the likelihood of obese patients requiring subsequent contralateral TKA is also significant. The need for contralateral TKA after unilateral TKA is 37% within 10 years in obese patients (McMahon and Block 2003; Zeni et al. 2010). In a 2018 review of 85,616 patients, obesity and index TKA were the strongest predictors of the 23.6% of patients requiring contralateral joint replacement 5–8 years later (Lamplot et al. 2018).

9.5.1 Associated Risks

Obesity infers a higher risk of perioperative complications including the following:

- Increased intraoperative blood loss
- Increased incidence of medial collateral ligament avulsions
- Higher risk of PJI
- Thrombotic events
- Falls
- Early failures
- Subsequent TKA revision surgery (Alvi et al. 2015; Gillespie and Porteous 2007; Mantilla et al. 2003; Memtsoudis et al. 2009; Winiarsky et al. 1998)

In a comparison of obese (BMI > 30 kg/m^2) and non-obese (BMI < 30 kg/m^2) patients undergoing TKA, Järvenpää et al. (2012) demonstrated significantly more postoperative complications in the obese group (Järvenpää et al. 2012). In a review of 1.7 million TKAs, D'Apuzzo et al. (2015) proved that morbid obesity was an independent risk factor for perioperative complications (D'Apuzzo et al. 2015). Additionally, having controlled for age, sex, and 28 other medical co-morbidities, morbid obesity resulted in the following:

- Prolonged operating times
- Increased component malpositioning
- Limited postoperative rehabilitation
- Increased likelihood of wound dehiscence
- Higher hospital costs
- Longer hospital stay (D'Apuzzo et al. 2015)

Furthermore, a dose-dependent relationship exists between obesity and an increased rate of complications after TKA.

> Each unit increase of BMI infers an additional 8% risk of surgically related complications (Dowsey et al. 2010).

This is both a consequence of obesity itself and the increased incidence of associated co-morbidities linked to obesity. The highest rate of adverse events following TKA subsequently occurs in super-obese patients (BMI > 50 kg/m^2). The complication rate in super-obese patients is not only double that of morbidly obese patients and four times more significant than non-obese patients, it is even higher than those patients undergoing revision TKA (Werner et al. 2015a).

> Prosthetic longevity may be compromised in obese patients due to exaggerated stresses on the underlying bone and implant material (Ayyar et al. 2012; Bagsby et al. 2016).

Implanted prostheses undergo greater mechanical strains in patients with higher BMI resulting in increased wear, poorer survivorship, and a higher demand for subsequent revision TKA for aseptic loosening. Implant survival is compromised in both primary and revision TKA in obese patients (Martin et al. 2017). Abdel et al. (2015) reported an exaggerated risk of tibial prostheses loosening in obese patients (BMI > 35 kg/m^2) after primary TKA that may be mitigated by the use of additional fixation such as stemmed implants (Abdel et al. 2015).

9.5.2 Functional Outcomes

The degree of functional improvement in obese patients after TKA is controversial. In a comparison of the clinical and radiographic outcomes of 326 TKAs in obese patients with 425 non-obese patients, Spicer et al. (2001) reported that no difference existed in both the 10-year survivorship and functional outcomes of the two groups (Spicer et al. 2001). Foran et al. (2004) showed that the functional outcome scores in 68 obese patients were inferior in comparison to a group of matched non-obese patients at a mean follow-up of 80 months (Foran et al. 2004). In a systematic review, Kerkhoffs et al. (2012) reported that Knee Society scores (KSS) in obese patients were significantly inferior to non-obese patients by almost 3.23 points on average (Kerkhoffs et al. 2012). Naziri et al. (2013) showed that both KSS and knee flexion was poorer in super-obese patients than non-obese patients at a 5-year follow-up (Naziri et al. 2013). In contrast, a retrospective review of the functional outcomes and complications of 402 TKAs using the same implant by Agarwala et al. (2020) showed no difference between obese and non-obese patients at a minimum of 1-year follow-up (Agarwala et al. 2020). Collins et al. (2017), similarly, demonstrated that the perception of pain and postoperative satisfaction was the same 2 years after TKA irrespective of preoperative BMI (Collins et al. 2017).

> The absolute functional outcomes of TKA in obese patients may be less than in non-obese patients but the relative improvement from preoperative to postoperative outcome scores and satisfaction rates are equivalent (Bookman et al. 2018).

However, the functional gains are far more moderate and more gradual as the BMI increases beyond 40 kg/m^2 and must be juxtaposed with the greater potential of postoperative complications (Workgroup of the American Association of Hip and Knee Surgeons Evidence Based Committee 2013).

> In morbidly obese patients the risk of focal osteolysis on postoperative radiographs is five times higher with an increased risk of revision.

Obesity is associated not only with poorer survivorship of primary TKA but also with a more rapid progression to early revision surgery (Bookman et al. 2018; Mulhall et al. 2010). Wagner et al. (2016) analyzed the prospectively collected data of 16,136 patients who underwent elective primary TKA and reported a significantly increased incidence of both re-operation and implant removal and revision (Wagner et al. 2016). A 3% increased risk of re-operation and a 5% increased rate of implant removal and revision accompanied each one-unit increase in BMI, respectively. An increased rate of revision for aseptic loosening was found in patients with a BMI > 35 kg/m^2 (Wagner et al. 2016). Functional outcomes are poorer and joint stiffness is more common in obese than in non-obese patients after revision TKA (Bookman et al. 2018; Mulhall et al. 2010).

9.5.3 Preoperative Optimization

Weight loss prior to TKA is recommended and may mitigate the need for TKA by improvement of clinically relevant symptoms (Martin et al. 2017; Pellegrini et al. 2017). A 10% decrease in body weight is associated with a reduction of pain and functional disability for patients with knee OA (Christensen et al. 2007; Flego et al. 2016).

> However, only 1 of 9 patients is able to preoperatively decrease body weight by more than 5% (Inacio et al. 2014).

Pellegrini et al. (2017) explored patient motives for weight loss and showed that improving physical appearance was most important followed by the need to alleviate knee symptoms and expedite TKA (Pellegrini et al. 2017).

> Significant hindrance to weight loss includes compromised mobility and debilitating pain associated with end-stage knee pathology (Pellegrini et al. 2017).

There is concern that strict preoperative weight loss may result in muscle weakness and impaired bone mineral density (Flego et al. 2016; Waters et al. 2013). There is limited data on the impact of preoperative weight loss on the outcomes of TKA.

Bariatric surgery (BS) has been suggested to complement diet and exercise to moderate the risks of TKA in obese patients.

> Bariatric surgery is indicated for morbidly obese patients and patients with a BMI > 35 kg/m^2 who have failed nonoperative weight loss strategies and have at least one clinically relevant co-morbidity (Liu et al. 2020; Zainul-abidin et al. 2019).

The potential to decrease BMI by 10–15 units and 50–70% of excess weight is possible after BS (Springer et al. 2017). Today, the safety of BS is equivalent to elective TJA with a mortality rate of 1% (Springer et al. 2017). BS may mitigate the impact of co-morbidities associated with obesity such as diabetes, hyperlipidemia, and obstructive sleep apnea (Buchwald et al. 2004; Liu et al. 2020; Zainul-abidin et al. 2019). The benefit of preoperative bariatric surgery prior to TKA remains contentious (Springer et al. 2017).

> Bariatric surgery has been associated with profound postoperative nutritional deficiencies including Vitamin D, iron, and albumin (Martin et al. 2017).

The timing of BS, before or after TKA, is controversial. Kulkarni et al. (2011) showed that patients who underwent BS before TJA were 3.5 times less likely to have wound infections and the incidence of hospital readmissions was 7 times lower than for patients with BS after TJA (Kulkarni et al. 2011). Werner et al. (2015b) reported that obese patients who had undergone bariatric surgery 2 years before TKA showed a rate of minor complications decreased by 40%, and the incidence of major complications halved in comparison with obese patients (Werner et al. 2015b). The rate of adverse events was still higher than compared with non-obese patients undergoing TKA (Werner et al. 2015b). The 2018 Proceedings of International Consensus on Orthopedic Infections do not recommend routine preoperative bariatric surgery as a result of inconclusive evidence (Zainul-abidin et al. 2019).

9.6 Rehabilitation TKA

There are big variations between the models of rehabilitation programs used across institutions and by clinicians worldwide. Rehabilitation programs should be designed to focus on the personal expectations, overall physical health, and preoperative baseline function of each patient. There are continued advances in surgery and between 2012 and 2018 the mean length of hospital stays has decreased from 2.3 days to 1.1 days in the USA (American Academy of Orthopaedic Surgeons, American Joint Replacement Registry (AJRR) 2018). There are undeniable positive short-term improvements in physical function and pain after TKA.

> However, there remains a recognized problem with medium- to long-term patient outcomes.

Despite similar clinical practice, improvement in surgical techniques, and surgeon experience between total hip arthroplasty (THA) and TKA, the global trend of patient satisfaction after TKA is more modest than after THA (Organisation for Economic Co-operation and Development (OECD) 2019).

> Although most patients receive early, supervised physiotherapy after TKA, there is a lack of evidence supporting the optimal type, duration or frequency of exercise that will ensure the best outcomes (Artz et al. 2015; Sattler et al. 2019).

A systematic review and meta-analysis by Sattler et al. (2019) assessed physiotherapy programs in the acute post-surgical phase after TKA (Sattler et al. 2019). There was no significant difference in functional outcomes across differing regimes after a follow-up at 6 weeks (Dujin et al. 2012; Hewitt and Shakespeare 2001; Kim et al. 2009; Pongkunakorn and Sawatphap 2014). There are several adjuncts to physiotherapy programs including electrical stimulation, acupuncture, cryotherapy, and various electrical modalities. Patients should be educated on these forms of therapy as an adjunct to an exercise regime offered on a personal preferential basis. However, the adjuncts to physiotherapy cannot be used in isolation and should be implemented in conjunction with an exercise routine (Artz et al. 2015). Various types of exercise such as hydrotherapy, cycling, or additional balancing movements have shown equivocal outcomes when compared to conventional physiotherapy. There are no significant differences in outcomes when outpatient physiotherapy was compared to a home-based exercise program (Artz et al. 2015; Dujin et al. 2012; Hewitt and Shakespeare 2001; Kim et al. 2009; Pongkunakorn and Sawatphap 2014; Sattler et al. 2019).

> After discharge even minimal physiotherapy has been shown to improve outcomes up to 6 months postoperatively when compared to a control group receiving no physiotherapy (Artz et al. 2015).

There is no evidence to suggest which exercise modality produces best outcomes and clinicians should consider patient motivation and preference when determining the most suitable exercise regime to recommend (Castrodad et al. 2019). The variation in short-term results across interventions indicates that further high-quality studies should be conducted to assess the impact of early rehabilitation after TKA over a longer follow-up interval. The length of hospital stay after TKA rates continues to decrease worldwide; however, activity during the proceeding days after surgery may have a crucial impact on long-term outcomes (Artz et al. 2015; Castrodad et al. 2019; Jahic et al. 2018; Sattler et al. 2019).

- **Conclusion**

Lifestyle-related risk factors demonstrated to negatively influence outcomes including younger age, smoking, and poor nutritional status. A younger population demographic is presenting for TKA with increased desires to RTW and RTS. There are no absolute restrictions on activities after TKA, and surgeons should consider each case on an individual basis to provide extensive counseling aimed at guiding patients. A multidisciplinary team approach should be implemented to ensure that patient expectations are met. The overall patient satisfaction after TKA is more modest than after THA and the vital role of perioperative rehabilitation and optimization of modifiable risk factors must be recognized.

Take-Home Messages

- There is increased demand for TKA in a younger demographic (<60 years) with increased expectations after TKA.
- Younger patients have shown the highest incidence of need for early revisions after TKA.
- RTW and RTS are now major expectations that have been strongly correlated with patient satisfaction.
- Smoking is a modifiable patient risk factor with an increased risk for revision TKA when compared to patients who have never smoked.
- Malnutrition, including both undernutrition and obesity, is implicated in a higher risk of overall complications, readmissions, and revisions.
- Undernutrition is often overlooked and underdiagnosed affecting between 40% and 60% of TJA patients.
- A low preoperative serum albumin of <3.5 g/dL may be an accurate indicator of postoperative infections.
- Although satisfaction rates are equivalent to non-obese patients, functional outcomes are lower in obese patients after TKA.
- Obesity may compromise prosthetic longevity due to exaggerated stresses on the underlying bone and implant material.
- Obesity is the strongest predictor of requiring contralateral joint replacement within 5 to 8 years after index TKA.
- Perioperative rehabilitation programs directly impact early and medium-term functional outcomes and a multidisciplinary team approach to optimize patient satisfaction after TKA.

References

Abdel MP, Bonadurer GF, Jennings MT, Hanssen AD (2015) Increased aseptic tibial failures in patients with a BMI ≥35 and well-aligned total knee arthroplasties. J Arthroplast 30(12):2181–2184. https://doi.org/10.1016/j.arth.2015.06.057

Agarwala S, Jadia C, Vijayvargiya M (2020) Is obesity a contra-indication for a successful total knee arthroplasty? J Clin Orthop Trauma 11(1):136–139. https://doi.org/10.1016/j.jcot.2018.11.016

Alito MA, de Aguilar-Nascimento JE (2016) Multimodal perioperative care plus immunonutrition versus traditional care in total hip arthroplasty: a randomized pilot study. Nutr J 15:34. https://doi.org/10.1186/s12937-016-0153-1

Alvi HM, Mednick RE, Krishnan V, Kwasny MJ, Beal MD, Manning DW (2015) The effect of BMI on 30 day outcomes following total joint arthroplasty. J Arthroplast 30(7):1113–1117. https://doi.org/10.1016/j.arth.2015.01.049

American Academy of Orthopaedic Surgeons, American Joint Replacement Registry (AJRR) (2018) Fifth AJRR annual report on hip and knee arthroplasty data. Downloaded from http://connect.ajrr.net/2019-ajrr-annual-report (7 Jan 2020)

Artz N, Elvers KT, Lowe CM, Sackley C, Jepson P, Beswick AD (2015) Effectiveness of physical therapy exercise following total knee replacement: systematic review and meta-analysis. BMC Musculoskelet Disord 16:15. https://doi.org/10.1186/s12891-015-0469-6

Ayyar V, Burnett R, Coutts FJ, van der Linden ML, Mercer TH (2012) The influence of obesity on patient reported outcomes following total knee replacement. Arthritis 2012:185208. https://doi.org/10.1155/2012/185208

Bagsby DT, Issa K, Smith LS, Elmallah RK, Mast LE, Harwin SF et al (2016) Cemented vs cementless total knee arthroplasty in morbidly obese patients. J Arthroplast 31(8):1727–1731. https://doi.org/10.1016/j.arth.2016.01.025

Bala A, Ivanov DV, Huddleston JI, Goodman SB, Maloney WJ, Amanatullah DF (2020) The cost of malnutrition in total joint arthroplasty. J Arthroplast 35(4):926–932, e1. https://doi.org/10.1016/j.arth.2019.11.018

Barber-Westin SD, Noyes FR (2016) Aerobic physical fitness and recreational sports participation after total knee arthroplasty: a systematic review. Sports Health 8(6):553–560. https://doi.org/10.1177/1941738116670090

Bardgett M, Lally J, Malviya A, Kleim B, Deehan D (2016) Patient-reported factors influencing return to work after joint replacement. Occup Med (Lond) 66(3):215–221

Blevins K, Aalirezaie A, Shohat N, Parvizi J (2018) Malnutrition and the development of periprosthetic joint infection in patients undergoing primary elective total joint arthroplasty. J Arthroplast 33(9):2971–2975. https://doi.org/10.1016/j.arth.2018.04.027

Bookman JS, Schwarzkopf R, Rathod P, Iorio R, Deshmukh AJ (2018) Obesity. Orthop Clin North Am 49(3):291–296. https://doi.org/10.1016/j.ocl.2018.02.002

Buchwald H, Avidor Y, Braunwald E, Jensen MD, Pories W, Fahrbach K et al (2004) Bariatric surgery. JAMA 292(14):1724–1737

Cao G, Huang Q, Xu B, Huang Z, Xie J, Pei F (2017) Multimodal nutritional management in primary total knee arthroplasty: a randomized controlled trial. J Arthroplast 32(11):3390–3395. https://doi.org/10.1016/j.arth.2017.06.020

Carli AV, Polascik BA, Stelmaszczyk K, Haas SB (2019) What is the status? A systematic review of nutritional status research in total joint arthroplasty. Tech Orthop 34(3):155–162

Castrodad IMD, Recai TM, Abraham MM, Etcheson JI, Mohamed NS, Edalatpour A et al (2019) Rehabilitation protocols following total knee arthroplasty: a review of study designs and outcome measures. Ann Transl Med 7(Suppl 7):S255. https://doi.org/10.21037/atm.2019.08.15

Changulani M, Kalairajah Y, Peel T, Field RE (2008) The relationship between obesity and the age at which hip and knee replacement is undertaken. J Bone Joint Surg Br 90(3):360–363. https://doi.org/10.1302/0301-620X.90B3.19782

Christensen R, Bartels EM, Astrup A, Bliddal H (2007) Effect of weight reduction in obese patients diagnosed with knee osteoarthritis: a systematic review and meta-analysis. Ann Rheum Dis 66(4):433–439

Collins JE, Donnell-Fink LA, Yang HY, Usiskin IM, Lape EC, Wright J et al (2017) Effect of obesity on pain and functional recovery following total knee arthroplasty. J Bone Joint Surg Am 99(21):1812–1818. https://doi.org/10.2106/JBJS.17.00022

Courtney PM, Rozell JC, Melnic CM, Sheth NP, Nelson CL (2016) Effect of malnutrition and morbid obesity on complication rates following primary total joint arthroplasty. J Surg Orthop Adv 25(2):99–104

D'Apuzzo MR, Novicoff WM, Browne JA (2015) The John Insall award: morbid obesity independently impacts complications, mortality, and resource use after TKA. Clin Orthop Relat Res 473(1):57–63

Dowsey MM, Liew D, Stoney JD, Choong PF (2010) The impact of pre-operative obesity on weight change and outcome in total knee replacement. J Bone Joint Surg Br 92(4):513–520. https://doi.org/10.1302/0301-620X.92B4.23174

Dujin P, Jeonghee K, Hyunok L (2012) Effectiveness of modified quadriceps Femoris muscle setting exercise for the elderly in early rehabilitation after Total knee arthroplasty. J Phys Ther Sci 24(1):27–30

Flego A, Dowsey MM, Choong PFM, Moodie M (2016) Addressing obesity in the management of knee and hip osteoarthritis-weighing in from an economic perspective. BMC Musculoskelet Disord 17:233. https://doi.org/10.1186/s12891-016-1087-7

Foran JRH, Mont MA, Etienne G, Jones LC, Hungerford DS (2004) The outcome of total knee arthroplasty in obese patients. J Bone Joint Surg Am 86(8):1609–1615

Garber CE, Blissmer B, Deschenes MR et al (2011) American College of Sports Medicine position stand. Quantity and quality of exercise for developing and maintaining cardiorespiratory, musculoskeletal, and neuromotor fitness in apparently healthy adults: guidance for prescribing exercise. Med Sci Sports Exerc 43:1334–1359

Gerhard P, Bolt R, Duck K, Mayer R, Friederich NF, Hirschmann MT (2013) Long-term results of arthroscopically assisted anatomical single-bundle anterior cruciate ligament reconstruction using patellar tendon autograft: are there any predictors for the development of osteoarthritis? Knee Surg Sports Traumatol Arthrosc 21:957–964

Gillespie GN, Porteous AJ (2007) Obesity and knee arthroplasty. Knee 14(2):81–86

Golant A, Christoforou DC, Slover JD, Zuckerman JD (2010) Athletic participation after hip and knee arthroplasty. Bull NYU Hosp Jt Dis 68:76–83

Granan LP, Bahr R, Lie SA, Engebretsen L (2009) Timing of anterior cruciate ligament reconstructive surgery and risk of cartilage lesions and meniscal tears: a cohort study based on the Norwegian National Knee Ligament Registry. Am J Sports Med 37:955–961

Greene KA, Wilde AH, Stulberg BN (1991) Preoperative nutritional status of total joint patients. Relationship to postoperative wound complications. J Arthroplast 6(4):321–325

Harding P, Holland AE, Delany C, Hinman RS (2014) Do activity levels increase after total hip and knee arthroplasty? Clin Orthop Relat Res 472:1502–1511

Haskell WL, Lee IM, Pate RR et al (2007) Physical activity and public health: updated recommendation for adults from the American College of Sports Medicine and the American Heart Association. Circulation 116:1081–1093

Healy WL, Sharma S, Schwartz B, Iorio R (2008) Athletic activity after total joint arthroplasty. J Bone Joint Surg Am 90: 2245–2252

Hewitt B, Shakespeare D (2001) Flexion vs. extension: a comparison of post-operative total knee arthroplasty mobilisation regimes. Knee 8(4):305–309

Hopper GP, Leach WJ (2008) Participation in sporting activities following knee replacement: total versus unicompartmental. Knee Surg Sports Traumatol Arthrosc 16:973–979

Huang R, Greenky M, Kerr GJ, Austin MS, Parvizi J (2013) The effect of malnutrition on patients undergoing elective joint arthroplasty. J Arthroplast 28(8):21–24

Inacio MCS, Kritz-Silverstein D, Raman R, Macera CA, Nichols JF, Shaffer RA et al (2014) The risk of surgical site infection and readmission in obese patients undergoing total joint replacement who lose weight before surgery and keep it off post-operatively. Bone Joint J 96-B(5):629–635. https://doi.org/10.1302/0301-620X.96B5.33136

Jahic D, Omerovic D, Tanovic AT, Dzankovic F, Campara MT (2018) The effect of prehabilitation on postoperative outcome in patients following primary total knee arthroplasty. Med Arch 72(6):439–443. https://doi.org/10.5455/medarh.2018.72.439-443

Jain NB, Higgins LD, Ozumba D et al (2005) Trends in epidemiology of knee arthroplasty in the United States, 1990–2000. Arthritis Rheum 52:3928–3933

Järvenpää J, Kettunen J, Soininvaara T, Miettinen H, Kröger H (2012) Obesity has a negative impact on clinical outcome after total knee arthroplasty. Scand J Surg 101(3):198–203

Johnston SS, Ammann E, Scamuffa R, Samuels J, Stokes A, Fegelman E et al (2020) Association of body mass index and osteoarthritis with healthcare expenditures and utilization. Obes Sci Pract 6(2):139–151. https://doi.org/10.1002/osp.398

Jones RE, Russell RD, Huo MH (2013) Wound healing in total joint replacement. Bone Joint J 95-B(11 Suppl A):144–147. https://doi.org/10.1302/0301-620X.95B11.32836

Kamath AF, McAuliffe CL, Kosseim LM, Hume E, Pio F (2016) Malnutrition in joint arthroplasty: prospective stud indicates risk of unplanned ICU admission. Arch Bone Jt Surg 4(2):128–131

Kerkhoffs GMMJ, Servien E, Dunn W, Dahm D, Bramer JAM, Haverkamp D (2012) The influence of obesity on the complication rate and outcome of total knee arthroplasty: a meta-analysis and systematic literature review. J Bone Joint Surg Am 94(20):1839–1844. https://doi.org/10.2106/JBJS.K.00820

Kievit AJ, van Geenen RC, Kuijer PP, Pahlplatz TM, Blankevoort L, Schafroth MU (2014) Total knee arthroplasty and the unforeseen impact on return to work: a cross-sectional multicenter survey. J Arthroplast 29(6):1163–1168

Kim T, Park K, Yoon S, Kim S, Chang C, Seong S (2009) Clinical value of regular passive ROM exercise by a physical therapist after total knee arthroplasty. Knee Surg Sports Traumatol Arthrosc 17(10):1152–1158

Kulkarni A, Jameson SS, James P, Woodcock S, Muller S, Reed MR (2011) Does bariatric surgery prior to lower limb joint replacement reduce complications? Surgeon 9(1):18–21. https://doi.org/10.1016/j.surge.2010.08.004

Lamplot JD, Bansal A, Nguyen JT, Brophy RH (2018) Risk of subsequent joint arthroplasty in contralateral or different joint after index shoulder, hip, or knee arthroplasty: association with index joint, demographics, and patient-specific factors. J Bone Joint Surg Am 100(20):1750–1756. https://doi.org/10.2106/JBJS.17.00948

Liu JX, Paoli AR, Mahure SA, Bosco J, Campbell KA (2020) Preoperative bariatric surgery utilization is associated with increased 90-day postoperative complication rates after total joint arthroplasty. J Am Acad Orthop Surg 28(5):e206–e212. https://doi.org/10.5435/JAAOS-D-18-00381

Mantilla CB, Horlocker TT, Schroeder DR, Berry DJ, Brown DL (2003) Risk factors for clinically relevant pulmonary embolism and deep venous thrombosis in patients undergoing primary hip or knee arthroplasty. Anesthesiology 99(3):552–560

Martin JR, Jennings JM, Dennis DA (2017) Morbid obesity and total knee arthroplasty. J Am Acad Orthop Surg 25(3):188–194. https://doi.org/10.5435/JAAOS-D-15-00684

McGonagle L, Convery-Chan L, DeCruz P et al (2019) Factors influencing return to work after hip and knee arthroplasty. J Orthop Traumatol 20:9. https://doi.org/10.1186/s10195-018-0515-x

McMahon M, Block JA (2003) The risk of contralateral total knee arthroplasty after knee replacement for osteoarthritis. J Rheumatol 30(8):1822–1824

Memtsoudis SG, Besculides MC, Gaber L, Liu S et al (2009) Risk factors for pulmonary embolism after hip and knee arthroplasty: a population-based study. Int Orthop 33(6):1739–1745. https://doi.org/10.1007/s00264-008-0659-z

Mulhall K, Ghomrawi H, Mihalko W, Cui Q, Saleh K (2010) Adverse effects of increased body mass index and weight on survivorship of total knee arthroplasty and subsequent outcomes of revision TKA. J Knee Surg 20(03):199–204

National Joint Registry 16th Annual Report (2019) Published 31 December 2019. NJR editorial board. Downloaded from https://reports.njrcentre.org.uk (7 Jan 2020)

Naziri Q, Issa K, Malkani AL, Bonutti PM, Harwin SF, Mont MA (2013) Bariatric orthopaedics: total knee arthroplasty in super-obese patients (BMI>kg/m^2). Survivorship and complications. Clin Orthop Relat Res 471(11):3523–3530. https://doi.org/10.1007/s11999-013-3154-9

Nishizaki K, Ikegami H, Tanaka Y, Imai R, Matsumura H (2015) Effects of supplementation with a combination of β-hydroxy-β-methyl butyrate, L-arginine, and L-glutamine on postoperative recovery of quadriceps muscle strength after total knee arthroplasty. Asia Pac J Clin Nutr 24(3):412–420. https://doi.org/10.6133/apjcn.2015.24.3.01

Odum SM, Springer BD, Dennos AC, Fehring TK (2013) National obesity trends in total knee arthroplasty. J Arthroplast 28(8 Suppl):148–151. https://doi.org/10.1016/j.arth.2013.02.036

Organisation for Economic Co-operation and Development (OECD) (2019) Health at a glance 2019: OECD indicators. OECD Publishing, Paris. https://doi.org/10.1787/4dd50c09-en

Pellegrini CA, Ledford G, Hoffman SA, Chang RW, Cameron KA (2017) Preferences and motivation for weight loss among knee replacement patients: implications for a patient-centered weight loss intervention. BMC Musculoskelet Disord 18(1):327. https://doi.org/10.1186/s12891-017-1687-x

Pongkunakorn A, Sawatphap D (2014) Use of drop and dangle rehabilitation protocol to increase knee flexion following total knee arthroplasty: a comparison with continuous passive motion machine. J Med Assoc Thail 97(Suppl 9):S16–S22

Ryan SP, Politzer C, Green C, Wellman S, Bolognesi M, Seyler T (2018) Albumin versus American society of anesthesiologists score: which is more predictive of complications following total joint arthroplasty? Orthopedics 41(6):354–362. https://doi.org/10.3928/01477447-20181010-05

Sahyoun NR, Hochberg MC, Helmick CG, Harris T, Pamuk ER (1999) Body mass index, weight change, and incidence of self-reported physician-diagnosed arthritis among women. Am J Public Health 89(3):391–394

Sattler LN, Hing WA, Vertullo CJ (2019) What is the evidence to support early supervised exercise therapy after primary total knee replacement? A systematic review and meta-analysis. BMC Musculoskelet Disord 20:42. https://doi.org/10.1186/s12891-019-2415-5

Sayeed Z, Anoushiravani AA, Simha S, Padela MT, Schafer P, Awad ME et al (2019) Markers for malnutrition and BMI status in total joint arthroplasty and pharmaconutrient therapy. JBJS Rev 7(5):1–9

Schroer WC, Diesfeld PJ, LeMarr AR, Morton DJ, Reedy ME (2018) Modifiable risk factors in primary joint arthroplasty increase 90-day cost of care. J Arthroplast 33(9):2740–2744

Sharma R, Ardebili MA, Abdulla IN (2019) Does rehabilitation before total knee arthroplasty benefit postoperative recovery? A systematic review. Indian J Orthop 53(1):138–147

Sloan M, Premkumar A, Sheth NP (2018) Projected volume of primary total joint arthroplasty in the U.S., 2014 to 2030. J Bone Joint Surg Am 100:1455–1460. https://doi.org/10.2106/JBJS.17.01617

Spicer DD, Pomeroy DL, Badenhausen WE, Schaper LA, Curry JI, Suthers KE et al (2001) Body mass index as a predictor of outcome in total knee replacement. Int Orthop 25(4):246–249

Springer BD, Carter JT, Mclawhorn AS, Scharf K, Roslin M, Kallies KJ et al (2017) Obesity and the role of bariatric surgery in the surgical management of osteoarthritis of the hip and knee: a review of the literature. Surg Obes Relat Dis 13(1):111–118. https://doi.org/10.1016/j.soard.2016.09.011

Sturm R (2007) Increases in morbid obesity in the USA: 2000–2005. Public Health 121(7):492–496

Sturm R, Hattori A (2013) Morbid obesity rates continue to rise rapidly in the United States. Int J Obes 37(6):889–891

Tappenden KA, Quatrara B, Parkhurst ML, Malone AM, Fanjiang G, Ziegler TR (2013) Critical role of nutrition in improving quality of care. JPEN J Parenter Enteral Nutr 37(4):482–497. https://doi.org/10.1177/0148607113484066

Tilbury C, Schaasberg W, Plevier JWM, Fiocco M, Nelissen RGHH, Vlieland V et al (2014) Return to work after total hip and knee arthroplasty: a systematic review. Rheumatology 53(3):512–525

Tobert CM, Mott SL, Nepple KG (2018) Malnutrition diagnosis during adult inpatient hospitalizations: analysis of a multi-institutional collaborative database of academic medical centers. J Acad Nutr Diet 118(1):125–131. https://doi.org/10.1016/j.jand.2016.12.019

Tsantes AG, Papadopoulos DV, Lytras T, Tsantes AE, Mavrogenis AF, Korompilias AV et al (2019) Association of malnutrition with periprosthetic joint and surgical site infections after total joint arthroplasty: a systematic review and meta-analysis. J Hosp Infect 103(1):69–77. https://doi.org/10.1016/j.jhin.2019.04.020

van Zaanen Y, van Geenen RCI, Pahlplatz TMJ (2019) Three out of ten working patients expect no clinical improvement of their ability to perform work-related knee-demanding activities after total knee arthroplasty: a multicenter study. J Occup Rehabil 29:585–594. https://doi.org/10.1007/s10926-018-9823-5

Vielgut I, Leitner L, Kastner N, Radl R, Leithner A, Sadoghi P (2016) Sports activity after low-contact stress total knee arthroplasty – a long term follow-up study. Sci Rep 6:24630. https://doi.org/10.1038/srep24630

Wagner ER, Kamath AF, Fruth K, Harmsen WS, Berry DJ (2016) Effect of body mass index on reoperation and complications after total knee arthroplasty. J Bone Joint Surg Am 98(24):2052–2060. https://doi.org/10.2106/JBJS.16.00093

Waters DL, Ward AL, Villareal DT (2013) Weight loss in obese adults 65years and older: a review of the controversy. Exp Gerontol 48(10):1054–1061. https://doi.org/10.1016/j.exger.2013.02.005

Werner BC, Evans CL, Carothers JT, Browne JA (2015a) Primary total knee arthroplasty in super-obese patients: dramatically higher postoperative complication rates even compared to revision surgery. J Arthroplast 30(5):849–853

Werner BC, Kurkis GM, Gwathmey FW, Browne JA (2015b) Bariatric surgery prior to total knee arthroplasty is associated with fewer postoperative complications. J Arthroplast 30(9 Suppl):81–85. https://doi.org/10.1016/j.arth.2014.11.039

Winiarsky R, Barth P, Lotke P (1998) Total knee arthroplasty in morbidly obese patients. J Bone Joint Surg Am 80(12):1770–1774

Workgroup of the American Association of Hip and Knee Surgeons Evidence Based Committee (2013) Obesity and total joint arthroplasty. J Arthroplast 28(5):714–721. https://doi.org/10.1016/j.arth.2013.02.011

World Health Organisation (WHO) (2018) [Internet] https://www.who.int/news-room/fact-sheets/detail/malnutrition (Last updated 16 February 2018) (Last accessed 28 March 2020)

Zainul-abidin S, Amanatullah DF, Anderson MB, Barretto M, Battenberg A, Austin M et al (2019) General assembly, prevention, host related general: proceedings of international consensus on orthopedic infections. J Arthroplast 34(2S):S13–S35. https://doi.org/10.1016/j.arth.2018.09.050

Zeni JA, Snyder-Mackler L, Snyder-Mackler L (2010) Most patients gain weight in the 2 years after total knee arthroplasty: comparison to a healthy control group. Osteoarthr Cartil 18(4):510–514. https://doi.org/10.1016/j.joca.2009.12.005

The Microbiome of the Joint

Samuel J. Clarkson, Karan Goswami, and Javad Parvizi

Contents

E. Hansen, K.-D. Kühn (eds.), *Essentials of Cemented Knee Arthroplasty*,
https://doi.org/10.1007/978-3-662-63113-3_10

10.1 Microbiome Overview

Over the past several decades, it has become clear that the microorganisms that reside in ecological niches of the human body play an important role in health and disease (Byrd et al. 2018; Cho and Blaser 2012; Davenport et al. 2017; Young 2017). This community of microorganisms comprises part of what is known as the human microbiome, a term that encompasses the composition of all microbial genes in a community, as well as host epithelium, immune components, and both host and microbe metabolites (Byrd et al. 2018; Young 2017). In all, the human microbiome is estimated to contain over 10^{13} cells, outnumbering human cells by 10:1 according to some estimates (Sender et al. 2016). Bacteria, especially in the digestive tract, have been by far the most studied component of the microbiome. However, other organisms including fungi, viruses, and protozoa all play important roles. Moreover, the specific composition of species differs vastly in different areas of the body (Cho and Blaser 2012).

The study of the microbiome has taken off in large part due to improvements in the ability of new technologies to characterize the diverse array of microorganisms. Prior to DNA sequencing technology, our ability to identify the multitude of species was limited as standard culturing techniques are unable to detect over 80% of the microorganisms within the human microbiome (Clemente et al. 2018; Eckburg et al. 2005). Utilizing the relative consistency of the 16S rRNA subunit of the bacterial genome, culture-independent approaches have allowed researchers to rapidly sequence the enormous amount of genetic data contained within a given sample (Clemente et al. 2018; Goswami and Parvizi 2020; Hodkinson and Grice 2015). For example, technologies based on polymerase chain reaction (PCR) were groundbreaking in detecting and classifying components of the human genome and microbiome, as well as diagnosing infections in a clinical context. However, PCR is limited by its relatively low sensitivity and reliance on preconceived primer targets. In more recent years, non-Sanger-based high throughput DNA sequencing methods, collectively referred to as next-generation sequencing (NGS), have shown promise in its ability to quickly and accurately characterize all microbial DNA in a given sample without suffering from the limitations inherent to PCR (Goswami et al. 2018; Goswami and Parvizi 2020).

10.2 Clinical Significance of Microbiome

The advances as described have begun to provide researchers with a more comprehensive picture of the human microbiome. This work has made it clear, in recent decades, that characteristics of specific components of the microbiome are linked to certain pathologies. In particular, the microbiome of the digestive tract has been studied extensively. Within the realm of infectious diseases, there is an increased understanding that the composition of the gut microbiome mediates resistance to colonization of invasive species.

> As such an indirect path to infection can be exploited by certain species when dysbiosis occurs.

A prominent example is the ability of *Clostridium difficile* to colonize and cause disease in individuals whose microbiome has been affected by the administration of antibiotics (Libertucci and Young 2019). There is also substantial evidence of the microbiome's role in oncogenesis within the digestive tract, including associations with the development of gastric adenocarcinoma (Atherton and Blaser 2009), esophageal adenocarcinoma (Atherton and Blaser 2009), and colorectal carcinoma (Castellarin et al. 2012; Kostic et al. 2012).

The effect of the gut microbiome is not limited to local organs. Through regulation of nutritional absorption, regulation of the gut's immune system, and translocation of microbes into the systemic circulation, the composition of the microbiome influences disease systemically and at specific distant organs (Hernandez 2017). Variations have been implicated in a wide array of diseases, including cardiovascular disease (Wang et al. 2011), obesity (Ley et al. 2005; Turnbaugh et al. 2006), psychiatric illness (Bravo et al. 2011; Dinan and Cryan 2013), multiple sclerosis (Clemente et al. 2018), and systemic lupus erythematosus (Clemente et al. 2018). Of note, there is also evidence to support the influence of the gut microbiome on bone and joint diseases such as inflammatory arthritis, osteoarthritis, and osteoporosis (Clemente et al. 2018; Hernandez 2017; Hernandez et al. 2019; Scher et al. 2016).

10.3 Microbiome in "Sterile" Compartments

> The microbiome of the digestive tract, skin, and other locations are considered to be commensal and consistent with normal physiology. Disruptions in the composition of the microbiome lead to disease, not the mere existence of organisms.

In contrast, there are many areas of the body, such as joints, that are traditionally considered to be sterile. Detection of microorganisms in these locations is often considered contaminants or markers of specific pathologies that have developed due to immune suppression or implantation of a foreign material (Rohde and Goswami n.d.).

> However, it is important to approach the concept of a "sterile" compartment with a degree of hesitation, as historically the concept has been challenged in various fields.

The idea that the bladder was devoid of any physiologic microorganisms was a dogma dating back to initial germ theory research in the mid-1800s. This was not challenged until the 1950s, and since then it has become accepted that the bladder contains a microbiome similar to the digestive tract. It is the overall composition and balance of this microbiome that confers pathology and disease, not simply a threshold of the number of bacteria (Thomas-White et al. 2016).

More recent work has also challenged assumptions of the sterility of other organs. Sequencing technologies have allowed researchers insight into the native microbiome of the subepidermal skin (Nakatsuji et al. 2013), cerebrospinal fluid (Perlejewski et al. 2016), breast tissue (Hieken et al. 2016; McGuire and McGuire 2017; Urbaniak et al. 2016), and the lung (Berger and Wunderink 2013; Charlson et al. 2011; Segal et al. 2013). Similar to investigations into the gut microbiome, these studies have identified associations of the composition of each microbiome to malignancies and other pathologies related to each organ.

10.4 Chronic Colonization of the Native Joint

> This assumption of sterility has also been challenged within orthopedics. Specifically, recent literature has suggested that there may be a reason to question the sterility of joint fluid and tissue.

One area of interest has been the microbial composition of the shoulder, stemming from investigations into periprosthetic joint infections caused by *Cutibacterium acnes*. *C. acnes* is a commensal species of skin flora and is a common cause of infection following shoulder arthroplasty. Data from revision cases estimate that *C. acnes* is found in 19% to 70% of infected shoulders (Hudek et al. 2014). However, it has been suggested that a proportion of these results represent false positives, leading researchers to investigate the microbial composition of non-infected shoulders (Frangiamore et al. 2015; Mook et al. 2015).

Multiple studies have identified *C. acnes* in the native joint of individuals who have never undergone shoulder surgery, suggesting that *C. acnes* is a commensal organism in this location, and infections may be a result of the opportunistic expansion of the organism (Hudek et al. 2014; Levy et al. 2013; Mook et al. 2015; Rao et al. 2020). This is complicated by the findings of Qiu et al. (Qiu et al. 2018), who found in a series of 23 patients undergoing primary shoulder arthroplasty, no *C. acnes* was found in shoulder tissue after stringent removal of contamination. They concluded that *C. acnes* infections are derived from skin contamination rather than opportunistic expansion. Interestingly, they did note DNA from *Acinetobacter*species and the Oxalobacteraceae family, indicating the possibility of a microbiome other than *C. acnes*.

In all, investigations into the shoulder have found the presence of a microbiome, although the possibility of skin contamination remains under question. Further complicating the picture, it must be noted that the samples obtained in these studies are not taken from individuals with healthy shoulders, but rather taken from patients with indications for primary arthroplasty. It is possible that an osteoarthritic shoulder contains microorganisms that a healthy shoulder does not, and some have postulated that the presence of bacteria, in fact, represents the pathogenesis of osteoarthritis (Hudek et al. 2014; Levy et al. 2013; Mook et al. 2015).

Alongside these studies examining the microbiome of the shoulder, recent literature in total knee arthroplasty (TKA) and total hip arthroplasty (THA) has identified organisms using molecular technologies in these native joints. In a 2018 study investigating the potential of NGS in diagnosing culture-negative PJI, Tarabichi et al. (Tarabichi et al. 2018a) noted organisms present in 35% of 17 control patients undergoing primary TKA or THA. Also using NGS, Torchia, et al. (Torchia et al. 2020) found that 30% of 40 patients undergoing primary TKA had at least one positive organism identified. Two further studies, both using PCR-based methods, found evidence of a microbiome in native hips and knees. Jacovides et al. (Jacovides et al. 2012) identified organisms from the knee joint in five out of seven patients undergoing TKA, and Témoin et al. (Témoin et al. 2012) detected organisms in 13.9% of 36 native knees and hips in patients with osteoarthritis and rheumatoid arthritis undergoing joint aspiration in an office setting.

Most recently, a multicenter study of 14 academic institutions recruited patients undergoing primary joint arthroplasty. Analyzing samples from 53 patients undergoing TKA and 30 patients undergoing THA, this multicenter workgroup found a rich diversity of microbes after removal of reagent contamination. The three most abundant genera identified in the hip samples were *Escherichia*, *Cutibacterium*, and *Acinetobacter*. Also of note, this microbial composition was present irrespective of the type of specimen sampled (synovial fluid vs. tissue vs. swabs; $p = 0.80$). Furthermore, while microbiota in hips versus knees were noted to be statistically different ($F = 2.86$; $p = 0.001$), the joint type explained <1% of overall compositional variation (Goswami 2019).

> The data supporting a microbiome of the hip and knee are convincing.

While skin contamination is a possibility, as in the discussion of the shoulder, the species found in studies of the hip and knee make this an unlikely explanation. All studies mentioned above report the identification of organisms present in the gut microbiome. For example, the two aforementioned studies (Goswami 2019; Torchia et al. 2020) recognized the most predominant organism as *E. Coli*—an intestinal commensal organism and unlikely to represent a contaminant.

As in the shoulder, the possibility remains that findings in the hip and knee do not represent a truly physiologic microbiome. Samples obtained from patients undergoing primary joint arthroplasty are invariably taken from joints with some amount of arthropathy. The native joint of a truly healthy individual may not be represented by this population, and therefore further study is needed.

10.5 Colonization of Native/Implanted Joint Without Evidence of Disease

The presence of a joint microbiome as suggested above needs to be examined in the context of our current understanding of chronic joint colonization. In the presence of an implanted device, chronic persistent colonization can often occur, and the hallmark of most periprosthetic joint infections is the infiltration of skin microbiota into the joint. The same properties that allow organisms such as *S. aureus* and *S. epidermitis* to flourish on the skin result in the formation of a biofilm that forms on the surface of many devices. Biofilm formation prevents penetration of antibiotics and host immune-mediated clearance, allowing the microorganisms to persist as a chronic and persistent infection (Scherr et al. 2014).

> Despite this clear mechanism involving the contamination by skin microbiota, the suggestion of a native joint microbiome as described above indicates that chronic colonization can exist without any signs of infection.

This is consistent with multiple studies that have detected biofilm formation on hardware explanted due to aseptic loosening, with a lack of a diagnosed infection (Bereza et al. 2017; Cazanave et al. 2013; Dempsey et al. 2007; Holinka et al. 2011; Rak et al. 2016). However, it remains unclear whether colonization of these implants can be considered truly asymptomatic colonization of a device. While not diagnosed as PJI based on our current standards of diagnosis, it has been postulated that aseptic loosening could represent an unrecognized low-grade infection that has simply not yet presented itself (Hudek et al. 2014; Levy et al. 2013). Further research should include patients who are fully asymptomatic with implants in situ (Rohde and Goswami n.d.). With that caveat, the established presence of chronic colonization in both native and presumably aseptic hardware indicates the possibility that a microbiome can exist physiologically without necessarily causing disease.

10.6 Implications for PJI

Periprosthetic joint infection (PJI) is the most common reason for revision of failed total knee arthroplasty, and the third most common reason for revision of failed total hip arthroplasty (Bozic et al. 2009; Bozic et al. 2010). Given the effects on morbidity and mortality as well as the associated healthcare costs, determining methods to accurately diagnose and treat PJI is of utmost importance (Goswami et al. 2018).

The same advances in molecular technologies that have made the study of the microbiome possible have demonstrated utility in diagnosing PJI. In particular, the increased sensitivity of next-generation sequencing can provide a much clearer picture of the microorganisms colonizing an infected joint (Tarabichi et al. 2018b). Current methods for diagnosing PJI rely on cultured tissue, but culture is unsuccessful in identifying an organism in 7–50% of PJI cases (Goswami and Parvizi 2020), causing patients to be subjected to unnecessary broad-spectrum antibiotics and worse outcomes (Mortazavi et al. 2011). Recent studies have shown that NGS can identify microorganisms in the hip and knee for culture-negative infections (Street et al. 2017; Tarabichi et al. 2018a; Tarabichi et al. 2018b). However, the possibility of a native joint microbiome as discussed in this chapter necessitates a cautioned approach when interpreting these results. It is plausible that some of the increased sensitivity of NGS is simply due to detecting organisms that are present in the native joint, and do not represent organisms causing disease.

The joint microbiome also has important implications on the prevention of PJI, particularly regarding the timing of steroid injections. While steroid injections in the hip and knee are a valuable treatment for symptomatic osteoarthritis (Jüni et al. 2015; Zhong et al. 2020), evidence points to an increased risk of PJI if performed shortly after administration (Richardson et al. 2019; Werner et al. 2016).

> As such, current recommendations suggest avoiding primary joint arthroplasty within a few months of ipsilateral steroid injection (Cizmic et al. 2019). The presence of a joint microbiome bolsters this recommendation.

There is evidence that steroids alter the microbiome in other niches of the body (Tetel et al. 2018), and recent evidence suggests that the joint microbiome is similarly altered. In 2015, Mook et al. (2015) found that an increased number of preoperative corticosteroid injections prior to shoulder arthroplasty is associated with a higher likelihood of bacterial growth in the native shoulder. Recent findings also suggest that the composition of the microbiome is altered when analyzed within 6 months following steroid injection (Goswami 2019). These findings strengthen the recommendation to avoid primary joint arthroplasty during this window and suggests a specific pathogenetic pathway as the cause.

▪ Conclusion

Emerging evidence suggests that a microbiome may exist in native, osteoarthritic, and implanted joints. NGS has shown potential in both characterizing this microbiome and identifying organisms when a true infection occurs. We now have a comprehensive means of identifying organisms in the native joint, infected joints with negative cultures, as well as implanted joints assumed to be non-infected. Continuing to identify the composition of the native joint microbiome will be crucial to our ability to differentiate signal from noise when an infection is suspected.

Take-Home Messages

- The human microbiome, which consists of all microorganisms residing in ecological niches of the human body, outnumbers human cells and plays an important role in health and disease.
- Technological advances in DNA sequencing have allowed researchers to rapidly characterize large amounts of genomic data and take an in-depth look into the composition of the microbiome.
- While the microbiome of the digestive tract, skin, and other locations are considered commensal and consistent with normal physiology, there are many areas of the body such as joints that are traditionally considered to be sterile.
- The assumption of the sterility of the native joint has been challenged, with recent literature demonstrating evidence of a commensal microbiome in the shoulder, hip, and knee.
- Recent literature suggests that disruptions in the native microbiome could play a role in the development of osteoarthritis, and a patient's susceptibility to periprosthetic joint infection.

References

Atherton JC, Blaser MJ (2009) Coadaptation of helicobacter pylori and humans: ancient history, modern implications. J Clin Invest 119:2475–2487

Bereza PL, Ekiel A, Auguściak-Duma A, Aptekorz M, Wilk I, Wojciechowski P et al (2017) Identification of asymptomatic prosthetic joint infection: microbiologic and operative treatment outcomes. Surg Infect 18:582–587

Berger G, Wunderink RG (2013) Lung microbiota: genuine or artifact? Isr Med Assoc J 15:3

Bozic KJ, Kurtz SM, Lau E, Ong K, Vail TP, Berry DJ (2009) The epidemiology of revision total hip arthroplasty in the United States. J Bone Joint Surg Am 91:128–133

Bozic KJ, Kurtz SM, Lau E, Ong K, Chiu V, Vail TP et al (2010) The epidemiology of revision total knee arthroplasty in the United States. Clin Orthop Relat Res 468:45–51

Bravo JA, Forsythe P, Chew MV, Escaravage E, Savignac HM, Dinan TG et al (2011) Ingestion of Lactobacillus strain regulates emotional behavior and central GABA receptor expression in a mouse via the vagus nerve. PNAS 108:16050–16055

Byrd AL, Belkaid Y, Segre JA (2018) The human skin microbiome. Nat Rev Microbiol 16:143–155

Castellarin M, Warren RL, Freeman JD, Dreolini L, Krzywinski M, Strauss J et al (2012) Fusobacterium nucleatum infection is prevalent in human colorectal carcinoma. Genome Res 22:299–306

Cazanave C, Greenwood-Quaintance KE, Hanssen AD, Karau MJ, Schmidt SM, Gomez Urena EO et al (2013) Rapid molecular microbiologic diagnosis of prosthetic joint infection. J Clin Microbiol 51:2280–2287

Charlson ES, Bittinger K, Haas AR, Fitzgerald AS, Frank I, Yadav A et al (2011) Topographical continuity of bacterial populations in the healthy human respiratory tract. Am J Respir Crit Care Med 184:957–963

Cho I, Blaser MJ (2012) The human microbiome: at the interface of health and disease. Nat Rev Genet 13:260–270

Cizmic Z, Feng JE, Huang R, Iorio R, Komnos G, Kunutsor SK et al (2019) Hip and knee section, prevention, host related: proceedings of international consensus on orthopedic infections. J Arthroplast 34:S255–S270

Clemente JC, Manasson J, Scher JU (2018) The role of the gut microbiome in systemic inflammatory disease. BMJ 360:j5145. Available from: https://www.bmj.com/content/360/bmj.j5145

Davenport ER, Sanders JG, Song SJ, Amato KR, Clark AG, Knight R (2017) The human microbiome in evolution. BMC Biol 15:127

Dempsey KE, Riggio MP, Lennon A, Hannah VE, Ramage G, Allan D et al (2007) Identification of bacteria on the surface of clinically infected and non-infected prosthetic hip joints removed during revision arthroplasties by 16S rRNA gene sequencing and by microbiological culture. Arthritis Res Ther 9:R46

Dinan TG, Cryan JF (2013) Melancholic microbes: a link between gut microbiota and depression? Neurogastroenterol Motil 25:713–719

Eckburg PB, Bik EM, Bernstein CN, Purdom E, Dethlefsen L, Sargent M et al (2005) Diversity of the human intestinal microbial flora. Science 308:1635–1638

Frangiamore SJ, Saleh A, Grosso MJ, Alolabi B, Bauer TW, Iannotti JP et al (2015) Early versus late culture growth of Propionibacterium acnes in revision shoulder arthroplasty. J Bone Joint Surg Am 97:1149–1158

Goswami K, Parvizi, Javad A (2019) Orthopedic genomic workgroup J. Microbiome of the osteoarthritic hip and knee joint: a prospective multicenter investigation. In: American Association of Hip and Knee Surgeons Annual Meeting, Dallas, TX
Goswami K, Parvizi J (2020) Culture-negative periprosthetic joint infection: is there a diagnostic role for next-generation sequencing? Expert Rev Mol Diagn 20:269–272
Goswami K, Parvizi J, Maxwell CP (2018) Current recommendations for the diagnosis of acute and chronic PJI for hip and knee—cell counts, alpha-defensin, leukocyte esterase, next-generation sequencing. Curr Rev Musculoskelet Med 11: 428–438
Hernandez CJ (2017) The microbiome and bone and joint disease. Curr Rheumatol Rep 19:77
Hernandez CJ, Yang X, Ji G, Niu Y, Sethuraman AS, Koressel J et al (2019) Disruption of the gut microbiome increases the risk of periprosthetic joint infection in mice. Clin Orthop Relat Res 477:2588–2598
Hieken TJ, Chen J, Hoskin TL, Walther-Antonio M, Johnson S, Ramaker S et al (2016) The microbiome of aseptically collected human breast tissue in benign and malignant disease. Sci Rep 6:1–10
Hodkinson BP, Grice EA (2015) Next-generation sequencing: a review of technologies and tools for wound microbiome research. Adv Wound Care (New Rochelle) 4(1):50–58. Available from: https://www.liebertpub.com/doi/abs/10.1089/wound.2014.0542
Holinka J, Bauer L, Hirschl AM, Graninger W, Windhager R, Presterl E (2011) Sonication cultures of explanted components as an add-on test to routinely conducted microbiological diagnostics improve pathogen detection. J Orthop Res 29:617–622
Hudek R, Sommer F, Kerwat M, Abdelkawi AF, Loos F, Gohlke F (2014) Propionibacterium acnes in shoulder surgery: true infection, contamination, or commensal of the deep tissue? J Shoulder Elb Surg 23:1763–1771
Jacovides CL, Kreft R, Adeli B, Hozack B, Ehrlich GD, Parvizi J (2012) Successful identification of pathogens by polymerase chain reaction (PCR)-based electron spray ionization time-of-flight mass spectrometry (ESI-TOF-MS) in culture-negative periprosthetic joint infection. J Bone Joint Surg Am 94: 2247–2254
Jüni P, Hari R, Rutjes AW, Fischer R, Silletta MG, Reichenbach S et al (2015) Intra-articular corticosteroid for knee osteoarthritis. Cochrane Database Syst Rev (10):CD005328. Available from: https://www.cochranelibrary.com/cdsr/doi/10.1002/14651858.CD005328.pub3/abstract
Kostic AD, Gevers D, Pedamallu CS, Michaud M, Duke F, Earl AM et al (2012) Genomic analysis identifies association of Fusobacterium with colorectal carcinoma. Genome Res 22:292–298
Levy O, Iyer S, Atoun E, Peter N, Hous N, Cash D et al (2013) Propionibacterium acnes: an underestimated etiology in the pathogenesis of osteoarthritis? J Shoulder Elb Surg 22:505–511
Ley RE, Bäckhed F, Turnbaugh P, Lozupone CA, Knight RD, Gordon JI (2005) Obesity alters gut microbial ecology. Proc Natl Acad Sci U S A 102:11070–11075
Libertucci J, Young VB (2019) The role of the microbiota in infectious diseases. Nat Microbiol 4:35–45
McGuire MK, McGuire MA (2017) Got bacteria? The astounding, yet not-so-surprising, microbiome of human milk. Curr Opin Biotechnol 44:63–68
Mook WR, Klement MR, Green CL, Hazen KC, Garrigues GE (2015) The incidence of Propionibacterium acnes in open shoulder surgery: a controlled diagnostic study. J Bone Joint Surg Am 97:957–963
Mortazavi SMJ, Vegari D, Ho A, Zmistowski B, Parvizi J (2011) Two-stage exchange arthroplasty for infected total knee arthroplasty: predictors of failure. Clin Orthop Relat Res 469:3049–3054
Nakatsuji T, Chiang H-I, Jiang SB, Nagarajan H, Zengler K, Gallo RL (2013) The microbiome extends to subepidermal compartments of normal skin. Nat Commun 4:1431
Perlejewski K, Bukowska-Ośko I, Nakamura S, Motooka D, Stokowy T, Płoski R et al (2016) Metagenomic analysis of cerebrospinal fluid from patients with multiple sclerosis. Adv Exp Med Biol 935:89–98
Qiu B, Al K, Pena-Diaz AM, Athwal GS, Drosdowech D, Faber KJ et al (2018) Cutibacterium acnes and the shoulder microbiome. J Shoulder Elb Surg 27:1734–1739
Rak M, KavčIč M, Trebše R, CőR A (2016) Detection of bacteria with molecular methods in prosthetic joint infection: sonication fluid better than periprosthetic tissue. Acta Orthop 87:339–345
Rao AJ, MacLean IS, Naylor AJ, Garrigues GE, Verma NN, Nicholson GP (2020) Next-generation sequencing for diagnosis of infection: is more sensitive really better? J Shoulder Elb Surg 29:20–26
Richardson SS, Schairer WW, Sculco TP, Sculco PK (2019) Comparison of infection risk with corticosteroid or hyaluronic acid injection prior to total knee arthroplasty. J Bone Joint Surg Am 101:112–118
Rohde H, Goswami K (n.d.) QUESTION 18: is there a distinct microbiome in the joints? 2
Scher JU, Littman DR, Abramson SB (2016) Review: microbiome in inflammatory arthritis and human rheumatic diseases. Arthritis Rheumatol 68:35–45
Scherr TD, Heim CE, Morrison JM, Kielian T (2014) Hiding in plain sight: interplay between staphylococcal biofilms and host immunity. Front Immunol 5:37. Available from: https://www.ncbi.nlm.nih.gov/pmc/articles/PMC3913997/
Segal LN, Alekseyenko AV, Clemente JC, Kulkarni R, Wu B, Chen H et al (2013) Enrichment of lung microbiome with supraglottic taxa is associated with increased pulmonary inflammation. Microbiome 1:19
Sender R, Fuchs S, Milo R (2016) Revised estimates for the number of human and bacteria cells in the body. PLoS Biol 14:e1002533
Street TL, Sanderson ND, Atkins BL, Brent AJ, Cole K, Foster D et al (2017) Molecular diagnosis of orthopedic-device-related infection directly from sonication fluid by metagenomic sequencing. J Clin Microbiol 55:2334–2347
Tarabichi M, Shohat N, Goswami K, Alvand A, Silibovsky R, Belden K et al (2018a) Diagnosis of Periprosthetic joint infection: the potential of next-generation sequencing. J Bone Joint Surg Am 100:147–154
Tarabichi M, Shohat N, Goswami K, Parvizi J (2018b) Can next generation sequencing play a role in detecting pathogens in synovial fluid? Bone Joint J 100-B:127–133
Témoin S, Chakaki A, Askari A, El-Halaby A, Fitzgerald S, Marcus RE et al (2012) Identification of oral bacterial DNA in synovial fluid of patients with arthritis with native and failed prosthetic joints. J Clin Rheumatol 18:117–121
Tetel MJ, de Vries GJ, Melcangi RC, Panzica G, O'Mahony SM (2018) Steroids, stress and the gut microbiome-brain axis. J Neuroendocrinol 30:e12548
Thomas-White K, Brady M, Wolfe AJ, Mueller ER (2016) The bladder is not sterile: history and current discoveries on the urinary microbiome. Curr Bladder Dysfunct Rep 11:18–24
Torchia MT, Amakiri I, Werth P, Moschetti W (2020) Characterization of native knee microorganisms using next-generation sequencing in patients undergoing primary total knee arthroplasty. Knee 27(3):1113–1119
Turnbaugh PJ, Ley RE, Mahowald MA, Magrini V, Mardis ER, Gordon JI (2006) An obesity-associated gut microbiome with increased capacity for energy harvest. Nature 444:1027–1031

Urbaniak C, Gloor GB, Brackstone M, Scott L, Tangney M, Reid G (2016) The microbiota of breast tissue and its association with breast cancer. Appl Environ Microbiol 82:5039–5048

Wang Z, Klipfell E, Bennett BJ, Koeth R, Levison BS, Dugar B et al (2011) Gut flora metabolism of phosphatidylcholine promotes cardiovascular disease. Nature 472:57–63

Werner BC, Cancienne JM, Browne JA (2016) The timing of total hip arthroplasty after intraarticular hip injection affects postoperative infection risk. J Arthroplast 31:820–823

Young VB (2017) The role of the microbiome in human health and disease: an introduction for clinicians. BMJ 356:j831. Available from: https://www.bmj.com/content/356/bmj.j831

Zhong H-M, Zhao G-F, Lin T, Zhang X-X, Li X-Y, Lin J-F et al (2020) Intra-articular steroid injection for patients with hip osteoarthritis: a systematic review and meta-analysis. Biomed Res Int 2020:e6320154. Available from: https://www.hindawi.com/journals/bmri/2020/6320154/

Radiographs and Outcomes

Contents

Radiographic Analysis of Knee Arthritis

Musa B. Zaid and Jeffrey Barry

Contents

E. Hansen, K.-D. Kühn (eds.), *Essentials of Cemented Knee Arthroplasty*,
https://doi.org/10.1007/978-3-662-63113-3_11

11.1 Introduction

As emphasized in this chapter, osteoarthritis (OA), and specifically OA of the knee, represents a growing global healthcare burden. OA of the knee encompasses a broad range of etiologies from primary (idiopathic) to secondary causes such as the following:
- Post-traumatic.
- Dysplastic.
- Infectious.
- Osteonecrosis.
- Inflammatory.

Because of this diverse pathogenesis, defining OA is often difficult but has broadly been defined as "a heterogenous group of conditions that leads to joint symptoms and signs which are associated with defective integrity of articular cartilage, in addition to related changes in the underlying bone and at the joint margins" (Altman et al. 1986). Diagnosis of knee OA is crucial to the delivery of appropriate treatment. Typically, a clinical diagnosis of OA synthesizes the patient-reported history with a physical exam and concordant radiographic findings.

Imaging plays a vital role in the entire care continuum of knee OA.

11

> Radiographs aid the physician in confirming the diagnosis, determining the compartments of the knee involved and severity, as well as assisting in presurgical planning and outcome prediction and postoperative implant surveillance.

Numerous imaging modalities are used diagnostically in knee OA including the following:
- Plain radiographs (XR).
- Magnetic resonance imaging (MRI).
- Computed tomography (CT) scans.

The purpose of this chapter is to highlight the uses of the aforementioned imaging modalities in the diagnosis and treatment and surveillance of knee arthritis as well as correlate preoperative imaging findings with postoperative total knee arthroplasty (TKA) outcomes.

11.2 Plain Radiographs

Plain radiographs are the mainstay of diagnostic imaging for knee OA. For the majority of cases, they should be the only imaging required throughout the care pathway.

> Plain radiographs are non-invasive, low-cost, low-radiation, readily obtainable, and have been validated as a diagnostic tool for determining cartilage wear and OA severity (Buckland-Wright et al. 1995).

Cartilage, being uncalcified, is radiolucent on conventional X-rays. XR imaging provides an indirect measurement of cartilage thickness and subsequently cartilage wear via the radiolucent joint space between the bone of two subchondral surfaces.

11.2.1 Technique

A knee OA plain radiograph series should include at a minimum the following *four standard views*:
- A weight-bearing anterior–posterior view.
- A 45-degreeposteroanterior flexion weight-bearing view.
- A lateral view.
- Apatellofemoral view (Fig. 11.1).

Each provides the clinician with different information that can guide treatment options and surgical decision-making.

Other views that are sometimes incorporated into clinical practice include the following:
- Full-extension anteroposterior.
- Varus/valgus stress.
- Full-limb alignment radiographs.

Consistent technique must be utilized when obtaining radiographs of the knee to allow for reproducibility in assessment and interpretation.

The *45-degree flexion weight-bearing posteroanterior view* (Fig. 11.1b) (also known as a Rosenberg view) is obtained with the patient standing upright with 45° of knee flexion (Rosenberg et al. 1988). The imaging beam should be angled 10–20° caudal, a small amount distal to the proximal pole of the patella, and centered on the knee joint. In this view, the tibial plateau should be clearly visualized without any superimposition and the intercondylar notch should be clearly visualized without any overlap of the femoral condyles. The *posteroanterior projection* should be used to determine the degree of medial and lateral joint space narrowing as well as tibiofemoral alignment. Weight-bearing PA radiographs allow for improved visualization of the anterior femoral condyle. This view can be useful in patients with isolated medial compartment osteoarthritis as the wear is predominantly located in the anteromedial femoral condyle (Weidow et al. 2002).

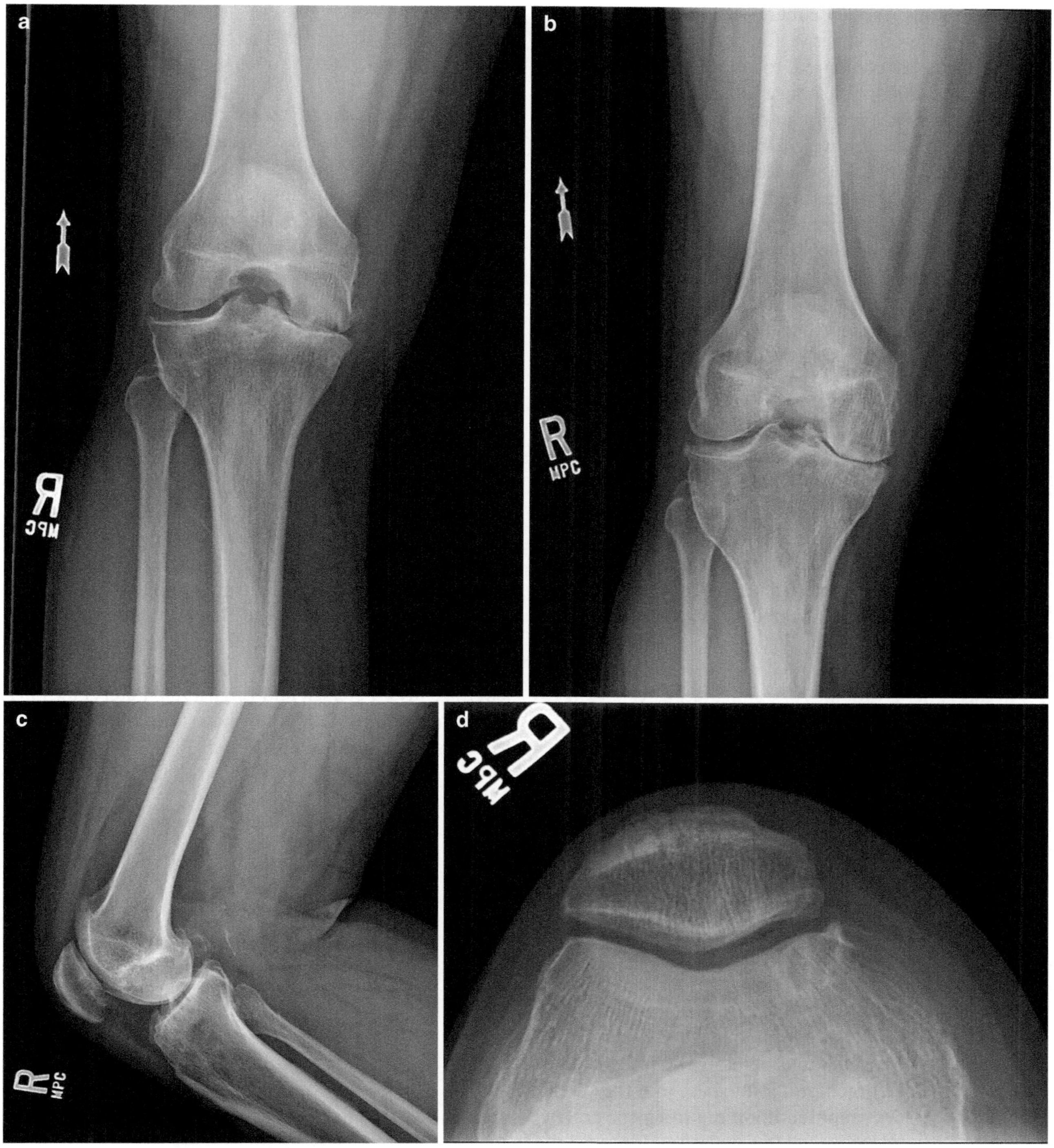

Fig. 11.1 Standard preoperative radiographs consisting of a weight-bearing PA view **a**, Rosenberg view **b**, lateral view **c**, and patello-femoral view **d**. Joint space narrowing, osteophyte formation, and cystic changes are characteristic of osteoarthritis

Placing the knee in flexion allows for improved visualization of the central and posterior aspects of the femoral condyles, which are more involved in advanced osteoarthritis as compared to the anterior medial femoral condyles (Bae et al. 2010), which are typically involved in isolated medial compartment osteoarthritis (Weidow et al. 2002). This flexed position allows for contact between the tibial plateau and the central to posterior aspect of the femoral condyles providing a true estimate of cartilage wear in the most commonly affected areas (Buckland-Wright 1995). Numerous studies have demonstrated that the degree of joint space narrowing can be significantly underestimated if the knee is locked in full extension as the femoral condyles can appear artificially elevated when sitting up on the anterior cartilage rim of the tibia (Messieh et al. 1990; Rueckl et al. 2018).

Because of this, the Rosenberg view has been demonstrated to be more sensitive for detecting tibiofemoral osteoarthritis as compared to an extension AP view (Ritchie et al. 2004; Fontboté et al. 2008).

The *lateral knee image* can be obtained in the supine position and be non-weight-bearing with the X-ray beam passing through the knee from medial to lateral. Alternatively, weight-bearing films can be utilized. In a well-performed lateral image of the knee, the medial and lateral femoral condyle should evenly overlap one another and the patellofemoral joint should be free of superimposition. The lateral projection is typically useful for assessing patellofemoral engagement, height, and osteoarthritis of the patellofemoral joint (Carrillon 2008).

Additionally, the lateral projection can be useful for surgical planning as it allows for the determination of the native posterior tibial slope.

The lateral radiograph can help diagnose anteromedial osteoarthritis of the knee, which is a common pattern of arthritis where posteromedial cartilage remains intact but the anteromedialtibial cartilage is eroded and worn (White et al. 1991).

In this pattern, with the ACL still intact a flexion lateral will demonstrate correction of the extension varus deformity as the femur rolls back onto the intact posterior tibial cartilage.

This pattern of arthritis can be successfully treated with unicompartmental knee replacements.

A *patellofemoral view* or tangential view of the patellofemoral joint can be performed in several ways. The most typical is the Merchant view which is done with the patient supine and the knee held in 45° of flexion. The X-ray beam is then positioned at a 45° angle relative to the tibia and shot inferior to the superior providing an axial view of the patellofemoral joint. A well-performed patellofemoral image should demonstrate clear visualization of the patellofemoral joint space and the patella should not be superimposed upon the trochlear groove. This view is useful for assessing patellar tracking and the degree of patellofemoral arthritis that may be present. The patellofemoral projection is more sensitive for judging the degree of severe patellofemoral joint arthritis as compared to the lateral X-ray, however, both are poor for detecting early stages of patellofemoral osteoarthritis (McDonnell et al. 2009). Furthermore, the patellofemoral view can also provide information with regard to patellar tracking and whether or not any subluxation is present. In addition to the Merchant view, the "sunrise" view also provides a tangential view of the patellofemoral joint.

The main distinguishing feature between the Merchant and sunrise views is the amount of knee flexion that the image is obtained with.

While the knee is usually at 45° of flexion in a Merchant view, which better allows subtle maltracking, a sunrise view is usually a prone hyperflexion view past 90° and is less accurate in finding subtle issues.

In addition to the posterior–anterior bent, lateral, and patellofemoral views, some surgeons routinely obtain *full-length standing weight-bearing X-rays* (◘ Fig. 11.2) to determine lower extremity alignment for presurgical planning; however, the routine use of these images is controversial. Standing alignment images are obtained by having the patient stand upright in front of a long X-ray cassette with their hips centered, feet forward, or rotated slightly inward to allow for the patellae to face directly forward, and the knees not touching. The beam is shot in an anterior to posterior direction. A good quality standing alignment X-ray should clearly show the femoral heads, have the patellae centered, and the ankles should be clearly visualized. From this image, the mechanical and anatomic axis can be measured and used for surgical planning. While some studies have found a significant difference in the degree of deformity as measured on a standard PA image of the knee as compared to full-length X-rays (Petersen and Engh 1988; Patel et al. 1991; Odenbring et al. 1993), others have found this difference to be insignificant (McGrory et al. 2002).

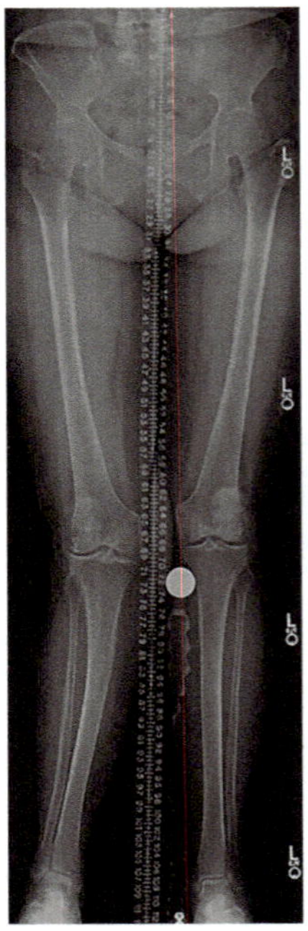

◘ **Fig. 11.2** Full-length standing alignment films can be useful in cases of deformity such as in the depicted image. Understanding the location and degree of deformity is critical to performing a well-functioning TKA

> Valgus stress radiographs of the knee have been described as a diagnostic option to assess the ability to correct varus knee deformity in patients with medial compartment osteoarthritis who may be candidates for medial unicompartmental knee arthroplasty (Argenson et al. 2002).

Similar to full-length standing radiographs, stress radiographs are not routinely obtained by all providers. To obtain this view, a firm valgus force is applied through the knee while the X-ray beam is shot from anterior to posterior (Waldstein et al. 2013). The utility of valgus stress radiographs is unknown as these radiographs do not significantly correlate to the amount of lateral compartment cartilage or the correctability of varus deformity (Waldstein et al. 2013). In theory, however, if the lateral compartment was to collapse on a valgus stress radiograph, the patient may not be an ideal candidate for medial unicompartmental knee arthroplasty.

11.3 Radiographic Grading

While a number of grading systems are utilized to quantify the severity of knee osteoarthritis as seen on plain radiographs, Kellgren–Lawrence (KL) is the most commonly used method to grade radiographic osteoarthritis severity (Braun and Gold 2011; Kellgren and Lawrence 1957). The KL system was first described in 1957 based on AP knee radiographs.

> The KL system combined their observed radiographic features of OA which included: osteophytes on the joint margin or tibial spines, narrowing of joint cartilage associated with sclerosis of subchondral bone, and small pseudocystic areas with sclerotic walls situated in subchondral bone (Kellgren and Lawrence 1957).

The system has become pervasive in orthopedic literature for research related to OA of many joints as well as useful in guiding clinical decision-making and outcome prediction. Even insurance companies will often require documentation of aspects of the KL classification prior to granting TKA and viscosupplementation injection authorization.

The KL grading system is shown in Table 11.1. Despite its wide adoption, studies have demonstrated a wide range of interobserver reliability of the KL grading system ranging from 0.51 to 0.89 (Wright 2014). Furthermore, a recent study found that the interclass correlation coefficient (ICC) of the KL grading system significantly varied based on the type of image that was being graded with a flexed posteroanterior X-ray having a higher ICC as compared to a fully extended anteroposterior X-ray (Wright et al. 2014).

Table 11.1 Kellgren–Lawrence grading system for knee osteoarthritis

Grade 0	No radiographic features of osteoarthritis are present.
Grade 1	Doubtful joint space narrowing and possible osteophyte formation
Grade 2	Definite osteophyte formation, possible joint space narrowing
Grade 3	Multiple osteophytes, definite joint space narrowing, sclerosis, possible deformity
Grade 4	Large osteophytes, marked joint space narrowing, severe sclerosis, definite deformity

In addition to the Kellgren–Lawrence grading system, a number of other radiographic grading systems exist (Table 11.2). Each of the grading systems assesses the degree of joint space narrowing as well as other identifiable characteristic osseous changes such as osteophytes. In a recent study, the International Knee Documentation Committee (IKDC) Classification had the most favorable combination of reliability and correlation to the severity of osteoarthritis as seen during arthroscopy (Wright et al. 2014).

11.4 Radiographic Assessment of Non-Osteoarthritic Arthritis

While the majority of patients who present to the arthroplasty clinic will have primary osteoarthritis, it is important for the provider to be able to critically assess radiographs to identify features that may suggest an alternative cause to the patient's arthritis such as an inflammatory process, trauma, or infection.

> The presence of bony erosions (Jacobson et al. 2008), which are a hallmark of inflammatory arthritis, can readily allow a clinician to differentiate between inflammatory and primary osteoarthritis.

Bony erosions in the setting of inflammatory arthritis typically occur at the margin of an inflamed joint in an area that is devoid of hyaline cartilage. In addition to bony erosions, inflammatory arthritis is also characterized by uniform joint space narrowing since cartilage destruction is uniform throughout the joint.

Rheumatoid arthritis is a common example of inflammatory arthritis. Radiographic features suggestive of rheumatoid arthritis include uniform joint space loss, bony erosions, soft tissue swelling, and periarticular osteopenia (Fig. 11.3) (Jacobson et al. 2008).

Table 11.2 Alternative radiographic grading systems for knee osteoarthritis

Grading system	Grade and characteristics				
IKDC	**A:** No JSN	**B:** Small osteophytes, slight sclerosis, > 4 mm joint space	**C:** 2–4 mm of joint space	**D:**< 2 mm joint space	
Fairbank	**0:** Normal	**1:** Squaring of tibia	**2:** Flattening of femoral condyles	**3:** Hypertrophic changes, JSN or both	**4:** Increased severity of all previously listed characteristics
Brandt	**0:**< 25% JSN	**1:**< 25% JSN with features (sclerosis, osteophytes) or 25–50% JSN without features	**2:** 25–50% JSN with features, 50–75% JSN without features	**3:** 50–75% JSN with features, or > 75% JSN without features	**4:**> 75% JSN with features
Ahlback	**0:** Normal	**1:** JSN without features	**2:** Obliteration of joint space	**3:** Bone loss <5 mm	**4:** Bone loss 5–10 mm
Jager–Wirth	**0:** Normal	**1:** Initial arthrosis, minimal JSN, small osteophytes	**2:** Moderate arthrosis, 50% JSN	**3:** Medium-grade arthrosis	**4:** Heavy-grade arthrosis

IKDC International Knee Documentation Committee, *JSN* joint space narrowing

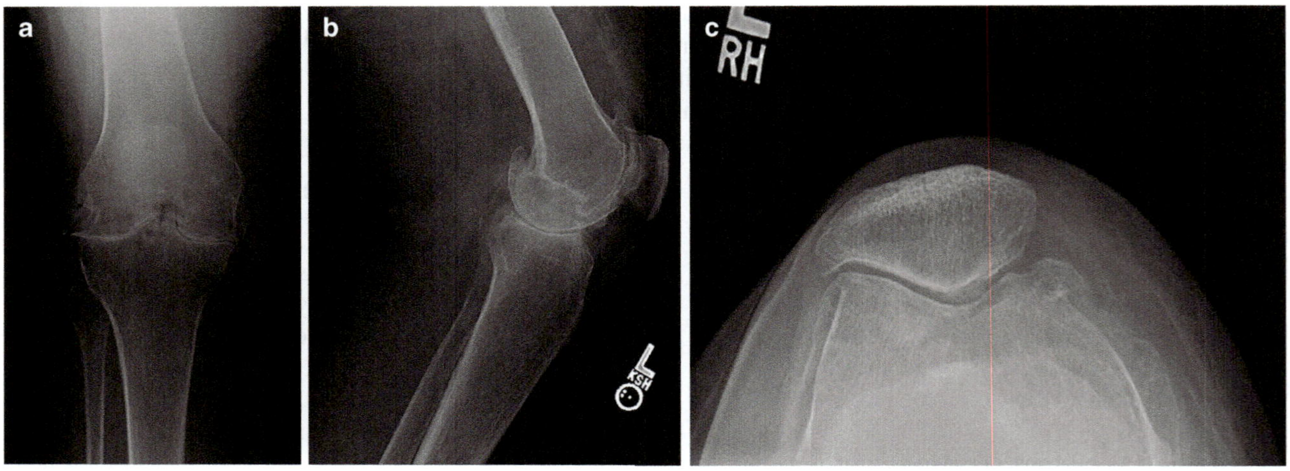

Fig. 11.3 **a–c** Radiographs demonstrating the characteristic appearance of rheumatoid arthritis with symmetric joint space narrowing, relatively minimal osteophyte formation, periarticular osteopenia, and cystic changes

Additionally, there tends to be a lack of bony proliferation (osteophyte formation) in patients with rheumatoid arthritis which may help further differentiate it from primary osteoarthritis (Jacobson et al. 2008).

Similar to rheumatoid arthritis, arthritis as the sequelae of a septic joint can be identified with uniform joint space narrowing, soft tissue swelling, and bony erosions. History is typically helpful in differentiating between rheumatoid and infectious arthritis as rheumatoid arthritis is polyarthritis while septic arthritis is typically monoarticular and the patient will describe a history of an infection.

A plain radiograph can offer diagnostic findings in addition to the standard patterns of wear. Clinicians should also be able to determine patterns of post-traumatic osteoarthritis of the knee on plain radiographs or ACL-deficient knee patterns (Johnson et al. 2017). Other diagnoses such as crystalline deposit disorders (calcium pyrophosphate disease [CPPD] or pseudogout and gout), retained hardware, bony and soft tissue tumors, avascular necrosis, osteochondral defects, vascular disease/calcifications, and congenital deformities are all apparent on plain radiographs.

11.5 Correlation of OA Severity and TKA Outcomes

Although TKA unquestionably can improve pain and function, there remains a subset of patients (up to 20%) who remain dissatisfied after TKA (Nilsdotter et al. 2009; Woolhead et al. 2005; Beswick et al. 2012). This group of unsatisfied patients remains an area of study within the arthroplasty community as we strive to maximize the benefit for our patients. Contributing factors that have been found to affect satisfaction postoperatively include patient-related (psychosocial and medical comorbidities), surgeon/healthcare-related (care access, rehabilitation, expectation management, and intraoperative technique such as soft tissue balancing and alignment), and disease-related (type of arthritis, preoperative severity, and deformity).

> Although there is a poor correlation between clinical symptoms and radiographic severity of knee osteoarthritis (Bedson and Croft 2008), recent literature may suggest that radiographic knee osteoarthritis severity correlates to postoperative outcomes after TKA.

A recent meta-analysis concluded that patients with worse radiographic preoperative knee osteoarthritis were more likely to be satisfied after surgery at final follow-up (Youlden et al. 2019). While patients with worse radiographic osteoarthritis were more satisfied after TKA, there was no significant difference in the postoperative pain or function scores in patients with KL 4 arthritis versus KL < 4 arthritis (Youlden et al. 2019). Understanding this possible relationship may play a role in counseling and the management of patient expectations following TKA. Additionally, a thorough preoperative evaluation of other possible pain generators and trial of conservative management options should be had with patients prior to undergoing TKA.

11.6 Radiographic Evaluation of TKA

Radiographs following TKA are routinely obtained at follow-up to assess implant position, wear, and fixation. A postoperative radiographic series is often similar to a preoperative series though variations in practice exist. For our practice, we typically obtain a standing AP, max flexion lateral, and patellofemoral view. For an accurate assessment, the entire component must be visualized including any augments or long stems.

> Images are individually assessed and compared to prior films for component alignment and position, implant–cement and cement–bone interfaces, polyethylene thickness, bone quality, and any progressive lesions such as osteolytic defects (◘ Fig. 11.4).

More detailed evaluation for aseptic loosening can be found in ▶ Chap. 52. Briefly, however, the greatest tool is the evaluation of serial radiographs to look for a change in implant position or progression of radiolucent lines (◘ Fig. 11.5).

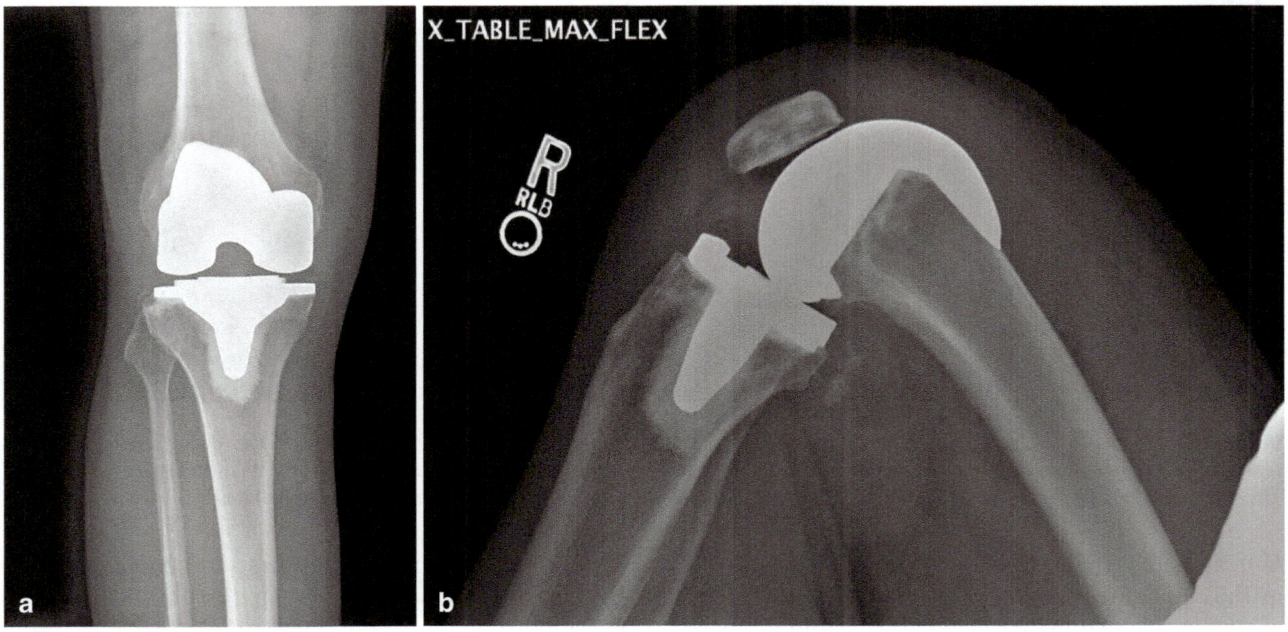

◘ **Fig. 11.4** **a**, **b** Standing PA and lateral views demonstrating a well-placed and well-fixed cemented TKA with an appropriate cement mantel

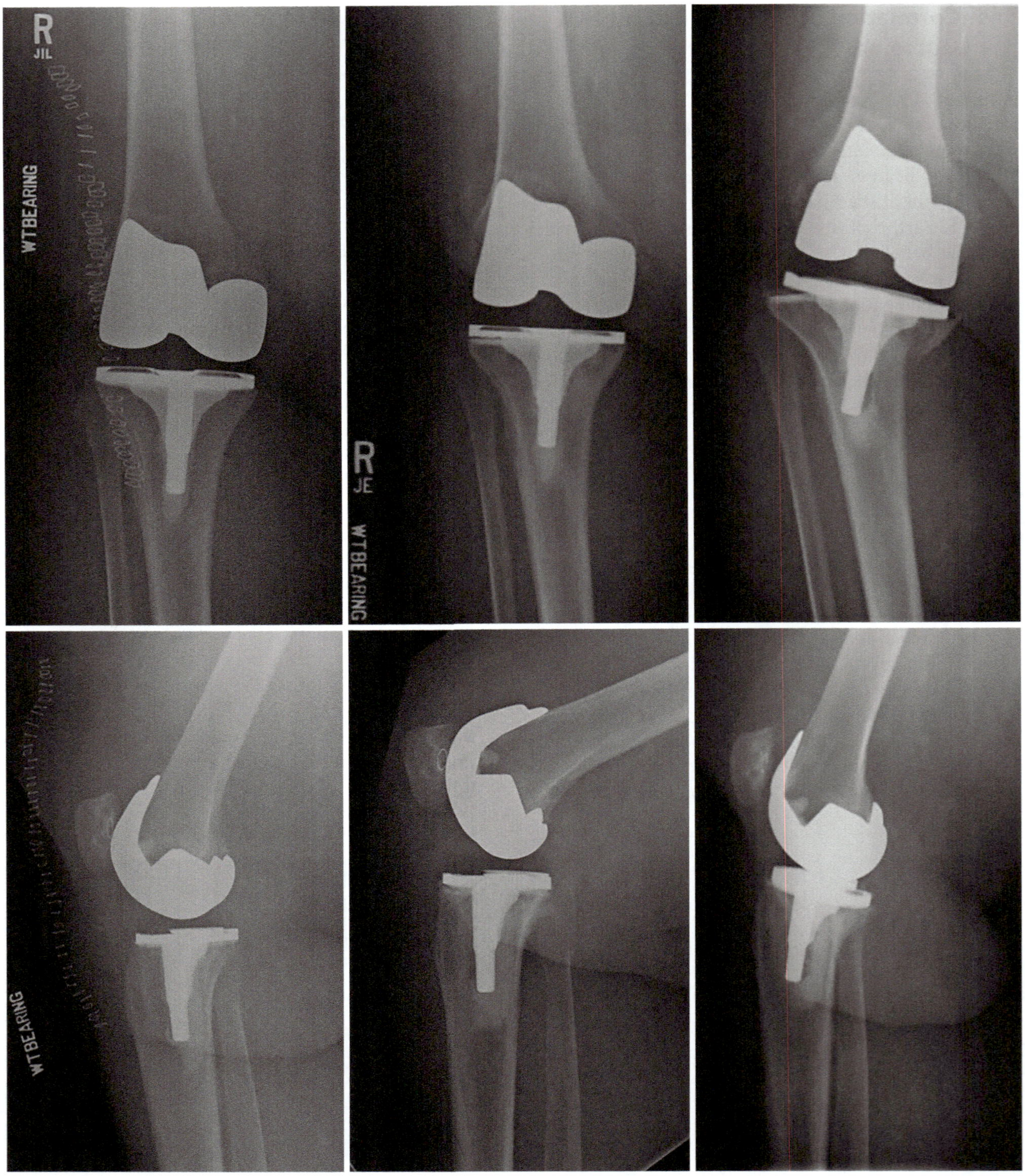

Fig. 11.5 A Series of standing PT and lateral X-rays of a cemented TKA demonstrating progressive loosening and failure. The immediate postoperative image *on the left side* demonstrates a well-fixed arthroplasty; subsequent images demonstrate the formation of radiolucent lines at the bone–implant interface indicative of loosening and then subsequent varus collapse

Unfortunately, there is a relative lack of standardization in the radiographic assessment of total knee implants postoperatively (Elmallah et al. 2015). Although classification systems were proposed in 1989 such as the Knee Society Total Knee Arthroplasty Roentgenographic Evaluation and Scoring System (Ewald 1989), many revision articles typically only report coronal, sagittal, and axial alignment and then bone loss at the time of revision. A more recent updated Knee Society scoring system has been created, which we encourage readers to utilize for standardization.

> The Modern Knee Society scoring system (Meneghini et al. 2015) provides a structured framework to evaluate the integrity of total knee prosthesis fixation.

Weight-bearing AP, lateral, and patellofemoral views are examined for radiolucent lines at cement–bone and implant–cement interfaces. Additionally, the significance of these radiolucencies depends on whether they are stable or progressive on serial imaging and if they involve the entire contact interface or just part of it. The Modern Knee Society scoring system assesses loosening of a cemented component by breaking the tibia and femur into five distinct zones and looking for the cumulative amount of radiolucency at the prosthetic interface (Table 11.3) (Meneghini et al. 2015). Additionally, component alignment and position are evaluated on each radiographic view. On the weight-bearing PA view, the coronal alignment can be evaluated relative to the anatomic axis of the femur; the coronal alignment of the tibial component can be judged by measuring the angle between the baseplate and the mechanical axis of the tibia. The lateral radiographs are used to evaluate the sagittal alignment of the component. Sagittal tibial component alignment can be determined by measuring the angle between the baseplate and the tibial shaft while the sagittal femoral component position can be measured from the angle between the femoral shaft and a line perpendicular to the most distal fixation point of the femoral component. Finally, patellofemoral component position is assessed by examining subluxation and tilt in the trochlear groove as seen on the Merchant view.

While cement fixation remains the gold standard for total knee arthroplasty, interest in cementless implants has been increasing.

> Overall, postoperative evaluation of cementless implants is similar to that of cemented implants; providers should assess serial radiographs for signs of implant loosening such as progressive migration or radiolucencies.

The appearance of a well-functioning cemented total knee implant may be significantly different than a well-functioning cementless implant; it is important that the provider be able to recognize these differences as cementless implants become more common. A recent series of modern cementless total knee implants demonstrated that all patients demonstrated peri-implant radiolucencies at the 6-week follow-up with the majority of these on the tibial side. These radiolucencies can persist as long as 1 year (the final follow-up in the study) and are typically small (<2 mm), incomplete, and nonprogressive (Costales et al. 2020).

11.7 Cross-Sectional and Advanced Imaging

11.7.1 Computed Tomography

Routine use of cross-sectional imaging techniques such as computed tomography and magnetic resonance imaging are not typically used for the diagnosis of knee osteoarthritis as X-ray can consistently provide a diagnosis in most cases and is more readily available and affordable at less radiation risk to the patient.

Table 11.3 Modern Knee Society radiographic grading

Zone	Tibial component		Femoral component	Patellofemoral component
	AP XR	Lateral XR	Lateral and AP XR	PF XR
1	Medial baseplate	Anterior baseplate	Anterior flange	Medial
2	Lateral baseplate	Posterior baseplate	Posterior flange	Lateral
3	Central keel/stem [a]	Central keel/stem [b]	Central box/pegs/distal fixation region [c]	Central peg/baseplate [a]
4	Revision TKA stem extension [a]	Revision TKA stem extension [b]	Revision TKA stem extension [b]	–
5	Inferior aspect of keel/stem	Inferior aspect of keel/stem	Superior aspect of revision TKA stem	–

[a] Can further be denoted with M (medial) and L (lateral)
[b] Can further be denoted with A (anterior) and P (posterior),
[c] can further be denoted with A (anterior chamfer) and P (posterior chamfer) if visible

Conventional CT scans offer no significant benefit over plain radiographs as cartilage is not readily visualized (Blackburn et al. 1996). To overcome this, arthrography with an iodized-based injection may be done to allow for improved visualization of intraarticular structures including cartilage (Carrillon 2008). With this technique, focal cartilage defects and thinning can readily be identified in each of the compartments. Little evidence exists in the current literature examining the efficacy of CT scans in the diagnosis of knee osteoarthritis.

> In the postoperative setting, CT scan is most often used to assess component rotation or to evaluate for fractures around the implant.

11.7.2 Magnetic Resonance Imaging

Similar to computed tomography, magnetic resonance imaging does not play a significant role in the routine diagnosis of knee osteoarthritis. Although unlike CT scans and plain radiographs, MRI is able to visualize cartilage, it is less readily available, relatively expensive, and does not offer significant benefit for routine diagnosis. Typically, cartilage is visualized on T2 weighted images with fat suppression where it appears grey in color and can readily be distinguished from subchondral bone which is dark, and synovial fluid, which is bright.

> Magnetic resonance imaging may play a role in preoperative planning for unicompartmental knee replacements where the clinician will need to determine if the patient truly has arthritis isolated to a single compartment and whether or not they have an intact anterior cruciate ligament.

Radiographic assessment of knee osteoarthritis is typically performed on plain radiographs. For the majority of cases, the standard osteoarthritis X-rays series should be sufficient enough to make a diagnosis and aid in presurgical planning. Advanced cross-sectional imaging techniques such as computed tomography and magnetic resonance imaging should be used sparingly and for specific cases.

11.7.3 Nuclear Medicine

Nuclear medicine studies including three-phase Technetium-99m bone scans and tagged white blood cell (WBC) scans are alternative diagnostic tools for implant loosening and infection that are typically used in conjunction with history, physical exam, and serologies in difficult diagnostic cases.

Technetium-99 m is a sensitive marker of bone turnover, however, since increased bone turnover is seen in cases of implant loosening, tumor, infection, and metabolic bone disease, the test is relatively non-specific (Hofmann et al. 1990; Rosenthall et al. 1987; Hill et al. 2019). A recent retrospective study found that Technetium-99 m bone scans had a positive predictive value of 2.5%, a negative predictive value of 100%, a specificity of 33%, and a sensitivity of 100%, making it relatively poor stand-alone test (Hill et al. 2019). Additionally, increased radionuclide uptake can persist for a year or even longer after an index procedure in patients who are completely asymptomatic (Rosenthall et al. 1987). This is especially true in cementless TKA.

> It has been demonstrated that in asymptomatic patients, increased Technetium-99 m take-up can be seen at the bone–implant interface in cementless total knees for up to 4 years following the index procedure; however, rates of uptake typically decrease as time progresses (Rubello et al. 1996).

Given the excellent negative predictive value of the bone scan, this tool can be useful in ruling out infection or implant loosening if it is negative.

Take-Home Messages

- Knee osteoarthritis is a clinical diagnosis that is confirmed on plain radiographs consisting of a series of a flexed weight-bearing PA views, lateral views, and patellofemoral views.
- Full-length standing radiographs may be useful for presurgical planning in patients with lower extremity deformity.
- Radiographic osteoarthritis severity poorly correlates to pain; however, preoperative radiographic osteoarthritis severity inversely correlates to postoperative TKA outcomes.
- Serial radiographs to check for changes in implant position or radiolucencies at the bone–cement or cement–implant interface can be useful for the diagnosis of implant loosening. Peri-implant radiolucency is common in cementless TKA; these lucencies can be persistent and asymptomatic.
- Technetium-99 m bone scans have poor specificity but high sensitivity for diagnosing loosening and possibly infection.

References

Altman R, Asch E, Bloch D et al (1986) Development of criteria for the classification and reporting of osteoarthritis: classification of osteoarthritis of the knee. Arthritis Rheum 29(8):1039–1049. https://onlinelibrary.wiley.com/doi/abs/10.1002/art.1780290816. https://doi.org/10.1002/art.1780290816

Argenson J, Chevrol-Benkeddache Y, Aubaniac J (2002) Modern unicompartmental knee arthroplasty with cement: a three to ten-year follow-up study. J Bone Joint Surg 84(12):2235–2239. http://ovidsp.ovid.com/ovidweb.cgi?T=JS&NEWS=n&CSC=Y&PAGE=fulltext&D=ovft&AN=00004623-200212000-00017. https://doi.org/10.2106/00004623-200212000-00017

Bae W, Payanal M, Chen A et al (2010) Topographic patterns of cartilage lesions in knee osteoarthritis. Cartilage 1(1):10–19. https://journals.sagepub.com/doi/full/10.1177/1947603509354991. https://doi.org/10.1177/1947603509354991

Bedson J, Croft PR (2008) The discordance between clinical and radiographic knee osteoarthritis: a systematic search and summary of the literature. BMC Musculoskelet Disord 9(1):116. https://www.ncbi.nlm.nih.gov/pubmed/18764949. https://doi.org/10.1186/1471-2474-9-116

Beswick AD, Wylde V, Gooberman-Hill R, Blom A, Dieppe P (2012) What proportion of patients report long-term pain after total hip or knee replacement for osteoarthritis? A systematic review of prospective studies in unselected patients. BMJ Open 2(1):e000435. https://doi.org/10.1136/bmjopen-2011-000435

Blackburn W, Chivers S, Bernreuter W (1996) Cartilage imaging in osteoarthritis. Semin Arthritis Rheum 25(4):273–281. https://www.sciencedirect.com/science/article/pii/S0049017296800370. https://doi.org/10.1016/S0049-0172(96)80037-0

Braun HJ, Gold GE (2011) Diagnosis of osteoarthritis: imaging. Bone 51(2):278–288. https://www.clinicalkey.es/playcontent/1-s2.0-S8756328211013585. https://doi.org/10.1016/j.bone.2011.11.019

Buckland-Wright C (1995) Protocols for precise radio-anatomical positioning of the tibiofemoral and patellofemoral compartments of the knee. Osteoarthr Cartil 3(Suppl A):71. https://www.ncbi.nlm.nih.gov/pubmed/8581753

Buckland-Wright JC, Macfarlane DG, Lynch JA, Jasani MK, Bradshaw CR (1995) Joint space width measures cartilage thickness in osteoarthritis of the knee: high resolution plain film and double contrast macroradiographic investigation. Ann Rheum Dis 54(4):263–268. https://doi.org/10.1136/ard.54.4.263

Carrillon Y (2008) Imaging knee osteoarthritis. In: Bonnin M and Chambat P (eds) Osteoarthritis of the knee. Springer-Verlag France, Paris, pp 3–14. https://doi.org/10.1007/978-2-287-74175-3

Costales TG, Chapman DM, Dalury DF (2020) The natural history of radiolucencies following uncemented total knee arthroplastyat 9 years. J Arthroplast 35(1):127–131. https://www.sciencedirect.com/science/article/pii/S0883540319307636. https://doi.org/10.1016/j.arth.2019.08.032

Elmallah RK, Scuderi GR, Jauregui JJ et al (2015) Radiographic evaluations of revision total knee arthroplasty: a plea for uniform assessments. J Arthroplasty 30(11):1981–1984. https://www.clinicalkey.es/playcontent/1-s2.0-S0883540315007342. https://doi.org/10.1016/j.arth.2015.08.013

Ewald FC (1989) The knee society total knee arthroplastyroentgenographic evaluation and scoring system. Clin Orthop Relat Res 248:9–12. https://www.ncbi.nlm.nih.gov/pubmed/2805502. https://doi.org/10.1097/00003086-198911000-00003

Fontboté RC, Nemtala UF, Contreras OO, Guerrero R (2008) Rosenberg projection for the radiological diagnosis of knee osteoarthritis. Revistamedica de Chile 136(7):880. https://www.ncbi.nlm.nih.gov/pubmed/18949164

Hill D, Kinsella D, Toms A (2019) Three-phase technetium-99m bone scanning in patients with pain in the knee region after cemented total knee arthroplasty. Eur J Orthop Surg Traumatol 29(5):1105–1113. https://www.ncbi.nlm.nih.gov/pubmed/30888518. https://doi.org/10.1007/s00590-019-02407-5

Hofmann AA, Wyatt RW, Daniels AU, Armstrong L, Alazraki N, Taylor J (1990) Bone scans after total knee arthroplasty in asymptomatic patients. Cemented versus cementless. Clin Orthop Relat Res 251(251):183–188. https://www.ncbi.nlm.nih.gov/pubmed/2295172. https://doi.org/10.1097/00003086-199002000-00031

Jacobson JA, Girish G, Jiang Y, Resnick D (2008) Radiographic evaluation of arthritis: inflammatory conditions. Radiology 248(2):378–389. https://www.ncbi.nlm.nih.gov/pubmed/18641245. https://doi.org/10.1148/radiol.2482062110

Johnson VL, Guermazi A, Roemer FW, Hunter DJ (2017) Comparison in knee osteoarthritis joint damage patterns among individuals with an intact, complete and partial anterior cruciate ligament rupture. Int J Rheum Dis 20(10):1361–1371. https://onlinelibrary.wiley.com/doi/abs/10.1111/1756-185X.13003. https://doi.org/10.1111/1756-185X.13003

Kellgren JH, Lawrence JS (1957) Radiological assessment of osteo-arthrosis. Ann Rheum Dis 16(4):494–502. https://doi.org/10.1136/ard.16.4.494

McDonnell SM, Bottomley NJ, Hollinghurst D et al (2009) Skyline patellofemoral radiographs can only exclude late stage degenerative changes. Knee 18(1):21–23. https://www.clinicalkey.es/playcontent/1-s2.0-S0968016009002099. https://doi.org/10.1016/j.knee.2009.10.008

McGrory J, Trousdale R, Pagnano M, Nigbur M (2002) Preoperative hip to ankle radiographs in total knee arthroplasty. Clin Orthop Relat Res 404(404):196–202. https://www.ncbi.nlm.nih.gov/pubmed/12439260. https://doi.org/10.1097/00003086-200211000-00032

Meneghini RM, Mont MA, Backstein DB, Bourne RB, Dennis DA, Scuderi GR (2015) Development of a modern knee society radiographic evaluation system and methodology for total knee arthroplasty. J Arthroplasty 30(12):2311–2314. https://www.clinicalkey.es/playcontent/1-s2.0-S0883540315004507. https://doi.org/10.1016/j.arth.2015.05.049

Messieh S, Fowler P, Munro T (1990) Anteroposterior radiographs of the osteoarthritic knee. J Bone Joint Surg 72(4):639–640. https://www.ncbi.nlm.nih.gov/pubmed/2380220. https://doi.org/10.1302/0301-620X.72B4.2380220

Nilsdotter AK, Toksvig-Larsen S, Roos EM (2009) Knee arthroplasty: are patients' expectations fulfilled? Acta Orthop 80(1):55–61. http://www.tandfonline.com/doi/abs/10.1080/17453670902805007. https://doi.org/10.1080/17453670902805007

Odenbring S, Berggren AM, Peil L (1993) Roentgenographic assessment of the hip-knee-ankle axis in medial gonarthrosis. A study of reproducibility. Clin Orthop Relat Res 289:195–196. https://www.ncbi.nlm.nih.gov/pubmed/8472414. https://doi.org/10.1097/00003086-199304000-00027

Patel D, Ferris B, Aichroth P (1991) Radiological study of alignment after total knee replacement. short radiographs or long radiographs? Int Orthop 15(3):209. https://www.ncbi.nlm.nih.gov/pubmed/1743835. https://doi.org/10.1007/BF00192296

Petersen T, Engh G (1988) Radiographic assessment of knee alignment after total knee arthroplasty. J Arthroplast 3(1):67–72. https://www.sciencedirect.com/science/article/pii/S0883540388800548. https://doi.org/10.1016/S0883-5403(88)80054-8

Ritchie JFS, Al-Sarawan M, Worth R, Conry B, Gibb PA (2004) A parallel approach: the impact of schuss radiography of the degenerate knee on clinical management. Knee 11(4):283–287. https://www.sciencedirect.com/science/article/pii/S0968016003001182. https://doi.org/10.1016/j.knee.2003.09.001

Rosenberg T, Paulos L, Parker R, Coward D, Scott S (1988) The forty-five-degree posteroanterior flexion weight-bearing radiograph of the knee. J Bone Joint Surg 70(10):1479–1483. http://ovidsp.ovid.com/ovidweb.cgi?T=JS&NEWS=n&CSC=Y&PAGE=fulltext&D=ovft&AN=00004623-198870100-00006. https://doi.org/10.2106/00004623-198870100-00006

Rosenthall L, Lepanto L, Raymond F (1987) Radiophosphate uptake in asymptomatic knee arthroplasty. J Nucl Med 28(10):1546. http://jnm.snmjournals.org/cgi/content/abstract/28/10/1546

Rubello D, Caricasulo D, Borsato N, Chierichetti F, Zanco P, Ferlin G (1996) Three-phase bone scan pattern in asymptomatic uncemented total knee arthroplasty. Eur J Nucl Med 23(10):1400–1403. https://www.ncbi.nlm.nih.gov/pubmed/8781147. https://doi.org/10.1007/BF01367598

Rueckl K, Boettner F, Maza N, Runer A, Bechler U, Sculco P (2018) The posterior–anterior flexed view is better than the anterior–posterior view for assessing osteoarthritis of the knee. Skelet Radiol 47(4):511–517. https://www.ncbi.nlm.nih.gov/pubmed/29159676. https://doi.org/10.1007/s00256-017-2815-2

Waldstein W, Monsef J, Buckup J, Boettner F (2013) The value of valgus stress radiographs in the workup for medial unicompartmental arthritis. Clin Orthop Relat Res 471(12):3998–4003. https://www.ncbi.nlm.nih.gov/pubmed/23917994. https://doi.org/10.1007/s11999-013-3212-3

Weidow J, Pak J, Kärrholm J (2002) Different patterns of cartilage wear in medial and lateral gonarthrosis. Acta Orthop Scand 73(3):326–329. http://www.tandfonline.com/doi/abs/10.1080/000164702320155347. https://doi.org/10.1080/000164702320155347

White SH, Ludkowski PF, Goodfellow JW (1991) Anteromedial osteoarthritis of the knee. J Bone Joint Surg Br 73:582–586

Woolhead GM, Donovan JL, Dieppe PA (2005) Outcomes of total knee replacement: a qualitative study. Rheumatology (Oxford) 44(8):1032–1037. https://www.ncbi.nlm.nih.gov/pubmed/15870149. https://doi.org/10.1093/rheumatology/keh674

Wright RW (2014) Osteoarthritis classification scales: Interobserver reliability and arthroscopic correlation. J Bone Joint Surg 96(14):1145–1151. http://ovidsp.ovid.com/ovidweb.cgi?T=JS&NEWS=n&CSC=Y&PAGE=fulltext&D=ovft&AN=00004623-201407160-00001. https://doi.org/10.2106/JBJS.M.00929

Wright R, Wright R, Ross J et al (2014) Osteoarthritis classification scales: Interobserver reliability and arthroscopic correlation. J Bone Joint Surg 96(14):1145–1151. https://doi.org/10.2106/JBJS.M.00929

Youlden DJ, Dannaway J, Enke O (2019) Radiographic severity of knee osteoarthritis and its relationship to outcome post total knee arthroplasty: a systematic review. ANZ J Surg. https://www.ncbi.nlm.nih.gov/pubmed/31338950. https://doi.org/10.1111/ans.15343

Patient-Reported Outcomes in Total Knee Arthroplasty

Anas Saleh and Denis Nam

Contents

E. Hansen, K.-D. Kühn (eds.), *Essentials of Cemented Knee Arthroplasty*,
https://doi.org/10.1007/978-3-662-63113-3_12

12.1 Introduction

Recent emphasis on demonstrating treatment outcomes and "value-based care" in total knee arthroplasty (TKA) has led to the development of multiple outcome measures and scoring systems. These may include performance-based objective assessments, patient-reported assessments, or both. As a result of honoring the relative importance of patient satisfaction as compared to surgeon satisfaction with treatment results, there has been a shift in orthopedic literature toward patient-reported outcomes (Wright 2009). These patient-reported outcome measures can be generic measures of quality of life or joint-specific. The general health measures evaluate a range of physical and mental parameters. A joint-specific measure is focused on issues that are related to a specific joint or injury.

> Most epidemiologists believe that studies should include general health outcomes in addition to joint-specific ones (Vangsness et al. 1995).

In general, a practical outcome measure should be easy to administer, reliable, valid, and responsive to clinical change (Roos et al. 1998).

- Reliability refers to the test's ability to give consistent and reproducible results under similar testing conditions.
- Validity is the ability of an outcome measure to evaluate what it is designed to measure.
- Responsiveness is the ability to detect change in condition when it occurs.
- The minimal clinically important difference (MCID) of an outcome measure is the smallest change in an outcome score that corresponds to a significant change in a patient's condition (Beaton et al. 2002; Smith et al. 2012).

The purpose of this chapter is to examine the more common patient-reported outcomes in TKA, including both general health outcome measures and knee-specific measures. It will also serve as an update on some of the newly developed outcome measures. Knowledge of these various patient-reported outcomes is critical for both researchers involved in designing clinical studies and clinicians evaluating the literature on TKA outcomes.

12.2 General Health Outcome Measures

The advantage of a general health outcome measure is that it can be used to compare diseases and conditions across the medical spectrum. This allows researchers to compare the relative impact of treatment on patients despite completely different diagnoses. Patients and clinicians may believe that the general health measure is less relevant to the disease condition in question and that any such measure should be combined with disease-specific outcome measures that have more content and validity for that specific condition (Giesinger et al. 2014).

12.2.1 Medical Outcomes Study Short-Form (SF-36 and SF-12)

The Medical Outcomes Study 36-Item Short-Form (SF-36)is one of the most popular general health outcome measures (Ware and Sherbourne 1992). It was developed to assist in health policy development, clinical practice, research, and general population surveys. The SF-36 has been extensively used in numerous publications to measure outcomes of over 130 diseases and conditions (Ware 2000).

This questionnaire consists of 35 questions in 8 subscale domains (4physical health domains and 4 mental health domains), and one general overall health status question (Table 12.1). Each subscale score is totaled, weighted, and transformed to fall between 0 (worst possible health and severe disability) and 100 (best possible health, no disability). This was designed so that an average US citizen would score 50 on a subscale. The SF-36 has been validated for a variety of ages and languages, and for patients aged 75 years and older (Weinberger et al. 1991; Jenkinson et al. 1994; Lyons et al. 1994; Perneger et al. 1995; Sullivan et al. 1995).

While the SF-36 has proved to be useful for a variety of diseases, it is too long for inclusion in some large-scale health measurements. Subsequently, the 12-Item Short-Form (SF-12) was developed (Table 12.1) (Ware et al. 1996). This represented a "downsizing" of the SF-36, including 12 items that reproduced more than 90% of the variance in SF-36 physical health and mental health components, and accurately reproduced the average scores of these measures. The length of this questionnaire reduced the original SF-36 to one to two pages, so that it is sufficient for self-administration in 2 minutes or less. In choosing between forms, Ware et al. recommended the use of SF-36 for smaller studies due to its reliability in measuring more levels of health, whereas the SF-12 is recommended in studies with large sample sizes having constraints on questionnaire length and in studies focusing on patient-based assessments of physical and mental health (Ware et al. 1996).

> Webster et al. compared the performance of SF-12 and SF-36 in 407 patients who underwent TKA and found a significant correlation between both versions for preoperative and 1-year postoperative measures (Webster and Feller 2016). The change in score from pre- to postoperative was also highly correlated.

Table 12.1 Short-Form subscales and 36- and 12-items

Summary measures	Scale	Items [a]
Physical component summary (PCS)	Physical functioning (PF)	Vigorous activities **Moderate activities** Lift, carry groceries **Climb several flights** Climb one flight Bend, kneel Walk mile Walk several blocks Walk one block Bathe, dress
	Role – Physical (RP)	Cut downtime **Accomplished less** **Limited in kind of work** Had difficulty
	Bodily pain (BP)	Pain magnitude **Paininterfere**
	General health (GH)	**General health rating** Sick easier As healthy Health to get worse Health excellent
Mental component summary (MCS)	Vitality (VT)	Pep/life **Energy** Worn out Tired
	Social functioning (SF)	Social extent **Social time**
	Role – Emotional (RE)	Cut downtime **Accomplished less** **Not careful**
	Mental health (MH)	Nervous Down in dumps **Peaceful** **Blue/sad** Happy

[a] SF-12 items are highlighted in bold

Clement et al. studied the minimally clinically important difference (MCID) for the SF-12 scores in TKA (Clement et al. 2019). They identified 2589 TKAs performed in a 10-year period, and collected SF-12 scores preoperatively and at one-year postoperatively. They found that the MCID for the physical component (PCS) to be 1.8, and for the mental component (MCS) to be 1.5. This indicated that in order to power a randomized controlled trial with 80% power and an alpha of 0.05, 394 patients would need to be randomized to each arm.

12.2.2 EuroQOL 5-Dimension Score (EQ-5D)

The EuroQol 5-dimension (EQ-5D) is one of the most commonly used generic measures of health status developed by the EuroQol Group (EuroQol Group 1990; Brooks 1996). Applicable to a wide range of health conditions and treatments, the EQ-5D is designed for self-completion by respondents and is ideally suited for use in postal surveys, in clinics, and in face-to-face interviews. It takes only a few minutes to complete. This survey consists of two pages: the EQ-5D descriptive system and the EQ visual analogue scale (EQ VAS) (EQ-5D instruments – EQ-5D 2021).

The descriptive system includes five health outcome domains or dimensions, which are the following:

- Mobility.
- Self-care.
- Usual activities.
- Pain/discomfort.
- Anxiety/depression.

In the original EQ-5D 3-level version (EQ-5D-3L), each dimension had three levels: No problems, some problems, extreme problems.

In 2005, a task force was established within the EuroQol Group to improve the instrument's sensitivity and reduce the ceiling effect. The group decided that the new version of the EQ-5D should include five levels of severity in each of the existing five domains, and was renamed EQ-5D-5L (Fig. 12.1) (Herdman et al. 2011). Each dimension has five levels of perceived problems:

- No problems.
- Slight problems.
- Moderate problems.
- Severe problems.
- Extreme problems.

The descriptive system defines health in a total of 3125 health states; each state is referred to in terms of a five-digit code. For example, state 11,111 indicates no problem in any of the five dimensions. These states are then converted into a single index value using a crosswalk link function (van Reenen and Janssen 2019).

The EQ VAS records the patient's self-rated health on a vertical visual analogue scale, where the endpoints are labeled "the best health you can imagine" and "the worst health you can imagine" (Fig. 12.1b).

Shim et al. studied the responsiveness of the EQ-5D questionnaire in patients undergoing TKA (Shim and Hamilton 2019). They used data from a prospective multicenter cohort study in the United Kingdom, including 721 patients. With regards to internal responsiveness, the EQ-5D showed significant change between preoperative and postoperative scores, with most improvement occurring during the first 3 months in all patients. There was a small but significant change between 3 and 6 months, and no further statistical

a

Under each heading, please tick the ONE box that best describes your health TODAY.

MOBILITY

I have no problems in walking about ☐

I have slight problems in walking about ☐

I have moderate problems in walking about ☐

I have severe problems in walking about ☐

I am unable to walk about ☐

SELF-CARE

I have no problems washing or dressing myself ☐

I have slight problems washing or dressing myself ☐

I have moderate problems washing or dressing myself ☐

I have severe problems washing or dressing myself ☐

I am unable to wash or dress myself ☐

USUAL ACTIVITIES *(e.g. work, study, housework, family or leisure activities)*

I have no problems doing my usual activities ☐

I have slight problems doing my usual activities ☐

I have moderate problems doing my usual activities ☐

I have severe problems doing my usual activities ☐

I am unable to do my usual activities ☐

PAIN / DISCOMFORT

I have no pain or discomfort ☐

I have slight pain or discomfort ☐

I have moderate pain or discomfort ☐

I have severe pain or discomfort ☐

I have extreme pain or discomfort ☐

ANXIETY / DEPRESSION

I am not anxious or depressed ☐

I am slightly anxious or depressed ☐

I am moderately anxious or depressed ☐

I am severely anxious or depressed ☐

I am extremely anxious or depressed ☐

Fig. 12.1 UK sample version of EuroQOL 5-Dimension Score (EQ-5D-5L Health Questionnaire). **a** The *first page* is descriptive, **b** the *second page* is showing a visual analogue scale. (© EuroQol Research Foundation. EQ-5D™ is a trademark of the EuroQol Research Foundation. Reproduced by permission of EuroQol Research Foundation. Reproduction of this version is not allowed. For reproduction, use, or modification of the EQ-5D [any version], please register your study by using the online EQ registration page: ▶ www.euroqol.org)

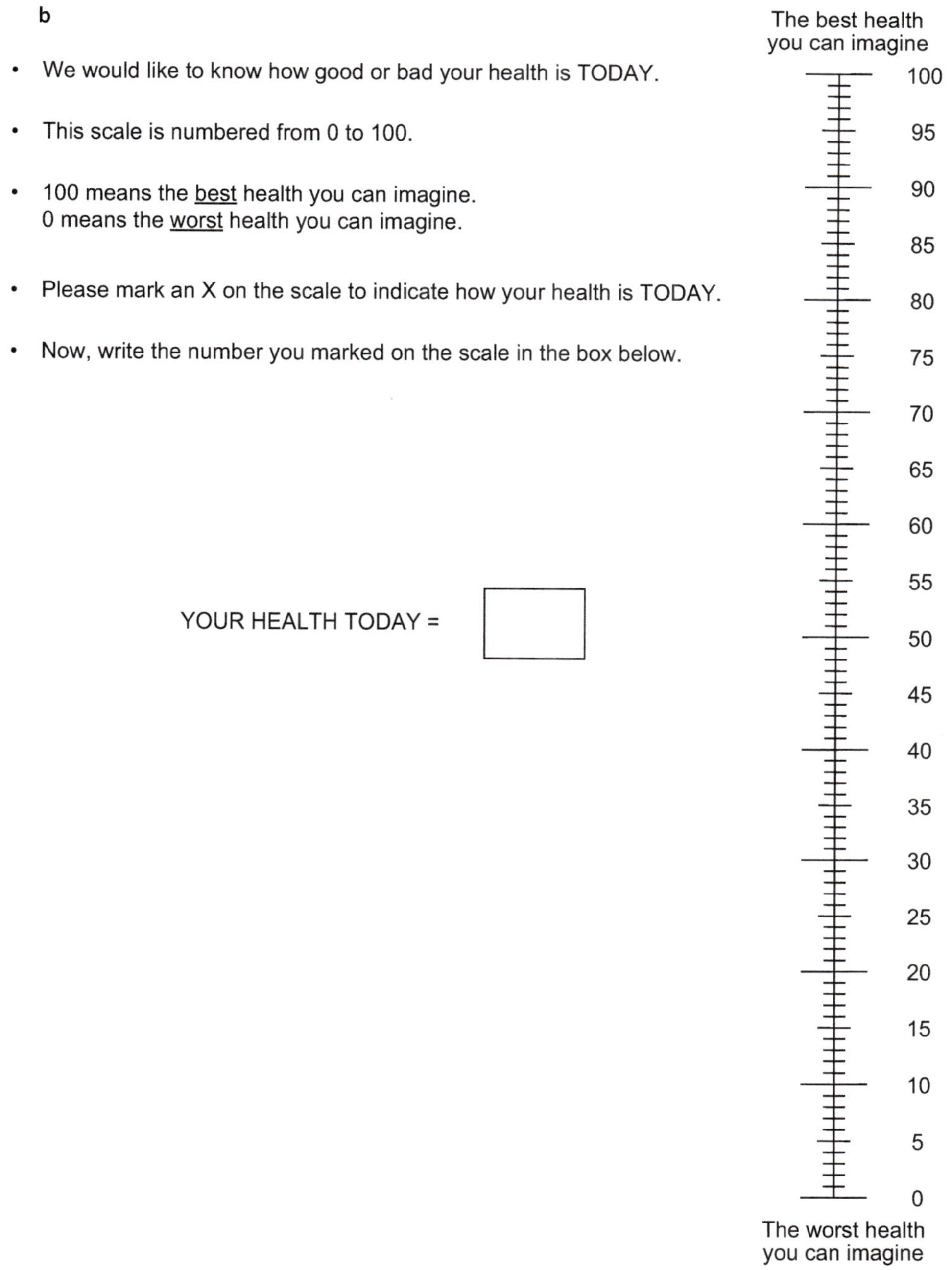

b

- We would like to know how good or bad your health is TODAY.
- This scale is numbered from 0 to 100.
- 100 means the <u>best</u> health you can imagine.
  0 means the <u>worst</u> health you can imagine.
- Please mark an X on the scale to indicate how your health is TODAY.
- Now, write the number you marked on the scale in the box below.

YOUR HEALTH TODAY =

The best health you can imagine

100
95
90
85
80
75
70
65
60
55
50
45
40
35
30
25
20
15
10
5
0

The worst health you can imagine

Fig. 12.1 (continued)

change between 6 and 12 months. External responsiveness was assessed by correlating change scores of the EQ-5D with the MCID of the Oxford Knee Score (OKS). Their study showed that the EQ-5D was able to discriminate between patients who achieved the OKS score MCID (>5) and those who did not.

> Both SF-12 and EQ-5D-5L tools are commonly used in total joint arthroplasty studies, and there are no strong advantages of one tool over the other.

Thus, the International Society of Arthroplasty Registries (ISAR) does not make specific recommendations about the preferred general health PROMs tool (Rolfson et al. 2016).

12.2.3 The Patient-Reported Outcomes Measurement Information System (PROMIS)

In 2004, a group of US scientists, statisticians, and psychometricians received funding from the National Institute of Health (NIH) and initiated a multicenter cooperative group referred to as the Patient-Reported Outcomes Measurement Information System (PROMIS)

(Cella et al. 2007). The goal of this initiative was to build and validate common, accessible item banks to measure key symptoms and health concepts applicable to a range of conditions, enabling efficient interpretation of clinical trials.

PROMIS consists of item banks organized into domains of health, such as physical health and mental health. PROMIS measures can be administered as static "short forms" similar to those available for other measures, but also can be administered dynamically on a computer (Fries et al. 2014). Administration via computer involves a highly accurate computerized format called computerized adaptive testing (CAT), in which a computer algorithm customizes item delivery to an examinee by selecting each subsequent item based on answers to previous items. This way the CAT software enables a high level of precision using fewer questions. This CAT provides a key advantage of PROMIS that distinguishes it from many conventional patient-reported measures. One study estimated the MCID for the physical function component of PROMIS CAT to be around 7.9 (Hung et al. 2018).

In relation to total joint arthroplasty, the most relevant components are physical function, pain intensity, and pain interference. The performance of PROMIS in TKA literature has shown mixed results. Shim et al. evaluated the responsiveness of PROMIS in five domains, which are as follows:

- Physical function.
- Fatigue.
- Pain.
- Emotional distress.
- Social health (Shim and Hamilton 2019).

They found the physical health domain to have the best internal and external responsiveness (positive correlation with OKS), but the mental health component showed poorer discriminatory ability. They concluded that the PROMIS-10 Physical health tool offers superior responsiveness to change compared with the EQ5D in TKA. Padilla et al. attempted to correlate PROMIS CAT to joint-specific outcome measures, such as the Knee Injury and Osteoarthritis Outcome Score (KOOS-JR) (Padilla et al. 2019). The authors found a modest to strong correlation (ranging from 0.56 to 0.71), indicating that the role of PROMIS in capturing joint-specific changes can be limited after TKA. Kagan et al. sought to characterize the recovery curve for TKA patients using the physical function and pain interference domains of PROMIS CAT (Kagan et al. 2018). In 91 patients enrolled in the study, they found the greatest magnitude of improvement in both physical function and pain interference had occurred within the first 3 months. After 6 months, patients might expect modest improvements (Fig. 12.2). Stiegel et al. reported their early experience with using PROMIS to predict patients who would achieve MCID (Stiegel et al.

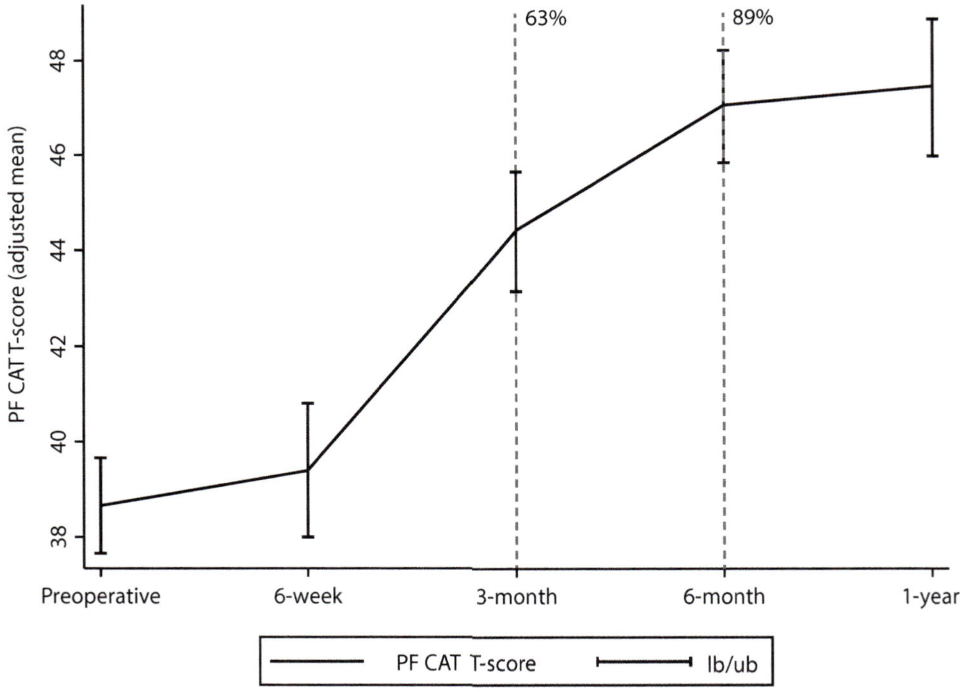

Fig. 12.2 **a** The change in PROMIS physical function (*PF*) computerized adaptive test (*CAT*) in the first year after TKA. **b** The change in PROMIS pain interference (*PI*) computerized adaptive test (*CAT*) in the first year after TKA. (Reproduced from Kagan et al. (2018), with permission from Elsevier)

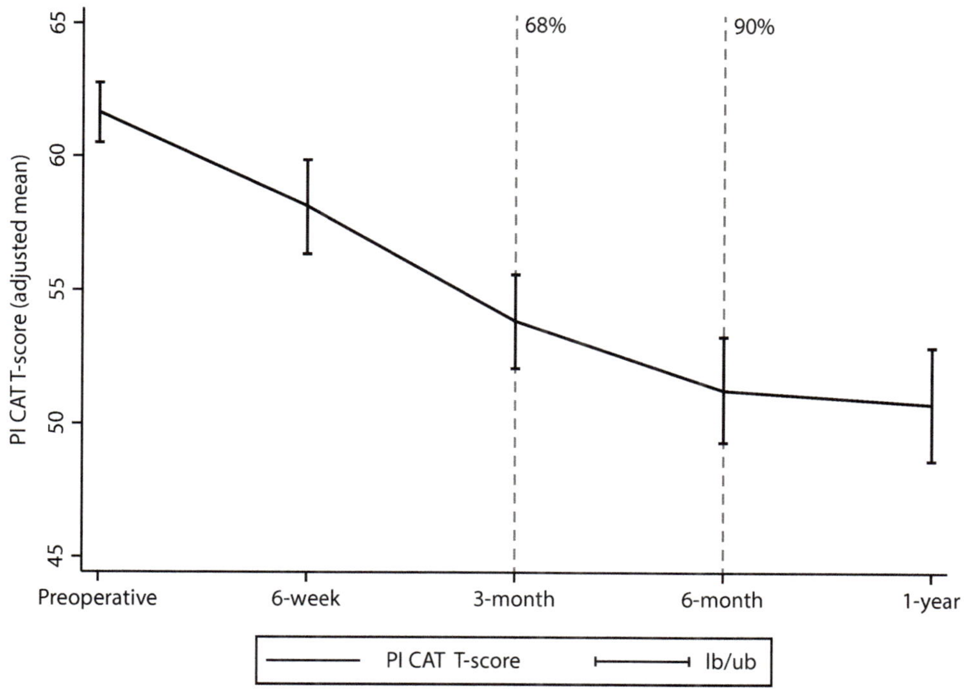

Fig. 12.2 (continued)

2019). Using the PROMIS short forms print-outs, they found that 68% of TKA patients met the MCID for pain interference, 28% for physical function, and 14% for depression at the 6-week postoperative visit. Although the authors concluded that preoperative PROMIS can reliably predict achieving the MCID after TKA, the area under the curve (AUC) for predicting physical function and pain interference was 0.7 and 0.68, respectively, indicating less than ideal accuracy.

> Further research is necessary to describe the reliability, validity, and responsiveness of PROMIS in TKA.

12.2.4 Press Ganey

Press Ganey is the nation's largest provider of tools for patient satisfaction measurement and analysis. The survey simply known as the "Press Ganey Survey" has become the most commonly used survey of outpatient satisfaction in the United States (Graham et al. 2015). The survey is used by health care administrations as a metric assessing various aspects of health care delivery such as wait times in clinic, and the patient–provider interaction. Care satisfaction surveys such as the Press Ganey Survey are increasingly being used as a metric in performance-based compensation for both hospitals and health care providers (Holzer and Minder 2011).

The Press Ganey Outpatient Medical Practice Survey consists of over 20 questions divided into several subdomains such as:

- Access.
- Moving through your visit.
- Nurse or assistant.
- Care provider.
- Personal issues.
- Overall assessment of the practice.

Each question measures responses on a Likert scale ranging from 1 (indicating very poor) to 5 (indicating very good). Responses are converted into a 0–100-point scale, and the mean overall score for all answered questions within an individual subdomain is used to calculate the score for that subdomain. The unweighted mean of the six subdomain scores is then used to calculate the mean overall care satisfaction score.

> It is important to understand the contrast between satisfaction as it relates to the outcome of care and satisfaction with the process of care (Graham et al. 2015).

Situations arise in which the outcome of a TKA is considered successful by both the patient and the surgeon, but the process of care is considered to be unsatisfactory because of cost, inconvenience, or hardship related to receiving that care.

> Care satisfaction scores, such as the Press Ganey, have yet to be validated as a true measure of health care quality in relation to actual patient outcomes.

Kohring et al. evaluated the correlation between Press Ganey Outpatient Medical Practice Survey collected from outpatient clinical encounters and PROMIS CAT collected preoperatively and postoperatively (Kohring et al. 2018). They found no correlation at all time points (Spearman correlation coefficient—0.13–0.18). The authors question the utility of these scores as surrogate measures of health care quality, especially when reimbursements become tied to these metrics. Chughtai et al. also found no correlation between Press Ganey Survey results with several validated patient-reported outcomes after TKA, such as SF-12, Knee Society Score, or Western Ontario and McMaster Universities Arthritis Index (Chughtai et al. 2017).

12.2.5 Prediction Model for Patient Satisfaction (PMPS)

A recent Prediction Model for Patient Satisfaction was developed by Van Onsem et al. with the goal of predicting patients' postoperative satisfaction with high sensitivity and positive-predictive value (Van Onsem et al. 2016). They analyzed five commonly used patient-reported outcomes (KOOS, EQ-5D, OKS, PCS, and KSS), and identified ten questions, which when answered preoperatively could predict patient satisfaction as measured by the 2011 Knee Society Score (KSS). Their model had a sensitivity of 97% and a positive-predictive value of 93%. Since their data came from 113 patients at a single center, Calkins et al. sought to externally validate their model in a new patient sample (Calkins et al. 2019). In this external validation cohort, PMPS failed to predict any of the 12 dissatisfied patients and falsely predicted dissatisfaction in 4 patients with maximum postoperative KSS.

12

> Further research is needed to refine and validate this prediction model.

12.3 Joint-Specific Outcome Measures

12.3.1 Western Ontario and McMaster Universities Osteoarthritis Index (WOMAC)

The Western Ontario and McMaster Universities Arthritis Index (WOMAC) is arguably the most widely used joint-specific outcome measure. It has been extensively validated and translated and linguistically validated in over 60 alternative-language forms (Angst et al. 2001; Wolfe and Kong 1999; Bae et al. 2001). The validity, reliability, and responsiveness of the WOMAC were originally demonstrated by Bellamy et al. in the context of a randomized controlled clinical trial of two nonsteroidal anti-inflammatory drugs in patients with hip and knee osteoarthritis (Bellamy et al. 1988).

The WOMAC consists of the following three subscales:

- Pain.
- Stiffness.
- Physical function.

The score is interpreted from a best-to-worst scale, in which lower values indicate less pain and higher function. The scores can be normalized, with 0 indicating severe symptoms, and 100 indicating no symptoms. The minimal clinically important difference for the WOMAC was reported to be 12% of the baseline score or 6% of the maximum score in a study that examined rehabilitation intervention in osteoarthritis (Angst et al. 2001). A minimal clinically important difference of 9–12 points (on a scale of 0–100) has also been reported (Ehrich et al. 2000).

> The use of WOMAC is recommended in all clinical studies evaluating TKA outcomes.

12.3.2 Knee Injury and Osteoarthritis Outcome Score (KOOS)

Since the WOMAC was mostly focused on the elderly, its utility in younger patients has been questioned as it is likely to have ceiling effects in this group. The KOOS was created from the WOMAC as a result of this proposition (Roos et al. 1998, 1999; Roos and Lohmander 2003). It was created for evaluating sports injuries as well as the short- and long-term sequelae of the injury including the risk of developing osteoarthritis after these injuries. The KOOS was the only joint-specific patient-reported outcome measure adopted by the Centers for Medicare and Medicaid Services (CMS) to meet their pay-for-performance measures (CMS 2019).

This outcome measure consists of 42 self-administered items distributed over the following 5 domains:

- Pain.
- Symptoms.
- Activities of daily living.
- Sport and recreation function.
- Knee-related quality of life.

Each domain is summed and transformed into a score from 0 (worst) to 100 (best). All WOMAC questions are included in KOOS in their original form to assess osteoarthritis in older individuals, and therefore a WOMAC score can be calculated.

> It is thought that the KOOS has utility in active and young patients undergoing unicompartmental knee arthroplasty or patellofemoral arthroplasty (Roos and Lohmander 2003; Paxton and Fithian 2005).

A short-form survey derived from the full KOOS questionnaire was developed by Lyman et al. in order to improve efficiency in reporting TKA outcomes and reduce questionnaire burden (Lyman et al. 2016). This KOOS Joint Replacement (KOOS-JR) survey sought to represent a single domain of "knee health," combining pain, symptoms, and functional ability into a single score. Their study included 2291 from their hospital knee replacement registry to reduce KOOS to 7 items using Rasch analysis. The KOOS-JR showed high internal validity against full KOOS, and also excellent external validity in the Function and Outcomes Research for Comparative Effectiveness in Total Joint Replacement (FORCE-TJR) (Lyman et al. 2016).

12.3.3 Oxford Knee Score (OKS)

The OKS was developed from interviews with patients to measure outcomes after TKA (Murray et al. 2007; Dawson et al. 1998). It is a 12-item survey, assessed on a Likert scale with values from 0 to 4; a summative score is then calculated where 48 is the best possible score. In the above-mentioned study by Shim et al., OKS had the greatest responsiveness to change after TKA when compared with general health outcome measures such as EQ-5D and PROMIS-10 (Shim and Hamilton 2019). Clement et al. reported an MCID of 5 (Clement et al. 2014).

12.3.4 Knee Society Score

In 1989, the original Knee Society Score (KSS) was developed as an objective tool to rate the patient's functional abilities (Insall et al. 1989). In an era where patient satisfaction is key, the original KSS was criticized as being a surgeon-assessed questionnaire, and its utility was challenged in contemporary patients who have expectations and demands. In 2012, the Knee Society published a new scoring system that is both physician- and patient-derived (Scuderi et al. 2012; Noble et al. 2012). The objective score is completed by the surgeon and includes alignment, instability, and range of motion. The patient-reported subscale includes symptoms, satisfaction, expectation, and functional activity items. The higher the score, the better the outcome in all subscales.

> What is unique regarding the patient-reported subscale is that it includes both advanced activities and three self-selected activities of greatest importance to the individual patient.

Giesinger et al. evaluated the responsiveness of the KSS (Giesinger et al. 2014). They reviewed prospective data from 98 patients and found the KSS to have the largest effect size from preoperative to 2-month and 1-year follow up, and therefore more responsive in comparison to generic health outcome tools. Scuderi et al. developed a short-form version of the new KSS using the same patient sample used in the long-form of KSS in 2012 (Scuderi et al. 2016). Their proposed short-form reduced satisfaction items from 5 to a single item, and reduced functional activities items from 17 to 6. This short-form correlated well with the original longer form and was capable of discriminating clinically different groups of patients before and after TKA with virtually the same estimated effect size.

Take-Home Messages

- Patient-reported outcomes are particularly crucial in measuring the results of "elective" procedures such as TKA because patient-reported outcomes take into account the more subjective issues of expectations and preferences.
- Patient-reported outcomes are generally described as generic quality-of-life measures (e.g., SF-12 and EQ-5D) or joint-specific measures (e.g., KOOS, OKS, or KSS).
- SF-36, SF-12, EQ-5D, WOMAC, KOOS, KSS, and OKS are among the most published and validated outcome measures.
- Further research is required to validate PROMIS in TKA.
- Arthroplasty surgeons should be familiar with the different measures available to help improve future study design and incorporate meaningful findings in their clinical practice.

References

Angst F, Aeschlimann A, Stucki G (2001) Smallest detectable and minimal clinically important differences of rehabilitation intervention with their implications for required sample sizes using WOMAC and SF-36 quality of life measurement instruments in patients with osteoarthritis of the lower ex.

Arthritis Rheum 45:384–391. https://doi.org/10.1002/1529-0131(200108)45:4<384::AID-ART352>3.0.CO;2-0
Bae SC, Lee HS, Yun HR et al (2001) Cross-cultural adaptation and validation of Korean Western Ontario and McMaster Universities (WOMAC) and Lequesne osteoarthritis indices for clinical research. Osteoarthr Cartil 9:746–750. https://doi.org/10.1053/joca.2001.0471
Beaton DE, Boers M, Wells GA (2002) Many faces of the minimal clinically important difference (MCID): a literature review and directions for future research. Curr Opin Rheumatol 14:109–114
Bellamy N, Buchanan WW, Goldsmith CH et al (1988) Validation study of WOMAC: a health status instrument for measuring clinically important patient relevant outcomes to antirheumatic drug therapy in patients with osteoarthritis of the hip or knee. J Rheumatol 15:1833–1840
Brooks R (1996) EuroQol: the current state of play. Health Policy 37:53–72
Calkins TE, Culvern C, Nahhas CR et al (2019) External validity of a new prediction model for patient satisfaction after total knee arthroplasty. United States
Cella D, Yount S, Rothrock N et al (2007) The Patient-Reported Outcomes Measurement Information System (PROMIS): progress of an NIH roadmap cooperative group during its first two years. Med Care 45:S3–S11. https://doi.org/10.1097/01.mlr.0000258615.42478.55
Chughtai M, Patel NK, Gwam CU et al (2017) Do press Ganey scores correlate with total knee arthroplasty-specific outcome questionnaires in postsurgical patients? J Arthroplast 32:S109–S112. https://doi.org/10.1016/j.arth.2017.01.007
Clement ND, MacDonald D, Simpson AHRW (2014) The minimal clinically important difference in the Oxford knee score and Short Form 12 score after total knee arthroplasty. Knee Surg Sports Traumatol Arthrosc 22:1933–1939. https://doi.org/10.1007/s00167-013-2776-5
Clement ND, Weir D, Holland J et al (2019) Meaningful changes in the Short Form 12 physical and mental summary scores after total knee arthroplasty. Knee 26:861–868. https://doi.org/10.1016/j.knee.2019.04.018
CMS (2019) Measure methodology. https://www.cms.gov/Medicare/Quality-Initiatives-Patient-Assessment-Instruments/HospitalQualityInits/Measure-Methodology.html. Accessed 26 Sep 2019
Dawson J, Fitzpatrick R, Murray D, Carr A (1998) Questionnaire on the perceptions of patients about total knee replacement. J Bone Joint Surg Br 80:63–69
Ehrich EW, Davies GM, Watson DJ et al (2000) Minimal perceptible clinical improvement with the Western Ontario and McMaster Universities osteoarthritis index questionnaire and global assessments in patients with osteoarthritis. J Rheumatol 27:2635–2641
EQ-5D instruments – EQ-5D. https://euroqol.org/eq-5d-instruments/. Accessed 12 May 2021
EuroQol Group (1990) EuroQol–a new facility for the measurement of health-related quality of life. Health Policy 16:199–208
Fries JF, Witter J, Rose M et al (2014) Item response theory, computerized adaptive testing, and PROMIS: assessment of physical function. J Rheumatol 41:153–158. https://doi.org/10.3899/jrheum.130813
Giesinger K, Hamilton DF, Jost B et al (2014) Comparative responsiveness of outcome measures for total knee arthroplasty. Osteoarthr Cartil 22:184–189. https://doi.org/10.1016/j.joca.2013.11.001
Graham B, Green A, James M et al (2015) Measuring patient satisfaction in orthopaedic surgery. J Bone Joint Surg Am 97:80–84. https://doi.org/10.2106/JBJS.N.00811
Herdman M, Gudex C, Lloyd A et al (2011) Development and preliminary testing of the new five-level version of EQ-5D (EQ-5D-5L). Qual Life Res 20:1727–1736. https://doi.org/10.1007/s11136-011-9903-x
Holzer BM, Minder CE (2011) A simple approach to fairer hospital benchmarking using patient experience data. Int J Qual Heal Care J Int Soc Qual Heal Care 23:524–530. https://doi.org/10.1093/intqhc/mzr047
Hung M, Bounsanga J, Voss MW, Saltzman CL (2018) Establishing minimum clinically important difference values for the patient-reported outcomes measurement information system physical function, hip disability and osteoarthritis outcome score for joint reconstruction, and knee injury and osteoarthritis ou. World J Orthop 9:41–49. https://doi.org/10.5312/wjo.v9.i3.41
Insall JN, Dorr LD, Scott RD, Scott WN (1989) Rationale of the Knee Society clinical rating system. Clin Orthop Relat Res:13–14
Jenkinson C, Wright L, Coulter A (1994) Criterion validity and reliability of the SF-36 in a population sample. Qual Life Res 3:7–12
Kagan R, Anderson MB, Christensen JC et al (2018) The recovery curve for the patient-reported outcomes measurement information system patient-reported physical function and pain interference computerized adaptive tests after primary total knee arthroplasty. J Arthroplast 33:2471–2474. https://doi.org/10.1016/j.arth.2018.03.020
Kohring JM, Pelt CE, Anderson MB et al (2018) Press Ganey outpatient medical practice survey scores do not correlate with patient-reported outcomes after primary joint arthroplasty. United States
Lyman S, Lee Y-Y, Franklin PD et al (2016) Validation of the KOOS, JR: a short-form knee arthroplasty outcomes survey. Clin Orthop Relat Res 474:1461–1471. https://doi.org/10.1007/s11999-016-4719-1
Lyons RA, Perry HM, Littlepage BN (1994) Evidence for the validity of the Short-form 36 Questionnaire (SF-36) in an elderly population. Age Ageing 23:182–184. https://doi.org/10.1093/ageing/23.3.182
Murray DW, Fitzpatrick R, Rogers K et al (2007) The use of the Oxford hip and knee scores. J Bone Joint Surg Br 89:1010–1014. https://doi.org/10.1302/0301-620X.89B8.19424
Noble PC, Scuderi GR, Brekke AC et al (2012) Development of a new Knee Society scoring system. Clin Orthop Relat Res 470:20–32. https://doi.org/10.1007/s11999-011-2152-z
Padilla JA, Rudy HL, Gabor JA et al (2019) Relationship between the patient-reported outcome measurement information system and traditional patient-reported outcomes for osteoarthritis. United States
Paxton EW, Fithian DC (2005) Outcome instruments for patellofemoral arthroplasty. Clin Orthop Relat Res:66–70. https://doi.org/10.1097/01.blo.0000171544.38095.77
Perneger TV, Leplege A, Etter JF, Rougemont A (1995) Validation of a French-language version of the MOS 36-Item Short Form Health Survey (SF-36) in young healthy adults. J Clin Epidemiol 48:1051–1060. https://doi.org/10.1016/0895-4356(94)00227-h
Rolfson O, Bohm E, Franklin P et al (2016) Patient-reported outcome measures in arthroplasty registries report of the Patient-Reported Outcome Measures Working Group of the International Society of Arthroplasty Registries Part II. Recommendations for selection, administration, and analysis. Acta Orthop 87(Suppl 1):9–23. https://doi.org/10.1080/17453674.2016.1181816
Roos EM, Lohmander LS (2003) The Knee injury and Osteoarthritis Outcome Score (KOOS): from joint injury to osteoarthritis. Health Qual Life Outcomes 1:64. https://doi.org/10.1186/1477-7525-1-64
Roos EM, Roos HP, Lohmander LS et al (1998) Knee Injury and Osteoarthritis Outcome Score (KOOS)–development of a self-administered outcome measure. J Orthop Sports Phys Ther 28:88–96. https://doi.org/10.2519/jospt.1998.28.2.88

Roos EM, Roos HP, Lohmander LS (1999) WOMAC Osteoarthritis Index–additional dimensions for use in subjects with post-traumatic osteoarthritis of the knee. Western Ontario and MacMaster Universities. Osteoarthr Cartil 7:216–221. https://doi.org/10.1053/joca.1998.0153

Scuderi GR, Bourne RB, Noble PC et al (2012) The new Knee Society Knee Scoring System. Clin Orthop Relat Res 470:3–19. https://doi.org/10.1007/s11999-011-2135-0

Scuderi GR, Sikorskii A, Bourne RB et al (2016) The knee society short form reduces respondent burden in the assessment of patient-reported outcomes. Clin Orthop Relat Res 474:134–142. https://doi.org/10.1007/s11999-015-4370-2

Shim J, Hamilton DF (2019) Comparative responsiveness of the PROMIS-10 Global Health and EQ-5D questionnaires in patients undergoing total knee arthroplasty. England

Smith MV, Klein SE, Clohisy JC et al (2012) Lower extremity-specific measures of disability and outcomes in orthopaedic surgery. J Bone Joint Surg Am 94:468–477. https://doi.org/10.2106/JBJS.J.01822

Stiegel KR, Lash JG, Peace AJ et al (2019) Early experience and results using patient-reported outcomes measurement information system scores in primary Total hip and knee arthroplasty. J Arthroplast. https://doi.org/10.1016/j.arth.2019.05.044

Sullivan M, Karlsson J, Ware JEJ (1995) The Swedish SF-36 Health Survey–I. Evaluation of data quality, scaling assumptions, reliability and construct validity across general populations in Sweden. Soc Sci Med 41:1349–1358. https://doi.org/10.1016/0277-9536(95)00125-q

Van Onsem S, Van Der Straeten C, Arnout N et al (2016) A new prediction model for patient satisfaction after total knee arthroplasty. J Arthroplasty 31:2660–2667.e1. https://doi.org/10.1016/j.arth.2016.06.004

van Reenen M, Janssen B (2019) EQ-5D-5L User Guide. https://euroqol.org/wp-content/uploads/2016/09/EQ-5D5L_UserGuide_2015.pdf. Accessed 8 Sep 2019

Vangsness CTJ, Mac P, Requa R, Garrick J (1995) Review of outcome instruments for evaluation of anterior cruciate ligament reconstruction. Bull Hosp Jt Dis 54:25–29

Ware JEJ (2000) Using generic measures of functional health and well-being to increase understanding of disease burden. Spine (Phila Pa 1976) 25:1467

Ware JEJ, Sherbourne CD (1992) The MOS 36-item short-form health survey (SF-36). I. Conceptual framework and item selection. Med Care 30:473–483

Ware JJ, Kosinski M, Keller SD (1996) A 12-Item Short-Form Health Survey: construction of scales and preliminary tests of reliability and validity. Med Care 34:220–233. https://doi.org/10.1097/00005650-199603000-00003

Webster KE, Feller JA (2016) Comparison of the short form-12 (SF-12) health status questionnaire with the SF-36 in patients with knee osteoarthritis who have replacement surgery. Knee Surg Sports Traumatol Arthrosc 24:2620–2626. https://doi.org/10.1007/s00167-015-3904-1

Weinberger M, Samsa GP, Hanlon JT et al (1991) An evaluation of a brief health status measure in elderly veterans. J Am Geriatr Soc 39:691–694. https://doi.org/10.1111/j.1532-5415.1991.tb03623.x

Wolfe F, Kong SX (1999) Rasch analysis of the Western Ontario MacMaster questionnaire (WOMAC) in 2205 patients with osteoarthritis, rheumatoid arthritis, and fibromyalgia. Ann Rheum Dis 58:563–568. https://doi.org/10.1136/ard.58.9.563

Wright RW (2009) Knee injury outcomes measures. J Am Acad Orthop Surg 17:31–39

Treatment

Contents

Fixation in Joint Arthroplasty

Michael Morlock, Sarah Fischer, and Elke Lieb

Contents

E. Hansen, K.-D. Kühn (eds.), *Essentials of Cemented Knee Arthroplasty*,
https://doi.org/10.1007/978-3-662-63113-3_13

13.1 Clinical History

The clinical history of total joint arthroplasty (TJA) started with implants fixed into the bone without cement. First pioneers in orthopedics concentrated rather on innovative prosthesis designs imitating the mechanical functions of natural joints than on their fixation method into the surrounding bone bed. In total hip arthroplasty (THA) milestone developments in implant fixation were introduced in the mid-nineteenth century by Judet with his artificial femoral head (Judet and Judet 1950), the Matchett Brown hemiarthroplasty (Emery and Gray 1996), and the Phillip Wiles design of a metal-on-metal prosthesis (Gomez and Morcuende 2005). Some impressively good long-term results exist for these prostheses. For example, for a Judet polymethylmethacrylate (PMMA) hip hemiprosthesisa time in situ of 51 years before revision was reported (◘ Fig. 13.1). This makes it the first implant to have survived for longer than 50 years. No signs of aggressive osteolysis were found on histologic analysis, which confirms good tissue tolerance for PMMA (Kovač et al. 2004). In 1890, already the outstanding work from Themistocles Gluck about mechanical principles has led to an important understanding of total knee arthroplasty (TKA) prosthesis designs, which came into clinical use quite sometime after the THA designs (Eynon-Lewis et al. 1992).

Based on these early biomechanical insights, it was Sir John Charnley who marked one of the crucial milestones in orthopedics with his "low friction" arthroplasty concept that prevented mechanical loosening and was associated with less wear debris due to a small head diameter of 22.225 mm (◘ Fig. 13.2) (Charnley 2012). The area of tribology research was born. For the fixation of his implant, he utilized an acrylate bone cement that was in surgical use for cranioplasty, which he modified in terms of adequate working time and the addition of a radio-opaque agent. He described the property of

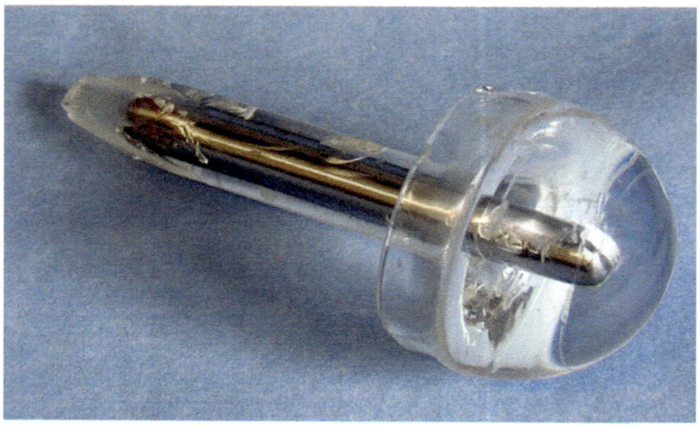

◘ **Fig. 13.1** Example of a Judet prosthesisexplant, revised at AK Eilbek in Hamburg after 27 years in situ

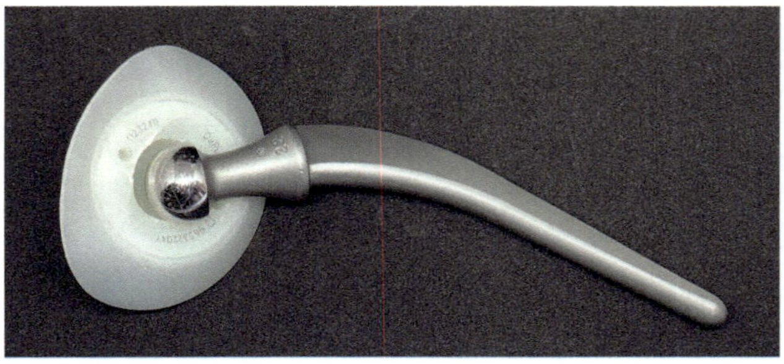

◘ **Fig. 13.2** The Charnley monoblock prosthesiswith a small head (diameter 22.225 mm) and a Charnley Ogee PE Cup

this bone cement as a grout and not as a glue, highlighting that it acts as a space-filler holding the implant against the bone due to its bounding to the adjacent surfaces by penetrating cavities and closely molding the surface asperities. This fixation method solved the initial problem for the mechanical stability of the prosthesis in the bone.

PMMA bone cement for TJA fixation was launched as a medical device. Initially, PMMA bone cement did not contain any antibiotics. At the same time, Buchholz and Engelbrecht were the first to introduce the concept of antibiotic-loaded bone cement (ALBC) in their cemented hip procedures by mixing gentamicin powder into their Palacos® bone cement (Buchholz and Engelbrecht 1970). The antibiotic powder was mixed into the cement first by hand without really knowing the right dosage and the release properties. This made it difficult to achieve an optimized combination aligned with the patient-specific systemic antibiotic therapy. Despite these shortcomings during the initial 10 years, an overall 77% success rate in controlling infections could be demonstrated by this use of ALBC in 583 patients and a 90% success rate after subsequent revisions (Buchholz et al. 1981). In the coming years, improvements in clinical success rates continued to rise with the market access of industrially mixed and certified off-the-shelf ALBC.

> Today, there is some evidence that ALBC significantly reduces the rate of infections in revision procedures (Kleppel et al. 2017; Leong et al. 2020).

Fixation philosophies in TJA, nowadays, vary not only greatly between countries (in Europe there is the phrase: The further you go south the less cement in THA) but also between different joints like hip, knee, shoulder, and ankle. In 2019, the German Arthroplasty Registry(EPRD) reported primary THA fixation methods: 78.6% for cementless, 5% for cemented, and 14.8% for hybrid cemented cases, whereas only 1.3% reverse-hybrid cemented implantations occurred. For TKA primary interventions, the situation was the opposite: Cemented implantations are dominant with 93.2% and only 1.2% for cementless fixations. Hybrid and reverse-hybrid cement fixation was reported in only about 5% of the cases (Endoprothesenregister Deutschland (EPRD) 2019). For the same year, the Swedish Knee Arthroplasty Register reported very similar data with only 7.3% cementless TKA surgeries. Between 1985 and 1995, Swedish surgeons experimented with cementless and hybrid fixations but came back to mainly all cemented implants soon after (Swedish Knee Arthroplasty Register 2019).

13.2 Clinical Outcome

> In all available national registries, the most frequent reason for revision is loosening of the prosthesis in the surrounding bone bed in both THA and TKA with 34% and 32% of all respective revision cases. The second reason is diagnosed infection with 19% for THA and 22% for TKA.

The EPRD reported loosening in 34% and infection in 19% of THA cases as a reason for revision and for TKA revision 32% loosening and 22% infection. Notable is that the national joint registries from Scandinavia, existing since the early 1970s—thus with the most matured data—expressed their doubts if the true incidence of infection is underestimated by about 40% (Gundtoft et al. 2015; Jämsen et al. 2009; Espehaug et al. 2006; Witso 2015).

> The clinical outcome of TJA depends on multiple factors.

Of all the factors responsible for the clinical outcome of TJA, the most important factor cannot be assessed directly: the implantation process performed by the operating surgeon. The influence of other factors can be assessed by comparing patient cohorts, even so a surgeon bias cannot be completely ruled out.

Fixation Method and Patient Age

Registries have started early in their development to report their data in addition to the whole data set separately for different age groups since age has a major influence. Most of the data show that THA patients younger than 75 years generally benefit more from cementless fixation, especially when considered on long-term follow-up. However, a significantly better and longer clinical success result is achieved with cementing fixation for patients older than 75 years (Endoprothesenregister Deutschland (EPRD) 2019). In TKA, the influence of age for the comparison between cemented and cementless fixation of the femur component in young patients does not show a significant difference with respect to function or revision rate (Franceschetti et al. 2017).

Patient Weight

Another factor that influences significantly the long-term survival of a joint implant is the patient's body mass index (BMI). Studies show, for instance in TKA, that the adjusted cumulative hazard of revision due to aseptic tibial loosening more than doubles when BMI passes more than 35 kg/m^2 (Abdel et al. 2015). Interestingly, some newer studies indicate that uncemented TKA in the obese and morbidly obese might be performing equal or better (Sinicrope et al. 2019). Again, such results are strongly influenced by the respective surgeon. In THA, body weight also comprises an important issue but the results are not coherent: Some publications quote a quite significant increase in complications with increased bodyweight; others do not (Haynes et al. 2017).

Prosthesis Design

Since the introduction of the Swedish Hip Arthroplasty Registry 40 years ago, the choice of prosthesis design has become less and less important. This does not mean that the prosthesis design is not important anymore, but rather that all registries and institutions (e.g., the Orthopaedic Data Evaluation Panel) together, have been very effective in identifying poor designs or materials and consequently removing them from the market. This statement accounts for cemented and for uncemented prostheses.

13.3 Fixation Method

> Uncemented and cemented designs are similarly successful in most registries with national differences with respect to preferred choices (Deere et al. 2019a; Deere et al. 2019b).

A recent analysis of a National Joint Registry comes to the conclusion that despite improved survivorship of uncemented fixation in TKA for osteoarthritis, cemented fixation remains the gold standard (Nugent et al. 2019). Several clinical studies are available, either demonstrating the advantage of certain designs or showing similarities. Clinical studies always have to be viewed under the limitation that surgeon influence might be a major factor for the results. As an example, just a single study comparing 200 cases of a cementless tibial mobile-bearing TKA design showing similar survival rates after 11 years compared with cemented similar tibial design is mentioned (Prudhon and Verdier 2017). Own TKA autopsy study demonstrated that the fixation strength of cemented designs decreases with time in situ and showed that cement pockets for increased cement bonding are advantageous (Gebert de Uhlenbrock et al. 2012). Again the age-related factor influences the long-term result hypothesizing that younger patients are more active and that the load factor does play a negative role for the bony interface loading.

13.3.1 Cement Type

There are *many different cements* from several companies available (■ Fig. 13.3). The handling differences mainly concern viscosity (low, medium, or normal, high). Depending on the cement type, work timings are different and penetration and interdigitation into the bone also vary with the application method (Kelly et al. 2018; Silverman et al. 2014). This makes it difficult for surgeons since they have to adapt to their respective cementing techniques depending on the kind of cement they use. A data summary from the National Joint Registry (NJR) concluded for cement type when extracted for brand name with endpoint as cemented component revision that Palacos® bone cement from Heraeus Medical resulted in a significantly lower cumulative revision rate after 12 years than all other cement brands (National Joint Registry 2020). Other registries indicate that the introduction of new bone cements led to survival rates as good as with "the old" bone cements (Birkeland et al. 2016), but that not all bone cements perform equally well (Trela-Larsen et al. 2017).

13.3.2 Cementing Technique

The introduction of innovative minimally invasive surgery (MIS) in 2016 represented a challenge for the correct cementing technique due to minimized access to the bone site. The unilateral knee arthroplasty design (UKA) introduced in parallel to MIS experienced early failure rates assumingly also linked to the limited access to the surgical site exposure which could result in poor or non-homogenous cement penetration into the bone (Hauptmann et al. 2008). Another complication associated with early failure could be posterior cement leakage when the implanted prosthesis was moved before the cement had hardened completely (Karataglis et al. 2012). This started discussions regarding the questions such as which patient is best for which prosthesis design (mobile or fixed bearing, constraint or unconstraint), which modern surgical technique (minimal invasive or computer-assisted), and which fixation technique is most suitable (cemented, uncemented, or special coatings). A multitude of studies performed at the University of Technology in Hamburg highlighted that preparation of the bone bed is one of the most crucial aspects for the fixation strength of TKA components (Nagel et al. 2017; Schlegel et al. 2015; Schlegel et al. 2014a; Schlegel et al. 2014; Schlegel et al. 2011).

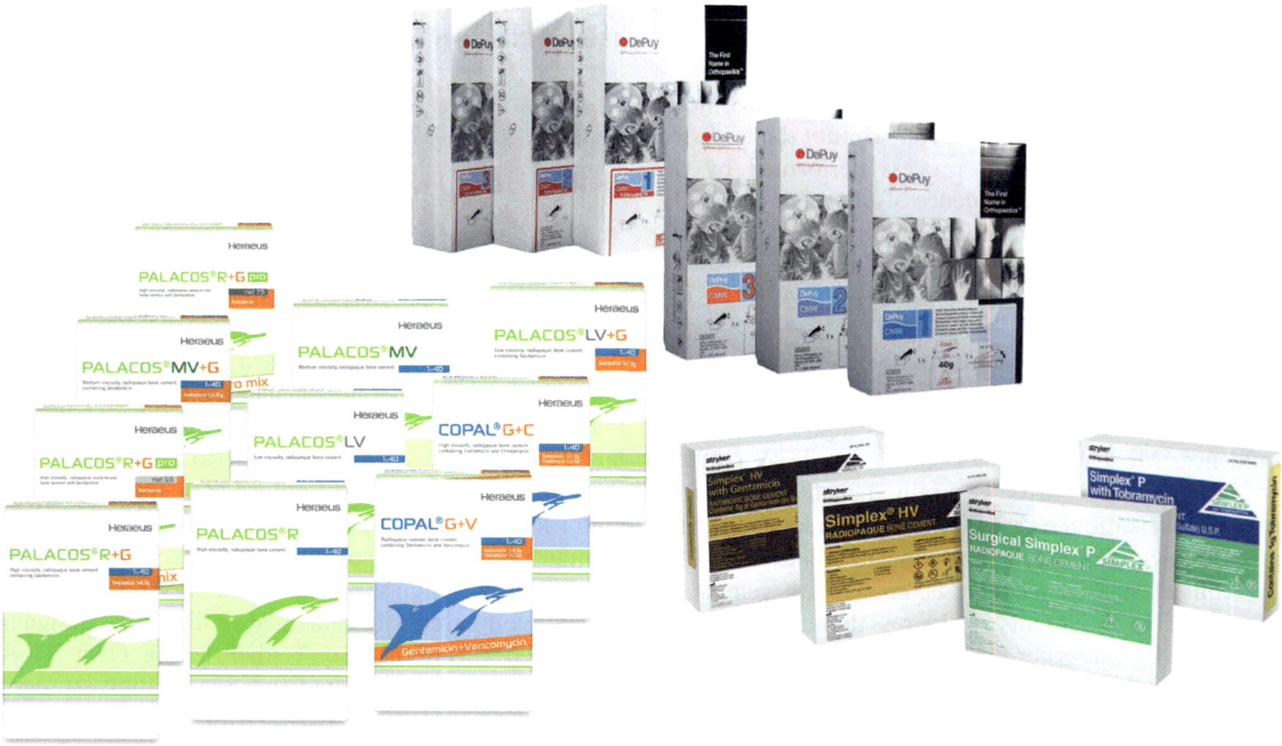

■ **Fig. 13.3** Examples for different cement types available

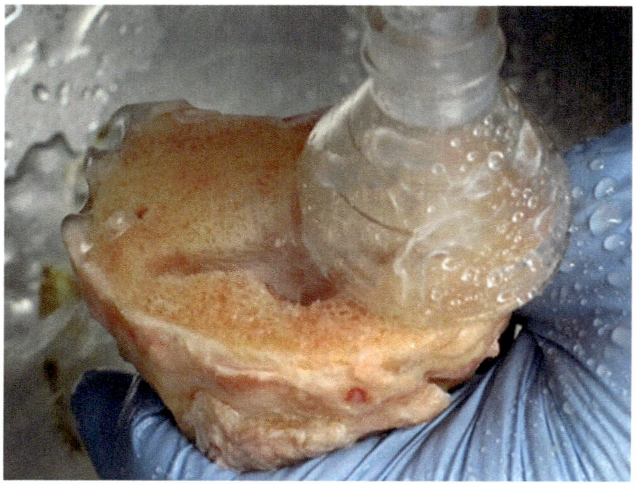

Fig. 13.4 Jet lavage as an effective way to improve cement-to-bone fixation strength

> The use of jet lavage seems to be a simple but very effective way of improving the interdigitation and strength of the initial cement–implant bond (Fig. 13.4).

Applying pressure to cement also improves the fixation strength (Pérez-Mañanes et al. 2011).

13.4 What Have We Learned?

TJA has become a very successful procedure; it should be considered as the operation of the century (Learmonth et al. 2007), especially in THA. In the past, improvements in outcomes were made possible by improvements in implant design and materials. As in other highly specialized performing fields, further improvement relying only on improvement of the "hardware" will hardly be possible anymore.

> "Big Data" available from the registries highlight more and more the dominating importance of the implantation process and the surgeon. The concentration on these factors will mark the twenty-first century.

Especially in TKA, surgeons still face a group of unhappy patients postoperatively despite the fact the surgery went well and the positioning of the implant was achieved as planned (Kahlenberg et al. 2018a; Klem et al. 2020). Up to one out of four patients is unhappy with the outcome of the TKA surgery after the rehab phase, which is in contrast to THA surgery, for which "the forgotten joint" is achieved in more than 90% of the patients (Puliero et al. 2019). It's paradoxical, that despite the higher percentage of unhappy patients, revision rates in TKA after 10 years are lower than in THA (Puliero et al. 2019; Deere et al. 2019b). Future research should focus on standardizing patient satisfaction reporting and defining ways to optimize patient satisfaction after TKA (Kahlenberg et al. 2018b) and the implementation of patient-reported outcome measures (PROMs) into national and even international common registries.

The final challenge to be solved is what Justin Cobb from Imperial College in London calls "epistemology—patient welfare and function versus Device survival". A revision or addition surgery might very well be justified and not collectively called a "failure", if every stage of the process has produced the desired outcome. UKA is a good example of this: The design with quite high overall revision rates in the registries performs very well if implanted by high-volume surgeons and can show better function than TKA (Endoprothesenregister Deutschland (EPRD) 2019; Deere et al. 2019a; Mohammad et al. 2018; Casper et al. 2019).

> The focus on further improving the cementing technique for cemented TJA and on improving the primary stability for uncemented TJA will prevail.

Take-Home Messages

- Fixation in total joint replacement has been greatly improved by improvement in design and materials over the last 50 years.
- Patient and surgical factors play an important role in long-term survival.
- Further improvement is only possible if all relevant factors are addressed: material, design, surgeon, and patient.
- Uncemented and cemented fixations perform equally well but benefits of one method over the other exist in certain patient cohorts.
- In cemented fixation, the preparation of the bone bed is crucial and the use of jet lavage is highly advised, especially in TKA.

References

Abdel MP, Bonadurer GF 3rd, Jennings MT, Hanssen AD (2015) Increased aseptic Tibial failures in patients with a BMI ≥35 and well-aligned total knee arthroplasties. J Arthroplast 30(12):2181–2184

Birkeland Ø, Espehaug B, Havelin LI, Furnes O (2016) Bone cement product and failure in total kneearthroplasty. Acta Orthop 88(1):75–81

Buchholz HW, Engelbrecht H (1970) Depot effects of various antibiotics mixed with Palacos resins. Chirurg 41(11):511–515

Buchholz HW, Elson RA, Engelbrecht E, Lodenkämper H, Röttger J, Siegel A (1981) Management of deep infection of total hip replacement. J Bone Joint Surg 63-B(3):342–353

Casper DS, Fleischman AN, Papas PV, Grossman J, Scuderi GR, Lonner JH (2019) Unicompartmental knee arthroplasty provides significantly greater improvement in function than total knee arthroplasty despite equivalent satisfaction for isolated medial compartment osteoarthritis. J Arthroplast 34(8): 1611–1616
Charnley J (2012) Low friction arthroplasty of the hip. Springer Publishing, New York
Deere KC, Whitehouse MR, Porter M, Blom AW, Sayers A (2019a) Assessing the non-inferiority of prosthesis constructs used in total and unicondylar knee replacements using data from the National Joint Registry of England, Wales, Northern Ireland and the Isle of Man: a benchmarking study. BMJ Open 9(4):e026736
Deere KC, Whitehouse MR, Porter M, Blom AW, Sayers A (2019b) Assessing the non-inferiority of prosthesis constructs used in hip replacement using data from the National Joint Registry of England, Wales, Northern Ireland and the Isle of Man: a benchmarking study. BMJ Open 9(4):e026685
Emery DP, Gray DH (1996) Matchett Brown hemiarthroplasty for displaced subcapital fractures of the hip. ANZ J Surg 66(3): 159–161
Endoprothesenregister Deutschland (EPRD) (2019) Annual report
Espehaug B, Furnes O, Havelin LI, Engesaeter LB, Vollset SE, Kindseth O (2006) Registration completeness in the Norwegian ArthroplastyRegister. Acta Orthop 77(1):49–56
Eynon-Lewis NJ, Ferry D, Pearse MF (1992) Themistocles Gluck: an unrecognised genius. The BMJ 305(6868):1534–1536
Franceschetti E, Torre G, Palumbo A, Papalia R, Karlsson J, Ayeni OR, Samuelsson K, Franceschi F (2017) No difference between cemented and cementless total knee arthroplasty in young patients: a review of the evidence. Knee Surg Sports Traumatol Arthrosc 25(6):1749–1756
Gebert de Uhlenbrock A, Püschel V, Püschel K, Morlock MM, Bishop NE (2012) Influence of time in-situ and implant type on fixation strength of cemented tibial trays – a post mortem retrieval analysis. Clin Biomech 27(9):929–935
Gomez PF, Morcuende JA (2005) Early attempts at hip arthroplasty-1700s to 1950s. Iowa Orthop J 25:25–29
Gundtoft PH, Overgaard S, Schønheyder HC, Møller JK, Kjærsgaard-Andersen P, Pedersen AB (2015) The "true" incidence of surgically treated deep prosthetic joint infection after 32,896 primary total hip arthroplasties. Acta Orthop 86(3):326–334
Hauptmann SM, Weber P, Glaser C, Birkenmaier C, Jansson V, Müller PE (2008) Free bone cement fragments after minimally invasive unicompartmental knee arthroplasty: an underappreciated problem. Knee Surg Sports Traumatol Arthrosc 16(8):770–775
Haynes J, Nam D, Barrack RL (2017) Obesity in total hip arthroplasty: does it make a difference? Bone Joint J 99-B(1 Supple A):31–36
Jämsen E, Huotari K, Huhtala H, Nevalainen J, Konttinen YT (2009) Low rate of infected knee replacements in a nationwide series—is it an underestimate? Acta Orthop 80(2):205–212
Judet J, Judet R (1950) The use of an artificial femoral head for arthroplasty of the hip joint. J Bone Joint Surg 32-B(2):166–173
Kahlenberg CA, Nwachukwu BU, McLawhorn AS, Cross MB, Cornell CN, Padgett DE (2018a) Patient satisfaction after total knee replacement: a systematic review. HSS J 14(2):192–201
Kahlenberg CA, Nwachukwu BU, McLawhorn AS, Cross MB, Cornell CN, Padgett DE (2018b) Patient satisfaction after total knee replacement: a systematic review. HSS J 14(2):192–201
Karataglis D, Agathangelidis F, Papadopoulos P, Petsatodis G, Christodoulou A (2012) Arthroscopic removal of impinging cement after unicompartmental knee arthroplasty. Hippokratia 16(1):76–79
Kelly MP, Illgen RL, Chen AF, Nam D (2018) Trends in the use of high-viscosity cement in patients undergoing primary total knee arthroplasty in the United States. J Arthroplast 33(11):3460–3464
Klem NR, Kent P, Smith A, Dowsey M, Fary R, Schütze R, O'Sullivan P, Choong P, Bunzli S (2020) Satisfaction after total knee replacement for osteoarthritis is usually high, but what are we measuring? A systematic review. Osteoarthritis Cartilage Open 2(1):100032
Kleppel D, Stirton J, Liu J, Ebraheim NA (2017) Antibiotic bone cement's effect on infection rates in primary and revision total knee arthroplasties. World J Orthop 8(12):946–955
Kovač S, Pišot V, Trebše R, Rotter A (2004) Fifty-one-year survival of a Judetpolymethylmethacrylate hip prosthesis. J Arthroplast 19(5):664–667
Learmonth ID, Young C, Rorabeck C (2007) The operation of the century: total hip replacement. Lancet 370(9597):1508–1519
Leong JW, Cook MJ, O'Neill TW, Board TN (2020) Is the use of antibiotic-loaded bone cement associated with a lower risk of revision after primary total hip arthroplasty? Bone Joint J 102-B(8):997–1002
Mohammad HR, Strickland L, Hamilton TW, Murray DW (2018) Long-term outcomes of over 8,000 medial Oxford phase 3 unicompartmental knees-a systematic review. Acta Orthop 89(1):101–107
Nagel K et al (2017) The influence of cement morphology parameters on the strength of the cement-bone Interface in Tibial tray fixation. J Arthroplast 32:563–569
National Joint Registry (2020) Implant Summary Report for: Heraeus Medical Hips using Palacos Antibiotic Cement. https://www.heraeus.com/media/media/hme/doc_hme/aboutheraeus/njr/Summary_Report_HP_Cement_Palacos_Antibiotic_17-02-20.pdf
Nugent M, Wyatt MC, Frampton CM, Hooper GJ (2019) Despite improved survivorship of uncemented fixation in total knee arthroplasty for osteoarthritis, cemented fixation remains the gold standard: an analysis of a National Joint Registry. J Arthroplast 34(8):1626–1633
Pérez-Mañanes R, Vaquero Martín J, Villanueva Martínez M (2011) Influence of the fixing technique on the quality of the cement mantle in knee arthroplasty. Experimental study on a synthetic model. Revista Espanola de CirugiaOrtopedica y Traumatologia 55(1):39–49
Prudhon JL, Verdier R (2017) Cemented or cementless total knee arthroplasty? – comparative results of 200 cases at a minimum follow-up of 11 years. SICOT-J 3:70
Puliero B, Blakeney WG, Beaulieu Y, Vendittoli PA (2019) Joint perception after total hip arthroplasty and the forgotten joint. J Arthroplast 34(1):65–70
Schlegel U et al (2011) Pulsed lavage improves fixation strength of cemented tibial components. Int Orthop 35:1165–1169
Schlegel U et al (2014) Effect of tibial tray design on cement morphology in total knee arthroplasty. J Orthop Surg Res 9:123
Schlegel U et al (2014a) An in vitro comparison of tibial tray cementation using gun pressurization or pulsed lavage. Int Orthop 38:967–971
Schlegel U et al (2015) Comparison of different cement application techniques for tibial component fixation in TKA. Int Orthop 39:47–54
Silverman EJ, Landy DC, Massel DH, Kaimrajh DN, Latta LL, Robinson RP (2014) The effect of viscosity on cement penetration in total knee arthroplasty, an application of the squeeze film effect. J Arthroplast 29(10):2039–2042
Sinicrope BJ, Feher AW, Bhimani SJ, Smith LS, Harwin SF, Yakkanti MR, Malkani AL (2019) Increased survivorship of Cementless versus cemented TKA in the morbidly obese. A minimum 5-year follow-up. J Arthroplast 34(2):309–314
Swedish Knee Arthroplasty Register (2019) Annual Report 2019
Trela-Larsen L, Sayers A, Blom AW, Webb JCJ, Whitehouse MR (2017) The association between cement type and the subsequent risk of revision surgery in primary total hip replacement. Acta Orthop 89(1):40–46
Witso E (2015) The rate of prosthetic joint infection is underestimated in the arthroplasty registers. Acta Orthop 86(3):277–278

Medial Unicompartmental Knee Arthroplasty

Asim Khan and Fares Haddad

Contents

E. Hansen, K.-D. Kühn (eds.), *Essentials of Cemented Knee Arthroplasty*,
https://doi.org/10.1007/978-3-662-63113-3_14

14.1 Introduction

Knee arthroplasty provides a predictable and reliable way of treating painful loss of mobility of the knee joint in patients with arthritis. There is a philosophical and surgical debate as to whether osteoarthritis of the knee can only affect individual compartments or whether the whole knee is inevitably affected, either primarily or secondarily. The belief that arthritis is a disease of the whole knee joint has led to a biased focus on improvements in total knee arthroplasty (TKA) design at the expense of innovations in unicompartmental knee arthroplasty (UKA; medial, lateral, or patellofemoral). At the turn of the century, the introduction of minimally invasive techniques (Repicci and Eberle 1999) resulted in renewed interest in UKA and its utilization has increased at a rate nearly triple that of TKA (Foran et al. 2013). Although the decision to undertake partial or total knee arthroplasty may depend in part on a surgeon's training, experience, or interpretation of literature, both partial and total knee arthroplasty are viable options for the treatment of osteoarthritis of the knee. The decision may ultimately be shaped by the ability of enhanced technologies to help with the execution of the procedure (Kayani et al. 2018a, b).

A recent synthesis of evidence from randomized trials, registries, and cohort studies suggested a shorter hospital stay, fewer early complications, and better functional outcome with unicompartmental arthroplasty. Following this procedure, patients can kneel better and have better patient-reported outcomes. Mortality rates may be reduced compared with TKA. The patients also need fewer manipulations under anesthesia.

Revision surgery, however, is much more commonly needed after unicompartmental versus total knee arthroplasty (NJR Online 2019). A higher perceived revision rate has led to the UKA falling out of favor in some centers and countries. While this should not be the only key metric to assess an implant, there is potentially a solution with the use of enhanced technologies that can avoid malalignment and other risks associated with UKA.

> In simple terms, hitting a target through a minimally invasive incision and with high accuracy because of the sensitivity and balance of the rest of the joint demands better instruments or enhanced technologies that are now available (Kayani et al. 2018a).

Authors from centers that perform high volumes of partial knee arthroplasty assert that for optimal outcomes, a surgeon's proportion of unicompartmental arthroplasty ought to be more than 20% to minimize the one disadvantage of this operation, namely its higher revision rate (Murray and Parkinson 2018). To add to the confusion, because UKA is perceived as being a lesser operation, some surgeons may be tempted to offer it to patients with less severe osteoarthritis. Unfortunately, this may lead to worse outcomes that may further tarnish the reputation of this procedure (Murray and Parkinson 2018). We must also recognize the potential for a lower threshold for revising a "painful" partial knee arthroplasty, as this is a relatively straightforward operation, whereas surgeons are less likely to advise revision of total knee arthroplasty for the same indication due to its perceived technical difficulty. In addition, because of the presence of early degenerative changes and osteophytes in the non-resurfaced compartments in a patient with a partial knee arthroplasty, a surgeon may more easily justify revision, which may have a poor functional outcome because the symptoms could have nothing to do with the arthroplasty. This is akin to secondary resurfacing of the patella in a patient with a TKA and a non-resurfaced patella, which, of course, is a very unpredictable operation. Comparison of revision rates as the only way of assessing outcome is, therefore, dangerous and we must look beyond registry data to cohort series, prospective studies, and other datasets to understand the pros and cons of UKA compared with TKA (Murray and Parkinson 2018; Murray et al. 2017; Goodfellow et al. 2010).

The communication of findings can only be effective if all authors refer to the same operation by the same name. Terms such as unicompartmental, unicondylar, bicondylar, and bicompartmental need to be defined and standardized so that readers of research articles can truly understand what is being referred to. More importantly, international registries need to agree on one nomenclature so that long-term results can be accurately understood and compared. Garner et al. (2019) proposed a simple classification system for combined partial knee arthroplasty in an attempt to address issues of nomenclature. There will doubtless be differing views within the orthopedic community, but the simplicity of the proposed classification system should enhance its widespread adoption, or at least the adoption of a modification that will be acceptable to all.

14.2 Patient Selection

Patient selection for UKA has remained a heavily debated topic in the literature.

> The ideal candidate for UKA is the symptomatic, unicompartmental osteoarthritic patient with an intact ACL, preserved range of motion, a correctable deformity, no inflammatory arthritis, and an intact medial collateral ligament (MCL).

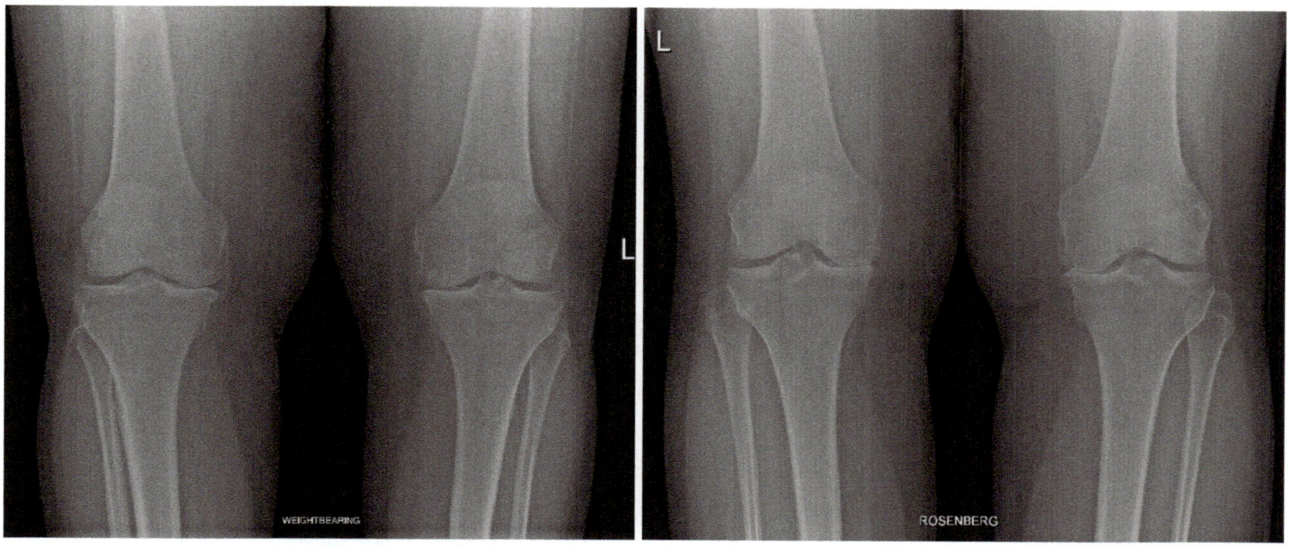

Fig. 14.1 Weight-bearing posteroanterior radiographs in extension (*left*) and flexion Rosenberg views (*right*)

We have moved on from the initial Kozinn and Scott's criteria, which recommended against UKA in patients who were under the following categories:

- Younger than 60 years of age.
- Weighed more than 82 kg.
- Extremely active or heavy laborers.
- Had chondrocalcinosis or exposed bone in the patellofemoral joint (PFJ) because of an early risk of failure (Kozinn et al. 1989; Kozinn and Scott 1989).

Pandit et al. have shown similar or better clinical outcomes with mobile-bearing UKA in patients with the potential contraindications proposed by Kozinn and Scott (Pandit et al. 2011). Furthermore, work by Scott and Goodfellow et al. challenged the thresholds previously reported and showed that weight, age, activity, the state of the PFJ, and chondrocalcinosis should not be considered contraindications to UKA (Deshmukh and Scott 2001; Scott 2003; Goodfellow 2006).

Special preoperative weight-bearing X-rays can be extremely useful. Standing PA views in extension and flexion (Rosenberg views) can be used to screen for unicompartmental disease (Fig. 14.1). Standing lateral X-rays will reveal the pattern of wear; posterior tibial bone loss indicates a disrupted or non-functional ACL (Fig. 14.2). Anterior tibial translation in ACL-deficient knees exposes the posterior tibia to contact stresses from the distal femoral condyles. Merchant or skyline views may demonstrate PFJ arthritis which is a relative contraindication to UKA.

Intraoperative assessment of unicompartmental disease can be made at the time of surgery with the option to proceed with TKA if there is significant lateral or patellofemoral compartment wear. Mild softening or fissuring of cartilage in the lateral compartment can be accepted. Konan et al. have shown that medial PFJ chondral lesions do not appear to affect outcomes after UKA; however significant (modified Outerbridge grade 3 or higher) lesions in the central or lateral PFJ are an indication to proceed with TKA (Konan and Haddad 2016). ACL deficiency is considered a significant (yet not absolute) contraindication to UKA. If the tibial plateau wear pattern is central or anterior, a fixed-bearing UKA may still be feasible and mobile-bearing implants should be avoided. Little or no posterior slope should be applied. The surgeon should bear in mind that lateral subluxation of the tibia may still lead to contralateral compartment arthritis. As varus osteoarthritis progresses, it may present with a kissing lesion or an “anvil osteophyte”. The former results from central tibial subluxation. The lateral tibial spine erodes the medial aspect of the lateral femoral condyle producing a chondral lesion. A lesion of significant size warrants a total or bicompartmental knee replacement. The anvil osteophyte is a tibial osteophyte that occurs just anterior to the footprint of the ACL and causes notch impingement. The resultant flexion contracture can be corrected on the removal of this osteophyte. Inflammatory arthritis in the form of a significant synovial reaction or diffuse chondrocalcinosis, as seen in gout or pseudogout, particularly involving hyaline cartilage as opposed to the menisci alone, are considered contraindications to UKA.

Although osteoarthritis limited to a single compartment of the knee is the most common indication for UKA, focal spontaneous osteonecrosis of the knee (SPONK) with articular surface collapse may be another indication. Osteonecrosis of the medial femoral condyle and rarely of the medial tibial plateau has anatomical

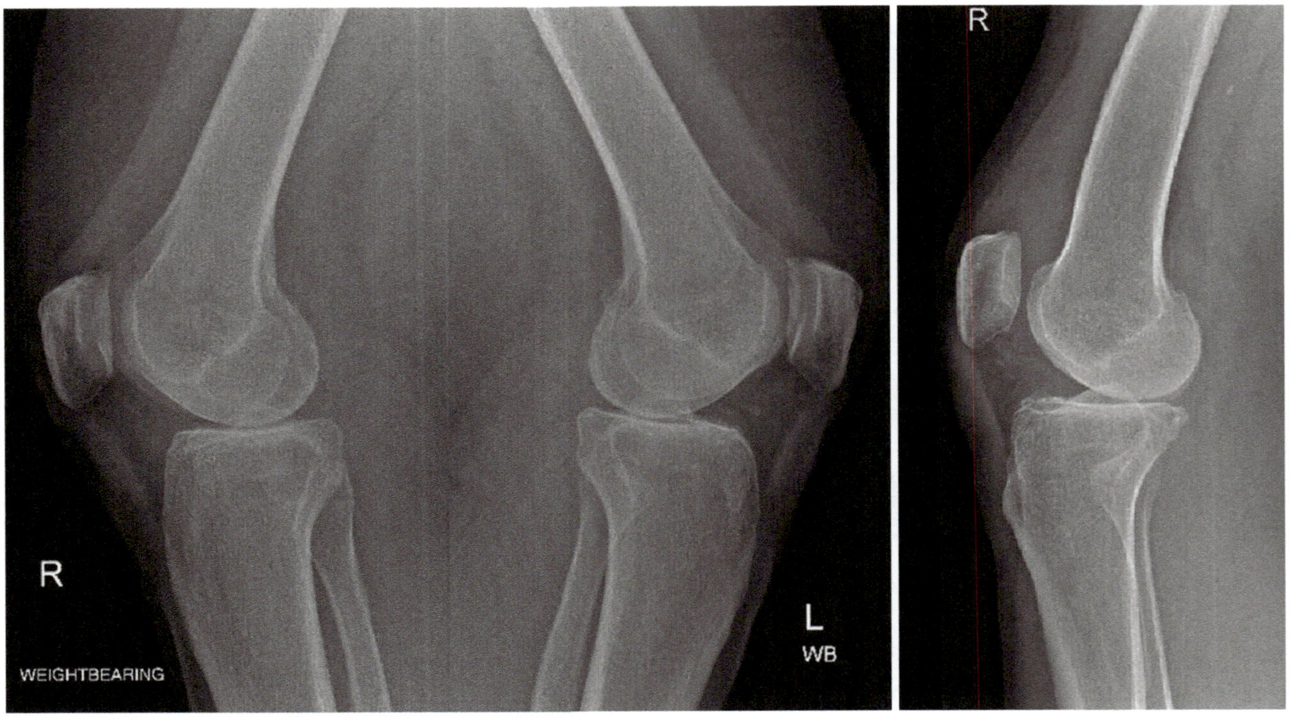

Fig. 14.2 Lateral weight-bearing views of both knees (*left*) of the patient in Fig. 14.1 showing a central pattern of wear in both knees. In contrast, standing lateral X-rays of a patient with posterior tibial bone loss (*right*) indicating ACL deficiency

features very similar to those of osteoarthritis and the surgical technique for UKA is very similar to that used for patients with medial osteoarthritis lesions (Radke et al. 2005).

14

> A deep femoral defect secondary to SPONK has to be dealt with carefully to ensure that not too much bone is milled off the femur and cemented techniques should be utilized whenever possible (Radke et al. 2005).

A meta-analysis of 273 patients undergoing UKA instead of TKA for SPONK has shown fewer complications, significant improvements in functional outcomes, and 95% survivorship at a mean follow-up of 6 years (Jauregui et al. 2018).

14.3 Implant Development

UKA has the advantage of being anatomic by design; preservation of both cruciate ligaments and restoration of the native tension in the collateral ligaments results in the reproduction of near-normal kinematics of the knee (Patil et al. 2005).

One of the earliest UKA designs, the polycentric, was developed in 1968 by Frank Guston, a Canadian surgeon, while on a fellowship at Wrightington Hospital in the UK. It involved replacing both the medial and lateral compartments of the knee while preserving the cruciate ligaments (Gunston 1971). Modular designs such as the St. Georg Sled (1969), the Manchester knee (1971), the Marmor (1972), the Liverpool knee (1972), and Insall's Unicondylar knee (1976) were all developed during a short period of time as interest in UKA was revived. The materials used in the development of these implants evolved over time and initial results were disappointing perhaps because of the learning curve associated with the introduction of a new technique.

The Oxford UKA designed by Goodfellow and O'Connor and first used clinically in 1982 (Phase 1, Fig. 14.3) was perhaps the most significant evolution in UKA design (Goodfellow and O'Connor 1978). Earlier designs had utilized a polyradial, convex metal femoral component based on the natural polycentric form of the femoral condyles. This is articulated with a non-confirming flat or slightly concave polyethylene tibial component. The rounded femoral component articulating with a flat tibia led to the reduced contact area and, therefore, increased contact pressures particularly in deep flexion where the radius of the posterior part of the femoral component was smaller. Designers of the Oxford UKA wanted to maximize the contact area between the two components of the prosthesis while allowing for the natural translation and axial rotation that occurs in the native knee during flexion and extension activities (Goodfellow and O'Connor 1978). The Oxford UKA was therefore designed with two

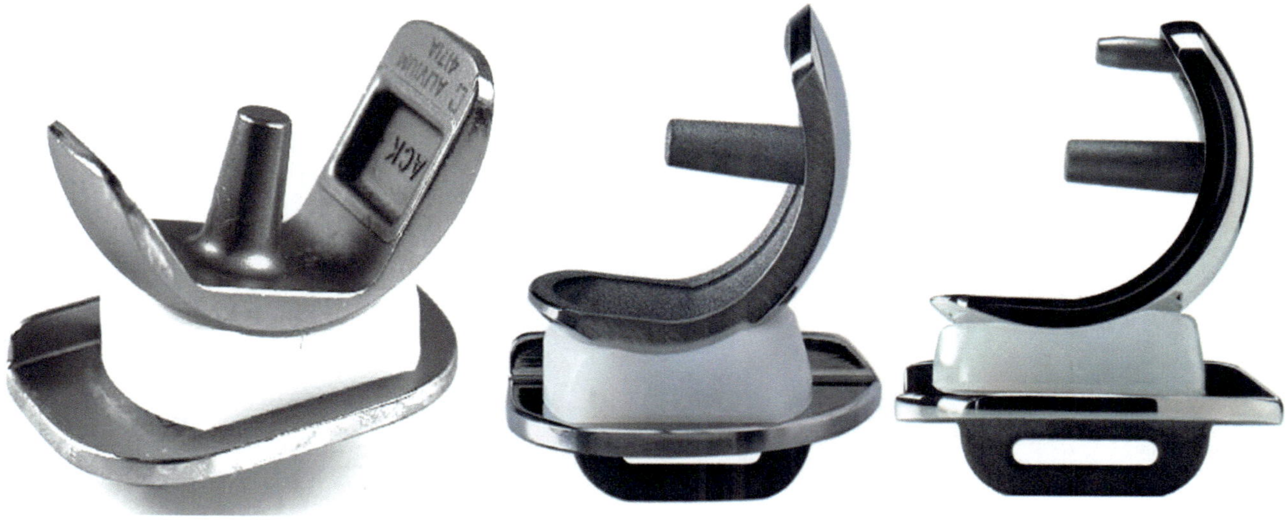

Fig. 14.3 The Oxford Phase 1 (*left*), Phase 2 (*center*), and Phase 3 designs (*right*)

mobile-bearing interfaces. It has a monoradial femoral component and a flat tibial component with a "meniscal" bearing composed of high-density polyethylene in between. The spherical femoral component conforms to the upper spherical surface of the polyethylene insert (ball in socket), thus reducing contact stresses and wear at the first joint interface. The flat lower surface of the insert is mobile on the flat metal tibial base plate (flat on flat) allowing for translation. Both interfaces allow some degree of axial rotation to occur. The unconstrained bearing is retained only by its shape and soft tissue tension (Murray et al. 1998).

Using a monoradial or spherical component to replace the posterior medial condyle resulted in the reproduction of the shape of all of the condyle except its most anterior part where impingement could occur. The anterior lip of the meniscal bearing was lowered amongst other adjustments in 1987 (Phase 2, Fig. 14.3) to prevent it from catching on the femur in extension (Weale et al. 1999). The Phase 3 Oxford UKA was introduced in 1998 with instrumentation to allow a minimally invasive approach and a range of component sizes(Price et al. 2001).

A timeline of key events showing developments in UKA design can be seen in Table 14.1.

The latest annual report from the National Joint Registry (NJR) for England and Wales shows that the majority (55%) of UKAs performed used the Oxford implant, however, the proportion of Physica ZUK (Lima Corporate, Udine, Italy) and Sigma HP (both fixed-bearing implants) are rising year on year. The ZUK has a polyradial femoral component made of cobalt–chrome alloy, twin pegs, a titanium tibial tray with two lugs and a keel, and a polyethylene insert which clicks into the tibial tray with anterior and posterior lips (Fig. 14.4). The liner is flat, resulting in a non-congruent, round-on-flat articulation. The same instrumentation can be used for both medial and lateral ZUK UKAs. UK-based figures show that the combined 10-year survival rate for ZUKs is 93.3%, which is the highest for all unicondylar prostheses. Medial UKA compromise approximately 90% of the total UKA procedures undertaken worldwide. We will, therefore, focus the content of this chapter on medial UKA design and surgical technique.

14.4 Implant Design

UKA design may be classified into two types based on bearing surface utilization (Fig. 14.4): fixed bearing (FB) and mobile bearing (MB). The metallic femoral component and tibial baseplates are similar in both types.

The *fixed-bearing* design has the polyethylene insert fixed to the tibial baseplate. This is a familiar concept to surgeons as it is similar to most TKA designs. TKA polyethylene inserts, however, are more conforming to the femoral component geometry and, therefore, guide knee motion. FB UKA inserts are relatively flat so the articular geometry offers no guided motion. Since FB designs are non-conforming, there are increased contact stresses at the articulating surface with the femoral component and higher rates of wear due to a spherical femoral component contacting a small area of the polyethylene liner (Collier et al. 2007).

The *mobile-bearing* design has a polyethylene insert with a curved upper surface that is highly conforming to the shape of the femoral component and a flat lower surface that freely slides on the tibial baseplate. The theoretical advantages of this design are reduced contact stresses at the femoral interface, compressive forces on

Table 14.1 Timeline of key events in the development of unicompartmental knee arthroplasty

Material used	Year	Inventor	Name
Acrylic	1954	MacIntosh	–
	1960s	McKeever	–
Vitallium	1964	MacIntosh	–
Vitallium	1968	Gunston	Polycentric knee prosthesis
	1969		St. Georg sled
Stainless steel High-density polyethylene	1971	Shaw and Chatterjee	Manchester
	1972	Cavendish and white	Liverpool
Polyethylene	1972	Marmor	Marmor modular
	1974	Cavendish and white	Mark II Liverpool
Vitallium	1976	Insall, Walker, and Ranawat	Insall
Cobalt–chrome	1982 1987 1998	Goodfellow and O'Connor	Oxford phase 1 Oxford phase 2 Oxford phase 3

Adapted from Johal et al. (2018)

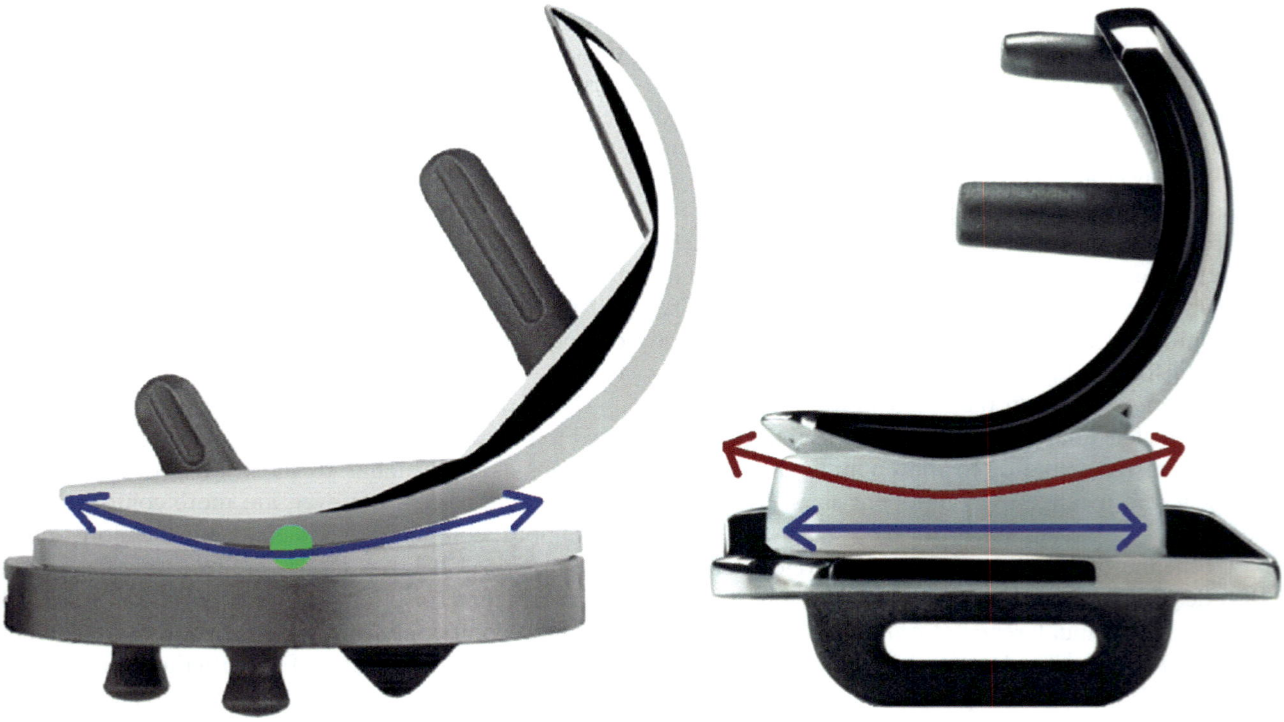

Fig. 14.4 Fixed-bearing (*left*, Physica ZUK) versus mobile-bearing (*right*, Oxford UKA) designs. In the FB design, all motion occurs between the femoral component and the polyethylene insert (*blue arrow*) which is fixed onto the tibial baseplate. Contact stresses are focused on a small area of the insert (*green circle*). In the MB design, motion occurs at the femoral component and bearing interface (*red arrow*) and the insert is free to glide on the tibial baseplate (*blue arrow*). The superior curvature of the insert matches the femoral component, thus increasing the contact area

14

the tibial component throughout the motion, and restoration of normal kinematics as it allows for rotation and translation. Disadvantages of the MB design include the addition of another articulating interface between the baseplate and the insert where backside wear can occur, the risk of poly dislocation, and soft tissue irritation due to excessive insert mobility. The MB articulation is attractive as it maximizes contact area and decreases contact stresses while avoiding excessive constraint (Dennis and Komistek 2005).

Conformity may be desirable to reduce wear, however, the surgeon must bear in mind the design type of UKA being employed. Ko et al. conducted a systematic review comparing complication rates following FB and MB UKA (Ko et al. 2015). The overall re-operation rate and incidence of complications were similar between the two designs, however, mobile bearings were more susceptible to re-operations due to progression of arthritis and bearing dislocation.

> These two causes of failure appear to be interrelated, such that prevention of one predisposes to the other.

In choosing to have a tight knee and avoid medial compartment laxity which would risk bearing dislocation, a surgeon may overcorrect the deformity leading to a valgus overload of the lateral compartment and progression to arthritis. The MB UKA requires fine-tuned ligament balance and limb alignment and is, therefore, a technically challenging operation. Ko et al. also noted that FB UKA were prone to re-operation for excessive wear of the polyethylene insert. This can be explained by the non-conforming design of the implant. Furthermore, a fixed bearing allows for undercorrection without the risk of dislocation, therefore is less prone to the progression of arthritis in the lateral compartment.

Component development continues to evolve with time as we aim to design the ideal prosthesis for UKA. Many lessons have been learned over the years. Early femoral implants were too narrow in the coronal plane to provide adequate condylar coverage and had large fixation pegs leading to high rates of subsidence and excess bone loss during removal, respectively (Padgett et al. 1991; Barrett and Scott 1987). The size of the femoral plugs can be relatively small as long as there are two or a fin to achieve rotational stability. Multiple femoral component sizes have been developed to accommodate for variations in patient anatomy. The aim is to provide adequate coverage of the resurfaced condyle and widely distributing forces.

> Lack of posterior femoral condylar coverage can lead to increased contact stresses in deep flexion whereas too prominent an anterior edge can lead to patellar impingement.

The latest iterations of implants have *a longer posterior condylar surface to maximally cover the condyle and avoid edge loading in deep flexion*. The anterior edge of the component has been tapered to sit below the subchondral bone to reduce patellar impingement. An additional 15° arc of metal added anteriorly allows for a second peg for improved femoral fixation and for the component to be flexed a further 15° to further improve contact area in high flexion (Phase 3 Oxford UKA, ▪ Fig. 14.3).

> The posterior condylar surface is divergent to the fixation pegs thus optimizing cement penetration and pressurization.

The thickness of the components determines bony resection so thinner components are preferred. With metal-backed tibial designs, resection depth is determined by the combined thickness of the tibial component and the bearing. The thinnest tibial component and bearing combination available is 6 mm (Oxford UKA). Advances in polyethylene technology may deliver better materials that would allow for thinner bearings and preserve the tibial bone stock.

The design of UKA prostheses has also been influenced by retrieval analyses of worn tibial inserts. Psychoyios et al. retrieved 16 failed Phase 2 Oxford bearings and found that impingement of the insert most commonly occurred anteriorly against the femoral condyle with the knee in extension (Psychoyios et al. 1998). When impingement was present, it led to a significantly higher rate of wear compared to inserts with no signs of impingement (penetration rate 0.05 vs. 0.01 mm/year, respectively). The pattern of wear tends to be similar to that of the native arthritic varus knee with loss of material anteriorly and peripherally on the medial side.

In the coronal plane, a mismatch between components' positions can lead to edge loading, impingement of soft tissues, and poly dislocation. In FB UKA, positioning the femoral component more laterally in the coronal plane may alter this wear pattern and decrease edge loading of the medial aspect of the tibial component. Since the meniscal bearing follows the femoral component in MB UKA, slight lateral placement of the femoral component keeps the bearing closer to the vertical wall of the tibial component. This avoids soft tissue irritation and potential spin out of a subluxing meniscal bearing.

Excessive bone resection, particularly on the tibial side, produces increased strain within the remaining cortical bone (Pegg et al. 2013). This can lead to pain and fractures postoperatively. Overhang of the tibial component is to be avoided as this can lead to impingement issues. The keel or fins of most tibial components should preserve the bone stock and not damage the posterior tibial cortex. The tibial component should be sized such that it covers as much of the cut surface as possible in order to maximize the area available for load transmission. Uneven load transmission due to underhang can lead to pain, subsidence, loosening, or fracture. Tibial cortical coverage is particularly important medially and posteriorly (Chau et al. 2009), so much so that overhang of up to 2 mm is preferable to any underhang.

The difficulty in achieving cortical coverage in UKA was demonstrated by Fitzpatrick et al. who studied medial and lateral tibial resection surfaces 5 mm below the joint surface in 34 CT-based models of the knee (Fitzpatrick et al. 2007). Despite using theoretically optimal implant designs a maximum of 76% of cortical coverage was achieved. With commercially available implants (Preservation and LCS Uni Systems), maximum coverage achieved was 67%. As an alternative to overhanging implants or ill-fitting designs, personalized implants probably will play a large role in the future.

14.5 Surgical Technique

With a multitude of UKA designs available on the market, surgeons should use the operative techniques recommended by individual manufacturers. The authors have traditionally utilized a mobile-bearing UKA (Oxford). We now use robotic-assisted arthroplasty and our current standard is a FB, robotic-arm-assisted UKA (Stryker Restoris MCK with metal-backed onlay tibial component), although both are used in our ongoing prospective randomized trial (▶ Clinicaltrials.gov Identifier NCR04095637). The Stryker Restoris UKA has twin 6.5 mm pegs, a polyradial femoral component made with cobalt–chrome alloy, and a titanium tibial tray with two pegs and a keel. Two tibial designs are available: an all-polyethylene onlay and a metal-backed onlay tibial component. The latter has been shown to have superior functional outcomes, improved biomechanics, and survivorship (van der List et al. 2017; Small et al. 2011; Walker et al. 2011; Hutt et al. 2015; Zambianchi et al. 2015). The general surgical principles based on the authors' experience are described here.

14

▪ Patient Position

The patient is positioned supine with a thigh tourniquet applied but only inflated during cementing. The knee is held flexed using side support and sandbag under the foot. Alternatively, a thigh holder or a specialized positioner such as the De Mayo or Robb Knee Positioner which allows for full extension and flexion can also be used.

▪ Incision and Approach

The availability of minimally invasive instrumentation allows for a smaller incision compared to that utilized for conventional TKA. A medial or lateral arthrotomy is used to expose the knee joint.

▪ Inspection

Utilizing retractors, inspection of the ACL, and lateral and patellofemoral compartments is carried out without everting the patella.

> **Soft Tissue and Osteophyte Management**
> Formal ligament releases should not be undertaken and overcorrection of the deformity is to be avoided. The UKA should perhaps be considered the equivalent of a resurfacing procedure; undercorrection of 2–3° of the mechanical axis is acceptable.

With MB designs, the tendency is to overstuff the medial compartment in order to reduce the risk of insert dislocation. Overcorrection would lead to stress transfer and accelerated progression of contralateral compartment arthritis. Release of the deep MCL would imply that the deformity is too severe for unicompartmental surgery to work. Osteophytes are resected peripherally without any significant soft tissue releases. This usually corrects any deformity in the coronal plane.

> Keep bone resection to a minimum. Care should be taken to avoid damage to chondral surfaces, the ACL, and the anterior horn of the lateral meniscus.

▪ Component Position and Bone Cuts

The position of the femoral component should be central over the femoral condyle in the coronal plane. Slight lateral positioning of the femoral component is preferable due to the reasons described above but significant overhang laterally results in impingement on the medial tibial spine.

> Aim for a size that reproduces the sagittal dimensions of the femoral condyle. If in-between sizes choose a larger implant to preserve more bone.

The femoral and tibial components should be well aligned and congruent throughout flexion and extension motion to avoid edge loading and impingement. The anterior edge of the femoral component should be flushed against or below the chondral surface to prevent patellar impingement during flexion.

The vertical tibial cut should be perpendicular to the anatomical axis of the tibia. A vertical cut that is too deep or medial, a horizontal cut that is too low, and damage to the back of the tibial keel significantly increase the risk of tibia plateau fractures and postoperative pain(Simpson et al. 2009; Pegg et al. 2013). The posterior slope of the tibial component varies between 3–7° depending on the manufacturer. Increasing the posterior slope places increased strain on the ACL and should be avoided. The components should be inserted so as to recreate the pre-disease level of the joint line by choosing a thickness of polyethylene that restores the height of the worn tibia.

Cementing Technique

Once implant preparation and trialing are complete, there is a *choice between cementing or* using *cementless implants*. With the mobile-bearing option, the authors have shifted to using cementless implants for the majority, but with the fixed bearing we are still using cemented implants. The tourniquet is only inflated for the cementing part of the procedure and then only if there is enough bleeding to warrant it. Surfaces are carefully washed with pulse lavage and dried. If there is sclerotic bone, multiple drill holes are used. Once a dry field is achieved, Palacos cement is mixed and the tibial component is cemented first and pressurized.

> One of the problems of unicompartmental arthroplasty is cement extrusion at the back of the tibial component which can be difficult to remove subsequently, particularly with more anatomical components and robotic-arm-assisted surgery where the gap is small.

The authors, therefore, implant the tibial component and then put on a femoral trial and a bearing to compress the tibia. The femoral trial and insert are subsequently removed at this stage so that the excess posterior cement can be removed. The same cement that was initially mixed can then be used to cement in the femoral component. Cement is then allowed to cure for at least 10–12 minutes and any further excess removed. Once all loose cement is removed, a further trial is undertaken and the definitive bearing is inserted.

14.6 New Technology in UKA

Three-dimensional imaging and computer-aided design have led to the development of patient-specific implants (PSI) for UKA. These allow for customization of the implants and instrumentation in order to control for variations in the geometry and size of the joint surfaces for individual patients, albeit with significant cost implications.

The proven advantages of PSI include the following:

- Lower contact stresses.
- Uniform stress distribution.
- Accurate restoration of the mechanical axis.
- Improved tibial cortical bone coverage.
- Avoidance of implant malposition (van den Heever et al. 2011; Steklov et al. 2010; Koeck et al. 2011).

Whether these improvements lead to longer implant survival remains to be seen.

Robotic-arm-assisted surgery (RAS) or "Makoplasty" was developed in 2006 by Mako Surgical Corporation (Fort Lauderdale, Florida, USA) and utilizes a CT scan of the patient's knee joint to generate a 3D virtual model of the unique anatomy of the patient. This virtual model is loaded into the Mako system software and is used to create the patient's personalized preoperative plan. A haptic-guided 6 mm burring device is used for bone resection following intraoperative mapping of the bony anatomy (Fig. 14.5). The robotic arm has tactile feedback and assists the surgeons' movements such that only bone within the defined boundaries of the preoperative plan can be removed. The system outputs data on flexion and extension gaps in real-time and allows for intraoperative adjustments to facilitate optimal implant position.

Work published by our unit has shown a short learning curve of six cases for operating time and surgical team confidence levels for UKA using robotic assistance.

No learning curve for implant positioning was noted (Kayani et al. 2018a).

> Robotic-arm-assisted UKA was associated with statistically significant reductions in postoperative pain scores, opioid analgesia requirements, time to straight leg raise, number of physiotherapy sessions, and time to discharge compared with conventional jig-based UKA (Kayani et al. 2019).

A systematic review looking at outcomes of UKA using RAS has shown 96% survival in6 years (Robinson et al. 2019).

14.7 Postoperative Rehabilitation

Optimizing pain control in the postoperative period is essential. A multimodal management approach including local anesthetic infiltration intraoperatively and avoidance of opioid use postoperatively aids earlier recovery and discharge. Use of tranexamic acid both

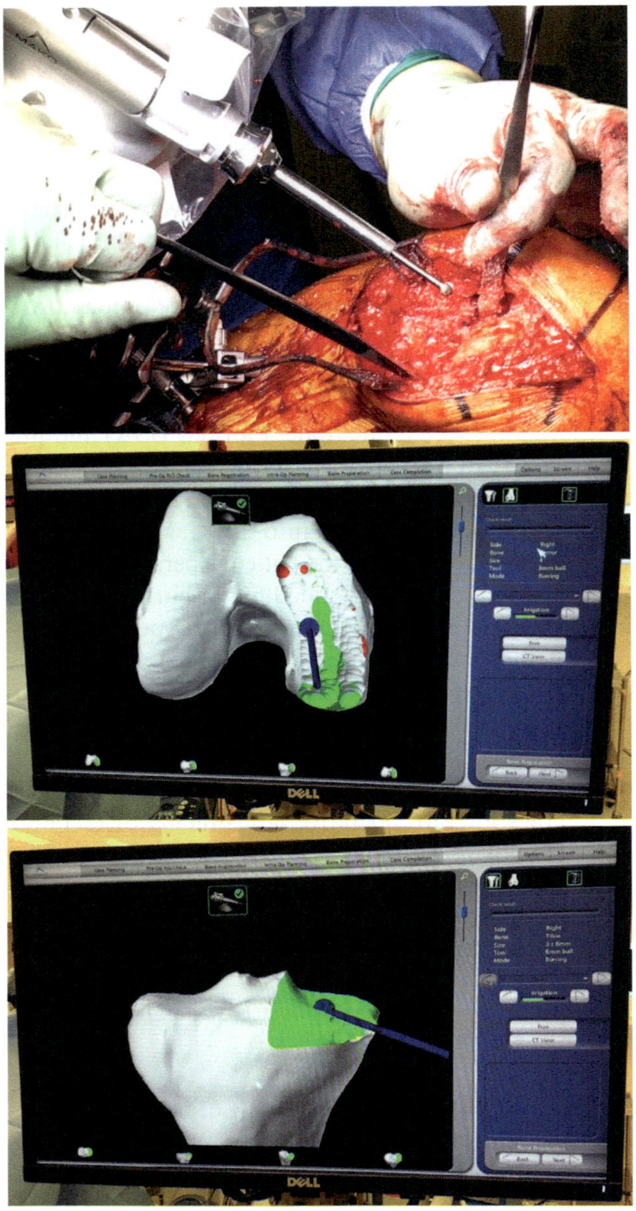

Fig. 14.5 Intra-op image of a haptic-guided burr connected to the Mako robotic arm (*top*) and computer-generated imaging (*bottom two images*) showing resection margins in *green*

locally and intravenously helps control blood loss. This usually avoids the need for a drain. Immediate postoperative straight leg raise and flexion should be encouraged while the local anesthetic is still working. No restrictions are placed on weight-bearing. Team education on the wards is key to differentiate these patients from those that have had conventional TKA. Enhanced recovery and early discharge protocols should be followed where possible, particularly in patients who are medically fit, live locally, and have a support system at home. Preoperative identification and education of such patients need to be set up by way of a local protocol and pathway for early or same-day discharge.

Take-Home Messages

- Unicompartmental knee replacement is a feasible first prosthetic treatment for selected patients with symptomatic single-compartment disease.
- It is an alternative to osteotomy or total joint arthroplasty and restores the natural kinematics of the knee joint while preserving host bone.
- Significant improvement in our understanding of the biomechanics of the knee joint and advances in implant design have made long-term UKA outcomes comparable to those of TKA.
- Cementing techniques should follow a predetermined plan of action and removal of all extruded cement, particularly behind the tibial component it is important to prevent impingement and third body wear.
- The use of robotics continues to improve the accuracy of component positioning. Whether this translates to improved outcomes in the long run remains to be seen.

References

Barrett WP, Scott RD (1987) Revision of failed unicondylar unicompartmental knee arthroplasty. J Bone Joint Surg Am 69:1328–1335

Chau R, Gulati A, Pandit H et al (2009) Tibial component overhang following unicompartmental knee replacement – does it matter? Knee 16:310–313

Collier MB, Engh CA Jr, McAuley JP, Engh GA (2007) Factors associated with the loss of thickness of polyethylene tibial bearings after knee arthroplasty. J Bone Joint Surg Am 89:1306–1314

Dennis DA, Komistek RD (2005) Kinematics of mobile-bearing total knee arthroplasty. Instr Course Lect 54:207–220

Deshmukh RV, Scott RD (2001) Unicompartmental knee arthroplasty: long-term results. Clin Orthop Relat Res 392:272–278

Fitzpatrick C, Fitzpatrick D, Lee J, Auger D (2007) Statistical design of unicompartmental tibial implants and comparison with current devices. Knee 14:138–144

Foran JR, Brown NM, Della Valle CJ et al (2013) Long-term survivorship and failure modes of unicompartmental knee arthroplasty. Clin Orthop Relat Res 471:102–108

Garner A, Van Arkel RJ, Cobb J (2019) Classification of combined partial knee arthroplasty. Bone Joint J 101-B:922–928

Goodfellow J (2006) Unicompartmental arthroplasty with the Oxford knee. Oxford University Press, Oxford, New York

Goodfellow J, O'Connor J (1978) The mechanics of the knee and prosthesis design. J Bone Joint Surg Br 60-B:358–369

Goodfellow JW, O'Connor JJ, Murray DW (2010) A critique of revision rate as an outcome measure: re-interpretation of knee joint registry data. J Bone Joint Surg Br 92:1628–1631

Gunston FH (1971) Polycentric knee arthroplasty. Prosthetic simulation of normal knee movement. J Bone Joint Surg Br 53:272–277

Hutt JR, Farhadnia P, Masse V et al (2015) A randomised trial of all-polyethylene and metal-backed tibial components in unicompartmental arthroplasty of the knee. Bone Joint J 97-B:786–792

Jauregui JJ, Blum CL, Sardesai N et al (2018) Unicompartmental knee arthroplasty for spontaneous osteonecrosis of the knee: a meta-analysis. J Orthop Surg (Hong Kong) 26:2309499018770925
Johal S, Nakano N, Baxter M et al (2018) Unicompartmental knee arthroplasty: the past, current controversies, and future perspectives. J Knee Surg 31:992–998
Kayani B, Konan S, Pietrzak JRT et al (2018a) The learning curve associated with robotic-arm assisted unicompartmental knee arthroplasty: a prospective cohort study. Bone Joint J 100-B:1033–1042
Kayani B, Konan S, Tahmassebi J et al (2018b) Robotic-arm assisted total knee arthroplasty is associated with improved early functional recovery and reduced time to hospital discharge compared with conventional jig-based total knee arthroplasty: a prospective cohort study. Bone Joint J 100-B:930–937
Kayani B, Konan S, Tahmassebi J et al (2019) An assessment of early functional rehabilitation and hospital discharge in conventional versus robotic-arm assisted unicompartmental knee arthroplasty: a prospective cohort study. Bone Joint J 101-B:24–33
Ko YB, Gujarathi MR, Oh KJ (2015) Outcome of unicompartmental knee arthroplasty: a systematic review of comparative studies between fixed and mobile bearings focusing on complications. Knee Surg Relat Res 27:141–148
Koeck FX, Beckmann J, Luring C et al (2011) Evaluation of implant position and knee alignment after patient-specific unicompartmental knee arthroplasty. Knee 18:294–299
Konan S, Haddad FS (2016) Does location of patellofemoral chondral lesion influence outcome after Oxford medial compartmental knee arthroplasty? Bone Joint J 98-B:11–15
Kozinn SC, Scott R (1989) Unicondylar knee arthroplasty. J Bone Joint Surg Am 71:145–150
Kozinn SC, Marx C, Scott RD (1989) Unicompartmental knee arthroplasty. A 4.5–6-year follow-up study with a metal-backed tibial component. J Arthroplast 4(Suppl):S1–S10
Murray DW, Parkinson RW (2018) Usage of unicompartmental knee arthroplasty. Bone Joint J 100-B:432–435
Murray DW, Goodfellow JW, O'Connor JJ (1998) The Oxford medial unicompartmental arthroplasty: a ten-year survival study. J Bone Joint Surg Br 80:983–989
Murray DW, Liddle AD, Judge A, Pandit H (2017) Bias and unicompartmental knee arthroplasty. Bone Joint J 99-B:12–15
NJR Online (2019) 16th Annual Report 2019. https://reports.njrcentre.org.uk/portals/0/pdfdownloads/njr16th annual report 2019.pdf
Padgett DE, Stern SH, Insall JN (1991) Revision total knee arthroplasty for failed unicompartmental replacement. J Bone Joint Surg Am 73:186–190
Pandit H, Jenkins C, Gill HS et al (2011) Unnecessary contraindications for mobile-bearing unicompartmental knee replacement. J Bone Joint Surg Br 93:622–628
Patil S, Colwell CW Jr, Ezzet KA, D'Lima DD (2005) Can normal knee kinematics be restored with unicompartmental knee replacement? J Bone Joint Surg Am 87:332–338
Pegg EC, Walter J, Mellon SJ et al (2013) Evaluation of factors affecting tibial bone strain after unicompartmental knee replacement. J Orthop Res 31:821–828
Price AJ, Webb J, Topf H et al (2001) Rapid recovery after oxford unicompartmental arthroplasty through a short incision. J Arthroplast 16:970–976
Psychoyios V, Crawford RW, O'Connor JJ, Murray DW (1998) Wear of congruent meniscal bearings in unicompartmental knee arthroplasty: a retrieval study of 16 specimens. J Bone Joint Surg Br 80:976–982
Radke S, Wollmerstedt N, Bischoff A, Eulert J (2005) Knee arthroplasty for spontaneous osteonecrosis of the knee: unicompartimental vs bicompartimental knee arthroplasty. Knee Surg Sports Traumatol Arthrosc 13:158–162
Repicci JA, Eberle RW (1999) Minimally invasive surgical technique for unicondylar knee arthroplasty. J South Orthop Assoc 8:20–27. discussion 27
Robinson PG, Clement ND, Hamilton D et al (2019) A systematic review of robotic-assisted unicompartmental knee arthroplasty: prosthesis design and type should be reported. Bone Joint J 101-B:838–847
Scott RD (2003) Unicondylar arthroplasty: redefining itself. Orthopedics 26:951–952
Simpson DJ, Price AJ, Gulati A et al (2009) Elevated proximal tibial strains following unicompartmental knee replacement – a possible cause of pain. Med Eng Phys 31:752–757
Small SR, Berend ME, Ritter MA et al (2011) Metal backing significantly decreases tibial strains in a medial unicompartmental knee arthroplasty model. J Arthroplast 26:777–782
Steklov N, Slamin J, Srivastav S, D'Lima D (2010) Unicompartmental knee resurfacing: enlarged tibio-femoral contact area and reduced contact stress using novel patient-derived geometries. Open Biomed Eng J 4:85–92
Van Den Heever DJ, Scheffer C, Erasmus P, Dillon E (2011) Contact stresses in a patient-specific unicompartmental knee replacement. Clin Biomech (Bristol, Avon) 26:159–166
van der List JP, Kleeblad LJ, Zuiderbaan HA, Pearle AD (2017) Mid-term outcomes of metal-backed unicompartmental knee arthroplasty show superiority to all-polyethylene unicompartmental and total knee erthroplasty. HSS J 13:232–240
Walker PS, Parakh DS, Chaudhary ME, Wei CS (2011) Comparison of interface stresses and strains for onlay and inlay unicompartmental tibial components. J Knee Surg 24:109–115
Weale AE, Murray DW, Crawford R et al (1999) Does arthritis progress in the retained compartments after 'Oxford' medial unicompartmental arthroplasty? A clinical and radiological study with a minimum ten-year follow-up. J Bone Joint Surg Br 81:783–789
Zambianchi F, Digennaro V, Giorgini A et al (2015) Surgeon's experience influences UKA survivorship: a comparative study between all-poly and metal back designs. Knee Surg Sports Traumatol Arthrosc 23:2074–2080

Lateral Unicompartmental Knee Arthroplasty

Neel R. Patel, Keith R. Berend, and Adolph V. Lombardi Jr.

Contents

E. Hansen, K.-D. Kühn (eds.), *Essentials of Cemented Knee Arthroplasty*,
https://doi.org/10.1007/978-3-662-63113-3_15

15.1 Introduction

Unicompartmental knee osteoarthritis (OA) represents up to 40% of knee OA.

> Although anteromedial signifies 25% of knee OA, lateral compartment disease may represent up to 10% of knee OA (Sah and Scott 2007; Scott 2005).

The unique challenges present to lateral compartment OA include insufficient diagnosis, implant selection, and surgical technique. Diagnosing lateral compartment OA begins with proper history and physical exam. Standard weight-bearing radiographs in addition to varus stress radiographs are critical to identifying patients with isolated lateral compartment OA.

> Lateral unicompartmental knee arthroplasty (UKA) is also considered a more technically demanding procedure than medial UKA or total knee arthroplasty (TKA) due to the more complex kinematic profile.

Finally, the evolution of implant designs plays a critical role in the survivorship of lateral UKA (literature review in ► Sect. 15.5). Therefore, choosing proper surgical indications, implant designs, and surgical techniques can lead to a successful outcome and survivorship that rivals TKA and medial UKA. The case and the surgical technique presented in this chapter illustrate these key concepts and provide guidelines for performing a successful lateral UKA.

15.2 Case Example

The patient is a 66-year-old male who presented to the office with intermittently moderate knee pain that was present for the past 1 year. He localizes the pain to the lateral and peripatellar region of his left knee. Additionally, he reports grating, popping, and instability with ambulation. He is currently retired and remains mainly semi-sedentary while ambulating between 5 and 10 blocks secondary to his knee pain. His past medical history was significant for hypertension, hyperlipidemia, and remote venous thromboembolism of the left leg. His prior treatments include home exercises, physical therapy, nonsteroidal anti-inflammatory drugs (NSAIDs), and topical medications.

On physical examination, he exhibits no effusion or tenderness to palpation of the left knee. He does not use any assistive devices; however, he requires a handrail to ascend and descend stairs. His tibiofemoral alignment is noted to be 7° of valgus. He does not exhibit flexion contracture or mediolateral/anteroposterior instability.

Initial radiographic evaluation includes standing anteroposterior, flexed posteroanterior, lateral, and sunrise axial patellar view (◘ Fig. 15.1a–d). As visualized, the patient's varus stress radiograph demonstrates a correctable deformity with the maintenance of the medial joint space (◘ Fig. 15.1e). Therefore, this patient's radiographs demonstrate an isolated lateral compartment disease. As such, patients that are being considered for lateral UKA should have isolated lateral compartment disease radiographically and by examination.

15.3 Evaluation, Indications, and Contraindications

Isolated lateral compartment osteoarthritis represents 10% of all knee OA (Sah and Scott 2007; Pandit et al. 2010). However, the incidence may be more common and diagnosis is often missed due to being a disease of flexion (Sah and Scott 2007; Pandit et al. 2010).

> Therefore, the flexed posteroanterior radiograph presents a critical piece of information in the evaluation and treatment of lateral compartment knee disease (◘ Fig. 15.1b).

Lateral UKA also represents less than 1% of all knee arthroplasties, partly due to technical difficulties and less reproducible results.

> The lateral compartment comprises a complex kinematic profile with the presence of a "screw-home mechanism" (Scott 2005; Fitz 2009; Ashraf et al. 2002).

Indications of lateral UKA include the following:

- Full-thickness articular cartilage loss in the lateral compartment.
- Maintenance of joint space in the medial compartment as depicted on varus stress radiograph.
- No significant radiographic or arthroscopic patellofemoral disease.

However, the patellofemoral disease can be ignored unless there is severe lateral patellar facet wear and grooving of the lateral trochlear ridge (Berend et al. 2012).

Contraindications for lateral UKA include the following:

- Significant disease in more than one compartment.
- A fixed valgus deformity greater than 10°.
- Ligamentous deficiency.
- Less than 90° of flexion.
- Inflammatory arthritis.

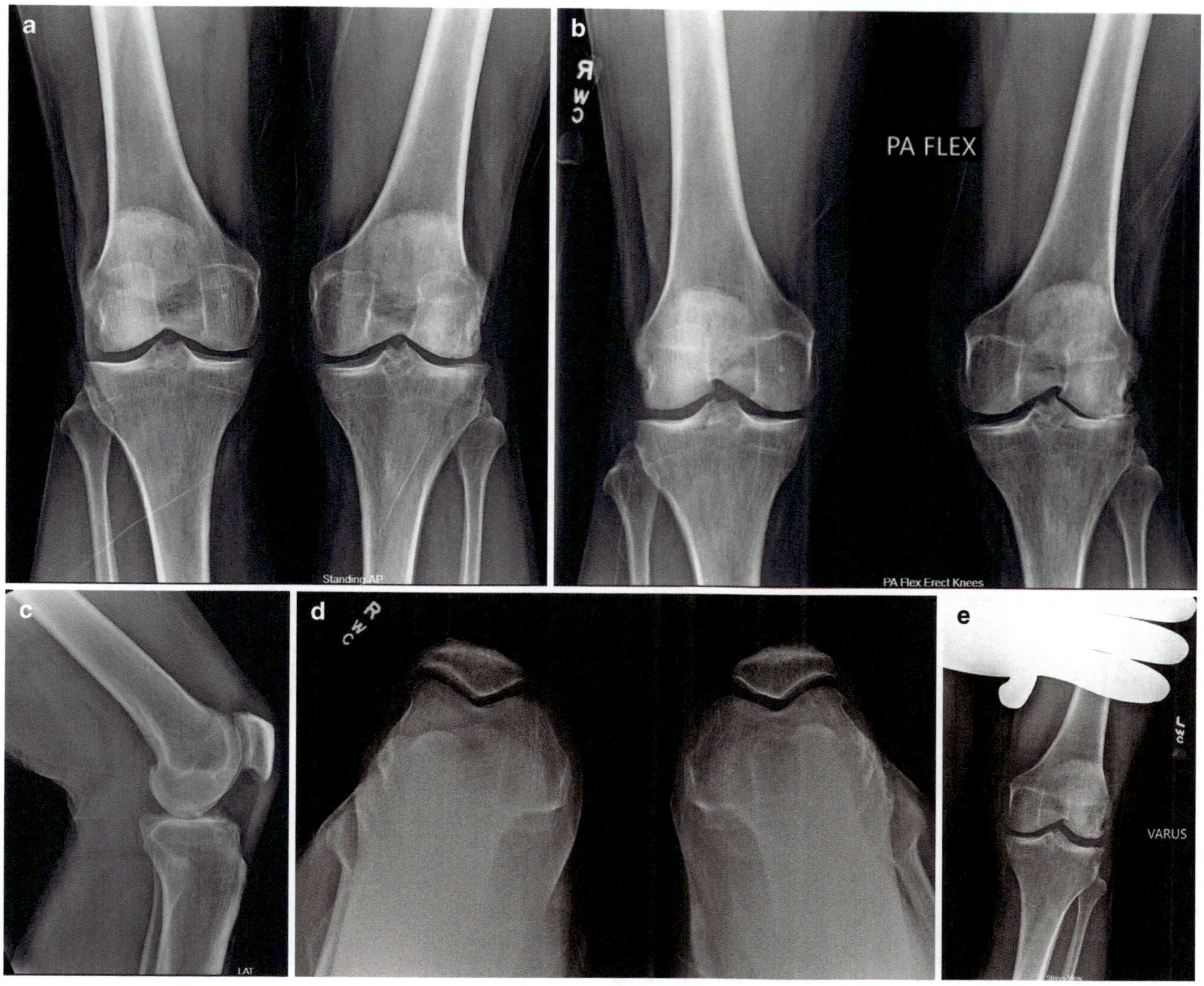

Fig. 15.1 a–e Preoperative radiographic views obtained include **a** standing anteroposterior, **b** posteroanterior flexed, **c** lateral, **d** Merchant axial patellar, and **e** varus stress radiographs. Varus stress radiograph demonstrates correctible deformity and maintenance of the medial joint space in this patient, which correlates with isolated lateral compartment disease. (Printed with permission of Joint Implant Surgeons, Inc., New Albany, Ohio)

Age, weight, activity, and degree of flexible deformity are not used as contraindications in any case (Berend et al. 2015).

15.4 Surgical Technique

15.4.1 Positioning and Lateral Exposure

Unlike positioning for a medial UKA at the authors' institution, patient positioningand draping for a lateral UKA is identical to a TKA. A proximal thigh tourniquet is utilized with the patient lying supine position on a standard operating. The patient is subsequently prepped and draped in a standard fashion (Fig. 15.2a). An Alvarado boot is secured to the operative foot with a self-adherent wrap (Coban, 3 M, St. Paul, MN) (Fig. 15.2b). The implant system and instrumentation currently used by the authors for lateral UKA is the Fixed Lateral Oxford (Zimmer Biomet), much of the technique described will be universal to other implant systems.

With the knee flexed to 90°, a lateralized incision is made from 1 cm proximal to the superior pole of the patella to the proximal, lateral border of the tibial tubercle (Fig. 15.3). After incising through the skin and subcutaneous fat, a lateral arthrotomy is performed from proximal to distal, staying lateral to the patellar tendon (Fig. 15.4a). Distally, the scalpel blade is redirected medially between the patellar tendon and the infrapatellar fat pad. This will preserve a portion of the infrapatellar fat pad and leave it attached to the lateral retinacular tissue. This tissue will augment the thin lateral retinacular tissue and eventually facilitate a watertight closure of the arthrotomy (Fig. 15.4b).

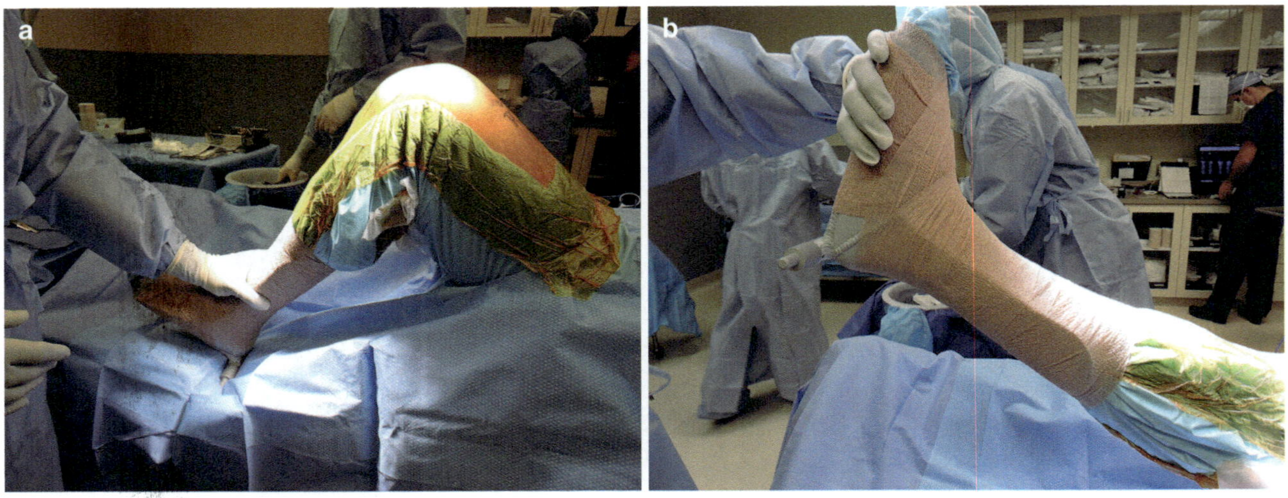

Fig. 15.2 a, b Draping. a Standard draping of the left extremity utilizing a thigh-high tourniquet and b an Alvarado boot. (Printed with permission of Joint Implant Surgeons, Inc., New Albany, Ohio)

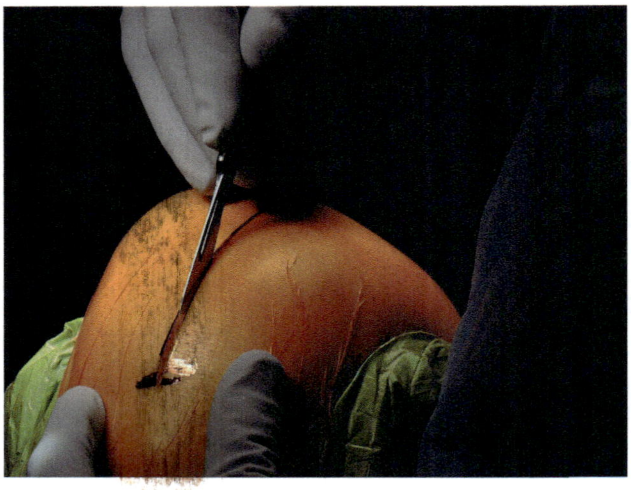

Fig. 15.3 Laterally based incision is made from 1 cm proximal to the superior pole of the patella to the proximal, lateral border of the tibial tubercle. (Printed with permission of Joint Implant Surgeons, Inc., New Albany, Ohio)

The intercondylar notch osteophytes, lateral tibial osteophytes, and the visible portion of the lateral meniscus are removed to allow for adequate exposure (Fig. 15.5). However, the lateral femoral osteophytes should be retained, as they help guide the positioning of the femoral component during femoral preparation. Next, the anterior tibia is exposed from the tibial tubercle to the rim of the plateau and Gerdy's tubercle. Once proper exposure is achieved, a Hohmann retractor is placed on the medial epicondyle to evaluate the patellofemoral and medial compartments for degeneration. Prior to tibial preparation, isolated lateral disease and an intact anterior cruciate ligament should be confirmed to achieve reproducible results.

15.4.2 Tibial Preparation

With the use of the extramedullary tibial guide, the varus/valgus is set at neutral alignment and the slope is built-in at 7° when the guide is parallel to the tibial crest.

> However, the tibial slope should match the patient's native slope. Since lateral compartment disease has a greater effect on femoral condyle than a tibial plateau, the tibial resection is minimal.

The extramedullary guide is typically set to resect around 1–2 mm below the tibial defect. The guide should be fixed to the tibia with one pin to prevent any risk of fracture (Fig. 15.6a). The amount of tibia resected varies for each patient but, once removed, the extension gap should have enough space to accommodate the tibial template and a 3 mm feeler gauge. If this is not the case, more bone should be excised.

The first tibial bone cut is the vertical tibial cut. It is completed with a stiff and narrow reciprocating saw blade. Care must be taken to saw in the flexion axis and parallel to the plate as lifting the hand may violate the posterior cortex and increase the risk of fracture. This cut sets the rotation of the tibial component.

> It should be in line with the medial border of the lateral femoral condyle and internally rotated 10–15° from the mid-sagittal plane of the tibia.

This amount of internal rotation will place the patellar tendon in the path of the reciprocating saw blade. Therefore, the tendon should be carefully retracted when making the vertical tibial cut (Fig. 15.6b).

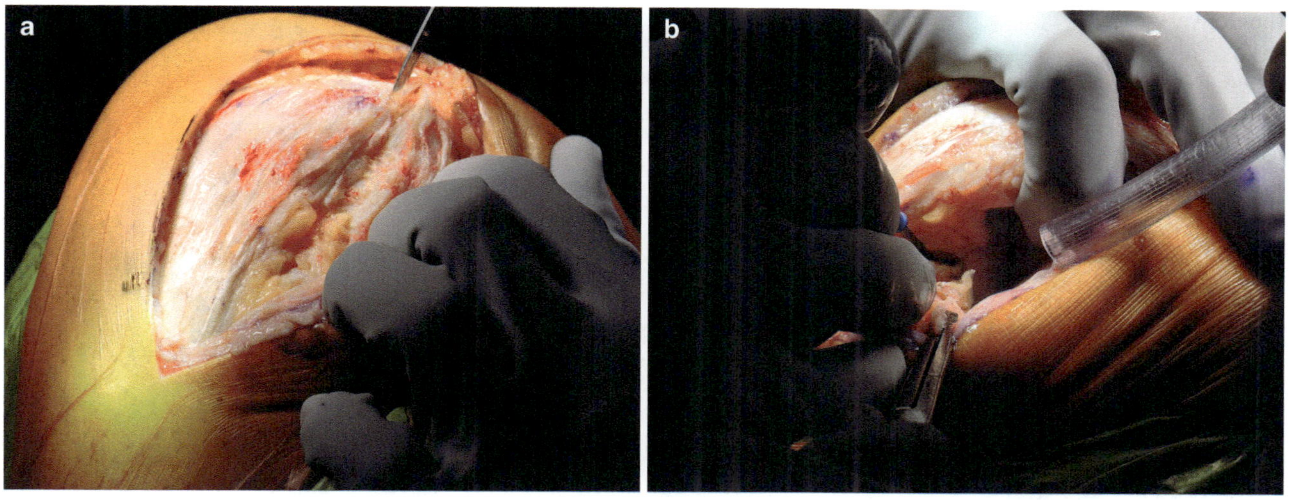

Fig. 15.4 **a** Arthrotomy. Lateral arthrotomy is performed from proximal to distal, staying lateral to the patellar tendon. **b** Infrapatellar fat pad preserved to augment thin lateral retinacular tissue to facilitate water-tight closure. (Printed with permission of Joint Implant Surgeons, Inc., New Albany, Ohio)

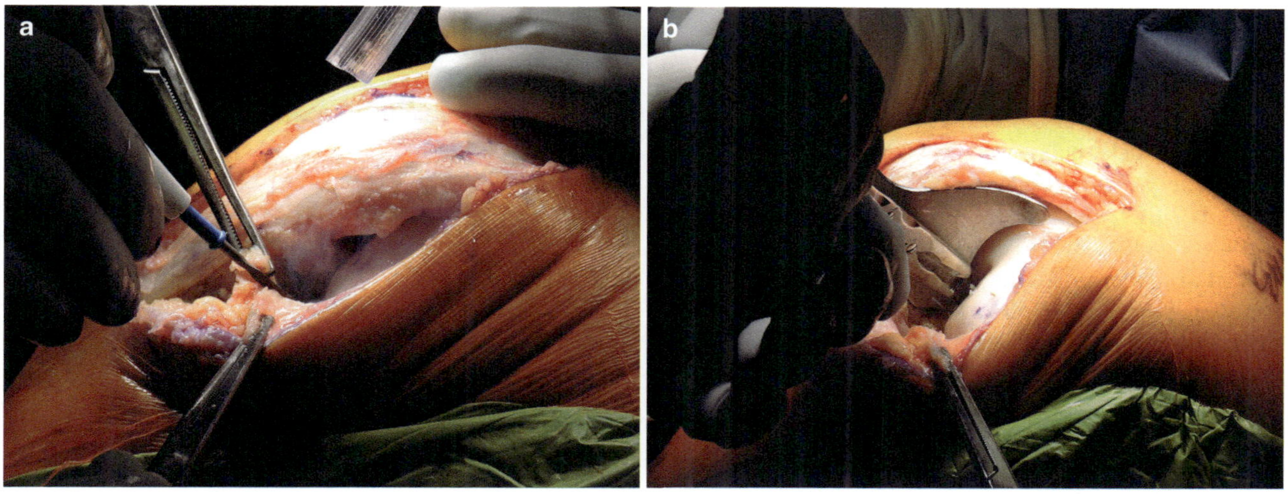

Fig. 15.5 **a**, **b** Exposure. The intercondylar notch osteophytes, lateral tibial osteophytes, and the visible portion of the lateral meniscus are removed to allow for adequate exposure. (Printed with permission of Joint Implant Surgeons, Inc., New Albany, Ohio)

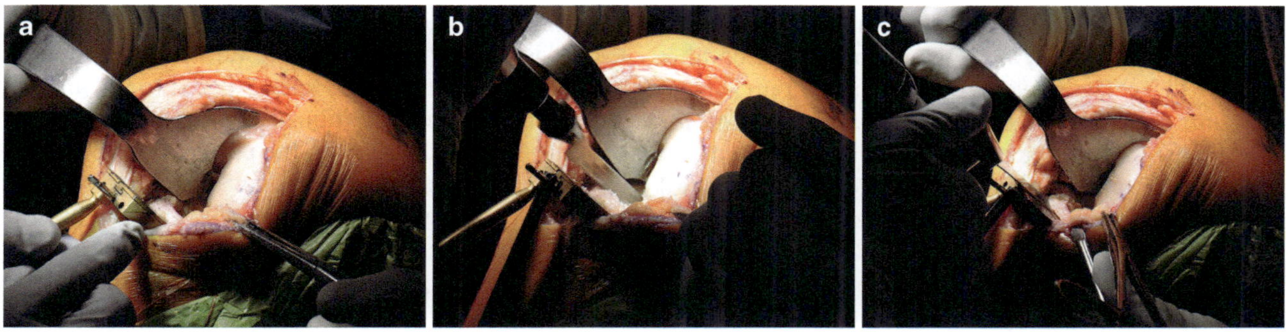

Fig. 15.6 **a–c** Tibial preparation. **a** The extramedullary tibial guide is fixed to the tibia with a single pin. **b** The patellar tendon is retracted medially and a vertical tibial resection is made with a stiff, narrow reciprocating saw blade. **c** With the patellar tendon retracted medially, and the iliotibial (IT) band and lateral collateral ligament (LCL) protected laterally, the horizontal tibial cut is made using 12-mm-wide oscillating saw blade. (Printed with permission of Joint Implant Surgeons, Inc., New Albany, Ohio)

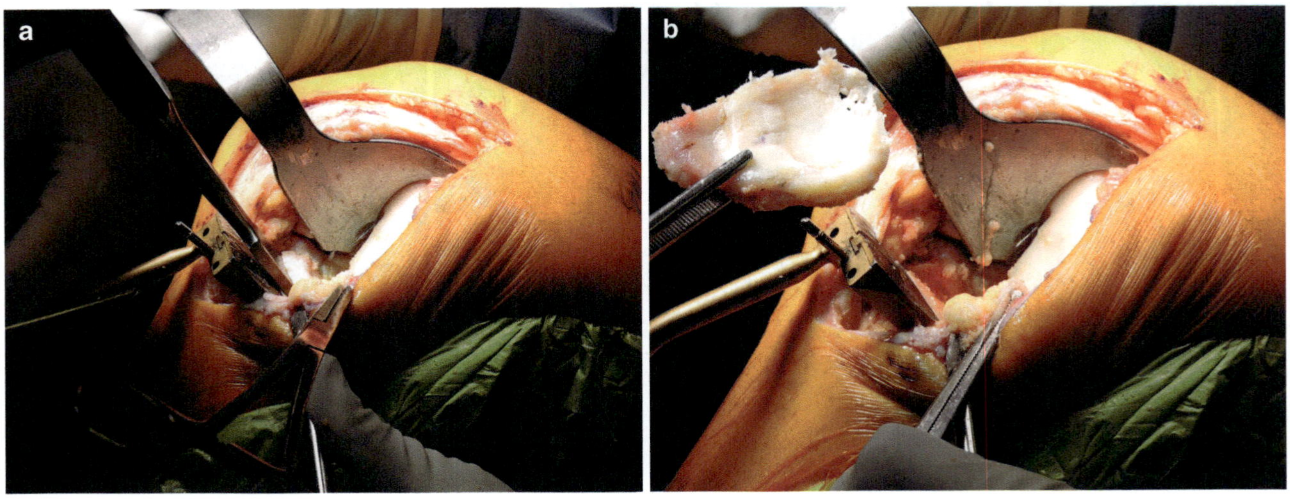

Fig. 15.7 **a** The resected tibia is released from soft tissue attachments and then excised. **b** The resected tibia is measured against a contralateral trial to determine appropriate sizing. (Printed with permission of Joint Implant Surgeons, Inc., New Albany, Ohio)

> This is a critical step, as the adequate amount of the tibial component's internal rotation not only ensures the femoral component articulate with the tibial polyethylene evenly throughout the screw-home mechanism but it also enlarges the implant surface area and helps to prevent subsidence.

A common mistake is to externally rotate the tibial component. Furthermore, the reciprocating saw should be handled along the flexion axis of the tibia because excessively lifting the hand will lead to violation of the posterior cortex and increased risk of fracture.

15

With the patellar tendon retracted medially, and the iliotibial (IT) band and lateral collateral ligament (LCL) protected laterally, the horizontal tibial cut is made using a 12-mm-wide oscillating saw blade (Fig. 15.6c). Again, the minimum amount of tibia resected should accommodate the tibial template and a 3 mm feeler gauge in the extension gap. Next, an osteotome is used to lever the resected tibia, which is then secured with a straight Kocher forceps. The soft tissue attachments are then excised, thereby removing the resected tibia (Fig. 15.7). The resected tibia is matched up against the contralateral tibial baseplate trials to evaluate for appropriate sizing. Once an appropriate size is determined, the keel-prep tibial trial is placed on the lateral tibia to assess implant rotation and size (Fig. 15.8).

15.4.3 Femoral Preparation

Femoral preparation begins with the introduction of the intramedullary (IM) guide into the femoral canal. An entrance drill hole is introduced in the distal femur 1 cm anterior to the anterolateral corner of the intercondylar notch with the knee at 45° of flexion (Fig. 15.9). The IM rod is inserted and directed toward the anterior inferior iliac spine (AIIS). The knee is flexed to 90° and the femoral drill guide is positioned against the distal femur with the foot in contact with the posterior femoral condyle. The IM link guide now connects the IM rod and the femoral drill guide (Fig. 15.10). This will flex the femoral component 5°. After coupling the IM rod with the femoral drill guide, the drill guide is positioned in the middle of the femoral condyle. This ultimately sets the position of the femoral component.

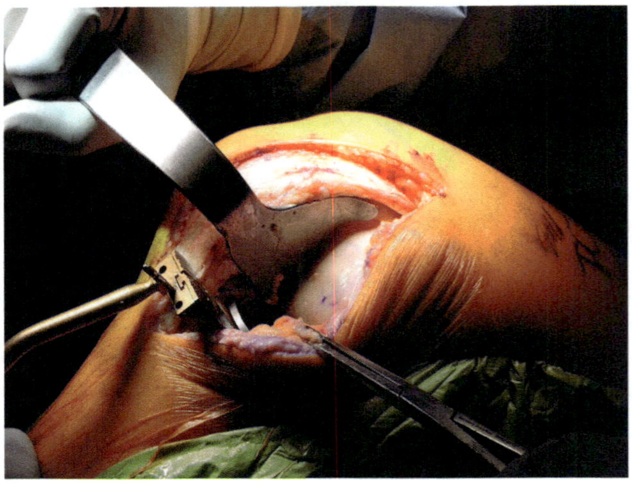

Fig. 15.8 The keel-prep tibial trial is placed on the lateral tibia to assess implant rotation and size. (Printed with permission of Joint Implant Surgeons, Inc., New Albany, Ohio)

> Just like medial UKA, the femoral guide has a tendency to migrate medially and care must be taken to center the guide on the lateral femoral condyle.

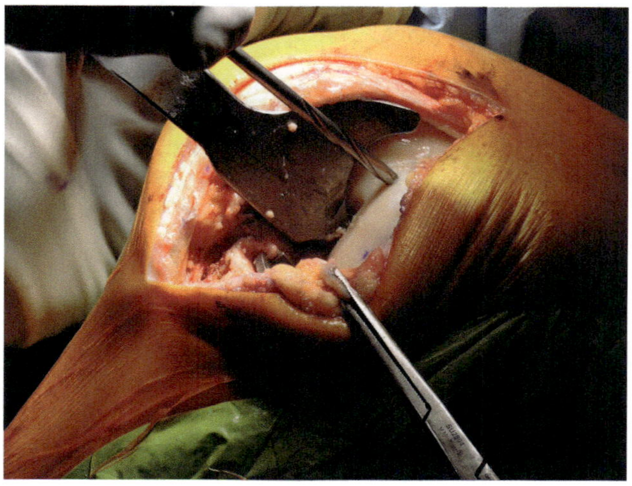

Fig. 15.9 Femoral preparation. With the knee in 45° flexion, the entrance hole is made 1 cm anterior to the anterolateral corner of the intercondylar notch and the rod is directed toward anterior inferior iliac spine (AIIS). (Printed with permission of Joint Implant Surgeons, Inc., New Albany, Ohio)

The screw-home mechanism of the knee describes the relative external rotation of the tibia with respect to the femur during extension.

> A femoral component placed too medial in flexion may seem appropriately positioned; however, with knee extension, the femoral component impinges against the tibial spine eminence or edge loads the tibial polyethylene.

This is a critical step as placing the drill guide in the middle of the lateral condyle or even slightly lateral will lead to a decrease in impingement.

After the drill guide is placed in the appropriate position, a 4 mm drill in passed through the upper drill slot, and a 6 mm drill is passed through the lower drill slot. The femoral drill guide and the linking guide are removed (Fig. 15.11). The femoral saw block is now placed into the drill holes; the IT band and LCL are protected with a laterally placed retractor. The posterior

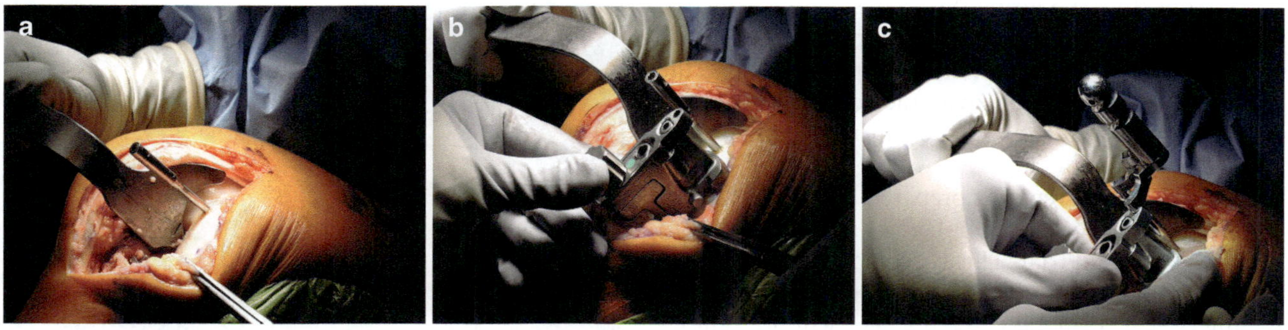

Fig. 15.10 **a** Intramedullary (IM) rod placement. **b** The knee is flexed to 90° and the femoral drill guide is positioned against the distal femur with the foot in contact with the posterior femoral condyle. **c** The IM link guide connects the IM rod and the femoral drill guide. (Printed with permission of Joint Implant Surgeons, Inc., New Albany, Ohio)

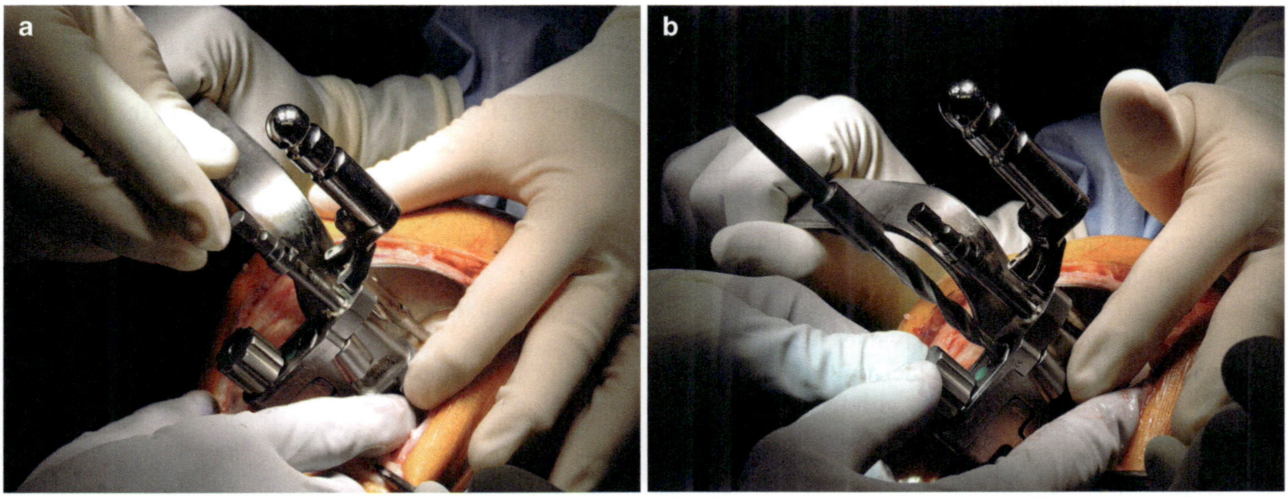

Fig. 15.11 **a** With the drill guide in appropriate position, a 4 mm drill is passed through the upper hole and **b** a 6 mm drill is passed through the lower hole. (Printed with permission of Joint Implant Surgeons, Inc., New Albany, Ohio)

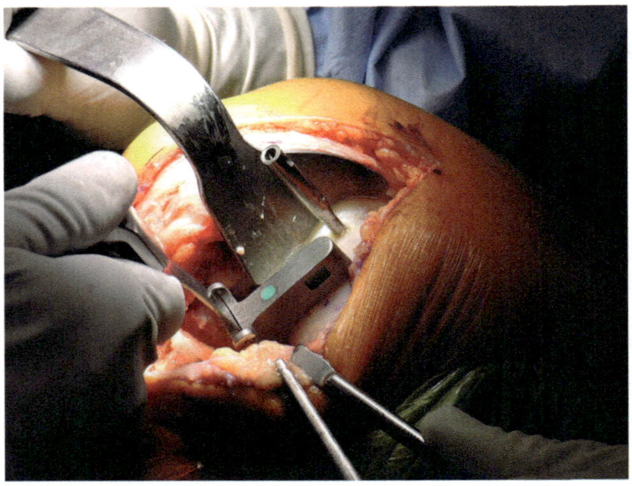

Fig. 15.12 The femoral saw block is now placed into the drill holes, the iliotibial band, and lateral collateral ligament are protected, and the posterior femoral resection is made using a broad sagittal saw. (Printed with permission of Joint Implant Surgeons, Inc., New Albany, Ohio)

femoral resection is made using a broad, thin sagittal saw (Fig. 15.12). During this step, slightly flexing the saw will lead to a cut that is planar with the cutting guide. Following the posterior femoral resection, the saw block is removed along with the bony fragment. The lateral meniscus and soft tissue can now be appropriately removed.

Next, the distal femur is prepared by milling the lateral condyle into a round, spherical shape in order to accept the femoral trial. This is accomplished by inserting the 0 spigot into the 6 mm (lower) drill hole and milling over it. Generally, the 0 spigot will not remove any distal femoral bone secondary to distal femoral hypoplasia. Once the mill stops advancing, the 0 spigot is removed. The residual protruding corners of bone are removed with an osteotome, which is directed tangentially to the milled surface (Fig. 15.13).

15.4.4 Balancing the Flexion and Extension Gaps

The femoral trial and the tibial template are placed to evaluate the flexion and extension gap. The flexion gap is measured at 95° of flexion with a feeler gauge (Fig. 15.14). The extension gap is measured in full extension with a feeler gauge that is at least 2 mm smaller than what was measured for the flexion gap.

After initial gap measurement with feeler gauges, the distal femur is sequentially milled in millimeter increments until the gaps are balanced in flexion and extension. With each size increase in the spigot, an additional 1 mm of distal femur is removed, thereby increasing the extension gap by 1 mm. After each milling, the distal

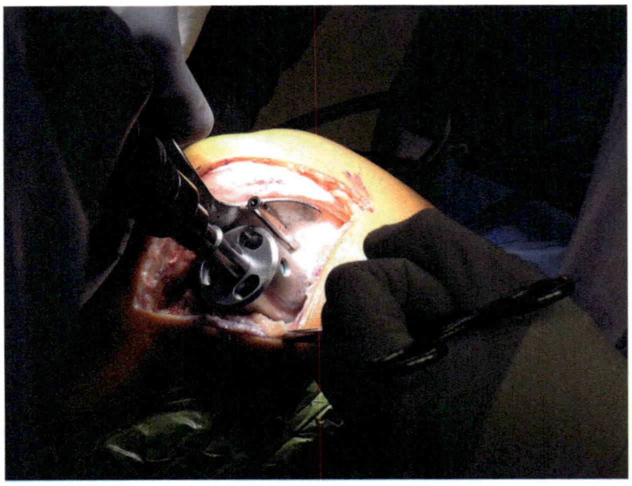

Fig. 15.13 The distal femur is initially milled with a 0 spigot. (Printed with permission of Joint Implant Surgeons, Inc., New Albany, Ohio)

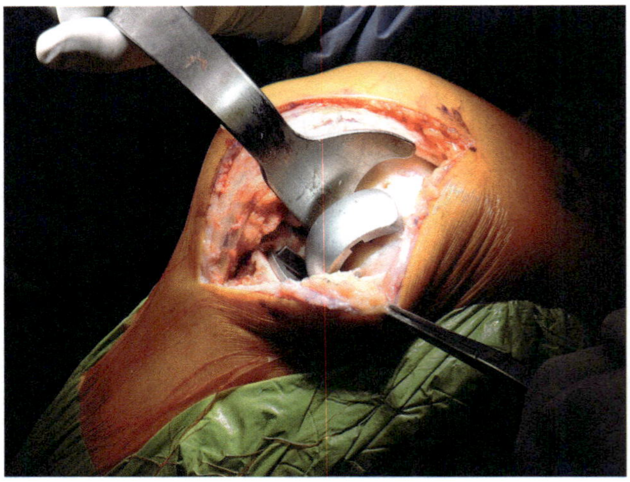

Fig. 15.14 The femoral trial and the tibial template are placed to evaluate the flexion and extension gap. (Printed with permission of Joint Implant Surgeons, Inc., New Albany, Ohio)

femur osteophytes are moved, the trials are placed, and the extension and flexion gaps are re-evaluated (Fig. 15.15). It is critical not to mallet in the spigots as the sizing is based on the depth created by the 6 mm drill.

> Balancing the gaps in the lateral compartment differs from a medial UKA or TKA. In the lateral compartment of a normal knee, the flexion gap is loose compared with the extension gap.

This normal disparity should be recreated without overcorrection.

> The authors' preference is to balance 2–3 mm lax at 90° of flexion and "tight" or 0 mm at full extension. This will allow for the tibiofemoral screw-home mechanism and translation.

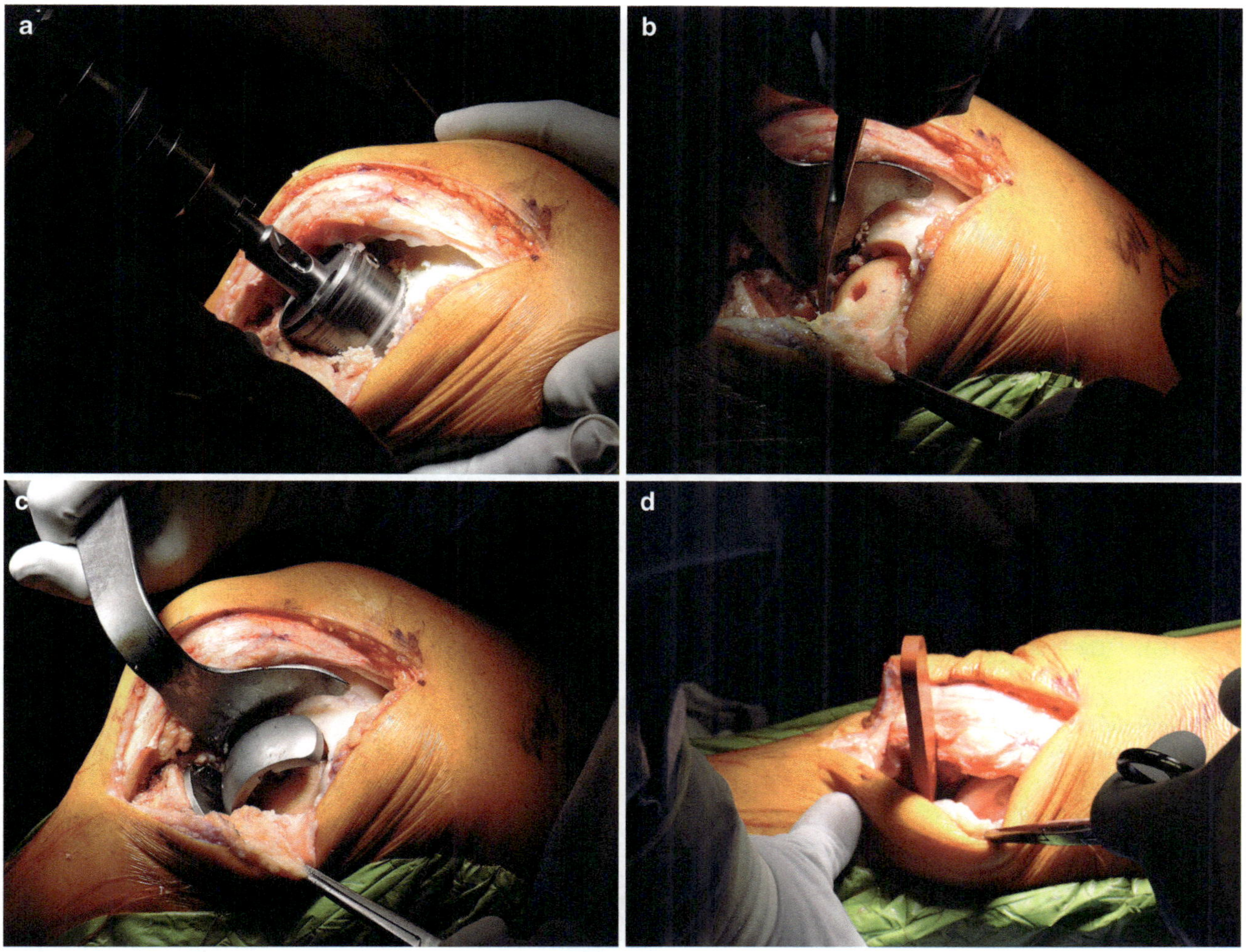

Fig. 15.15 **a–d** Balancing gaps. **a** After each milling, **b** the distal femur osteophytes are moved, **c** the trials are placed, and **d** the extension and flexion gaps are re-evaluated. (Printed with permission of Joint Implant Surgeons, Inc., New Albany, Ohio)

Once the gaps are adequately balanced, the trials are removed and a tibial template is placed on the tibia. The tibial keel slot is prepared with a keel cut saw (Fig. 15.16). The template is forced medially against the vertical border and held in place with a tibial template nail. The keel cut saw is introduced in the template slot and advanced anterior to posterior. Once the saw cut is complete, the groove is excavated with a cemented tibial groove cutter to allow for proper cementation of the keel. The final trial is subsequently performed with a trial bearing (Fig. 15.17).

15.4.5 Cementation and Component Fixation

The trials are removed and the bony surfaces are prepared with pulsatile lavage to provide a dry and clean surface for cement interdigitation. Drill holes are placed circumferentially around the femur and tibia utilizing a short segment drill (Fig. 15.18).

> Care is taken not to drill deep holes into the tibia.

The authors' preference is the use of high-viscosity bone cement with Biomet Bone Cement (Zimmer-Biomet, Warsaw, IN). The cement is prepared in a standard fashion with 1 g of vancomycin and subsequently placed on the implants. The cement is placed on the undersurface of both the tibial and femoral implants (Fig. 15.19).

During the tibial preparation, a thin layer of cement is placed into the prepared tibial bone with a curved osteotome to ensure pressurization and limit posterior extrusion of the cement (Fig. 15.20). The tibial component with a small amount of cement is inserted first and malleted from posterior to anterior direction. This will limit the amount of cement that is extruded into the posterior capsule (Fig. 15.21a). Next, a 90-degree Woodson curette is utilized to remove extruded cement from the posterior to anterior direction (Fig. 15.21b). The leg is subsequently extended to tighten the posterior capsule and compress the remaining posterior cement onto the implant. The Woodson elevator is utilized again to remove any remaining cement.

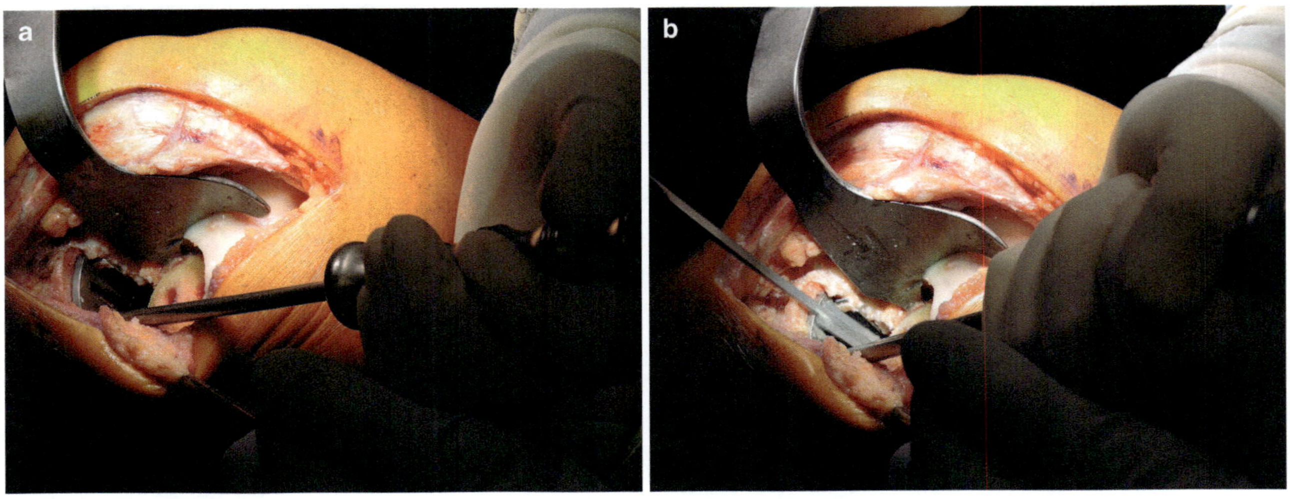

Fig. 15.16 **a** Once the gaps are adequately balanced, the trials are removed and a tibial template is placed on the tibia. **b** The tibial keel slot is prepared with a keel cut saw. (Printed with permission of Joint Implant Surgeons, Inc., New Albany, Ohio)

Fig. 15.17 The final trial is subsequently performed with a trial bearing. (Printed with permission of Joint Implant Surgeons, Inc., New Albany, Ohio)

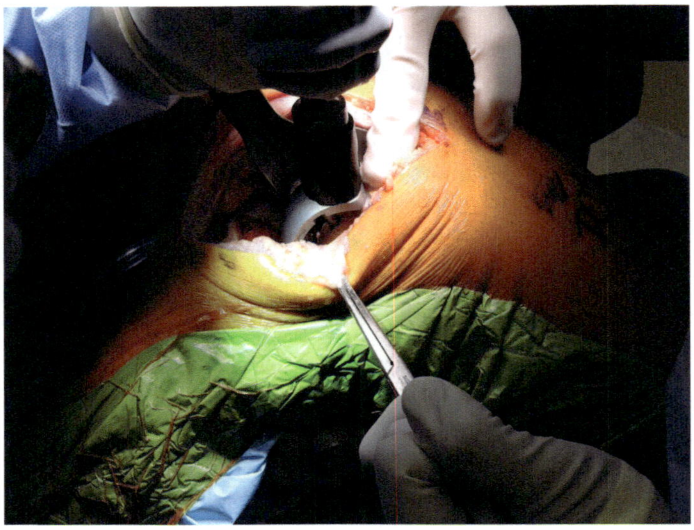

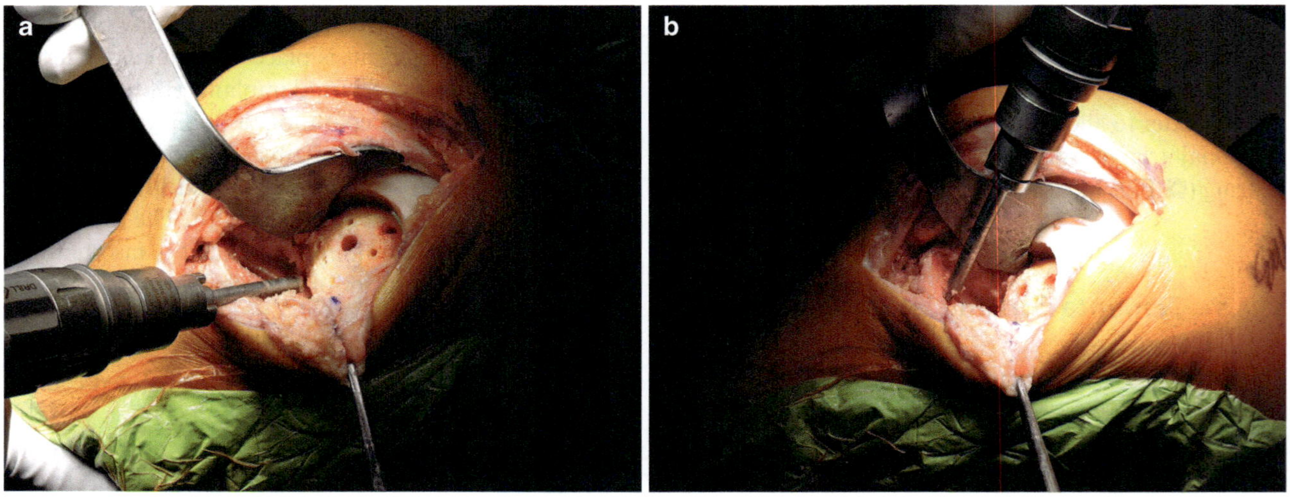

Fig. 15.18 Cementation and component fixation. Drill holes are placed circumferentially around the femur (**a**) and tibia (**b**) utilizing a short segment drill. (Printed with permission of Joint Implant Surgeons, Inc., New Albany, Ohio)

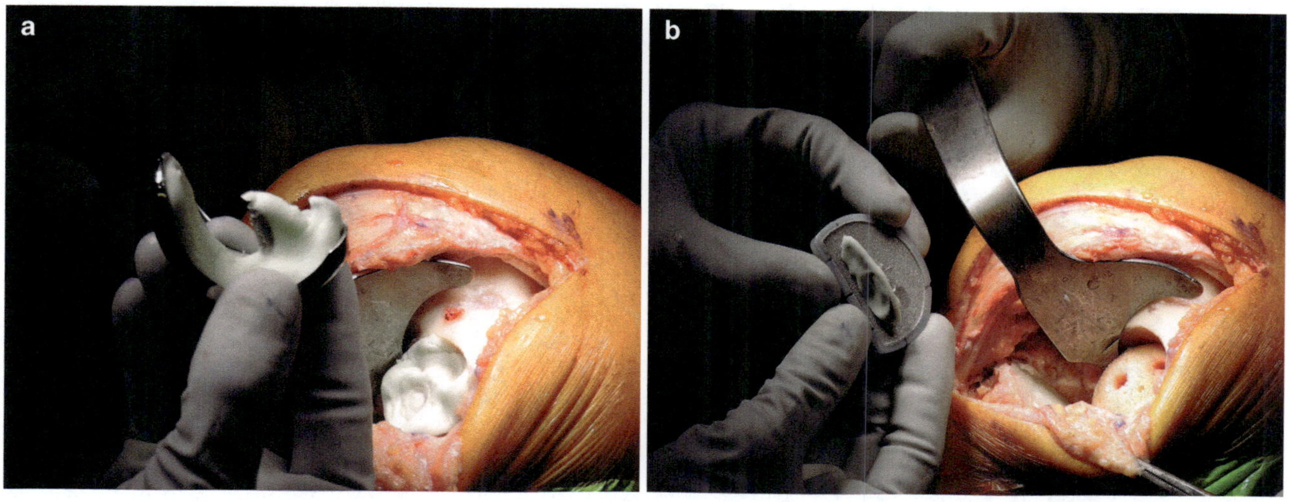

Fig. 15.19 Cementation and component fixation. The cement is placed on the undersurface of both the femoral (**a**) and tibial (**b**) implants (Printed with permission of Joint Implant Surgeons, Inc., New Albany, Ohio)

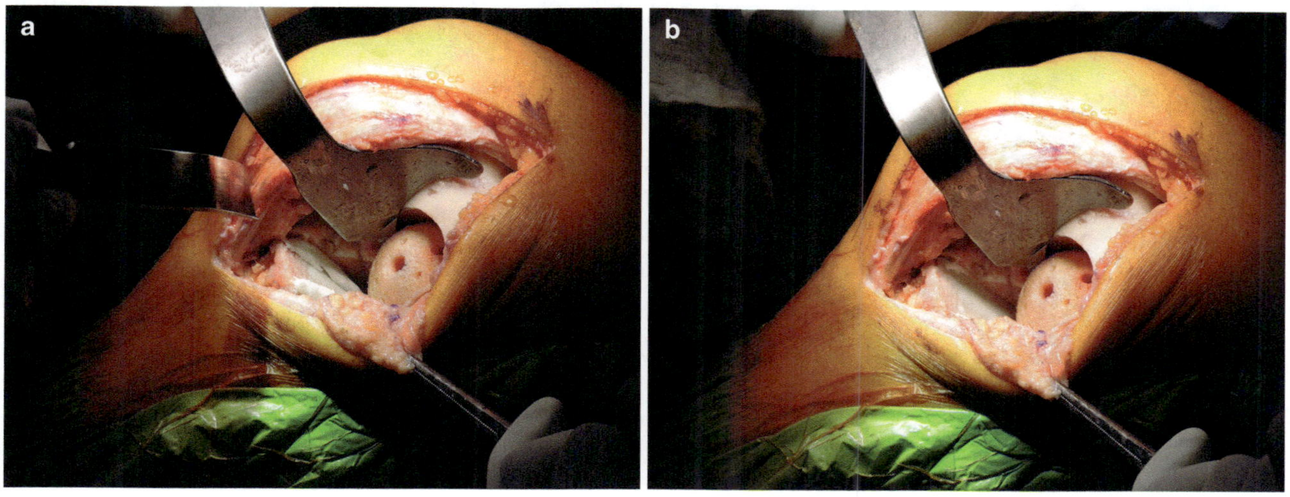

Fig. 15.20 **a, b** Tibial cementation preparation. A thin layer of cement is placed into the prepared tibial bone with a curved osteotome to ensure pressurization and limit posterior extrusion of the cement. (Printed with permission of Joint Implant Surgeons, Inc., New Albany, Ohio)

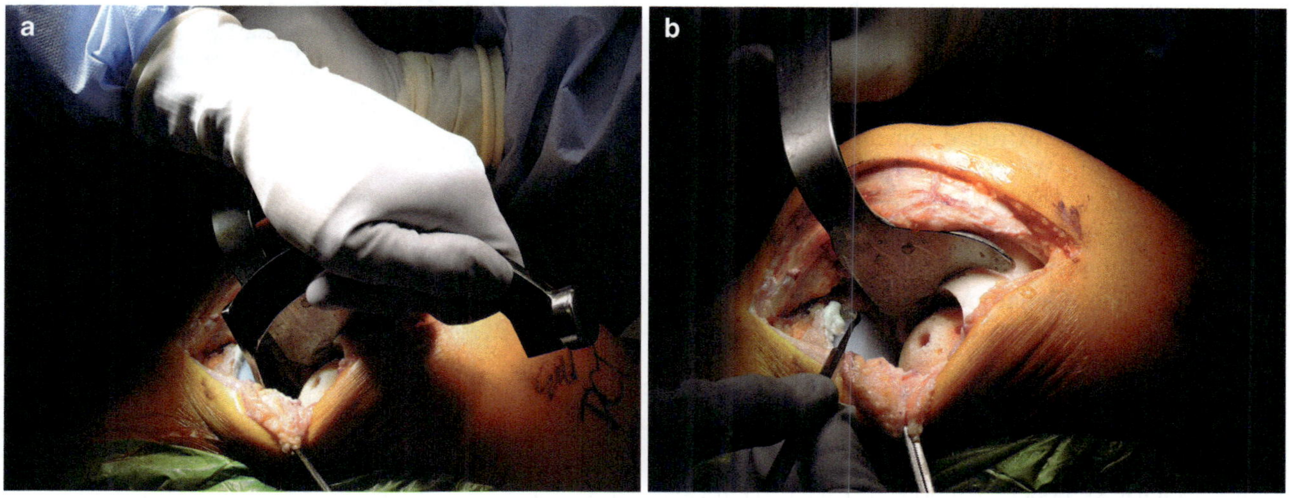

Fig. 15.21 Tibial cement fixation. **a** With a small amount of cement,the tibial component is inserted first and malleted from posterior to anterior direction. **b** A 90-degree Woodson curette is utilized to remove extruded cement from posterior to anterior direction. (Printed with permission of Joint Implant Surgeons, Inc., New Albany, Ohio)

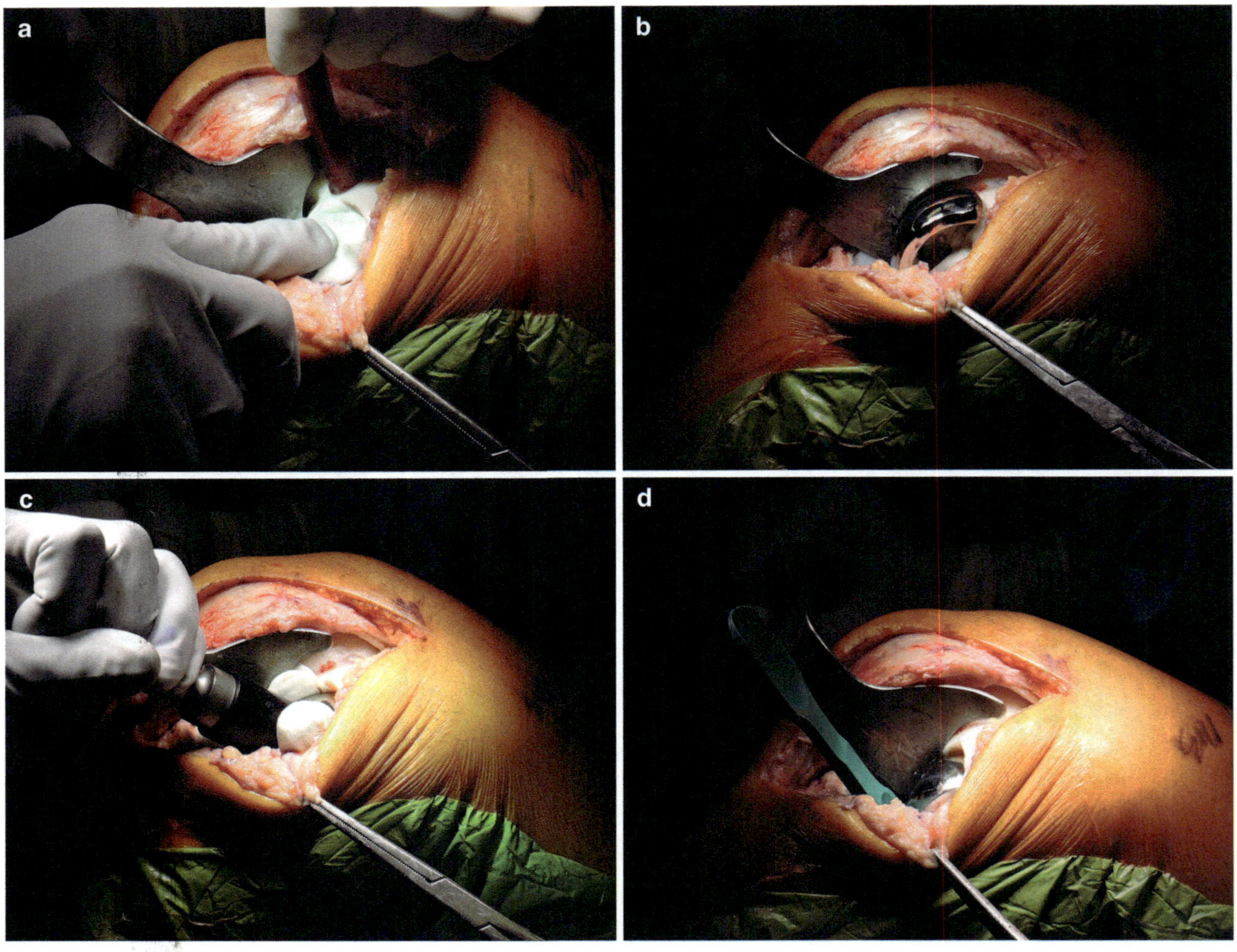

■ Fig. 15.22 **a** A suction tip is placed on the prior 4 mm drill hole to induce negative pressure within the bone and finger pressurized into distal femur. **b**, **c** The femoral component loaded with cement is impacted into the bone with an impactor. **d** Both components are compressed at 45° of knee flexion with a 2 mm feeler gauge and extruded cement is removed from both components. (Printed with permission of Joint Implant Surgeons, Inc., New Albany, Ohio)

Once the tibial component is set, attention is now placed on the femoral component. A suction tip is placed on the prior 4 mm drill hole to induce negative pressure within the bone. An adequate amount of cement is finger pressurized into the prepared distal femur (■ Fig. 15.22a). Next, the femoral component loaded with cement is impacted into the bone with an impactor (■ Fig. 15.22b, c). At this point, the extruded cement is removed from the margins with the Woodson curette. Both components are compressed at 45° of knee flexion with a 2 mm feeler gauge; and, any extruded cement is subsequently removed from both components (■ Fig. 15.22d). The wound is irrigated with warm saline and prepared for closure.

15.4.6 Closure

The capsular tissue is approximated with 2 Quill™PDO(RX-2066Q, Angiotech Pharmaceuticals, Vancouver, BC, Canada) (■ Fig. 15.23), subcutaneous-

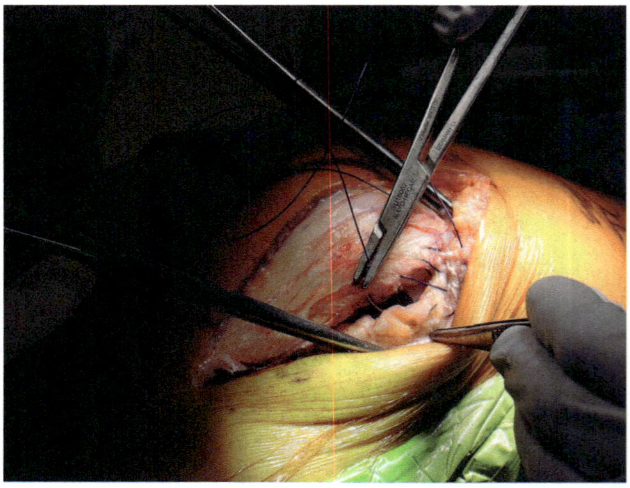

■ Fig. 15.23 The arthrotomy and capsular tissue are closed with 2 Quill™ PDO. (Printed with permission of Joint Implant Surgeons, Inc., New Albany, Ohio)

tissue with 0 Quill™Monoderm™ (YA-1029Q, Angiotech Pharmaceuticals, Vancouver, BC, Canada), and the skin is closed with 2–0 Quill™Monoderm™(YA-2024Q, Angiotech Pharmaceuticals, Vancouver, BC, Canada), and Dermabond® Skin Adhesive (DNX12, Ethicon Inc., Somerville, NJ).

15.5 Discussion of Current Literature

In the past, various surgical techniques and devices have been utilized in the treatment of lateral compartment arthritis with varying degrees of survivorship (Table 15.1).

> In recent years, multiple studies have demonstrated a significant increase in survivorship as devices and surgical techniques continue to improve (Table 15.1).

In one of the largest series, Berend et al. reported 99% survivorship in 100 lateral UKA presented with 3-year follow-up (Berend et al. 2012). Smith et al. reported 95.5% survivorship for 101 lateral UKA at 5 years (Smith et al. 2014). Berend et al. reported similar survivorship on a non-modular, fixed-bearing, metal-backed tibial component utilizing a lateral parapatellar approach at a 2.3-year follow-up (Berend et al. 2015). Recently, Greco et al. reported on similar survivorship and clinical outcomes utilizing a lateral-specific fixed-bearing implant at 2.7 years follow-up (Greco et al. 2019).

Van der List et al. performed the largest systemic review with 96 eligible studies and reported the survivorship in medial and lateral UKA. With regard to lateral UKA survivorship, 15 cohort studies and a single registry's data were analyzed. This study reported 93.2% survivorship at 5 years, 91.4% survivorship at 10 years, and 89.4% survivorship at 15 years (van der List et al. 2015).

Although isolated lateral compartment osteoarthritis exhibits decrease incidence relative to medial compartment osteoarthritis, it still presents with relative frequency and is amenable to appropriate treatment. With proper patient diagnosis and surgical technique, multiple studies have demonstrated excellent survivorship.

Table 15.1 Published results of lateral unicompartmental knee arthroplasty

Authors	Year	# Knees	Type of implant (manufacturer)	Follow-up (years)	Survivorship (# Revisions)
Scott and Santore (1981)	1981	12	Brigham I & II (DePuy); cemented, all-poly tibia	3.5 (2–6)	83.3% at 3.5 years (2)
Mallory and Danyi (1983)	1983	4	Polycentric 17% (Stryker); Marmor 83% (Smith & Nephew); both cemented, all-poly tibia	5.6 (5.1–8.1)	50% survival at 5.6 years (2)
Marmor (1984)	1984	14	Marmor (Smith & Nephew), cemented, all-poly tibia	7.4 (2.5–9.83)	85.7% at 7.4 years (2)
Kozinn et al. (1989)	1989	11	Brigham Mod (DePuy), cemented, metal-backed	5.5 (4.5–6)	100% at 5.5 years (0)
Magnussen and Bartlett (1990)	1990	9	PCA (Stryker), cementless, metal-backed	(2–3.3)	100% at 2 years (0)
Christensen (1991)	1991	54	St. Georg Sled (Link), cemented, all-poly tibia	3.9 (1–9)	98.4% at 3.9 years (na)
Rougraff et al. (1991)	1991	14	Compartmental I & II (Zimmer), cemented, all-poly	6.5 (0.7–13.5)	92.9% at 6.5 years (1)
Scott et al. (1991)	1991	12	Brigham I & II (Stryker); cemented, all-poly tibia	(8–12)	83.3% at 9 years (2)
Capra Jr. and Fehring (1992)	1992	4	Marmor (Richards)	11.1 (8–14)	100% at 11.1 years (0)
		8	Compartmental II (Zimmer)	6.3 (4–11)	100% at 6.3 years (0)
Heck et al. (1993)	1993	39	Marmor (Smith & Nephew); compartmental I & II (Zimmer)	6 (maximum 14.8)	97.4% at 6 years (1)

(continued)

Table 15.1 (continued)

Authors	Year	# Knees	Type of implant (manufacturer)	Follow-up (years)	Survivorship (# Revisions)
Swank et al. (1993)	1993	7	5 Fibermesh (Zimmer); 2 Microloc (DePuy); cementless & cemented	5.5 (4–8)	87.8% at 5.5 years (na)
Lewold et al. (1995)	1995	36	Oxford (Biomet), cemented, mobile bearing	6 (1–10)	86.1% at 6 years (5)
Tabor Jr. and Tabor (1998)	1998	6	Marmor-style, cemented, all-poly tibia	9.7 (5–20)	66.7% at 9.7 years (2)
Ohdera et al. (2001)	2001	18	Four different designs	8.25 (5–15.75)	NA (2)
Ashraf et al. (2002)	2002	83	St. Georg Sled (Link), cemented all-poly tibia	9 (2–21)	74% at 15 years (15)
Keblish and Briard (2004)	2004	19	LCS (DePuy), cemented, mobile bearing	11 (5–19)	84.2% at 11 years (3)
Saxler et al. (2004)	2004	46	AMC Uniglide (Corin), 72% cemented, 25% cementless, 3% hybrid, mobile bearing	5.5 (2.3–12.5)	89% at 5.5 years (5)
O'Rourke et al. (2005)	2005	14	Marmor (Smith & Nephew), cemented all-poly tibia	24 (17–28)	72% at 25 years (2)
Carlsson et al. (2006)	2006	29	Miller-Galante (Zimmer), cemented, metal-backed (75%); all-poly tibia (25%)	12.4 (3.1–15.6)	100% at 12.4 years (0)
Cartier et al. (2007)	2007	30	< age 60, Genesis (Smith & Nephew); 20% cementless; 43% all-poly	(5–14)	94% at 10 years; 92% at 11 years; 88% at 12 years
Forster et al. (2007)	2007	30	Preservation (DePuy), cemented, 13 mobile bearing; 17 all-poly fixed	2	Mobile-77% at 2 years (3); fixed-100% at 2 years (0)
Sah and Scott (2007)	2007	49	Four different designs	5.2 (2–14)	100% at 5.4 years (0)
Argenson et al. (2008)	2008	38	Four different designs	12.6 (3–23)	84% at 16 years (5)
Bertani et al. (2008)	2008	35	Four different designs	9 (2–22)	85.7% at 9 years (5)
Lustig et al. (2009)	2009	60	HLS Evolution (Tornier), cemented, all-poly tibia	5.2 (2.1–13.3)	98.3% at 5 years; 98.3% at 10 years (11/144)
John et al. (2011)	2010	9	Miller-Galante (Zimmer), cemented, metal-backed, fixed bearing	10.8 (2–16)	97% at 5 years; 41% at 8 years
Pandit et al. (2010)	2010	53	Oxford I&II (Biomet)	5.2	82% at 4 years (11)
		65	Oxford III flat tibia	4.7 (3–9)	91% at 4 years (9)
		101	Oxford III domed tibia	2.3 (1–4)	98% at 4 years (1)
Lustig et al. (2011)	2011	54	HLS Evolution, all-poly tibia	8.4 (5–16)	98.1% (1)
Berend et al. (2012)	2012	132	Vanguard M (Biomet), cemented, metal-backed	2.4 (1–5.8)	100% at 2 years (0)
Heyse et al. (2012)	2012	50	Genesis (now Accuris; Smith & Nephew), 20 uncemented, 23 all-poly	10.8 (5–16)	94.0% (3)
Lustig et al. (2012)	2012	13	All post-traumatic; 6 HLS Evolution all-poly; 2 Marmor II (Richards) metal-backed; 5 Miller-Galante metal-backed	10.2 (3–22)	92.3% (1)

Table 15.1 (continued)

Authors	Year	# Knees	Type of implant (manufacturer)	Follow-up (years)	Survivorship (# Revisions)
Panni et al. (2012)	2012	9	Zimmer High Flex (Zimmer)	4.5 (3–6)	100% (0)
Schelfaut et al. (2013)	2013	25	Oxford III domed mobile bearing	Min 1	96% (1)
Streit et al. (2012)	2012	50	Oxford III domed mobile bearing	3 (2–4)	94% (3)
Xing et al. (2012)	2012	31	Preservation (DePuy)	4.5 (2–6)	100% (0)
Altuntas et al. (2013)	2013	64	Oxford III domed mobile bearing	3.2 (2–5)	96.9% (2)
Sebilo et al. (2013)	2013	82	Implants from 30 companies	5.2 (<1–23)	84% at 10 years
Thompson et al. (2013)	2013	30	Miller-Galante, Zimmer ZUK, Smith & Nephew Journey, Mako	2	96.4%
Marson et al. (2014)	2014	15	Oxford domed mobile bearing	2.9 (1–4)	93.3% (1)
		12	Zimmer High-flex fixed bearing	2.7 (1–6)	100% (0)
Smith et al. (2014)	2014	101	AMC Uniglide fixed bearing (Corin)	3.9	98.7% at 2 years 95.5% at 5 years
Walker et al. (2014)	2014	22	Oxford III domed mobile bearing	1.8	96% at 2 years (1)
Weston-Simons et al. (2014)	2014	265	Oxford III domed mobile bearing	4 (0.5–8.3)	92.1% at 8 years (4)
Berend et al. (2015)	2015	104	Vanguard M fixed bearing	2.3 (<1–6.2)	98.1% (2)
Demange et al. (2015)	2015	33	iUni G1 (ConforMIS)	2–4.4	97% at 3.1 years (2)
		19	Miller-Galante	6.3 (2–9)	85% at 2.8 years (3)
Newman et al. (2017)	2017	61	Oxford III domed mobile bearing	7	87% at 7 years 13% reoperation
Fornell et al. (2018)	2018	41	Oxford III domed mobile bearing	Min 2	97.6% at 2 years (1)
Edmiston et al. (2018)	2018	67	Zimmer Unicompartmental knee system or the Zimmer Miller-Galante Unicompartmental knee before 2004	Min 2 years; mean: 7 years	94% at min 2 years
Walker et al. (2020)	2019	52	Oxford fixed lateral prosthesis	2	100% at 2 years
Zambianchi et al. (2020)	2019	67	Robotic assisted Stryker Restoris MCK	Min 2	100% at 2 years
Gill and Nicolai (2019)	2019	14	Physica Zuk	1.5	100% at 1.5 years
Greco et al. (2019)	2019	56	Oxford fixed lateral prosthesis	2.7	96% at min 2 years

Take-Home Messages

- Isolated lateral compartment knee osteoarthritis occurs in 5–10% of individuals with knee osteoarthritis.
- Varus stress and flexed posteroanterior radiographs are critical to identifying patients with isolated lateral compartment arthritis.
- Lateral parapatellar approach limits incision size, but care must be taken to preserve the inferior fat pad with thin lateral retinacular tissue to provide adequate closure.
- Care must be taken during the vertical tibial saw cut to ensure proper rotation and limit any violation of the posterior cortex.
- The normal knee kinematics and flexion/extension ligamentous laxity should be taken into consideration when balancing the knee. The lateral compartment has greater laxity in flexion than extension and should be reproduced when performing lateral UKA.
- Cementation techniques include drilling holes to increase surface area, limiting posterior extrusion of the cement, and using a 90-degree Woodson curette to remove any additional cement.
- Lateral UKA has excellent results and early survivorship with proper patient selection, implant selection, and proper surgical technique.

References

Altuntas AO, Alsop H, Cobb JP (2013) Early results of a domed tibia, mobile bearing lateral unicompartmental knee arthroplasty from an independent centre. Knee 20(6):466–470

Argenson JN et al (2008) Long-term results with a lateral unicondylar replacement. Clin Orthop Relat Res 466(11):2686–2693

Ashraf T et al (2002) Lateral unicompartmental knee replacement survivorship and clinical experience over 21 years. J Bone Joint Surg Br 84(8):1126–1130

Berend KR et al (2012) Lateral unicompartmental knee arthroplasty through a lateral parapatellar approach has high early survivorship. Clin Orthop Relat Res 470(1):77–83

Berend KR et al (2015) The current trends for lateral unicondylar knee arthroplasty. Orthop Clin North Am 46(2):177–184

Bertani A et al (2008) Unicompartmental-knee arthroplasty for treatment of lateral gonarthrosis: about 30 cases. Midterm results. Rev Chir Orthop Reparatrice Appar Mot 94(8):763–770

Capra SW Jr, Fehring TK (1992) Unicondylar arthroplasty. A survivorship analysis. J Arthroplast 7(3):247–251

Carlsson LV, Albrektsson BE, Regner LR (2006) Minimally invasive surgery vs conventional exposure using the Miller-Galante unicompartmental knee arthroplasty: a randomized radiostereometric study. J Arthroplast 21(2):151–156

Cartier P et al (2007) Unicondylar knee arthroplasty in middle-aged patients: a minimum 5-year follow-up. Orthopedics 30(8 Suppl):62–65

Christensen NO (1991) Unicompartmental prosthesis for gonarthrosis. A nine-year series of 575 knees from a Swedish hospital. Clin Orthop Relat Res 273:165–169

Demange MK et al (2015) Patient-specific implants for lateral unicompartmental knee arthroplasty. Int Orthop 39(8): 1519–1526

Edmiston TA et al (2018) Clinical outcomes and survivorship of lateral unicompartmental knee arthroplasty: does surgical approach matter? J Arthroplast 33(2):362–365

Fitz W (2009) Unicompartmental knee arthroplasty with use of novel patient-specific resurfacing implants and personalized jigs. J Bone Joint Surg Am 91(Suppl 1):69–76

Fornell S et al (2018) Mid-term outcomes of mobile-bearing lateral unicompartmental knee arthroplasty. Knee 25(6):1206–1213

Forster MC, Bauze AJ, Keene GC (2007) Lateral unicompartmental knee replacement: fixed or mobile bearing? Knee Surg Sports Traumatol Arthrosc 15(9):1107–1111

Gill JR, Nicolai P (2019) Clinical results and 12-year survivorship of the Physica ZUK unicompartmental knee replacement. Knee 26(3):750–758

Greco NJ et al (2019) Lateral unicompartmental knee arthroplasty utilizing a modified surgical technique and specifically adapted fixed-bearing implant. Surg Technol Int 34:371–378

Heck DA et al (1993) Unicompartmental knee arthroplasty. A multicenter investigation with long-term follow-up evaluation. Clin Orthop Relat Res 286:154–159

Heyse TJ et al (2012) Survivorship of UKA in the middle-aged. Knee 19(5):585–591

John J, Mauffrey C, May P (2011) Unicompartmental knee replacements with Miller-Galante prosthesis: two to 16-year follow-up of a single surgeon series. Int Orthop 35(4):507–513

Keblish PA, Briard JL (2004) Mobile-bearing unicompartmental knee arthroplasty: a 2-center study with an 11-year (mean) follow-up. J Arthroplast 19(7 Suppl 2):87–94

Kozinn SC, Marx C, Scott RD (1989) Unicompartmental knee arthroplasty. A 4.5-6-year follow-up study with a metal-backed tibial component. J Arthroplast 4 Suppl:S1–S10

Lewold S et al (1995) Oxford meniscal bearing knee versus the Marmor knee in unicompartmental arthroplasty for arthrosis. A Swedish multicenter survival study. J Arthroplast 10(6):722–731

Lustig S et al (2009) Cemented all polyethylene tibial insert unicompartimental knee arthroplasty: a long term follow-up study. Orthop Traumatol Surg Res 95(1):12–21

Lustig S et al (2011) 5- to 16-year follow-up of 54 consecutive lateral unicondylar knee arthroplasties with a fixed-all polyethylene bearing. J Arthroplast 26(8):1318–1325

Lustig S et al (2012) Lateral unicompartmental knee arthroplasty relieves pain and improves function in posttraumatic osteoarthritis. Clin Orthop Relat Res 470(1):69–76

Magnussen PA, Bartlett RJ (1990) Cementless PCA unicompartmental joint arthroplasty for osteoarthritis of the knee. A prospective study of 51 cases. J Arthroplast 5(2):151–158

Mallory TH, Danyi J (1983) Unicompartmental total knee arthroplasty. A five- to nine-year follow-up study of 42 procedures. Clin Orthop Relat Res 175:135–138

Marmor L (1984) Lateral compartment arthroplasty of the knee. Clin Orthop Relat Res 186:115–121

Marson B et al (2014) Lateral unicompartmental knee replacements: early results from a District General Hospital. Eur J Orthop Surg Traumatol 24(6):987–991

Newman SDS et al (2017) Up to 10 year follow-up of the Oxford domed lateral partial knee replacement from an independent centre. Knee 24(6):1414–1421

Ohdera T, Tokunaga J, Kobayashi A (2001) Unicompartmental knee arthroplasty for lateral gonarthrosis: midterm results. J Arthroplast 16(2):196–200

O'Rourke MR et al (2005) The John Insall award: unicompartmental knee replacement: a minimum twenty-one-year followup, end-result study. Clin Orthop Relat Res 440:27–37

Pandit H et al (2010) Mobile bearing dislocation in lateral unicompartmental knee replacement. Knee 17(6):392–397

Panni AS et al (2012) Unicompartmental knee replacement provides early clinical and functional improvement stabilizing over time. Knee Surg Sports Traumatol Arthrosc 20(3):579–585

Rougraff BT, Heck DA, Gibson AE (1991) A comparison of tricompartmental and unicompartmental arthroplasty for the treatment of gonarthrosis. Clin Orthop Relat Res 273:157–164

Sah AP, Scott RD (2007) Lateral unicompartmental knee arthroplasty through a medial approach. Study with an average five-year follow-up. J Bone Joint Surg Am 89(9):1948–1954

Saxler G, Temmen D, Bontemps G (2004) Medium-term results of the AMC-unicompartmental knee arthroplasty. Knee 11(5): 349–355

Schelfaut S et al (2013) The risk of bearing dislocation in lateral unicompartmental knee arthroplasty using a mobile biconcave design. Knee Surg Sports Traumatol Arthrosc 21(11):2487–2494

Scott RD (2005) Lateral unicompartmental replacement: a road less traveled. Orthopedics 28(9):983–984

Scott RD, Santore RF (1981) Unicondylar unicompartmental replacement for osteoarthritis of the knee. J Bone Joint Surg Am 63(4):536–544

Scott RD et al (1991) Unicompartmental knee arthroplasty. Eight- to 12-year follow-up evaluation with survivorship analysis. Clin Orthop Relat Res 271:96–100

Sebilo A et al (2013) Clinical and technical factors influencing outcomes of unicompartmental knee arthroplasty: retrospective multicentre study of 944 knees. Orthop Traumatol Surg Res 99(4 Suppl):S227–S234

Smith JR et al (2014) Fixed bearing lateral unicompartmental knee arthroplasty--short to midterm survivorship and knee scores for 101 prostheses. Knee 21(4):843–847

Streit MR et al (2012) Mobile-bearing lateral unicompartmental knee replacement with the Oxford domed tibial component: an independent series. J Bone Joint Surg Br 94(10):1356–1361

Swank M et al (1993) The natural history of unicompartmental arthroplasty. An eight-year follow-up study with survivorship analysis. Clin Orthop Relat Res 286:130–142

Tabor OB Jr, Tabor OB (1998) Unicompartmental arthroplasty: a long-term follow-up study. J Arthroplast 13(4):373–379

Thompson SA et al (2013) Factors associated with poor outcomes following unicompartmental knee arthroplasty: redefining the "classic" indications for surgery. J Arthroplast 28(9):1561–1564

van der List JP, McDonald LS, Pearle AD (2015) Systematic review of medial versus lateral survivorship in unicompartmental knee arthroplasty. Knee 22(6):454–460

Walker T et al (2014) Total versus unicompartmental knee replacement for isolated lateral osteoarthritis: a matched-pairs study. Int Orthop 38(11):2259–2264

Walker T et al (2020) Minimally invasive lateral unicompartmental knee replacement: early results from an independent center using the Oxford fixed lateral prosthesis. Knee 27(1):235–241.

Weston-Simons JS et al (2014) An analysis of dislocation of the domed Oxford lateral unicompartmental knee replacement. Knee 21(1):304–309

Xing Z, Katz J, Jiranek W (2012) Unicompartmental knee arthroplasty: factors influencing the outcome. J Knee Surg 25(5): 369–373

Zambianchi F et al (2020) Clinical results and short-term survivorship of robotic-arm-assisted medial and lateral unicompartmental knee arthroplasty. Knee Surg Sports Traumatol Arthrosc 28(5):1551–1559

Lateral Unicompartmental Knee Arthroplasty: A French Perspective

Axel Schmidt, Christophe Jacquet, Matthieu Ollivier, and Jean-Noël Argenson

Contents

E. Hansen, K.-D. Kühn (eds.), *Essentials of Cemented Knee Arthroplasty*,
https://doi.org/10.1007/978-3-662-63113-3_16

16.1 Introduction

Lateral unicompartmental knee arthroplasty (UKA) represents a minority, around 10% (Scott 2005), of all UKA performed for osteoarthritis (OA) (Parratte et al. 2015; Berend et al. 2015). Lateral UKA is a challenging surgical procedure, more than medial UKA due to its rarity (low incidence of genu valgum in the population (Ranawat et al. 2005; Rossi et al. 2014) and better tolerance in the long term of lateral compartment osteoarthritis), to the specificity of the indications, and the characteristics of the lateral knee compartment (anatomy and kinematics).

The surgical procedure is performed through a lateral parapatellar approach. An orthogonal tibial cut to the mechanical axis is performed which has to be as minimal as possible. The lateral tibial slope is less important than in the medial compartment and should be reproduced. The sagittal tibial cut is realized close to the tibial spines and in the internal rotation due to the constitutional external rotation of the lateral tibial plateau (screw-home mechanism). The distal femoral cut should be as conservative as possible allowing to "distalize" the femoral implant and compensate for the congenital hypoplasia and the wear. In genu valgum, OA affects preferentially the posterior part of the femoral condyle explaining why there may be intact cartilage on the distal part of the condyle which has to be removed before positioning the distal femoral cutting guide. Due to the divergence of the lateral condyle, it is crucial to avoid excessive internal rotation in flexion, which will create an impingement in extension with the tibial spines.

The tibial implant should be close to the tibial spines with 15°–20° of internal rotation. The femoral implant is placed on a flexed knee with external rotation and as lateral as possible, sometimes it may rest on lateral condyle osteophytes.

Clinical and radiological results of lateral UKA are similar to medial UKA with 90% survival at medium term and 80% at long term. The main cause of failure for lateral UKA is OA progression (87.5%), especially in the medial compartment, followed by aseptic loosening (12.5%).

16.2 Case Example

A 64-year-old woman suffered from isolated lateral knee pain for 2 years. The clinical examination found a valgus morphotype completely reducible with no sagittal laxity, no stiffness, and no medial tibiofemoral or patellofemoral pain. Standard radiographic investigations (Fig. 16.1) showed isolated joint space narrowing of the lateral tibiofemoral joint with condensation of the lateral sub-chondral tibial plateau and osteophytes. The OA was confirmed with the Rosenberg view (Fig. 16.2) showing complete joint space loss (stage 3 of Ahlback's classification) indicating that cartilage wear is predominately posterior. Complete X-ray investigations were realized with varus/valgus stress and leg-length views (Fig. 16.3). They confirmed the complete reducibility of the knee (varus stress), no medial collateral ligament laxity (valgus stress), and quantified the importance of the valgus deformity and the origin of the deformation (leg-length view): valgus deformation of 10° (HKA angle = 190°) with hypoplasia of the lateral condyle (mechanical femoral angle = 98°) (Moreland et al. 1987).

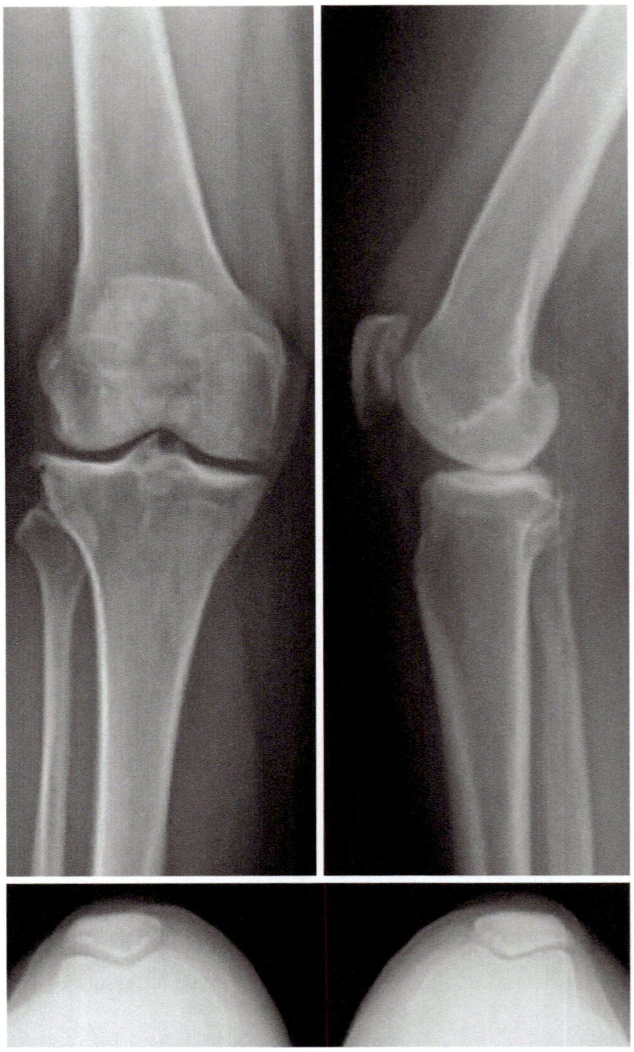

Fig. 16.1 Standard X-ray. Lateral OA stage 2 with lateral tibial osteophytes

A lateral UKA was performed (Fig. 16.4). Varus femoral osteotomy was not recommended for this case because of the advanced OA stage. A UKA was preferred over TKA because the pain was limited to lateral knee compartment with preserved medial and patello-

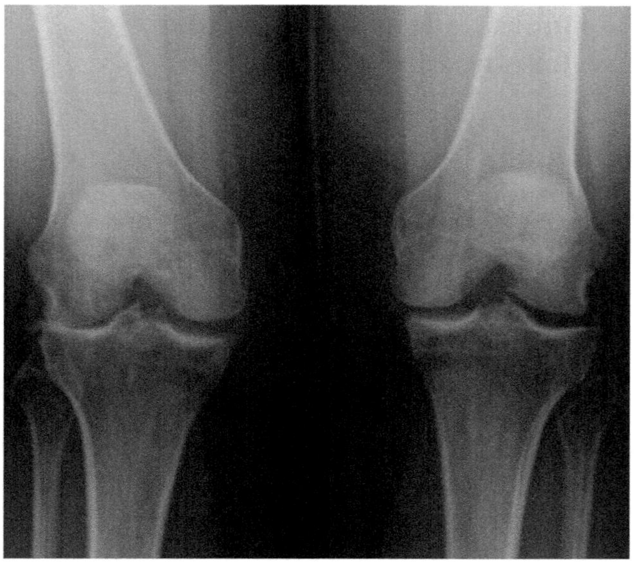

Fig. 16.2 Narrowing of the lateral joint line with lateral OA stage 3 in Rosenberg view

femoral joint spaces. A tibial implant was positioned as close as possible to the tibial spines with internal rotation. The femoral implant was positioned very lateral and vertical to have optimal contact with the tibial implant during all range of motion and avoid any impingement with the patella and the tibial spines. Attention should be paid to avoid any overhanging and altering of the tibial slope.

16.3 Anatomy

Asymmetries between the medial and the lateral tibiofemoral spaces are explained by their proper anatomical characteristics (Miyatake et al. 2016).

The lateral tibial plateau has four characteristics (Weinberg et al. 2017):

- The cartilage surface is convex.
- The articular surface is smaller than the medial tibial plateau (anteroposterior and mediolateral axis).

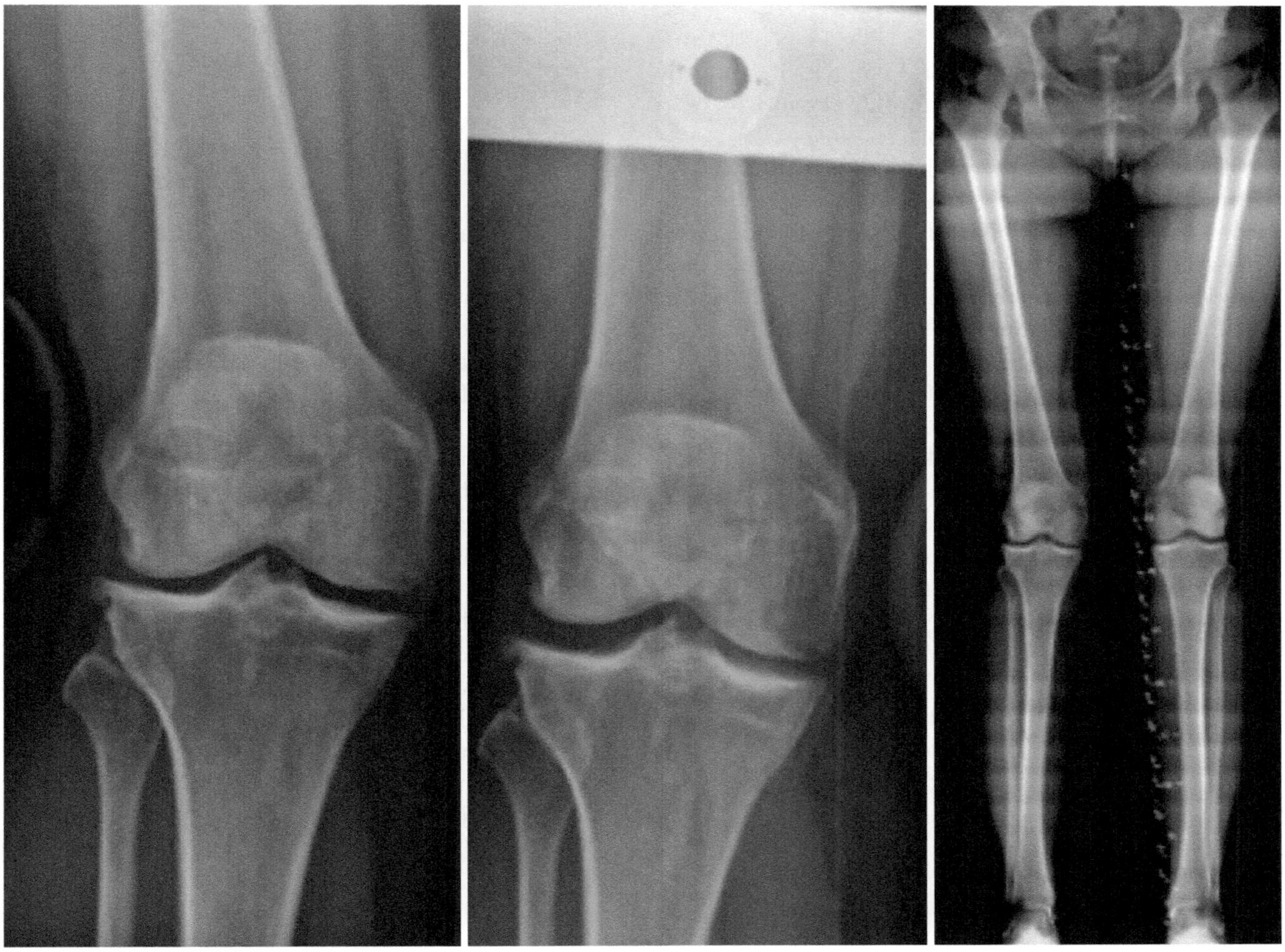

Fig. 16.3 Complete X-ray investigation with varus/valgus stress and leg-length X-ray. A good reduction of the deformity with varus stress can be observed

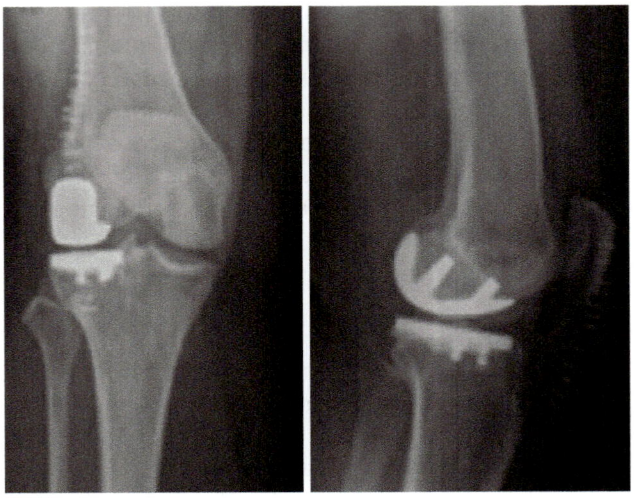

Fig. 16.4 Postoperative X-ray after lateral cemented UKA

- The anteroposterior axis has an internal rotational axis of 10–15°.
- The posterior tibial slope is reduced on the lateral side compared to the medial side (4° vs. 7°) (Karimi et al. 2017).

Regarding the lateral femoral condyle, it is mostly hypoplastic in genu valgum with a divergent axis from the anteromedial to the posterolateral side.

The congruency between the femoral condyle and the tibial plateau is closely related to the lateral meniscus: its shape and its mobility. In the case of prior lateral meniscectomy, the stability of the lateral compartment is altered leading to degenerative tears explaining the high rate of lateral OA in young patients after meniscectomy (Longo et al. 2019).

All these anatomical characteristics of the lateral tibiofemoral compartment will impact the surgical technique, implant positioning, and the choice of prosthesis (Demange et al. 2015; Greco et al. 2019).

16

> While in the medial compartment, the cartilage wear is preferentially developing in the anterior part of the joint, in the lateral compartment, OA starts in the posterior part of the joint (Gulati et al. 2009).

This is particularly important and will influence the radiological investigations, especially with the Rosenberg posteroanterior view required to see the posterior wear and appreciate the stage of OA.

16.4 Indications and Preoperative Investigations

Indications and Contraindications of Lateral UKA

Indications:

- Primary lateral OA secondary to a constitutional genu valgum
- Avascular osteonecrosis of the femoral condyle or tibial plateau
- Post-traumatic OA secondary to tibial plateau fracture or a femoral condyle fracture
- Post-meniscectomy OA

Contraindications:

- OA in other compartments are as follows:
  - Medial tibiofemoral compartment
  - Patellofemoral compartment (especially on the lateral facet)
- Chronic anterior laxity
- Medial or lateral laxity due to collateral ligament insufficiency
- Valgus deformity >15° or non-reducible valgus deformity (Kozinn and Scott 1989)
- Preoperative flexion contracture >15°
- Stiffness with flexion limited to 100°
- Previous history of distal femoral osteotomy or high tibial osteotomy
- Inflammatory disease

The clinical exam has to demonstrate concordanceregarding the location of the pain which has to be limited to the lateral compartment and eliminate other contraindications. Testing of the collateral ligaments and the cruciate ligament is crucial to estimate their integrity. Confirmation with radiographic stress exams varus/valgus and anteroposterior plane may be helpful. The ACL evaluation may be difficult to interpret due to the pain and the effusion.

The standard preoperative radiological investigations will confirm the localization in the lateral compartment of the OA, without medial tibiofemoral or patellofemoral degeneration and can be graded according to Ahlback's classification. The stress X-rays in varus/valgus will evaluate the reducibility of the deformity and the thickness of the cartilage in the contralateral compartment. The full leg-length X-rays are necessary to appreciate the global deformity of the lower limbs and analyze the origin of the valgus deformity.

Origins of Valgus Knee Deformity

- Lateral femoral condyle dysplasia (Feldman et al. 2016)
- Post-traumatic valgus secondary to a tibial plateau or lateral condyle fracture (Lustig et al. 2012)
- OA after lateral meniscectomy (Pengas et al. 2017)
- Avascular osteonecrosis of the femoral condyle or lateral tibial plateau
- Valgus secondary to a hip pathology (Barrios et al. 2016)
- Congenital tibial deformity (van Lieshout et al. 2019)

Hypoplasia of the lateral femoral condyle is the most frequent cause of valgus deformity (Rossi et al. 2014). In this case, the position of the femoral component has to be adapted to the severity of the dysplasia: distally and posteriorly to restore a normal intra-articular joint space in sagittal and coronal planes.

In cases of post-traumatic OA (Lustig et al. 2012), the challenge is not due to bone dysplasia but rather poor bone quality or a malunion which has to be anticipated and addressed with one option being bone graft with screw fixation. Although this indication is rare, lateral UKA is an efficient procedure with good results on knee pain and a good survival rate in the long term (Lustig et al. 2012).

16.5 Kinematics of a Native Knee and After UKA

Kinematics of a native knee consists of external femoral rotation on the tibia during knee flexion associated with posterior femoral roll-back, more important for the lateral condyle (10 mm) than for the medial condyle (2 mm). This is the concept of "medial pivot of the knee": the medial compartment is the compartment of knee stability, while the lateral compartment is the compartment of mobility (Argenson et al. 2002). The translation of the medial femoral condyle seems to be correlated to ACL integrity (Du et al. 2018) while the mobility of the lateral condyle on the lateral tibial plateau seems to be independent of the osteoarthritis and ACL status. The femur will progressively pass from its neutral position at 0° of rotation in full extension to 7° of external rotation during flexion. At the end of the extension, between 0° and 20° of flexion, both cruciate ligaments exert tension on the tibia, putting it in external rotation and locking the knee. The tibia is then in the position of maximal stability with the femur. This mechanism, called "the screw-home mechanism" is the key to knee stability in terminal extension (Kim et al. 2015).

> Appropriate understanding of this tibial external rotation during extension explains why the femoral implant has to be placed as lateral as possible and the tibial implant has to be positioned in internal rotation to avoid any impingement with the tibial spines in extension.

16.6 Surgical Technique

Classically, a lateral parapatellar approach is preferentially used for this procedure even if some authors publish on the possibility of performing it through a medial approach (Berend et al. 2012; Sah and Scott 2008).

The skin incision starts from the superior border of the patella and finishes 2 cm distally to the lateral border of the ATT (Fig. 16.5). After a lateral arthrotomy, an articular exploration confirms ACL integrity and confirms the limitation of OA in the lateral compartment. Sometimes, to improve the exposure a lateral vertical facet osteotomy of the patella is required.

> To maintain appropriate ligament tension, it is important to respect the peripheral structures around the lateral tibial plateau (lateral collateral ligament and

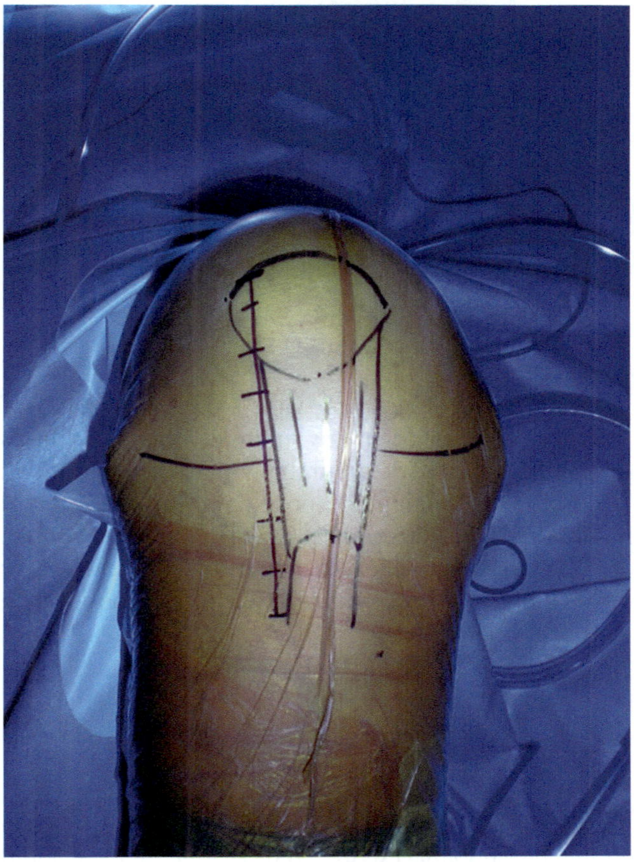

Fig. 16.5 Skin incision and cutaneous landmarks

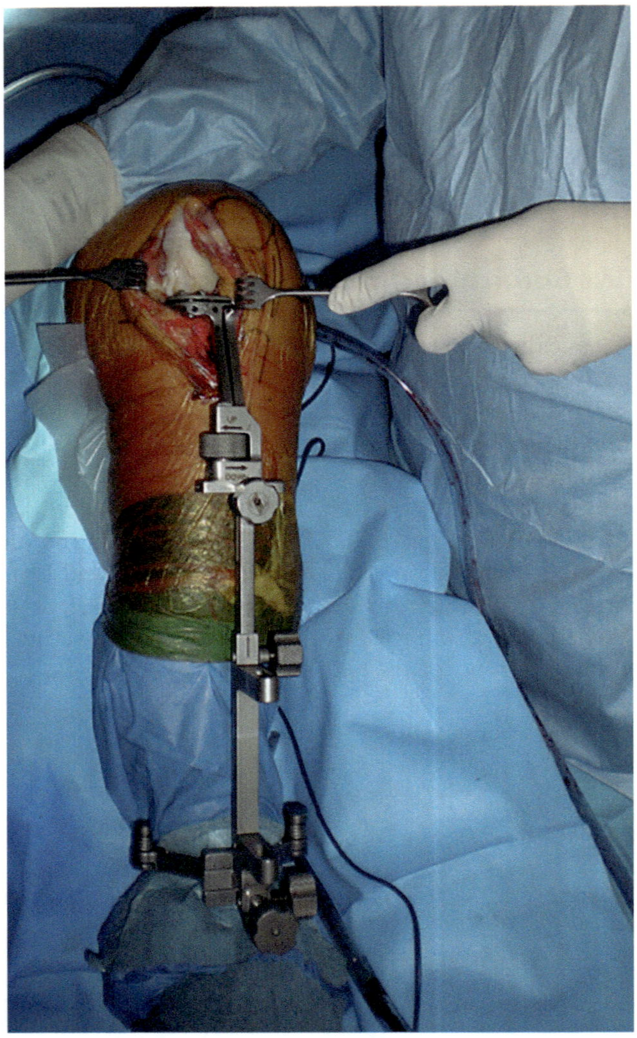

■ **Fig. 16.6** Tibial cut with an extra-medullary guide placed orthogonal to the mechanical tibial axis

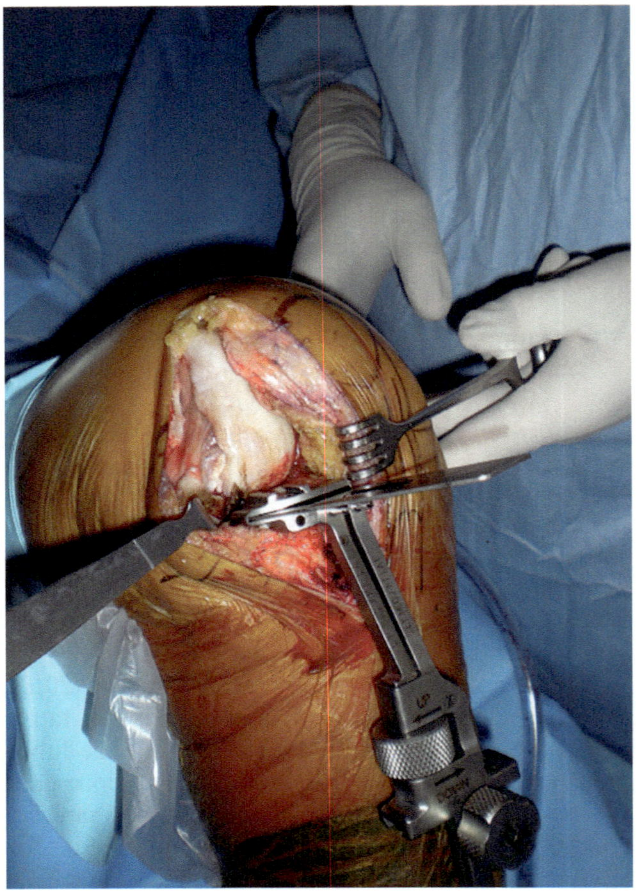

■ **Fig. 16.7** Tibial cut with an extra-medullary guide. Preview of the cut with the palpator

16

fascia lata), while keeping a final undercorrection of coronal alignment (Ollivier et al. 2014).

To avoid any impingement with ACL, osteophytes of the intercondylar notch are removed while osteophytes of the lateral condyle are initially preserved. They will be useful for helping the positioning of the femoral implant (Argenson et al. 2008). The anterior contact point in extension between femur and tibia has to be noticed and will be a landmark for implant positioning (size and orientation).

16.6.1 Tibial Cut

With an extra-medullary guide, an orthogonal tibial cut to the mechanical axis is performed which has to be as minimal as possible (Scott 2005) (■ Figs. 16.6, 16.7 and 16.8). An economic bone resection will insure a bigger bone surface area for the component and a better cortical support.

In the lateral compartment, the tibial slope is less important than in the medial compartment (Weinberg et al. 2017), and should be reproduced with the prosthesis to avoid any flexion laxity or stiffness (Lustig et al. 2014; Randall et al. 2019). An excessive posterior tibial slope will increase the anterior tibial translation and the tension on the ACL (Dejour and Bonnin 1994).

The sagittal tibial cut is realized close to the tibial spines and will determine the rotation of the tibial implant. The two landmarks of this anteroposterior cut are as follows:

- In extension: the medial point of the anterior lateral tibial plateau, in front of ACL insertion.
- In flexion: the medial point of the lateral tibial plateau, behind the ACL insertion.

Due to the constitutional external rotation of the lateral tibial plateau (screw-home mechanism (Kim et al. 2015)), this line will cross the patellar ligament which has to be carefully retracted to perform the bone cut (■ Fig. 16.9).

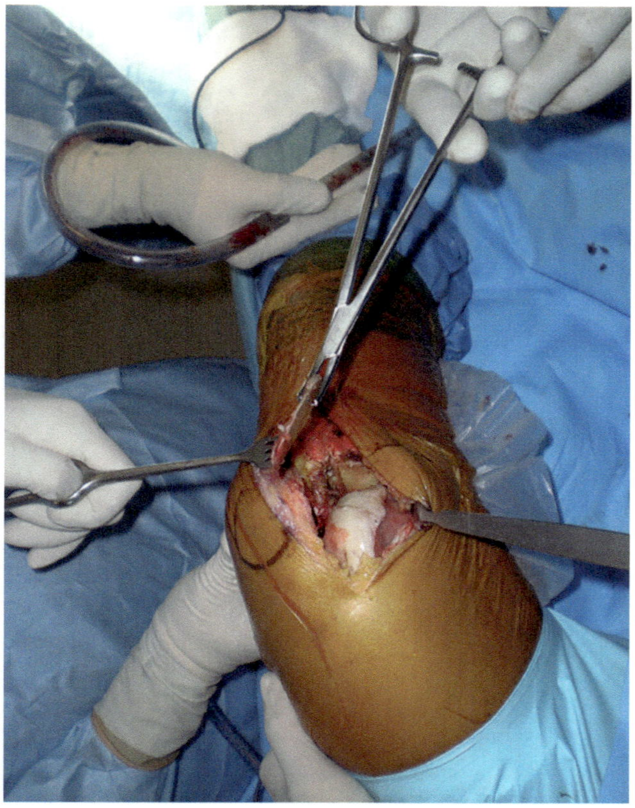

Fig. 16.8 Minimal bone resection during the tibial cut

16.6.2 Femoral Cuts

The distal femoral cut should also be as conservative as possible allowing to"distalize"the femoral implant and compensate for the congenital hypoplasia and the wear (Fig. 16.10). In genu valgum, OA affects preferentially the posterior part of the femoral condyle (Ollivier et al. 2014) explaining why there may be intact cartilage on the distal part of the condyle which has to be removed before positioning the distal femoral cutting guide (Scott 2005).

> If the surgeon desires to conserve a valgus deformity, it can be adjusted for at this step depending on the level of the cut. It should not be performed previously during the tibial cut.

There are two ways to perform the distal femoral cut depending on the prosthesis characteristics and the manufacturing:

- Dependent cut: in extension, the cutting-guide is placed in the tibiofemoral space like a spacer. The level of the cut corresponds to the thickness of the component and will depend on the tibial cut level.

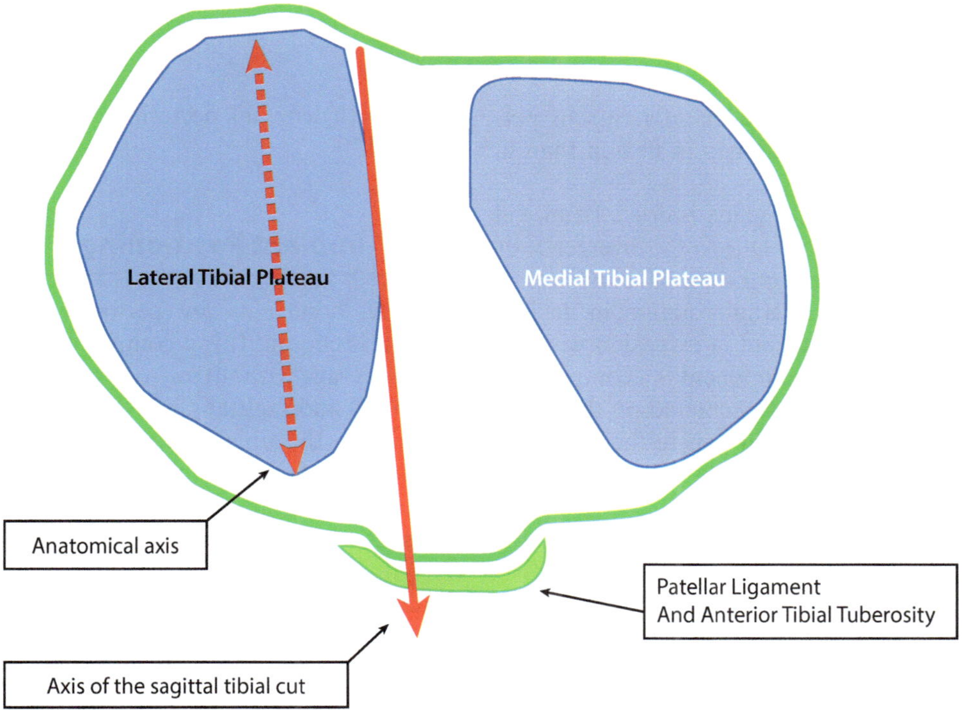

Fig. 16.9 Direction of the sagittal tibial cut in internal rotation

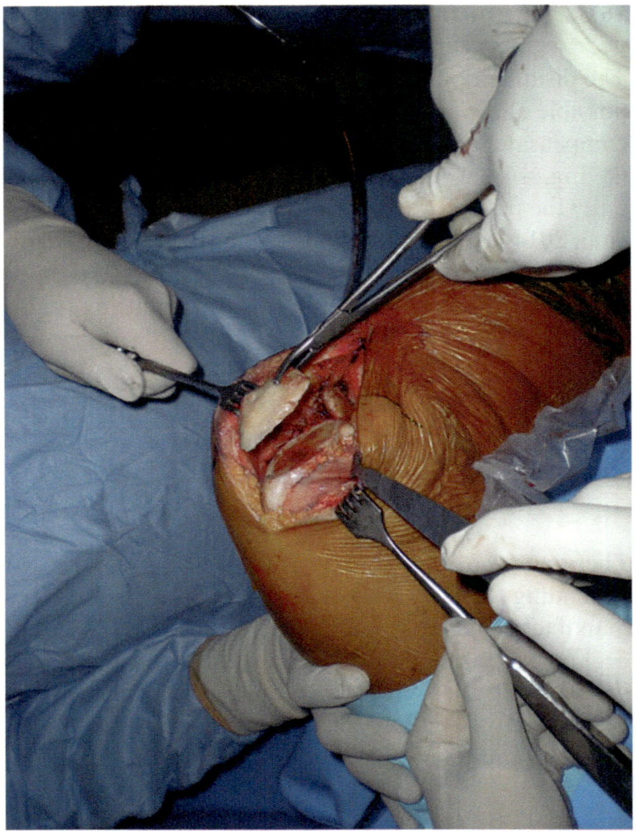

■ **Fig. 16.10** Distal femoral cut

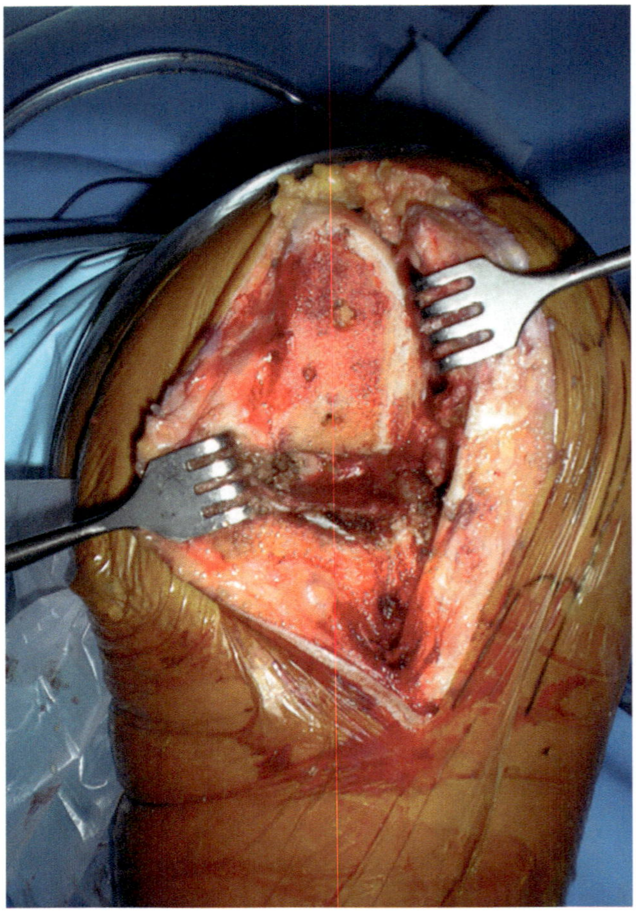

■ **Fig. 16.11** Posterior femoral and chamfer cuts performed on a flexed knee. The objective is to reproduce the same gap in flexion and extension

- Independent cut: thanks to an intra-medullary guide, the distal cut is performed according to the HKS angle (between 4° and 6°).

Second, posterior femoral and chamfer cuts are performed and reproduce the same gap in flexion than in extension (■ Fig. 16.11).

The rotation in the cutting-guide is crucial and will influence the implant rotation. Due to the divergence of the lateral condyle compared to the medial condyle, it is crucial to avoid excessive internal rotation in flexion, which will create an impingement in extension with the tibial spines. The size of the component is a compromise between the anatomical position centered on the femoral condyle and the perpendicular axis to the tibial plateau.

> It is important not to oversize the femoral implant and preferentially to undersize it if necessary.

The anterior border of the prosthesis has to be at the level of the landmark point contact between the femur and tibia. This has to be 1 or 2 mm under the border between cartilage and cancellous bone created by the bone cut. To avoid any impingement in full flexion with the polyethylene, all posterior osteophytes have to be removed.

16.6.3 Implant Positioning

After all bone cuts are performed, the size of the implant is chosen. It is a compromise between the best bone coverage without any overhanging of the implant in coronal and sagittal plans. The tibial implant should be close to the tibial spines with 15°–20° of internal rotation. The femoral implant is placed on a flexed knee with external rotation and as lateral as possible, and at times it may rest on lateral condyle osteophytes (Argenson et al. 2008). This positioning allows the ideal contact between the two implants preventing any impingement between the femoral condyle with the tibial spines during extension. The knee is then placed in full flexion and internal rotation to improve exposition on the tibial plateau and finish the preparation of the implant.

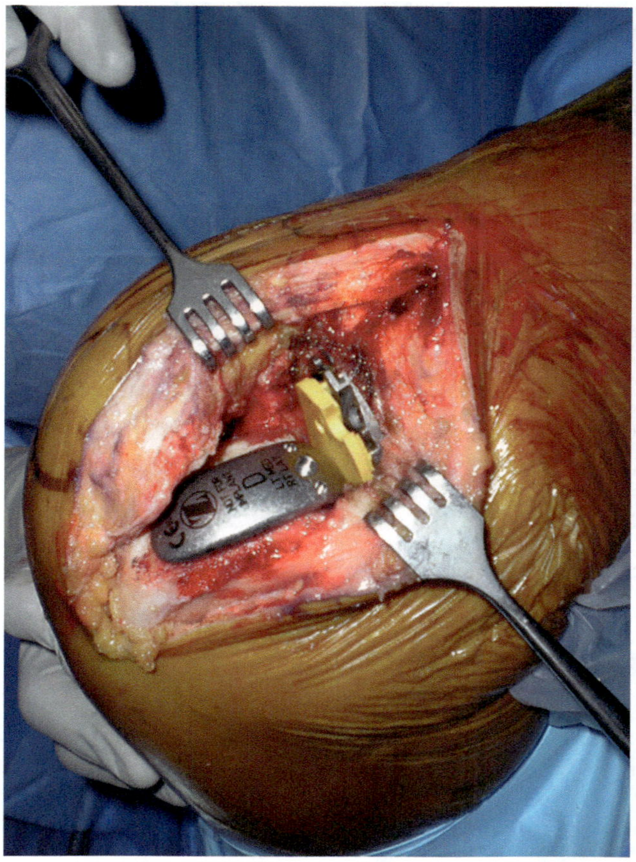

Fig. 16.12 Knee stability and implant positioning are tested with trial components in flexion

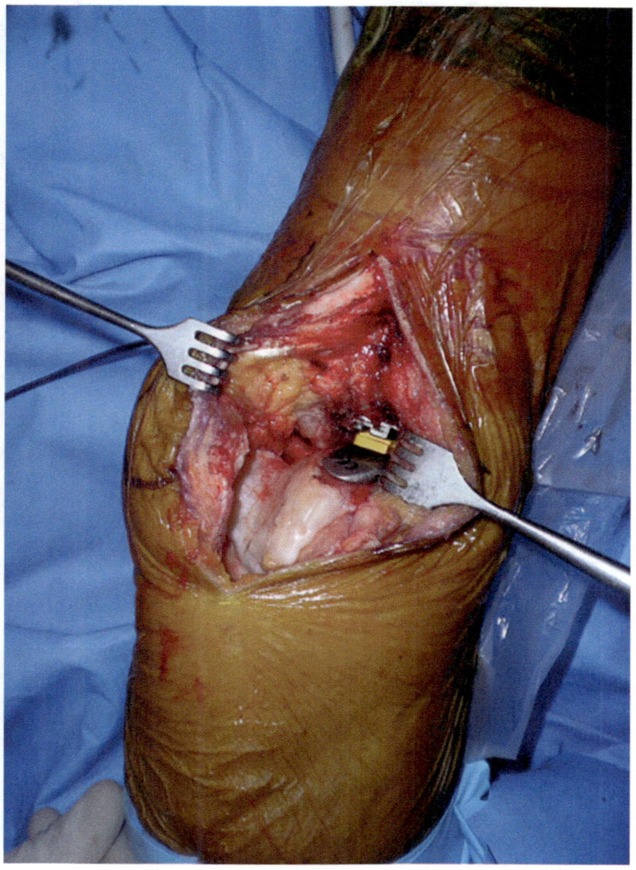

Fig. 16.13 Kneestabilityandimplantpositioningaretestedwithtrialcomponents in extension

With trial components, the stability of the knee is tested (Figs. 16.12 and 16.13). During flexion/extension movements, the medial part of the femoral implant should stay in front of the center of the tibial implant.

> At this step, it is important to detect any impingement between the femoral implant and tibial spines in extension as well as impingement between the patella and femoral implant in extension due to the lack of external rotation of the femoral component.

The testing in flexion and extension will evaluate the residual frontal laxity and the thickness of the polyethylene insert which is generally more important after lateral UKA than medial UKA due to femoral dysplasia.

The ligament balancing is evaluated with the trial components. The goal is to maintain slight lateral laxity on the unlocked knee (at 15° of flexion).

> In lateral UKA, it is crucial to undercorrect the deformity to avoid any excess pressure in the medial compartment and the development of medial OA in the long term (Lustig et al. 2014).

Lateral UKA is a resurfacing procedure of the lateral part of the knee joint and will only correct the deformity due to the wear (intra-articular deformation) and will respect the extra-articular deformity.

Finally, the definitive prosthesis is implanted. The tibial implant is placed and cemented with the knee in complete flexion and internal rotation to improve exposition of the lateral compartment (Figs. 16.14 and 16.15). Second, the femoral implant is cemented, placing the knee in full flexion, impacting the posterior part first and then anteriorly. The knee is then moved close to extension in order to remove all cement particles from the back of the knee. The polyethylene insert is placed after cleaning off the metal-back (Figs. 16.16 and 16.17), this can be also realized after placing temporally a trial insert while the cement is setting in order to make a final check of all remaining cement particles. It is important to place the knee at 45° of flexion during the time when the cement is curing (Figs. 16.18 and 16.19).

Good cementation has to respect some rules to improve implant fixation (Randall et al. 2019). It is mandatory to prepare and clean the bone surface using

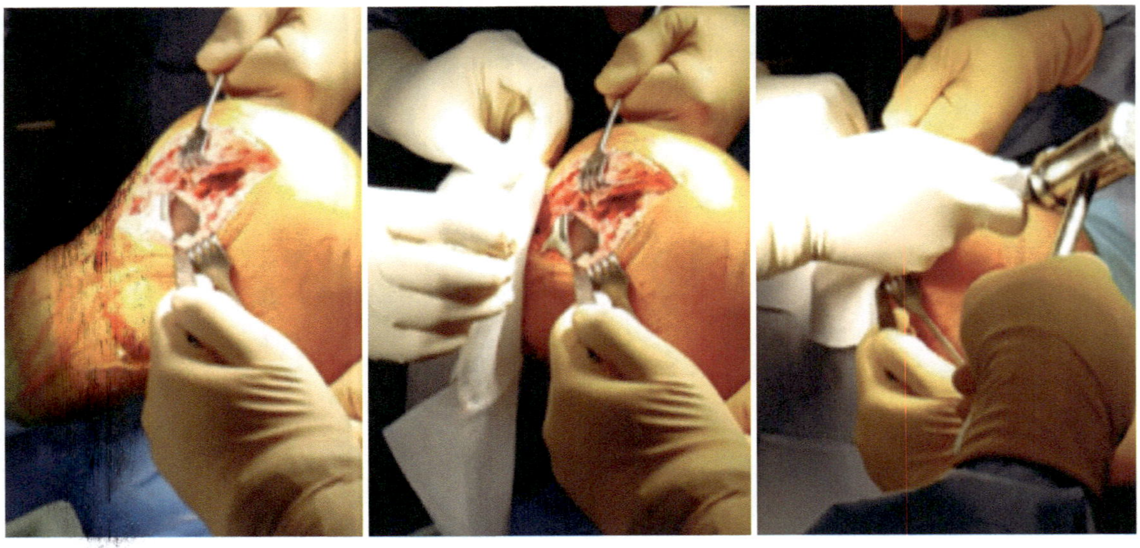

Fig. 16.14 Double cementation of the tibial component and impaction in the cancellous bone

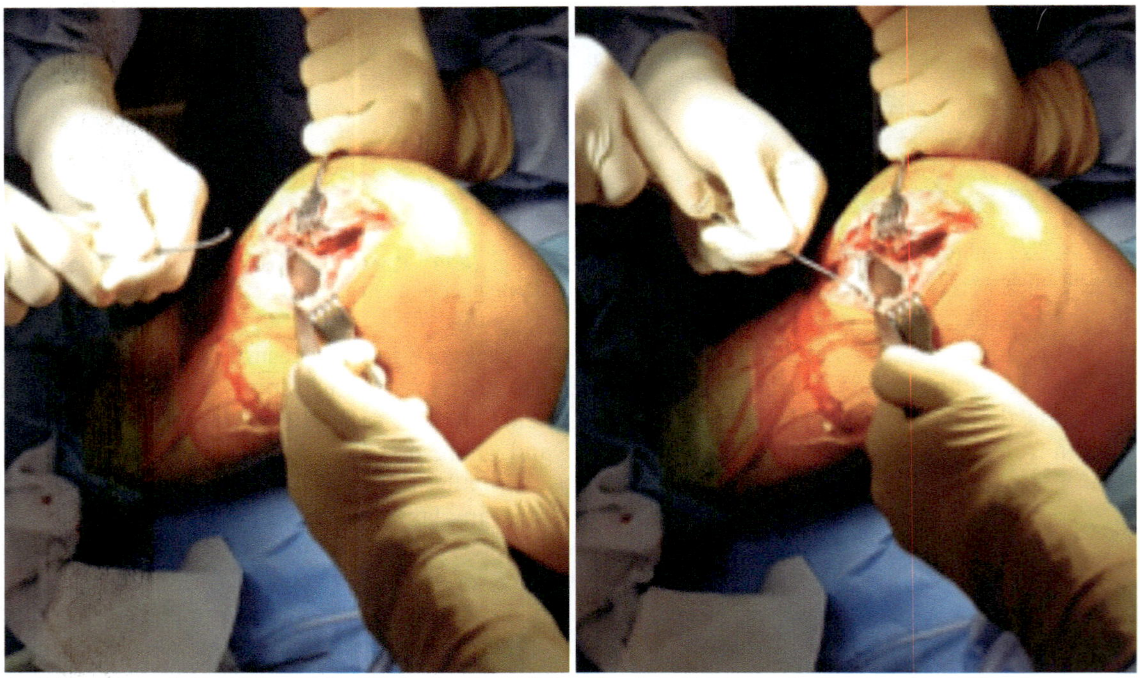

Fig. 16.15 Removal of excess cement around the implant with a specific curette to avoid any cemented foreign bodies, especially in the posterior part of the knee

a pulsed lavage to remove all foreign bodies and dry the blood of the trabecular bone (Schlegel et al. 2015). Using a tourniquet or doing a double cementation (Refsum et al. 2019)is not obligatory but is highly recommended. Several studies confirm that draining and cleaning the cancellous bone alveolus will allow good penetration of the cement and increase the implant fixation (Scheele et al. 2017; Schlegel et al. 2014; Jaeger et al. 2013, 2014; Clarius et al. 2009, 2012; Seeger et al. 2013).

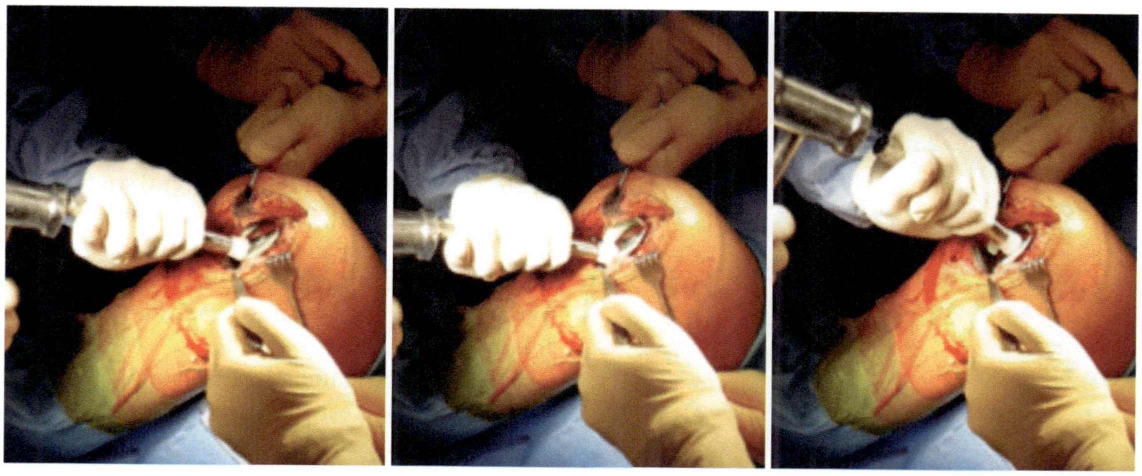

Fig. 16.16 Cementation of the femoral component. The impaction is performed at 90° of flexion and concerns all parts of the implant (anterior, distal, and posterior)

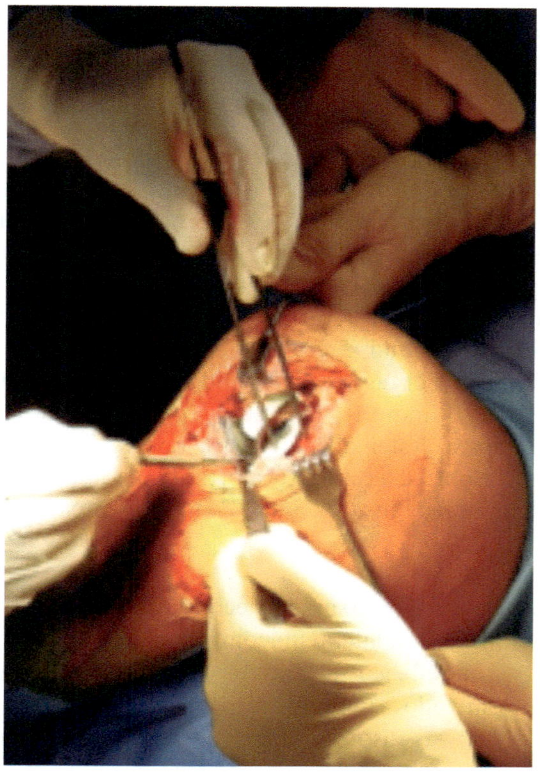

Fig. 16.17 Removal of excess cement close to the femoral implant to avoid any impingement with soft tissues

> The objective of good cementation is to decrease the long-term risk of aseptic loosening of the tibial component due to implant–cement–bone interface fatigue.

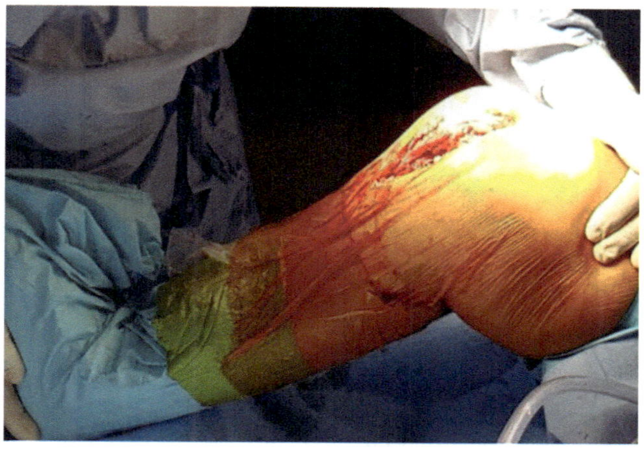

Fig. 16.18 The knee is placed at 45° of flexion during the curing time of the cement

16.6.4 Common Mistakes and Operating Difficulties

Overcorrection with postoperative varus deformity leads to increased load in the medial compartment and the development of medial OA. A postoperative varus deformity could be secondary to insufficient bone cut or to a thick polyethylene insert. Conversely, undercorrection with persistence of a valgus deformity more than 7° is associated with a higher revision rate (Perkins and Gunckle 2002).

Concerning femoral implant positioning, the divergence axis of the condyle in flexion should not be reproduced with the prosthesis to avoid any impingement in

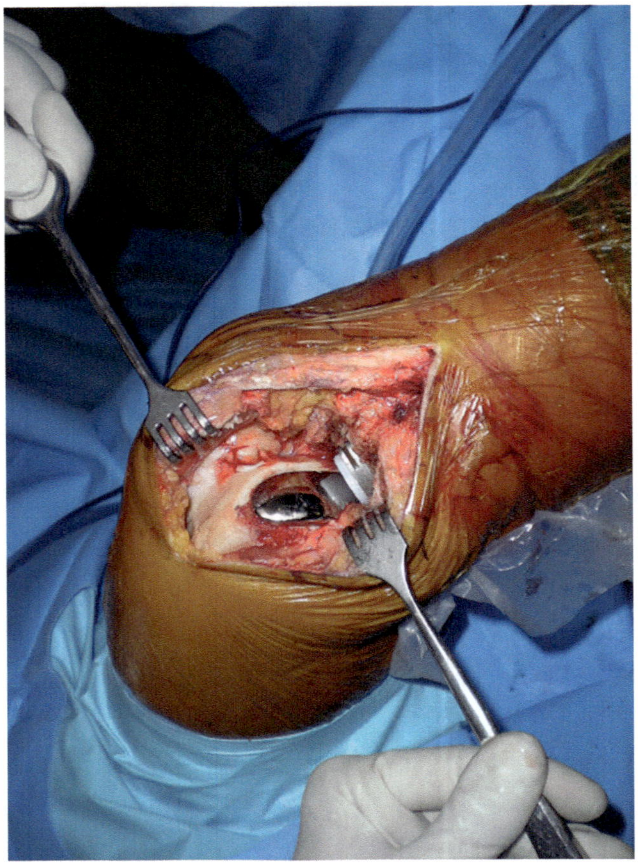

Fig. 16.19 Final view of the definitive prosthesis

extension with the tibial spines and with the patella in flexion.

During the tibial cut, it is important to prevent an excessive posterior tibial slope which will increase tension on ACL and impact the ligament balancing with laxity in flexion. The tibial implant should be positioned with an internal rotation of 15–20° and aligned with the natural tibial slope.

16

16.7 Results and Revision

Outcomes of modern UKA are excellent with 90% of survivorship at medium and long term (Greco et al. 2019; Vasso et al. 2015; Pandit et al. 2011; Walker et al. 2017). In case of failure, revision UKA with TKA is easier with better results than revision TKA with TKA (Lunebourg et al. 2015). Clinical and radiological results of lateral UKA are similar to medial UKA (Argenson et al. 2008).

Recent studies report lower revision rates with the modern implant than previous studies on lateral UKA. In 2002, Ashraf et al. (Ashraf et al. 2002) found a survival rate of 83% at 10 years follow-up and 74% at 15 years. More recent studies reported better survivorship of lateral UKA with 90% at medium term and 80% at long term (Deroche et al. 2019; Fornell et al. 2018). Better patient selection criteria, surgical technique, and implant manufacturing could explain the improvement of the results of lateral UKA. Several studies as Deroche et al. (Deroche et al. 2019) or Lustig et al. (Lustig et al. 2014)analyzed cemented all-polyethylene tibial implants and found excellent results at long term with 94.4% survival at 10 years, 91.4% at 15 years, and 79.4% at 20 years follow-up.

The cause of main failure of lateral UKA is OA progression (87.5%), especially in the medial compartment (Deroche et al. 2019), followed by aseptic loosening (12.5%). Deroche et al. (Deroche et al. 2019) reported a mean revision rate of 20.5% at 17.9 years follow-up. For patients not requiring revision surgery, the satisfaction scores were excellent with 90.5% good results. Concerning cemented metal-back implants, excellent results were also reported at short (Kim et al. 2016) and long term (Argenson et al. 2008). Argenson et al. (2008) found these implants showed good survivorship of 92% at 10 years and 84% at 16 years for lateral UKA. For mobile-bearing UKA, Fornell et al. (2018) reported a survival rate of 97.5% at 5 years with a revision rate of 2.4% at 49 months follow-up. The main cause of failure of mobile-bearing in lateral UKA was the dislocation of the polyethylene (Pandit et al. 2010).

Concerning the return to physical activity, Canetti et al. (2018) found a return to sports with the low and medium impact between 94% and 100% after a delay of 4.2 to 10.5 months in a study of cemented lateral UKA. In a systematic literature review, Witjes et al. (2017), reported a return to sports at high impact in 8%, medium impact in 22%, and 70% for low impact sport.

Conclusion

With an appropriate surgical technique and good patient selection criteria, lateral unicompartmental knee arthroplasty is an efficient procedure with good outcomes in long-term follow-up similar to medial UKA (Ollivier et al. 2014; Argenson et al. 2008). Due to the anatomical and biomechanical differences between the lateral and medial compartments, some technical specificities have to be known when performing lateral UKA, which has to be considered as a resurfacing procedure without any correction of the frontal deformity to avoid any early failure due to medial OA. Positioning of implants should respect some general rules, including internal rotation of the tibia component and positioning the femoral component as lateral as possible with external rotation to avoid any impingement with the tibial spines in extension or with the patella in flexion. Respecting the importance and increased mobility of the lateral compartment due to normal knee kinematics, it seems to be preferential to use fixed-bearing tibial components. In order to limit the risk of aseptic loosening, it is recommended to implant cemented prostheses and have a strict cementation technique with pulsed lavage.

Take-Home Messages

- The anteroposterior axis of the lateral tibial plateau has an internal rotational axis of 10–15°.
- The posterior tibial slope is reduced on the lateral side compared to the medial side (4° vs. 7°).
- Due to the constitutional external rotation of the lateral tibial plateau ("screw-home mechanism" (Kim et al. 2015)), the sagittal tibial cut will be performed in internal rotation and will cross the patellar ligament.
- The distal femoral cut should also be as conservative as possible allowing to "distalize" the femoral implant and compensate for the congenital hypoplasia and the wear.
- Due to the divergence of the lateral condyle compared to the medial condyle, it is crucial to avoid excessive internal rotation in flexion, which will create an impingement in extension with the tibial spines.
- The tibial implant should be close to the tibial spines with 15–20° of internal rotation.
- The femoral implant is placed on a flexed knee with external rotation and as lateral as possible, sometimes it may rest on lateral condyle osteophytes.

References

Argenson J-NA, Komistek RD, Aubaniac J-M et al (2002) In vivo determination of knee kinematics for subjects implanted with a unicompartmental arthroplasty. J Arthroplast 17(8):1049–1054

Argenson J-NA, Parratte S, Bertani A, Flecher X, Aubaniac J-M (2008) Long-term results with a lateral unicondylar replacement. Clin Orthop 466(11):2686–2693

Ashraf T, Newman JH, Evans RL, Ackroyd CE (2002) Lateral unicompartmental knee replacement survivorship and clinical experience over 21 years. J Bone Joint Surg Br 84(8):1126–1130

Barrios JA, Heitkamp CA, Smith BP, Sturgeon MM, Suckow DW, Sutton CR (2016) Three-dimensional hip and knee kinematics during walking, running, and single-limb drop landing in females with and without genu valgum. Clin Biomech Bristol Avon. 31:7–11

Berend KR, Kolczun MC, George JW, Lombardi AV (2012) Lateral unicompartmental knee arthroplasty through a lateral parapatellar approach has high early survivorship. Clin Orthop 470(1):77–83

Berend KR, Turnbull NJ, Howell RE, Lombardi AV (2015) The current trends for lateral unicondylar knee arthroplasty. Orthop Clin North Am 46(2):177–184

Canetti R, Batailler C, Bankhead C, Neyret P, Servien E, Lustig S (2018) Faster return to sport after robotic-assisted lateral unicompartmental knee arthroplasty: a comparative study. Arch Orthop Trauma Surg 138(12):1765–1771

Clarius M, Hauck C, Seeger JB, James A, Murray DW, Aldinger PR (2009) Pulsed lavage reduces the incidence of radiolucent lines under the tibial tray of Oxford unicompartmental knee arthroplasty: pulsed lavage versus syringe lavage. Int Orthop 33(6):1585–1590

Clarius M, Seeger JB, Jaeger S, Mohr G, Bitsch RG (2012) The importance of pulsed lavage on interface temperature and ligament tension force in cemented unicompartmental knee arthroplasty. Clin Biomech Bristol Avon 27(4):372–376

Dejour H, Bonnin M (1994) Tibial translation after anterior cruciate ligament rupture. Two radiological tests compared. J Bone Joint Surg Br 76(5):745–749

Demange MK, Von Keudell A, Probst C, Yoshioka H, Gomoll AH (2015) Patient-specific implants for lateral unicompartmental knee arthroplasty. Int Orthop 39(8):1519–1526

Deroche E, Batailler C, Lording T, Neyret P, Servien E, Lustig S (2019) High survival rate and very low wear of lateral unicompartmental arthroplasty at long term: a case series of 54 cases at a mean follow-up of 17 years. J Arthroplast 34(6):1097–1104

Du PZ, Markolf KL, Boguszewski DV, McAllister DR (2018) Femoral contact forces in the anterior cruciate ligament deficient knee: a robotic study. Arthrosc J Arthrosc Relat Surg 34(12):3226–3233

Feldman DS, Goldstein RY, Kurland AM, Sheikh Taha AM (2016) Intra-articular osteotomy for genu Valgum in the knee with a lateral compartment deficiency. J Bone Joint Surg Am 98(2):100–107

Fornell S, Prada E, Barrena P, García-Mendoza A, Borrego E, Domecq G (2018) Mid-term outcomes of mobile-bearing lateral unicompartmental knee arthroplasty. Knee 25(6):1206–1213

Greco NJ, Cook GJE, Lombardi AV, Adams JB, Berend KR (2019) Lateral unicompartmental knee arthroplasty utilizing a modified surgical technique and specifically adapted fixed-bearing implant. Surg Technol Int 34:371–378

Gulati A, Chau R, Beard DJ, Price AJ, Gill HS, Murray DW (2009) Localization of the full-thickness cartilage lesions in medial and lateral unicompartmental knee osteoarthritis. J Orthop Res 27(10):1339–1346

Jaeger S, Seeger JB, Schuld C, Bitsch RG, Clarius M (2013) Tibial cementing in UKA: a three-dimensional analysis of the bone cement implant interface and the effect of bone lavage. J Arthroplast 28(9 Suppl):191–194

Jaeger S, Rieger JS, Bruckner T, Kretzer JP, Clarius M, Bitsch RG (2014) The protective effect of pulsed lavage against implant subsidence and micromotion for cemented tibial unicompartmental knee components: an experimental cadaver study. J Arthroplast 29(4):727–732

Karimi E, Norouzian M, Birjandinejad A, Zandi R, Makhmalbaf H (2017) Measurement of posterior Tibial slope using magnetic resonance imaging. Arch Bone Jt Surg 5(6):435–439

Kim HY, Kim KJ, Yang DS, Jeung SW, Choi HG, Choy WS (2015) Screw-home movement of the Tibiofemoral joint during normal gait: three-dimensional analysis. Clin Orthop Surg 7(3):303–309

Kim KT, Lee S, Kim J, Kim JW, Kang MS (2016) Clinical results of lateral unicompartmental knee arthroplasty: minimum 2-year follow-up. Clin Orthop Surg 8(4):386–392

Kozinn SC, Scott R (1989) Unicondylar knee arthroplasty. J Bone Joint Surg Am 71(1):145–150

Longo UG, Ciuffreda M, Candela V et al (2019) Knee osteoarthritis after arthroscopic partial meniscectomy: prevalence and

progression of radiographic changes after 5 to 12 years compared with contralateral knee. J Knee Surg 32(5):407–413
Lunebourg A, Parratte S, Ollivier M, Abdel MP, Argenson J-NA (2015) Are revisions of unicompartmental knee arthroplasties more like a primary or revision TKA? J Arthroplast 30(11):1985–1989
Lustig S, Parratte S, Magnussen RA, Argenson J-N, Neyret P (2012) Lateral Unicompartmental knee arthroplasty relieves pain and improves function in posttraumatic osteoarthritis. Clin Orthop 470(1):69–76
Lustig S, Lording T, Frank F, Debette C, Servien E, Neyret P (2014) Progression of medial osteoarthritis and long term results of lateral unicompartmental arthroplasty: 10 to 18 year follow-up of 54 consecutive implants. Knee 21(Suppl 1):S26–S32
Miyatake N, Sugita T, Aizawa T et al (2016) Comparison of intraoperative anthropometric measurements of the proximal tibia and tibial component in total knee arthroplasty. J Orthop Sci 21(5):635–639
Moreland JR, Bassett LW, Hanker GJ (1987) Radiographic analysis of the axial alignment of the lower extremity. J Bone Joint Surg Am 69(5):745–749
Ollivier M, Abdel MP, Parratte S, Argenson J-N (2014) Lateral unicondylar knee arthroplasty (UKA): contemporary indications, surgical technique, and results. Int Orthop 38(2):449–455
Pandit H, Jenkins C, Beard DJ et al (2010) Mobile bearing dislocation in lateral unicompartmental knee replacement. Knee 17(6):392–397
Pandit H, Jenkins C, Gill HS, Barker K, Dodd C (2011) a. F, Murray DW. Minimally invasive Oxford phase 3 unicompartmental knee replacement: results of 1000 cases. J Bone Joint Surg Br 93(2):198–204
Parratte S, Ollivier M, Lunebourg A, Abdel MP, Argenson J-N (2015) Long-term results of compartmental arthroplasties of the knee: long term results of partial knee arthroplasty. Bone Jt J 97-B(10 Suppl A):9–15
Pengas IP, Nash W, Khan W, Assiotis A, Banks J, McNicholas MJ (2017) Coronal knee alignment 40 years after total meniscectomy in adolescents: a prospective Cohort study. Open Orthop J 11:424–431
Perkins TR, Gunckle W (2002) Unicompartmental knee arthroplasty: 3- to 10-year results in a community hospital setting. J Arthroplast 17(3):293–297
Ranawat AS, Ranawat CS, Elkus M, Rasquinha VJ, Rossi R, Babhulkar S (2005) Total knee arthroplasty for severe valgus deformity. J Bone Joint Surg Am 87 Suppl 1(Pt 2):271–284
Randall DJ, Anderson MB, Gililland JM, Peters CL, Pelt CE (2019) A potential need for surgeon consensus: cementation techniques for total knee arthroplasty in orthopedic implant manufacturers' guidelines lack consistency. J Orthop Surg Hong Kong 27(3):2309499019878258
Refsum AM, Nguyen UV, Gjertsen J-E et al (2019) Cementing technique for primary knee arthroplasty: a scoping review. Acta Orthop 90(6):582–589
Rossi R, Rosso F, Cottino U, Dettoni F, Bonasia DE, Bruzzone M (2014) Total knee arthroplasty in the valgus knee. Int Orthop 38(2):273–283
Sah AP, Scott RD (2008) Lateral unicompartmental knee arthroplasty through a medial approach. Surgical technique. J Bone Joint Surg Am 90 Suppl 2 Pt 2:195–205
Scheele C, Pietschmann MF, Schröder C et al (2017) Effect of lavage and brush preparation on cement penetration and primary stability in tibial unicompartmental total knee arthroplasty: an experimental cadaver study. Knee 24(2):402–408
Schlegel UJ, Püschel K, Morlock MM, Nagel K (2014) An in vitro comparison of tibial tray cementation using gun pressurization or pulsed lavage. Int Orthop 38(5):967–971
Schlegel UJ, Bishop NE, Püschel K, Morlock MM, Nagel K (2015) Comparison of different cement application techniques for tibial component fixation in TKA. Int Orthop 39(1):47–54
Scott RD (2005) Lateral unicompartmental replacement: a road less traveled. Orthopedics 28(9):983–984
Seeger JB, Jaeger S, Bitsch RG, Mohr G, Röhner E, Clarius M (2013) The effect of bone lavage on femoral cement penetration and interface temperature during Oxford unicompartmental knee arthroplasty with cement. J Bone Joint Surg Am 95(1):48–53
van Lieshout WAM, van Ginneken BJT, Kerkhoffs GMMJ, van Heerwaarden RJ (2019) Medial closing wedge high tibial osteotomy for valgus tibial deformities: good clinical results and survival with a mean 4.5 years of follow-up in 113 patients. Knee Surg Sports Traumatol Arthrosc 28:2798
Vasso M, Del Regno C, Perisano C, D'Amelio A, Corona K, Schiavone PA (2015) Unicompartmental knee arthroplasty is effective: ten year results. Int Orthop 39:2341
Walker T, Aldinger PR, Streit MR, Gotterbarm T (2017) Lateral unicompartmental knee arthroplasty - a challenge. Oper Orthopadie Traumatol 29(1):17–30
Weinberg DS, Williamson DFK, Gebhart JJ, Knapik DM, Voos JE (2017) Differences in medial and lateral posterior Tibial slope: an osteological review of 1090 Tibiae comparing age, sex, and race. Am J Sports Med 45(1):106–113
Witjes S, Van Geenen RCI, Koenraadt KLM (2017) Expectations of younger patients concerning activities after knee arthroplasty: are we asking the right questions? Qual Life Res 26(2):403–417

Patellofemoral Arthroplasty

Simon Garceau, William J. Long, and Ran Schwarzkopf

Contents

E. Hansen, K.-D. Kühn (eds.), *Essentials of Cemented Knee Arthroplasty*,
https://doi.org/10.1007/978-3-662-63113-3_17

17.1 Introduction

Arthritis, isolated to the patellofemoral joint (PFJ), is a well-described entity that can result in significant disability and pain (Lonner 2007; Hofmann et al. 2013). Epidemiological studies suggest that nearly 10% of individuals over the age of 40 may have isolated PF arthritis (Davies et al. 2002). Furthermore, females appear to be at significantly greater risk with one study by McAlindon et al. suggesting a >2:1 female-to-male predisposition in individuals over the age of 55 (McAlindon et al. 1992).

Non-surgical management represents the initial mainstay of treatment and consists of a combination of the following:

- Activity modification.
- Weight reduction.
- Targeted physical therapy.
- Oral anti-inflammatory medication.
- Intra-articular injections (Lonner 2018; Lonner and Bloomfield 2013).

Physical therapy regimens should focus on optimizing patellar tracking through a low-impact quadriceps strengthening exercise program (Witvrouw et al. 2003). Non-operative management can reduce symptoms and delay the need for surgical intervention. When non-operative management fails, surgical treatment options can be considered.

Surgical options that have been described in the treatment of patellofemoral arthritis with varying degrees of success, include the following:

- Arthroscopic irrigation and debridement.
- Tibial tubercle offloading osteotomy (i.e., Fulkerson anteromedialization and Maquet elevation).
- Cartilage grafting.
- Patellectomy.
- Patellar resurfacing.
- Patellofemoral arthroplasty (PFA).
- Total knee arthroplasty (TKA) (Federico and Reider 1997; Heatley et al. 1986; Mont et al. 2002; Parvizi et al. 2001; Hangody and Füles 2003; Minas and Bryant 2005; Pidoriano et al. 1997).

In the short term, fair to good results have been described in 20–75% of patients (Federico and Reider 1997; Heatley et al. 1986; Mont et al. 2002; Parvizi et al. 2001; Hangody and Füles 2003; Minas and Bryant 2005; Pidoriano et al. 1997; Paletta and Laskin 1995). In this chapter, a focused discussion of PFA as a treatment modality will be conducted. To optimize surgical outcomes, careful patient selection, PFA design choice, and meticulous surgical technique are essential.

17.2 Clinical Evaluation

17.2.1 Patient History

An attentive collection of the patient history is necessary for the identification and treatment of patients with a painful knee secondary to PF arthritis. The clinician should identify any history of PF dislocation which can be indicative of PF malalignment. In such cases, re-alignment procedures may be required prior to surgical intervention (Lonner 2004). Similarly, recurrent PFJ dislocations may be associated with significant joint dysplasia. Prior conservative and surgical treatment measures should be documented as part of a comprehensive assessment. Characterization of the location, quality, and onset of pain as well as aggravating and alleviating factors is important for both accurate diagnosis and treatment. Classically, pain associated with degenerative changes within the PFJ is situated directly anteriorly, within the retropatellar region, and/or in the peripatellar region (Lonner 2007, 2018).

Furthermore, painful symptoms are typically exacerbated by activities that load the PFJ such as squatting, ascending and descending stairs, kneeling, and prolonged sitting with the knee in a flexed position (Lonner 2004, 2007). Activities that allow the knee to remain in a more extended position such as ambulating on level ground and being seated with the knee extended, offload the PFJ and are generally better tolerated.

> Any history of pain located in the medial or lateral compartments of the tibiofemoral articulation should be identified as this may be indicative of more diffuse degenerative changes which are important for indicating the appropriate treatment.

17.2.2 Physical Examination

Initial physical examination commences with having the patient standing facing the examiner. Special attention should be placed on the overall alignment of the lower extremity, specifically the Q-angle. This is characterized by the angle subtended by a line drawn from the anterior superior iliac spine (ASIS) to the center of the patella, and a second line from the center of the patella to the middle of the tibial tubercle.

> For Q-angles measuring greater than 15° in males and greater than 20° in females, consideration for an anteromedializing tibial tubercle osteotomy should be entertained prior to PFA to ensure satisfactory PF tracking (Lonner 2007; Lonner and Bloomfield 2013).

Second, attention should be placed on observing overall patellar tracking throughout range of motion (ROM). With the patient's knee over the edge of the bed, the knee can be ranged from 90° of flexion to full extension while actively contracting the quadriceps musculature. The presence of a J-sign, which is characterized by lateral subluxation of the patella during the final 20° of extension, is indicative of patellofemoral malalignment and/or muscular imbalance. In scenarios where such a sign is present, an emphasis on a strenuous physical therapy program is necessary, and assessment for PF malalignment is mandatory.

Third, assessment for crepitus and pain during ROM is indicative of PF arthritis and can be further elicited through the PF grind test. Tenderness on palpation of the medial and lateral joint lines can be indicative of more diffuse arthritic pathology which would not be addressed through singular PFA.

Finally, a screening neurovascular examination and assessment of both the hip joint and the foot and ankle should be performed to identify potential sources of referred pain. Assessment of the feet is of particular interest as the presence of planovalgus foot deformity can predispose to PF maltracking, and such a position of the foot can potentially be corrected through the use of a medial arch support orthotic (Lonner 2007). However, this has not been supported as a treatment for PF arthritis.

17.2.3 Imaging

At the time of assessment, standing anteroposterior (AP), lateral, and axial patellar view radiographs of the affected joint should be obtained to confirm the diagnosis of PF arthritis (◘ Fig. 17.1). Careful observation of AP X-rays along the medial and lateral joint line should be performed to assess for possible arthritic involvement in other compartments. Midflexion (Rosenberg view) posteroanterior radiographs may be obtained and can help to identify posterior condylar wear, which should be a contraindication to proceeding with isolated PFA.

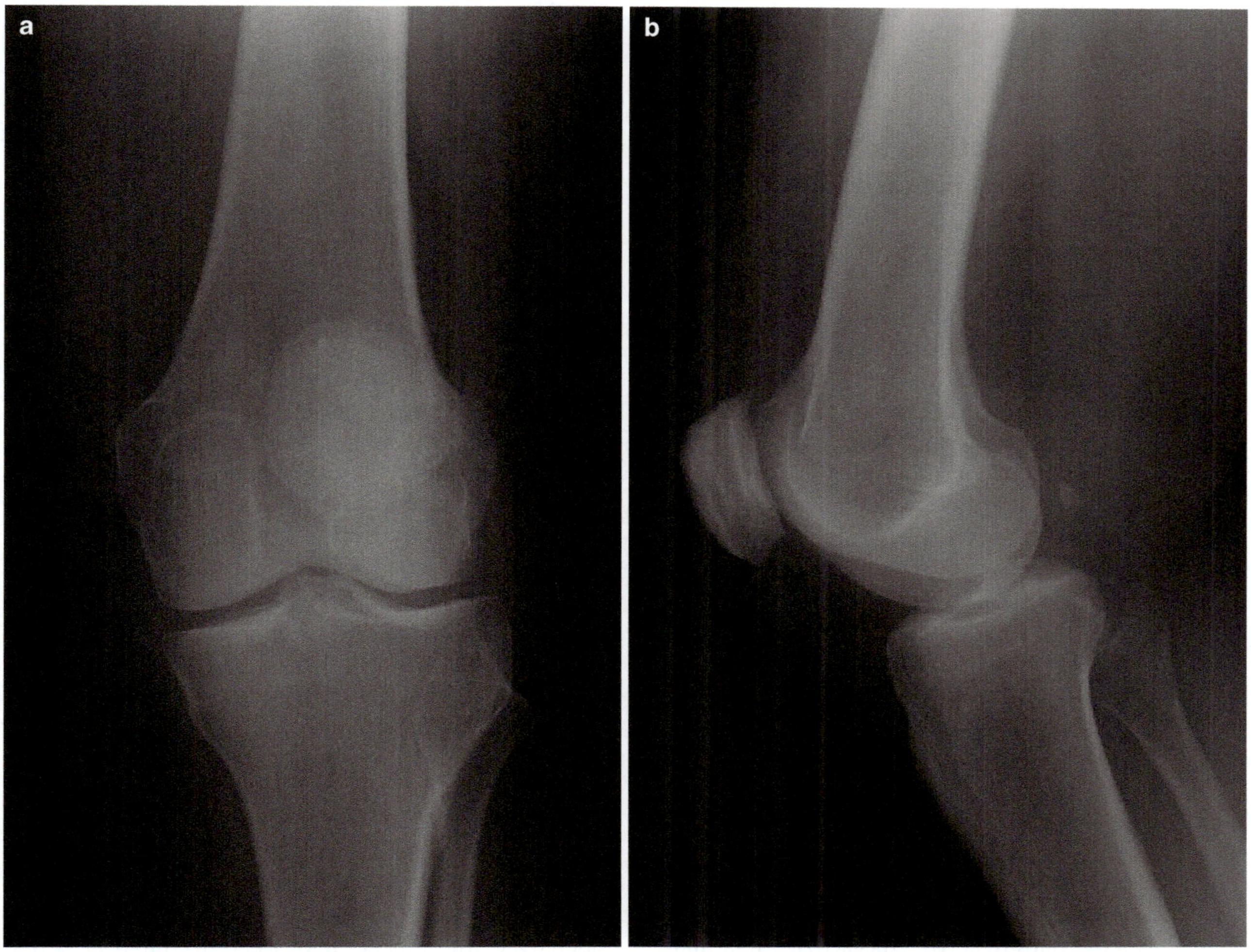

◘ **Fig. 17.1** **a**, **b** Anteroposterior and lateral radiographs of a patient presenting with isolated anterior knee pain. Moderate osteoarthritic changes are noted in the PFJ with general preservation of the tibiofemoral articulation

Moreover, recent advancements in magnetic resonance imaging (MRI) provide a useful adjunct in the assessment of cartilage quality in the PFJ (Novakofski et al. 2016). More importantly, however, MRI can aid in the identification of chondral wear within the medial and lateral compartments of the tibiofemoral articulation. Lateral radiographic views are useful both to confirm degenerative changes within the PFJ, and to identify the presence of patella alta or baja. Additionally, axial radiographic views, skyline, and Merchant should be obtained to detect the presence of trochlear dysplasia, patellar tilt, and subluxation or dislocation. Axial computer tomography scans may complement standard axial radiographs for further characterization of PFJ tracking, but are rarely necessary (Lonner 2007).

Finally, if available, previous arthroscopic images should be obtained to further depict the pathology.

17.3 Patellofemoral Arthroplasty

> To ensure optimal results after PFA, stringent patient selection criteria should be applied (► Sect. 17.3.1, overview on Contraindications to Patellofemoral Arthroplasty).

17.3.1 Contraindications to Patellofemoral Arthroplasty (Leadbetter et al. 2005)

Contraindications to Patellofemoral Arthroplasty

- No attempt at nonoperative care or to rule out other sources of pain.
- Arthritis of greater than Kellgren–Lawrence Grade 1 involving the tibiofemoral articulation.
- Systemic inflammatory arthropathy.
- Osteoarthritis/chondrosis of the patellofemoral joint of Grade 3 or less.
- Osteoarthritis/chondrocalcinosis of the PFJ ≤ Grade 3.
- Patella infera.
- Uncorrected patellofemoral instability or malalignment.
- Uncorrected tibiofemoral mechanical malalignment (valgus >8° or varus >5°).
- Active infection.
- Evidence of chronic regional pain syndrome.
- Fixed loss of knee range of motion (−10° of extension to 110° of flexion at a minimum).
- Psychogenic pain.
- Adapted courtesy of Dr. Michael A. Mont and Wolters Kluwer publishing company.

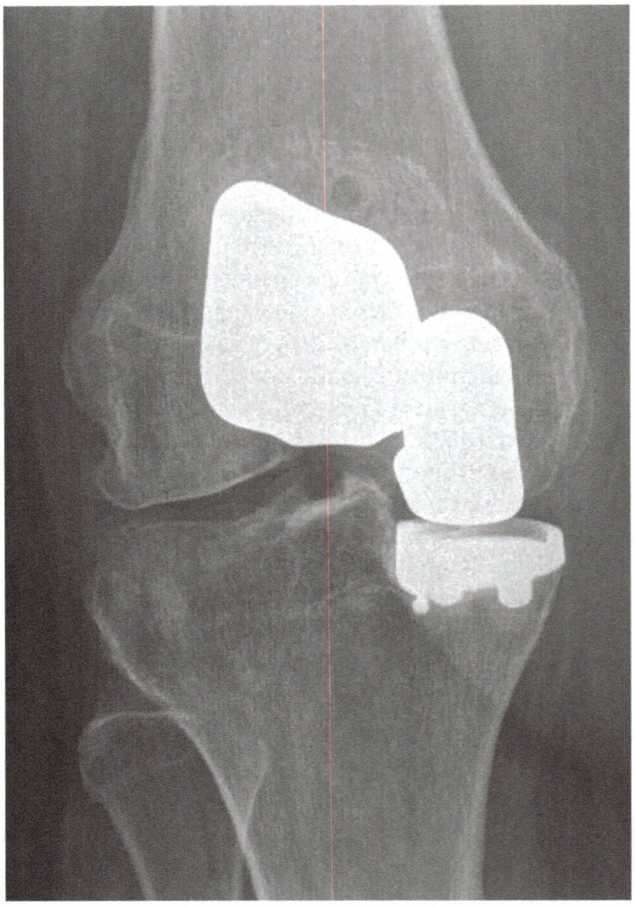

Fig. 17.2 Anteroposterior radiograph of a patient having previously undergone combined Mako™PFA and unicondylar knee arthroplasty (Stryker, Mahwah, NJ). Note the development of osteoarthritis in the lateral compartment of the knee

The procedure should be limited to those suffering from *isolated* PFJ osteoarthritis, post-traumatic arthritis, severe chondrosis on either joint surface, and PF degeneration secondary to dysplasia/malalignment (Leadbetter et al. 2006). Even focal chondral lesions involving the tibiofemoral articulation can affect the outcome of PFA (Leadbetter et al. 2006; Lonner et al. 2007). In such situations, TKA should be considered (Lonner 2007, 2018). Alternatively, PFA may be combined with UKA (Fig. 17.2), or autologous chondral grafting for small, well-defined lesions (Lonner et al. 2007). PFA should not be performed in patients suffering from inflammatory arthritis, avascular necrosis, or chondrocalcinosis involving the structures surrounding the tibiofemoral articulation (Leadbetter et al. 2006).

Additionally, history and physical examination findings should corroborate with the diagnosis of PF arthritis with an absence of discomfort to the medial or lateral joint lines. As such, pain in other areas should be considered a contraindication for PFA. In equivocal scenarios, MRI may serve as a more sensitive adjunct to standard radiographs in the identification of chondral

17

wear (Novakofski et al. 2016). Similarly, other pathology such as tendonitis and pain referred from the hip, ankle, or lower back should be excluded.

Although effective treatment of patients with trochlear dysplasia with PFA is well-described, the avoidance of this procedure in those with significant PF maltracking and malalignment is recommended unless it is corrected preoperatively (Lonner 2007; Leadbetter et al. 2006). In individuals with mild to moderate PF maltracking or observed patellar tilt on axial radiographic views, PFA can usually be performed safely through proper orientation of newer prostheses using an onlay technique with or without lateral release (Lonner and Bloomfield 2013). This is usually sufficient to ensure central tracking of the patellar button on the trochlear prosthesis. In patients noted to have excessive Q-angles, a staged approach should be selected, commencing with an anteromedializing tibial tubercle osteotomy to correct the abnormal force vectors across the PFJ (Hofmann et al. 2013; Lonner 2018; Lonner and Bloomfield 2013).

> Failure to correct the Q-angle prior to PFA can lead to persistence of patellar subluxation causing painful snapping and asymmetric wear of the patellar button (Dy et al. 2012; Lustig 2014; Oni et al. 2014).

Although some have advocated for the avoidance of PFA in patients with more advanced age, there are no specific age criteria for this procedure if no other contraindications are present (Bohu et al. 2019).

Lastly, although data regarding failure rates and outcomes of PFA in patients with obesity and cruciate deficiency is lacking, concern remains regarding the outcomes of this procedure for this patient population (van Jonbergen et al. 2010; Burger et al. 2020).

17.3.2 Design Features

Over the last several decades, PFA has evolved significantly. In its infancy, original designs consisted of simple patellar resurfacing without the insertion of a trochlear implant (McKeever 1955). As one might expect, ongoing pain and PF instability were an issue (Harrington 1992). Until recently, significant controversy regarding the use of PFA remained due to historically high failure rates (Harrington 1992).

> Modern designs, however, have led to significantly improved results and can generally be categorized into two design styles: inlay and onlay (Roussot and Haddad 2018; Bunyoz et al. 2019; Odgaard et al. 2018).

Table 17.1 Generalized design characteristics of inlay and onlay designed patellofemoral prostheses (Lonner and Bloomfield 2013)

Design characteristic	Inlay	Onlay
Positioning	Inset flush with native trochlea	Replaces entire trochlea, perpendicular to AP axis
Rotation	Determined by native trochlea	Set by surgeon, perpendicular to AP axis
Width	Narrower	Wider
Proximal extension	No further than native trochlear surface	Extends further proximal than native trochlea

Adapted courtesy of Dr. Jess Lonner and Elsevier publishing company

Key differences between these two design types can be summarized as follows:
- Positioning.
- Rotation.
- Width.
- Proximal trochlear extension (Table 17.1) (Lonner and Bloomfield 2013).

Inlay Design

Earlier PFA designs employed trochlear prostheses that were designed to be inset into the native trochlea. The premise with such inlay designs was to position the trochlear component in such a way as to have it sitting flush with the surrounding articular cartilage. Unfortunately, difficulties are frequently encountered (Hofmann et al. 2013; Lonner and Bloomfield 2013; Lonner 2004). First, accurately matching the component contour to the shape of the trochlear surface is often challenging. This can result in the component not sitting flush with the articular surface. This is especially true in cases where trochlear dysplasia is present which can lead to component malpositioning. Additionally, several inlay trochlear prostheses have large radii of curvature. This feature can lead to the component being placed in a flexed position to avoid impingement of the prosthesis at the level of intercondylar notch. Consequent to such positioning, however, the anterior flange will rest in an elevated position relative to the anterior cortex of the femur. This can lead to catching and subluxation of the patellar component at the commencement of knee flexion from an extended position. Another issue that can arise with the inlay design is its propensity for malrotation. In such cases, a predilection for internal rotation results from the fact that component rotation is determined by the native trochlear orientation. With malrotation, effective medialization of the trochlear groove occurs which equates to an increase in Q-angle (Lonner and Bloomfield 2013). Once again, this appears to be especially problematic in cases of dysplasia where trochlear inclination is often reduced, and thus predisposing to patellar maltracking and subluxation. Third, inlay design trochlear prostheses are often narrow in width and can employ a deeper and more constrained sulcus (Hofmann et al. 2013; Lonner and Bloomfield 2013). Such features leave little room for error or accommodation of patellar tracking which can predispose to PF instability. Lastly, due to its attempt at reproducing the native trochlear surface, inlay-style trochlear components do not extend proximal to the native articular margin. Such a characteristic, especially in cases of patella alta, can result in problematic engagement of the patellar button within the trochlea when nearing a terminal extension.

> As such, proper insertion of inlay-style PFA components is associated with significant challenges, the constellation of which can result in issues of catching and subluxation.

Onlay Design

Onlay-style trochlear components are broader in nature and essentially replace the entire trochlear surface (Fig. 17.3). Such a design feature allows for greater excursion throughout ROM and makes for a more forgiving implant that can be utilized in all situations (Lonner 2018; Lonner and Bloomfield 2013). The onlay design is particularly useful in scenarios where native anatomy is distorted, as in the case of trochlear dysplasia. Second, most prostheses utilizing this design style have an anatomic radius of curvature (Lonner and Bloomfield 2013; Lonner 2004). This allows the proximal aspect of the component to sit flush with the anterior femoral surface while preventing excessive excursion distally into the intercondylar notch. Third, a significant benefit of the onlay design is the independence of component rotation from native anatomy (Lonner 2018). Appropriate component rotation is set by the treating physician referencing local intraoperative landmarks (perpendicular to Whiteside's line and parallel to the transepicondylar axis). As such, modern onlay prostheses can allow the treating surgeon to correct for mild to moderate abnormality in local anatomy and often obviates the need for additional corrective procedures such as an anteromedializing tibial tubercle osteotomy. Lastly, onlay-style trochlear prostheses, unlike the inlay-style, often extend proximally, past the native articular cartilage, and sit flush with the anterior femoral cortex.

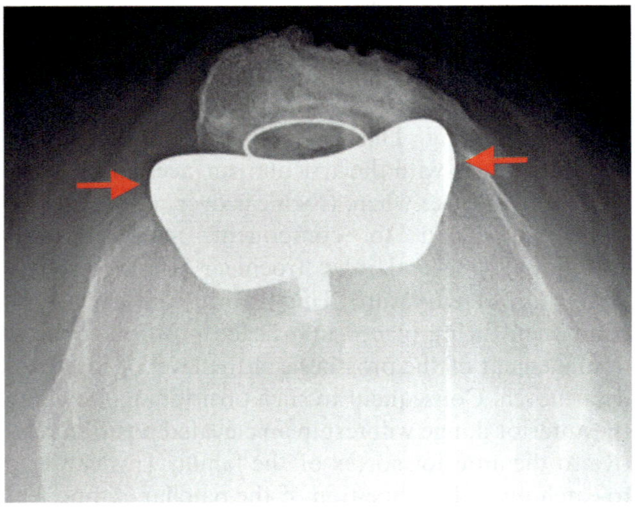

Fig. 17.3 Skyline view radiograph demonstrating an onlay design Journey trochlear prosthesis (Smith & Nephew, London, UK). Note the broad (*red arrows*) and relatively unconstrained nature of the design

> This thus ensures capture the patellar button within the trochlear sulcus in full knee extension, and as such may prevent catching.

17.3.3 Surgical Technique

> Prior to surgery, informed consent should be reviewed with the patient.

All possible interventions should be outlined as the plan to proceed with PFA may change during intraoperative assessment of the articular surfaces of the knee. As such, after careful assessment of the tibiofemoral articulation, a decision to proceed with PFA alone or in conjunction with cartilage grafting to focal chondral lesions of the femoral condyle(s) is made. In scenarios of more defuse arthritic changes, a low threshold for conversion to TKA should be maintained and clearly discussed with the patient preoperatively and documented.

As such, due to the possibility of conversion to a TKA in the future, the skin incision (i.e., midline) should be adaptable to such a procedure. The arthrotomy is then performed in the standard fashion for a TKA which is most familiar to the treating surgeon (i.e., medial parapatellar, midvastus, or subvastus). During the arthrotomy, special attention should be paid to protect normal articular cartilage, menisci, intermeniscal ligaments, and cruciates. Ensuring adequate exposure and visualization should be prioritized over less invasive techniques (Lonner 2003).

> Although differences in technique vary to some degree based on both system instrumentation and implant design (inlay vs. onlay), the basic technical principles remain the same.

Prior to commencement, osteophytes bordering the intercondylar notch should be removed to prevent impingement with the PF prosthesis. Visualization of rotational landmarks is then performed. To ensure optimal patellar tracking, the trochlear prosthesis should be perpendicular to Whiteside's line and parallel to the transepicondylar axis (Fig. 17.4) (Lonner 2018). Although both landmarks are effective, the transepicondylar axis may be difficult to visualize due to the limited exposure, and as such Whiteside's line is the most commonly used reference.

Selection of an appropriately sized trochlear component is critical (Lonner 2004). The ideal component maximizes coverage of the anterior femur, yet does not overhang either medially or laterally. Additionally, it is important that the prosthesis does not extend too far distally into the intercondylar notch, and encroach on the tibiofemoral articulation or menisci. Intrusion in this region can lead to articular impingement and pain. Finally, the trochlear component should be positioned such that it is either flush with the surrounding articular cartilage of the femoral condyles or recessed 1 mm.

Patellar resurfacing should follow a similar surgical technique to that performed for TKA (Roussot and Haddad 2018). Resection should be performed such that restoration of native patellar thickness is achieved after patellar button application. Similar to TKA, superomedial positioning of the patellar button is advisable to optimize patellar tracking. Excess bone remaining along the lateral border of the patella should be resected and beveled to prevent potentially painful articulation with the trochlear prosthesis (Valoroso et al. 2017).

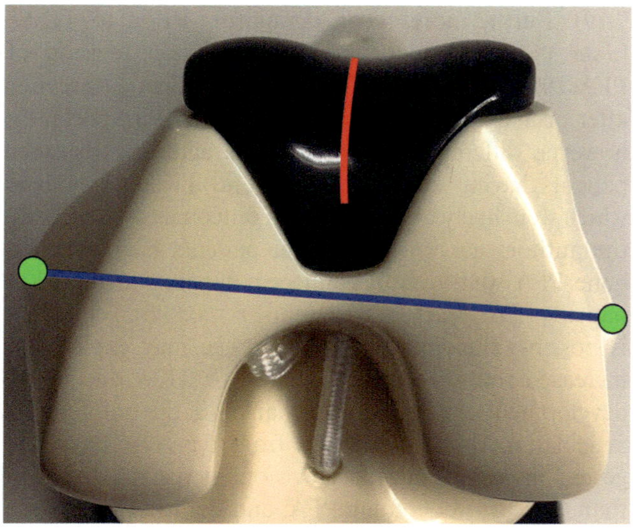

Fig. 17.4 Journey patellofemoral arthroplasty implant model (Smith & Nephew, London, UK) demonstrating correct trochlear component rotation, perpendicular to Whiteside's line (*red line*) and parallel to the transepicondylar axis (*blue line*)

Upon insertion of the trial prosthesis, careful attention to overall patellar tracking throughout ROM for evidence of patellar button subluxation, tilting, and catching is required. In scenarios where mild subluxation or tilting is observed, a lateral retinacular release can be performed and is generally sufficient (Lonner 2003). If maltracking persists, reassessment of component position and rotation should be performed. This underlines the importance of careful preoperative examination for more significant maltracking in the presence of Q-angle elevation. In such scenarios, a staged approach with anteromedialization of the tibial tubercle prior to PFA is advised, or alternatively TKA can be performed (Hofmann et al. 2013; Lonner and Bloomfield 2013).

> Once final implants are selected and inserted, excess cement surrounding the trochlear implant should be removed. Furthermore, copious irrigation can be beneficial to prevent thermal damage to the surrounding cartilage which can result from the exothermal process during PMMA polymerization.

17.3.4 Clinical Results

Most recent studies have reported good short- and mid-term follow-up outcomes after PFA. In a recent study by Odgaard et al. a total of 100 PFA and TKAs were randomized for comparison of early postoperative clinical outcomes (Odgaard et al. 2018). Throughout the first 2 years postoperatively, the authors reported both superior patient-reported outcome scores and ROM for those having undergone PFA. Similarly, recent advents in minimally invasive techniques and the emergent use of robotic-arm-assisted surgery, although early, appear promising (Fig. 17.5) (Burger et al. 2020).

Additionally, the use of PFA in younger patients has demonstrated promise as a more conservative approach to TKA in patients with isolated PFJ osteoarthritis. A recent study by Kamikovski et al. compared patient-reported outcomes (PROs) in 19 individuals (23 PFAs) younger than 55 years undergoing PFA or TKA for isolated PFJ osteoarthritis (Kamikovski et al. 2019). At a minimum 2-year follow-up, the authors noted no difference in the Western Ontario and McMaster Osteoarthritic Index, Knee injury and Osteoarthritis Outcome scores, Tegner, and the University of California, Los Angeles activity scores. Moreover, Chawla et al. demonstrated the cost-effectiveness of PFA compared to TKA as a joint-preserving procedure in this younger patient popu-

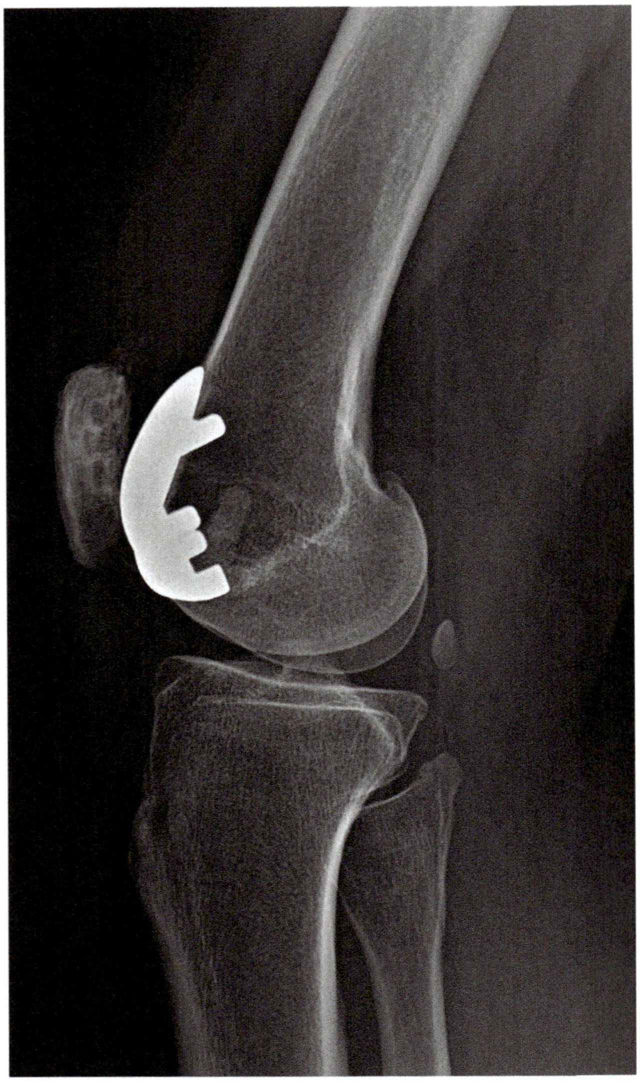

Fig. 17.5 Lateral radiograph demonstrating an appropriately positioned inlay design Gender Solutions™PFA trochlear component (Zimmer, Warsaw, IN) sitting flush with the anterior cortex

lation (Chawla et al. 2017). Other studies, however, suggest that although a significant improvement in PROs may be observed, significant patient dissatisfaction may be present after PFA. In a study by Kazarian et al., the authors assessed the clinical outcomes of 70 PFAs using a modern onlay trochlear design at a mean follow-up of 4.9 years (Kazarian et al. 2016). The authors noted that although significant improvements in Knee Society scores were observed, fewer than two-thirds of patients were satisfied or had their expectations met. Furthermore, such dissatisfied patients were noted to have significantly lower Mental Health scores according to the Short-Form-36.

As such, thorough preoperative patient counseling with regard to postoperative expectations is paramount.

Although promising results have been observed, current joint registry data has reported higher rates of failure. Such results highlight the importance of rigorous patient selection criteria, implant design characteristics, and attentive surgical technique on postoperative outcomes and revision rates.The National Joint Registry for England, Wales, Northern Ireland, and the Isle of Man (NJR) reported a 9.82% overall revision rate at 5 years, 18.86% at 10 years, and increasing to 26.93% at 15-year follow-up (National Joint Registry for England 2019). In the Australian Joint Registry (AJR), greater rates of revision were noted at similar time points with rates of 13.8% and 46.1% at 5- and 16-years follow-up in patients with osteoarthritis, respectively ((AOANJRR) AOANJRR 2019).Complete assessment of such general results, however, requires a more in-depth analysis of factors likely to influence post-surgical outcomes.

Numerous studies suggest that the principal cause for failure of PFA results from the progression of OA in the tibiofemoral joint (Dy et al. 2012; Dahm et al. 2014; Baker et al. 2012). This is followed by mechanical complications (subluxation, dislocation, catching, etc.) (Dy et al. 2012; Lustig 2014; Oni et al. 2014). Woon et al. performed a systematic review of 1738 PFAs with mean follow-up of 4.5 years comparing revision rates after primary PFA for osteoarthritis versus TKA (Woon et al. 2019). Importantly, only studies utilizing modern onlay-type PFA prostheses were included. Inlay PFA designs were excluded. Comparing weighted rates, the authors noted that patients undergoing PFA were more likely to return to the operating room for conversion to TKA, and/or revision surgery (6.34, 95% CI: 4.77–8.07 vs. 0.11, 95% CI: 0–1.38) compared to primary TKA. Of note, however, a significant proportion of PFA patients underwent revision for conversion to TKA (5.47, 95% CI: 3.94–7.19). Furthermore, when comparing PFAs to TKAs, fewer patients underwent non-conversion revision of PFAs (0.05, 95% CI: 0–0.38) compared to patients revised after primary TKA (0.11, 95% CI: 0–1.38). Importantly, however, differences in baseline characteristics between patients having undergone PFA and TKA were noted which were likely to have affected outcomes. In this study, the authors acknowledged that patients having undergone PFA were overall younger compared to the TKA patients (59.2 years vs. 67.3 years, $p = 0.006$). As such, it is possible that this difference in age may explain the increased rate of PFA conversion to TKA due to the development of degenerative changes in the tibiofemoral articulation. In fact, findings from the AJR have suggested increased rates of revision in patients younger than 65 years undergoing PFA, and slightly greater rates of revision in males. Such risk factors for revision appear similar to those observed in the AJR for primary TKA.

In another study by Argenson et al., 66 onlay-type uncemented PFAs were assessed at a mean of 16 years postoperatively (Argenson et al. 2005). Although improvement in pain and function was observed, significant rates of failure were noted; 25% were revised for progression of the disease to the tibiofemoral articulation at a mean of 7.3 years, and 14% were revised for aseptic loosening at a mean of 4.5 years after PFA. The authors stress the importance of stringent selection criteria for patients undergoing PFA, and suggest that superior results can be expected for patients with the principal diagnosis of post-traumatic PF arthritis or patellar subluxation. In those with primary PF osteoarthritis, careful observation of the tibiofemoral articulation for signs of osteoarthritis is critical and can be supplemented with MRI if diagnostic uncertainty persists (Lonner 2018). Furthermore, caution regarding the use of uncemented PFA implants may be warranted due to the risk of aseptic loosening.

> Implant design characteristics, specifically inlay versus onlay design, are important elements to consider when assessing the current body of literature on outcomes after PFA.

Similarly, as previously discussed, implant radius of curvature, width, thickness, and degree of constraint should be considered. In a study by Blazina et al. the authors assessed 55 PFAs at a mean follow-up of less than 2 years using an early inlay-type PFA characterized by a narrow, constrained design (Blazina et al. 2005). Although the authors noted good results at short-term follow-up, 30 subsequent re-alignment procedures were required due to PFA maltracking. Conversely, Lonner et al. compared a consecutive series of first-generation inlay PFAs to 25 second-generation onlay implants and noted poorer results with the former. In fact, 17% of patients with an inlay-style prosthesis compared to 4% with the more accommodating onlay trochlear component experienced PFA dysfunction, subluxation, catching, and/or pain. Both the increased constraint and resultant internal rotation inherent to many inlay designs are important factors to consider and should be avoided (Ackroyd et al. 2007). Ensuring adequate external rotation of the trochlear component is necessary to ensure adequate patellar tracking (Cho et al. 2016).

Revision of patellofemoral arthroplasty has demonstrated positive clinical results (Fig. 17.6). Parratte et al. assessed 21 PFAs revised to TKA with a minimum 5-year follow-up period (Parratte et al. 2015). The authors concluded that revision of PFA to TKA was comparable to primary TKA with regard to both surgical characteristics and clinical outcomes. Furthermore, they noted that the majority of patients could be treated with standard implants, although a greater number of perioperative complications was noted compared to primary TKA. Another study by Lewis et al. however, portends caution (Lewis et al. 2019). The authors assessed 482 cases of PFAs revised to TKA over a 17-year period. They observed an increased rate of repeat revision surgery in patients having been revised from a PFA to a TKA, compared to the risk of patients having undergone primary TKA requiring first revision surgery (HR, 2.39 [1.77–3.24]; $p < 0.001$). As such, the authors recommend that a possible increased risk of repeat revision surgery be included in the preoperative discussion with patients considering PFA.

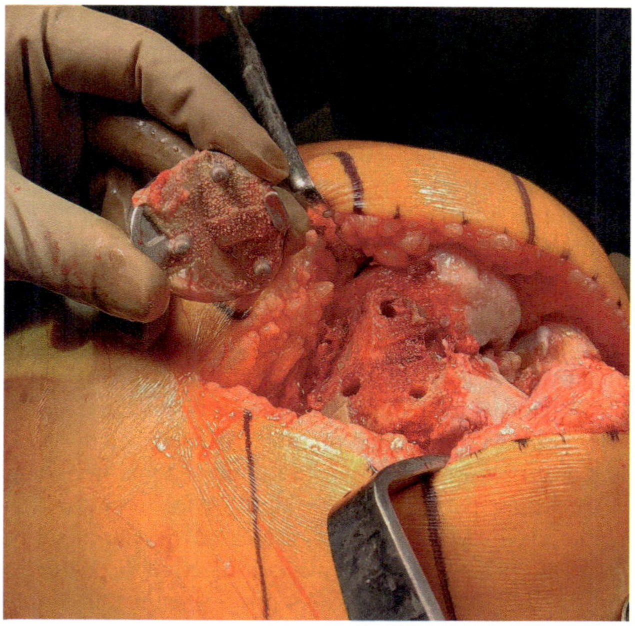

Fig. 17.6 Intraoperative image of a conversion patellofemoral arthroplasty to a TKA secondary to the development of osteoarthritis of the tibiofemoral articulation. Note the conservation of native bone and the integrity of surrounding ligamentous structures

17.4 Complications

Complications specific to PFA can broadly be classified as either early or late, with most early complications related to issues of catching and PF maltracking. A recent study by Rezzadeh et al. assessed early complications (<30 days) in 1069 patients from the American College of Surgeons National Surgical Quality Improvement Program (NSQIP) database (Rezzadeh et al. 2019). The authors noted that re-admission and re-operation rates after PFA were <5%. Both older age and elevated BMI were identified as risk factors for adverse perioperative outcomes, notably longer operative times, longer hospital stays, and transfusion requirements. It should be noted, however, that overall, such adverse outcomes are infrequent with most patients being discharged early and very rarely requiring transfusion secondary to blood loss. Conversely, late complications requiring revision surgery occur in the context of a previously well-functioning PFA and appear to be especially elevated in those with obesity (van Wagenberg et al.

2009). By far, the most common reason for late revision surgery is development of degenerative changes in the tibiofemoral articulation. Kooijman et al. noted that 25% of patients in their series required revision surgery due to the development of osteoarthritis in other compartments at 15 years postoperatively (Kooijman et al. 2003). Similarly, Nicol et al. noted a 12% revision rate for the development of tibiofemoral arthritic disease at a mean of 55 months postoperatively (Nicol et al. 2006). Moreover, it is interesting to note that in the latter study, all patients revised for development of osteoarthritis in other compartments underwent PFA for the indication of osteoarthritis. None of the patients revised had the primary diagnosis of trochlear dysplasia at the time of PFA. As such, this study as well as others appears to suggest improved long-term survivorship for patients undergoing PFA for trochlear dysplasia (likely as a result of decreased development of disease to other compartments) compared to those treated for primary osteoarthritis. Aseptic loosening, although observed, is relatively infrequent (Konan and Haddad 2016; Clement et al. 2019). In a series by Argenson et al. 14% of patients undergoing PFA were revised for aseptic loosening at a mean of 16 years postoperatively (Argenson et al. 2005). In this series, however, most components having loosened were of a cementless design.

> As such, to avoid higher rates of loosening, a cemented prosthesis may be preferable.

Take-Home Messages

- To ensure optimal results, PFA should be limited to patients suffering from isolated PFJ osteoarthritis, post-traumatic arthritis, severe chondrosis on either joint surface, and PF degeneration secondary to dysplasia/malalignment.
- Anteromedializing tibial tubercle osteotomy should be considered prior to performing PFA in patients with observed PFJ maltracking and concurrent Q-angle elevation.
- Modern PFA designs can be categorized into two styles: inlay and onlay. Key differences between these design types are related to positioning, rotation, width, and proximal trochlear extension.
- Key technical principles in PFA include ensuring appropriate trochlear prosthesis rotation (perpendicular to Whiteside's line), positioning (flush with the surrounding articular cartilage or 1 mm recessed), and sizing.
- Progression of arthritic disease in other compartments of the knee is the most common reason for revision surgery after PFA.
- Due to the risk of aseptic loosening observed with cementless PFA designs, cemented prostheses may be preferable.

References

(AOANJRR) AOANJRR (2019) Hip, knee & shoulder arthroplasty: 2019 annual report. AOA, Adelaide

Ackroyd CE, Newman JH, Evans R, Eldridge JD, Joslin CC (2007) The Avon patellofemoral arthroplasty: five-year survivorship and functional results. J Bone Joint Surg Br 89(3):310–315. https://doi.org/10.1302/0301-620X.89B3.18062

Argenson JN, Flecher X, Parratte S, Aubaniac JM (2005) Patellofemoral arthroplasty: an update. Clin Orthop Relat Res 440:50–53. https://doi.org/10.1097/01.blo.0000187061.27573.70

Baker PN, Refaie R, Gregg P, Deehan D (2012) Revision following patello-femoral arthoplasty. Knee Surg Sports Traumatol Arthrosc 20(10):2047–2053. https://doi.org/10.1007/s00167-011-1842-0

Blazina ME, Fox JM, Del Pizzo W, Broukhim B, Ivey FM (2005) Patellofemoral replacement. 1979. Clin Orthop Relat Res 436:3–6

Bohu Y, Klouche S, Sezer HB, Gerometta A, Lefevre N, Herman S (2019) Hermes patellofemoral arthroplasty: annual revision rate and clinical results after two to 20 years of follow-up. Knee 26(2):484–491. https://doi.org/10.1016/j.knee.2019.01.014

Bunyoz KI, Lustig S, Troelsen A (2019) Similar postoperative patient-reported outcome in both second generation patellofemoral arthroplasty and total knee arthroplasty for treatment of isolated patellofemoral osteoarthritis: a systematic review. Knee Surg Sports Traumatol Arthrosc 27(7):2226–2237. https://doi.org/10.1007/s00167-018-5151-8

Burger JA, Kleeblad LJ, Laas N, Pearle AD (2020) Mid-term survivorship and patient-reported outcomes of robotic-arm assisted partial knee arthroplasty. Bone Joint J 102-B(1):108–116. https://doi.org/10.1302/0301-620X.102B1.BJJ-2019-0510.R1

Chawla H, Nwachukwu BU, van der List JP, Eggman AA, Pearle AD, Ghomrawi HM (2017) Cost effectiveness of patellofemoral. Bone Joint J 99-B(8):1028–1036. https://doi.org/10.1302/0301-620X.99B8.BJJ-2016-1032.R1

Cho KJ, Erasmus PJ, Müller JH (2016) The effect of axial rotation of the anterior resection plane in patellofemoral arthroplasty. Knee 23(5):895–899. https://doi.org/10.1016/j.knee.2016.04.006

Clement ND, Howard TA, Immelman RJ, MacDonald D, Patton JT, Lawson GM, Burnett R (2019) Patellofemoral arthroplasty versus total knee arthroplasty for patients with patellofemoral osteoarthritis: equal function and satisfaction but higher revision rate for partial arthroplasty at a minimum eight years' follow-up. Bone Joint J 101-B(1):41–46. https://doi.org/10.1302/0301-620X.101B1.BJJ-2018-0654.R2

Dahm DL, Kalisvaart MM, Stuart MJ, Slettedahl SW (2014) Patellofemoral arthroplasty: outcomes and factors associated with early progression of tibiofemoral arthritis. Knee Surg Sports Traumatol Arthrosc 22(10):2554–2559. https://doi.org/10.1007/s00167-014-3202-3

Davies AP, Vince AS, Shepstone L, Donell ST, Glasgow MM (2002) The radiologic prevalence of patellofemoral osteoarthritis. Clin Orthop Relat Res 402:206–212. https://doi.org/10.1097/00003086-200,209,000-00020

Dy CJ, Franco N, Ma Y, Mazumdar M, McCarthy MM, Gonzalez Della Valle A (2012) Complications after patello-femoral versus total knee replacement in the treatment of isolated patellofemoral osteoarthritis. A meta-analysis. Knee Surg Sports Traumatol Arthrosc 20(11):2174–2190. https://doi.org/10.1007/s00167-011-1677-8

Federico DJ, Reider B (1997) Results of isolated patellar debridement for patellofemoral pain in patients with normal patellar alignment. Am J Sports Med 25(5):663–669. https://doi.org/10.1177/036354659702500513

Hangody L, Füles P (2003) Autologous osteochondral mosaicplasty for the treatment of full-thickness defects of weight-bearing joints: ten years of experimental and clinical experience. J Bone Joint Surg Am 85-A(Suppl 2):25–32. https://doi.org/10.2106/00004623-200,300,002-00004

Harrington KD (1992) Long-term results for the McKeever patellar resurfacing prosthesis used as a salvage procedure for severe chondromalacia patellae. Clin Orthop Relat Res 279:201–213

Heatley FW, Allen PR, Patrick JH (1986) Tibial tubercle advancement for anterior knee pain. A temporary or permanent solution. Clin Orthop Relat Res 208:215–224

Hofmann AA, McCandless JB, Shaeffer JF, Magee TH (2013) Patellofemoral replacement: the third compartment. Bone Joint J 95-B(11 Suppl A):124–128. https://doi.org/10.1302/0301-620X.95B11.32985

Kamikovski I, Dobransky J, Dervin GF (2019) The clinical outcome of patellofemoral arthroplasty vs total knee arthroplasty in patients younger than 55 years. J Arthroplasty 34(12):2914–2917. https://doi.org/10.1016/j.arth.2019.07.016

Kazarian GS, Tarity TD, Hansen EN, Cai J, Lonner JH (2016) Significant functional improvement at 2 years after isolated patellofemoral arthroplasty with an Onlay Trochlear implant, but low mental health scores predispose to dissatisfaction. J Arthroplasty 31(2):389–394. https://doi.org/10.1016/j.arth.2015.08.033

Konan S, Haddad FS (2016) Midterm outcome of Avon patellofemoral arthroplasty for posttraumatic unicompartmental osteoarthritis. J Arthroplasty 31(12):2657–2659. https://doi.org/10.1016/j.arth.2016.06.005

Kooijman HJ, Driessen AP, van Horn JR (2003) Long-term results of patellofemoral arthroplasty. A report of 56 arthroplasties with 17 years of follow-up. J Bone Joint Surg Br 85(6):836–840

Leadbetter WB, Ragland PS, Mont MA (2005) The appropriate use of patellofemoral arthroplasty: an analysis of reported indications, contraindications, and failures. Clin Orthop Relat Res 436:91–99

Leadbetter WB, Seyler TM, Ragland PS, Mont MA (2006) Indications, contraindications, and pitfalls of patellofemoral arthroplasty. J Bone Joint Surg Am 88(Suppl 4):122–137. https://doi.org/10.2106/JBJS.F.00856

Lewis PL, Graves SE, Cuthbert A, Parker D, Myers P (2019) What is the risk of repeat revision when patellofemoral replacement is revised to TKA? An analysis of 482 cases from a large national arthroplasty registry. Clin Orthop Relat Res 477(6):1402–1410. https://doi.org/10.1097/CORR.0000000000000541

Lonner JH. Patellofemoral arthroplasty. Techniques in Knee Surgery. Lippincott, Williams & Wilkins. 2003;2:144–152.

Lonner JH (2004) Patellofemoral arthroplasty: pros, cons, and design considerations. Clin Orthop Relat Res 428:158–165

Lonner JH (2007) Patellofemoral arthroplasty. J Am Acad Orthop Surg 15(8):495–506. https://doi.org/10.5435/00124635-200,708,000-00006

Lonner JH (2018) Patellofemoral Arthroplasty. Insall & Scott Surgery of the Knee, vol vol 2, 6th edn. Elsevier, Philadelphia

Lonner JH, Bloomfield MR (2013) The clinical outcome of patellofemoral arthroplasty. Orthop Clin North Am 44(3):271–280., vii. https://doi.org/10.1016/j.ocl.2013.03.002

Lonner JH, Mehta S, Booth RE (2007) Ipsilateral patellofemoral arthroplasty and autogenous osteochondral femoral condylar transplantation. J Arthroplasty 22(8):1130–1136. https://doi.org/10.1016/j.arth.2005.08.012

Lustig S (2014) Patellofemoral arthroplasty. Orthop Traumatol Surg Res 100(1 Suppl):S35–S43. https://doi.org/10.1016/j.otsr.2013.06.013

McAlindon TE, Snow S, Cooper C, Dieppe PA (1992) Radiographic patterns of osteoarthritis of the knee joint in the community: the importance of the patellofemoral joint. Ann Rheum Dis 51(7):844–849. https://doi.org/10.1136/ard.51.7.844

McKeever DC (1955) Patellar prosthesis. J Bone Joint Surg Am 37-A(5):1074–1084

Minas T, Bryant T (2005) The role of autologous chondrocyte implantation in the patellofemoral joint. Clin Orthop Relat Res 436:30–39. https://doi.org/10.1097/01.blo.0000171916.40245.5d

Mont MA, Haas S, Mullick T, Hungerford DS (2002) Total knee arthroplasty for patellofemoral arthritis. J Bone Joint Surg Am 84(11):1977–1981. https://doi.org/10.2106/00004623-200,211,000-00011

National Joint Registry for England, Wales, Northern Ireland and the Isle of Man: 16th Annual Report (2019). https://reports.njrcentre.org.uk/Portals/0/PDFdownloads/NJR%2016th%20Annual%20Report%202019.pdf. Accessed January 19, 2019

Nicol SG, Loveridge JM, Weale AE, Ackroyd CE, Newman JH (2006) Arthritis progression after patellofemoral joint replacement. Knee 13(4):290–295. https://doi.org/10.1016/j.knee.2006.04.005

Novakofski KD, Pownder SL, Koff MF, Williams RM, Potter HG, Fortier LA (2016) High-resolution methods for diagnosing cartilage damage in vivo. Cartilage 7(1):39–51. https://doi.org/10.1177/1947603515602307

Odgaard A, Madsen F, Kristensen PW, Kappel A, Fabrin J (2018) The Mark Coventry award: patellofemoral arthroplasty results in better range of movement and early patient-reported outcomes than TKA. Clin Orthop Relat Res 476(1):87–100. https://doi.org/10.1007/s11999.0000000000000017

Oni JK, Hochfelder J, Dayan A (2014) Isolated patellofemoral arthroplasty. Bull Hosp Jt Dis 72(1):97–103

Paletta GA, Laskin RS (1995) Total knee arthroplasty after a previous patellectomy. J Bone Joint Surg Am 77(11):1708–1712. https://doi.org/10.2106/00004623-199,511,000-00010

Parratte S, Lunebourg A, Ollivier M, Abdel MP, Argenson JN (2015) Are revisions of patellofemoral arthroplasties more like primary or revision TKAs. Clin Orthop Relat Res 473(1):213–219. https://doi.org/10.1007/s11999-014-3756-x

Parvizi J, Stuart MJ, Pagnano MW, Hanssen AD (2001) Total knee arthroplasty in patients with isolated patellofemoral arthritis. Clin Orthop Relat Res 392:147–152. https://doi.org/10.1097/00003086-200,111,000-00018

Pidoriano AJ, Weinstein RN, Buuck DA, Fulkerson JP (1997) Correlation of patellar articular lesions with results from anteromedial tibial tubercle transfer. Am J Sports Med 25(4):533–537. https://doi.org/10.1177/036354659702500417

Rezzadeh K, Behery OA, Kester BS, Dogra T, Vigdorchik J, Schwarzkopf R (2019) Patellofemoral arthroplasty: short-term complications and risk factors. J Knee Surg. https://doi.org/10.1055/s-0039-1,688,960

Roussot MA, Haddad FS (2018) The evolution and role of patellofemoral joint arthroplasty: the road less travelled, but not forgotten. Bone Joint Res 7(12):636–638. https://doi.org/10.1302/2046-3758.712.BJR-2018-0303

Valoroso M, Saffarini M, La Barbera G, Toanen C, Hannink G, Nover L, Dejour DH (2017) Correction of patellofemoral malalignment with patellofemoral arthroplasty. J Arthroplasty 32(12):3598–3602. https://doi.org/10.1016/j.arth.2017.06.048

van Jonbergen HP, Werkman DM, Barnaart LF, van Kampen A (2010) Long-term outcomes of patellofemoral arthroplasty. J Arthroplasty 25(7):1066–1071. https://doi.org/10.1016/j.arth.2009.08.023

van Wagenberg JM, Speigner B, Gosens T, de Waal MJ (2009) Midterm clinical results of the Autocentric II patellofemoral prosthesis. Int Orthop 33(6):1603–1608. https://doi.org/10.1007/s00264-009-0719-z

Witvrouw E, Cambier D, Danneels L, Bellemans J, Werner S, Almqvist F, Verdonk R (2003) The effect of exercise regimens on reflex response time of the vasti muscles in patients with anterior knee pain: a prospective randomized intervention study. Scand J Med Sci Sports 13(4):251–258. https://doi.org/10.1034/j.1600-0838.2003.00311.x

Woon CYL, Christ AB, Goto R, Shanaghan K, Shubin Stein BE, Gonzalez Della Valle A (2019) Return to the operating room after patellofemoral arthroplasty versus total knee arthroplasty for isolated patellofemoral arthritis-a systematic review. Int Orthop 43(7):1611–1620. https://doi.org/10.1007/s00264-018-04280-z

Bicompartmental Knee Arthroplasty

Michael D. Ries

Contents

E. Hansen, K.-D. Kühn (eds.), *Essentials of Cemented Knee Arthroplasty*,
https://doi.org/10.1007/978-3-662-63113-3_18

18.1 Introduction

Bicompartmental knee arthroplasty or selective replacement of the patellofemoral and either the medial or lateral tibiofemoral compartment is an alternative to total knee arthroplasty (TKA) for treatment of osteoarthritis involving one tibiofemoral compartment and the patellofemoral joint. Bicompartmental knee arthroplasty preserves the anterior cruciate ligament and is associated with more favorable knee function and kinematics than TKA. However, early failure after bicompartmental arthroplasty can develop from a number of causes including progression of arthritis in the unreplaced tibiofemoral compartment, patellar tracking problems, mechanical loosening, and unexplained pain. Survivorship of bicompartmental arthroplasty is less favorable than TKA.

18.2 Case Example

An active 61-year-old woman who had undergone successful medial right unicompartmental arthroplasty developed medial and anterior left knee pain which restricted her activity. She had undergone prior left knee ACL reconstruction. Exam of the left knee demonstrated tenderness over the medial joint line and pain on patellar compression. The knee was stable to anterior draw and varus/valgus stress. Radiographs demonstrated good overall limb alignment and medial compartment joint space narrowing (◘ Fig. 18.1a, b). Patellar views also demonstrated arthritic changes (◘ Fig. 18.1c). TKA was recommended since the arthritic involvement included both medial and patellofemoral compartments, and the patient had prior ACL reconstruction. However, the patient requested a partial knee replacement based on the favorable experience she had with right knee medial UKA and preservation of the right knee ACL.

Medial bicompartmental knee arthroplasty was performed using a monolithic one-piece femoral component (Duece, Smith and Nephew, Memphis, TN) (◘ Fig. 18.2). At 2 years after surgery, range of motion was 0–135° in both knees. The patient had no knee pain and resumed all routine and recreational activities. She considered the clinical result of both knees to be equivalent.

18

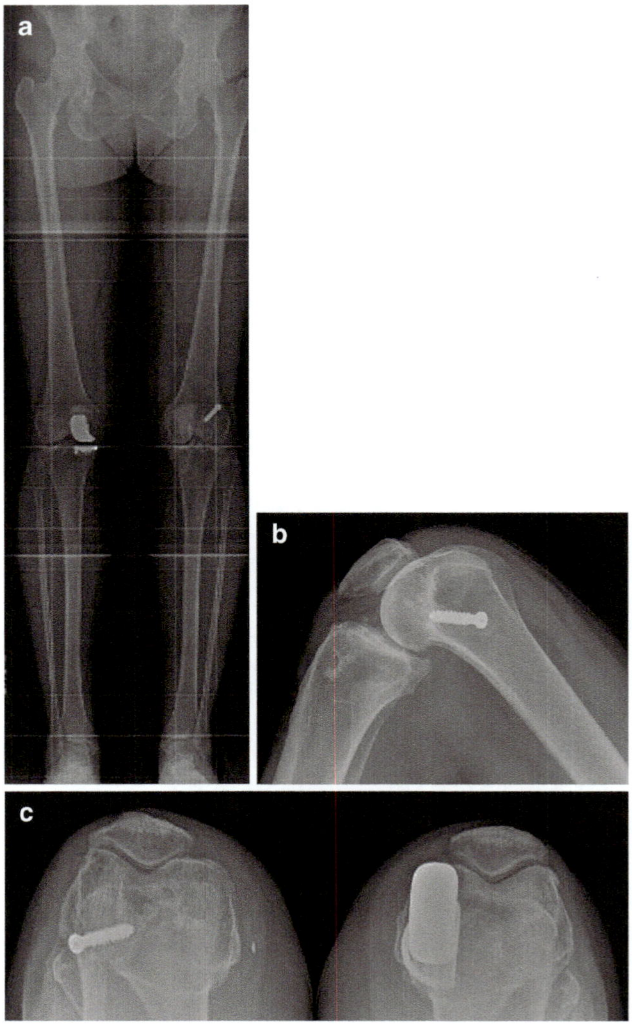

◘ **Fig. 18.1** **a** Long-standing alignment radiograph demonstrates medial right UKA, mild left knee medial joint space narrowing, and minimal coronal deformity. **b** Lateral left knee radiograph demonstrates prior ACL hardware and minimal deformity. **c** Axial radiographic views demonstrate patellofemoral arthritis of the left knee

18.3 Classification

Bicompartmental knee arthroplasty is a term used to describe combined medial tibiofemoral unicompartmental and patellofemoral arthroplasty (medial bicompartmental arthroplasty) or combined lateral tibiofemoral unicompartmentaland patellofemoral arthroplasty (lateral bicompartmental arthroplasty) (Garner et al. 2019).Replacement of both medial and lateral tibiofemoral compartments with two independent tibiofemoral unicompartmental arthroplasties could also be considered "bicompartmental arthroplasty", but has been termed bi-unicondylar arthroplasty (Bi-UKA) (Garner et al. 2019).

> Since combined medial and patellofemoral OA is more common than combined lateral and patellofemoral OA, most bicompartmental arthroplasties replace the medial tibiofemoral and patellofemoral compartments, while preserving the lateral tibiofemoral compartment and anterior cruciate ligament.

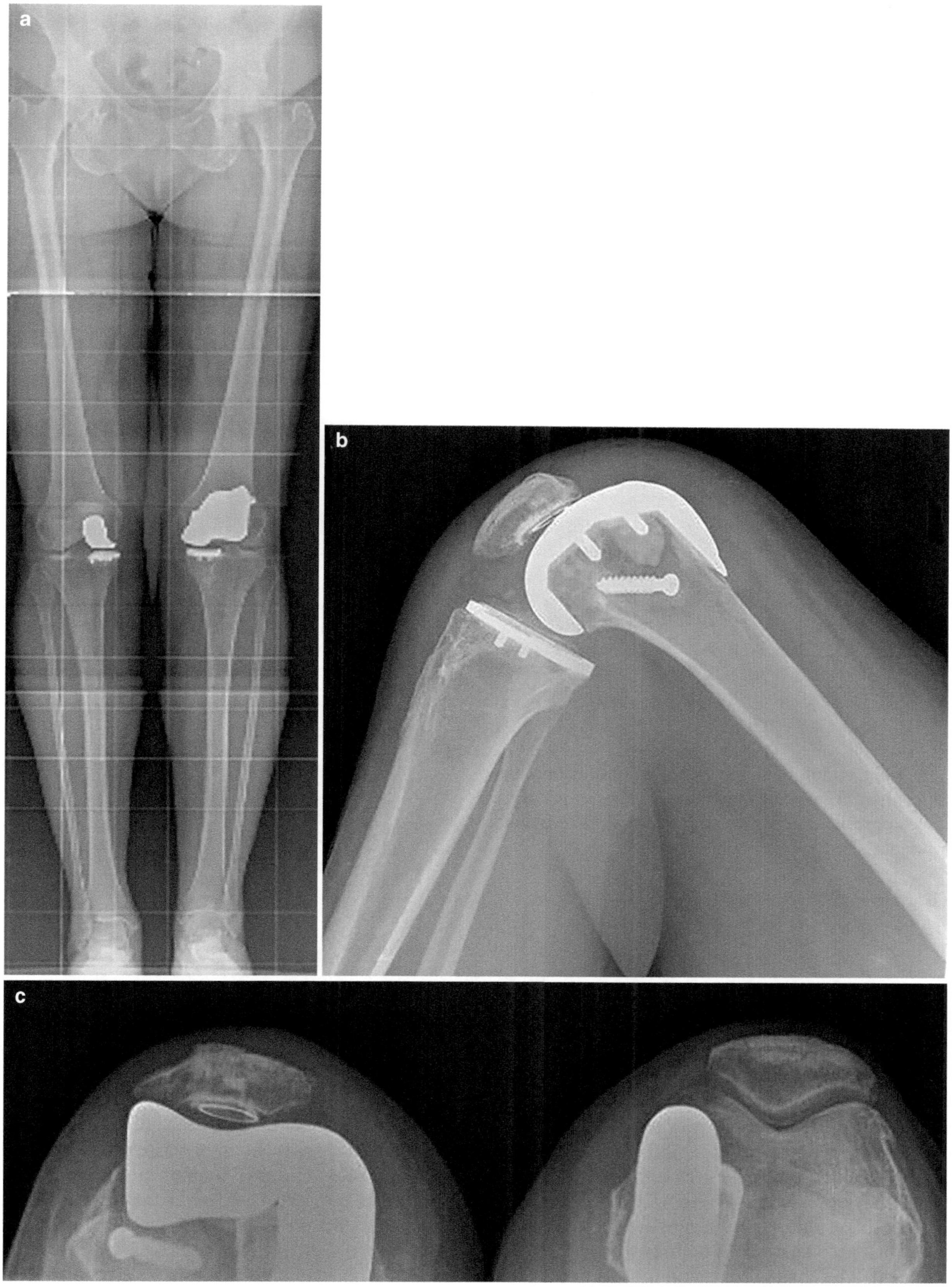

Fig. 18.2 **a** Long alignment radiograph after medial bicompartmental left knee arthroplasty. **b** Lateral radiograph after medial bicompartmental arthroplasty with monolithic femoral component. **c** Axial radiographic views demonstrate patellofemoral replacement of left knee

18.4 Indications

Bicompartmental arthroplasty is an alternative to total knee arthroplasty.It is indicated to treat medial or lateral OA combined with patellofemoral OA in which patellofemoral OA is considered severe enough that medial or lateral unicompartmental arthroplasty (UKA) is not a viable option.

> The ACL should be intact and the knee should be minimally deformed in terms of flexion contracture and coronal alignment.

The non-replaced tibiofemoral compartment should be well preserved without arthritic changes.

18.5 Implant Options and Surgical Technique

> Femoral implant options for bicompartmental arthroplasty include a one-piece "off-the-shelf" femoral component, a one-piece custom femoral component, and two-piece separate conventional femoral unicompartmental and patellofemoral implants (Rolston et al. 2007; Rolston 2009; Palumbo et al. 2011; Tria Jr. 2013; Arnholdt et al. 2018; Steinert et al. 2017; Tamam et al. 2015; Biazzo et al. 2019; Yeo et al. 2015; Kanna 2017; Kamath et al. 2014).

The tibial component consists of a conventional unicompartmental implant and the patella is either unresurfaced or resurfaced with a conventional TKA patellar component.

> The surgical technique for bicompartmental arthroplasty depends on the type of femoral component used.

For a one-piece off-the-shelf femoral component, the technique is based on a tibial cut first to assess the flexion and extension gaps prior to making the femoral bone cuts (Fig. 18.3). The femoral AP position is based on an anterior referencing technique (Fig. 18.4). The medial distal femoral condylar resection is based on a measured resection technique (Fig. 18.5). The AP femoral cut block determines the amount of posterior medial condylar resection (Fig. 18.6).

If the flexion and extension gaps are asymmetric, the gaps are balanced by upsizing or downsizing the femoral component. The chamfer cuts and transition cut at the junction of the intact lateral cartilage surface and femoral component are made through the femoral AP block to complete the femoral preparation (Fig. 18.7). The location of the femoral trochlear groove is determined by the mediolateral position of the femoral component. For one-piece custom component, patient-specific instruments are used based on a pre-op CT scan and measured resection technique (Arnholdt et al. 2018; Steinert et al. 2017). For two-piece nonlinked femoral unicompartmental and patellofemoral implants, each compartment is replaced independently using techniques specific to the tibiofemoral unicompartmental and patellofemoral implants selected. These include gap

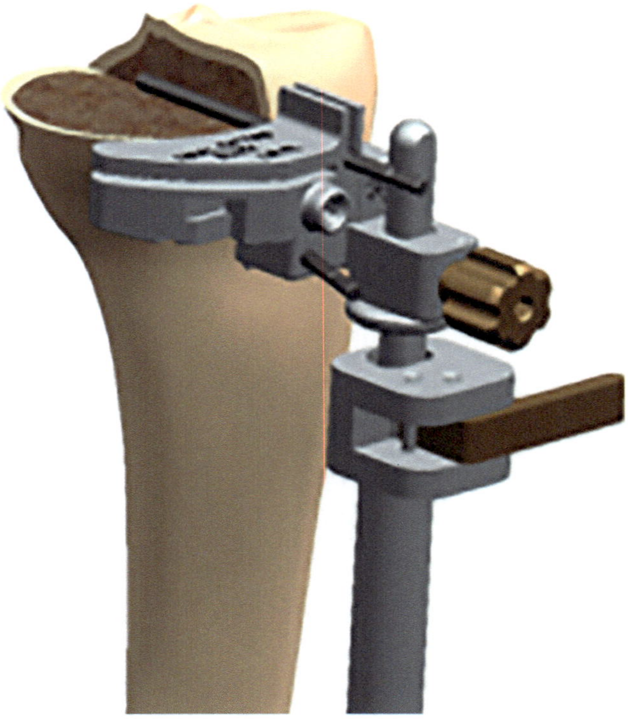

Fig. 18.3 The medial tibial plateau resection is made with extramedullary alignment used in UKA. Then the flexion and extension gaps are checked using spacer blocks at 0 and 90° of flexion. (Reproduced with permission from Smith and Nephew, Memphis, TN)

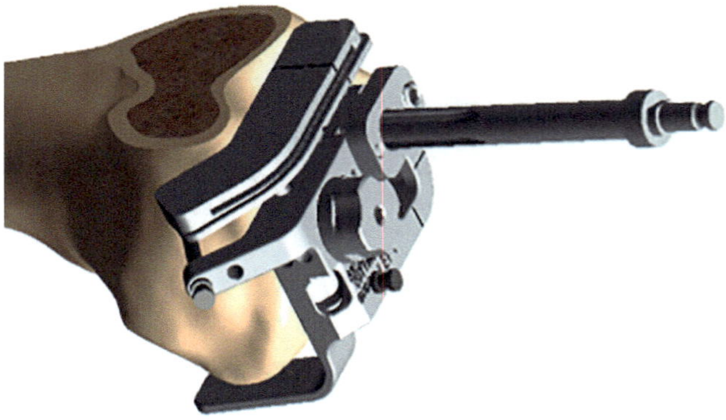

Fig. 18.4 The femoral anterior cut block is positioned using an intramedullary alignment rod and rotational position based on the AP axis of the trochlear groove. (Reproduced with permission from Smith and Nephew, Memphis, TN)

balancing, measured resection, patient-specific instrumentation, navigation, and robotics (Tamam et al. 2015; Biazzo et al. 2019; Yeo et al. 2015; Kanna 2017; Kamath et al. 2014).

The two independent femoral components of a modular bicompartmental knee arthroplasty can be identified on a lateral radiograph (Fig. 18.8).Revision to a TKA may require stems and augments (Fig. 18.9).

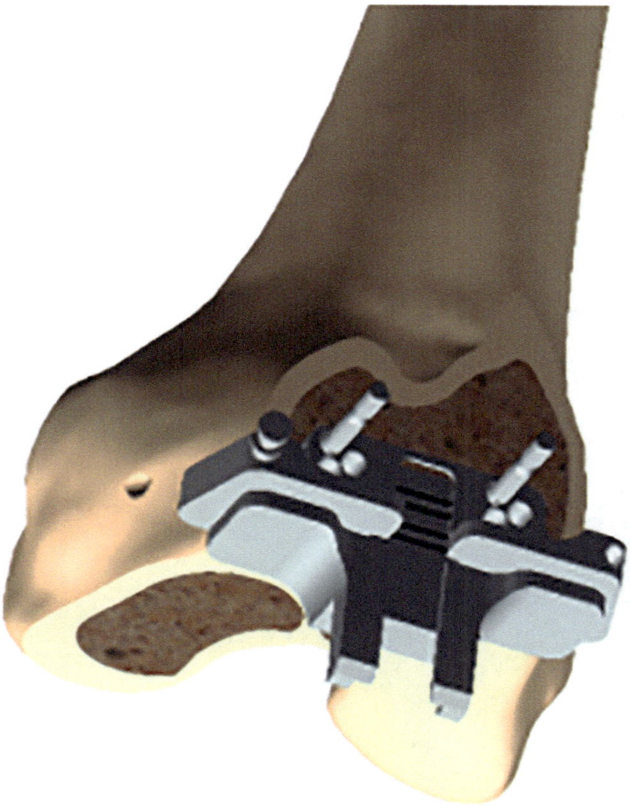

Fig. 18.5 The medial distal condylar resection is based on a measured resection technique so that the thickness of the femoral component matches the thickness of the resected distal femoral condyle. (Reproduced with permission from Smith and Nephew, Memphis, TN)

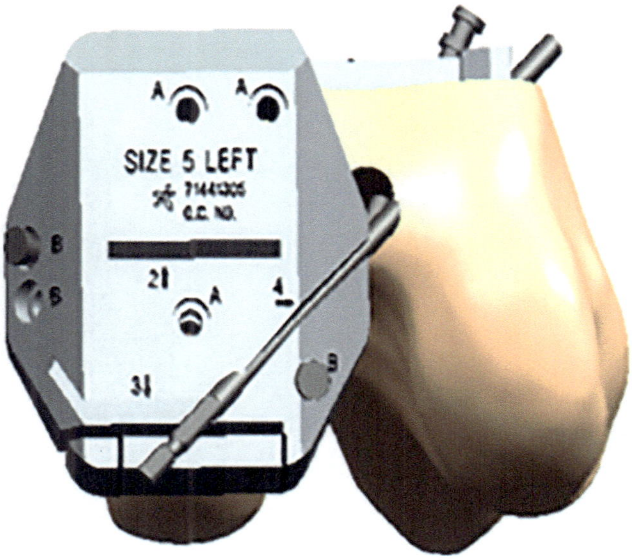

Fig. 18.6 The posterior medial condylar resection is determined by the size of the AP cutting block. (Reproduced with permission from Smith and Nephew, Memphis, TN)

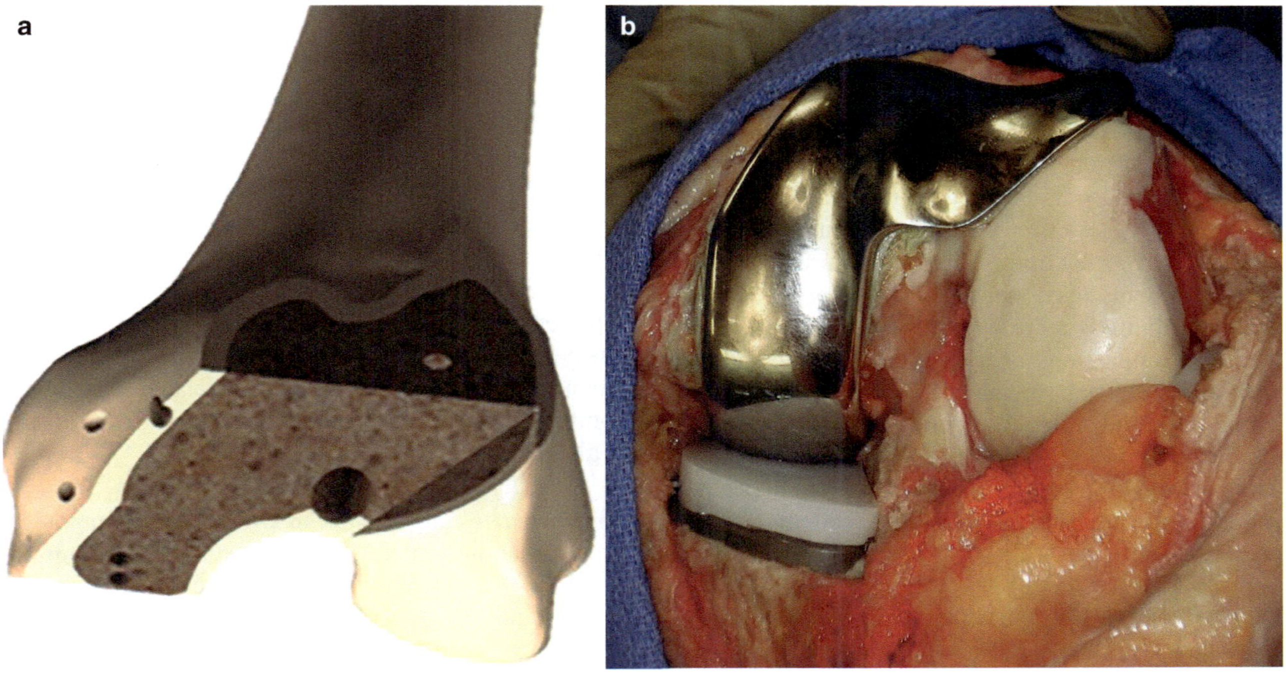

Fig. 18.7 **a** The chamfer cuts and transition cut at the junction of the intact lateral cartilage are made through the AP block to complete the femoral bone cuts. (Reproduced with permission from Smith and Nephew, Memphis, TN). **b** The measured distal reception technique is intended to provide a smooth transition between the femoral component articular surface and intact lateral cartilage

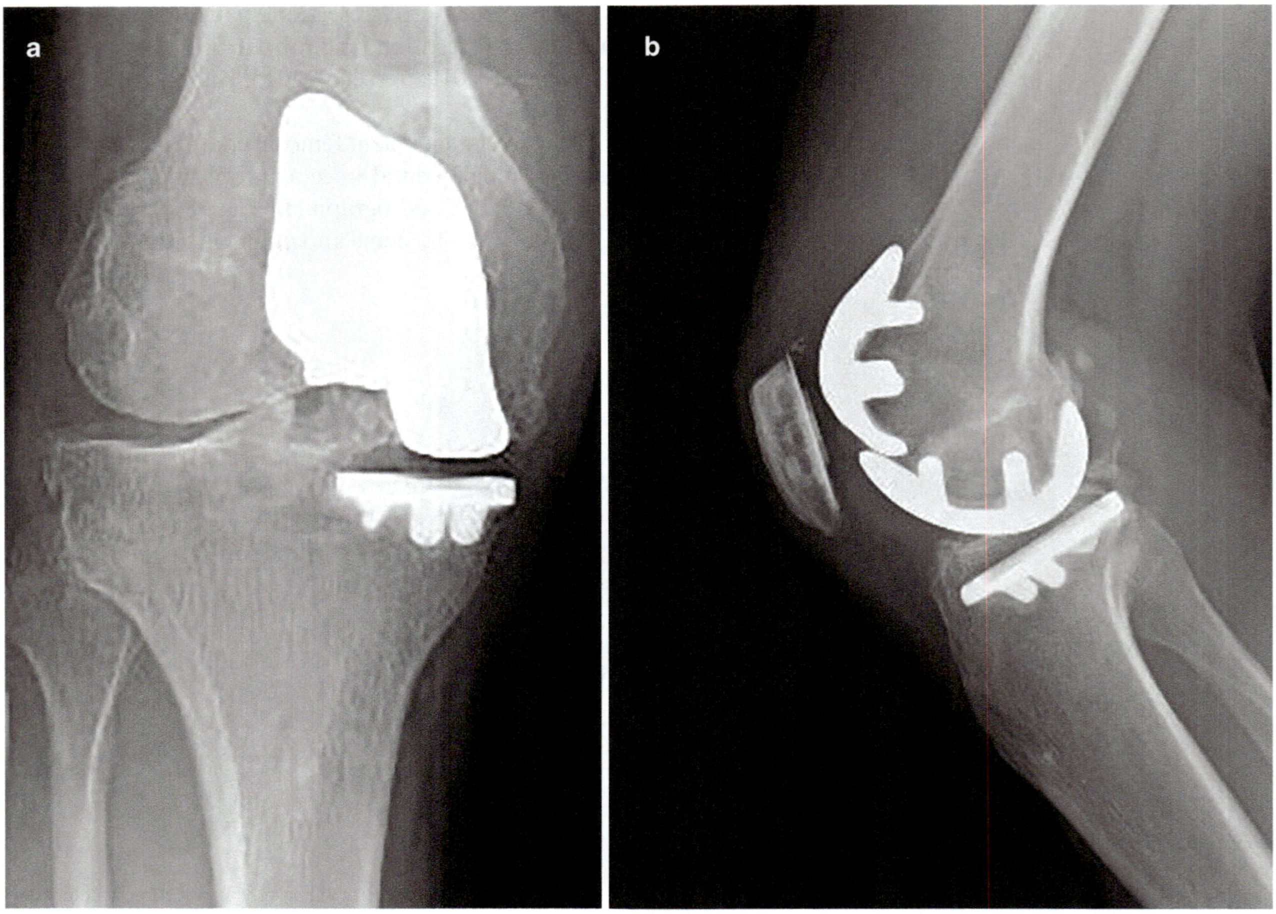

Fig. 18.8 **a** A 63-year-old male 4 years after modular bicompartmental knee arthroplasty developed pain limiting activity. AP radiograph demonstrates the progression of arthritis into the lateral tibiofemoral compartment. **b** Lateral radiograph shows that the two-part modular femoral component results in four independently cemented components (trochlear femoral component, medial femoral component, medial tibial component, and patellar component)

18.6 Results

The clinical outcome of partial and total knee arthroplasties can be assessed in terms of functional results and durability. Function is usually measured using knee scoring systems (e.g., Knee Society Score, KOOS Jr) while durability is represented by implant survivorship studies. Comparisons of unicompartmental and total knee arthroplasty have generally demonstrated equivalent or more favorable function after UKA, but better durability after TKA (Wilson et al. 2019).More favorable function after partial knee replacement in comparison to total knee replacement has been attributed to the preservation of the ACL.

> Meta-analyses of prior studies comparing bicompartmental and TKA have found more favorable knee function scores and range of motion after bicompartmental compared to TKA, but more complications and less survivorship than TKA (Amit et al. 2020; Ma et al. 2017) (Table 18.1).

More favorable knee function after partial knee replacement in comparison to total knee replacement has been attributed to preservation of the ACL. Bicompartmental arthroplasty is also associated with better comfort during everyday activities than TKA (Parratte et al. 2015a).

> Comparative fluoroscopic in vivo kinematics appear more normal after bicompartmental knee arthroplasty than TKA which is consistent with the proprioception and stability provided by an intact ACL (Park et al. 2015; Leffler et al. 2012).

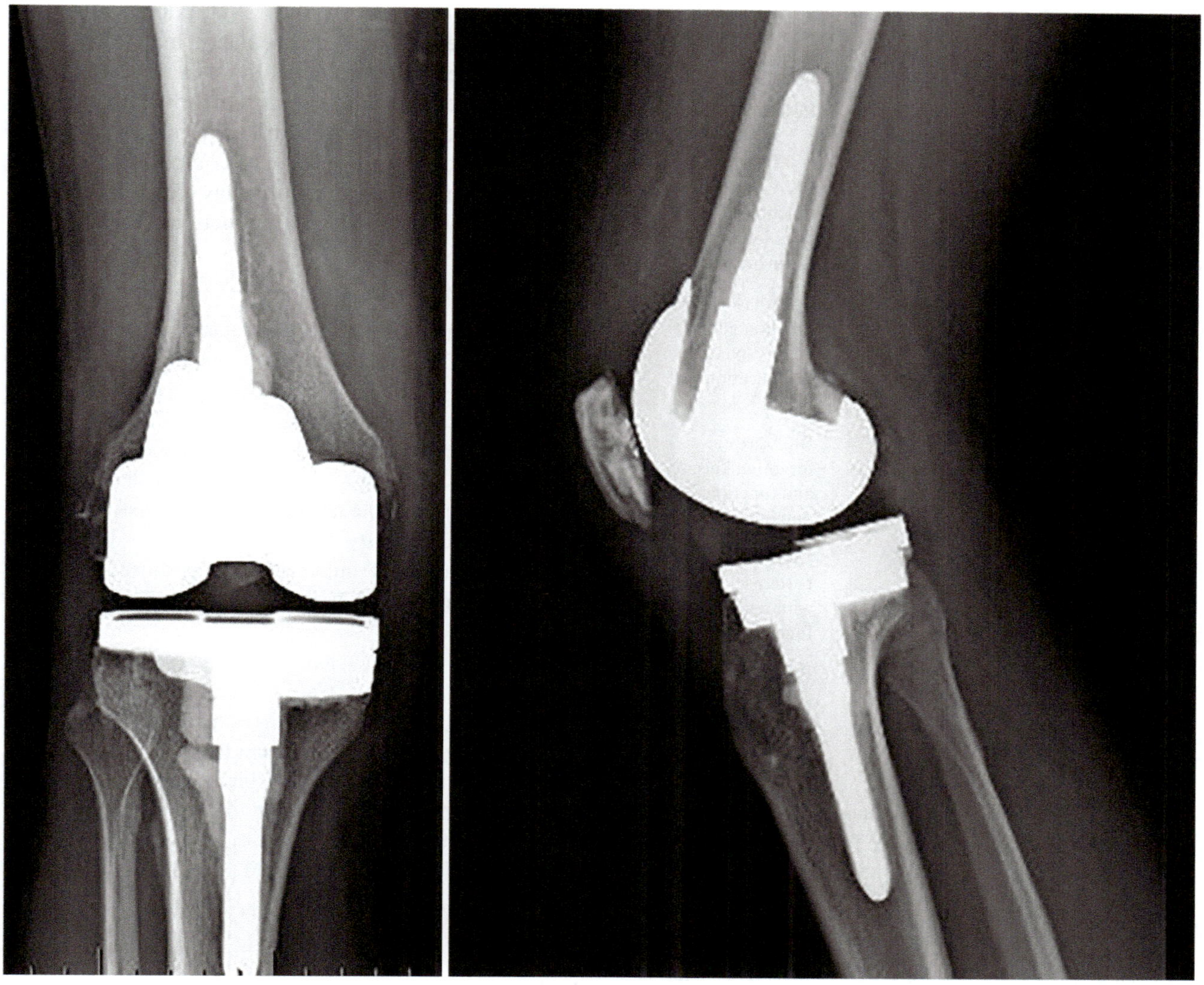

Fig. 18.9 **a** The patient was treated with revision TKA. AP radiograph demonstrates revision of the femoral and tibial components with a medial tibial augment and stemmed implants to accommodate bone loss. **b** Lateral radiograph demonstrates revision of the bicompartmental arthroplasty with retention of the original patellar component

> However, an unacceptably high revision rate after bicompartmental knee arthroplasty using a monolithic design has been identified (Kooner et al. 2017; Dudhniwala et al. 2016; Morrison et al. 2011).

The reasons for the failure of monolithic designs are not clear, but may be related to the link between the formal condylar and trochlear parts of the implant which restricts independent positioning and sizing of the tibiofemoral and patellofemoral components. Modular bicompartmental knee arthroplasty requires implantation of four independent components (medial or lateral femoral, trochlear femoral, patellar, and tibial components), each of which may result in mechanical failure.

Long-term studies with modular two-piece designs have also demonstrated less favorable survivorship than TKA (Parratte et al. 2010, 2015b).

> The relatively high failure and complication rate after modular bicompartmental knee arthroplasty has been attributed to the technical difficulty of the procedure, use of mechanical instrumentation, and various implant design factors (Parratte et al. 2010).

Use of more modern techniques such as robotics, navigation, and custom implants may mitigate the risk of mechanical failure.

Table 18.1 Published results of bicompartmental knee arthroplasty

Publication	Methods	Number of Patients	Results
Amit et al. (2020)	Systematic review	9 studies, 331 patients (341 knees)	BKA comparable function to TKA, but poor long-term survivorship
Ma et al. (2017)	Meta-analysis	5 studies, 261 patients	BKA has better knee function and life quality, but higher complication rate than TKA
Parratte et al. (2015a)	Comparative cohort study	34 BKA, 34 TKA	BKA greater forgotten knee score and functional outcomes than TKA
Park et al. (2015)	Kinematic fluoroscopic	10 BKA	BKA motion patterns consistent with retained ACL function
Leffler et al. (2012)	Kinematic gait analysis	10 BKA	BKA kinematics similar to contralateral normal knee
Kooner et al. (2017)	Systematic review	6 studies, 274 patients (277 knees)	No significant differences in knee function, length of stay, complication rate, or revision rate between BKA and TKA
Dudhniwala et al. (2016)	Retrospective review	15 BKA	BKA revision rate of 60% at follow-up of 54 months
Morrison et al. (2011)	Comparative cohort	21 BKA, 33 TKA	BKA had higher complication rate than TKA
Parratte et al. (2010)	Retrospective review	71 patients, (77 medial UKA/PFJ knees)	BKA survivorship at 17 years 54%
Parratte et al. (2015b)	Review article	5325 medial UKA, 408 lateral UKA, 107 BKA	BKA less favorable survivorship than UKA

TKA total knee arthroplasty, *BKA* bicompartmental knee arthroplasty, *UKA* unicompartmental knee arthroplasty

Conclusion

Bicompartmental knee arthroplasty may offer more favorable knee function than TKA as a result of preservation of the ACL and the non-arthritic tibiofemoral compartment. However, the limited durability of bicompartmental knee arthroplasty in comparison to TKA and risk of mechanical failure may not outweigh the potential benefit of better knee function than TKA.

Take-Home Messages

- Bicompartmental knee arthroplasty is an alternative to TKA when arthritis is limited to either the medial or lateral tibiofemoral compartment and the patellofemoral joint.
- Bicompartmental knee arthroplasty retains the ACL. Kinematics and knee function have been found to be more favorable after bicompartmental knee arthroplasty than TKA.
- A high rate of failure of bicompartmental knee arthroplasty has been reported at mid-term follow-up.
- Monolithic (one-piece) bicompartmental femoral component designs are associated with a higher failure rate than modular (two-part) trochlear and femoral condylar component designs.
- The limited durability of bicompartmental knee arthroplasty in comparison to TKA may not outweigh the potential benefit of ACL retention and better knee function than TKA.

References

Amit P, Singh N, Soni A, Bowman NK, Maden M (2020) Systematic review of modular bicompartmental knee arthroplasty for Medio-patellofemoral osteoarthritis. J Arthroplast 35:893–899

Arnholdt J, Kamawal Y, Holzapfel BM, Ripp A, Rudert M, Steinert AF (2018) Evaluation of implant fit and frontal plane alignment after bi-compartmental knee arthroplasty using patient-specific instruments and implants. Arch Med Sci 14:1424–1431

Biazzo A, Silvestrini F, Manzotti A, Confalonieri N (2019) Bicompartmental (uni plus patellofemoral) versus total knee arthroplasty: a match-paired study. Musculoskelet Surg 103:63–68

Dudhniwala AG, Rath NK, Joshy S, Forster MC, White SP (2016) Early failure with the Journey-Deuce bicompartmental knee arthroplasty. Eur J Orthop Surg Traumatol 26:517–521

Garner A, van Arkel RJ, Cobb J (2019) Classification of combined partial knee arthroplasty. Bone Joint J 101-B:922–928

Kamath AF, Levack A, John T, Thomas BS, Lonner JH (2014) Minimum two-year outcomes of modular bicompartmental knee arthroplasty. J Arthroplast 29:75–79

Kanna R (2017) Modular bicompartmental knee arthroplasty: indications, technique, prosthetic design, and results. Acta Orthop Belg 83:124–131

Kooner S, Johal H, Clark M (2017) Bicompartmental knee arthroplasty vs total knee arthroplasty for the treatment of medial compartment and patellofemoral osteoarthritis. Arthroplasty Today 29:309–314

Leffler J, Scheys L, Planté-Bordeneuve T, Callewaert B, Labey L, Bellemans J, Franz A (2012) Joint kinematics following bicompartmental knee replacement during daily life motor tasks. Gait Posture 36:454–460

Ma JX, He WW, Kuang MJ, Sun L, Lu B, Wang Y, Ma XL (2017) Efficacy of bicompartmental knee arthroplasty (BKA) for bicompartmental knee osteoarthritis: a metaanalysis. Int J Surg 46:53–60

Morrison TA, Nyce JD, Macaulay WB, Geller JA (2011) Early adverse results with bicompartmental knee arthroplasty: a prospective cohort comparison to total knee arthroplasty. J Arthroplast 26(6 Suppl):35–39

Palumbo BT, Henderson ER, Edwards PK, Burris RB, Gutiérrez S, Raterman SJ (2011) Initial experience of the Journey-Deuce bicompartmental knee prosthesis: are view of 36 cases. J Arthroplast 26(6 Suppl):40–45

Park BH, Leffler J, Franz A, Dunbar NJ, Banks SA (2015) Kinematics of mono block bicompartmental knee arthroplasty during weight-bearing activities. Knee Surg Sports Traumatol Arthrosc 23:1756–1762

Parratte S, Pauly V, Aubaniac JM, Argenson JN (2010) Survival of bicompartmental knee arthroplasty at 5 to 23 years. Clin Orthop Relat Res 468:64–72

Parratte S, Ollivier M, Opsomer G, Lunebourg A, Argenson JN, Thienpont E (2015a) Iskneefunctionbetterwithcontemporary-modularbicompartmentalarthroplastycomparedto total knee arthroplasty? Short-term outcomes of a prospective matched study including 68 cases. Orthop Traumatol Surg Res 101:547–552

Parratte S, Ollivier M, Lunebourg A, Abdel MP, Argenson JN (2015b) Long-term results of compartmental arthroplasties of the knee: long term results of partial knee arthroplasty. Bone Joint J 97-B(10 Suppl A):9–15

Rolston L (2009) Bicompartmental knee arthroplasty using a monolithic implant design. Sem Arthroplasty 20:161–163

Rolston L, Bresch J, Engh G, Franz A, Kreuzer S, Nadaud M, Puri L, Wood D (2007) Bicompartmental knee arthroplasty: a bone-sparing, ligament-sparing, and minimally invasive alternative for active patients. Orthopedics 30(8 Suppl):70–73

Steinert AF, Beckmann J, Holzapfel BM, Rudert M, Arnholdt J (2017) Bicompartmental individualized knee replacement : use of patient-specific implants and instruments (iDuo™). Oper Orthop Traumatol 29:51–58

Tamam C, Plate JF, Augart M, Poehling GG, Jinnah RH (2015) Retrospective clinical and radiological outcomes after robotic assisted bicompartmental knee arthroplasty. Adv Orthop 2015:747309. https://doi.org/10.1155/2015/747309. Epub 2015 Sep 3

Tria AJ Jr (2013) Bicompartmental knee arthroplasty: the clinical outcomes. Orthop Clin North Am 44:281–286

Wilson HA, Middleton R, Abram SGF, Smith S, Alvand A, Jackson WF, Bottomley N, Hopewell S, Price AJ (2019) Patient relevant outcomes of unicompartmental versus total knee replacement: systematic review and meta-analysis. BMJ 364:l352

Yeo NE, Chen JY, Yew A, Chia SL, Lo NN, Yeo SJ (2015) Prospective randomised trial comparing unlinked, modular bicompartmental knee arthroplasty and total knee arthroplasty: a five years follow-up. Knee 22:321–327

Total Knee Arthroplasty

Alex Lencioni and Craig A. Hogan

Contents

E. Hansen, K.-D. Kühn (eds.), *Essentials of Cemented Knee Arthroplasty*,
https://doi.org/10.1007/978-3-662-63113-3_19

19.1 Introduction

Surgical treatment of osteoarthritis (OA) of the knee can vary from implant design to surgical technique. This chapter provides a surgical case with the surgical technique developed at the authors' institution. The role of total knee arthroplasty for the treatment of knee OA, including measured resection and gap balancing techniques along with their comparative outcomes, are also discussed. The goal of maintaining mechanical versus kinematic alignment with regard to technique and outcomes in relation to each other is illustrated. In addition, the use of unicompartmental, bicompartmental, and tricompartmental knee arthroplasty with comparative outcomes for the treatment of unicompartmental and tricompartmental knee OA is covered.

19.2 Case Example

We present a case of a 66-year-old male who presented to our clinic with advanced right knee arthritis (◘ Figs. 19.1 and 19.2). He had a long standing history of right knee pain. Prior to presentation in our clinic, he underwent extensive conservative treatment with physical therapy, activity modifications, anti-inflammatories, cortisone, and viscosupplementation. At the time of evaluation, the patient elected to pursue operative management of his knee arthritis. This case highlights our surgical technique for total knee arthroplasty.

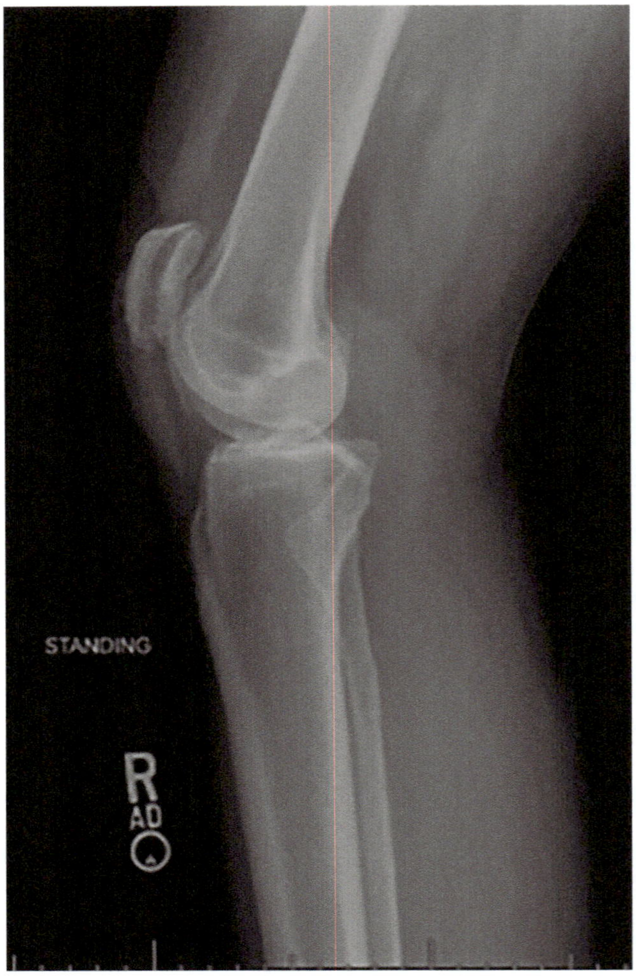

◘ **Fig. 19.2** Lateral X-ray demonstrating tibiofemoral arthritis mentioned above but also posterior femoral osteophytes and degenerative changes of the patellofemoral compartment

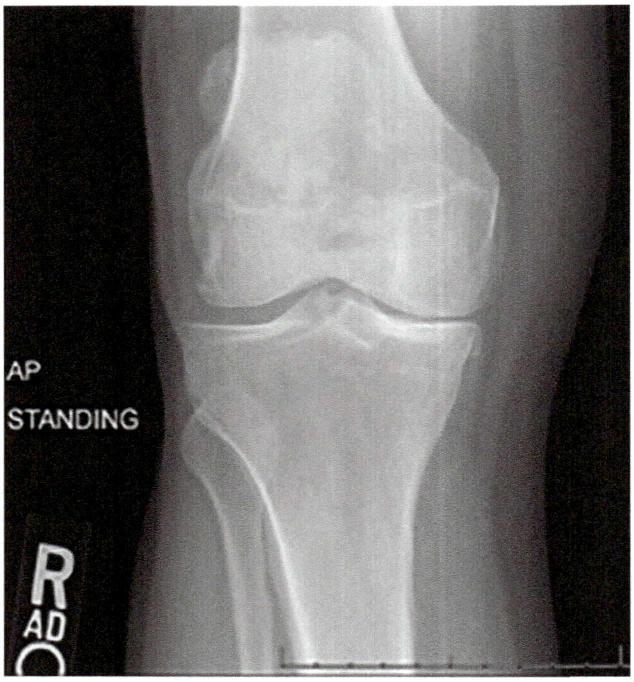

◘ **Fig. 19.1** Weight-bearing AP X-ray demonstrating advanced medial compartment degenerative changes including joint space narrowing, subchondral sclerosis, and marginal osteophytes

19.3 Surgical Technique

At our institution, we use the following preparation, positioning, and surgical technique for cemented total knee arthroplasty. If possible, all patients undergo a single-shot adductor canal block with the regional anesthesia team in the preoperative bay. Once complete, the patient is moved to the operating room and a single-shot short acting spinal is performed. The patient is then placed in a supine position, a formal time-out is held, and the patient is prepped and draped is a standard fashion. We use a double prep with chlorhexidine and a tourniquet is placed but typically not used. Once the drapes are in place, a De-Mayo surgical knee positioner is placed onto the field.

A standard midline incision is used for the surgical approach. Effort is made to ensure that the distal portion of the incision is medial to the tibial tubercle (potentially helps with kneeling pain). Next, a standard medial para-patella arthrotomy is used. Once the arthrotomy is complete we perform a subtotal synovectomy along the medial side and the supra-patellar pouch, and remove the retro-patellar fat pad in its entirety. Then, a complete subperiosteal dissection medially on the proximal tibia is performed to release the deep medial capsule, deep MCL back to the mid-coronal plane (note this release is significantly less for valgus knees).

> Note this is done in flexion with 90° Homan retractors protecting the collateral ligaments.

Next, using a *measured resection* technique we prepare the femur. Using an intramedullary guide, the distal femur cut is made either in 5° of valgus or 4° of valgus (for a valgus knee). The thickness of this cut is 9 mm for our system. Following this and using a *posterior referencing* system, the femur is sized and rotation is set to be parallel to the transepicondylar axis and perpendicular to Whiteside's axis (◘ Fig. 19.3). The order of these cuts is anterior, posterior, posterior chamfers, anterior chamfers. The box cut is made using the box-cut guide for a posterior stabilized knee system (◘ Fig. 19.4). After all the femoral cuts are made, the tibia is then subluxed forward with a posterior retractor. Medial and lateral 90° Homan retractors protect the collaterals.

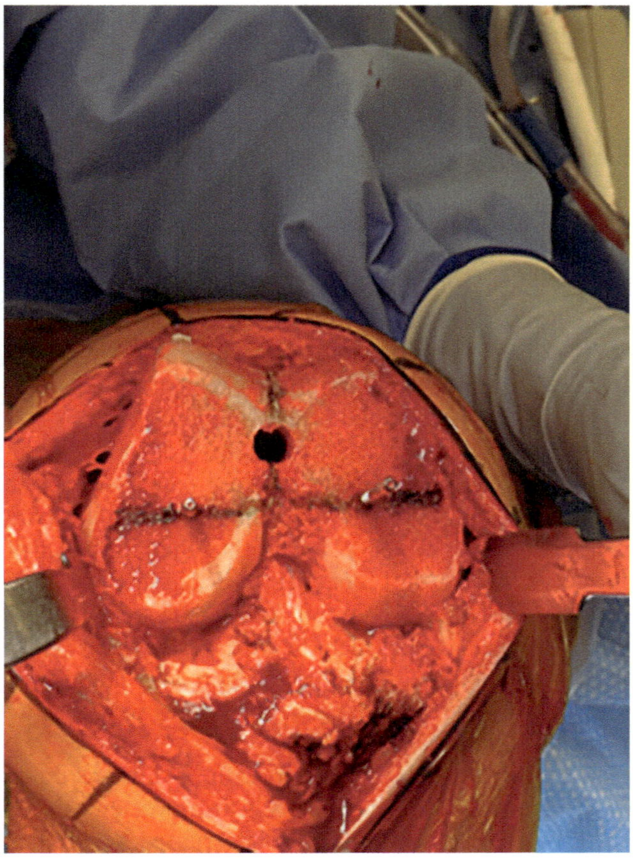

◘ Fig. 19.3 A bovie is used to mark out the Whiteside's (anteroposterior) and transepicondylar axis. Note these lines should be perpendicular to one another

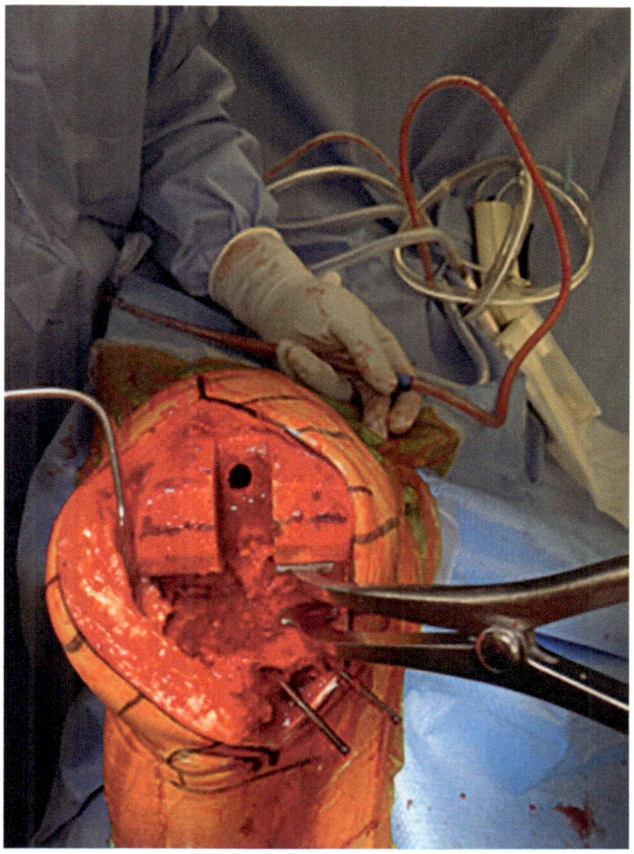

◘ Fig. 19.4 The box cut is made for a posterior stabilized femoral component. This will set the medial-lateral position of the femoral component, and in general a more lateral position optimizes patellar tracking

> Please ensure the lateral retractor is anterior to the midline of the tibia to protect the common peroneal nerve.

Next, using an extramedullary tibia guide set perpendicular to the mechanical axis of the tibia and in 3° of posterior slope, the tibia cut is made (◘ Fig. 19.5). This bony fragment and the medial and lateral menisci are removed (◘ Fig. 19.6). The knee is then brought to 90° of flexion and a laminar spreader is used to assess the flexion gap (◘ Fig. 19.7). Additionally, this allows access to the posterior compartment to remove osteophytes. A portion of our peri-articular joint cocktail is then infiltrated into the posterior medial capsule. Once adequate flexion balance is obtained the tibia is then

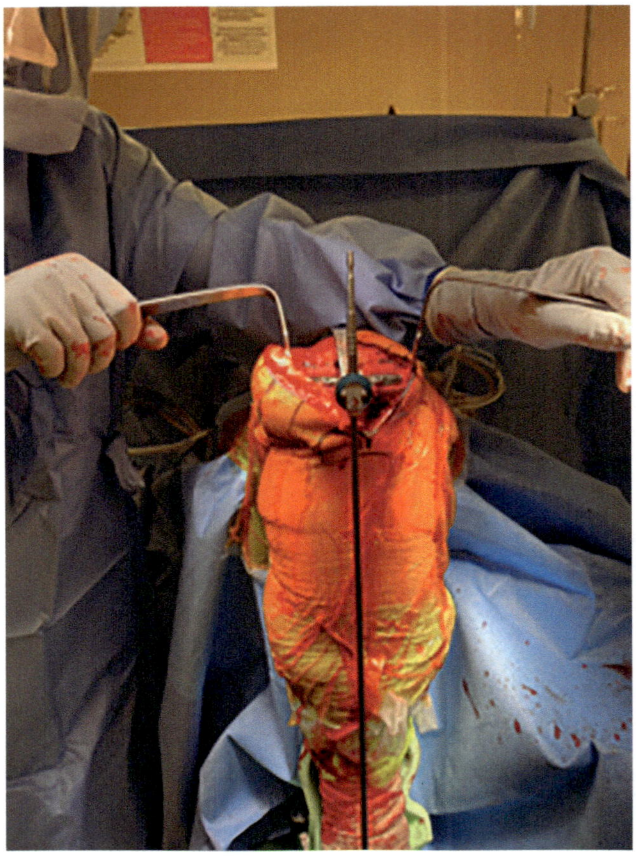

Fig. 19.5 An extramedullary guide is used to make the proximal tibial resection with attention placed on both coronal and sagittal alignment as well as depth of resection

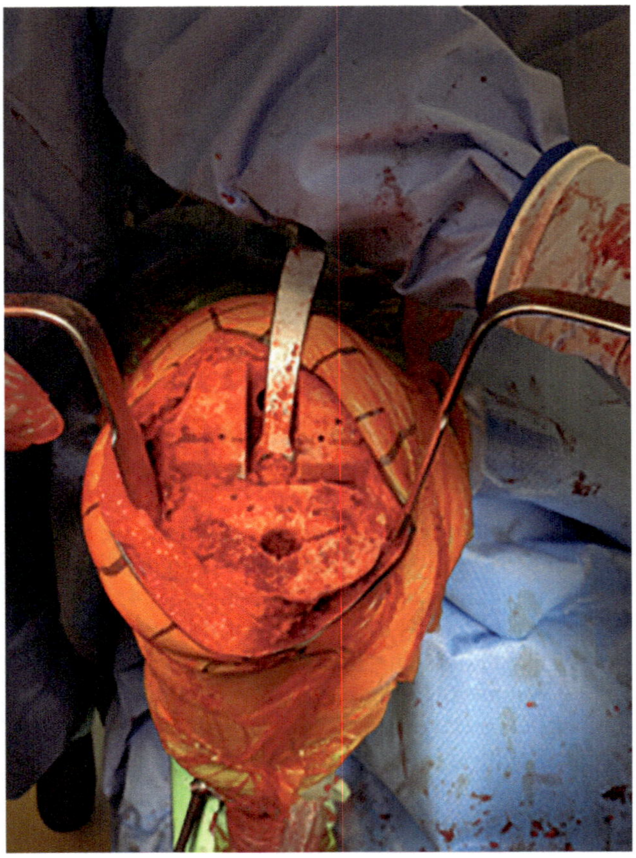

Fig. 19.6 After proximal tibial resection, the menisci are removed

sized and prepped. Rotational alignment of the tibia is set to the medial third of the tibial tubercle. At this point, trial implants are used to assess motion and stability in flexion and extension, varus and valgus instability. At this point, if stability is not adequate, further soft tissue releases are performed to obtain excellent stability. The patella is addressed last. The patella is everted and measured for composite thickness. The patellar cut is then made again using *measured resection*. This allows to prevent overstuffing the patellar femoral compartment.

> Ensure that a residual thickness of minimum 12 mm is left to protect against fracture.

At times I will accept slightly increased composite thickness if the cut necessary would leave less than 12 mm of residual thickness. All attempts are made not to change the initial thickness more than 20%. At this point, patellar tracking is checked with trials in place. This is done with a freehand technique.

Once the correct component size is set, balance has been determined and trialed, all trial implantsare removed. The bony surfaces are copiously irrigated with a pulse lavage and sterile saline (Fig. 19.8). The cement is prepared in standard vacuum environment and I use a medium-viscosity cement which has been prewarmed to speed curing time. We first cement the tibial component (Figs. 19.9 and 19.10) and then cement the femoral component (Figs. 19.11 and 19.12), inset the formal polyethylene and fully extend the knee while the patellar button is cemented. All excess cement is removed in standard fashion.

During cement curing, I place the foot on my stomach and apply a constant pressure. I feel this helps to prevent the slight changes that can occur during expansion of a curing cement. During this, the remainder of the peri-articular joint cocktail is placed in the synovium, medial/lateral periosteum of the femur, retropatellar area, and medial tibia including the pes complex. Once fully cured a final range of motion and stability is checked to ensure no changes. The knee is brought into flexion for closure.

The arthrotomy is closed with a unidirectional barbed suture (number 1). This is also oversewn at the same time by an assistant with interrupted #1 braided suture in figure-of-eight fashion. The subcutaneous tissues are closed with a 2.0 buried monocryl and the skin is approximated with standard skin staples. The dressing

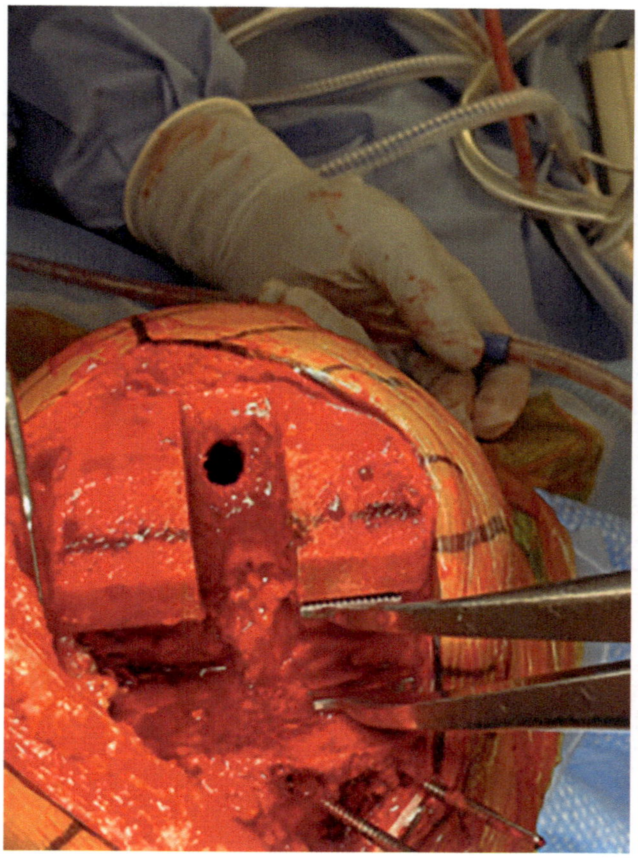

Fig. 19.7 The flexion gap is assessed using a laminar spreader. Ideally, if the bones have been resected appropriately, this will create a rectangle that will accept at least the minimum composite thickness of the tibial tray and smallest insert

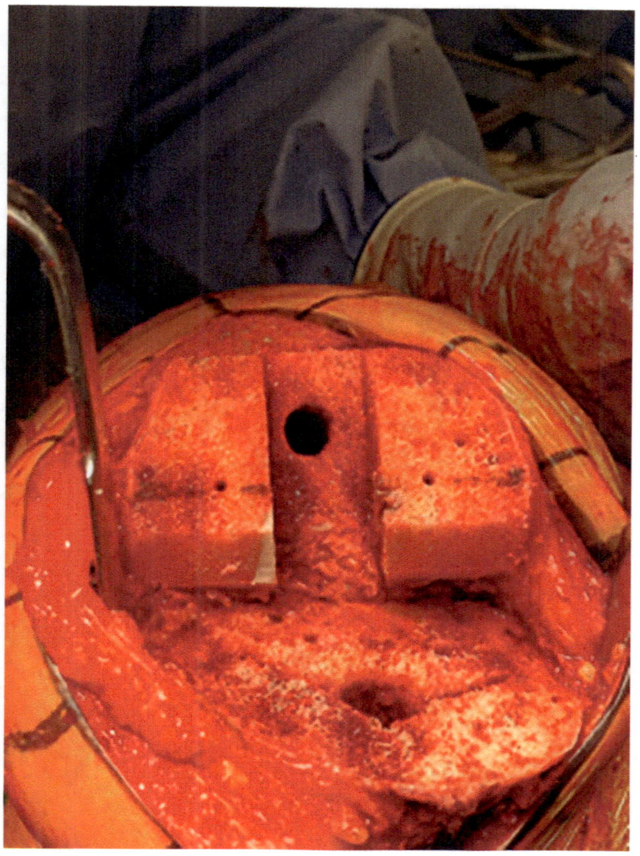

Fig. 19.8 The bony surfaces are irrigated clean of all blood and bone marrow to maximize cement interdigitation

consisted of adaptic, gauze, cast padding, and a bias wrap from ankle to mid-thigh. This allows some mild compression.

19.4 Gap Balancing Versus Measured Resection

When treating patients with end-stage knee OA the goal is to get patients to return to activities that their arthritis has been preventing them from participating in. Over time TKA engineers have modified the materials and designs of TKA to achieve this goal with the hopes to achieve stable knee implants with full flexion and extension. Two approaches for the implementation of TKA implants, *gap balancing* and *measured resection*, have been developed and popularized to achieve soft-tissue balance along with implant alignment, size, and rotation in hopes to help patients achieve their goals. While many surgeons will say they use one or the other, most surgeons actually will fall somewhere in the middle of the two methodologies. Surgeons have started using more of a hybrid technique in hopes to avoid the individual pitfalls of each specific technique (Sheth et al. 2017).

19.4.1 Gap Balancing

Gap balancing is a technique using the tension of the soft tissue to make bony cuts with the goal to have symmetric, rectangular flexion, and extension gaps. Making the assumption that the soft tissue tension of the patient's knee is "normal" and "un-altered", the goal is to cut the femur parallel to the tibial cut. This relies on a precise tibia cut which is typically perpendicular to the anatomic and mechanical axis of the tibia. The initial tibial cut acts as the foundation for soft tissue tensioning which allows one to place the guide for the posterior and distal femoral cuts. Before any femoral cut is made all tensioning is completed, including posterior osteophyte removal and soft tissue releases (Jaffe et al. 2018).

When using gap balancing for TKA implantation you want to have symmetric tension of the soft tissues in extension before setting femoral rotation and creating your flexion gap. Once extension tensioning is achieved with soft tissue release and osteophyte removal; the

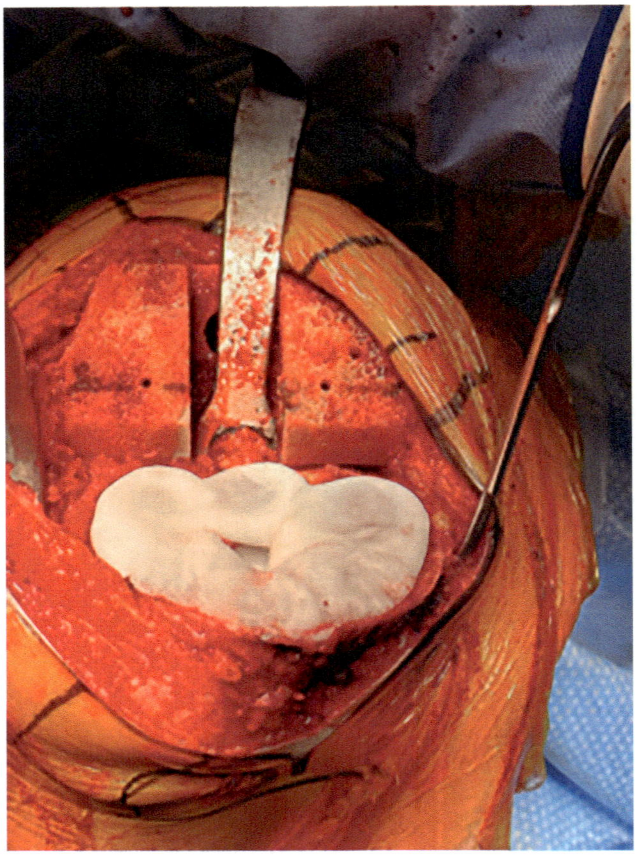

Fig. 19.9 First, cement is applied to the proximal tibia w/ finger packing of the tibial keel. It is important to avoid blood and cement on this surface

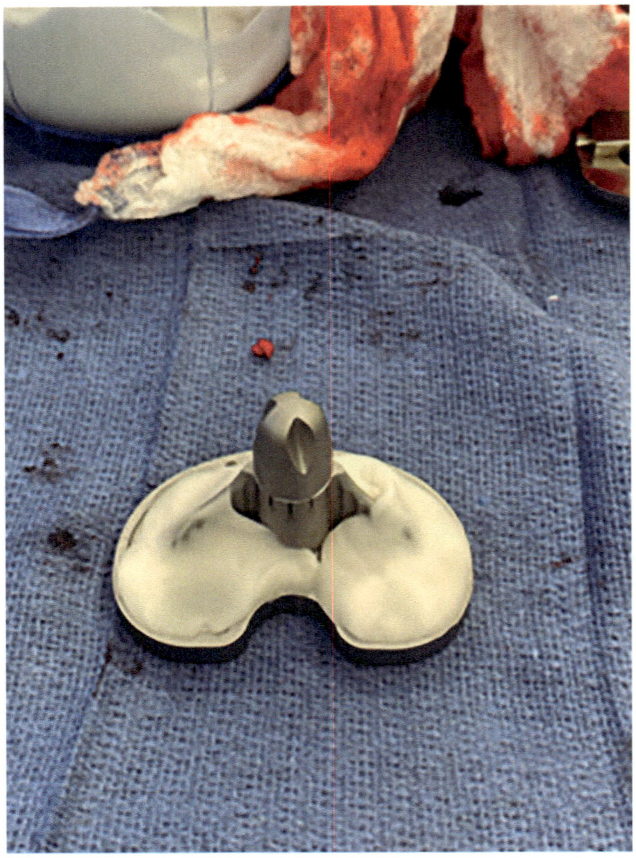

Fig. 19.10 Cement is applied to the undersurface of the tibial component to improve cement-to-cement bond and avoid fat interposition

proximal tibia and distal femur cut can be made using the tibia and femur mechanical axis as your guide. This allows you to make the proximal tibia and distal femur cuts and then using soft tissue releases to create a balanced extension gap (Sheth et al. 2017). Next, you set the femoral rotation and flexion gap by balancing the soft tissue in 90° of flexion using laminal spreaders or a system-specific soft tissue tensioner device to assist in measuring the posterior femoral condyle cut and distal femur rotation. This creates a rectangle with the bone removed from your posterior femoral condyles. Gap balancing and soft tissue tensioning will ideally restore the anatomic rotation of the knee and make balanced flexion and extension gaps.

As with measured resection, gap balancing is not perfect. The gap balancing technique has been criticized for incorrect condylar offset, and impingement leading to diminished knee flexion (Sheth et al. 2017).

While attempting to balance the flexion and extension gaps surgeons can incidentally raise the joint line, or alter the anatomic femoral rotation, which can lead to instability to mid-range motion (Sheth et al. 2017; Babazadeh et al. 2014; Lee et al. 2010; Martin and Whiteside 1990; Tigani et al. 2010). Elevation of the joint line in gap balancing technique occurs when the surgeon is attempting to balance the extension gap and will resect more distal femur and then insert a bigger implant in hopes to improve the extension gap tension. Mid-flexion instability occurs with an elevated joint line because of an altered patella femoral mechanics. Additionally, surgeons can sacrifice femoral rotation for balanced flexion gaps which will lead to internal rotation of the distal femur and mal-tracking of the patella, increasing the risk of patella fracture and other complications (Sheth et al. 2017).

Making any alteration to the soft tissue tension, including removing osteophytes, releasing IT band and popliteus, does not alter the flexion and extension gaps symmetrically. Also, anything done after the femoral cuts can ultimately affect final balancing of the knee and riskinstability.

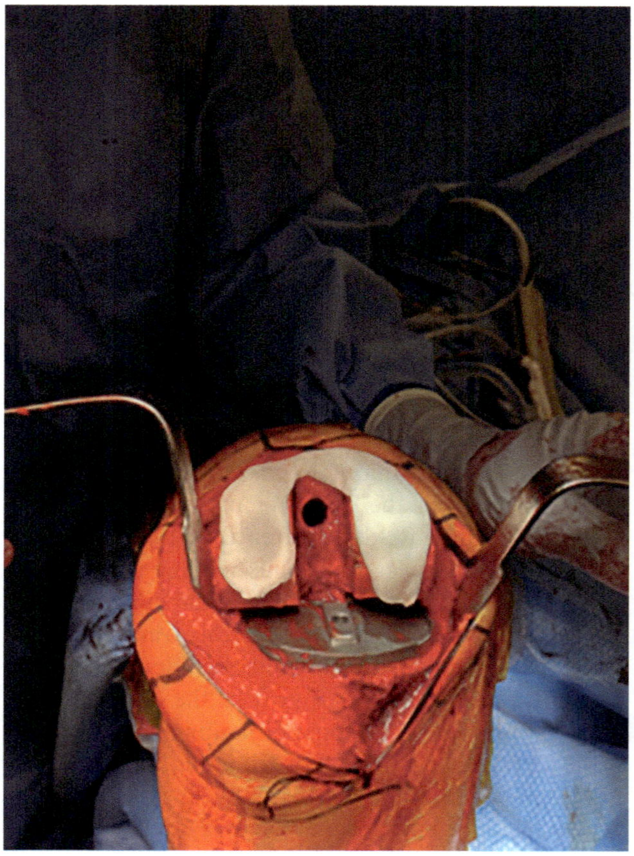

Fig. 19.11 A horseshoe-shaped layer of cement is placed on distal and anterior femoral surfaces. Note, cement is not applied to the posterior condylar surfaces so as to avoid excess posterior cement, which is more difficult to remove

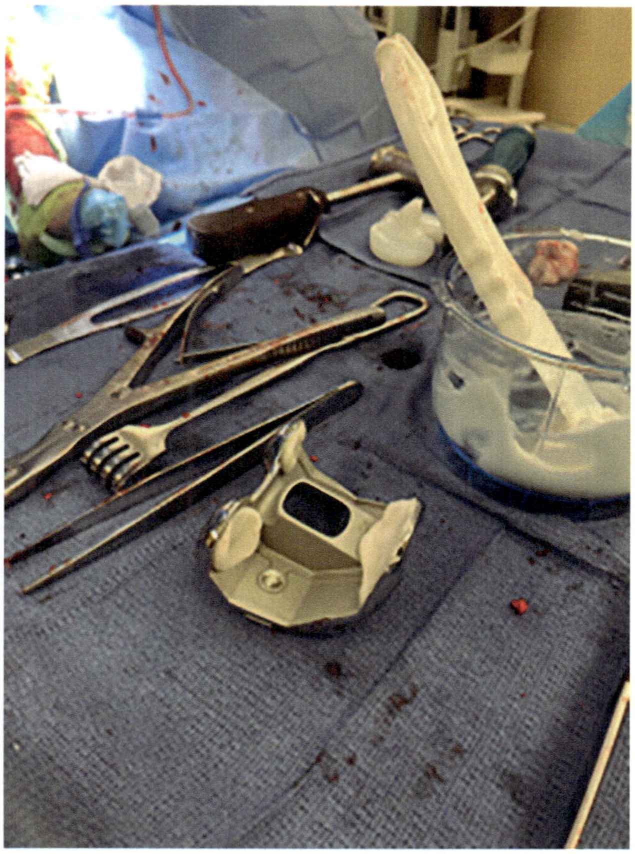

Fig. 19.12 Cement is applied to the anterior and posterior surfaces of the femoral component. This helps prevent cement–bone interface gaps anteriorly and minimizes the occurrence of excess cement posteriorly

19.4.2 Measured Resection

On the other hand, the goals of the measured resection technique are to replace the amount of bone resected with an equal thickness of prosthesis implanted and use anatomic landmarks to determine appropriate component position and rotation (Sheth et al. 2017). This technique relies on the ability of the surgeon to appropriately identify anatomic landmarks and size the implants. Measured resection allows for maintenance of the joint line, restoration of posterior condylar offset, and optimization of knee kinematics (Sheth et al. 2017). Using measured resection, the surgeon must rely on anatomic landmarks including the transepicondylar axis (TEA), the AP axis (Whiteside's line), and the posterior condylar axis to set the correct femoral rotation. When correctly identified, this technique allows for maintenance of the joint line, neutral femoral rotation, and appropriate flexion–extension gaps.

> Similar to gap balancing, measured resection has been criticized for some of the pitfalls associated with the technique, most notably relying on the anatomic landmarks for setting rotation of the femoral component (Sheth et al. 2017).

Given the wide range of femoral anatomy between patients, this results in a wide range of femoral component final rotation. In addition to variability of the anatomy, critics point out the poor interobserver reliability to correctly identify the anatomy (Sheth et al. 2017).

The TEA is traditionally described as the line connecting the prominence of the lateral epicondyle to the sulcus of the medial epicondyle (Sheth et al. 2017) and is thought to be the most reliable landmark for assessing the femoral rotation (Sheth et al. 2017; Jaffe et al. 2018). Intraoperatively the TEA is not easily identified, or reproducible, most notably difficulty identifying the medial epicondylar sulcus, where the MCL originates from (Sheth et al. 2017; Jaffe et al. 2018), and proper identification may require more soft tissue dissection. Whiteside's line has been described as the AP axis and is a line starting anterior at the trochlear sulcus and runs posterior through the deepest part of the trochlea to the midpoint of the intercondylar notch. In studies, the AP axis has been shown to be a more consistent predictor of the patient's natural external rotation than the PCA (Jaffe et al. 2018; Arima et al. 1995). Lastly, and according to critics as the least reliable landmark is the posterior condylar axis, connecting the posterior aspects of the femoral condyles. Traditionally the TEA and Whiteside's lines are perpendicular and the posterior condylar axis is thought to be 3–6° of internal rotation in relation to the TEA (Sheth et al. 2017; Jaffe et al. 2018).

When placing the femoral guides using the measured resection technique, the guide can be anterior- or posterior-referenced. With *anterior referencing* the surgeon will fix the guide to the anterior femur to ensure that femoral component sizing changes will not remove any additional anterior bone, while a differential amount of bone is cut from the posterior femoral condyles, which can affect the flexion gap. *Posterior referencing* sets the posterior femoral condyle cut with the jig pinned in place, and sizing changes take more or less bone from the anterior femur which could lead to notching and the risk of stress-riser fracture or overstuffing the patellofemoral joint, respectively (Jaffe et al. 2018).

Finally, proponents of gap balancing have pointed out the difficulty of adequate ability to perform soft tissue release to balance the flexion and extension gaps which can lead to coronal instability, and variability of the bony anatomy and difficulty identifying landmarks can lead to internal rotation of the femoral components which effectively lateralize the patella tracking.

19.4.3 Comparison of Outcomes

> At this time, there is no clear conclusion on which technique provides better patient outcomes.

In one study looking at TKA in patients who had both knees replaced, one using gap balancing and the other measured resection had no difference on 2-year outcomes (Tapasvi et al. 2020). Another study looked at prosthesis survivorship, patient outcomes, and complications, and in 214 patients both techniques provided excellent survivorship at 3 years along with excellent patient outcomes (Churchill et al. 2018).

19

19.5 Mechanical Versus Kinematic Alignment

While the type of implant and surgical approach is important to the surgery, so is the way the surgeon decides to ensure proper alignment of the knee after implantation to restore function and prevent eccentric wear on the implant leading to better surgical outcomes. Mechanical and Kinematic (anatomic) alignment are the two main ways surgeons have approached TKA alignment.

19.5.1 Mechanical Alignment

> Mechanical alignment in TKA is based on the thought that restoring the normal mechanical alignment will provide better outcomes.

To do this the surgeon will make the bone cuts in the femur and tibia perpendicular to the mechanical axis and parallel to each other removing the 3° of valgus and varus, respectively. The femur is cut with an intramedullary guide using the anatomic axis as a reference and the guide is set to cut the distal femur, an angle (usually 3–6°) that represents the difference of the mechanical and anatomic axis on plain films making a cut that is perpendicular to this axis. On the other side, the tibia's mechanical and anatomic axis are the same. The tibial cut is made using an extramedullary guide placed in the anatomic/mechanical axis and then the cut is perpendicular to this axis. The hopes of making the cuts parallel is to produce equal load distribution across the new joint line (Schiraldi et al. 2016). While making the tibial cut perpendicular to this axis there is a worry that this will remove too much lateral tibia and cause laxity which is managed with soft tissue balancing.

19.5.2 Kinematic Alignment

> Surgeons utilizing kinematic alignment,on the other hand, focus on restoring the anatomic alignment of the knee unlike in the mechanical axis approach.

So instead of femur and tibial bone cuts that ignore the anatomic access, these surgeons focus on recreating the 3° of femoral valgus and 3° of tibial varus in the hope to create a more balance knee throughout the entire arc of motion (Schiraldi et al. 2016).

19.5.3 Comparison of Outcomes

When historically looking at postoperative TKA alignment the literature supports the notion that greater than 3° of tibial varus leads to rapid failure due to implant wear, loosening, and decreased function (Schiraldi et al. 2016; Lad et al. 2013). Additionally, studies have shown that in 70–80% of patients we were successful in placing the final implants with less than 3° of error in the coronal plan thus placing a fair amount of patients at risk for rapid failure and less functioning implants (Lad et al. 2013).

Postoperatively, patients with less tibial varus had higher Knee Society scores than patients with more varus (Schiraldi et al. 2016). Schiraldi et al. began to look at long-term follow-up of these patients and found that those who had mechanical alignment with <3° of variation compared to those with >3° of variation from the mechanical axis had no statistically different 15-year implant survival rate, or revision rates when coronal plane alignment was used to compare groups (Schiraldi et al. 2016; Hadi et al. 2015). When Dossett et al. preformed a randomized control trial using kinematic and mechanical alignment as the two groups they found that patients randomized to the patient-specific kinematic group reported better pain relief, and better restoration of function than mechanically aligned TKA (Dossett et al. 2014). They reported the kinematically aligned group had WOMAC score 16 points higher ($p < .000$) and KSS 25 points better ($P = .001$) (Dossett et al. 2014). Additionally, Howell et al. found no difference in Oxford Knee scores and WOMAC scores in patients with kinematic-aligned knees regardless of their postoperative varus or valgus alignment (Howell et al. 2013).

While mechanical alignment is still the gold standard; many of the mentioned studies show promising results coming from small data cohorts and radiographic reporting of malalignment with noted observer bias. When the bias was removed, only one known study was found to have shown that worsening malalignment increased the risk of revisions (Hadi et al. 2015).

At this time, more studies on larger scales will need to be conducted as both methods have shown in recent literature to have successful outcomes and similar revision rates.

19.6 Unicompartmental, Bicompartmental, and Tricompartmental Knee Arthroplasty

While the TKA design was developed for tricompartmental OA treatment for patients who exhibited osteoarthritis in a single or two compartments, implants were developed as well. Traditionally, patients who were thought to be candidates for a unicompartmental knee arthroplasty (UKA) were patients with unicondylar osteoarthritis or osteonecrosis; frontal deformity <15°; flexion contracture <15°; functional integrity of the anterior cruciate ligament (ACL) and peripheral ligaments of the knee as well as the absence of inflammatory arthropathy (Vasso et al. 2018; Kim et al. 2018).

In a study of 106 cases of unicompartmental knee arthroplasty, evaluating the 10-year outcomes in patients <60 the implant survival rate was 89.3% when using all revision surgery as a failure with only 20 cases having documented complications (Kim et al. 2018). In addition, patients who underwent UKA in this study went from an average of 130.7° to 132.8° of ROM with a p-value of .045, and at the last follow-up 69.2% of patients reported Knee Society scores (KSS) of 85 or greater and an additional 26.4% with scores between 70 and 84 (Kim et al. 2018).

In the patients aged 80–89, one study found good outcomes for UKA for patients with tricompartmental OA (TCOA), with predominant medial compartment OA (MCOA) (Marya and Thukral 2013). Forty-five patients with TCOA and predominant MCOA underwent UKA with symptomatic relief and implant survival in 96.4% and 94.9% good or excellent outcomes (Marya and Thukral 2013). At 1-year follow-up the patients had an average of 115° of ROM, (100–125), KSS clinical scores improved from average of 46 (26–70) preoperatively to 81 (66–90) at the final follow-up. KSS functional scores improved from 24 (0–50) to 82 (55–90) (Marya and Thukral 2013).

In a meta-analysis comparing UKA to TKA, 60 studies were evaluated in patients with unicompartmental OA (Wilson et al. 2019). This study found both were viable options for these patients with higher venous thromboembolism and mortality rates with TKA, and higher revision rates with UKA (Wilson et al. 2019). There was a significant difference in hospital stay for UKA, but no significant difference in pain patient-reported outcome measures (PROM), but patients who underwent UKA reported significantly better functional PROMs than TKA patients, which included a combined score of consisting of the Oxford Knee score, Bristol Knee score, Western Ontario and McMaster Universities index, KSS, and Japanese Orthopaedic Association score (Wilson et al. 2019). In addition, they looked at 17 studies looking at the revision rate at 5 years and they found a risk ratio ranging from 1.29 to 5.95 with UKA requiring revision when compared to TKA. Again at 10 years, they evaluated 13 studies with similar results having UKA with higher revision rates and risk ratios ranging from .64 for 3.53, with 11/13 groups having higher rates of UKA revision (Wilson et al. 2019).

Isolated lateral compartment OA is much less common only compromising about 5–10% of people who have isolated unicompartmental OA. Lateral UKA has been preformed successfully in 98% of patients reporting return to recreational activities (Imarisio and Trecci 2017). Reported postoperative functional outcomes for lateral UKA have not been proven to be significantly different when compared to TKA for the same indications. Lateral UKA has been shown to have survivorship of around 96% at 10 years (Imarisio and Trecci 2017).

Bicompartmental Knee Arthroplasty (BKA) was also developed for patients with medial and patellofemoral compartmental OA. A study looking at a single-bicompartmental implant system used in 15 patients noted a 60% revision rate at 54-month follow-up (Dudhniwala et al. 2016). The study also found tibial component bone–cement interface radiolucency in 73.3% of patients and knee pain in 46.6% of patients at an average of 18 months postoperatively (Dudhniwala et al. 2016). BKA knee kinematic studies were also preformed and noted slower motor task cadence compared to control patients, and that overall knee joint kinematics following BKA replicate the knee kinematics in the non-operated contralateral limb (Leffler et al. 2012). Additionally, BKA was found to correct varus deformity in 130/137 patients (Rolston and Siewert 2009) with the mechanical axis passing through the center of the knee.

While, as shown in the current literature, in selected patient populations UKA can be a successful alternative which may decrease cost, hospitalization time, and shorten recovery time. There have not been many studies showing statistically significant clinical reported improved outcome scores for UKA or BKA when compared to TKA.

In addition, TKA has a lower revision rate at 5 and 10 years than UKA (Vasso et al. 2018; Kim et al. 2018; Marya and Thukral 2013; Wilson et al. 2019; Imarisio and Trecci 2017; Dudhniwala et al. 2016; Leffler et al. 2012; Rolston and Siewert 2009) and still is the gold standard for treating degenerative tricompartmental OA as anything less would not address the potential pain generator from arthritis in the unresurfaced compartment.

Take-Home Messages

- Today there are many options for the orthopedic surgeon to choose from with regard to TKA in a patient with primary knee OA.
- They have the options of implant design, surgical technique, and preoperative templating methods to provide the patient with improved ROM, function, and longevity of the implant.
- When looking at the literature there has been no significant difference with regard to outcomes or revision rates for gap balancing or measured resection, or with mechanical or kinematic alignment.
- When comparing UKA and BKA for knee OA, there have been some recent studies in the elderly population with tricompartmental OA; UKA for the medial compartment has been shown to provide some symptomatic relief with decreased morbidity related to the surgery but should not be used in younger active patients as this implant design does not address all the underlying pathology in these patients.

References

Arima J, Whiteside LA, McCarthy DS, White SE (1995) Femoral rotational alignment, based on the anteroposterior axis, in total knee arthroplasty in a valgus knee. A technical note. J Bone Joint Surg Am 77(9):1331–1334

Babazadeh S, Dowsey MM, Stoney JD, Choong PF (2014) Gap balancing sacrifices joint-line maintenance to improve gap symmetry: a randomized controlled trial comparing gap balancing and measured resection. J Arthroplast 29(5):950–954

Churchill JL, Khlopas A, Sultan AA, Harwin SF, Mont MA (2018) Gap-balancing versus measured resection technique in total knee arthroplasty: a comparison study. J Knee Surg 31(1):13–16

Dossett HG, Estrada NA, Swartz GJ, LeFevre GW, Kwasman BG (2014) A randomised controlled trial of kinematically and mechanically aligned total knee replacements: two-year clinical results. Bone Joint J 96-b(7):907–913

Dudhniwala AG, Rath NK, Joshy S, Forster MC, White SP (2016) Early failure with the Journey-Deuce bicompartmental knee arthroplasty. Eur J Orthop Surg Traumatol 26(5):517–521

Hadi M, Barlow T, Ahmed I, Dunbar M, McCulloch P, Griffin D (2015) Does malalignment affect revision rate in total knee replacements: a systematic review of the literature. Springerplus 4:835

Howell SM, Howell SJ, Kuznik KT, Cohen J, Hull ML (2013) Does a kinematically aligned total knee arthroplasty restore function without failure regardless of alignment category? Clin Orthop Relat Res 471(3):1000–1007

Imarisio D, Trecci A (2017) Lateral unicompartmental knee arthroplasty: a review of literature. Ann Joint 2:28.

Jaffe WL, Dundon JM, Camus T (2018) Alignment and balance methods in total knee arthroplasty. J Am Acad Orthop Surg 26(20):709–716

Kim KT, Lee S, Lee JS, Kang MS, Koo KH (2018) Long-term clinical results of unicompartmental knee arthroplasty in patients younger than 60 years of age: minimum 10-year follow-up. Knee Surg Relat Res 30(1):28–33

Lad DG, Thilak J, Thadi M (2013) Component alignment and functional outcome following computer assisted and jig based total knee arthroplasty. Indian J Orthop 47(1):77–82

Lee DH, Park JH, Song DI, Padhy D, Jeong WK, Han SB (2010) Accuracy of soft tissue balancing in TKA: comparison between navigation-assisted gap balancing and conventional measured resection. Knee Surg Sports Traumatol Arthrosc 18(3):381–387

Leffler J, Scheys L, Planté-Bordeneuve T, Callewaert B, Labey L, Bellemans J, Franz A (2012) Joint kinematics following bi-compartmental knee replacement during daily life motor tasks. Gait Posture 36(3):454–460

Martin JW, Whiteside LA (1990) The influence of joint line position on knee stability after condylar knee arthroplasty. Clin Orthop Relat Res 259:146–156

Marya SK, Thukral R (2013) Outcome of unicompartmental knee arthroplasty in octogenarians with tricompartmental osteoarthritis: a longer followup of previously published report. Indian J Orthop 47(5):459–468

Rolston L, Siewert K (2009) Assessment of knee alignment after bicompartmental knee arthroplasty. J Arthroplast 24(7):1111–1114

Schiraldi M, Bonzanini G, Chirillo D, de Tullio V (2016) Mechanical and kinematic alignment in total knee arthroplasty. Ann Translat Med 4(7):130–130

Sheth NP, Husain A, Nelson CL (2017) Surgical techniques for total knee arthroplasty: measured resection, gap balancing, and hybrid. J Am Acad Orthop Surg 25(7):499–508

Tapasvi SR, Shekhar A, Patil SS, Dipane MV, Chowdhry M, McPherson EJ (2020) Comparison of gap balancing vs measured resection technique in patients undergoing simultaneous bilateral total knee arthroplasty: one technique per knee. J Arthroplast 35(3):732–740
Tigani D, Sabbioni G, Ben Ayad R, Filanti M, Rani N, Del Piccolo N (2010) Comparison between two computer-assisted total knee arthroplasty: gap-balancing versus measured resection technique. Knee Surg Sports Traumatol Arthrosc 18(10):1304–1310
Vasso M, Antoniadis A, Helmy N (2018) Update on unicompartmental knee arthroplasty: current indications and failure modes. EFORT Open Rev 3(8):442–448
Wilson HA, Middleton R, Abram SGF, Smith S, Alvand A, Jackson WF, Bottomley N, Hopewell S, Price AJ (2019) Patient relevant outcomes of unicompartmental versus total knee replacement: systematic review and meta-analysis. BMJ 364:l352

Patellar Resurfacing in Cemented Total Knee Arthroplasty

Sachin Allahabadi and Derek Ward

Contents

E. Hansen, K.-D. Kühn (eds.), *Essentials of Cemented Knee Arthroplasty*,
https://doi.org/10.1007/978-3-662-63113-3_20

20.1 Introduction

Patellar resurfacing in total knee arthroplasty (TKA) continues to be an area of controversy in modern orthopedics and is an important consideration for the arthroplasty surgeon. Multiple studies have shown similar outcomes for patients with and without resurfacing but with increased revision rates for unresurfaced patellae. Complications associated with patellar resurfacing, although rare, can be devastating. Technique is critical for successful resurfacing and surgeons should carefully consider their chosen method.

20.2 Case Example and Surgical Technique

The patient is a 67-year-old female presenting with knee pain refractory to conservative management and radiographs showing medial and patellofemoral osteoarthritis with varus alignment (◘ Figs. 20.1, 20.2, and 20.3). A standard total knee replacement is undertaken with postoperative radiographs shown in ◘ Figs. 20.4, 20.5, and 20.6.

The authors' *preferred surgical technique* for the patella is as follows:

- The patella is everted (◘ Fig. 20.7) and measured using a caliper (◘ Fig. 20.8). The starting thickness (with assumptions made for cartilage loss and knowledge of the implant thickness options) will determine the appropriate resection depth to adequately restore the patella thickness. Care must be taken not to leave the patella too thin and risk fracture or too thick and risk over-stuffing the joint.
- The resection is made freehand with the patella everted and stabilized. A relatively short, wide, and flexible saw blade allows for good control.
- The resected piece and remaining patella (◘ Fig. 20.9) are checked for an even resection and appropriate thickness.
- The patella is then measured and a trial placed. Once adequate tracking is tested, the button is drilled. To optimize tracking, the button may be placed in a superomedial position without overhang. The residual lateral facet may be resected back with a rongeur or burr. Optimally, the patella should be centrally tracking without subluxation or impingement throughout range of motion.
- During cementing, the bone is thoroughly washed and dried and cement is manually pressurized into the lug holes (◘ Fig. 20.10).
- The patella is then clamped and the excess cement removed. The cement is allowed to fully harden before the clamp is removed (◘ Fig. 20.11).

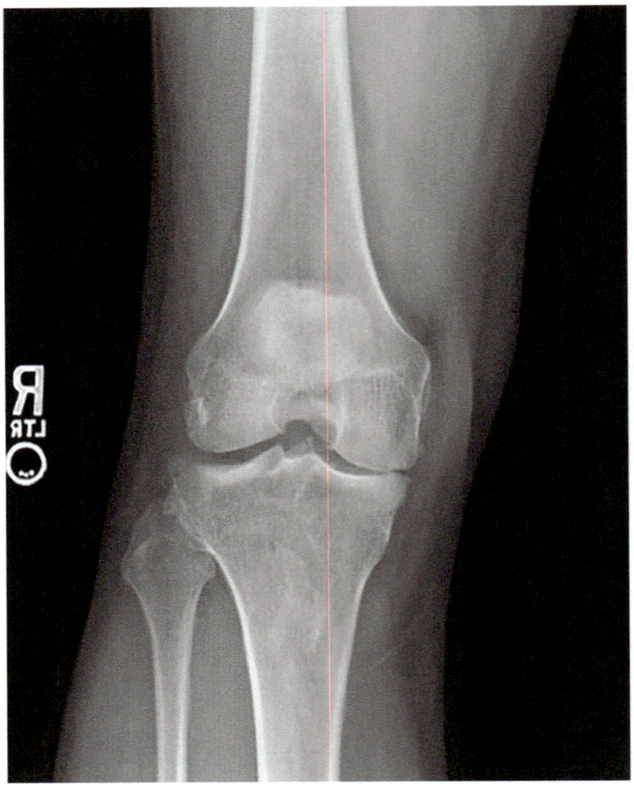

◘ **Fig. 20.1** Anteroposterior radiograph of the right knee demonstrating medial more than lateral tibiofemoral compartment degenerative changes, including subchondral sclerosis, joint space narrowing, and osteophytosis

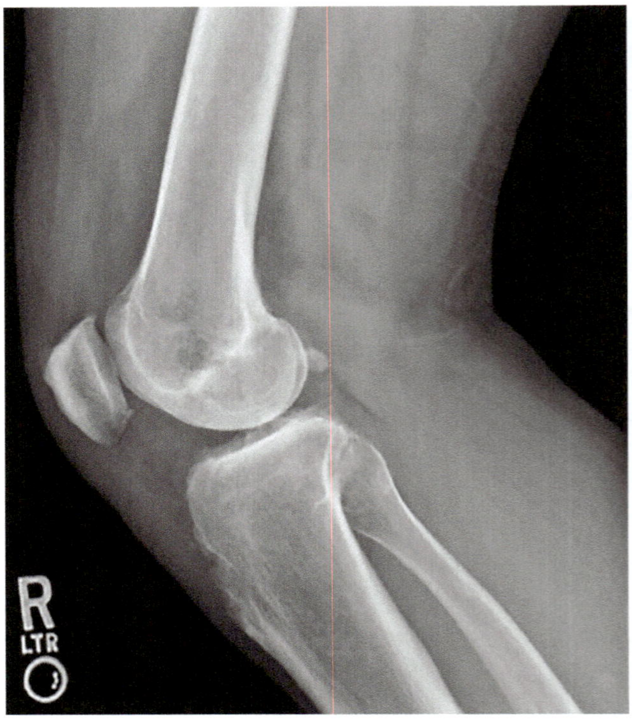

◘ **Fig. 20.2** Lateral radiograph of the right knee demonstrating joint space narrowing in patellofemoral and tibiofemoral compartments with patellar osteophytes and subchondral sclerosis

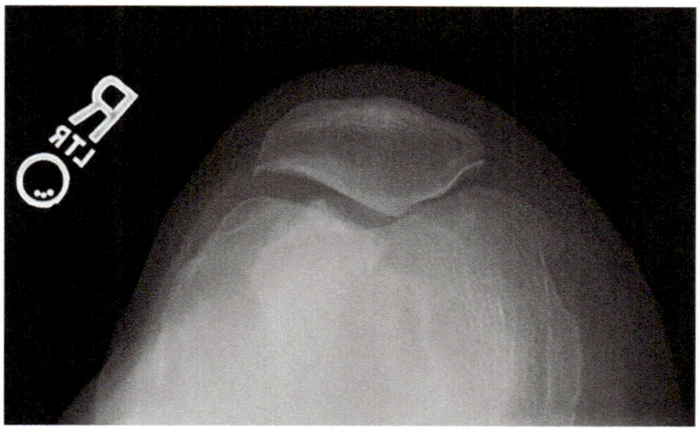

Fig. 20.3 Patellofemoral radiograph of the right knee demonstrating patellofemoral compartment joint space narrowing and osteophytosis

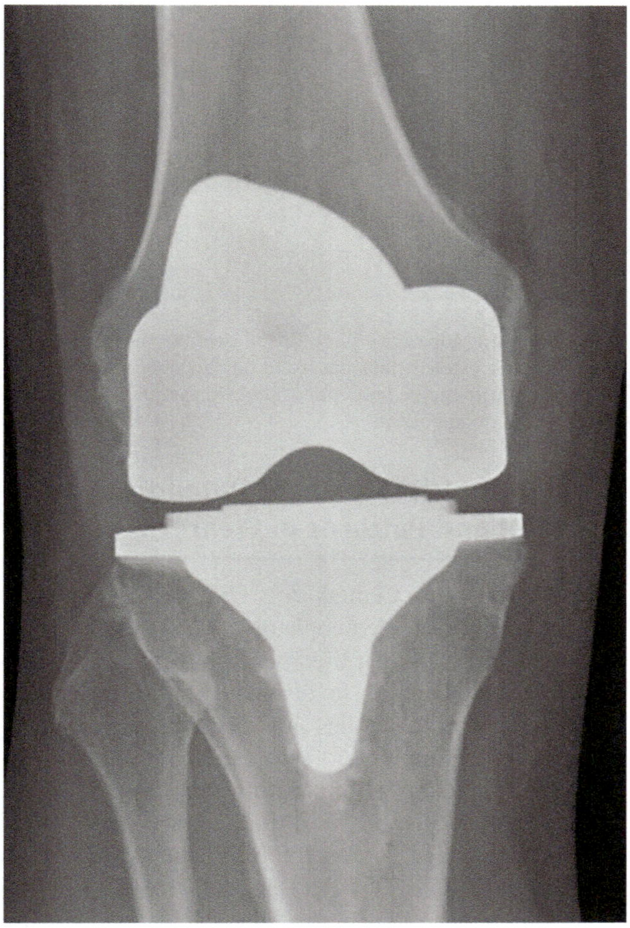

Fig. 20.4 Anteroposterior radiograph of the right knee demonstrating a cemented total knee arthroplasty of appropriate size without lateral overhang, appropriate mechanical alignment, and without loosening

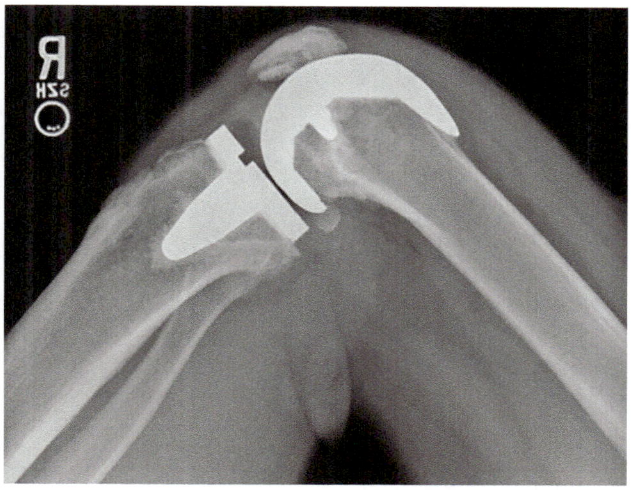

Fig. 20.5 Lateral bent knee radiograph of the right knee demonstrating a cemented cruciate-retaining total knee arthroplasty design of appropriate size without anteroposterior overhang with a cemented resurfaced patella

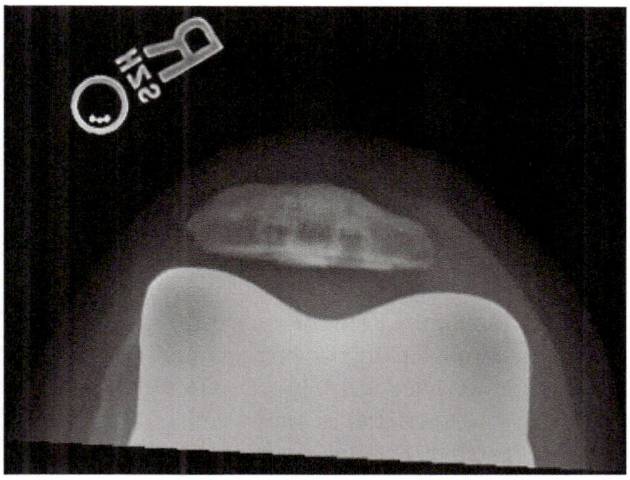

Fig. 20.6 Patellofemoral radiograph of the right knee demonstrating a cemented total knee arthroplasty with a resurfaced patellar component

20.3 History of Controversy

Patellar resurfacing has been controversial since the genesis of modern TKA. In 1986, John Insall published a series of 27 knee replacements from 1974 to 1980 where the patella was not resurfaced (Soudry et al. 1986). The study noted very similar outcomes for those patients compared with 100 patients with resurfaced patellae,

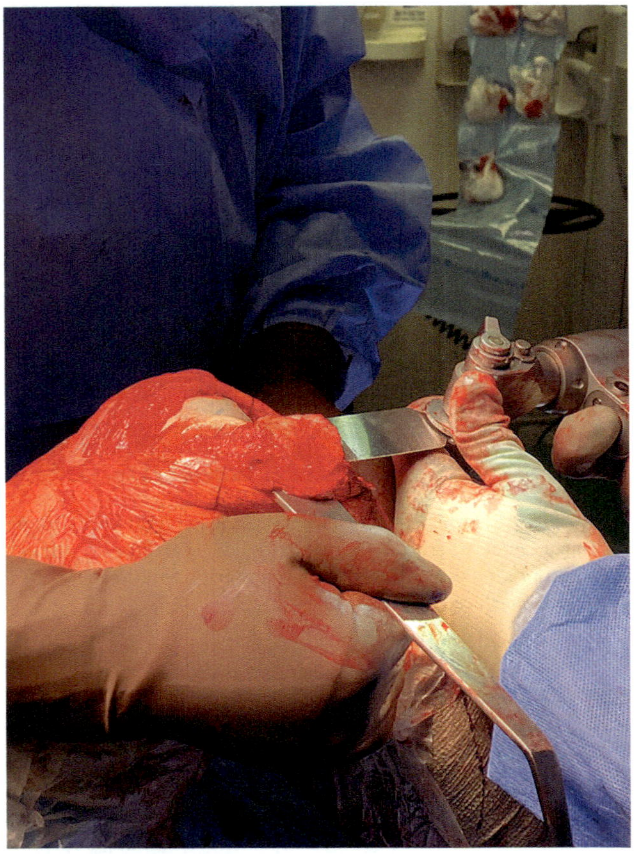

Fig. 20.7 Intraoperative photo demonstrating an everted patella. The patella must first be everted prior to resurfacing. Full visualization is important to avoid damage to the extensor mechanism

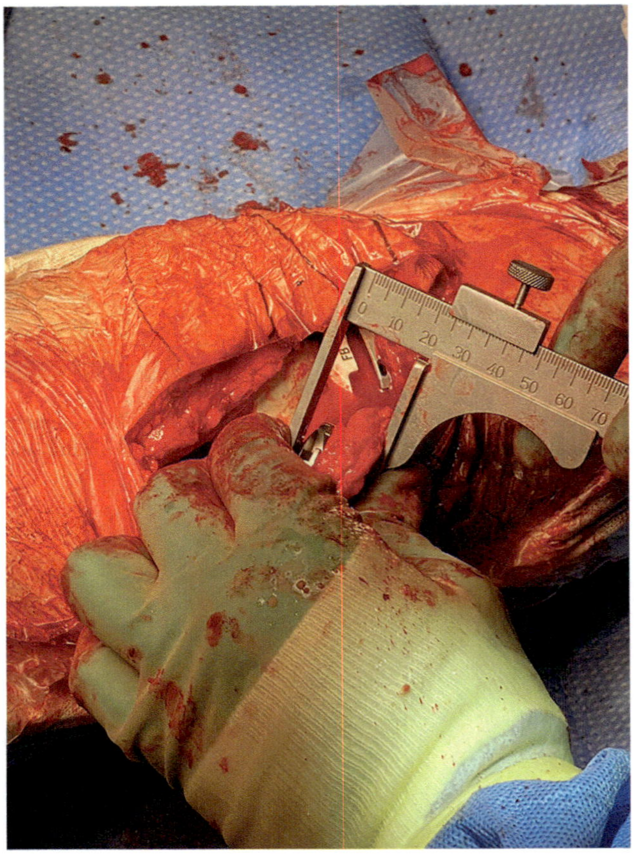

Fig. 20.8 Intraoperative photo demonstrating measurement of pre-resurfacing patellar thickness using calipers. Knowing the starting thickness helps guide the depth of resection as guided by the specific patellar implant design

thus questioning the need for resurfacing. This controversy has continued to the present day with rates of resurfacing varying widely (11–76%) in registry studies. Currently, multiple studies show similar outcomes in cases of patellar resurfacing versus non-resurfacing; however, the incidence of reoperation is consistently higher in patients without resurfacing. This may be largely due to the fact that an unresurfaced patella allows for a surgical option for anterior knee pain after total knee replacement, despite the fact that only half of the patients had an improvement of symptoms after secondary resurfacing (Parvizi et al. 2012). Although the risks of reoperation are higher for patients without patellar resurfacing, the complications associated with resurfacing can be devastating, particularly that of patellar fracture with concomitant extensor mechanism disruption.

> Given the excellent outcomes possible with and without resurfacing, thoughtful consideration should be employed when deciding the fate of the patella.

20.4 Natural History of the Patellofemoral Joint and Patterns of Wear

According to the Centers for Disease Control and Prevention, half of the people (46%) will develop painful knee arthritis in their lifetime, with varying wear patterns. Compartmental involvement of osteoarthritis vary in population studies, however, the incidence of isolated, radiographic tibiofemoral arthritis was as high as 23% in the Framingham study population with a combined patellofemoral and tibiofemoral incidence of 19.3% (the isolated patellofemoral incidence was 5.3%) (McAlindon et al. 1996). Another study by McAlindon et al. found that isolated medial compartment disease occurred in 21% of men and 12% of women in a cohort of 513 patients, while combined medial and patellofemoral disease occurred in 7% of men and 6% of women (McAlindon et al. 1992). Based on these studies, it appears that the patellofemoral joint may be spared in a significant portion of arthritic population.

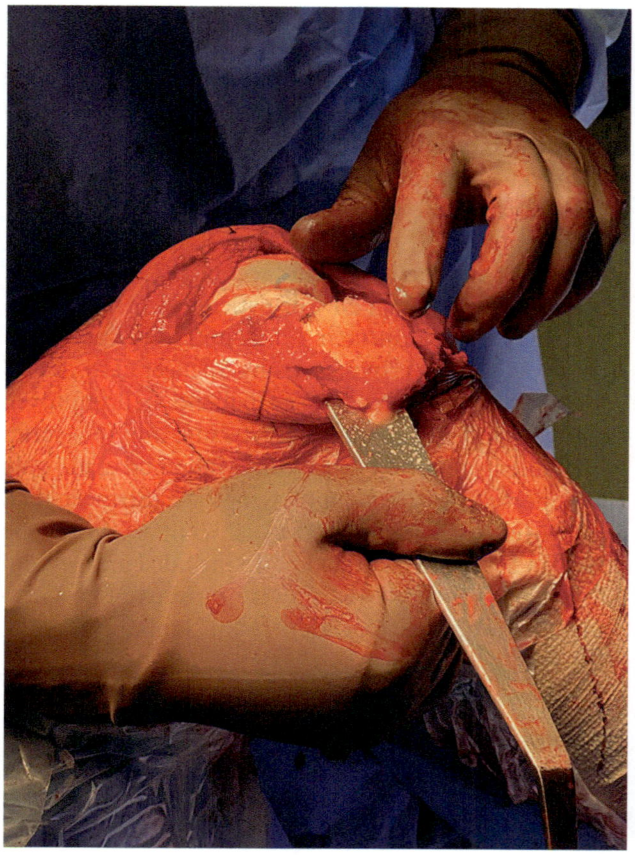

Fig. 20.9 Intraoperative photo demonstrating the patellar articular surface after resection with a thin saw blade using freehand technique. The articular cartilage has been removed with the cut depth. After resection, thickness of the patella should be remeasured to evaluate the symmetry of the cut and to gauge if additional resection is necessary or if too much resection was performed

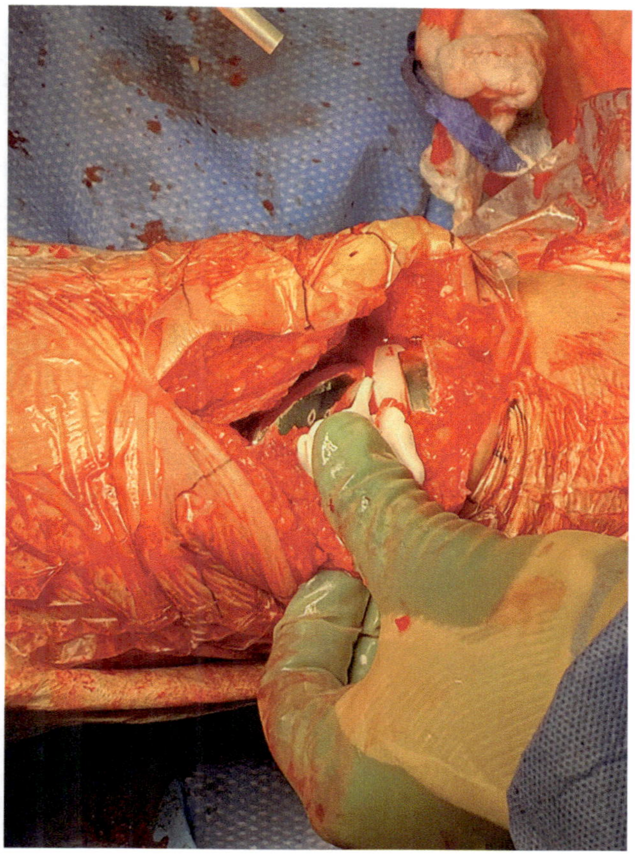

Fig. 20.10 Intraoperative photo demonstrating cement application onto the previously cut patella. The cement is manually applied to the patellar surface and pressurized into the previously drilled lug holes

20.5 Indications for Resurfacing or Not Resurfacing

There are certain populations for whom patellar resurfacing is generally indicated. Inflammatory arthritis is often reported as an indication to resurface the patella, however, this is not universally the case for all surgeons. Certain studies have shown that obese patients have an increased rate of patellofemoral pain after TKA and a higher rate of patellofemoral complications have been reported with increased weight in unresurfaced patellae (Wood et al. 2002; Berend et al. 2007). The ideal BMI or weight is not known as an absolute indication for patella resurfacing, but these factors should likely be an integral part of surgical decision-making.

The degree of patellofemoral arthritis present is an important component of selective resurfacing with the greater degree of arthritis warranting resurfacing. In a prospective, randomized study of 500 TKAs, patients with Outerbridge grade IV arthritis had a significantly higher secondary resurfacing rate, whereas patients with grade I to III arthritis had a very low rate of revision surgery (Rodríguez-Merchán and Gómez-Cardero 2010).

Given the suggestion of lower durability of resurfaced patellae in the literature, younger patients may be considered for patella retention (Robertsson et al. 2000). Tracking and congruency are important issues as well and if the unresurfaced patella does not track well (despite appropriate component rotation) or is not congruent with the chosen prosthesis, then resurfacing should be considered. If the patella is too thin to be safely resurfaced the surgeon should consider retention, although there is no clear agreement as to the specific thickness required for resurfacing.

The literature has classically described 12 mm or less of remaining bone as a risk factor for periprosthetic fracture, however, this has been disputed (Koh et al. 2002; Lie et al. 2005). Some authors describe the change in thickness or amount of bony resection as a risk factor for fracture, with one retrospective analysis with a fracture group having a change in thickness of −0.5 mm compared to the non-fracture group of +1.05 mm and bony resection greater in the fracture group (average

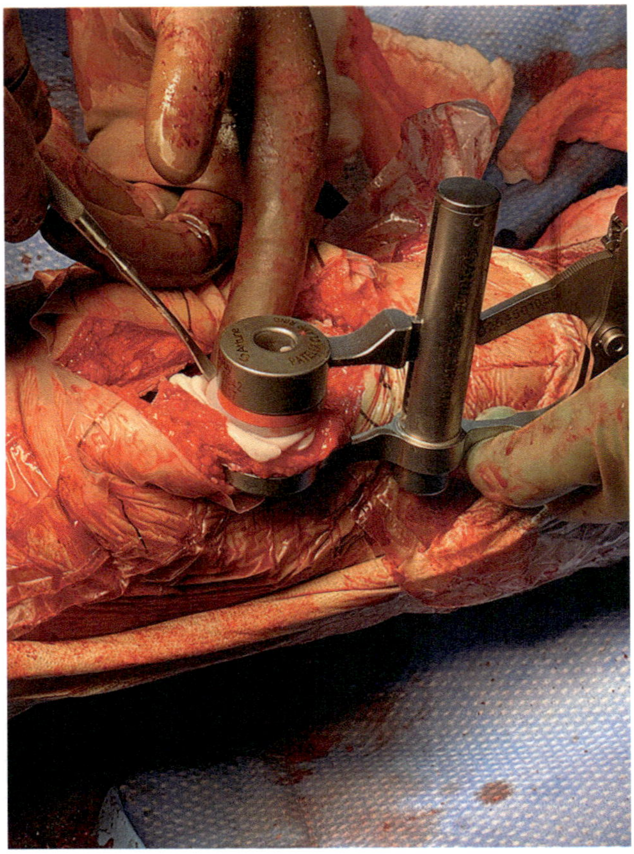

Fig. 20.11 Intraoperative photo demonstrating the final step of cementation—application of the patellar clamp. The clamp is used to maintain pressure on the patellar component while the cement hardens. Excess cement is removed along the edges of the component. Only after the cement is fully hardened should the clamp be released

9.5 mm, 43%) compared to the non-fracture group (average 8.1 mm, 38%) (King et al. 2015). Another assessment of 3655 TKAs demonstrated no difference in fractures of residual thickness <12 mm or >12 mm, but there was a significant increase in fracture risk based on native patellar pre-resection thickness <18 mm (Hamilton et al. 2017).

20.6 Risks of Patellar Non-resurfacing and Outcomes of Secondary Resurfacing

It well-documented that the risk of revision surgery is higher for the patient with a non-resurfaced patella. A meta-analysis in 2011 by Argawal et al., included 16 randomized controlled trials involving 2041 knees finding a relative risk of reoperation for the patellofemoral articulation in resurfaced knees to be 0.52 (1.8 vs 6.2%, 95% CI, $p = 0.012$) with no difference in anterior knee pain (Agrawal et al. 2011). Several other meta-analyses reached the same conclusions (Pakos et al. 2005; He et al. 2011). This type of revision surgery to resurface the patella is most often performed for anterior knee pain, however a large percentage (approximately 10%) of patients with resurfaced patellae have residual anterior knee pain and secondary resurfacing has a poor track record of alleviating such pain.

Of import is the fact that several studies have shown patient dis-satisfaction with secondary resurfacing. Parvizi et al. found that 20% of patients were unsatisfied after secondary resurfacing for anterior knee pain (Parvizi et al. 2012). In a series by Spencer et al., of 28 patients with 29 TKAs, 59% of patients had improved satisfaction after secondary resurfacing, and in a series of 27 patients reported by Munoz-Mahamud et al., only 63% reported improvement of symptoms (Spencer et al. 2010; Muñoz-Mahamud et al. 2011). A systematic review in 2016 demonstrated of 15 included articles and 232 patients, only 148 (64%) were satisfied after a secondary resurfacing procedure (van Jonbergen et al. 2016).

> Interpretation of increased rates of revision for unresurfaced patellae might be approached with caution as non-resurfacing gives the surgeon an option for revision of the painful TKA, thus artificially increasing the rate without truly alleviating the cause of residual pain.

20.7 Risks of Patellar Resurfacing

Patellar resurfacing is not without downsides. Biomechanical studies have shown a significant increase in retropatellar contact forces concomitant with the decreased contact area in several different patellar designs (Wurm et al. 2013). This increased force may account, in part for the increased risk of patellar fracture after resurfacing and possible osteonecrosis.

> The complications associated with extensor mechanism disruption in particular can be devastating.

Other complications associated with patellar resurfacing include the following:
- Over-stuffing the patellofemoral joint
- Creating too thin of a resurfacing and subsequent extensor mechanism weakness
- Patellar clunk syndrome
- Aseptic loosening
- Malpositioning
- Maltracking
- Excessive tilt
- Instability

- Osteonecrosis, and
- Catastrophic failure of the implant

Many of these may require reoperation with unpredictable results (Burnett and Bourne 2004). Patellofemoral complications have been cited around 7–8% after total knee arthroplasty (Dalury et al. 2013; Schiavone Panni et al. 2014).

20.8 Comparison Studies of Resurfacing

20.8.1 Randomized Controlled Trials

Multiple randomized controlled trials exist that show equivocal functional outcomes, a clear increased risk of reoperation for unresurfaced patellae, but a questionable increase in anterior knee pain for those same patients. In a meta-analysis by Argawal et al., 16 RCTs (6925 TKAs) were analyzed for incidence of anterior knee pain. Seven of these trials reported no difference between the two groups, five supported resurfacing the patella, while one favored no resurfacing of the patella. Overall, anterior knee pain was present in 12.9% of cases in the resurfaced group, while 24.1% in the patellar unresurfaced group with the RR of 0.56 (95% CI, $P < 0.00001$). However, when the analysis was limited to the high-quality RCTs with random allocation and observer blinding, there was no significant difference between the two groups (RR = 1.03, 95% CI, $P = 0.90$) (Agrawal et al. 2011).

A subsequent decision-analysis paper by Helmy et al., which argued in favor of resurfacing, used the RR-generated looking at all studies, though not the highest quality studies (Helmy et al. 2008). It is unclear what the results of this decision analysis would have been if the incidence of anterior knee pain in the parameters was set as equal. Another larger meta-analysis of 7075 knees by Pavlou et al. did not show any statistical difference in anterior knee pain or function, but again confirmed a higher risk of reoperation. This meta-analysis also attempted to determine if "patellar-friendly" implant designs impacted pain or function but was unable to show a difference (Pavlou et al. 2011). One of the largest randomized controlled trials found slightly contradictory results in 198 TKAs in 180 patients followed for a minimum of 3 years. The authors found no significant increase in the risk of revision but did find an increased incidence in the rate of anterior knee pain in the unresurfaced group. Weight was found to be the only predictor of anterior knee pain, however, this was not significant when adjusted for sex and age (Wood et al. 2002).

An important note is that most randomized controlled trials do not include selective resurfacing, with all degrees of patellofemoral arthritis randomized to each treatment arm. In a recently published randomized controlled trial by Roberts et al., all patients with exposed subchondral bone on the undersurface of the patella were excluded and the remaining patients were randomized. In their RCT of 350 patients without significant preexisting patellofemoral arthritis, they found a statistically significant, but likely clinically irrelevant improvement in patient satisfaction with an average of 7.8 years follow-up. In a subgroup of 110 patients followed for 10 years, there was no difference. Importantly, there was also no difference in revision rate (Roberts et al. 2015).

> This trial is important in demonstrating that selective resurfacing may not only have equivalent outcomes but may also have equivalent secondary surgery rates.

20.8.2 Registry Data

The Swedish Knee Arthroplasty Registry is an important source of data to consider regarding decision-making for patellar resurfacing. A review of 27,372 knees operated between 1981 and 1995 and followed longitudinally had several interesting findings (Robertsson et al. 2000). In general, patients with a resurfaced patella were more satisfied than patients without resurfacing (19% versus 15% for patients with osteoarthritis and 15% versus 12% for patients with rheumatoid arthritis), however, the satisfaction of the unresurfaced group was more durable over time with a greater percentage of patients with resurfaced patellae reporting lower satisfaction over time.

20.8.3 Bilateral Comparisons

A theoretically ideal comparison exists in patients with bilateral total knee arthroplasty with one patella resurfaced. In the highest quality trial, Barrack et al. reported after a randomized controlled trial with 86 patients that they found no difference in pain and function. Thirty (94%) of the patients were satisfied with the unresurfaced knee and 31 (97%) were satisfied with the resurfaced knee. When the patients were asked which side they preferred, 11 (34%) said the resurfaced side, 12 (38%) said the unresurfaced side (Barrack et al. 1997). In a series by Levitsky et al., there were 13 patients who had bilateral mixed TKA. When asked what knee they preferred six (46%) rated the knees as equal, six(46%) preferred the resurfaced patella, and one (7.7%) preferred the unresurfaced patella (Levitsky et al. 1993). In a series by Enis et al., 25 patients undergoing bilateral TKA had the right knee patellar resurfaced and the left was unresurfaced. The resurfaced knees had superior isokinetic measures and less patellofemoral pain and were preferred by patients (Enis et al. 1990).

20.9 Cost-Effectiveness

Recent studies have begun to evaluate the cost-effectiveness of resurfacing the patella. However, study outcomes on costs are mixed, perhaps due to differences in length of follow-up, cost profiles, and complication and revision rates. In the United States, Medicare reimbursements do not differ with or without patellar resurfacing, as the common CPT code for TKA (27447) does not distinguish the decision to resurface (Meijer and Dasa 2015). Meijer and Dasa in 2015 evaluated randomized controlled trials and concluded that the cost at 5 years postoperatively was $227.92 more in Medicare dollars for unresurfaced patellae compared to those that were resurfaced. This cost estimate model favors more cost-effectiveness for resurfacing as long as revision rates after patellar resurfacing remain less than 3.54% and revision rates after not resurfacing remain greater than 0.77% (Meijer and Dasa 2015). In another 5-year analysis in the United Kingdom, 1715 patients were randomized to resurfacing or not and no significant difference existed in total healthcare costs, including those associated with revision surgeries (Breeman et al. 2011). An evaluation of procedure costs based in Canada (reported in US Dollars), however, noted that not resurfacing the patella resulted in higher costs by $379.62. This model utilized data including revisions and complications of 14 years compared to the aforementioned studies of 5 years, though these revision rates were derived from an Australian Registry and were assumed to be similar in Canada (Weeks et al. 2018). Furthermore, Zmistowski et al. evaluated prospective randomized studies and found that resurfacing patella without significant patellofemoral arthritis was not cost-effective, perhaps suggesting that selective resurfacing may ultimately be a way to optimize costs (Zmistowski et al. 2019).

20

20.10 Technique for Cemented Patella Resurfacing

When resurfacing the patella, several factors should be considered. The amount of resection should be adequate to minimize over-stuffing of the joint (which may impact flexion and extensor mechanism mechanics) after patellar implant placement, but should not be so extensive to leave minimal bone stock (Bengs and Scott 2006). Optimally, the angle of resection of the patella is parallel to the anterior femoral cut to minimize patellar tilt.

Patellar resurfacing may be performed through freehand technique or with the assistance of cutting guides. Exposure of the articular surface of the patella is necessary and synovial tissue around the patellar should be excised circumferentially to allow for full visualization and evaluation of the patellar and quadriceps insertions (Lombardi et al. 1998).

First, patellar thickness should be assessed utilizing calipers. It is important to evaluate the thickness throughout the patella, as varying thicknesses are not uncommon particularly with patellofemoral arthritis associated with patellar subluxation.

> When evaluating patellar thickness, care should be taken to avoid rotation of the patella, as the patella has a median ridge that is off-center and resection may be excessive laterally and insufficient medially (Anglin et al. 2009).

Asymmetric resurfacing is associated with worse outcomes including patellar component loosening, patellofemoral pain, and revision surgery (Pagnano and Trousdale 2000). Preoperative knowledge of the surgeon's preferred system patellar component sizes is critical to understand the amount of resection required.

> When performing the resection, disruption of the extensor mechanism proximally and distally should be avoided at all costs.

If using freehand technique, the surgeon may use a non-offset oscillating sawblade with an aim to cut symmetrically across the articular surface of the patella for the desired thickness. Freehand resection has been described utilizing both haptic feedback and four-quadrant measurements on the posterior patellar surface (Camp et al. 2015). Utilizing haptic feedback, measurements of anterior to posterior patellar thickness may be taken centrally and assessment of symmetry is performed with haptic evaluation. The four-quadrant technique involves caliper measurements in the center of each of the four sections of the patella, with the assessment of symmetry based on these caliper readings (Camp et al. 2015). Surgeons may use either or a combination of these techniques. After passing the saw, remaining posterior to the quadriceps and patellar tendon attachments, the calipers and/or haptic feedback are again used to reevaluate patellar thickness and symmetry. The saw may be passed again in an iterative process until the optimal thickness and symmetry are created.

Similar concepts are applied to the use of cutting guides; however, after measurement of the patella with calipers, the guide allows for setting the goal depth of resection. After utilizing the oscillating saw through the guide, the surgeon should still reassess patellar thickness and symmetry, and reapply the guide or utilize freehand technique for additional cutting if desired.

After appropriate resection is achieved, a patellar clamp is used to place the patellar drill button guide on the patella. Care should be taken to medialize the patellar component and to secure the clamp to avoid shifting during drilling. Medialization of the patellar component assists with lateral movement of the extensor mechanism, which will theoretically improve tracking with a reduced Q-angle (Camp et al. 2013; Dennis et al. 2011; Anglin et al. 2010). The associated drill is used in the guide lug holes to drill and a trial component may be placed. The component selected should maximize bone coverage, which is often limited by the proximal and distal axis of the patella which tends to be smaller than the medial to lateral width (Dennis et al. 2011).

Residual parapatellar osteophytes should be removed if not already done. Once the patellar trial is in place in addition to the femoral and tibial trials, the knee is taken through a range of motion in flexion and extension and the tracking of the patella is carefully evaluated for lateral subluxation or tilt. If maltracking of the patella is noted, bone cuts and component rotation should be reassessed and if these are found to be appropriate, soft-tissue balancing may be needed, which may include lateral retinacular release. It is also important to check patellar component position or resection symmetry as this can also affect tracking. The thickness of the patellar trial component plus patellar bone should be measured and be similar to that of the bony thickness prior to resection accounting for cartilage loss (Lombardi et al. 1998; Marmor 1988; Hurson et al. 2010).

> Cement works best via interdigitation in cancellous spaces.

Therefore, in areas of sclerotic bone, the surgeon should consider placing small holes with either a thin drill or k-wire in areas of sclerosis to expose the healthy cancellous bone and allow increased area for cement to settle. When drilling sclerotic surfaces, avoid over drilling to the anterior cortex of the patella to reduce stress-risers that may theoretically increase the risk of fracture. The patella should be irrigated thoroughly and dried prior to cementation.

When it is time to cement and implant the patellar component, the cement is prepared through standard technique. The cement is placed with a spatula and clean gloves onto the posterior, resurfaced aspect of the patella.

> Using his or her fingers, the surgeon pressurizes cement into the previously established drill lug holes for the patellar pegs. The patellar component is pressed into its position and the clamp is applied and held throughout the duration of cement hardening.

Excess cement that extrudes beyond the edges of the patellar component should be promptly removed. Once the cement has dried, the clamp may be removed. At this time, patellar tracking should be revisited, and the knee should be taken through a range of motion with the final components in place.

Various studies have been done evaluating outcomes with the differing patellar resection techniques. A randomized trial performed by Yuan et al. demonstrated no significant differences in anterior knee pain between freehand technique or cutting guide technique groups, in addition to no differences in functional measures, patient-reported outcomes, or clinical examination results postoperatively (Yuan et al. 2019). The major difference noted in the study between the freehand and cutting guide technique groups for patellar resection was that the freehand group had significantly more outliers with lateral patellar tilt >10°, though the average tilt did not vary between groups (Yuan et al. 2019). This suggests perhaps improved reliability in measure with a cutting guide. Camp et al. performed a prospective trial comparing freehand technique with haptic feedback, freehand technique as evaluated with four-quadrant measurements, and cutting guide techniques (Camp et al. 2015). In this study, freehand techniques were more reliable with less asymmetry and less deviation from goal thickness compared to cutting guide, although accuracy of measurements was assessed with a quadrant method similar to one of the freehand techniques (Camp et al. 2015).

> It is important that when using a cutting guide to ensure proper application in terms of security and depth and when utilizing the saw within the guide, it is important to be parallel to the slot.

20.11 Conclusion

Patellar resurfacing is an important consideration of total knee arthroplasty that remains controversial. Excellent outcomes are achievable with and without resurfacing, and selective resurfacing is a reasonable option. The arthroplasty surgeon should carefully weigh the risks and benefits of resurfacing specific to each patient in order to provide the most-durable TKA with the lowest risk of complication. Specific attention should be paid to resurfacing techniques to minimize complications.

Take-Home Messages

- Patellar resurfacing is controversial, and excellent outcomes have been shown with or without resurfacing.
- Complications of resurfacing can be devastating, including extensor mechanism disruption or patellar fracture.
- Selective resurfacing may be considered, but regardless of surgeon preference, understanding patient-specific risks with and without resurfacing may impact outcomes.
- Various techniques for patellar resurfacing exist, including freehand techniques and use of cutting guides.
- It is critical to understand the surgeon's selected implant design and accurately measure the pre-resection thickness to determine the appropriate depth of resection.
- To achieve symmetry of the patellar cut, remeasurement and recutting may be necessary.
- Placement of the trial patellar component should be done to evaluate patellar alignment and tracking prior to implantation of the final component.
- The cement may be placed on the articular side of the resurfaced patella with a spatula or freehand and should be manually pressurized into the lug holes with constant pressure being applied with a patellar clamp until the cement has fully hardened.

References

Agrawal M, Jain V, Yadav VP, Bhardwaj V (2011) Patellar resurfacing in total knee arthroplasty. J Clin Orthop Trauma 2:77–81. https://doi.org/10.1016/S0976-5662(11)60048-9

Anglin C, Fu C, Hodgson AJ et al (2009) Finding and defining the ideal patellar resection plane in total knee arthroplasty. J Biomech 42:2307–2312. https://doi.org/10.1016/j.jbiomech.2009.06.021

Anglin C, Brimacombe JM, Wilson DR et al (2010) Biomechanical consequences of patellar component medialization in total knee arthroplasty. J Arthroplast 25:793–802. https://doi.org/10.1016/j.arth.2009.04.023

Barrack RL, Wolfe MW, Waldman DA et al (1997) Resurfacing of the patella in total knee arthroplasty. A prospective, randomized, double-blind study. J Bone Joint Surg Am 79:1121–1131. https://doi.org/10.2106/00004623-199708000-00002

Bengs BC, Scott RD (2006) The effect of patellar thickness on intraoperative knee flexion and patellar tracking in total knee arthroplasty. J Arthroplast 21:650–655. https://doi.org/10.1016/j.arth.2005.07.020

Berend KR, Lombardi AV, Adams JB (2007) Obesity, young age, patellofemoral disease, and anterior knee pain: identifying the unicondylar arthroplasty patient in the United States. Orthopedics 30:19–23

Breeman S, Campbell M, Dakin H et al (2011) Patellar resurfacing in total knee replacement: five-year clinical and economic results of a large randomized controlled trial. J Bone Joint Surg Am 93:1473–1481. https://doi.org/10.2106/JBJS.J.00725

Burnett RS, Bourne RB (2004) Indications for patellar resurfacing in total knee arthroplasty. Instr Course Lect 53:167–186

Camp CL, Bryan AJ, Walker JA, Trousdale RT (2013) Surgical technique for symmetric patellar resurfacing during total knee arthroplasty. J Knee Surg 26:281–284. https://doi.org/10.1055/s-0032-1330056

Camp CL, Martin JR, Krych AJ et al (2015) Resection technique does affect resection symmetry and thickness of the patella during Total knee arthroplasty: a prospective randomized trial. J Arthroplast 30:2110–2115. https://doi.org/10.1016/j.arth.2015.05.038

Dalury DF, Pomeroy DL, Gorab RS, Adams MJ (2013) Why are total knee arthroplasties being revised? J Arthroplast 28:120–121. https://doi.org/10.1016/j.arth.2013.04.051

Dennis DA, Kim RH, Johnson DR et al (2011) The John Insall Award: control-matched evaluation of painful patellar Crepitus after total knee arthroplasty. Clin Orthop Relat Res 469:10–17. https://doi.org/10.1007/s11999-010-1485-3

Enis JE, Gardner R, Robledo MA et al (1990) Comparison of patellar resurfacing versus nonresurfacing in bilateral total knee arthroplasty. Clin Orthop Relat Res:38–42

Hamilton WG, Ammeen DJ, Parks NL et al (2017) Patellar cut and composite thickness: the influence on postoperative motion and complications in total knee arthroplasty. J Arthroplast 32:1803–1807. https://doi.org/10.1016/j.arth.2016.12.033

He J-Y, Jiang L-S, Dai L-Y (2011) Is patellar resurfacing superior than nonresurfacing in total knee arthroplasty? A meta-analysis of randomized trials. Knee 18:137–144. https://doi.org/10.1016/j.knee.2010.04.004

Helmy N, Anglin C, Greidanus NV, Masri BA (2008) To resurface or not to resurface the patella in total knee arthroplasty. Clin Orthop Relat Res 466:2775–2783. https://doi.org/10.1007/s11999-008-0420-3

Hurson C, Kashir A, Flavin R, Kelly I (2010) Routine patellar resurfacing using an inset patellar technique. Int Orthop 34:955–958. https://doi.org/10.1007/s00264-009-0831-0

King AH, Engasser WM, Sousa PL et al (2015) Patellar fracture following patellofemoral arthroplasty. J Arthroplast 30:1203–1206. https://doi.org/10.1016/j.arth.2015.02.007

Koh JSB, Yeo SJ, Lee BPH et al (2002) Influence of patellar thickness on results of total knee arthroplasty: does a residual bony patellar thickness of <or=12 mm lead to poorer clinical outcome and increased complication rates? J Arthroplast 17:56–61. https://doi.org/10.1054/arth.2002.29320

Levitsky KA, Harris WJ, McManus J, Scott RD (1993) Total knee arthroplasty without patellar resurfacing. Clinical outcomes and long-term follow-up evaluation. Clin Orthop Relat Res:116–121

Lie DTT, Gloria N, Amis AA et al (2005) Patellar resection during total knee arthroplasty: effect on bone strain and fracture risk. Knee Surg Sports Traumatol Arthrosc 13:203–208. https://doi.org/10.1007/s00167-004-0508-6

Lombardi AV, Mallory TH, Maitino PD et al (1998) Freehand resection of the patella in total knee arthroplasty referencing the attachments of the quadriceps tendon and patellar tendon. J Arthroplast 13:788–792. https://doi.org/10.1016/s0883-5403(98)90032-8

Marmor L (1988) Technique for patellar resurfacing in total knee arthroplasty. Clin Orthop Relat Res:166–167

McAlindon TE, Snow S, Cooper C, Dieppe PA (1992) Radiographic patterns of osteoarthritis of the knee joint in the community: the importance of the patellofemoral joint. Ann Rheum Dis 51:844–849. https://doi.org/10.1136/ard.51.7.844

McAlindon T, Zhang Y, Hannan M et al (1996) Are risk factors for patellofemoral and tibiofemoral knee osteoarthritis different? J Rheumatol 23:332–337

Meijer KA, Dasa V (2015) Is resurfacing the patella cheaper? An economic analysis of evidence based medicine on patellar resurfacing. Knee 22:136–141. https://doi.org/10.1016/j.knee.2014.12.009

Muñoz-Mahamud E, Popescu D, Nuñez E et al (2011) Secondary patellar resurfacing in the treatment of patellofemoral pain after total knee arthroplasty. Knee Surg Sports Traumatol Arthrosc 19:1467–1472. https://doi.org/10.1007/s00167-011-1402-7

Pagnano MW, Trousdale RT (2000) Asymmetric patella resurfacing in total knee arthroplasty. Am J Knee Surg 13:228–233

Pakos EE, Ntzani EE, Trikalinos TA (2005) Patellar resurfacing in total knee arthroplasty. A meta-analysis. J Bone Joint Surg Am 87:1438–1445. https://doi.org/10.2106/JBJS.D.02422

Parvizi J, Mortazavi SMJ, Devulapalli C et al (2012) Secondary resurfacing of the patella after primary total knee arthroplasty. Does the anterior knee pain resolve? J Arthroplasty 27:21–26. https://doi.org/10.1016/j.arth.2011.04.027

Pavlou G, Meyer C, Leonidou A et al (2011) Patellar resurfacing in total knee arthroplasty: does design matter?: a meta-analysis of 7075 cases. J Bone Joint Surg Am Vol 93:1301–1309. https://doi.org/10.2106/JBJS.J.00594

Roberts DW, Hayes TD, Tate CT, Lesko JP (2015) Selective patellar resurfacing in total knee arthroplasty: a prospective, randomized, double-blind study. J Arthroplast 30:216–222. https://doi.org/10.1016/j.arth.2014.09.012

Robertsson O, Dunbar M, Pehrsson T et al (2000) Patient satisfaction after knee arthroplasty: a report on 27,372 knees operated on between 1981 and 1995 in Sweden. Acta Orthop Scand 71:262–267. https://doi.org/10.1080/000164700317411852

Rodríguez-Merchán EC, Gómez-Cardero P (2010) The outerbridge classification predicts the need for patellar resurfacing in TKA. In: Clinical orthopaedics and related research, pp 1254–1257

Schiavone Panni A, Cerciello S, Del Regno C et al (2014) Patellar resurfacing complications in total knee arthroplasty. Int Orthop (SICOT) 38:313–317. https://doi.org/10.1007/s00264-013-2244-3

Soudry M, Mestriner LA, Binazzi R, Insall JN (1986) Total knee arthroplasty without patellar resurfacing. Clin Orthop Relat Res:166–170

Spencer SJ, Young D, Blyth MJG (2010) Secondary resurfacing of the patella in total knee arthroplasty. Knee 17:187–190. https://doi.org/10.1016/j.knee.2009.08.003

van Jonbergen H-PW, Boeddha AV, van Raaij JJA M (2016) Patient satisfaction and functional outcomes following secondary patellar resurfacing. Orthopedics 39:e850–e856. https://doi.org/10.3928/01477447-20160509-05

Weeks CA, Marsh JD, MacDonald SJ et al (2018) Patellar resurfacing in total knee arthroplasty: a cost-effectiveness analysis. J Arthroplast 33:3412–3415. https://doi.org/10.1016/j.arth.2018.07.001

Wood DJ, Smith AJ, Collopy D, et al (2002) Patellar resurfacing in total knee arthroplasty: a prospective, randomized trial

Wurm S, Kainz H, Reng W, Augat P (2013) The influence of patellar resurfacing on patellar kinetics and retropatellar contact characteristics. J Orthop Sci 18:61–69. https://doi.org/10.1007/s00776-012-0326-5

Yuan F, Sun Z, Wang H et al (2019) Clinical and radiologic outcomes of two patellar resection techniques during total knee arthroplasty: a prospective randomized controlled study. Int Orthop 43:2293–2301. https://doi.org/10.1007/s00264-018-4264-5

Zmistowski BM, Fillingham YA, Salmons HI et al (2019) Routine patellar resurfacing during total knee arthroplasty is not cost-effective in patients without patellar arthritis. J Arthroplast 34:1963–1968. https://doi.org/10.1016/j.arth.2019.04.040

Patella Replacement in Knee Arthroplasty: A Japanese Perspective

Atsushi Takahashi

Contents

E. Hansen, K.-D. Kühn (eds.), *Essentials of Cemented Knee Arthroplasty*,
https://doi.org/10.1007/978-3-662-63113-3_21

21.1 Introduction

The use of patellar resurfacing versus retention in total knee arthroplasty (TKA) has long been controversial. There are significant differences in the rates of patellar resurfacing among countries (Fig. 21.1) (Fraser and Spangehl 2017). Hence, whether this procedure should be performed remains unclear. Patellar retention is advantageous because it is less invasive to the extensor mechanism, can preserve the bone, and has a short operative time. Moreover, it is beneficial for revision surgery particularly in cases of infection. The treatment of patellar fracture after patellar resurfacing is challenging, with a high complication rate and low satisfaction outcome (Chalidis et al. 2007; Ortiguera and Berry 2002). However, patellar retention has disadvantages, which include anterior knee pain and a high rate of revision surgery (Fig. 21.2). Grassi et al. revealed that a higher risk of re-surgery after patellar retention should be interpreted with caution due to the methodological limitations of previous meta-analyses on search criteria, heterogeneity, and inherent bias of the indication for reoperation when the patella is not resurfaced (Grassi et al. 2018). Considering these factors, patellar retention could be a better option if anterior knee pain is managed.

21.2 Patellofemoral Contact Stress in TKA

21.2.1 Factors Correlated with Patellofemoral Contact Stress after TKA

> High-contact pressure in the patellofemoral joint causes postoperative anterior knee pain (Becher et al. 2009; Whiteside and Nakamura 2003).

Moreover, it induces degenerative changes in the patella, which may be associated with pain around the patellofemoral joint (Rodriguez-Merchan and Gomez-Cardero 2009; Sawaguchi et al. 2010). To date, several studies have reported about numerous factors affecting patellofemoral contact pressure which include the following:

- The design of the femoral component (Whiteside and Nakamura 2003; Browne et al. 2005)
- Rotational alignment (Kessler et al. 2008; Merican et al. 2011; Verlinden et al. 2010) and
- Use of either a mobile-bearing insert (Sawaguchi et al. 2010) or highly conforming inlays (Heyse et al. 2010)

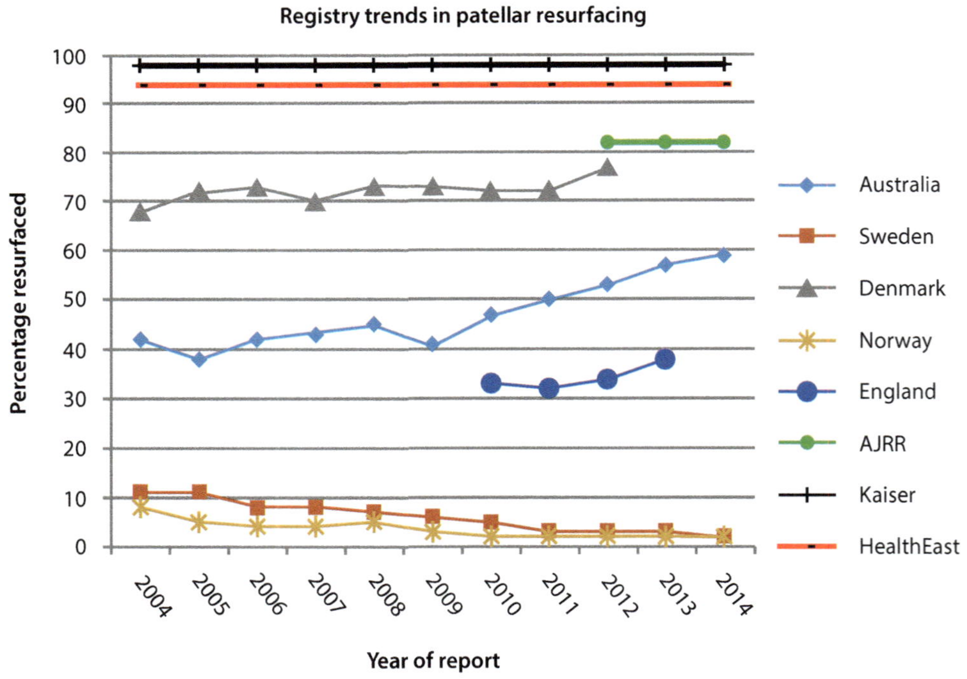

Fig. 21.1 International rates of patellar resurfacing in primary total knee arthroplasty (Fraser and Spangehl 2017) based on the American Joint Replacement Registry

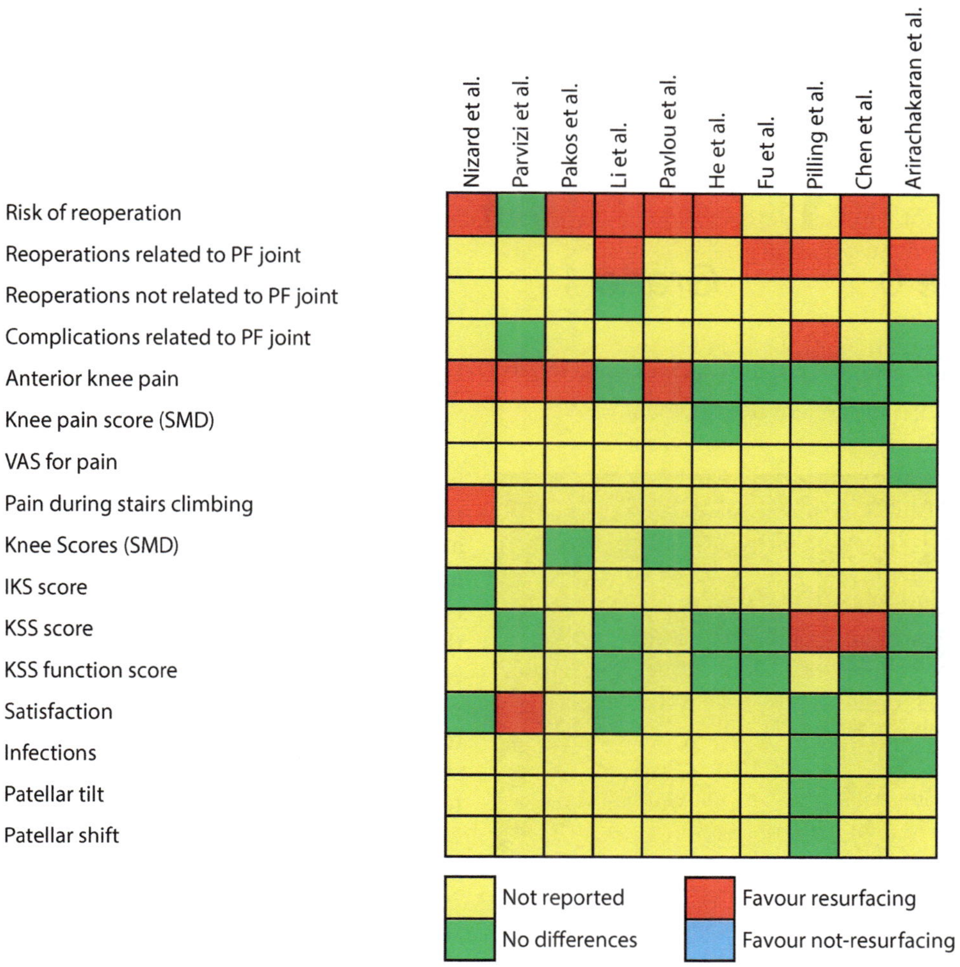

Fig. 21.2 Use of the Jadad algorithm to select the best quality of evidence (Grassi et al. 2018)

> Patellar morphology and femoral component geometry are significant factors correlated with patellofemoral contact stress in total knee arthroplasty without patellar resurfacing (Takahashi et al. 2012).

21.2.2 Effect of Patellar Morphology on Postoperative Patellofemoral Contact Stress

In general, the mineral density of the subchondral bone reflects the distribution of stress caused by joint contact over a long period of time (Noble and Alexander 1985). The measurement of mineral density is a convenient method for assessing biomechanical stress within the bone in clinical practice. Hence, subchondral bone mineral density can be used as a clinical indicator of patellofemoral joint contact stress. Based on this point of view, osteosclerosis was classified to assess patellofemoral contact stress after TKA without patellar resurfacing (Takahashi et al. 2012). Pre- and postoperative axial radiograph images obtained 1 year after surgery were compared. Then, they were evaluated according to the grade of newly diagnosed osteosclerosis, which were as follows:

- None (grade 0)
- Slight (grade 1)
- Moderate (grade 2)
- Severe (grade 3) (Fig. 21.3)

The patellae significantly vary in terms of morphology. Some have a steep facet angle and others are flat. The medial-to-lateral facet length ratio also varies. The patellar facet angle is a radiographic parameter that expresses patellar flatness (Fig. 21.4). The Wiberg classification is the most well-known classification system for patellar shape (Wiberg 1941). However, it is not correlated with the occurrence of osteosclerosis of the patella after surgery. Osteosclerosis is commonly observed in patellae with a small facet angle, and the results were statistically significant (Fig. 21.5). Moreover, patient-specific finite element analyses revealed a negative correlation between the patellar facet angle and the peak von Mises stress inside the patella (Fig. 21.6).

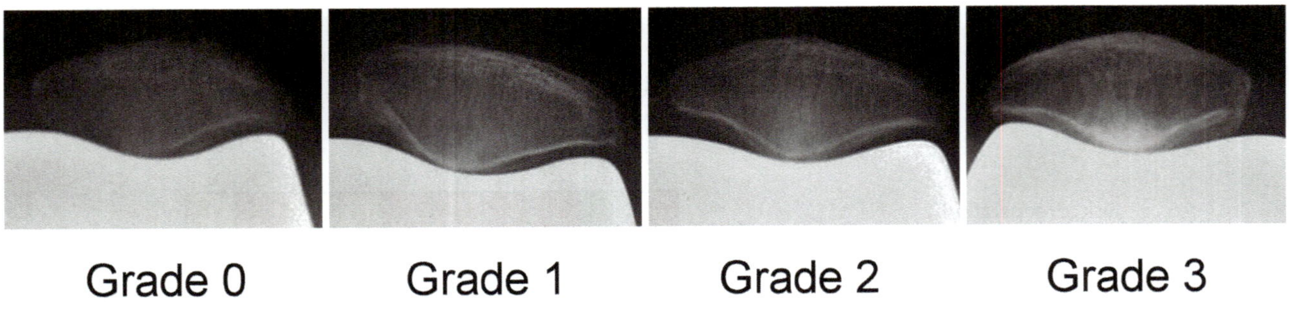

Fig. 21.3 Grade of newly diagnosed osteosclerosis after surgery (Takahashi et al. 2012)

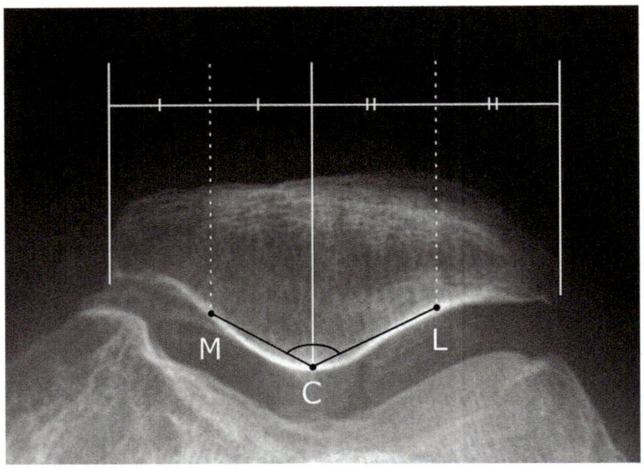

Fig. 21.4 Measurement of the patellar facet angle (Takahashi et al. 2012). *C* is a point on the central ridge, *M* is a point bisecting the medial facet, and *L* is a point bisecting the lateral facet. The patellar facet angle is the angle formed using lines *MC* and *LC*

> Based on these findings, patellae with a large facet angle (flat patellae) do not require patellar resurfacing. Hence, the preoperative patellar facet angle can be used as an indicator for selective patellar resurfacing.

21.2.3 Effect of Component Geometry on Postoperative Patellofemoral Contact Stress

As mentioned in ▶ Sect. 21.1, previous studies comparing patellar resurfacing and retention have different results. One possible explanation for this discrepancy is that these studies used various implants with different geometries. For example, Montonen et al. reported that Triathlon cruciate retaining (CR) had a higher risk for patellar revision than Nexgen CR Flex (Montonen et al. 2018). Moreover, Wyatt et al. showed that the rate of revision for secondary resurfacing of the patella in the fixed-bearing posterior-stabilized (PS) TKA designs was higher than that in either fixed-bearing CR or mobile-bearing designs (Wyatt et al. 2013). Some authors reported that the prosthetic design did not influence the patellofemoral clinical outcome in TKA (Johnson et al. 2012; Pavlou et al. 2011). However, in their studies, most of the new prostheses were considered as patella-friendly. In contrast, our study compared new prostheses with different designs of the femoral trochlea (Fig. 21.7). Results showed that the significance of the patellofemoral contact stress patterns differed even in modern implants (Takahashi et al. 2012). In this study, the maximum von Mises stress values were significantly lower in both the LCS and NexGen groups than in the Genesis II group, and the stress distribution pattern within the patella coincided with the localization of osteosclerosis, which was confirmed on radiography (Fig. 21.8). To date, several studies have used the term "patella-friendly". However, it does not have a clear definition (Montonen et al. 2018; Wyatt et al. 2013; Johnson et al. 2012; Pavlou et al. 2011; Atzori et al. 2015; Koh et al. 2018; Roessler et al. 2018).

> The result of our study showed that a deep trochlea could be patella-friendly.

21.3 Complications Associated with the Patellofemoral Joint in TKA

21.3.1 Patellar Fracture

Chlidis et al. showed that the incidence rate of patellar fracture was 1.19% (range: 0.15–12%) (Chalidis et al. 2007). Moreover, approximately 99% of patellar fractures occurred after patellar resurfacing, and 88% were not associated with a traumatic event and identified during the follow-up examination within the first 2 years after TKA. Bone thickness <12 mm after patellar resurfacing was considered a risk factor for patellar fracture

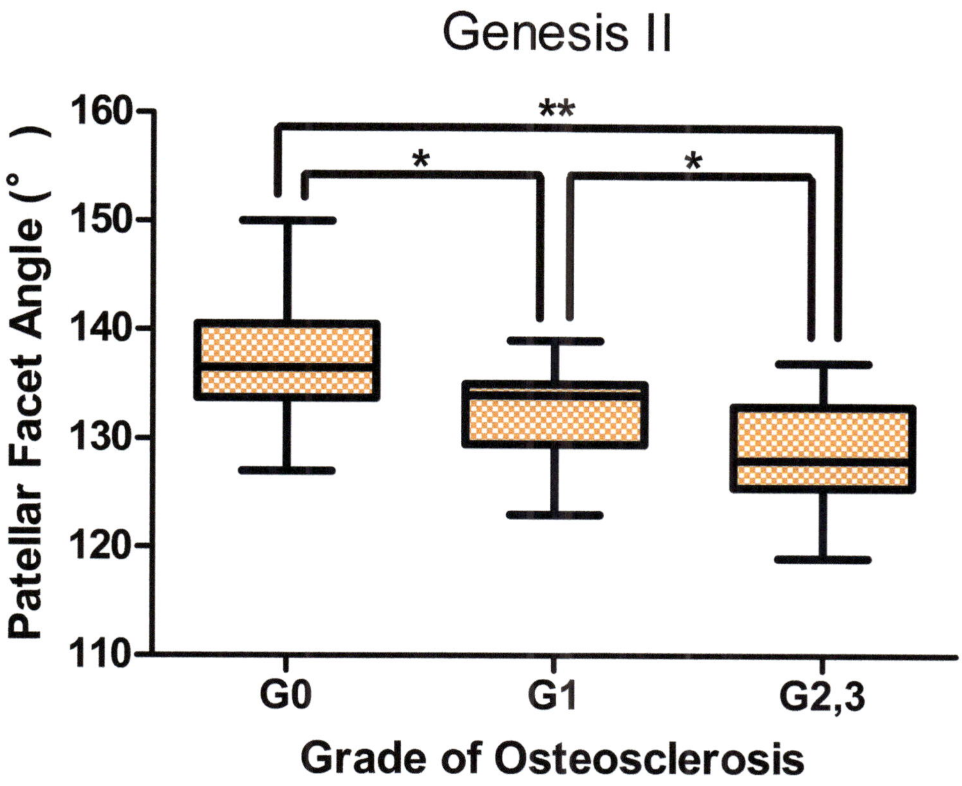

Fig. 21.5 Relationship between postoperative osteosclerosis grade and patellar facet angle. Patients with high-grade osteosclerosis had a small facet angle (**$p < 0.01$, *$p < 0.05$)

regardless of preoperative patellar thickness (Hamilton et al. 2017). Moreover, other risk factors include body mass index >30 kg/m^2, male gender, large preoperative varus, and intraoperative lateral release (Meding et al. 2008). Ortiguera and Berry classified patellar fracture as follows (Ortiguera and Berry 2002):

Classification of Patellar Fractures (Ortiguera and Berry 2002)

- Type 1: Stable implant and intact extensor mechanism
- Type 2: Disruption of the extensor mechanism
- Type 3: Loose patellar component with an intact extensor mechanism
  - Type 3a: Indicated reasonable remaining bone stock
  - Type 3b: Poor bone stock

Patellar fracture after TKA often occurs without trauma, and lateral retinacular release is considered a risk factor for patellar fracture (Chalidis et al. 2007; Meding et al. 2008). Thus, hypovascularity or osteonecrosis of the patella has been considered the etiology of this type of fracture. Chalidis et al. reported that open reduction and internal fixation (ORIF) was not successful in 92% of cases, and the final outcome was poor (Chalidis et al. 2007). Avascular fracture fragments have minimal healing potential, and the surgical complication rate is extremely high.

> Hence, simple ORIF should not be routinely recommended.

Considering these factors, Putman et al. summarized the management of post-TKA patellar fractures as follows (Putman et al. 2019):

Management of Post-TKA Patellar Fractures (Putman et al. 2019)

- Type 1: Nonoperative treatment (splint, cast) is used.
- Type 2 with a stable implant: In this condition, the fracture involves either the proximal or the distal pole of the patella. The implant is left in place to prevent the fragilization of the residual bone, and the extensor apparatus is reconstructed.
- Type 2 with a loose implant: Surgery is usually required, with the primary objective of restoring a continuous extensor apparatus (trans-osseous suture, hamstring graft augmentation, and allogeneic graft). The patellar implant must be removed.
- Type 3: Removal of the patellar implant is sufficient.

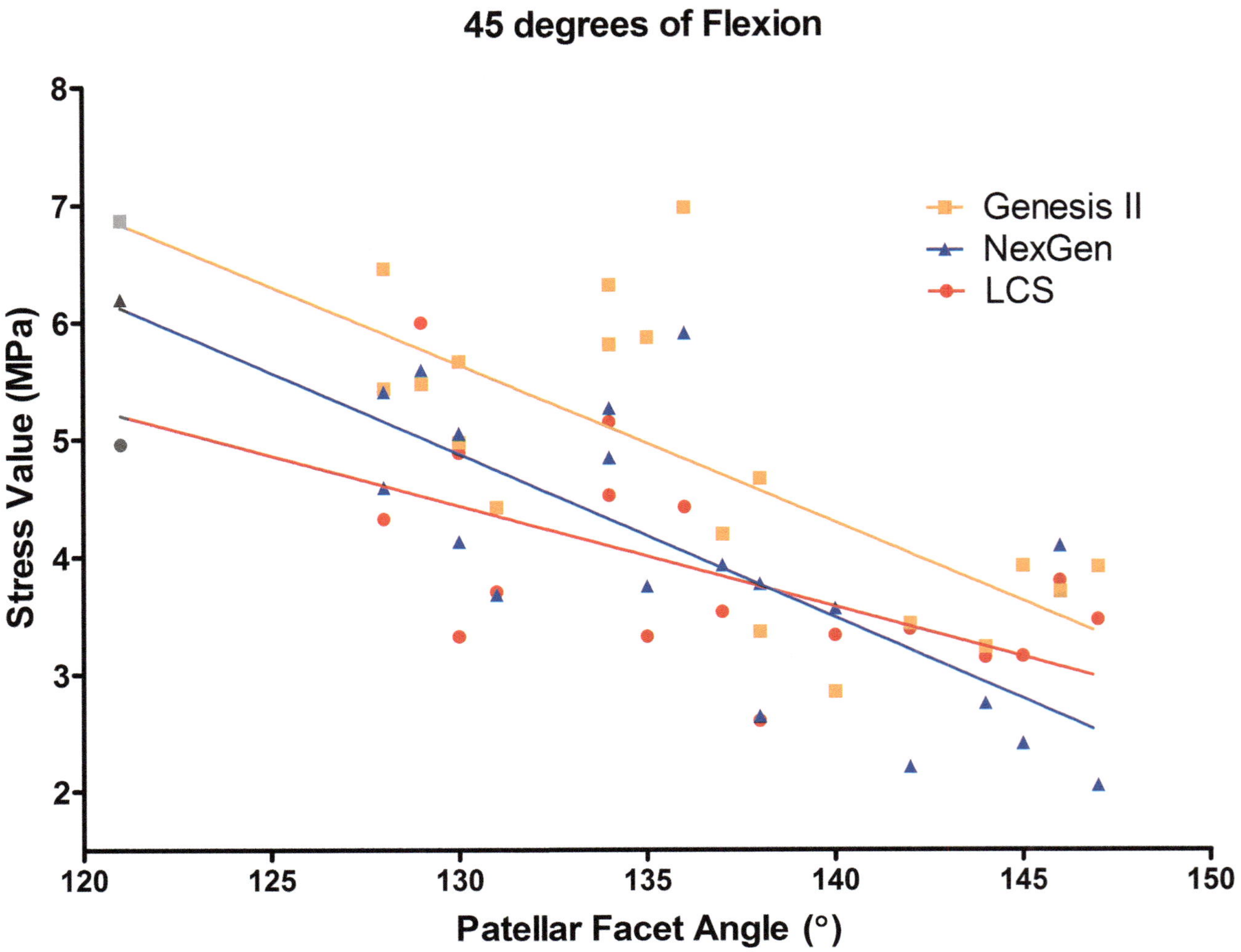

Fig. 21.6 Relationship between von Mises stress inside the patella and patellar facet angle (Takahashi et al. 2012)

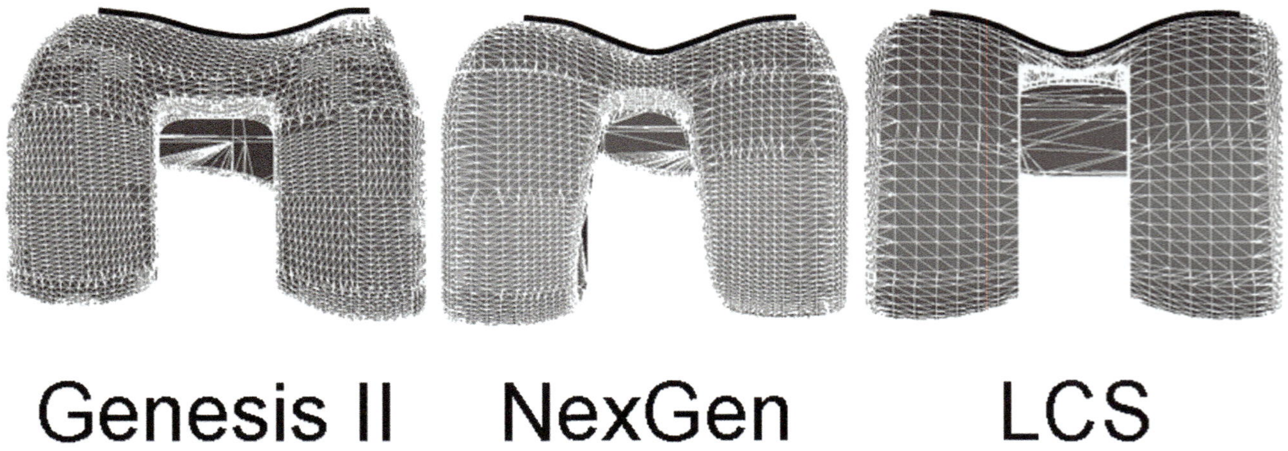

Fig. 21.7 Comparison of the femoral trochlea of different prostheses. Genesis II has a relatively shallow trochlea whereas LCS has a deep trochlea

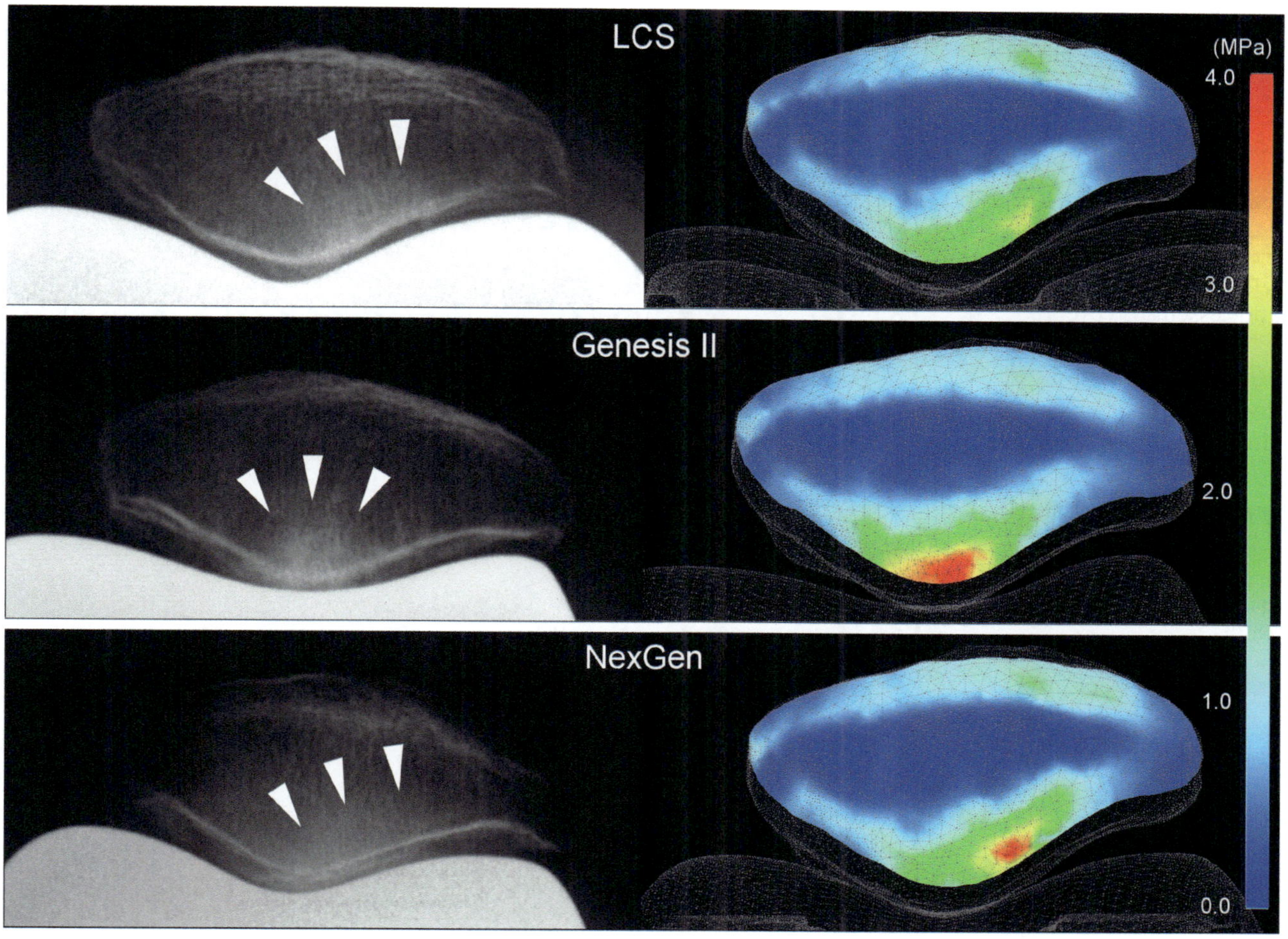

Fig. 21.8 Osteosclerosis confirmed on radiography and simulated stress distribution within the patella. The *right column* shows an equivalent stress distribution within the patella model created using the data of the same patient. In the finite element analysis, both the LCS and NexGen implants had a high stress concentration on the lateral facet where osteosclerosis was observed (*arrowhead*). Both high stress concentration and osteosclerosis are observed on the central ridge in the Genesis II implant

21.3.2 Osteonecrosis of the Patella

As described ▶ Sect. 21.3.1, most patellar fractures after patellar resurfacing is associated with hypovascularity or osteonecrosis of the patella. Osteonecrosis-like lesion after TKA was also observed in non-resurfaced patellae, which had radiological similarities to those of spontaneous osteonecrosis of the knee (Fig. 21.9) (Takahashi et al. 2014). In this study, the major osteoporotic fracture risk assessed using the World Health Organization fracture risk assessment tool was significantly higher in the osteonecrosis group than in the control group. In addition, the average patellar facet angle in the radiolucent group was significantly smaller than that in the control group (Fig. 21.10). As described in ▶ Sect. 21.3.1, a small patellar facet angle was associated with stress concentration (Fig. 21.6).

Therefore, both underlying osteoporosis and stress concentration may play an important role in the pathogenesis of the radiolucent zones in the patellae after TKA without patellar resurfacing.

Based on the author's experience, this condition might cause mild-to-moderate anterior knee pain. However, it can be treated conservatively.

21.3.3 Patellar Clunk Syndrome and Crepitus

Hozack et al. firstly proposed the patellar clunk syndromeas patellofemoral pain due to an unusual suprapatellar fibrous nodule after posterior-stabilized (PS) TKA, which is characterized by catch or clunk on extension of

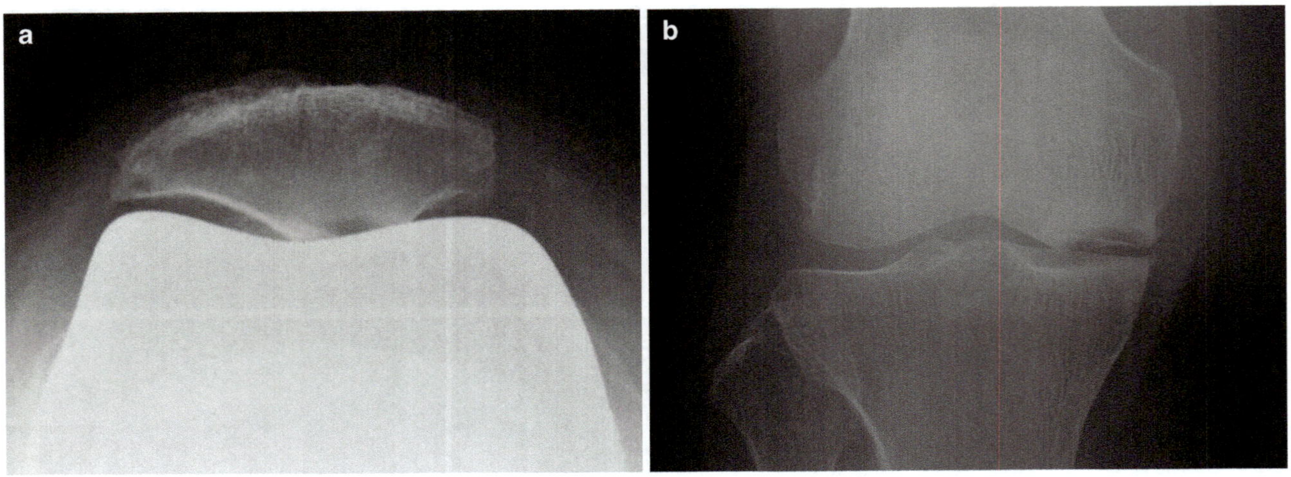

Fig. 21.9 The radiolucent zone of the patella **a** has a radiological similarity to that of spontaneous osteonecrosis of the knee **b** (Takahashi et al. 2014)

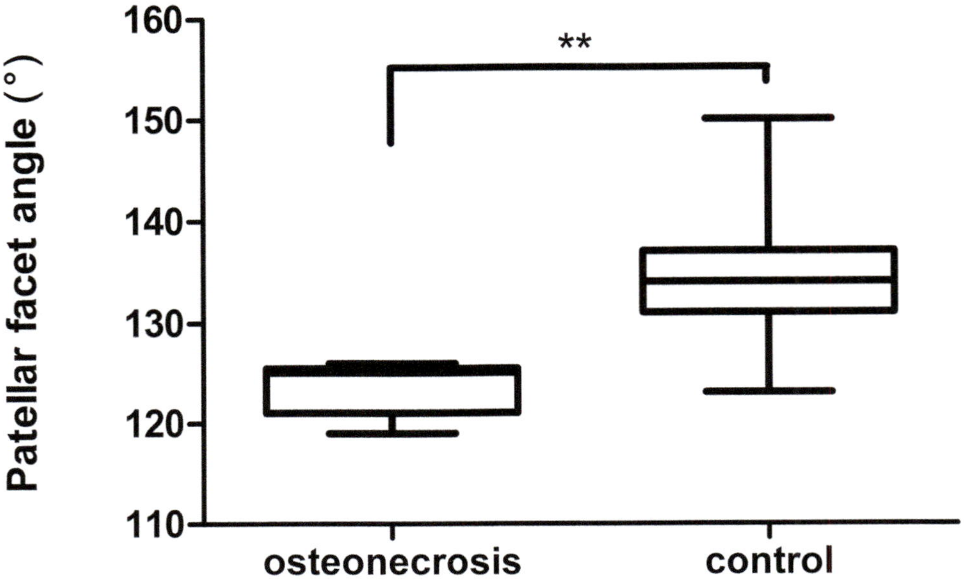

Fig. 21.10 Comparison between patients with and without osteonecrosis. Patients with osteonecrosis had a small facet angle (** $p < 0.01$)

the knee (Hozack et al. 1989). The synovial entrapment is caused by hypertrophic synovial tissue at the superior pole of the patella (Fig. 21.11) (Pollock et al. 2002). This condition is commonly observed in PS knees particularly when prostheses have an intercondylar box ratio >0.7 (Fukunaga et al. 2009). Other risk factors are previous surgeries, small femoral component size, thick polyethylene bearing, and patella baja (Conrad and Dennis 2014).

To prevent patellar crepitus and clunk, the removal of fibrosynovial tissues at the border of the superior pole of the patella and distal quadriceps tendon was recommended at the time of primary TKA (Conrad and Dennis 2014).

> When treating patellar clunk syndrome, more than half will improve with time under conservative treatment (Ip et al. 2004; Gholson et al. 2017).

Arthroscopic resection of the suprapatellar nodule has good outcomes, with a low rate of recurrence (Costanzo et al. 2014).

21.3.4 Anterior Knee Pain after TKA

Anterior knee pain after TKA is a multifactorial problem. When treating anterior knee pain, known causes such as patellar fracture, patellar clunk, loosening of the

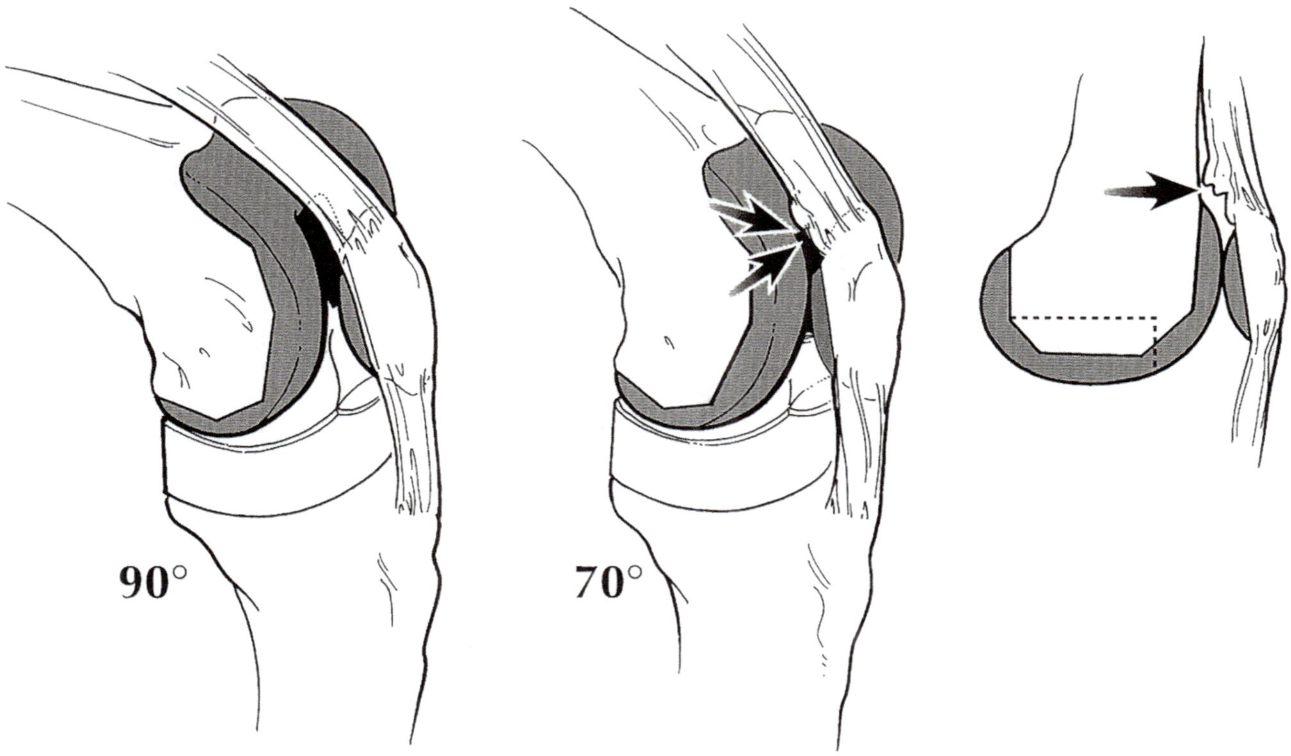

Fig. 21.11 Knees with synovial entrapment syndromehave hypertrophic tissue proximal to the patella (*arrows*) (Pollock et al. 2002)

patellar implant, asymmetric patellar cut, lateral patellar facet impingement, and component malrotation, should be ruled out (Putman et al. 2019; Antinolfi et al. 2018). Lateral patellofemoral impingement or lateral patellar facet impingement is a cause of treatable pain after TKA (Nikolaus et al. 2014; Cercek et al. 2011). An axial weight-bearing radiographic view (Fig. 21.12) while the patient is in semi-squatting position is occasionally useful to detect impingement (Baldini et al. 2007).

> Lateral patellar facet impingement after TKA could be treated with lateral facetectomy, with relatively good outcomes (Nikolaus et al. 2014; Cercek et al. 2011). Lateral facetectomy is a useful preparation method of the patella in primary TKA with patellar retention (Kim et al. 2017).

Moreover, patellar denervation and patelloplasty are techniques used to reduce anterior knee pain in patellar-retaining TKA. Xie et al. showed that patellar denervation can significantly reduce the incidence of anterior knee pain and improve early clinical outcomes after TKA (Xie et al. 2015). However, after a prolonged follow-up period, this advantage may not be observed. Cerciello et al. reported that the outcome of patelloplastyis superior to that of isolated osteophyte removal and denervation, with a lower rate of anterior knee pain (Cerciello et al. 2016).

> Importantly, successful repair of the MPFL after using the medial parapatellar approach in TKA could reduce anterior knee pain (Keshmiri et al. 2017).

21.4 Surgical Technique and Strategies that Can Reduce Anterior Knee Pain

> Although there are some cementless patellar components available, cement fixation is the gold standard for patellar replacement.

When resurfacing the patella, a flat surface during bone resection should be made. The patellar thickness should be similar to or slightly thinner than the original thickness. Multiple small anchor holes are necessary only when the patella is eburnated. An adequate component size must be selected, and the position slightly should be medialized. Lateral partial facetectomy is recommended to prevent lateral patellar facet impingement. Dry the bone surface before starting cement fixation. Apply cement on to both the implant and bony surfaces, and compression force should be applied until cement polymerization is complete.

The author used the following strategies to reduce anterior knee pain in primary TKA:

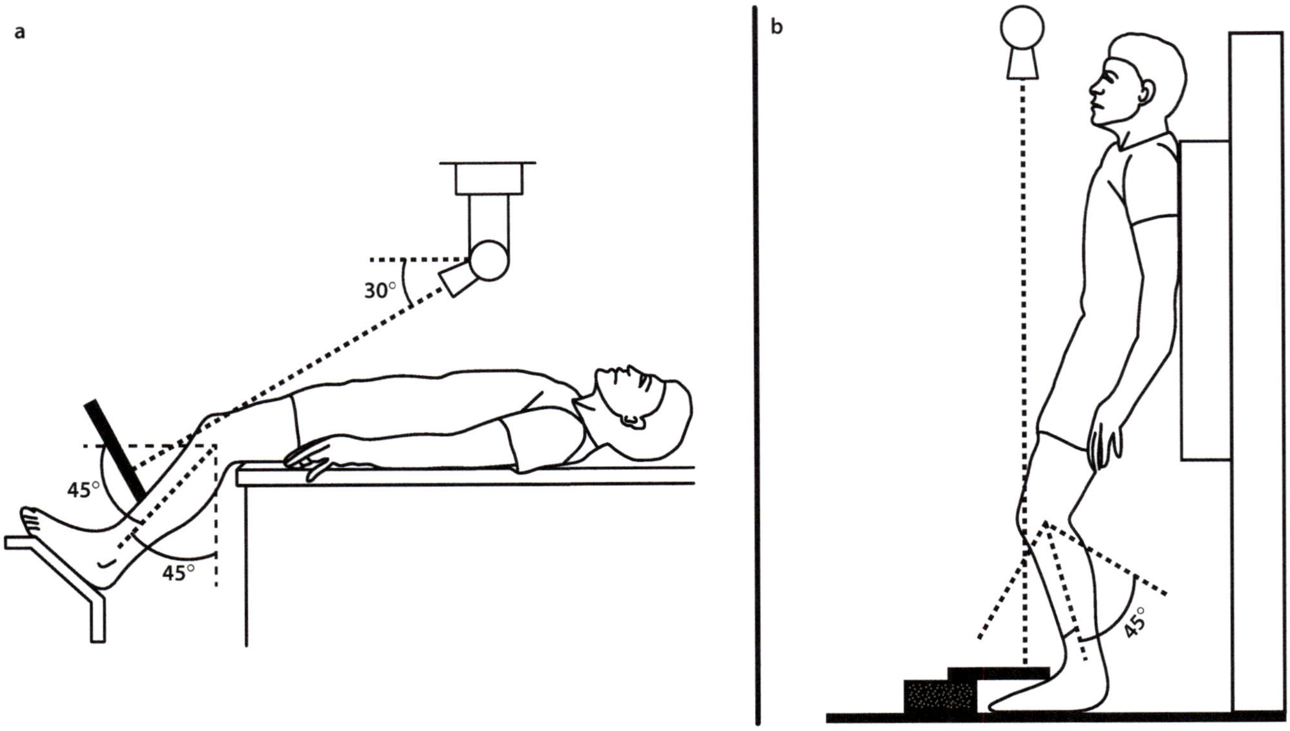

Fig. 21.12 Patient positioning for the Merchant **a** and modified weight-bearing **b** axial views (Baldini et al. 2007)

Strategies for Anterior Knee Pain Reduction in Primary TKA

- Preventing axial malrotation of the components via detailed preoperative planning
- Proper cementing technique when resurfacing
- Firm capsular closure particularly around MPFL
- Rheumatoid arthritis: patellar resurfacing with lateral facetectomy
- Degenerative arthritis when using components with the deep trochlea (Takahashi et al. 2012): patellar retention with patelloplasty
- Degenerative arthritis when using components with a shallow trochlea:
  - Patellar facet angle (Takahashi et al. 2012) ≥133° (flat patella): patellar retention with patelloplasty
  - Patellar facet angle <133° (projecting patella): patellar resurfacing with lateral facetectomy

Take-Home Messages

- The use of patellar resurfacing versus retention in TKA has long been a controversy since there are significant variations in the rates of patellar resurfacing among countries, whether it should be performed remains unclear.
- Patellar retention is advantageous as it is less invasive to the extensor mechanism, can preserve the bone, and has a shorter operative time. However, patellar retention has disadvantages, which include anterior knee pain and a high rate of revision surgery for patellofemoral joint fracture.
- High-contact pressure in the patellofemoral joint causes postoperative anterior knee pain.
- Axial malrotation of the components could cause patellofemoral high-contact pressure; thus, this should be avoided via detailed preoperative planning.

- Steep facet angle and component trochlea are associated with patellofemoral high-contact stress. Hence, they could be indicators for selective patellar resurfacing.
- Lateral patellar facet impingement after TKA could be treated with lateral facetectomy, with relatively good outcomes.
- Successful repair of the MPFL after using the medial parapatellar approach in TKA could reduce the incidence of anterior knee pain.
- When resurfacing the patella with cement fixation, multiple small anchor holes are necessary only when the patella is eburnated. The bone surface should be dried before starting cement fixation. Moreover, cement must be placed on both the implant and bony surfaces, and compression force should be applied until cement polymerization is completed.

References

Antinolfi P et al (2018) The challenge of managing the "third-space" in total knee arthroplasty: review of current concepts. Joints 6(3):204–210

Atzori F et al (2015) Evaluation of anterior knee pain in a PS total knee arthroplasty: the role of patella-friendly femoral component and patellar size. Musculoskelet Surg 99(1):75–83

Baldini A et al (2007) Patellofemoral evaluation after total knee arthroplasty. Validation of a new weight-bearing axial radiographic view. J Bone Joint Surg Am 89(8):1810–1817

Becher C et al (2009) Posterior stabilized TKA reduce patellofemoral contact pressure compared with cruciate retaining TKA in vitro. Knee Surg Sports Traumatol Arthrosc 17(10):1159–1165

Browne C et al (2005) Patellofemoral forces after total knee arthroplasty: effect of extensor moment arm. Knee 12(2):81–88

Cercek R et al (2011) Lateral patellofemoral impingement: a cause of treatable pain after TKA. J Knee Surg 24(3):181–184

Cerciello S et al (2016) The role of patelloplasty in total knee arthroplasty. Arch Orthop Trauma Surg 136(11):1607–1613

Chalidis BE et al (2007) Management of periprosthetic patellar fractures. A systematic review of literature. Injury 38(6):714–724

Conrad DN, Dennis DA (2014) Patellofemoral crepitus after total knee arthroplasty: etiology and preventive measures. Clin Orthop Surg 6(1):9–19

Costanzo JA et al (2014) Patellar clunk syndrome after total knee arthroplasty; risk factors and functional outcomes of arthroscopic treatment. J Arthroplast 29(9 Suppl):201–204

Fraser JF, Spangehl MJ (2017) International rates of patellar resurfacing in primary total knee arthroplasty, 2004-2014. J Arthroplast 32(1):83–86

Fukunaga K et al (2009) The incidence of the patellar clunk syndrome in a recently designed mobile-bearing posteriorly stabilised total knee replacement. J Bone Joint Surg Br 91(4):463–468

Gholson JJ et al (2017) Management of painful patellar clunk and crepitance: results at a mean follow-up of five years. Iowa Orthop J 37:171–175

Grassi A et al (2018) Patellar resurfacing versus patellar retention in primary total knee arthroplasty: a systematic review of overlapping meta-analyses. Knee Surg Sports Traumatol Arthrosc 26(11):3206–3218

Hamilton WG et al (2017) Patellar cut and composite thickness: the influence on postoperative motion and complications in total knee arthroplasty. J Arthroplast 32(6):1803–1807

Heyse TJ et al (2010) Patellofemoral pressure after TKA in vitro: highly conforming vs. posterior stabilized inlays. Arch Orthop Trauma Surg 130(2):191–196

Hozack WJ et al (1989) The patellar clunk syndrome. A complication of posterior stabilized total knee arthroplasty. Clin Orthop Relat Res 241:203–208

Ip D et al (2004) Natural history and pathogenesis of the patella clunk syndrome. Arch Orthop Trauma Surg 124(9):597–602

Johnson TC et al (2012) Revision surgery for patellofemoral problems: should we always resurface? Clin Orthop Relat Res 470(1):211–219

Keshmiri A et al (2017) Stability of capsule closure and postoperative anterior knee pain after medial parapatellar approach in TKA. Arch Orthop Trauma Surg 137(7):1019–1024

Kessler O et al (2008) The effect of femoral component malrotation on patellar biomechanics. J Biomech 41(16):3332–3339

Kim CW et al (2017) Clinical and radiologic outcomes of partial lateral patellar facetectomy in total knee arthroplasty. J Knee Surg 30(2):185–192

Koh IJ et al (2018) Patients undergoing total knee arthroplasty using a contemporary patella-friendly implant are unaware of any differences due to patellar resurfacing. Knee Surg Sports Traumatol Arthrosc

Meding JB et al (2008) Predicting patellar failure after total knee arthroplasty. Clin Orthop Relat Res 466(11):2769–2774

Merican AM et al (2011) The effect of femoral component rotation on the kinematics of the tibiofemoral and patellofemoral joints after total knee arthroplasty. Knee Surg Sports Traumatol Arthrosc 19(9):1479–1487

Montonen E et al (2018) What is the long-term survivorship of cruciate-retaining TKA in the finnish registry? Clin Orthop Relat Res 476(6):1205–1211

Nikolaus OB et al (2014) Lateral patellar facet impingement after primary total knee arthroplasty: it does exist. J Arthroplast 29(5):970–976

Noble J, Alexander K (1985) Studies of tibial subchondral bone density and its significance. J Bone Joint Surg Am 67(2):295–302

Ortiguera CJ, Berry DJ (2002) Patellar fracture after total knee arthroplasty. J Bone Joint Surg Am 84-A(4):532–540

Pavlou G et al (2011) Patellar resurfacing in total knee arthroplasty: does design matter? A meta-analysis of 7075 cases. J Bone Joint Surg Am 93(14):1301–1309

Pollock DC, Ammeen DJ, Engh GA (2002) Synovial entrapment: a complication of posterior stabilized total knee arthroplasty. J Bone Joint Surg Am 84-A(12):2174–2178

Putman S et al (2019) Patellar complications after total knee arthroplasty. Orthop Traumatol Surg Res 105(1S):S43–S51

Rodriguez-Merchan EC, Gomez-Cardero P (2009) The outerbridge classification predicts the need for patellar resurfacing in TKA. Clin Orthop Relat Res

Roessler PP et al (2018) Predictors for secondary patellar resurfacing after primary total knee arthroplasty using a "patellafriendly" total knee arthroplasty system. Int Orthop

Sawaguchi N et al (2010) Mobile-bearing total knee arthroplasty improves patellar tracking and patellofemoral contact stress:

in vivo measurements in the same patients. J Arthroplast 25(6):920–925
Takahashi A et al (2012) Patellar morphology and femoral component geometry influence patellofemoral contact stress in total knee arthroplasty without patellar resurfacing. Knee Surg Sports Traumatol Arthrosc 20(9):1787–1795
Takahashi A et al (2014) Radiolucent zone of the patella following total knee arthroplasty without patellar resurfacing. J Orthop Sci 19(4):558–563
Verlinden C et al (2010) The influence of malrotation of the femoral component in total knee replacement on the mechanics of patellofemoral contact during gait: an in vitro biomechanical study. J Bone Joint Surg Br 92(5):737–742
Whiteside LA, Nakamura T (2003) Effect of femoral component design on unresurfaced patellas in knee arthroplasty. Clin Orthop Relat Res 410:189–198
Wiberg G (1941) Roentgenographs and anatomic studies on the femoropatellar joint: with special reference to chondromalacia patellae. Acta Orthop Scand 12(1):319–410
Wyatt MC et al (2013) Mobile- versus fixed-bearing modern total knee replacements- which is the more patella-friendly design?: the 11-year New Zealand Joint Registry study. Bone Joint Res 2(7):129–131
Xie X et al (2015) Does patellar denervation reduce post-operative anterior knee pain after total knee arthroplasty? Knee Surg Sports Traumatol Arthrosc 23(6):1808–1815

Knee Arthroplasty: An Asian Perspective

Wilson Wang, Bryan T. H. Koh, and Vikaesh Moorthy

Contents

E. Hansen, K.-D. Kühn (eds.), *Essentials of Cemented Knee Arthroplasty*,
https://doi.org/10.1007/978-3-662-63113-3_22

22.1 Introduction

22.1.1 Demographics of Knee OA in Western Versus Asian Populations

Knee osteoarthritis (OA) is the most common joint disorder affecting the elderly throughout the world. It is the leading cause of disability stemming from chronic pain and immobility with an incredible impact on public health (Kim et al. 2008). The downstream effects of knee OA include reduced quality of life from an individual's and caregiver's perspective (Fransen et al. 2011) to increased healthcare cost and reduced productivity. Total knee arthroplasty (TKA) is known to be the most effective intervention for advanced-stage knee OA for pain control and functional improvement (Lin et al. 2018).

Knee OA occurs in 12% of American adults aged 65 years or older, and in 13% of women and 10% of men 60 years or older in the United States (Kim et al. 2008; Lin et al. 2018; Zhang et al. 2001). The prevalence of knee OA for females in East Asian countries has been reported to be higher than the equivalent prevalence for females reported in the US Caucasian population, while for males the figure is slightly lower comparatively (Kim et al. 2008; Zhang et al. 2001). In one report (Beijing Osteoarthritis Study), the prevalence of knee OA was found to be 15% in women and 5.6% in men aged 60 years or older in Beijing, China, and that among those over 50 years old in Taiwan was about 37% (Zhang et al. 2001). A population-based epidemiological study conducted in Vietnam, which involved 170 men and 488 women over 40 years of age also found that 31% of men and 35% of women had radiographic OA of the knee (Ho-Pham et al. 2014). As such the prevalence of knee OA in Asia is comparable with Caucasian populations (Nguyen 2014).

In 2012, OA affected 27% of the population aged over 45 years in industrialized countries and this rate is expected to increase by 11% by 2032 when an additional 26,000 individuals per one million population will be affected (Pabinger et al. 2015). Among these patients, the highest incidence of OA is found in the knee joint, which is affected twice as often as the hip joint. This is especially the case in Asia where people have the habit of squatting or sitting on the floor, and it has been postulated that squatting may in fact protect against OA of the hip (Nguyen 2014). It is estimated that 6% of those aged 30 years and older and 15% of those aged 45 years and older experience knee OA, with a lifetime risk of 45% (Murphy et al. 2008). In view of these trends, it is unsurprising that the need for TKAs is also expected to grow exponentially in the coming years (Pabinger et al. 2015).

22.1.2 TKA in Western Versus Asian Countries

TKA is one of the most successful clinical interventions for patients with debilitating hip and knee diseases (Kumar et al. 2015) and is currently the international standard of care for treating degenerative and rheumatologic knee disorders (Kurtz et al. 2011). TKA is the treatment of choice in the most severe forms of knee OA and has even been described as a surrogate marker of severe OA (Jonsson et al. 2016). Previous studies of knee replacement have shown substantial improvements in patients' health-related quality of life (HRQoL) scores after the surgery, especially in terms of the pain dimension (Ko et al. 2011), suggesting high utility and benefit of TKA as the treatment of choice for severe knee OA.

Given that both population aging and economic growth have taken place at a fast pace in many Asian countries, it is expected that knee OA will become a major public health problem and that utilization of TKA will increase in many Asian countries as well, where over 60% of the world population lives (Kim et al. 2008; Ko et al. 2011). Apart from aging, there is much evidence from mostly Western cohorts that obesity or heavy-occupational physical activity, such as that carried out by many people in rural communities in Asia, are clear risk factors for symptomatic knee OA (Fransen et al. 2011). These further support the view of a rapidly rising rate of TKAs across Asia in the coming years.

In fact, primary TKA rates have increased by 407% in South Korea from 2001 to 2010, according to data from the Health Insurance Review Agency (HIRA) from South Korea (Koh et al. 2013). Also using the national data collected by HIRA in South Korea, Kim et al. (2008) found that from 2002 to 2005, 103,601 TKA surgeries were performed in South Korea, with the rate of TKA increasing over the years from 2002 to 2005 and being significantly higher in women than in men. Likewise, in Taiwan, a retrospective study by Lin et al. (2018) using Taiwan's National Health Insurance Research Database, showed that 154,553 TKA surgeries were performed in Taiwan during the 15-year study period from 1996 to 2010, with the number of TKAs increasing from 5303 in 1996 to 17,368 in 2010 (an increase of 202.56%), while the rate of TKAs tripled, from 24.64 to 74.55 per 100,000 between 1996 and 2010. This trend of a rapid increase in the rate of TKAs in recent years is expected to continue in Asia, in view of the aforementioned factors.

Most studies to date have also reported that satisfaction following TKA is high. Mahomed et al. (2011) evaluated 857 patients 1 year following TKA and reported an overall satisfaction score of 88%. A study on 25,275 patients from the Swedish Joint Arthroplasty

Registry showed a satisfaction score of 81% (Dunbar 2001). While these figures have to be quoted from studies performed on a predominantly Western population, there are no large-scale studies that have evaluated satisfaction rates on Asian patients undergoing TKA.

> However, of note, TKA in Asian populations involves a few unique challenges, especially that of higher demands of postoperative flexion among Asians (Bin AbdRazak and Yeo 2015).

As such, further improving patient satisfaction following TKA is certainly a challenge, especially in the Asian context. In fact, Thambiah et al. (2015) also concluded that although there was a high level of patient satisfaction (92.8%) following TKA in their cohort of 103 Asian patients in Singapore, a significant minority was dissatisfied, likely due to reasons of patient expectations and inadequate postoperative flexion as deemed by the patients.

22.1.3 Predictors of Knee OA and Knee Arthroplasty

Risk factors for knee OA have been studied mostly in Caucasian populations residing in high-income countries and include age, female gender, obesity, a history of knee surgery or significant trauma, or having an occupation requiring heavy lifting, kneeling, or squatting (Jensen 2008). Less epidemiological research in chronic musculoskeletal conditions has been conducted in countries in Asia (Fransen et al. 2011).

> While it is reasonable to extend some of these risk factor findings to Asian countries, there are also likely to be a significant demographic, cultural, lifestyle, and environmental differences influencing the onset and progression of knee OA in Asian populations.

Kim et al. (2008) have suggested that both kneeling and squatting are strong risk factors for knee OA, and this lifestyle factor might account for greater functional disability as well as the prevalence of knee OA in Asians due to greater use of the squatting posture by Asians in daily activities, such as toileting. Compared with Western countries in which stability for walking is important, in Asian countries, knee flexion for squatting and kneeling may be more important in the decision to undergo surgery, accounting for the increase of OA and TKA rates among Asians.

Using functional data from 120 persons with end-stage knee OA, Zeni Jr. et al. (2010) determined clinical factors which predict the decision to undergo TKA in individuals with end-stage knee OA. Logistic regression revealed that age, Knee Outcome Survey–Activities of Daily Living Subscale (KOS-ADLS), Timed Up and Go (TUG), Stair Climbing Task (SCT), quadriceps strength, and knee extension range of motion (ROM) significantly predicted TKA within 2 years ($p \leq 0.001$, $R^2 = 0.412$). Conversely, younger age, higher KOS-ADLS scores, faster TUG and SCT times, stronger quadriceps, and full knee extension predicted those who do not undergo TKA. Using backward regression, age, knee extension ROM and KOS-ADLS together significantly predicted whether or not a person would undergo TKA ($p \leq 0.001$, $R^2 = 0.403$).

Lin et al. (2018) also identified year, female gender, increased age, and OA as key risk factors and predictors of TKA. The relative risk ratio (RR) was as follows:

- 1.09 (95% CI: 1.08–1.09) per year
- 1.66 (95% CI:1.63–1.69) for females compared with males
- 5.45 (95% CI: 5.16–5.75) for the 50 to 59 age group
- 15.21 (95% CI: 14.45–16.00) for the 60 to 69 age group
- 21.23 (95% CI: 20.17–22.34) for the 70 to 79 age group
- 16.24 (95% CI: 15.30–17.25) for the ≥80 age group, when compared with the <50 age group

Patients with rheumatoid arthritis (RA) and avascular necrosis (AVN) as their primary diagnoses were also found to have a lower risk for TKA (RR = 0.15, 95% CI:15.30–17.25 and RR = 0.007, 95% CI:15.30–17.25, respectively) than those with OA.

22.1.4 Unicompartmental and Patellofemoral Arthroplasty

Apart from TKA, current surgical treatments for knee OA patients also include unicompartmental knee arthroplasty (UKA). Previous studies have shown that TKA and UKA are both safe and effective (Callahan et al. 1994, 1995). Although UKA is effective in patients with knee OA restricted to a single compartment, TKA is generally recommended for patients with more extensive knee OA (Zhang et al. 2008). Of note, in comparison to TKA, UKA has the additional benefits of lower costs, shorter hospitalization, less invasiveness, quicker rehabilitation, and a potentially better cost-effectiveness profile (Ko et al. 2011; Slover et al. 2006).

More recent studies on US patients suggest that 12–26% of patients might qualify for UKA according to the Kozinn and Scott criteria (Woolson et al. 2010). In contrast, He et al. (2018) suggest that a smaller percentage of Chinese patients undergoing knee arthroplasty are candidates for UKA: Of the 300 knees with OA that were studied, they found that 241 knees were excluded from UKA because of the extent of deformity ($n = 156$), decreased range of motion ($n = 119$), advanced patellofemoral arthritis with bone loss ($n = 11$), and AP instability ($n = 1$). Of the remaining 63 knees, only 54 knees (18%) met the modified Oxford criteria for mobile UKA and only 25 knees (8%) met the Kozinn and Scott criteria for fixed UKA.

> The authors concluded that in comparison to Caucasian population only a smaller percentage of patients in a Chinese cohort meet the UKA indication criteria and therefore propose that it might make more sense to concentrate UKA surgeries in high volume centers for predominantly Asian communities.

The patellofemoral (PF) joint is the most incongruent joint in the body and problems of the PF joint in Asian populations are distinct enough from the tibiofemoral joint to warrant separate attention, including patellofemoral osteoarthritis (PFOA), which occurs due to the loss of cartilage of the patella and the trochlear groove of the femur.

A high prevalence of PFOA has been observed in studies conducted in the Middle East and Asia, whereas lower prevalence rates were reported in Estonia and Sweden (Kobayashi et al. 2016; Wise et al. 2012). These findings were consistent with Pereira et al. (2011) who found that studies conducted in Europe, particularly Northern Europe, reported a lower prevalence of PFOA. A previous study by Muraki et al. (2009) has also suggested that the culture of kneeling, particularly in Asian countries, could lead to a higher prevalence of knee OA. However, there has been no conclusive evidence to suggest any cultural link with PFOA. In fact, conflicting evidence has suggested that the increased contact area between the patella and femoral trochlear during kneeling could be a protective mechanism from developing patellofemoral OA (Rytter et al. 2009).

Certain genes have also been reported to have high associations with knee OA in some ethnic populations but not others. For instance, variants in the expression of genes responsible for cartilage and bone growth (such as DVWA, DQB1, and BTNL2) have been shown to increase the risk of developing knee OA in Asian cohorts (Japanese, Chinese and Korean), but not in European cohorts (Valdes and Spector 2011). Therefore, it is reasonable to believe that ethnic groups have different genetic predispositions for developing OA, accounting for the geographic variability of PFOA. It has also been suggested that identification of individuals at a high risk of OA and of TKA failure might be facilitated by the use of combinations of such genetic markers, allowing for the application of preventive and disease management strategies in knee OA and TKAs (Valdes and Spector 2011).

22.2 Ethnic Differences in Knee Morphology

22.2.1 Asian Versus Western Knee Anatomy

TKA is a precise procedure, requiring accurate soft-tissue balancing and resection of bone thickness equal to the thickness of the implanted prosthetic component. A properly shaped prosthesis can provide the best coverage and avoid soft-tissue impingement. Therefore, TKA prostheses based on accurate morphologic data of the knee, taking into account morphologic differences between gender and ethnicity would give better surgical and postoperative results (Hosseinzadeh et al. 2013).

> Recent anthropometric studies have suggested that the current design of TKA prostheses does not fully cater to racial anthropometric differences and that most of the commercially available TKA prostheses are designed according to the anthropometric data of Caucasian knees.

This has been suspected as the cause of the component mismatch in Asian patients (Yue et al. 2011).

Iorio et al. (2007) showed that Japanese patients had a significantly lower postoperative ROM than Caucasian patients after TKA and that 4.1% of Japanese patients required revision after primary posterior cruciate-retaining TKA within an average follow-up of 6.6 years, whereas only 2.6% of their American counterparts needed revision within an average follow-up of 9 years. The authors suggested that the racial morphologic differences in knee anatomy and resultant component mismatch might be a key contributing factor, causing this significant difference in outcomes (Hosseinzadeh et al. 2013).

Studies have also shown that the dimensions of Chinese knees are generally smaller than Caucasian knees, with Chinese females having a significantly narrower distal femur than Caucasian females, and Chinese males having a wider proximal tibia than their Caucasian counterparts. Morphological measurements of Chinese knees have also shown that both Chinese males and females have smaller femoral aspect ratio (mediolateral [fML]/anteroposterior [fAP]) dimensions than their Caucasian counterparts (Hosseinzadeh et al. 2013; Yue et al. 2011; Mahfouz et al. 2012).

The findings on TKA component mismatch have led some researchers to suggest that Asians should have special designs of the TKA prosthesis system (Yue et al.

2011). With the higher prevalence of knee OA and lower preoperative knee function in Asian populations than Caucasian populations (Zhang et al. 2001; Inoue et al. 2001; Joshy et al. 2006) and the increasing use of TKA in Asia,(Kim et al. 2008) it has become essential to understand the differences in knee morphology and anatomy between Asian and Caucasian populations, so as to improve TKA prostheses and the outcomes of TKA in Asians.

22.2.2 Lower Extremity Axial Alignment in Asian Versus Caucasian Adults

Achieving normal axial alignment of the lower extremity is important to surgeons who perform reconstructive surgery of the knee. The normal alignment of the lower extremity in Caucasians has been documented by Moreland et al. (1987) with the use of radiographs of the lower extremity and currently, there are several known differences in the axial alignment of the lower extremities between Asians and Caucasian populations.

The inferolateral angle between the knee joint surface and the mechanical axis of the tibia is an index of knee joint obliquity. This angle in subjects, as reported by Tang et al. (2005) was 95.4 ± 2.5° in women and 94.9 ± 2.3° in men which is significantly larger than that in Caucasian subjects, as reported by Hsu et al. (1990) with a mean of 91.0 ± 1.4° in Caucasian men and a mean of 90.1 ± 1.9° in Caucasian women.

- These findings suggest agreater medial inclination of the knee joint in Chinese as compared to Caucasian people (Hosseinzadeh et al. 2013).

- According to Shao et al. (2018) East Asian individuals also have a more lateral tibial shaft axis than Caucasians.

The study found that East Asian individuals had a −9.9 ± 2.7 mm (range −16.2 to −4.6 mm) offset from the tibial shaft axis to Akagi's line in the mediolateral direction, compared to −7.7 ± 3.1 mm (range −13.4 to −0.3 mm) for Caucasians. However, there was no significant difference in the femoral diaphysis offset between the East Asian and Caucasian groups.

- In general, existing studies have shown that the Asian knee tends to be more varus than Caucasian knees, although there are some discrepancies seen in the literature.

Hovinga and Lerner (2009)) found that the mechanical alignment in Caucasians was slightly varus in 57% (0.55 ± 0.338), while 78% of Japanese subjects exhibited a more varus alignment (1.64 ± 0.438). Tang et al. (2005) also showed that the lower extremities of the Chinese women had a mean of 2.2 ± 2.5° of varus alignment, and those of Chinese men had a mean of 2.2 ± 2.7° of varus alignment, suggesting that the knees of Chinese female subjects, were in more varus alignment than were those in the Caucasian female subjects in the study by Hsu et al. (1990)

The mean anatomic axis angle, condyle angle, and condyle–plateau angle were also significantly different in the Beijing Osteoarthritis Study (BOA) (n = 173) when compared with the Framingham Osteoarthritis Study (FOA) (n = 134). Although the mean anatomic axis angle was valgus in both cohorts, the BOA cohort was 1.35° more valgus ($p = 0.01$) in men and 2.01° more valgus ($p < 0.001$) in women, as compared to their counterparts in the FOA cohort (Harvey et al. 2008). Considering the distribution for the anatomic axis angle in the Framingham and Beijing subjects before adjusting for age and BMI, the difference in the mean anatomic axis was more valgus in Beijing subjects, with the standard deviation of this measure in the Beijing subjects being larger compared with the Framingham subjects (F-test for equality of variances $p < 0.0001$) (Harvey et al. 2008). However, examination of the anatomic axis is a small sample of the cohort of the Beijing and Framingham populations did not explain the higher lateral tibiofemoral OA prevalence in Chinese and no clear conclusions could be made (Harvey et al. 2008).

Currently, most TKA systems recommend prosthesis placement such that the transverse axis of the artificial knee joint is perpendicular to the mechanical axes of the tibia and the femur. This results in an alignment of the lower extremity which is most similar to the alignment documented by Moreland et al. and Hsu et al. Unsurprisingly, the mechanical axes of the femur and the tibia did not form a straight line in either Chinese males or females (Hosseinzadeh et al. 2013).

- Further studies are required to conclusively characterize the axial alignment of the lower extremities in Asians and how it differs from that of Caucasians, and such data need to be used to develop new and updated guidelines and TKA prostheses systems that better accommodate and suit the Asian knee.

22.2.3 Differences in Distal Femoral Morphology

Recent studies have suggested that the current design of total knee arthroplasty does not cater to racial anthropometric differences, causing a component mismatch in

Asian patients,(Yue et al. 2011) due to poor fit and compatibility of the femoral component of the prosthesis for the Asian knee. Ho et al. (2006) found that three of five TKA systems used in China tended to overhang across the mediolateral width of resected femurs from Chinese patients. Cheng et al. (2009) also found that the femoral component overhang was more obvious in Chinese females than males and suggested that the prostheses that were designed for Caucasian patients may be too large for Chinese patients,(Yue et al. 2011) due to morphological differences between the Chinese and Caucasian knee. Thus, it is crucial to characterize the distal femoral morphology and differences in this morphology between Asian and Western populations.

The mediolateral (fML) and anteroposterior (fAP) size of the femur, measured using a viewing plane set perpendicular to the femoral long axis have revealed significant differences in the dimensions and morphology of Asian versus Caucasian knees. Several studies (Ho et al. 2006; Cheng et al. 2009; Urabe et al. 2008) have compared the morphology of Asian knees to that of TKA prostheses currently used in Asia and found that the general size and femoral aspect ratio (mediolateral [fML]/anteroposterior [fAP]) of these prostheses were not suitable for Asian patients.

> In general, the femoral volume of East Asians (466.5 ± 95.0 cm^3) is significantly smaller than that of Caucasians (540.2 ± 117.3 cm^3) (Shao et al. 2018).

The height-adjusted ratios of the half metaphyseal femur ($p < 0.001$), the whole condyle ($p = 0.03$), the anterior condyle ($p < 0.001$), and the resected condyle ($p = 0.004$) have also been found to be significantly lower in Japanese women compared to their Caucasian counterparts. However, the height-adjusted ratio of the posterior condyle was significantly smaller in Caucasian women ($p = 0.02$) (Urabe et al. 2008).

The fML dimension of Chinese females (72.8 ± 2.6 mm; range, 70.0–79.1 mm) was significantly smaller than that of Caucasian females (76.4 ± 4.0 mm; range, 70.3–82 mm) ($P = 0.002$). Chinese males had an average fML dimension of 82.6 ± 3.6 mm (range, 72.6–87.1 mm), which was significantly smaller than that of Caucasian males (86.0 ± 5.6 mm; range, 74.9–100.2 mm) ($P = 0.028$) (Yue et al. 2011).

Chinese females also had a significantly smaller average fML/fAP ratio than Caucasian females (1.239 ± 0.042 vs. 1.286 ± 0.063). While a progressive decline in the fML/fAP ratio with increasing fAP dimension was noted for both races, there was a distinct offset between the corresponding regression lines for Chinese and Caucasian knees, indicating that Chinese females had a smaller fML/fAP ratio than Caucasian females for the same fAP dimension. Thus, the differences in average values of femoral aspect ratio between Chinese and Caucasian females cannot be explained by differences in knee size alone, and this may point to a distinct variation in femoral shape between the two races (Yue et al. 2011).

22.2.4 Differences in Proximal Tibial Morphology

In general, the tibial volume of East Asians (293.1 ± 61.1 cm^3) has been found to be smaller than that of Caucasians (327.0 ± 74.7 cm^3) (Shao et al. 2018). The tibial dimension of Chinese males is generally smaller than that of Caucasian males and measurements of tibia have also shown that the tibial size of Chinese females is generally smaller than that of Caucasian females (Yue et al. 2011).

A significant difference has been noted for the tibial aspect ratio, with that of Chinese males being significantly larger than that of Caucasian males (1.82 ± 0.07 vs. 1.75 ± 0.11) ($P = 0.033$) (Yue et al. 2011). Mahfouz et al. (2012) also found that East Asian males had a smaller tibial mediolateral/tibial anteroposterior (tML/tAP) ratio than Caucasian males (1.33 ± 0.12 vs. 1.4 ± 0.06), with normalized ratios and nonlinear shape analysis in support of differences between East Asians and Caucasians independent of any scale factor.

Based on the study by Hovinga and Lerner (2009) a lower tibial torsion was also found in Japanese as compared to Caucasian populations. The average torsion angle was 37.58° for all subjects and showed significant differences with ethnicity ($p < 0.01$) with Caucasians demonstrating a higher torsion angle than Japanese (Hovinga and Lerner 2009). Tamari et al. (2006) also found that the Japanese patients had significantly greater femoral torsion angles (FTA) and femoral antetorsion than Australian Caucasians, more so in females than males and more so in the younger than older age group.

The coronal tibial slope, which measures the mediolateral slope of the tibial plateau, has recently been appreciated as a factor associated with accelerated development of knee OA, in a study based on follow-up of 4796 individuals of both genders from ages 45 to 79 in the Osteoarthritis Initiative (OAI), a longitudinal observational study of adults with or at risk for knee osteoarthritis at four clinical sites in the United States [Driban] (Driban et al. 2016). The study showed that the coronal slope ranged from 3.0° valgus to 9.0° varus, and a greater varus coronal slope was associated with an increased risk of incident accelerated knee osteoarthritis (OR = 1.15, 95% CI = 1.01 to 1.32), and that for every degree of increase in varus coronal slope, the odds of developing accelerated knee osteoarthritis increased by 15%. This study did not discuss racial differences in their findings, but the increased incidence in Asian populations may be hypothesized from other related alignment reports,(Hosseinzadeh et al. 2013; Tang et al. 2005; Hsu et al. 1990) and this feature is a frequent finding in the authors' clinical experience (◘ Fig. 22.1).

22.2.5 Differences in Patella Morphology and Others

Little work has been done comparing the anthropometric patella morphology of Asians to that of Caucasians. However, unsurprisingly, in line with the differences in the tibial and femoral dimensions, current studies show that the patella of Asians is generally smaller than that of their Western counterparts.

Kim et al. (2016) found that in Koreans, mean heights and widths of the patella were smaller than corresponding measurements in Westerners for both men (36.2 mm and 45.6 mm vs. 39.4 mm and 49.5 mm) and women (33.1 mm and 41.0 mm vs. 35.0 mm and 42.7 mm). However, the width/height ratios and ridge positions were similar in both Koreans and Westerners. Koreans were also found to have thinner patellae than Westerners. The mean central ridge thickness was 21.2 mm (range 17 to 26 mm) in women and 23.1 mm (range 20 to 26 mm) in men, whereas corresponding reported mean thicknesses in Western patients were 21.8 to 22.5 mm and 23.9 to 26.1 mm.

The general principle of resecting patellar bone equivalent to the height of the patellar button (usually around 8 to 9 mm) means that the thinner the patella, the less the residual bone thickness. This measurement is of significance in TKA as thinner patellae are less amenable to patellar resurfacing, particularly if the resected residual thickness is 11 mm or less, which may entail a fracture risk (Kim 2013). Thinner patellae of less than 21 mm preoperatively or less than 12 mm of residual thickness after resurfacing seem to be associated with less satisfactory results and ROM, even without patellar fracture or implant loosening (Chung et al. 2015).

> Thin patellae may be overlooked in preoperative radiographs due to variable and often increased magnifications in patellar views, and in Asian knees, patellar thickness should always be measured carefully before any step towards patellar resurfacing.

In our experience, native patellae of 14 to 15 mm thickness have been encountered in Asian female patients which are not amenable to current patellar resurfacing techniques (◘ Fig. 22.2). Strategies to develop thinner patellar resurfacing components have been adopted recently to address the problems of resurfacing thin patellae and these may be of benefit in Asian TKAs,(Ha and Na 2012) but longer term results regarding tribology and long-term survivorship are awaited (◘ Fig. 22.2).

Hovinga et al. also found higher ACL laxity in Japanese compared to Caucasian populations (Hovinga and Lerner 2009). ACL laxity measurement for Caucasian females was 6.4 ± 0.36 mm (n = 22), and for males was 4.9 ± 0.35 mm (n = 20). For Japanese females, the laxity was 8.1 ± 0.65 mm (n = 12), and for males 6.9 ± 0.56 mm (n = 11). Significant differences were found for both gender (p = 0.003) and ethnicity (p = 0.0002) (Hovinga and Lerner 2009).

Concluding Remarks

Almost all prosthetic implants have been designed and manufactured to accommodate the knee anatomy of Caucasians, and there is some doubt about the application of these TKA prostheses systems in Asians, as even the smallest size from each Western prosthesis company may be too big for some Asian patients.

Beyond the mere size, as reviewed in the above paragraphs, there are many differences in various anatomic parameters between Asian and Caucasian knees, affecting the fit of current prostheses in Asian knees.

As such, it is clearly necessary to have specifically designed TKA prostheses systems for Asian populations, accommodating not only the smaller Asian knee but also the variations in aspect ratios and size parameters. Another consideration in Asian knee prostheses is their need for more flexion than their western counterparts, given the differences in cultural and lifestyle factors necessitating greater flexions in Asians for functionality and operative satisfaction. As such, achieving deep flexion after TKA, although not as important as the technical consideration, is also a significant point to consider in prosthesis design.

22.3 Prevailing Knee Arthroplasty Techniques

22.3.1 Special Considerations in Asian Knee Arthroplasty

Generally, the strategies currently used to manage joint deformities in Asian patients are similar to those used when treating other ethnic groups (Kim et al. 2016). Some experts believe that any type of Western- or Asian-manufactured TKA prosthesis system can accommodate subtle differences in anthropometric knee anatomy between Asians and Westerners, regardless of differ-

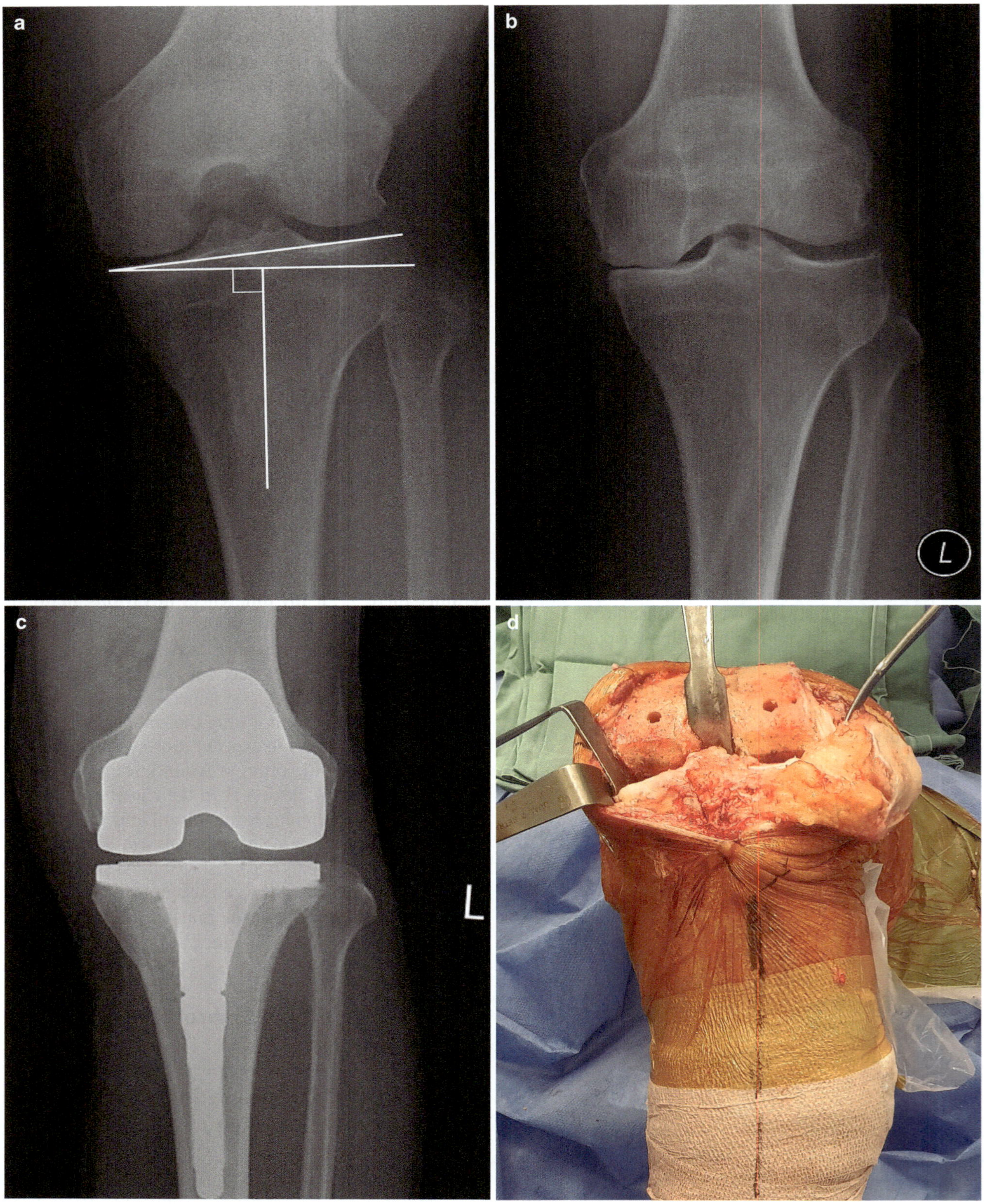

Fig. 22.1 **a** Coronal varus tibial slope of 6.2° in a Chinese male aged 57. **b** Accelerated medial knee OA in the same patient after 8 years. **c** X-ray of TKA for left knee in the same patient. **d** Intraoperative photograph of the same patient, demonstrating varus coronal slope compared to line marking tibial crest

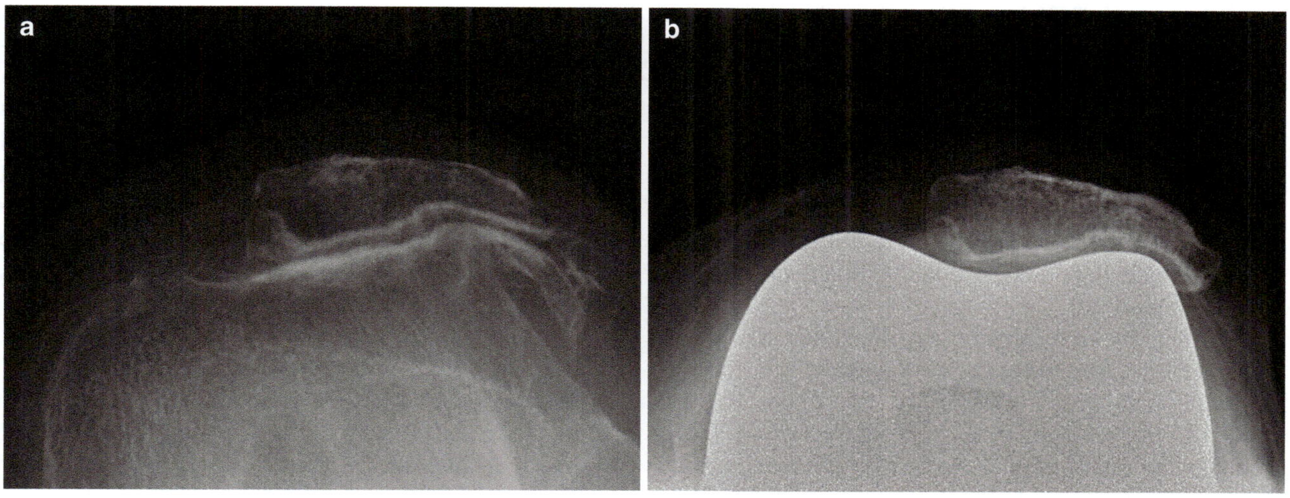

Fig. 22.2 **a** Thin patella in an 80-year-old Chinese female, measuring 14 mm thickness. **b** X-ray of the same patient 9 years after TKA. Patella resurfacing was not possible in this patient with conventional implants, despite her patellofemoral symptoms. Care was taken to position the patella on the femoral component by adjusting component rotation to ensure the best fit for the patellar profile

ences in culture, gender, activity level, or ethnicity (Kim et al. 2016).

But despite the generally successful results of contemporary TKAs, many patients' still remain unsatisfied with the performance of their replaced knees. This may be especially the case among Asian patients, since their lifestyle factors such as floor-based practices call for frequent high-flexion movement, causing them to demand greater postoperative flexion for higher satisfaction (Kim et al. 2008; Kim 2013). Furthermore, if Asian patients undergoing TKA have unique demographic and anatomic features known to influence the surgical outcome, these should also be taken into consideration at the level of patient selection, prosthesis design, and surgical technique (Kim 2013). Many studies (Chung et al. 2015; Ha and Na 2012; Ishimaru et al. 2014) have compared the structure of the Asian knee (Japanese, Chinese, Indian, and Korean) to existing Western-designed TKA prostheses systems and these anthropometric studies have suggested that Western-designed knee prostheses may not be suitable for Asian knees.

> Therefore, some researchers have suggested that Asian patients should have specially designed TKA prostheses systems (Kim et al. 2016) to better accommodate differences in knee morphology between Asians and Caucasians.

Considering the rapidly increasing number of TKAs performed in Asia, scientific data on Asian patients undergoing TKA will prove more important in the coming years. Current studies of Asian populations reporting the presence of unique anatomic characteristics of their patient population can be accommodated in designing prostheses and optimizing surgical techniques for Asian patients (Kim 2013). Furthermore, if Asian patients have certain demographic and anatomical characteristics known to affect clinical outcomes, special strategies to accommodate the unique nature of Asian patients may be required for preoperative patient counseling, prosthesis design, surgical technique, and postoperative rehabilitation (Kim et al. 2016).

For instance, high-flexion (HF) knee prostheses were designed to accommodate flexion of up to 155° through modification of posterior condylar geometry and cam design. Unlike in the Western world, limited flexion less than 130°reportedly impairs patient satisfaction in Asian populations (Kim et al. 2009b) because it limits common activities of daily living such as squatting or kneeling. Lee et al. (2013) reported the performance of these HF prostheses in Korean patients and showed that they improve function of TKA (52% could achieve >135° maximum flexion) in Asian patients without decreasing early survivorship (0.9%). Furthermore, such HF prostheses might also be associated with less polyethylene wear and subsequent osteolysis.

Based on the observation of a two times higher failure rate for fracture of the gliding surfaces of a multidirectional floating platform knee design (FP) in Asian countries compared to European countries, Maas et al. (2014) suggested that it is likely due to a combination of anatomy-driven internally rotated tibia components and a higher range of active knee flexion, producing a loading scenario which generates tensile stress levels above the yield strength of the ultrahigh-molecular-weight polyethylene (UHMWPE) material.

The authors also suggested that an improved posterior stabilized rotating platform design (RPS) would be more suitable for Asian patients. They found that at neutral tibia position the occurring maximum stress value at the FP system is 36% lower than the value determined for the RPS design. But at a tibia rotation of 10° off the neutral position, the maximum stress value determined at the FP system is 44% higher than the value computed for the RPS system (FP = 26 MPa vs. RPS = 18 MPa) and first exceeds the material yield strength of 25 MPa with a deformation of the lateral compartment, suggesting that such modifications to current TKA prostheses systems might have some value and significance to the Asian population.

Further research into the customization and development of prostheses to accommodate the morphological differences and intricacies of the Asian Knee is needed to improve outcomes and satisfaction of TKAs in this subpopulation of patients with unique anatomy, degree, and patterns of deformities, as well as cultural aspects, such as a traditional floor-based lifestyle and frequent high-flexion activities in daily living, which necessitate a substantially higher ROM as compared to Caucasian patients (Maas et al. 2014).

22.3.2 UKA Utility in Asia

UKA has gained popularity recently because of several studies (Amin et al. 2006; Lyons et al. 2012; Noticewala et al. 2012) which have shown that it is less invasive and has a reduced operative time, larger postoperative ROM, improved pain relief, earlier return to daily activities and sports, and cost reduction, in comparison to TKA. Furthermore, recent advancements in surgical instruments have contributed to decreasing the learning curve of the once technically challenging procedure (Kim et al. 2017). National and annual registries show similar trends, with increasing usage of UKA over the past 10 years, currently ranging from 5% to 11% globally in 2014 (Kleeblad et al. 2017).

Kim et al. (2017) retrospectively reviewed the mid-term results of minimally invasive Oxford medial UKA and followed 82 knees in 78 relatively young Asian patients. The authors found that Oxford medial UKA was reliable and effective in young active Asian patients providing good clinical results and survival rates in the mid-term follow-up, with a low complication rate and the 10-year cumulative survival rate using the Kaplan–Meier survival method being 94.7% (95% CI: 88.7%–100%). These mid-term results of UKA in <60-year-old Asian patients, with a different lifestyle from Western patients, have not been reported before and support the existing views that the <60-year-old contraindication for UKA should be modified,(Bruni et al. 2013; Thompson et al. 2013) especially so in the Asian context.

UKA has also been shown to give excellent results in Asian patients. Wong et al. (2014) found that the overall clinical outcomes of the knee showed the functional outcome of the knee to be normal in 51%, nearly normal in 37%, abnormal in 8%, and severely abnormal in only 4% in a study of 48 patients with 51 UKA knees in Taiwan. Based on their results, the authors concluded that UKA provides excellent pain relief and restoration of knee function including kneeling, squatting, and sit-to-stand activities that perfectly fit the oriental lifestyle and high patient satisfaction in Asian patients at medium-term follow-up.

> As such, UKA is a promising option in the Asian population as well, given its high utility in the restoration of the functional status even among Asians with high flexion demands. However, bearing dislocation is the most common cause of failure.

Bearing dislocation requires reoperation after UKA and the risk of bearing dislocation is three times higher in Asian patients than in their Western counterparts, with an incidence of 3/82 (3.6%), in a South Korean cohort studied by Kim et al. (2017). As such, mobile-bearing UKA may not be the best solution for knee OA in most Asian patients living in cultures where high flexion of the knee is essential (Bruni et al. 2013). At the very least, bearing dislocation should be considered as a potential complication for Asian patients undergoing mobile-bearing UKA (Kim et al. 2017) considering their lifestyle that necessitates high flexion postures such as kneeling and squatting.

22.4 Cementless TKA

22.4.1 Background of Cementless TKA

For the most part, cemented tibial fixations have been applied and excellent long-term results have been reported and while cemented fixation remains the gold standard for TKA, aseptic loosening continues to be a common failure mechanism, particularly in young patients (Pap et al. 2018). TKA with cementless fixation was thus developed to decrease cement-related complications, to potentially preserve the native bone stock, and to prolong implant survivorship. Even though the original designs were associated with early failures, innovations in technology have led to newer implants and biomaterials that accelerate implant osseointegration, which could eventually lead to improved long-term survivorship of cementless implants (Mont et al. 2017).

Pap et al. (2018) used the combination of titanium plasma spray and the hydroxyapatite porous-coating technique in cementless prostheses and the results showed that the novel SanatSwing cementless total knee prosthesis could be a good alternative to cemented TKA. The authors found normal osseointegration with the formation of a biological interface between the bone and the prosthetic components and a significantly shorter operation time (likely due to sparing of the cementing time) with low complication rates that were almost similar in both groups without any significant difference, suggesting the promising applications and utility of cementless TKA.

22.4.2 Cementless Versus Cemented TKA

Cementless TKA has been shown to have implant survivorshipof 10 and 20 years, which is comparable to cemented TKA (odds ratio [OR], 1.1; 95% confidence interval [CI], 0.62–2.00) (Mont et al. 2017). In a recent review of 37 studies by Mont et al. (2017) of the outcomes of cementless TKA in patients <50 years, the cohort of patients had aseptic survivorship of 100%, with no periprosthetic complications noted clinically or radiographically. In contrast, the cemented fixation has been shown to present a greater risk of future aseptic loosening Nakama et al. 2012).

Furthermore, using cementless TKA is undoubtedly time-saving, it reduces the pneumatic ischemia time (there is no need for complete exposure of the trabecular bone ready to receive the cement), and allows an easier bone-sparing revision in the event of failure (Wong et al. 2014).

In vitro studies have also demonstrated that the use of rotating platforms in cementless TKA is associated with better tribological performance and survival of the implant, related to the reduction of stresses at the bone–metal interface (Aprato et al. 2016).

However, cementless tibial baseplates may migrate early (in the first 3 months postoperatively), while cemented tibial components do not migrate in the immediate postoperative period, although they may show micromotion over 60 months.

- No differences have been demonstrated in the migration pattern of cemented with respect to cementless femoral components (Aprato et al. 2016).

Nakama et al. (2012) in their systematic review concluded that there was a smaller displacement of the cemented tibial component as compared to cementless fixation in studies with OA and RA participants who underwent primary TKA with a follow-up of 2 years. Likewise, similar results in terms of migration, clinical outcomes, and survival rates in young patients (<60 years) undergoing knee replacement were found in a study by Gao et al. (2009).

- Carlsson et al. (Chockalingam and Scott 2000) compared three types of fixation (cemented, uncemented porous, and uncemented porous hydroxyapatite fixation) and reported that cementing of the tibial component offers more stable bone-implant contact for 5 years postoperatively compared to uncemented fixation.

When cemented and cementless cases were amalgamated to form two groups, there was a significant improvement in survival ($P < 0.05$, log rank test) in favor of cemented fixation at year 6.

The majority of cementless TKA systems have endured limited success predominantly due to failed metal-backed patellar components with subsequent metallosis (Thompson et al. 2013). Osteolysis secondary to tibial and patellar failures (due to wear debris such as polyethylene, metal or both) have typically required removal and revision of all three components in the knee replacement in cementless TKA (Berry et al. 1993). In fact, the United Kingdom, Australia, Sweden, and New Zealand registry data have shown lower failure rates and greater usage of cemented than cementless fixation, with level I and II evidence strongly supporting cemented fixation (Aprato et al. 2016).

Beaupre et al. (2007) performed a prospective, randomized clinical trial where the subjects were randomized to be treated with either cementless tibial fixation with hydroxyapatite or cemented tibial fixation. At 5-year follow-up, there was no difference between cementless tibial fixation with hydroxyapatite and cemented tibial fixation in terms of self-reported pain, function, HRQoL, postoperative complications, or radiographic scores. In a prospective, randomized controlled study of cemented versus uncemented TKA, Fricka et al. (2015) reported the following findings:

- At 2 years, KSS functional scores, Oxford scores, and self-reported questions for satisfaction, less pain, and better function were similar; the cemented group had higher KSS clinical scores (96.4 vs. 92.3, $P = 0.03$) and more radiolucencies were seen in knees with cementless fixation ($P < 0.001$).

To date, there is a lack of research into a comparison of cemented and cementless TKA specifically in Asian populations.

> However, of note, anatomical variations in the lower limb are frequently seen in patients with arthritic knees, more frequently in Asian populations, including excessive bowing of the femoral shaft and metaphyseal bowing of the proximal tibia.

Mullaji et al. (2009, 2013) have also suggested the need for cemented stems in Asia where distorted anatomy in the form of sagittal and coronal bowing of the femur, a larger valgus correction angle (2–12°), and tibial bowing are often seen, while cementless stems can only provide 5–7°of valgus. Such excessive bowing may put the patient at increased risk for end-of-stem pain and periprosthetic fractures with a long, thick, press-fit uncemented stem, due to malalignment of the components, throwing the femoral component forward and resulting in a large flexion gap. In these situations, a shorter cemented stem (with a cement restrictor) has been suggested to be a better option (Beaupre et al. 2007) which is worth considering, especially in Asian patients.

Notably, cementation of the patellar component is crucial as it is now clear that cementless patellas are associated with a high risk of failure due to early loosening of the component (Aprato et al. 2016).

> Compared to cemented fixation, uncemented fixation has been shown to involve more PF complications, including increased susceptibility to wear due to a thinner polyethylene bearing on the cementless metal-backed component.

Concluding Remarks on Cementless TKA

In conclusion, prosthesis systems for cementless TKA should be customized to the Asian knee (such as the use of shorter cemented stems) and assessed using further research into differential outcomes in Asians between cemented and various cementless TKA prosthesis systems. Such data should be used, instead of extrapolating outcomes and results identified in Western populations, which may not be entirely applicable to Asians, given the differences in knee morphology.

22.5 Patellofemoral Arthroplasty and Background and Utility of Patellar Resurfacing

As described in the earlier sections, patellar dimensions are also different between Asians and Caucasians, with the Asian patella being smaller and thinner than that of Caucasians (Kim et al. 2016). So although specific considerations in RP techniques for Asians are necessary, a specifically designed thinner patella prosthesis has also been suggested to be essential to accommodate the thinner patella in the Asian knee (Hosseinzadeh et al. 2013). The challenge of restoring preoperative patellar thickness is also greater in Asian patients, in whom it is common to find a patella of less than 20 mm in thickness (Hosseinzadeh et al. 2013; Kim et al. 2016; Dy et al. 2012). Jhurani et al. (2018b) recently also found that the 6.2 mm thin patellar button is useful to restore the native thickness in such patients with a patellar thickness of less than 20 mm, without risk of button fracture, loosening, or overstuffing, which is especially applicable in Asians undergoing RP.

> Yet, while some implant manufacturers have recently taken Asian anthropometric data into consideration when designing implants for this population which has smaller and narrower bone sizes, the patellar button thickness has not been revised.

Sulaiman and Nordin (2005) also reported that in a cross-sectional study on patella thickness using plain radiographs of 56 patients in Malaysia, the average thickness of the bony part of the patella was 20.05 mm (range 17–23 mm) and the actual thickness of cartilage varied from 2.0 to 5.5 mm (mean 3.2 mm). The authors concluded that since the majority of the patients in their cohort (73%) had patellar thickness of 24 mm or less, the majority of their patients in Malaysia are not suitable for RP as a patella of 25 mm or less in thickness is not suitable for resurfacing using the currently available total knee systems. This further suggests the limited utility of current RP systems in Asian patients and supports the need for further development and adapting of knee replacement systems to suit the thinner and smaller Asian patella.

Summary and Conclusion

Total knee arthroplasty is one of the most successful clinical interventions for severe, end-stage OA and substantially improves the patients' quality of life after surgery, especially in terms of pain reduction, suggesting the high utility and benefit of TKA as the treatment of choice for severe knee OA. Given both population aging and the rapid economic growth Asia, it is likely that knee OA will become a more prevalent problem and that the utilization of TKA will increase in many Asian countries as well, with many Asian countries already showing a rapid rise in TKA rates, including South Korea, Taiwan, Vietnam, and China.

However, of note, TKA in Asian populations involves a few unique challenges, especially that of higher demands of postoperative flexion among Asians. Special considerations in TKA for Asians are also required. Recent anthropometric studies have suggested that the current design of TKA does not cater to racial anthropometric differences and most of the commercially available TKA prostheses are designed according to the anthropometric data of Caucasian knees, causing component mismatch when used in Asian patients.

Almost all prosthetic implants have been designed and manufactured to accommodate the knee anatomy of Caucasians, resulting in TKA component mismatch. This has led some researchers to suggest that Asians should have special designs of the TKA prostheses system based on accurate morphologic data of the Asian knee. With the higher prevalence of knee OA and the increasing use of TKA in Asia, it has become essential to understand the differences between knee morphology and anatomy of the Asian and Caucasian population to improve TKA prostheses and the outcomes of TKA in Asian populations.

Furthermore, if Asian patients have certain demographic and anatomical characteristics known to affect clinical outcomes, special strategies to cater to these, in terms of modified prosthesis design, surgical technique, and postoperative rehabilitation, would be greatly beneficial. For instance, high-flexion (HF) knee prostheses in Korean patients improve function of TKA in Asian patients without decreasing early survivorship (0.9%). Modifications to current TKA prostheses systems such as an improved posterior stabilized rotating platform design (RPS) might also have some value and significance to the Asian population who have lifestyle factors that demand higher flexion.

Based on the mid-term results of minimally invasive Oxford medial UKA in <60-year-old Asian patients with a different lifestyle from Western patients (which have not been reported thus far), the view that the <60-year-old contraindication for UKA should be modified, especially so in the Asian context, is one that is worth considering and that requires further research and data in this area. But at the same time, bearing dislocation is three times higher in Asian patients than in their Western counterparts and should be considered as a potential complication for Asian patients undergoing mobile-bearing UKA.

Moreover, with the growing number of younger, more active patients requiring TKA in Asia, cementless fixation may be the best modality that is most suitable for those who have an active lifestyle; thereby, decreasing the risk for revision surgery. As such, more prospective, randomized trials are needed to clearly delineate any differences between cemented and cementless fixation options and their utility in Asian populations.

PFA has also been shown to be a viable option for the treatment of isolated PFOA and modern PFA designs which onlay style, strict patient selection, and improvement in surgical techniques have produced satisfactory results in the past decades.

However, current treatment paradigms for PFOA are inadequate and published guidelines are based exclusively on research utilizing tibiofemoral OA, instead of evidence for PFOA. As such, future studies assessing the long-term results of new designs and technologies of PFA as well as comparison studies to TKA are necessary to evaluate patient outcomes and implant performance.

Clearly, the Asian knee must be given special consideration in the context of TKA regarding the various differences that exist between the anatomy and functional factors of Asian versus Western knees. As such, future research into TKA should consider stratification by ethnicity to better delineate how the Asian knee differs from Western knees, and therefore, how current TKA systems can be modified to accommodate these differences to further improve knee replacement surgeries in this patient population. This will allow for further improvements in postoperative function, satisfaction, and reduction in complication rates in this subgroup of patients undergoing TKA.

Take-Home Messages

- There is an increasing evidence delineating clinically significant anatomical differences between the Caucasian and Asian knee. These factors should play a role in implant design for purposes of TKA.
- Cementless TKA, which is increasingly used especially for young active patients, has the benefit of a lower risk of aseptic loosening. However, improvements to the design to account for angular and length disparities between implants of the Asian lower limb should be accounted for.
- Implant design should also cater to lifestyle factors of the Asian population, such as the need for a high-flexion prosthesis.

References

Amin AK, Patton JT, Cook RE, Gaston M, Brenkel IJ (2006) Unicompartmental or total knee arthroplasty?:Results from a matched study. Clin Orthop Relat Res 451:101–106

Aprato A, Risitano S, Sabatini L, Giachino M, Agati G, Masse A (2016) Cementless total kneearthroplasty. Ann TranslMed 4(7):129

Beaupre LA, al-Yamani M, Huckell JR, Johnston DW (2007) Hydroxyapatite-coated tibial implants compared with cemented tibial fixation in primary total knee arthroplasty. A randomized trial of outcomes at five years. J Bone Joint Surg Am 89(10):2204–2211

Berry DJ, Wold LE, Rand JA (1993) Extensive osteolysis around an aseptic, stable, uncemented total knee replacement. Clin Orthop Relat Res. 293:204–207

Bin AbdRazak HR, Yeo SJ (2015) Meeting patient expectations and ensuring satisfaction in total knee arthroplasty. Ann Transl Med 3(20):315

Bruni D, Akkawi I, Iacono F et al (2013) Minimum thickness of all-poly tibial component unicompartmentalkneearthroplasty in patients youngerthan 60 yearsdoes not increaserevision rate for

asepticloosening. Knee Surg Sports Traumatol Arthrosc. 21(11):2462–2467
Callahan CM, Drake BG, Heck DA, Dittus RS (1994) Patient outcomesfollowingtricompartmental total knee replacement. A meta-analysis. Jama 271(17):1349–1357
Callahan CM, Drake BG, Heck DA, Dittus RS (1995) Patient outcomesfollowingunicompartmental or bicompartmentalkneearthroplasty. A meta-analysis. J Arthroplasty 10(2):141–150
Cheng FB, Ji XF, Lai Y et al (2009) Three dimensional morphometry of the knee to design the total knee arthroplasty for Chinese population. Knee 16(5):341–347
Chockalingam S, Scott G (2000) The outcome of cemented vs. cementless fixation of a femoral component in total knee replacement TKR with the identification of radiological signs for the prediction of failure. The Knee 7:233–238
Chung BJ, Kang JY, Kang YG, Kim SJ, Kim TK (2015) Clinical implications of femoral anthropometrical features for total knee arthroplasty in Koreans. J Arthroplast 30(7):1220–1227
Driban JB, Stout AC, Duryea J, Lo GH, Harvey WK, Price LL, Ward RJ, Eaton CB, Barbe MF, Lu B, McAlindon TE (2016) Coronal tibial slopeis associated with accelerated kneeosteoarthritis: data from the Osteoarthritis Initiative. BMC Musculoskelet Disord 17:299
Dunbar MJ (2001) Subjective outcomes after knee arthroplasty. Acta Orthop Scand Suppl 72(301):1–63
Dy CJ, Franco N, Ma Y, Mazumdar M, McCarthy MM, Gonzalez Della Valle A (2012) Complications after patello-femoral versus total knee replacement in the treatment of isolatedpatellofemoralosteoarthritis. A meta-analysis. Knee Surg Sports Traumatol Arthrosc 20(11):2174–2190
Fransen M, Bridgett L, March L, Hoy D, Penserga E, Brooks P (2011) The epidemiology of osteoarthritis in Asia. Int J Rheum Dis 14(2):113–121
Fricka KB, Sritulanondha S, McAsey CJ (2015) To cement or not? Two-year results of a prospective, randomized study comparing cemented vs. cementless Total Knee Arthroplasty (TKA). J Arthroplast 30(9 Suppl):55–58
Gao F, Henricson A, Nilsson KG (2009) Cemented versus uncemented fixation of the femoral component of the NexGen CR total knee replacement in patients youngerthan 60 years: a prospective randomisedcontrolled RSA study. Knee 16(3):200–206
Ha CW, Na SE (2012) The correctness of fit of current total knee prostheses compared with intra-operative anthropometric measurements in Korean knees. J Bone Joint Surg Br 94(5):638–641
Harvey WF, Niu J, Zhang Y et al (2008) Knee alignment differences between Chinese and Caucasian subjects without osteoarthritis. Ann Rheum Dis 67(11):1524–1528
He Y, Xiao L, Zhai W, Kasparek MF, Ouyang G, Boettner F (2018) What percentage of patients is a candidate for unicompartmental knee replacement at a Chinese arthroplasty center? Open Orthop J 12:17–23
Ho WP, Cheng CK, Liau JJ (2006) Morphometrical measurements of resected surface of femurs in Chinese knees: correlation to the sizing of current femoral implants. Knee 13(1):12–14
Ho-Pham LT, Lai TQ, Mai LD, Doan MC, Pham HN, Nguyen TV (2014) Prevalence of radiographic osteoarthritis of the knee and its relationship to self-reported pain. PLoS One 9(4):e94563
Hosseinzadeh, Hossein G, Masoudi A et al (2013) Special considerations in Asian knee arthroplasty. In: Arthroplasty – update
Hovinga KR, Lerner AL (2009) Anatomic variations between Japanese and Caucasian populations in the healthy young adult knee joint. J Orthop Res. 27(9):1191–1196
Hsu RW, Himeno S, Coventry MB, Chao EY (1990) Normal axial alignment of the lower extremity and load-bearing distribution at the knee. Clin Orthop Relat Res. 255:215–227
Inoue K, Hukuda S, Fardellon P et al (2001) Prevalence of large-joint osteoarthritis in Asian and Caucasian skeletal populations. Rheumatology (Oxford) 40(1):70–73
Iorio R, Kobayashi S, Healy WL, Cruz AI Jr, Ayers ME (2007) Primary posterior cruciate-retaining total knee arthroplasty: a comparison of American and Japanese cohorts. J Surg Orthop Adv 16(4):164–170
Ishimaru M, Hino K, Onishi Y, Iseki Y, Mashima N, Miura H (2014) A three-dimensional computed tomography study of distal femoral morphology in Japanese patients: gender differences and component fit. Knee 21(6):1221–1224
Jensen LK (2008) Knee osteoarthritis: influence of work involving heavy lifting, kneeling, climbing stairs or ladders, or kneeling/squatting combined with heavy lifting. Occup Environ Med 65(2):72–89
Jhurani A, Agarwal P, Aswal M, Saxena P, Singh N (2018b) Safety and efficacy of 6.2 mm patellar button in resurfacing less than 20 mm thin patella: a matched pair analysis. Knee Surg Relat Res. 30(2):153–160
Jonsson H, Olafsdottir S, Sigurdardottir S et al (2016) Incidence and prevalence of total joint replacements due to osteoarthritis in the elderly: riskfactors and factorsassociatedwithlate life prevalence in the AGES-Reykjavik Study. BMC Musculoskelet Disord 17:14
Joshy S, Datta A, Perera A, Thomas B, Gogi N, Kumar SB (2006) Ethnic differences in preoperative function of patients undergoing total knee arthroplasty. Int Orthop 30(5):426–428
Kim TK (2013) Specialconsiderations for TKA in Asian patients: editorial comment. Clin Orthop Relat Res. 471(5):1439–1440
Kim HA, Kim S, Seo YI et al (2008) The epidemiology of total knee replacement in South Korea: national registry data. Rheumatology (Oxford) 47(1):88–91
Kim TK, Chang CB, Kang YG, Kim SJ, Seong SC (2009b) Causes and predictors of patient's dissatisfaction after uncomplicated total knee arthroplasty. J Arthroplast 24(2):263–271
Kim YH, Matsuda S, Kim TK (2016) ClinicalFaceoff: do we need special strategies for Asian patients with TKA? Clin Orthop Relat Res. 474(5):1102–1107
Kim YJ, Kim BH, Yoo SH, Kang SW, Kwack CH, Song MH (2017) Mid-term results of Oxford medial unicompartmental knee arthroplasty in young Asian patients Less than 60 years of age: a minimum 5-year follow-up. Knee Surg Relat Res 29(2):122–128
Kleeblad LJ, Zuiderbaan HA, Hooper GJ, Pearle AD (2017) Unicompartmental knee arthroplasty: state of the art. J ISAKOS 2(2):97–107
Ko Y, Narayanasamy S, Wee HL et al (2011) Health-relatedquality of life after total knee replacement or unicompartmentalkneearthroplasty in an urbanasian population. Value Health 14(2):322–328
Kobayashi S, Pappas E, Fransen M, Refshauge K, Simic M (2016) The prevalence of patellofemoral osteoarthritis: a systematic review and meta-analysis. Osteoarthr Cartil 24(10):1697–1707
Koh IJ, Kim TK, Chang CB, Cho HJ, In Y (2013) Trends in use of total kneearthroplasty in Koreafrom 2001 to 2010. Clin Orthop Relat Res 471(5):1441–1450
Kumar A, Tsai WC, Tan TS, Kung PT, Chiu LT, Ku MC (2015) Temporal trends in primary and revision total knee and hip replacement in Taiwan. J Chin Med Assoc 78(9):538–544
Kurtz SM, Ong KL, Lau E et al (2011) International survey of primary and revision total knee replacement. Int Orthop 35(12):1783–1789
Lee BS, Chung JW, Kim JM, Kim KA, Bin SI (2013) High-flexion prosthesis improves function of TKA in Asian patients without decreasing early survivorship. Clin Orthop Relat Res. 471(5):1504–1511

Lin FH, Chen HC, Lin C et al (2018) The increase in total knee replacement surgery in Taiwan: a 15-year retrospective study. Medicine (Baltimore) 97(31):e11749
Lyons MC, MacDonald SJ, Somerville LE, Naudie DD, McCalden RW (2012) Unicompartmental versus total knee arthroplasty database analysis: is there a winner? Clin Orthop Relat Res. 470(1):84–90
Maas A, Kim TK, Miehlke RK, Hagen T, Grupp TM (2014) Differences in anatomy and kinematics in Asian and Caucasian TKA patients: influence on implant positioning and subsequent loading conditions in mobile bearing knees. Biomed Res Int 2014:612838
Mahfouz M, Abdel Fatah EE, Bowers LS, Scuderi G (2012) Three-dimensional morphology of the knee reveals ethnic differences. Clin Orthop Relat Res. 470(1):172–185
Mahomed N, Gandhi R, Daltroy L, Katz JN (2011) The self-administered patient satisfaction scale for primary hip and knee arthroplasty. Arthritis 2011:591253
Mont MA, Gwam C, Newman JM et al (2017) Outcomes of a newer-generation cementless total knee arthroplasty design in patients less than 50 years of age. Ann Transl Med. 5(Suppl 3):S24
Moreland JR, Bassett LW, Hanker GJ (1987) Radiographic analysis of the axial alignment of the lower extremity. J Bone Joint Surg Am 69(5):745–749
Mullaji AB, Sharma AK, Marawar SV, Kohli AF, Singh DP (2009) Distal femoral rotational axes in Indian knees. J Orthop Surg (Hong Kong) 17(2):166–169
Mullaji AB, Shetty GM, Kanna R, Vadapalli RC (2013) The influence of preoperative deformity on valgus correction angle: an analysis of 503 total knee arthroplasties. J Arthroplast 28(1):20–27
Muraki S, Oka H, Akune T et al (2009) Prevalence of radiographic knee osteoarthritis and its association with knee pain in the elderly of Japanese population-based cohorts: the ROAD study. Osteoarthr Cartil 17(9):1137–1143
Murphy L, Schwartz TA, Helmick CG et al (2008) Lifetimerisk of symptomatickneeosteoarthritis. Arthritis Rheum 59(9):1207–1213
Nakama GY, Peccin MS, Almeida GJ, Lira Neto Ode A, Queiroz AA, Navarro RD (2012) Cemented, cementless or hybrid fixation options in total knee arthroplasty for osteoarthritis and other non-traumatic diseases. Cochrane Database Syst Rev 10:CD006193
Nguyen TV (2014) Osteoarthritis in Southeast Asia. Int J Clin Rheum 9(5):405–408
Noticewala MS, Geller JA, Lee JH, Macaulay W (2012) Unicompartmental knee arthroplasty relieves pain and improves function more than total knee arthroplasty. J Arthroplast 27(8 Suppl):99–105
Pabinger C, Lothaller H, Geissler A (2015) Utilization rates of knee-arthroplasty in OECD countries. Osteoarthr Cartil 23(10):1664–1673
Pap K, Vasarhelyi G, Gal T et al (2018) Evaluation of clinical outcomes of cemented vs uncemented knee prostheses covered with titanium plasma spray and hydroxyapatite: a minimum two years follow-up. Eklem Hastalik Cerrahisi 29(2):65–70
Pereira D, Peleteiro B, Araujo J, Branco J, Santos RA, Ramos E (2011) The effect of osteoarthritis definition on prevalence and incidence estimates: a systematic review. Osteoarthr Cartil 19(11):1270–1285
Rytter S, Egund N, Jensen LK, Bonde JP (2009) Occupational kneeling and radiographic tibiofemoral and patellofemoral osteoarthritis. J Occup Med Toxicol 4:19
Shao H, Chen C, Scholl D, Faizan A, Chen AF (2018) Tibial shaft anatomy differs between Caucasians and East Asian individuals. Knee Surg Sports Traumatol Arthrosc. 26(9):2758–2765
Slover J, Espehaug B, Havelin LI et al (2006) Cost-effectiveness of unicompartmental and total kneearthroplasty in elderlylow-demand patients. A Markov decisionanalysis. J Bone Joint Surg Am 88(11):2348–2355
Sulaiman AS, Nordin S (2005) Measurement of patellar thickness in relation to patellar resurfacing. Med J Malaysia 60 Suppl C:41–44
Tamari K, Tinley P, Briffa K, Aoyagi K (2006) Ethnic-, gender-, and age-relateddifferences in femorotibial angle, femoralantetorsion, and tibiofibular torsion: cross-sectional studyamonghealthyJapanese and AustralianCaucasians. Clin Anat 19(1):59–67
Tang WM, Chiu KY, Kwan MF, Ng TP, Yau WP (2005) Sagittal bowing of the distal femur in Chinese patients who require total knee arthroplasty. J Orthop Res 23(1):41–45
Thambiah MD, Nathan S, Seow BZ, Liang S, Lingaraj K (2015) Patient satisfaction after total knee arthroplasty: an Asian perspective. Singap Med J 56(5):259–263
Thompson SA, Liabaud B, Nellans KW, Geller JA (2013) Factorsassociatedwithpooroutcomesfollowingunicompartmentalkneearthroplasty: redefining the "classic" indications for surgery. J Arthroplast 28(9):1561–1564
Urabe K, Mahoney OM, Mabuchi K, Itoman M (2008) Morphologic differences of the distal femur between Caucasian and Japanese women. J Orthop Surg 16(3):312–315
Valdes AM, Spector TD (2011) Genetic epidemiology of hip and knee osteoarthritis. Nat Rev Rheum 7(1):23–32
Wise BL, Niu J, Yang M et al (2012) Patterns of compartment involvement in tibiofemoral osteoarthritis in men and women and in whites and African Americans. Arthritis Care Res (Hoboken) 64(6):847–852
Wong T, Wang CJ, Wang JW, Ko JY (2014) Functional outcomes of uni-knee arthroplasty for medial compartment knee arthropathy in asian patients. Biom J 37(6):406–410
Woolson ST, Shu B, Giori NJ (2010) Incidence of radiographic unicompartmental arthritis in patients under going knee arthroplasty. Orthopedics 33(11):798
Yue B, Varadarajan KM, Ai S, Tang T, Rubash HE, Li G (2011) Differences of knee anthropometry between Chinese and white men and women. J Arthroplast 26(1):124–130
Zeni JA Jr, Axe MJ, Snyder-Mackler L (2010) Clinicalpredictors of elective total joint replacement in personswith end-stage kneeosteoarthritis. BMC Musculoskelet Disord 11:86
Zhang Y, Xu L, Nevitt MC et al (2001) Comparison of the prevalence of knee osteoarthritis between the elderly Chinese population in Beijing and whites in the United States: the Beijing Osteoarthritis Study. Arthritis Rheum 44(9):2065–2071
Zhang W, Moskowitz RW, Nuki G et al (2008) OARSI recommendations for the management of hip and kneeosteoarthritis, Part II: OARSI evidence-based, expert consensus guidelines. Osteoarthr Cartil 16(2):137–162

Clinical Care Pathways

Contents

Preoperative Optimization in Total Joint Arthroplasty

Vignesh K. Alamanda and Bryan D. Springer

Contents

E. Hansen, K.-D. Kühn (eds.), *Essentials of Cemented Knee Arthroplasty*,
https://doi.org/10.1007/978-3-662-63113-3_23

23.1 Introduction

23.1.1 Scope of the Problem—Periprosthetic Joint Infections

Total joint arthroplasties represent some of the most commonly performed surgeries in the United States. However, periprosthetic joint infection (PJI) is a significant problem associated with increased morbidity and healthcare costs. The incidence of PJI after primary total hip and knee replacements has been reported in the literature to range from 0.5% to up to 2% (Bozic and Ries 2005; Sculco 1993).

PJI has a significant impact on the patient, the surgeon, and the healthcare system (Bozic and Ries 2005).

> The economic burden of PJI is expected to be in excess of 1.62 billion $ by the year 2020 (Kurtz et al. 2012).

This is crucial to address as current estimates project large increases in demand for total hip (growth of 174% by 2030) and knee arthroplasties (growth of 673% by 2030) (Kurtz et al. 2007). Similar trends are also anticipated with revision arthroplasty surgery.

23.1.2 Modifiable Versus Non-modifiable Risk Factors

It is imperative to appropriately recognize risk factor variables as modifiable versus non-modifiable. While the scope of this chapter is limited to identifying and acting on modifiable risk factors to improve rates of PJI, non-modifiable risk factors have also been recognized to affect rates of PJI. Specifically, revision surgery and non-same day surgery, i.e., surgery performed >24 h after admission, have been identified as negatively affecting rates of PJI by Maoz et al. (2015). While it is important to recognize, these risk factors are unfortunately beyond the control of the surgeon and their patients.

23.1.3 Currently Available Guidelines on Surgical Site Infections

The Centers for Disease Control and Prevention (CDC) provided new guidelines that have important updates and recommendations for the prevention of surgical site infections(SSI). These include guidelines from the use of antiseptic soap the night before surgery to maintaining appropriate oxygenation and glycemic control in the perioperative period (Berrios-Torres et al. 2017). However, as noted by Parvizi et al., the lack of evidence in many of the areas prevents it from being a comprehensive guide (Parvizi et al. 2017).

Thus, it is essential that we attempt to further understand and minimize the risk factors that can affect rates of PJI. In this review, the effects of both patient as well as perioperative modifiable risk factors that can affect PJI are analyzed.

23.2 Patient-Modifiable Risk Factors and Current Evidence

23.2.1 Diabetes

Diabetes and poor glycemic control have not only been associated with increased risk of surgical site infection in a variety of procedures but are also negatively implicated in PJI in multiple studies. Analysis of these studies has shown diabetes to increase the odds ratio by 2.28 times in one of the largest series (Marchant Jr. et al. 2009).

Hemoglobin A1c (Hgb A1c) has been regularly used as a prognostic indicator of long-term glycemic control in patients and may take 3 months to reflect significant changes. Patients with good glycemic control should ideally have Hgb A1C levels <7.0. Hgb A1c, a simple test, has frequently been used as a routine screening test which allows the provider to gain insight into the patient's glycemic control over the past 3 months (Stryker et al. 2013).

> However, perioperative glucose levels may serve as a better adjunct in predicting PJI as opposed to Hgb A1c alone (Iorio et al. 2012). Additionally, other markers such as serum fructosamine have also been proposed to serve as an adjunct to measuring glycemic control (Shohat et al. 2017).

The stress due to surgery results in an increased production of hormones antagonizing insulin and predisposes patients to hyperglycemia. Thus, it is important that perioperative glycemic control be strictly enforced. Surgical stress-related postoperative hyperglycemia, even in patients without a diagnosis of diabetes, can increase the risk of developing surgical site infection in a dose-related manner.

> Thus, the authors recommend that blood glucose levels be maintained between 110 and 180 mg/dL (optimal cutoff of around137 mg/dL) (Kheir et al. 2018) in the perioperative period through frequent blood sugar checks and initiation of diabetic management protocols postoperatively (Gallagher et al. 2017).

23.2.2 Obesity

Obesity has been correlated with higher rates of osteoarthritis and eventual increased use of arthroplasty (Workgroup of the American Association of H, Knee Surgeons Evidence Based C 2013). Studies have shown that patient satisfaction and functional improvement in the obese patient population is similar to the nonobese group; however, obese patients are at higher risk of postoperative complications, specifically PJI (Mason et al. 2014).

Obesity predisposes patients to increased surgical dissections needed for exposure which results in higher surgical times. The poor vascularity of adipose tissue further compounds this problem. The consensus opinion from the workgroup of the American Association of Hip and Knee Surgeons (AAHKS) evidence-based committee emphasized delaying total joint arthroplasty in a patient with a BMI >40, especially when associated with other comorbid conditions such as poorly controlled diabetes or malnutrition (Workgroup of the American Association of H, Knee Surgeons Evidence Based C 2013).

Furthermore, a small minority of obese patients may develop metabolic syndrome. This is composed of a cluster of conditions arising from insulin resistance that impairs normal leukocyte function. It is defined as having a BMI >30 kg/m^2 with central obesity, as well as two of the following conditions: hyperlipidemia, hyperglyceridemia, hypertension, or diabetes (Gage et al. 2014). Zmistowski et al. have shown an increased risk of PJI (14.3% vs. 0.8%) in patients with uncontrolled metabolic syndrome compared to patients with controlled disease/the healthy cohort (Zmistowski et al. 2013).

> Patients with obesity should be screened for other characteristics that may define metabolic syndrome.

23.2.3 Malnutrition

A frequently unrecognized aspect of obesity involves malnutrition and is associated with high caloric but nutritionally poor diets.

> Malnutrition was found to be present in 42.9% of obese patients in a prospective study evaluating the role of malnutrition in total joint arthroplasty patients (Huang et al. 2013).

Laboratory tests are easily available and can help to identify patients at risk for malnutrition.

> These include a total lymphocyte count of <1500 cells/mm^3, a serum albumin of <3.5 g/dL, or a transferrin level of <200 mg/dL. Of these, preoperative albumin has been found to be highly specific with a high positive predictive value for PJI (Blevins et al. 2018).

Patients with preoperative malnutrition should be encouraged to work with a dietician to help improve their nutritional intake and help prepare them for the catabolic demands required in the postsurgical period.

23.2.4 Smoking

Smoking, and its principal ingredient, nicotine, has been associated with decreased oxygen delivery to tissues secondary to microvascular constriction. Duchman et al. reported an increased risk of wound complications with both current and former smokers in a large national database study. Specifically, they found current smokers to have higher rates of wound complications than former smokers as it pertains to PJI (Duchman et al. 2015). The deleterious effects, in particular PJI, seen with smoking have also been confirmed by multiple other studies (Teng et al. 2015).

> Studies have shown that smoking cessation programs may help decrease complications associated with the use of nicotine, even if introduced as late as just 4 weeks before surgery (Lindstrom et al. 2008).

Thus, the authors recommend that patients undergoing total joint arthroplasty have a minimum period of 4 weeks of smoking cessation prior to their surgery. Smoking cessation can be confirmed via easily available laboratory tests such as the serum cotinine assay (normal value of ≤10 μg/L).

23.2.5 Vitamin D

Vitamin D has long been identified as playing a crucial role in bone health. Vitamin D deficiency, as defined by a serum 25-hydroxyvitamin D concentration ≤ 20 ng/mL, is unfortunately prevalent in the population of the United States with an overall reported rate of 41.6% (Forrest and Stuhldreher 2011). Studies have shown patients with PJI to have low levels of Vitamin D. Animal models have also demonstrated that reversal of Vitamin D deficiency can help improve rates of PJI (Hegde et al. 2017).

> Thus, the authors recommend that Vitamin D levels be obtained preoperatively and if deficient, i.e.,< 20 ng/mL, supplementation be instituted.

23.2.6 *Staphylococcus Aureus* Screening

Nasal swab rapid polymerase chain reaction has allowed physicians to identify patients who are colonized with methicillin-resistant *Staphylococcus aureus* (MRSA). This helps eliminate the bacteria from the patient's nasal flora prior to surgery. Implementation of an institution-wide prescreening program allows for the identification of the carrier status of *S. aureus* among patients; this can then lead to a significant reduction in postoperative rates of surgical site infections (Kim et al. 2010).

It is the authors'recommendation that patients undergoing elective total joint arthroplasty undergo screening for *S. aureus* through nasal swabs.

- The authors recommend that patients undergo application of mupirocin nasal ointment twice daily to both nares and a daily bath with chlorhexidine for 5 days immediately prior to the scheduled surgery if the nasal swab testing is positive.

- Additionally, patients screened positive for MRSA should also receive a single dose of vancomycin along with standard perioperative antibiotics during their surgery.

23.2.7 Inflammatory Arthropathies

Patients afflicted with inflammatory arthropathies such as rheumatoid arthritis and lupus are at increased risk of postoperative infection. Multiple systematic reviews have validated the correlation between inflammatory arthropathies and periprosthetic infection. Pooled studies such as that by Kong et al. have shown that rheumatoid arthritis can increase the odds of PJI by 1.57 (Kong et al. 2017).

Many of these patients are on multiple-drug regimens that may include immunomodulators. These medications often have significant effects on wound healing and infections. For example, tumor necrosis factor alpha (TNFα) inhibitors are frequently used as a powerful agent in the management of these diseases. However, by modulating the immune system, they place patients at significant risk for developing infections. Momohara et al. reported that patients on TNFα inhibitors were found to be at higher risk for surgical site infections (Momohara et al. 2011).

Guidelines jointly published by the American College of Rheumatology (ACR) and the American Association of Hip and Knee Surgeons (AAHKS) used available evidence to make recommendations on which medications should be continued and which medications should be stopped in elective total joint arthroplasty (Goodman et al. 2017). In general, traditional disease-modifying antirheumatic medications (DMARDS) do not need to be withheld prior to surgery.

- However, immunomodulating agents such as TNFα inhibitors place patients at an increased risk for the development of PJI and should be withheld one dosing cycle prior to surgery.

23.2.8 Urinary Tract Infections

A common type of nosocomial infection, urinary tract infections (UTI), creates a reservoir of pathogens and potentially increases patient morbidity during surgical intervention. The role of UTI in the development of PJI, however, remains controversial. Some authors have noted the development of PJI in patients with UTI (David and Vrahas 2000) while others have shown no association between UTI and PJI (Koulouvaris et al. 2009).

- It is the authors' recommendation that if the patient has symptoms of UTI such as dysuria, urgency, and frequency and has $>1 \times 10^5$ colony forming units (CFU)/mL of urine, surgery should be postponed.

- However, if the patient is asymptomatic but has 1×10^5 or more CFU/mL of urine, the authors recommend not withholding surgery and treating his UTI with a routine course of postoperative oral antibiotics.

23.2.9 Poor Oral Health

Total joint replacement patients tend to have good dental hygiene in general (Wood et al. 2016). However, there is not a lot of literature on the role of preoperative screening as well as the association between poor dental hygiene and PJI. Recent studies have questioned the need to obtain routine preoperative dental screening for hip and knee arthroplasty patients (Lampley et al. 2014).

- In general, the authors recommend a common-sense approach—patients should have a dental exam and clearance if they have evidence of decayed teeth, abscess, gingivitis, or periodontitis and should have routine cleanings done prior to surgical intervention.

23.2.10 Antibiotic Prophylaxis

Preoperative antibiotic prophylaxis is effective in reducing rates of surgical site infections and has been incorporated in many surgical checklists (Fernandez et al. 2001). Routine prophylactic antibiotics should be dosed in accordance with the patient's weight and should include a first-generation cephalosporin such as cefazolin. Patients allergic to β-lactam antibiotics should receive vancomycin or clindamycin in a timely fashion. Prophylactic antibiotics should ideally be administered as close to the time of the incision as possible.

- First-generation cephalosporin and clindamycin should be administered within 1 h and vancomycin within 2 h of incision.

- The authors recommend that a single dose of vancomycin be considered in addition to standard preoperative antibiotics for those who have been shown to be colonized with MRSA or those who had a prior infection with MRSA.

23.3 Conclusion

The well-known saying, a stitch in time saves nine, is certainly applicable to PJI. Targeting modifiable risk factors in the preoperative setting can help alter the risk profile for PJI postoperatively. While enacting on these variables may not completely eliminate the risk of PJI, it can certainly help improve the odds.

Take-Home Messages

- Periprosthetic joint infections pose high morbidity; however, modifiable risk factors can be optimized preoperatively to decrease risks.
- Diabetic patients should have their glycemic control optimized preoperatively, and frequent blood sugar checks and diabetic management protocols should be implemented postoperatively.
- Consideration should be given to delaying total joint arthroplasty in patients with a BMI >40, especially when associated with other comorbid conditions such as poorly controlled diabetes or malnutrition.
- Patients undergoing total joint arthroplasty should have a minimum period of 4 weeks of smoking cessation prior to their surgery.
- Strict antibiotic prophylaxis should be adhered to including the use of first-generation cephalosporins such as cefazolin. Patients with true allergies to cefazolin should receive vancomycin or clindamycin in a timely fashion.

Disclosure The authors have no funding sources and no conflicts of interest to report for this study.

References

Berrios-Torres SI, Umscheid CA, Bratzler DW, Leas B, Stone EC, Kelz RR et al (2017) Centers for disease control and prevention guideline for the prevention of surgical site infection, 2017. JAMA Surg 152(8):784–791

Blevins K, Aalirezaie A, Shohat N, Parvizi J (2018) Malnutrition and the development of periprosthetic joint infection in patients undergoing primary elective total joint arthroplasty. J Arthroplast

Bozic KJ, Ries MD (2005) The impact of infection after total hip arthroplasty on hospital and surgeon resource utilization. J Bone Joint Surg Am 87(8):1746–1751

David TS, Vrahas MS (2000) Perioperative lower urinary tract infections and deep sepsis in patients undergoing total joint arthroplasty. J Am Acad Orthop Surg 8(1):66–74

Duchman KR, Gao Y, Pugely AJ, Martin CT, Noiseux NO, Callaghan JJ (2015) The effect of smoking on short-term complications following total hip and knee arthroplasty. J Bone Joint Surg Am 97(13):1049–1058

Fernandez AH, Monge V, Garcinuno MA (2001) Surgical antibiotic prophylaxis: effect in postoperative infections. Eur J Epidemiol 17(4):369–374

Forrest KY, Stuhldreher WL (2011) Prevalence and correlates of vitamin D deficiency in US adults. Nutr Res 31(1):48–54

Gage MJ, Schwarzkopf R, Abrouk M, Slover JD (2014) Impact of metabolic syndrome on perioperative complication rates after total joint arthroplasty surgery. J Arthroplast 29(9):1842–1845

Gallagher JM, Erich RA, Gattermeyer R, Beam KK (2017) Postoperative hyperglycemia can be safely and effectively controlled in both diabetic and nondiabetic patients with use of a subcutaneous insulin protocol. JB JS Open Access 2(1):e0008

Goodman SM, Springer B, Guyatt G, Abdel MP, Dasa V, George M et al (2017) 2017 American College of Rheumatology/American Association of Hip and Knee Surgeons Guideline for the Perioperative Management of Antirheumatic Medication in Patients With Rheumatic Diseases Undergoing Elective Total Hip or Total Knee Arthroplasty. J Arthroplast 32(9):2628–2638

Hegde V, Dworsky EM, Stavrakis AI, Loftin AH, Zoller SD, Park HY et al (2017) Single-dose, preoperative vitamin-D supplementation decreases infection in a mouse model of periprosthetic joint infection. J Bone Joint Surg Am 99(20):1737–1744

Huang R, Greenky M, Kerr GJ, Austin MS, Parvizi J (2013) The effect of malnutrition on patients undergoing elective joint arthroplasty. J Arthroplast 28(8 Suppl):21–24

Iorio R, Williams KM, Marcantonio AJ, Specht LM, Tilzey JF, Healy WL (2012) Diabetes mellitus, hemoglobin A1C, and the incidence of total joint arthroplasty infection. J Arthroplast 27(5):726–729. e1

Kheir MM, Tan TL, Kheir M, Maltenfort MG, Chen AF (2018) Postoperative blood glucose levels predict infection after total joint arthroplasty. J Bone Joint Surg Am 100(16):1423–1431

Kim DH, Spencer M, Davidson SM, Li L, Shaw JD, Gulczynski D et al (2010) Institutional prescreening for detection and eradication of methicillin-resistant Staphylococcus aureus in patients undergoing elective orthopaedic surgery. J Bone Joint Surg Am 92(9):1820–1826

Kong L, Cao J, Zhang Y, Ding W, Shen Y (2017) Risk factors for periprosthetic joint infection following primary total hip or knee arthroplasty: a meta-analysis. Int Wound J 14(3):529–536

Koulouvaris P, Sculco P, Finerty E, Sculco T, Sharrock NE (2009) Relationship between perioperative urinary tract infection and deep infection after joint arthroplasty. Clin Orthop Relat Res 467(7):1859–1867

Kurtz S, Ong K, Lau E, Mowat F, Halpern M (2007) Projections of primary and revision hip and knee arthroplasty in the United States from 2005 to 2030. J Bone Joint Surg Am 89(4):780–785

Kurtz SM, Lau E, Watson H, Schmier JK, Parvizi J (2012) Economic burden of periprosthetic joint infection in the United States. J Arthroplast 27(8 Suppl):61–5 e1

Lampley A, Huang RC, Arnold WV, Parvizi J (2014) Total joint arthroplasty: should patients have preoperative dental clearance? J Arthroplast 29(6):1087–1090

Lindstrom D, Sadr Azodi O, Wladis A, Tonnesen H, Linder S, Nasell H et al (2008) Effects of a perioperative smoking cessation intervention on postoperative complications: a randomized trial. Ann Surg 248(5):739–745

Maoz G, Phillips M, Bosco J, Slover J, Stachel A, Inneh I et al (2015) The Otto Aufranc Award: modifiable versus nonmodifiable risk factors for infection after hip arthroplasty. Clin Orthop Relat Res 473(2):453–459

Marchant MH Jr, Viens NA, Cook C, Vail TP, Bolognesi MP (2009) The impact of glycemic control and diabetes mellitus on perioperative outcomes after total joint arthroplasty. J Bone Joint Surg Am 91(7):1621–1629

Mason JB, Callaghan JJ, Hozack WJ, Krebs V, Mont MA, Parvizi J (2014) Obesity in total joint arthroplasty: an issue with gravity. J Arthroplast 29(10):1879

Momohara S, Kawakami K, Iwamoto T, Yano K, Sakuma Y, Hiroshima R et al (2011) Prosthetic joint infection after total hip or knee arthroplasty in rheumatoid arthritis patients treated with nonbiologic and biologic disease-modifying antirheumatic drugs. Mod Rheumatol 21(5):469–475

Parvizi J, Shohat N, Gehrke T (2017) Prevention of periprosthetic joint infection: new guidelines. Bone Joint J 99-B(4 Supple B):3–10

Sculco TP (1993) The economic impact of infected total joint arthroplasty. Instr Course Lect 42:349–351

Shohat N, Tarabichi M, Tischler EH, Jabbour S, Parvizi J (2017) Serum fructosamine: a simple and inexpensive test for assessing preoperative glycemic control. J Bone Joint Surg Am 99(22):1900–1907

Stryker LS, Abdel MP, Morrey ME, Morrow MM, Kor DJ, Morrey BF (2013) Elevated postoperative blood glucose and preoperative hemoglobin A1C are associated with increased wound complications following total joint arthroplasty. J Bone Joint Surg Am 95(9):808–814, S1–2

Teng S, Yi C, Krettek C, Jagodzinski M (2015) Smoking and risk of prosthesis-related complications after total hip arthroplasty: a meta-analysis of cohort studies. PLoS One 10(4):e0125294

Wood TJ, Petruccelli D, Piccirillo L, Staibano P, Winemaker M, de Beer J (2016) Dental hygiene in maintaining a healthy joint replacement: a survey of Canadian total joint replacement patients. Curr Orthop Pract 27(5):515–519

Workgroup of the American Association of H, Knee Surgeons Evidence Based C (2013) Obesity and total joint arthroplasty: a literature based review. J Arthroplast 28(5):714–721

Zmistowski B, Dizdarevic I, Jacovides CL, Radcliff KE, Mraovic B, Parvizi J (2013) Patients with uncontrolled components of metabolic syndrome have increased risk of complications following total joint arthroplasty. J Arthroplast 28(6):904–907

Outpatient Total Knee Arthroplasty

Joshua A. Greenspoon, Charles P. Hannon, and Craig Della Valle

Contents

E. Hansen, K.-D. Kühn (eds.), *Essentials of Cemented Knee Arthroplasty*,
https://doi.org/10.1007/978-3-662-63113-3_24

24.1 Introduction

There has been an increased interest in performing total joint arthroplasty (TJA) in the outpatient setting over the past decade (Berger et al. 2009; Kelly et al. 2018; Kolisek et al. 2009; Meneghini and Ziemba-Davis 2017; Springer et al. 2017). Advances in surgical technique and pain management protocols have allowed for many surgical cases to be safely and successfully performed in the outpatient setting. Surgeons have been motivated to perform procedures in an outpatient setting by several factors including the ability to control more aspects of patient care and the surgical environment, increased patient satisfaction, and potential economic savings for the patient and the healthcare system (Meneghini et al. 2018). As outpatient procedures have become more prevalent, there is also a growing patient demand for outpatient TJA. In order to achieve optimal patient outcomes and safety, a multidisciplinary approach led by the surgeon must be utilized to create an outpatient TJA program.

24.2 Outpatient Total Knee Arthroplasty

The American Association of Hip and Knee Surgeons (AAHKS) released a consensus statement identifying the following elements as key to successfully performing outpatient TJA:

- Patient selection
- Patient education
- Social support system
- Clinical and surgical expertise
- Evidence-based protocols for perioperative management (Meneghini et al. 2018)

> Patient selection from both a medical and a social perspective is key to safely and effectively perform joint replacement surgery in the outpatient setting.

The patient as a whole is considered with regard to the following:

- Past medical history
- Age
- Body mass index (BMI)
- Physical fitness
- Mental capacity
- Social support system
- Environmental factors

Scoring systems such as the outpatient arthroplasty risk assessment (OARA) score or American Society of Anesthesiologists (ASA) can be utilized (Ziemba-Davis et al. 2019). The complexity of the surgical case is also evaluated and outpatient surgery is typically reserved for straightforward procedures that do not require extended operative times or complex equipment. Ultimately, the decision to perform surgery as an inpatient or an outpatient is a shared decision between patient and surgeon.

In general, patients selected for outpatient total joint replacements tend to be healthier, younger, and more physically fit. The authors do not employ an absolute cut-off for age or BMI.

> Particular attention is paid to cardiac history, history of anticoagulation, sleep apnea, prior prostate surgery or history of urinary retention, and preoperative narcotic use.

History of prostate surgery or urinary retention can pose a challenge with discharge after surgery due to the inability to void and preoperative narcotic use raises concerns about the ability to effectively control pain after surgery (Meneghini et al. 2018). All patients are required to see an internist for preoperative medical evaluation and clearance prior to surgery. If there are any modifiable risk factors, these are optimized prior to surgical intervention. There is a low threshold to indicate a patient for inpatient total joint replacement if concerns exist.

> As part of patient selection, the patient's social situation is carefully evaluated. This includes type of residence, presence of stairs in the house, location of bedrooms, and presence of a family member/caregiver that can assist in the postoperative setting.

Patients who must be able to go up several flights of stairs to get into their home or to their bedroom within the home may need additional physical therapy and thus may be better suited for an inpatient procedure. Detailed preoperative teaching is performed with both the patient and caregiver in either a group or individual setting. The teaching includes setting expectations for the day of surgery and postoperatively, outpatient-specific issues including transportation after surgery, and perioperative pain management.

A strong working relationship with anesthesia colleagues is needed to design and implement an appropriate multimodal analgesic regimen. Our current pain protocol is outlined in ◘ Table 24.1. In multimodal anesthesia and analgesia, multiple analgesic medications are delivered in different routes and timing that synergistically and additively target different aspects of the pain pathway. Multimodal analgesia has been associated with better pain control, rapid recovery, and shorter hospitalizations after surgery (Golladay et al. 2017; Kehlet and Dahl 1993).

Table 24.1 Multimodal analgesia protocol at our institution

Preoperative	1. Acetaminophen (Tylenol) 1000 mg PO 2. Celecoxib (Celebrex) 400 mg PO 3. Pregabalin (Lyrica) 100 mg PO
Intraoperative	1. Periarticular injection (PAI) consisting of ropivicaine 300 mg, epinephrine 0.2 mg, ketorolac 30 mg, clonidine 100 mcg 2. Acetaminophen (Ofirmev) 1 g IV 3. Ketorolac (Toradol) 15 mg IV 4. Dexamethasone (Decadron) 10 mg IV
Postoperative	1. Acetaminophen (Tylenol) 1 g PO every 8 hours scheduled 2. Celecoxib (Celebrex) 200 mg PO every 12 hours scheduled 3. Gabapentin (Neurontin) 200 mg PO every 8 hours 4. Tramadol (Ultram) 100 mg PO every 6 hours scheduled 5. Oxycodone (OxyIR) 5 mg PO every 4 hours as needed

> Multimodal analgesia starts before surgery with pre-emptive analgesia to blunt the sensitization of the peripheral and central nervous system from tissue injury induced during surgery (Kissin 2000).

We utilize a spinal anesthetic and adductor canal block, which have been shown to lead to improved ambulation and pain control compared to an epidural alone (Kayupov et al. 2018).

> For many of our outpatient TKAs, we use a general anesthetic to avoid any lower extremity weakness and reduce the risk of urinary retention (Kayupov et al. 2018).

Intraoperatively, we administer a periarticular injection, which provides pain relief and reduces opioid consumption after TJA (Ma et al. 2019). We also administer intravenous acetaminophen, ketorolac, and dexamethasone intraoperatively (Murata-Ooiwa et al. 2017; Tammachote and Kanitnate 2020). Postoperatively, we use a multimodal analgesic program to minimize the use of opioids. Acetaminophen, celecoxib, and gabapentin are given as scheduled medications and tramadol is the first breakthrough pain medication. Oxycodone immediate release is the last resort breakthrough pain medication. After discharge, we historically prescribed 90–120 opioid pills, however, reevaluated this quantity, given the need to reduce overprescribing.

We conducted a prospective randomized controlled trial evaluating the quantity of opioid pills prescribed after surgery and found that patients who received 30 oxycodone pills as opposed to 90 oxycodone pills had significantly fewer leftover pills (15 versus 73) (Hannon et al. 2019). In addition, patients who received 30 oxycodone pills were associated with taking fewer oxycodone pills.

> Today, all patients including inpatient and outpatient patients receive 30 oxycodone immediate release pills upon discharge.

Clinical and surgical expertise including preoperative planning is required to be successful in an outpatient setting. Ambulatory surgery centers have inherent limitations with respect to inventory and sterile processing capabilities relative to the hospital. Therefore, it is crucial to plan cases and communicate effectively with your vendor and surgery center to ensure the necessary equipment is ready and available on the day of surgery. Strict discharge criteria must be met prior to discharge including the following:

- Hemodynamic stability
- Ability to tolerate oral fluids
- Adequate pain control with oral pain medications
- Voiding without difficulty, and
- Safe ambulation and clearance from physical therapy

> If a patient fails to meet these criteria, pathways must be in place to escalate care appropriately to an overnight-care suite or facility.

In our practice, a *team meeting* is held *every week* to review cases and radiographs for the following week to ensure that all members of the clinical team are on the same page and aware of all the details pertaining to the patients and surgeries for the upcoming week.

In a traditional hospital setting, there is a large network of individuals participating in perioperative patient care and education including social workers, physicians, nurses, nursing aides, physical and occupational therapists, dieticians, and other medical providers.

> When performing TJA in the outpatient setting the responsibility of perioperative care is placed onto the family and surgeon (Shah et al. 2019).

When comparing the time and encounters between patients that underwent outpatient to inpatient surgeries, Shah et al. found that each patient undergoing outpatient surgery required an additional 48.4 minutes of staff time to prepare for surgery and care for in the first 7 days postoperatively (Shah et al. 2019).

> Surgeons starting to perform outpatient total joints should anticipate the additional resources required to care for patients and ensure that the team is adequately staffed to do so.

In our practice, a *phone call* is made from the attending surgeon to the patient *in the evening after surgery as well as the following morning* to check in with the patient and address additional questions, concerns, or problems. Physician extenders are utilized and readily available to answer and address concerns that arise in the postoperative period. An extensive effort is made to encourage patients to contact our office initially with any questions or issues that arise in the immediate postoperative period, as opposed to presenting to the emergency department or seeking the advice of their primary care provider. We have a very low threshold to bring patients into the clinic in the postoperative period for further evaluation.

24.3 Clinical Outcomes

Several studies have been published recently pertaining to cost, safety, and clinical outcomes, with a general consensus that outpatient arthroplasty can be performed safely and in a cost-effective manner in the appropriately selected patient (Courtney et al. 2018; Darrith et al. 2019; Huang et al. 2017; Kelly et al. 2018; Lovald et al. 2014)

> Potential decreases in cost on a per-case basis result from decreased staffing needs, decreased resource utilization, and increased efficiency in the outpatient setting as compared to the traditional hospital setting (Huang et al. 2017).

Savings have been reported up to $8500 or 30% per case for a primary total knee arthroplasty (Huang et al. 2017; Lovald et al. 2014).

A matched single-surgeon cohort analysis consisting of 486 primary arthroplasties performed in either an inpatient or outpatient setting was investigated looking at complications between the two groups in the first 90 days postoperatively (Darrith et al. 2019); 243 consecutive patients who underwent outpatient total joint replacements were matched to similar patients in the inpatient setting with respect to gender, age, ASA score, and BMI. Results demonstrated that there were no statistically significant differences in rates of major complications, minor complications, reoperations, emergency department visits, readmission rates, or unplanned clinic visits.

> The authors concluded that in the appropriate patient population, outpatient TJA had no difference in outcomes with regard to complications compared to the traditional inpatient hospital setting (Darrith et al. 2019).

Patient satisfaction has been a focus in evaluating healthcare delivery with the Centers for Medicare and Medicaid services starting to tie financial reimbursement to high-quality care. Kelly et al. investigated patient satisfaction in the inpatient and outpatient TJA population using specific questions from the Hospital Consumer Assessment of Healthcare Providers and Systems (HCAHPS) survey and a satisfaction scale of 0–10 (Kelly et al. 2018). Overall satisfaction scores were similarly high in the outpatient (9.7/10) and inpatient group (9.5/10) (Kelly et al. 2018). However, outpatient TJA patients were more satisfied with courtesy and respect from nurses, assistance getting to bathroom or bedpan, assistance with pain management, staff explanation of medications received, and information concerning symptoms or health problems upon discharge (Kelly et al. 2018).

24.4 Conclusion

Outpatient TJA can successfully be performed if careful attention is paid to patient selection and establishing a care pathway focusing on pain management, patient education, and evidence-based protocols for perioperative management. Performing surgery in the outpatient setting has the potential to increase patient satisfaction without compromising the quality of patient care and patient safety.

Take-Home Messages

- Outpatient total joint arthroplasty can be safely performed in the properly selected patient in both a freestanding ambulatory surgery center or in a hospital setting.
- Special attention must be given to patient selection and education for outpatient procedures.
- A multidisciplinary effort between surgeon, clinical staff, patient, caregiver, physical therapy, and anesthesia is required to achieve optimal outcomes.
- Outpatient arthroplasty has the potential to increase patient and surgeon satisfaction.

References

Berger RA, Kusuma SK, Sanders SA et al (2009) The feasibility and perioperative complications of outpatient arthroplasty. Clin Orthop Relat Res 467:1443–1449

Courtney PM, Froimson MI, Meneghini RM et al (2018) Can total knee arthroplasty be performed safely as an outpatient in the medicare population? J Arthroplast 33:S28–S31

Darrith B, Firsch NB, Tetreault MW et al (2019) Inpatient versus outpatient arthroplasty: a single-surgeon, matched cohort analysis of 90 day complications. J Arthroplast 34:221–227

Golladay GJ, Balch KR, Dalury DF et al (2017) Oral multimodal analgesia for total joint arthroplasty. J Arthroplast 32:S69–S73

Hannon CP, Calkins TE, Li J et al (2019) The James A. Rand Young Investigator's Award: large opioid prescriptions are unnecessary after total joint arthroplasty: a randomized controlled trial. J Arthroplasty 34:S4–S10

Huang A, Ryu JJ, Dervin G (2017) Cost savings of outpatient versus standard inpatient total knee arthroplasty. Can J Surg 60:57–62

Kayupov E, Okroj K, Young AC et al (2018) Continuous adductor canal blocks provide superior ambulation and pain control compared to epidural analgesia for primary knee arthroplasty: a randomized, controlled trial. J Arthroplast 33:1040–1044

Kehlet H, Dahl JB (1993) The value of "multimodal" or "balanced analgesia" in postoperative pain treatment. Anesth Analg 77:1048–1056

Kelly MP, Calkins TE, Culvern C et al (2018) Inpatient versus outpatient hip and knee arthroplasty: which has higher patient satisfaction? J Arthroplast 33:3402–3406

Kissin I (2000) Preemptive analgesia. Anesthesiology 93:1138–1143

Kolisek FR, McGrath MS, Jessup NM et al (2009) Comparison of outpatient versus inpatient total knee arthroplasty. Clin Orthop Relat Res 467:1438–1442

Lovald ST, Ong KL, Malkani AL et al (2014) Complications, mortality, and costs for outpatient and short-stay total knee arthroplasty patients in comparison to standard-stay patients. J Arthroplast 29:510–515

Ma H-H, Chou T-FA, Tsai S-W et al (2019) The efficacy of intraoperative periarticular injection in Total hip arthroplasty: a systematic review and meta-analysis. BMC Musculoskelet Disord 20:269

Meneghini RM, Ziemba-Davis M (2017) Patient perceptions regarding outpatient hip and knee arthroplasties. J Arthroplast 32:2701–2705

Meneghini R, Gibson W, Halsey D et al (2018) The American Association of Hip and Knee Surgeons, hip society, knee society, and American academy of orthopaedic surgeons position statement on outpatient joint replacement. J Arthroplast 33:3599–3601

Murata-Ooiwa M, Tsukada S, Wakui M (2017) Intravenous acetaminophen in multimodal pain management for patients undergoing total knee arthroplasty: a randomized, double-blind, placebo-controlled trial. J Arthroplast 32:3024–3028

Shah RP, Karas V, Berger RA (2019) Rapid discharge and outpatient total joint arthroplasty introduce a burden of care to the surgeon. J Arthroplast 34:1307–1311

Springer BD, Odum SM, Vegari DN et al (2017) Impact of inpatient versus outpatient total joint arthroplasty on 30-day hospital readmission rates and unplanned episodes of care. Orthop Clin North Am 48:15–23

Tammachote N, Kanitnate S (2020) Intravenous dexamethasone injection reduces pain from 12 to 21 hours after total knee arthroplasty: a double-blind, randomized, placebo-controlled trial. J Arthroplast 35:394–400

Ziemba-Davis M, Caccavallo P, Meneghini RM (2019) Outpatient joint arthroplasty-patient selection: update on the outpatient arthroplasty risk assessment score. J Arthroplast 34:S40–S43

Perioperative Pain Management in Total Knee Arthroplasty

Matthew A. Harb, John P. Taliaferro, and James A. Browne

Contents

E. Hansen, K.-D. Kühn (eds.), *Essentials of Cemented Knee Arthroplasty*,
https://doi.org/10.1007/978-3-662-63113-3_25

25.1 Introduction

Total knee arthroplasty(TKA) is a highly successful procedure for reducing pain and restoring function to patients with arthritis and debilitating joint disease.

> However, TKA is associated with moderate to severe pain, and poorly controlled pain in the perioperative period can hamper both the short- and long-term success of the procedure.

Pain management is an important concern for patients undergoing total knee arthroplasty and the recent shift to enhanced recovery after surgery and shorter length of stay has made perioperative pain management increasingly important (Barlow et al. 2015). Inadequate control of postoperative pain can lead to significant problems with rehabilitation and recovery as well as unnecessary patient discomfort, worse clinical outcomes, restricted range of motion, arthrofibrosis, patient frustration, and can lead to chronic and neuropathic pain (Dalury et al. 2011; Parvizi et al. 2011; Smith et al. 2017; Harden et al. 2003).

Currently, there are many approaches to perioperative analgesia for patients undergoing TKA. The primary focus of this chapter is on multimodal pain control and contemporary methods that surgeons can use to improve patient care and outcomes. Classically, analgesia following total knee arthroplasty was mainly delivered through intravenous and oral opioids. However, opioids have been associated with multiple undesirable side effects including over-sedation, constipation, nausea, and dependence.

> One of the main goals of multimodal pain control is to shift the reliance away from opioids and decrease the undesirable side effects.

Fundamentals of Multimodal Pain Control in TKA (Parvizi et al. 2011)

- Spinal analgesia
- Peripheral nerve blocks
- Cryotherapy
- Acetaminophen
- NSAIDs/COX-2 specific inhibitors
- Tramadol
- Local periarticular injections
- Limited use of opioids

Pain management strategies in TKA include a variety of these techniques in combination to provide the best possible pain relief, minimize complications, facilitate patient satisfaction, decrease length of stay, and improve the speed and outcome of the recovery process.

Pain management prior to TKA is increasingly being recognized as a key component of perioperative pain management.

> Preoperative opioid use can influence TKA outcomes; patients chronically exposed to opioids prior to surgery have been shown to experience more difficult recoveries and less pain relief from the operation compared to those who were not prescribed opioids.

The phenomena of opioid-induced hyperalgesia appears to be a state of nociceptive sensitization caused by exposure to opioids. The condition is characterized by a paradoxical response for which patients receiving opioids for the treatment of pain become more sensitive to painful stimuli (Smith et al. 2017). Risk for chronic pain has been noted to be as high as 12.7% in patients 6 months postoperatively with poorly controlled pain (Harden et al. 2003). Consideration for the limited use of preoperative opioid prescriptions should be made to optimize surgical outcomes.

25.2 Multimodal Analgesia

Multimodal analgesia includes the following:

- Preemptive analgesia
- Oral and intravenous analgesics from two or more different drug classes
- Periarticular injection
- Regional anesthesia

The focus is on using a variety of agents to act at different points in the pain pathway. Combining analgesics can maximize synergistic effects while reducing side effects (Kehlet and Dahl 1993).

> Multimodal analgesia has been associated with improved pain control, shorter hospitalization, and enhanced functional recovery after surgery (Buvanendran et al. 2003; American Society of Anesthesiologists Task Force on Acute Pain Management 2004).

25.3 The Pain Pathway

The current physiological understanding of the pain pathway suggests that perceived stimulus of pain causes a recruitment phenomenon in which initial painful stimuli leads to hyperpolarization of adjacent neural pathways. This makes subsequent pain more difficult to control.

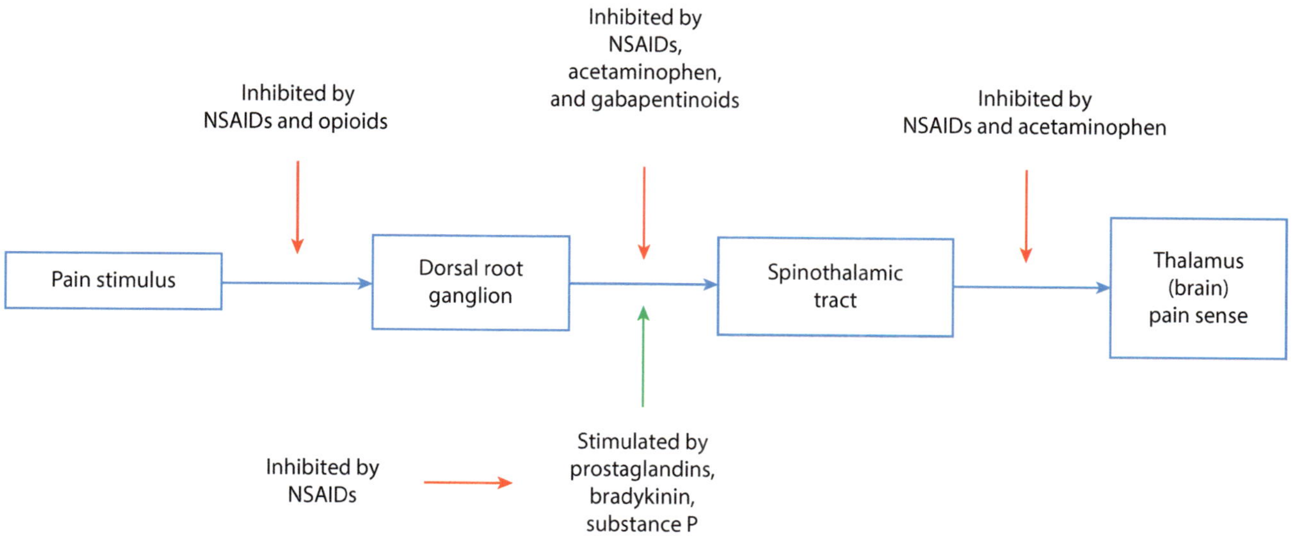

Fig. 25.1 The pain pathway. Pain can be inhibited or stimulated

> The target of pain control should thus be preventative and preemptive.

If the pain response can be dampened prior to the initial pain stimulus being experienced, then subsequent pain control can be achieved more reliably. This is the principle of "preemptive analgesia" (Wang et al. 2002; Bridenbaugh 1994).

The cause of pain after arthroplasty is related to mechanical, thermal, and chemical damage. This leads to the release of mediators at the cellular level such as prostaglandins, bradykinins, and histamine. The release of these signals leads to pain receptor sensitization, which lowers the amount of stimulation needed to trigger a pain response (Carr and Goudas 1999). This neurogenic and inflammatory pathway of pain can be targeted by implementing multimodal pain management techniques to target all aspects of the pain pathway (Fig. 25.1).

25.4 Preoperative Analgesia

Preemptive analgesia is defined as medication that has been administered before the onset of surgical stimuli.

> It has been shown that medications administered before surgery or trauma can blunt the response of the peripheral and central nervous system to sensitization from injury.

These medications can help mitigate early postoperative pain and decrease the risk of chronic neuropathic pain. Oral medications that have been given preemptively include acetaminophen, cyclooxygenase-2 (COX-2) inhibitors, and gabapentinoids (Golladay et al. 2017).

- At our institution, oral acetaminophen 975 mg is administered 2 h before incision if there are no contraindications.
- COX-2 specific inhibitors such as Celecoxib 200 mg can be given 2 h before incision if there are no contraindications such as renal insufficiency or prior gastric ulcers.
- Oral pregabalin75mg may also be given 2 h before incision but should be avoided in patients over 65 years of age and patients with sleeping disorders such as obstructive sleep apnea. Sedation and respiratory depression can occur when gabapentinoids are combined with opioids, and gabapentin for preemptive pain control is off-label use of this medication (Cavalcante et al. 2017).

> Pregabalin is preferable to gabapentin as it is more readily absorbed by the gut at a three-time faster rate and reaches peak blood concentration levels 1 h after ingestion (Athanasakis et al. 2013).

Although benzodiazepines had been given preemptively in the past, this practice is no longer recommended. Prior perceived benefits of anxiolysis and improved patient satisfaction are outweighed by the adverse effects of postoperative amnesia, drowsiness, and cognitive dysfunction (Rogers et al. 2002).

Similarly, we no longer administer opioids preoperatively due to concerns with nausea and confusion. Preoperative opioids have also been shown to have a significant association with inferior patient reported outcomes, high complication rate, increasing opioid consumption after surgery, and an increased risk for chronic opioid usage (Goplen et al. 2019). Long-acting opioid usage has also been shown to independently predict perioperative complications in total knee arthroplasty (Sing et al. 2016).

- **Preoperative Regional Anesthesia**

> Preoperative regional anesthesia can be used to decrease the initial peripheral pain signal and also aid to prevent central pain hypersensitivity.

Peripheral nerve blocks have also been shown to aid in postoperative pain management. Multiple regional techniques exist and have been shown to be efficacious.

The adductor canal block is an excellent peripheral nerve block that is commonly used and is the technique of choice at our institution. It is generally performed in the preoperative holding area using ultrasound guidance before the patient is transported to the operating room. The target of the adductor canal block is the largest sensory contributors from the femoral nerve to the knee, the saphenous nerve, the branch to the vastus medialis and the periarticular branches of the obturator nerve. It has been well documented in the literature that adductor canal block results in less postoperative analgesia consumption and less pain and rest during activity, when compared to no regional block (Jiang et al. 2016).

Another block that can be used in isolation or in combination with the adductor canal block is a block performed between the interspace between the popliteal artery and the capsule of the posterior knee (the so-called IPACK block). The goal of this block is to target the areas that may not be covered by the adductor canal block. Ultrasound-guided local infiltration can be performed by anesthesia in the preoperative holding area. Studies have shown that visual analog pain scores were significantly better in patients that received IPACK block plus adductor canal block versus adductor canal block in isolation (Lund et al. 2011). This block has become a routine part of perioperative pain control at our institution.

A femoral nerve block was routinely used in the past and provides excellent pain control. However, we no longer routinely use this block due to postoperative quadriceps weakness. This block targets both the motor and sensory branches of the femoral nerve and prevents early mobilization due to inability to fire the quadriceps muscles and the risk of falling. It has also been suggested that adductor canal block is superior to femoral nerve block in terms of pain management (Jiang et al. 2016). If a femoral nerve block is employed, a knee immobilizer in the early postoperative period should be used to reduce the risk of falls.

Although not used at our institution, cryoneurolysis is another potential technique for pain control. Cryoneurolysis or percutaneous freezing of sensory nerves targeting the infrapatellar branch of the saphenous nerve and anterior femoral cutaneous nerve is a newer innovation that has some early literature looking at efficacy. The goal is to temporarily block sensory conduction without causing permanent damage to the peripheral nerves. High-quality studies are needed to look at the use of cryoneurolysis to and determine if it can be efficacious for perioperative pain control for TKA without increasing adverse outcomes (Dasa et al. 2016).

25.5 Intraoperative Periarticular Injection

> Perioperative pain management is augmented with the use of a periarticular injection.

The injection is used to decrease pain at the central and peripheral levels while minimizing side effects to improve overall patient outcomes. The goal of these injections is to safely improve pain control while decreasing narcotic usage and the associated side effects of opioid medications.

Periarticular injections may include one single local anesthetic or may involve a mixture of multiple medications. There are a number of different drug "cocktails" that surgeons have developed and used over the years. The most common ingredients include morphine, epinephrine, ketorolac, depomedrol, bupivacaine, and lidocaine. Liposomal bupivacaine has also been used for this purpose. There have been multiple studies trying to determine the medication (or mix of medications) to inject, but at this time the data shows no clear superiority of one approach over another. A gold standard has yet to be established.

> Randomized placebo-controlled trials have shown that patients who received periarticular injections used less patient-controlled analgesia at 6, 12, and 24 h postoperatively and had lower postoperative pain scores in the recovery unit (Busch et al. 2006).

Studies have been conducted in patients undergoing simultaneous bilateral total knee injection in which patients reported significantly lower pain scores in the knee that received periarticular injection up to 4 weeks after surgery (Mullaji et al. 2010). In an effort to potentiate the analgesic effects, corticosteroids can be added to the mixture to be injected, although studies have failed to show improved pain control or Knee Society scores postoperatively (Christensen et al. 2009).Conversely, one newer study looking at visual analog pain scores suggested that adding ketorolac with ropivacaine and epinephrine to the periarticular injection could improve scores versus ropivacaine and epinephrine alone (Kelley et al. 2013).One example of a periarticular injection that has been described in the literature includes ropivacaine 5 mg/mL(49.25 mL), epinephrine 1 mg/mL, (0.5 mL), ketorolac 30 mg/mL (1 mL), clonidine 100 mg/mL (0.8 mL), and normal saline (48.45 mL) for a total volume of 100 mL. This mixture has been shown to improve patient satisfaction and outcomes, and has reduced recovery times (Kelley et al. 2013; Dalury et al. 2011).

Extended-release liposomal bupivacaine has also been considered for periarticular injection. One randomized control trial comparing extended release liposomal bupivacaine to standard bupivacaine as part of a multimodal pain strategy showed no difference in pain scores but a 100-times increase in the cost with liposomal medication. Extended-release liposomal bupivacaine and standard bupivacaine delivered with an intra-articular infusion pump compared with placebo yielded equal decreases in pain scores and opioid consumption in TKA patients (Sankineani et al. 2018). Other similar studies and a recent meta-analysis have also concluded that there does not appear to be a clear clinical benefit of liposomal bupivacaine compared to traditional local anesthetics (Yayac et al. 2019). We no longer use this medication for periarticular injection.

> A critical step to the efficacy of the periarticular injection appears to be the technique used to inject the medication. Technique is critical to providing a safe and appropriate result.

Injections should be given in a control syringe that allows for both aspiration and injection. Prior to injection the surgeon should aspirate before injection into areas of concern. A smaller size gauge spinal needle will ensure that liquid is relieved with minimal tissue trauma. The overall goal is to place as much medication into the soft tissues without seepage into the joint or intravascular injection.

The periosteum of both the femur and tibia is the primary target of injection due to its innervation. Flexion of the knee will facilitate protection of the neurovascular bundle. The surgeon must be aware of the location of the peroneal nerve laterally to prevent any neuropraxia and postoperative foot drop. Medial and lateral periosteum of the femur can be injected creating a wheel to form under the periosteal tissue. The posterior capsule of the knee is heavily innervated and is a common target for injection although the clinical importance of injecting the posterior capsule is unclear (Krenzel et al. 2009). The easiest and safest access to the posterior capsule is prior to implantation of components. One half of the injection should be placed into the posterior capsule medial, lateral, and central locations.

> Plunging the needle laterally should be avoided to prevent neurovascular injury or transient postoperative foot drop.

Palpation of the posterior aspect of the femur with the needle and aspiration allow for safe administration of the medication. The remaining medication can be injected into the medial soft tissue sleeve, remaining periosteum, subcutaneous tissue, fascia, retinaculum, and both sides of the extensor mechanism, tendon, and muscle. Careful injection technique can improve the outcomes of periarticular injections for pain control and have been shown to be well tolerated and safe (Kelley et al. 2013; Dalury et al. 2011).

25.6 Intraoperative Medications

> Dexamethasone is frequently administered in the perioperative period to reduce postoperative nausea and vomiting and may have analgesia effects as well.

Various methods of administration have been reported. Dexamethasone may be given in the preoperative holding area 1 h before incisions in a dosage amount of 10 mg. It has also been described as being given intraoperatively at a dosage of 0.15 mg/kg IV or 4–10 mg IV at the start of the surgical procedure. A second dosage of 10 mg postoperatively at 6 h after surgery can be given. It has also been described as being given for 1–3 weeks in oral dosage of 5 mg for postoperative pain control and to decrease inflammation.

While there is no consensus protocol for the usage of dexamethasone at this time, there is literature to support its usage. A recent study compared patients who were given no steroids versus a single dosage of 10 mg 1 h preoperative versus a dosage of 10 mg 1 h preoperatively and a second dosage of 10 mg at hours postoperatively. The study showed a significantly lower rise in CRP and IL-6 levels, a decrease in postoperative pain and visual analog scores, as well as a decrease of postoperative nauseas and vomiting and total opioid consumption in patients who received steroids pre- and postoperatively.

It is worth noting that at this time the relative dosage and optimal route of dexamethasone has yet to be established (Kelley et al. 2013; Wu et al. 2018). There has been some concern about the associated increased glucose levels with steroid administration, although a recent study demonstrated that administration of 6 or 12 mg IV dexamethasone before skin incision did not cause an increase in serum glucose in either diabetic or non-diabetic patients postoperatively compared with their baseline postoperative elevation (Godshaw et al. 2019).

Tranexamic acid(TXA) is widely used in total knee arthroplasty and has been proven to decrease blood loss and transfusion rate after surgery. One study looking at visual analog scores and morphine usage at 48 h postoperatively of no TXA, intra-articular TXA, and IV TXA. The study concluded that there was a significant decrease in pain scores at 6, 12, and 24 h in the intra-articular group compared with the no TXA group and IV TXA group. There was a significantly less morphine usage noted in the intra-articular TXA group. Currently this topic is controversial and more research is needed to determine if TXA influences perioperative pain control (Fan et al. 2018).

Intravenous acetaminophen has also been used as an approach to multimodal pain control. It has been shown that patients receiving IV acetaminophen had a significant decrease in visual analog scale pain scores between 16 and 24 h and a significant decrease in overall opioid consumption versus patients not receiving intravenous acetaminophen (Laoruengthana et al. 2019). When directly comparing oral versus IV acetaminophen the literature shows that both groups benefit with lower pain scores, limited opioid usage, and minimal opioid side effects, but there does not appear to be a clinically meaningful difference in pain or opioid usage between the two groups (Westrich et al. 2019; Sun et al. 2018).

25.7 Postoperative Analgesia

> Enhanced recovery after surgery protocols advocate for multimodal opioid-sparing techniques as the basis for postoperative pain control (Huang et al. 2018).

For this reason the use of neuraxial anesthesia, peripheral nerve block, acetaminophen, and non-steroidal anti-inflammatory drugs are featured prominently. General anesthesia monotherapy with intravenous opioids are not thought to be conducive to optimal outcomes after TKA (Lassen et al. 2009).

25.7.1 Gabapentinoids

Gabapentinoids are indicated to treat seizures and neuropathic pain but are often used off-label in the management of surgical pain. Although the exact mechanism of action of these medications is unknown, gabapentinoids may act on the calcium channels of neurons to reduce central sensitization of nociception and inflammation. The use of gabapentinoids has been an expanding area of interest for multimodal pain management.

> Recently published prospective randomized control trails have shown that in the perioperative period after primary total knee arthroplasty, gabapentinoids do not reduce immediate visual analogue pain scores although pregabalin has been associated with reduced postoperative opioid consumption.

Patients taking pregabalin after discharge have been shown to have lower rates of neuropathic pain and over all opioid consumption. Patients taking gabapentin did not show any reduction in pain or opioid consumption. When looking at low and high dosages of gabapentinoids, it has been shown that there are no differences in postoperative pain score opioid consumption with differing doses of gabapentinoids, although it is important to understand that gabapentinoids may increase the risk of confusion in elderly patients (Buvanendran et al. 2010; Clarke et al. 2009, 2014, 2015; Eloy et al. 2017; Petersen et al. 2018; Lee et al. 2015; Lunn et al. 2015; Mathiesen et al. 2008; Paul et al. 2013, 2015; Singla et al. 2014; Yik et al. 2019).

> Respiratory depression is also a concern, particularly with patients who are also taking an opioid.

At this point, the literature contains limited high-quality studies looking at gabapentinoids and TKA and it remains unclear as to whether the risks outweigh any potential benefits.

25.7.2 Nonsteroidal Anti-Inflammatory Drugs

Nonsteroidal anti-inflammatory drugs (NSAIDs) decrease inflammation by non-selectively diminishing cyclooxygenase production and also have an antinociceptive effect (Maund et al. 2011).

> Systematic reviews have shown that NSAIDs after major surgery decrease morphine consumption and reduce postoperative nausea and vomiting.

By targeting COX-1 and COX-2 this leads to a decreased production of prostaglandins which are involved in the sensitization of nerve fibers to arachidonic acid. COX-1 is located throughout the body while COX-2 enzymes are focused in areas of inflammation. It should also be noted that blocking the COX-1 pathway can lead to increased adverse events such as renal impairment, increased bleeding, and gastrointestinal ulcerations (Vadivelu et al. 2017).

Due to these side effects, the majority of focus for multimodal pain control protocols is targeted to COX-2 inhibitors. Celecoxib is the medication typically used at our institution for COX-2 blockade. Etoricoxib and parecoxib are other options which are of the same drug class. Prospective studies looking at COX-2 specific inhibitors have demonstrated superiority of the medication over placebo with regard to postoperative analgesia in TKA (Zhu et al. 2014; Rawal et al. 2013). It has also been shown that the optimal administration is preoperative initiation of COX-2 therapy, which leads to better pain control and improved functional outcomes when compared with postoperative initiation of therapy alone (Spreng et al. 2010). Ketorolac has also proven to be an excellent non-selective COX-1 and COX-2 inhibitor which has been shown to reduce postoperative pain and opioid consumption in total knee arthroplasty but should be avoided in patients with impaired renal function and gastrointestinal bleeding (Schwinghammer et al. 2017).

25.7.3 Opioids

Traditionally, pain control after TKA was primarily delivered with oral and intravenous opioid medication through patient-controlled analgesia or bolus.

> The downside of this approach are significant side effects that can range from vomiting, confusion, lethargy, nausea, depression, urinary retention, ileus, and pruritis, which are the most commonly reported.

These side effects associated with overreliance on narcotics for pain control can contribute to prolonged hospitalization and increased readmission rates, and decreased patient satisfaction scores (Lamplot et al. 2014; Oderda 2012). Long-term use of opioids and addiction are also a major public health concern.

> While opioids still play a large role in multimodal pain management postoperatively, the focus should be to reduce opioid consumption as much as reasonably possible (Horlocker et al. 2006; Rothwell et al. 2011).

Long-acting oral opioids can maintain stable serum concentrations by combining rapid onset with prolonged duration of action. In the past there has been some literature to support the use of long-acting oral opioids given on a scheduled basis as providing superior therapeutic concentrations, better bioavailability, and improved pain control compared with immediate acting opioids (Golladay et al. 2017). However, it is unlikely that these benefits outweigh the risks of adverse events.

> Caution should be used with the administration of extended-release opioids in elderly patients because of a high risk for side effects such as delirium.

It is important to be aware that opioids pose a risk to all patients when not safely administered. Patients who receive excess opioids are at significant risk for adverse events and our approach is to avoid extended release opioids to help mitigate this risk.

Tramadol is an opioid thought to have a lower potential for abuse and a lower risk for dependence. Tramadol does not typically provide the same quantitative pain relief as stronger opioids but it has been shown to have a more favorable side effect profile and demonstrated less systemic side effects (Golladay et al. 2017). This medication may be a useful option for less severe pain or for those patients at the highest risk for opioid side effects or addiction. Two studies comparing tramadol to non-opioid pain control demonstrated no difference regards to pain scores but did demonstrate a reduction in overall opioid consumption (Stiller et al. 2007; Stubhaug et al. 1995).

> The opioid epidemic is a national crisis and surgeons are working diligently to improve prescribing habits.

Patients with ongoing chronic pain problems and those who have taken opioids for prolonged periods are at greater risk of addiction. To curtail this risk of addiction the CDC recommends limiting prescriptions opioids. It has been shown that the risk of addiction is 125% with patients who take opioids for more than 8 days (Lespasio et al. 2019). A prospective cohort study found that a majority of primary total knee arthroplasty patients were able to successfully wean off narcotics 2–3 weeks after surgery or an average of 16.8 days. On average, 52.8% of patients are off narcotics at 2 weeks and 74.2% of patient no longer required narcotics after 3 weeks postoperatively (Fig. 25.2).

One recent study showed that an average of 105 narcotic pills are prescribed to patients following TKA although the average number of pills actually taken was 52. This left an excess of narcotic pills of over 50 pills per patient. Based on this data, reducing the quantity of pills prescribed to patients is advisable and the surgeon should be wary of patients who continue to request opioids past 4 weeks postoperatively. Management of expectations and education could promote weaning from narcotics postoperatively to take the least amount possible to keep TKA patients mobile (Runner et al. 2020).

25

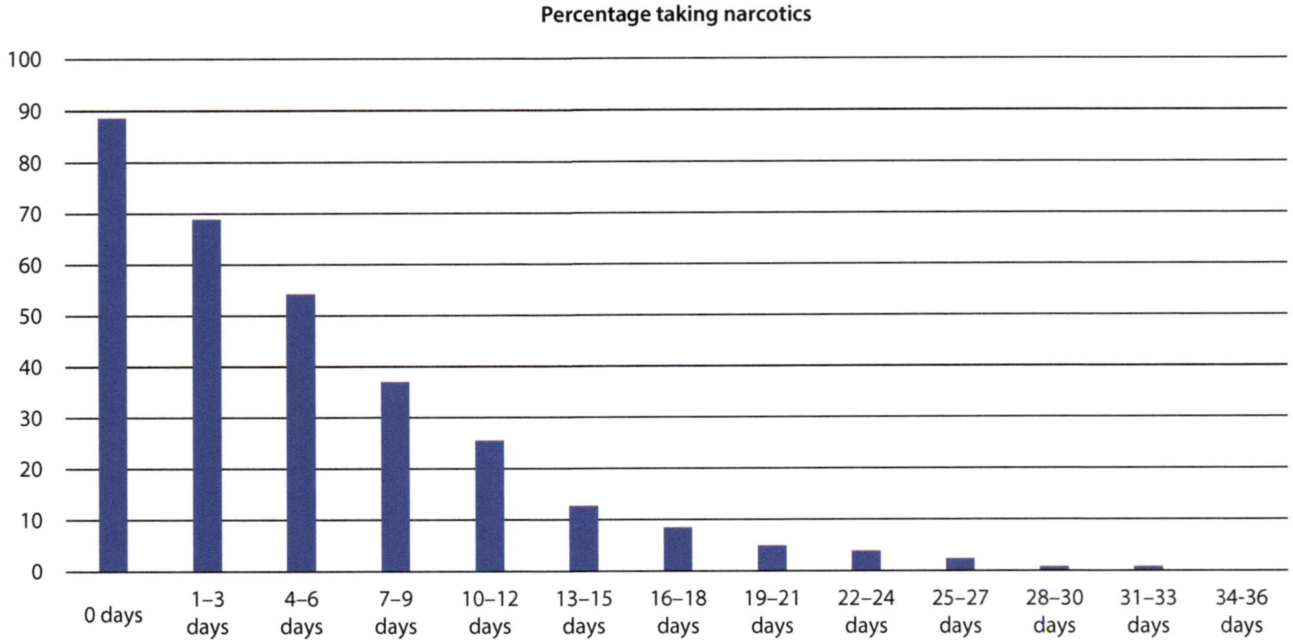

Fig. 25.2 Postoperative opioid use following TKA. The distribution of days taking narcotics was right shifted with 52.8% of patients having stopped narcotics after 2 weeks, and 74.2% of patients were off narcotics by 3 weeks postoperatively (Runner et al. (2020), with permission from Elsevier)

25.7.4 Intravenous Opioids Via Patient-Controlled Analgesia

The use of patient-controlled analgesia(PCA) pain pumps were once in widespread use and constituted the primary method of postoperative pain control following TKA.

> However, over the past 10 years, this practice has largely been abandoned.

Oral opioids have been shown to provide equal pain control compared with IV and have fewer side effects. Randomized controlled trials comparing PCA with multimodal pain management not including intravenous opioids found that multimodal group had fewer adverse effects, less narcotic usage, higher satisfaction rates, and earlier times to achieve physical therapy milestones. Two recent randomized controlled trials compared oral oxycodone with PCA pumps undergoing TKA again showed superior pain control with oral medications with less opioid consumption and better functional outcomes. Given the lack of evidence to support use of the PCA, oral administration of opioids is recommended at this time whenever possible following TKA (Barletta 2012).

Conclusion

Implementing a comprehensive approach to pain management after total knee arthroplasty is key to a successful outcome. Many approaches exist and the optimal protocol remains to be defined. Our current approach based on our institutional protocol to multimodal pain management around TKA is outlined in the following overview:

Example of a Multimodal Anesthesia Protocol for TKA

- *Preoperative:*
  - Celebrex 200 mg PO
  - Acetaminophen 975 mg PO
  - Pregabalin 75 mg PO (*caution* in elderly patients, respiratory depression!)
- *Intraoperative*:
  - Regional block—adductor canal and IPAC
  - Spinal anesthesia (unless contraindication or patient refusal)
  - Periarticular local injection
  - Dexamethasone 10 mg IV (caution in diabetic patients!)
- *Postoperative*:
  - Acetaminophen 975 mg PO TID
  - Celebrex 100 mg PO BID

- Pregabalin 75 mg PO (to be avoided in patients age >65, respiratory depression)
- Ketorolac 15 mg IV Q6H prn breakthrough severe pain (to be avoided in renal dysfunction)
- Dexamethasone 10 mg IV ONCE AM POD1 (caution in diabetic patients!)
- Oxycodone 5–10 mg PO Q4H prn severe pain (patients age >75: 5 mg PO)

This approach continues to be refined as new approaches and new data become available. Efforts to reduce opioid consumption, control pain, andenhance recovery through a multimodal analgesic approach have been proven to work and should be a part of every TKA pathway. Multimodal pain management and enhanced recovery after surgery approaches should be considered the new standard of care of pain management for TKA.

Take-Home Messages

- Multimodal pain control is used to improve pain control, decrease patient complications, shorten length of stay, and improve functional recovery.
- Peripheral nerve blocks and periarticular injections are an important part of multimodal pain control.
- Surgeons have shifted away from intravenous and extended duration opioid medications post operatively.
- Multimodal pain management strategies may include medications such as acetaminophen, NSAIDs, dexamethasone, and pregabalin; the use of these medications should be weighed against the risk of side effects or harm in an individual patient.
- Surgeons have an important role to play in the opioid crisis through maximizing pain control using non-opioid medications and being responsible with prescribing habits.

References

American Society of Anesthesiologists Task Force on Acute Pain Management (2004) Practice guidelines for acute pain management in the perioperative setting: an updated report by the American Society of Anesthesiologists Task Force on acute pain management. Anesthesiology 100:1573

Athanasakis K, Petrakis I, Karampli E, Vitsou E, Lyras L, Kyriopoulos J (2013) Pregabalin versus gabapentin in the management of peripheral neuropathic pain associated with post-herpetic neuralgia and diabetic neuropathy: a cost effectiveness analysis for the Greek healthcare setting. BMC Neurol 13:56. https://doi.org/10.1186/1471-2377-13-56. PubMed PMID: 23731598; PubMed Central PMCID: PMC3674934

Barletta JF (2012) Clinical and economic burden of opioid use for postsurgical pain: focus on ventilatory impairment and ileus. Pharmacotherapy 32(9 Suppl):12S–18S. https://doi.org/10.1002/j.1875-9114.2012.01178.x. Review. PubMed PMID: 22956490

Barlow T, Griffin D, Barlow D, Realpe A (2015) Patients' decision making in total knee arthroplasty: a systematic review of qualitative research. Bone Joint Res 4(10):163–169. https://doi.org/10.1302/2046-3758.410.2000420. PubMed PMID: 26450640; PubMed Central PMCID: PMC4649683

Bridenbaugh PO (1994) Preemptive analgesia—is it clinically relevant? Anesth Analg 78(2):203–204. https://doi.org/10.1213/00000539-199402000-00001. PubMed PMID: 8311268

Busch CA, Shore BJ, Bhandari R et al (2006) Efficacy of periarticular multimodal drug injection in total knee arthroplasty. A randomized trial. J Bone Joint Surg Am 88:959

Buvanendran A, Kroin JS, Tuman KJ, Lubenow TR, Elmofty D, Moric M, Rosenberg AG (2003) Effects of perioperative administration of a selective cyclooxygenase 2 inhibitor on pain management and recovery of function after knee replacement: a randomized controlled trial. JAMA 290(18):2411–2418. https://doi.org/10.1001/jama.290.18.2411. PubMed PMID: 14612477

Buvanendran A, Kroin JS, Valle CJ, Kari M, Moric M, Tuman KJ (2010) Perioperative oral pregabalin reduces chronic pain after total knee arthroplasty: a prospective, randomized, controlled trial. Anesth Analg 110:199–207. https://doi.org/10.1213/ane.0b013e3181c4273a

Carr DB, Goudas LC (1999) Acute pain. Lancet 353(9169):2051–2058. https://doi.org/10.1016/S0140-6736(99)03313-9. Review PubMed PMID: 10376632

Cavalcante AN, Sprung J, Schroeder DR, Weingarten TN (2017) Multimodal analgesic therapy with gabapentin and its association with postoperative respiratory depression. Anesth Analg 125(1):141–146. https://doi.org/10.1213/ANE.0000000000001719. PubMed PMID: 27984223

Christensen CP, Jacobs CA, Jennings HR (2009) Effect of periarticularcorticosteroid injections during total knee arthroplasty. A double-blind randomized trial. J Bone Joint Surg Am 91:2550

Clarke H, Pereira S, Kennedy D, Andrion J, Mitsakakis N, Gollish J et al (2009) Adding Gabapentin to a multimodal regimen does not reduce acute pain, opioid consumption or chronic pain after total hip arthroplasty. Acta Anaesthesiol Scand 53:1073–1083. https://doi.org/10.1111/j.1399-6576.2009.02039.x

Clarke H, Katz J, McCartney C, Stratford P, Kennedy D, Pagé M et al (2014) Perioperative gabapent inreduces 24 h opioid consumption and improves in-hospital rehabilitation but not post-discharge outcomes after total knee arthroplasty with peripheral nerve block. Br J Anaesth 113:855–864. https://doi.org/10.1093/bja/aeu202

Clarke H, Pagé G, McCartney C, Huang A, Stratford P, Andrion J et al (2015) Pregabalin reduces postoperative opioid consumption and pain for 1 week after hospital discharge, but does not affect function at 6 weeks or 3 months after total hip arthroplasty. Br J Anaesth 115:903–911. https://doi.org/10.1093/bja/aev363

Dalury DF, Lieberman JR, MacDonald SJ (2011) Current and innovative pain management techniques in total knee arthroplasty. J Bone Joint Surg Am 93(20):1938–1943

Dasa V, Lensing G, Parsons M, Harris J, Volaufova J, Bliss R (2016) Percutaneous freezing of sensory nerves prior to total knee arthroplasty. Knee 23(3):523–528. https://doi.org/10.1016/j.knee.2016.01.011. Epub 2016 Feb 10. PubMed PMID: 26875052

Eloy J, Anthony C, Amin S, Caparó M, Reilly MC, Shulman S (2017) Gabapentin does not appear to improve postoperative pain and sleep patterns in patients who concomitantly receive regional anesthesia for lower extremity orthopedic surgery: a randomized control trial. Pain Res Manag 2017:2310382. https://doi.org/10.1155/2017/2310382

Fan Z, Ma J, Kuang M, Zhang L, Han B, Yang B, Wang Y, Ma X (2018) The efficacy of dexamethasone reducing postoperative pain and emesis after total knee arthroplasty: a systematic review and meta-analysis. Int J Surg 52:149–155. https://doi.org/10.1016/j.ijsu.2018.02.043. Epub 2018 Feb 23. Review. PubMed PMID: 29481989

Godshaw BM, Mehl AE, Shaffer JG, Meyer MS, Thomas LC, Chimento GF (2019) The effects of peri-operative dexamethasone on patients undergoing total hip or knee arthroplasty: is it safe for diabetics? J Arthroplasty 34(4):645–649. https://doi.org/10.1016/j.arth.2018.12.014. Epub 2018 Dec 18. PubMed PMID: 30612830

Golladay GJ, Balch KR, Dalury DF, Satpathy J, Jiranek WA (2017) Oral multimodal analgesia for total joint arthroplasty. J Arthroplasty 32(9S):S69–S73. https://doi.org/10.1016/j.arth.2017.05.002. Epub 2017 May 11. PubMed PMID: 28705543

Goplen CM, Verbeek W, Kang SH et al (2019) Preoperative opioid use is associated with worse patient outcomes after total joint arthroplasty: a systematic review and meta-analysis. BMC Musculoskelet Disord 20(1):234. Published 2019 May 18. https://doi.org/10.1186/s12891-019-2619-8

Harden RN, Bruehl S, Stanos S, Brander V, Chung OY, Saltz S, Adams A, Stulberg SD (2003) Prospective examination of pain-related and psychological predictors of CRPS-like phenomena following total knee arthroplasty: a preliminary study. Pain 106(3):393–400. https://doi.org/10.1016/j.pain.2003.08.009. PubMed PMID: 14659522

Horlocker TT, Kopp SL, Pagnano MW, Hebl JR (2006) Analgesia for total hip and knee arthroplasty: a multimodal pathway featuring peripheral nerve block. J Am Acad Orthop Surg 14(3):126–135. https://doi.org/10.5435/00124635-200603000-00003. PubMed PMID: 16520363

Huang PS, Gleason SM, Shah JA, Buros AF, Hoffman DA (2018) Efficacy of intravenous acetaminophen for postoperative analgesia in primary total knee arthroplasty. J Arthroplasty 33(4):1052–1056. https://doi.org/10.1016/j.arth.2017.10.054. Epub 2017 Nov 10. PubMed PMID: 29174762

Jiang X et al (2016) Analgesic efficacy of adductor canal block in total knee arthroplasty: a meta-analysis and systematic review. Orthop Surg 8(3):294–300. https://doi.org/10.1111/os.12268

Kehlet H, Dahl JB (1993) The value of "multimodal" or "balancedanalgesia" in postoperative pain treatment. Anesth Analg 77(5):1048–1056. https://doi.org/10.1213/00000539-199311000-00030. Review. PubMed PMID: 8105724

Kelley TC, Adams MJ, Mulliken BD, Dalury DF (2013) Efficacy of multimodal perioperative analgesia protocol with periarticular medication injection in total knee arthroplasty: a randomized, double-blinded study. J Arthroplasty 28(8):1274–1277. https://doi.org/10.1016/j.arth.2013.03.008. Epub 2013 Apr 20. PubMed PMID: 23608085

Krenzel BA, Cook C, Martin GN, Vail TP, Attarian DE, Bolognesi MP (2009) Posterior capsular injections of ropivacaine during total knee arthroplasty: a randomized, double-blind, placebo-controlled study. J Arthroplasty 24(6 Suppl):138–143

Lamplot JD, Wagner ER, Manning DW (2014) Multimodal pain management in total knee arthroplasty: a prospective randomized controlled trial. J Arthroplasty 29(2):329–334. https://doi.org/10.1016/j.arth.2013.06.005. Epub 2013 July 11. PubMed PMID: 23850410

Laoruengthana A, Rattanaprichavej P, Rasamimongkol S, Galassi M, Weerakul S, Pongpirul K (2019) Intra-articular tranexamic acid mitigates blood loss and morphine use after total knee arthroplasty. A randomized controlled trial. J Arthroplasty 34(5):877–881. https://doi.org/10.1016/j.arth.2019.01.030. Epub 2019 Jan 23. PubMed PMID: 30755381

Lassen K, Soop M, Nygren J et al (2009) Consensus review of optimal perioperative care in colorectal surgery. Enhanced Recovery After Surgery (ERAS) Group recommendations. JAMA Surg 144:961–969

Lee J, Chung K-S, Choi C (2015) The effect of a single dose of preemptive pregabalin administered with COX-2 inhibitor: a trial in total knee arthroplasty. J Arthroplasty 30:38–42. https://doi.org/10.1016/j.arth.2014.04.004

Lespasio MJ, Guarino AJ, Sodhi N, Mont MA (2019) Pain management associated with total joint arthroplasty: a primer. Perm J 23:18–169. https://doi.org/10.7812/TPP/18-169

Lund J, Jenstrup MT, Jaeger P et al (2011) Continuous adductor-canal-blockade for adjuvant post-operative analgesia after major knee surgery: preliminary results. Acta Anaesthesiol Scand 55:14–19

Lunn T, Husted H, Laursen M, Hansen L, Kehlet H (2015) Analgesic and sedative effects of perioperative gabapentin in total knee arthroplasty. Pain 156:2438–2448. https://doi.org/10.1097/j.pain.0000000000000309

Mathiesen O, Jacobsen L, Holm H, Randall S, Adamiec-Malmstroem L, Graungaard B et al (2008) Pregabalin and dexamethasone for postoperative pain control: a randomized controlled study in hip arthroplasty. Br J Anaesth 101:535–541. https://doi.org/10.1093/bja/aen215

Maund E, McDaid C, Rice S, Wright K, Jenkins B, Woolacott N (2011) Paracetamol and selective and non-selective non-steroidal anti-inflammatory drugs for the reduction in morphine-related side-effects after major surgery: a systematic review. Br J Anaesth 106(3):292–297. https://doi.org/10.1093/bja/aeq406. Epub 2011 Feb 1. Review. PubMed PMID: 21285082

Mullaji A, Kanna R, Shetty GM et al (2010) Efficacy of periarticular injection of bupivacaine, fentanyl, and methylprednisolone in total kneearthroplasty: a prospective, randomized trial. J Arthroplasty 25:851

Oderda G (2012) Challenges in the management of acute postsurgical pain. Pharmacotherapy 32(9 Suppl):6S–11S. https://doi.org/10.1002/j.1875-9114.2012.01177.x. Review. PubMed PMID: 22956493

Parvizi J, Miller AG, Gandhi K (2011) Multimodal pain management after total joint arthroplasty. J Bone Joint Surg Am 93(11):1075–1084. https://doi.org/10.2106/JBJS.J.01095. Review. PubMed PMID: 21655901

Paul JE, Nantha-Aree M, Buckley N, Cheng J, Thabane L, Tidy A et al (2013) Gabapentindoes not improve multimodal analgesia outcomes for total knee arthroplasty: a randomized controlled trial. Can J Anesth 60:423–431. https://doi.org/10.1007/s12630-013-9902-1

Paul JE, Nantha-Aree M, Buckley N, Shahzad U, Cheng J, Thabane L et al (2015) Randomized controlled trial of gabapentin as an adjunct to perioperative analgesia in total hip arthroplasty patients. Can J Anesth 62:476–484. https://doi.org/10.1007/s12630-014-0310-y

Petersen K, Lunn T, Husted H, Hansen L, Simonsen O, Laursen M et al (2018) The influence of pre- and perioperative administration of gabapentin on pain 3–4 years after total knee arthroplasty. Scand J Pain 18:237–245. https://doi.org/10.1515/sjpain-2018-0027

Rawal N, Viscusi E, Peloso PM, Minkowitz HS, Chen L, Shah S, Mehta A, Chit-kara DK, Curtis SP, Papanicolaou DA (2013) Evaluation of etoricoxib in patients undergoing total knee replacement surgery in a double-blind, randomized controlled trial. BMC Musculoskelet Disord 14:300

Rogers JF, Morrison AL, Nafziger AN, Jones CL, Rocci ML Jr, Bertino JS Jr (2002) Flumazenil reduces midazolam-induced cognitive impairment without altering pharmacokinetics. Clin Pharmacol Ther 72(6):711–717. https://doi.org/10.1067/mcp.2002.128866. PubMed PMID: 12496752

Rothwell MP, Pearson D, Hunter JD, Mitchell PA, Graham-Woollard T, Goodwin L, Dunn G (2011) Oral oxycodone offers equivalent analgesia to intravenous patient-controlled analgesia after total hip replacement: a randomized, single-centre, non-blinded, non-inferiority study. Br J Anaesth 106(6):865–872. https://doi.org/10.1093/bja/aer084. Epub 2011 Apr 13. PubMed PMID: 21490024

Runner RP, Luu AN, Thielen Z, Patel J, Barnett S, Gorab R (2020) Opioid use after discharge following primary unilateral total knee arthroplasty: how much are we over-prescribing? J Arthroplasty 35(6S):S158–S162

Sankineani SR, Reddy ARC, Eachempati KK, Jangale A, GuravaReddy AV (2018) Comparison of adductor canal block and IPACK block (interspace between the popliteal artery and the capsule of the posterior knee) with adductor canal block alone after total knee arthroplasty: a prospective control trial on pain and knee function in immediate postoperative period. Eur J Orthop Surg Traumatol 28(7):1391–1395. https://doi.org/10.1007/s00590-018-2218-7. Epub 2018 May 2. PubMed PMID: 29721648

Schwinghammer AJ, Isaacs AN, Benner RW, Freeman H, O'Sullivan JA, Nisly SA (2017) Continuous infusion ketorolac for postoperative analgesia following unilateral total knee arthroplasty. Ann Pharmacother 51(6):451–456. https://doi.org/10.1177/1060028017694655. Epub 2017 Feb 1. PubMed PMID: 28478713

Sing DC, Barry JJ, Cheah JW, Vail TP, Hansen EN (2016) Long-acting opioid use independently predicts perioperative complication in total joint arthroplasty. J Arthroplasty 31(9 Suppl):170–174.e1. https://doi.org/10.1016/j.arth.2016.02.068. Epub 2016 Mar 16. PubMed PMID: 27451080

Singla N, Chelly J, Lionberger D, Gimbel J, Sanin L, Sporn J et al (2014) Pregabalin for the treatment of postoperative pain: results from three controlled trials using different surgical models. J Pain Res 8:9–20. https://doi.org/10.2147/jpr.s67841

Smith SR, Bido J, Collins JE, Yang H, Katz JN, Losina E (2017) Impact of preoperative opioid use on total knee arthroplasty outcomes. J Bone Joint Surg Am 99(10):803–808. https://doi.org/10.2106/JBJS.16.01200. PubMed PMID: 28509820; PubMed Central PMCID: PMC5426402

Spreng UJ, Dahl V, Hjall A, Fagerland MW, Ræder J (2010) High-volume local infiltration analgesia combined with intravenous or local ketorolac1morphine compared with epidural analgesia after total knee arthroplasty. Br J Anaesth 105(5):675–682. Epub 2010 Aug 24

Stiller CO, Lundblad H, Weidenhielm L, Tullberg T, Grantinger B, Lafolie P et al (2007) The addition of tramadol to morphine via patient-controlled analgesia does not lead to better post-operative pain relief after total knee arthroplasty. Acta Anaesthesiol Scand 51:322–330. https://doi.org/10.1111/j.1399--6576.2006.01191.x

Stubhaug A, Grimstad J, Breivik H (1995) Lack of analgesic effect of 50 and 100 mg oral tramadol after orthopaedic surgery: a randomized, double-blind, placebo and standard active drug comparison. Pain 62:111–118. https://doi.org/10.1016/0304-3959(95)00056-x

Sun L, Zhu X, Zou J, Li Y, Han W (2018) Comparison of intravenous and oral acetaminophen for pain control after total knee and hip arthroplasty: a systematic review and meta-analysis. Medicine (Baltimore) 97(6):e9751. https://doi.org/10.1097/MD.0000000000009751. Review. PubMed PMID: 29419667; PubMed Central PMCID: PMC5944691

Vadivelu N, Chang D, Helander EM, Bordelon GJ, Kai A, Kaye AD, Hsu D, Bang D, Julka I (2017) Ketorolac, oxymorphone, tapentadol, and tramadol: a comprehensive review. Anesthesiol Clin 35(2):e1–e20

Wang H, Boctor B, Verner J (2002) The effect of single-injection femoral nerve block on rehabilitation and length of hospitalstay-after total knee replacement. Reg Anesth Pain Med 27(2):139–144. https://doi.org/10.1053/rapm.2002.29253. PubMed PMID: 11915059

Westrich GH, Birch GA, Muskat AR, Padgett DE, Goytizolo EA, Bostrom MP, Mayman DJ, Lin Y, YaDeau JT (2019) Intravenous vs oral acetaminophen as a component of multimodal analgesia after total hip arthroplasty: a randomized, blinded trial. J Arthroplasty 34(7S):S215–S220. https://doi.org/10.1016/j.arth.2019.02.030. Epub 2019 Mar 6. PubMed PMID: 30948288

Wu Y, Lu X, Ma Y, Zeng Y, Bao X, Xiong H, Shen B (2018) Perioperative multiple low-dose Dexamethasones improves postoperative clinical outcomes after total knee arthroplasty. BMC Musculoskelet Disord 19(1):428. https://doi.org/10.1186/s12891-018-2359-1. PubMed PMID: 30501618; PubMed Central PMCID: PMC6271578

Yayac M, Li WT, Ong AC, Courtney PM, Saxena A (2019) The efficacy of liposomal bupivacaine over traditional local anesthetics in periarticular infiltration and regional anesthesia during total knee arthroplasty: a systematic review and meta-analysis. J Arthroplasty 34(9):2166–2183

Yik J, Tham W, Tay K, Shen L, Krishna L (2019) Perioperative pregabalin does not reduce opioid requirements in total knee arthroplasty. Knee Surg Sports Traumatol Arthrosc 27:2104–2110. https://doi.org/10.1007/s00167-019-05385-7

Zhu Y, Wang S, Wu H, Wu Y (2014) Effect of perioperative parecoxib on postoperative pain and local inflammation factors PGE2 and IL-6 for total knee arthroplasty: a randomized, double-blind, placebo-controlled study. Eur J Orthop Surg Traumatol 24(3):395–401. Epub 2013 Mar 13

Implant Design

Contents

Loosening of Total Knee Arthroplasty: An Australian Perspective

Ruben A. Mazzucchelli and Piers J. Yates

Contents

E. Hansen, K.-D. Kühn (eds.), *Essentials of Cemented Knee Arthroplasty*,
https://doi.org/10.1007/978-3-662-63113-3_26

26.1 Introduction

The latest data from the Australian registry (Australian Orthopaedic Association National Joint Replacement Registry (AOANJRR) 2018) describes that total knee replacement (TKR) has been increasingly implanted. In 2017 in Australia, more than 600,000 primary knee replacements have been recorded on the registry. This is 55,000 more procedures than in 2016; 55% of the patients are female. The age at primary implantation has been stable over the years, with only 6% of the patients being younger than 55 years.

Fully cemented implants are used in 68% of the cases, whereas fully cementless fixation has decreased to 11%; 21% of the implants have hybrid fixation. The patellar components are cemented in nearly all cases.

26.2 Illustrative Cases

26.2.1 Patient 1

A 57-year-old male patient with aseptic loosening of a hybrid right total knee arthroplasty 5 years after primary implantation. Infection has been previously excluded with blood tests and joint aspiration.

On the preoperative radiographs, osteolysis can be observed around the tibial component medially and anterior to the keel. In addition to that, radiolucent lines suggestive of loosening are noted behind the femoral component (◘ Fig. 26.1).

Revision TKR is performed (◘ Fig. 26.2). On the tibial side a metaphyseal sleeve achieves fixation in Zone 2 and a short, undersized, uncemented stem is used to

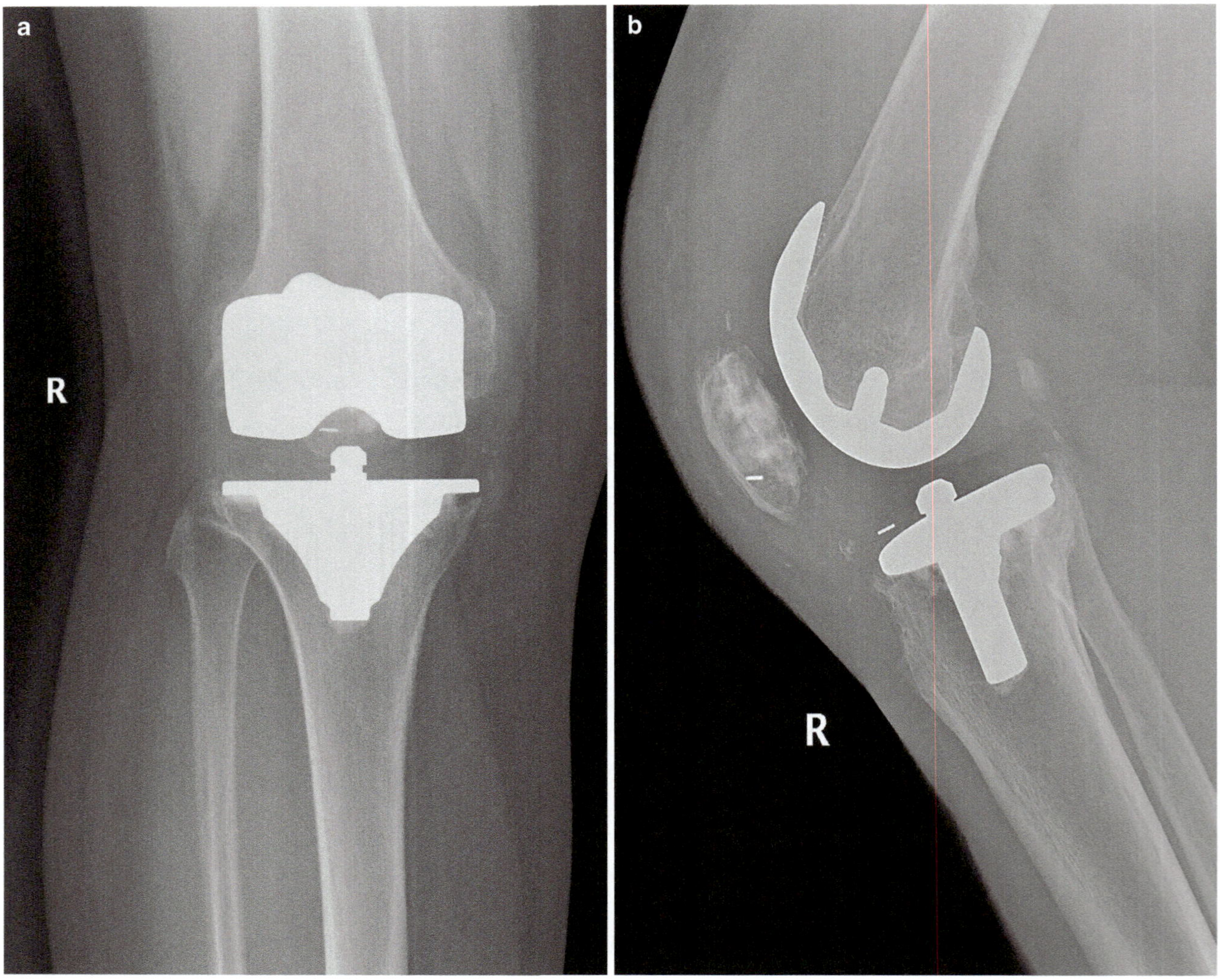

◘ **Fig. 26.1** Pre-revision X-rays of an aseptically loose hybrid right total knee replacement 5 years after primary implantation. **a** AP X-ray demonstrates radiolucencies around the medial tibial bone–implant interface. **b** Lateral X-ray demonstrates similar findings anterior to the tibial keel and around the femoral component

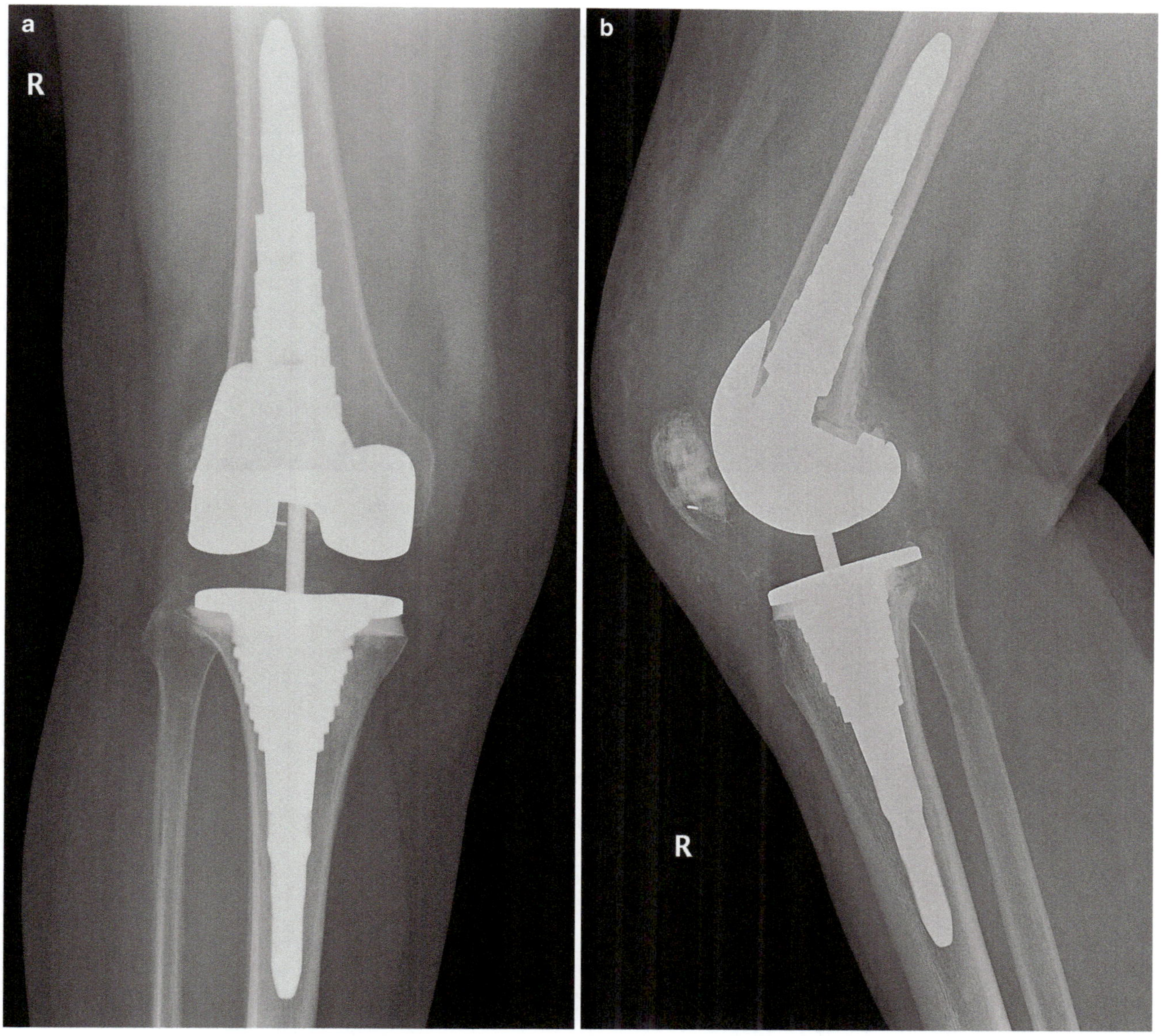

Fig. 26.2 Post-revision X-rays. **a** AP view and **b** lateral view demonstrate the revision rotating platform total knee replacement performed. Metaphyseal fixation is utilized with PMMA cement used only at the joint surface (zone 1)

ensure alignment. Antibiotic-loaded PMMA cement is used only on the joint zones (Zone 1) to deliver some antibiotics and help seal the interfaces. A rotating platform is used to further reduce the chances of loosening through decoupling of rotation and flexion motion, and to eliminate the chance of tibial malrotation. It also maximizes tibial bone coverage.

26.2.2 Patient 2

A 69-year-old obese female patient suffering from severe bilateral tricompartmental osteoarthritis of the knees with varus deformity (Fig. 26.3). The patient's weight is 120 kg with a BMI of 55 kg/m^2. The patient is active and independent in her daily activities.

Primary-cemented TKR is performed on the right side using a PS implant with rotating platform. The patella is resurfaced. On the tibial side, considering patients risk factors for loosening (weight and activity) we optimize fixation with a primary uncemented sleeve (Fig. 26.4).

26.3 Overview of the Australian Registry

26.3.1 Revision

Cumulative revision rates of primary TKR for osteoarthritis at 17 years is 8.4%.

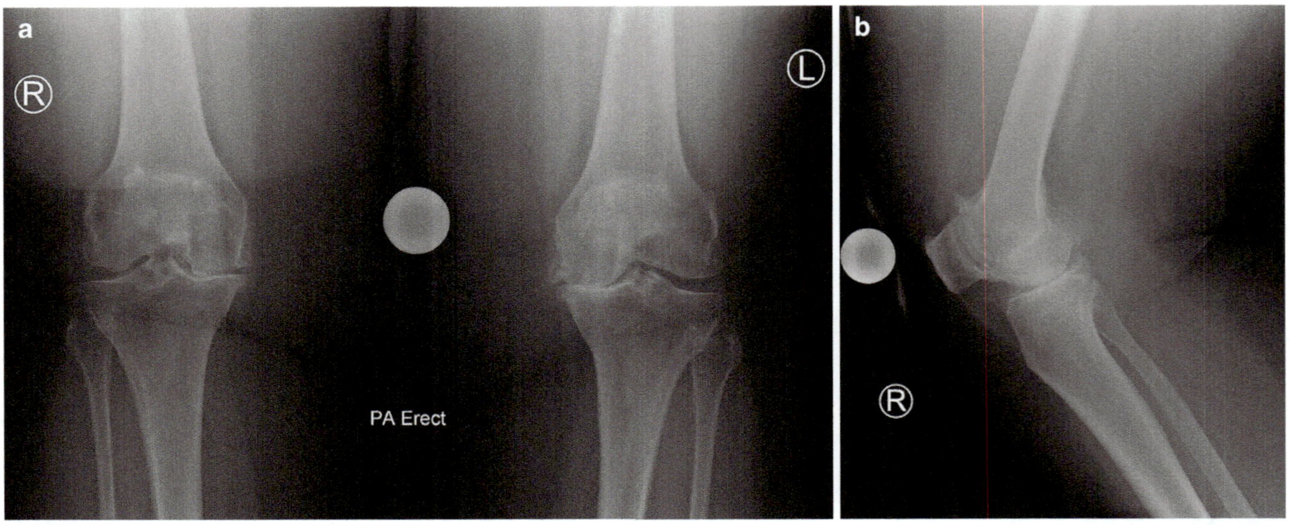

Fig. 26.3 **a** AP and **b** lateral X-rays of a 69-year-old obese female with severe bilateral tricompartmental osteoarthritis of the knees with varus deformity

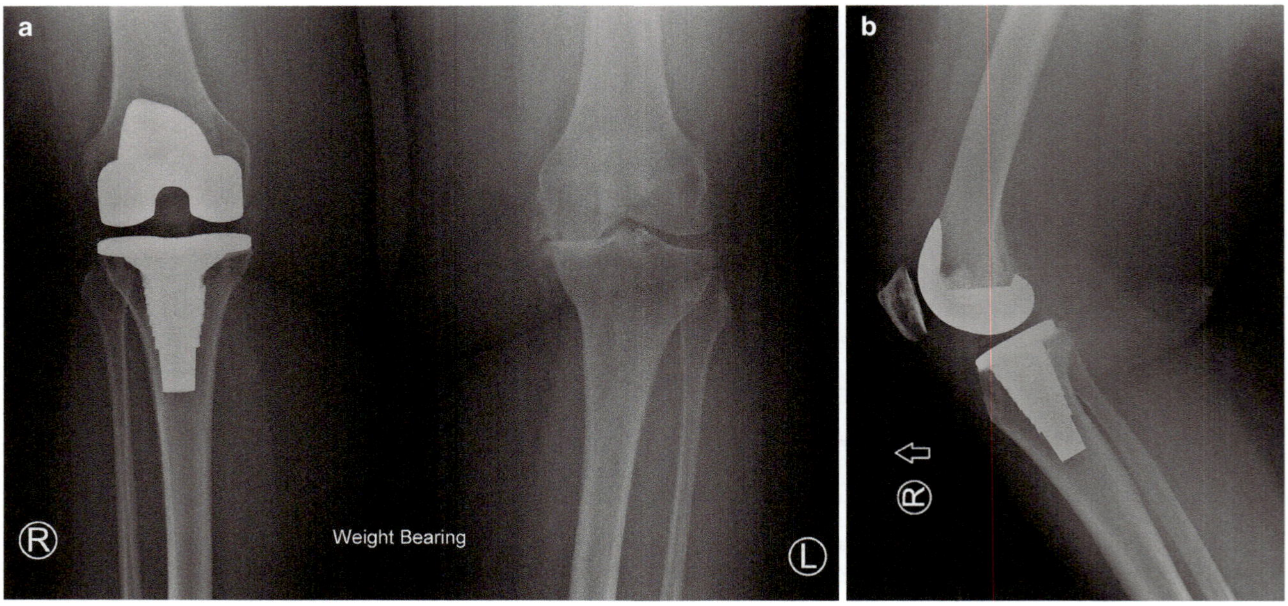

Fig. 26.4 **a** AP and **b** lateral X-rays of the primary cemented posterior-stabilized rotating platform total knee replacement used in this patient. A primary uncemented sleeve was utilized to optimize fixation considering patient's risk factors for loosening (weight and activity)

In Australia, loosening is the most frequent cause of revision (25.3%), followed by infection (22.9%) and patellofemoral pain (10.4%). Infection is the most common cause for revision in the first 6 years, after this time loosening predominates.

26.3.2 Implant Design and Bearing Mobility

The registry defines three major categories of implant design: minimally stabilized (CR), medial pivot design, and posterior-stabilized (PS). CR knees are the most commonly implanted in 2017 at 69%, PS prostheses account for 23%, and medial pivot for 7%.

PS implants have a slightly higher cumulative revision rate if compared to CR prostheses (at 17 years 8% vs. 9%). By looking specifically at loosening rates for different implant designs it is noted that CR knees are less prone to loosening at the 17-year mark (just below 2%) compared to PS implants (2.3%) (Fig. 26.5).

Considering the bearing mobility there are two major groups: "mobile" and fixed bearings. However, "mobile" combines rotating platforms and true mobile bearings, which behave differently. Of all the TKR implanted since the introduction of the registry 80% are fixed bear-

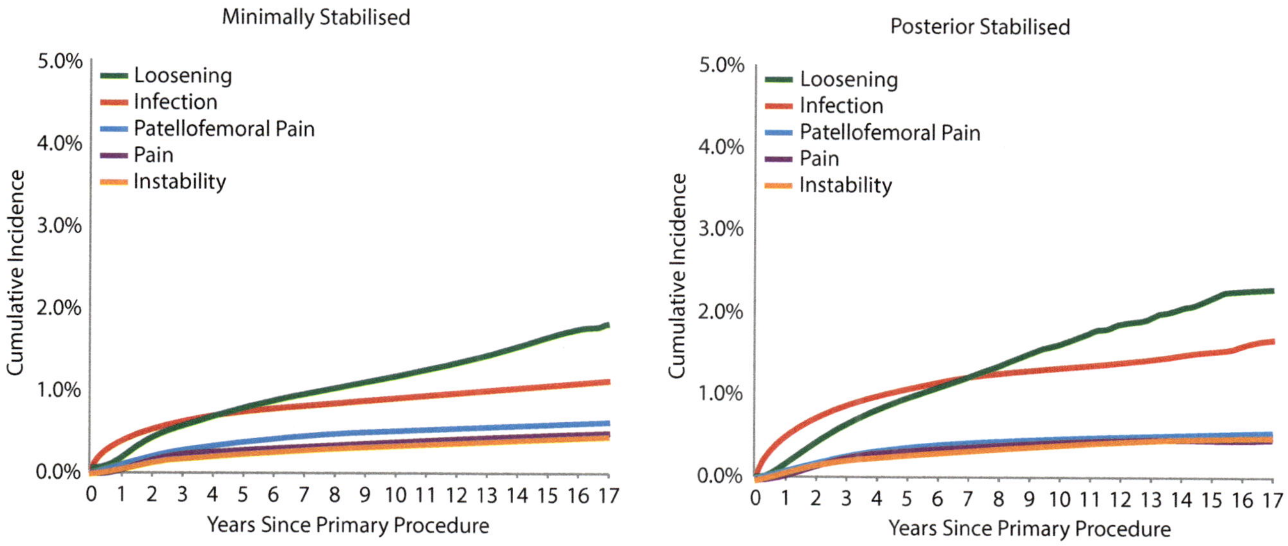

Fig. 26.5 Cumulative incidence revision diagnosis of total knee replacement by stability (primary diagnosis OA)

ing and 20% are "mobile" bearing. Looking at the cumulative revision rates fixed-bearing implants have a lower revision rate after 17 years compared to mobile-bearing TKR (8.1% vs. 9.5%). Although fixed bearings perform better in the first 7 years, after this time mobile-bearing TKR have the lower rate of revision if adjusted for age and gender.

> This said, it must be added that it can be difficult to compare results of CR and PS implants since there is always a selection-bias component due to the fact that some surgeons prefer to use PS design for less stable knees or anatomically more challenging situations.

Also, the use of PS knees is more common in certain brands.

26.3.3 Patella

The use of patella resurfacing is increasing (67% in 2017). Cumulative revision rates are higher when patella is not resurfaced for all implant designs. The worst-performing knees without patellar resurfacing is the PS design (11% at 17 years). No information can be found in the registry about loosening of the patellar component.

26.3.4 Fixation

> CR prostheses perform better if cemented (or hybrid) compared to cementless use.

Cemented CR implants have a 7.6% cumulative revision rate at 17 years, cementless get revised in 9.4% of the cases.

PS implants with cemented fixation lead to a lower revision rate compared to uncemented and hybrid fixation. Medial pivot design cemented prostheses perform better in the registry compared to cementless implants.

26.3.5 Patient Age, Gender, and BMI

Revision rate of TKR clearly decreases with increasing patient age. Patients younger than 55 years have more than seven times the rate of revision after 10 years than patients older than 75 years. One of the reasons for this is probably activity related. Males also have a higher revision rate than female patients due to their higher incidence of infection (1.7% in 17 years compared to 0.9%).

The Australian joint registry has only recently started collecting data about BMI. In the available dataset, revision rates are increased for BMI >40. What can be observed is a constant increase in revision for infection with increasing BMI. No clear registry data is available at the moment for loosening in this group.

Patients Older Than 80 Years

In patients aged 80 years or older, loosening is a less frequent reason for revision. The most common reason for implant failure is infection. According to the latest data, infection accounts for 35% of the revisions in patients aged 80–89 years and 61% of the revisions in patients older than 90 years. In fact, most of the revisions performed in these age groups are changes of the polyethylene insert whereas tibial and femoral components get revised in only 30% of the cases. This can also be explained by the fact that being faced with a frailer patient cohort, major revision surgery is more frequently avoided.

In the most-aged patient group (>80 years) (CR) implants are preferred (73%) compared to posterior-stabilized (PS) prostheses. Revision rates are almost equal, with cruciate-retaining implants having a slightly lower revision rate (2.3% compared to 2.7%). Fixation method has no influence on the revision rate of the different implant designs in this age group. Fixation type does influence the reason for failure: while cementless fixation was associated with a higher revision rate for loosening, cemented fixation increased revisions for infection. Patella resurfacing significantly reduced the revision rate for all implant designs regardless of fixation technique.

26.4 Other National Joint Registries (UK and Scandinavia)

The UK National Joint Registry(National Joint Registry for England, Wales Northern Ireland and the Isle of Man 2018) has even less uncemented fixation, with about 85% of fully cemented prostheses and less than 5% cementless and hybrid procedures.

Design-wise the trend is similar: in the cemented group 70% of the implants are CR, 25% are PS, whereas in the uncemented/hybrid group more than 90% of the prostheses used are CR design.

Preference of bearing mobility in the UK is heavily toward fixed bearing when using cemented implants (91%) and is 50% when cementless/hybrid procedures are performed.

Looking at the revision rates in the UK the best-performing implants at the 14-year mark are cemented CR fixed bearing (revision rate below 4%) whereas cemented PS implants and CR with mobile bearing have revision rates around 5%. The worst-performing appear to be uncemented or hybrid PS/FB prostheses with revision rates of 9% at 14 years.

The Norwegian arthroplasty register (Norwegian National Advisory Unit on Arthroplasty and Hip Fractures 2018) shows 70% fully cemented primary TKR, 15% hybrid procedures (cementless femur only), and 15% fully cemented. The patellar component is always cemented in Norway. From 1994 to 2017, cemented and hybrid perform better than uncemented implants, but the difference is apparent only later, after 10 years. Hybrid implants are the ones with the best survival rate.

Particularly interesting is the inverse trend compared to the UK and Australia to not resurface the patella. The Norwegian registry shows only 8% of the total knee replacements to have patellar resurfacing.

In the time period between 2013 and 2017 looking at the seven most commonly used implants, 28% of the TKR were rotating platforms. The vast majority of the surgeons preferred CR designs, these accounting for 95% of the implants used.

A recent study based on the Norwegian registry (Gothesen et al. 2017) shows an increased relative risk for aseptic loosening up to almost 7% in rotating-platform knees compared to fixed bearings in the time between 2003 and 2014.

In the Swedish arthroplasty registry (The Swedish Knee Arthroplasty Register 2018), a very high incidence of fully cemented TKR with rates around 95%is observed. Leaving the patella un-resurfaced is also common in Sweden, as it is in Norway (>m95% of TKR without patella). Posterior-stabilized implants are less commonly used in Sweden, with CR being used in 91% of the cases across the country. Loosening accounts for approximately 30% of the revisions performed, similar to the Australian cohort.

26.5 Loosening: The Most Common Cause of Failure

Aseptic loosening and infection are the most common reasons for a TKR to be revised (Sharkey et al. 2013). Furthermore, it is accepted that an unknown proportion of aseptic loosening cases are in fact undiagnosed low-grade septic cases not identified at the time of revision. Septic loosening is usually observed in low-grade periprosthetic joint infections with low virulence pathogens (e.g., *Cutibacterium acnes*) causing a chronic inflammatory process. This leads to an activation of a bone resorptive cascade ultimately resulting in component loosening. It is one of the most common causes of late TKR failures and must always be considered before revision surgery is performed.

Aseptic loosening affects more commonly the tibial component; it has multiple etiologies and can be grossly differentiated into early and late loosening. Early loosening can be understood as failure to achieve primary stability and is, therefore, linked to implant type (cemented vs. uncemented) and correct preparation and cementing technique whereas late loosening is a result of bone resorption and/or failure at the bone–implant or cement–bone interface. Osteolysis is bone loss from the result of a harmful combination of mechanical and biological events (Gallo 2013).

Many factors can contribute to loosening of an initially well-fixed implant.

26.5.1 Implant Type (Cemented vs. Uncemented)

Ideal fixation of TKR is still controversial. Historically TKR were designed to be cemented to the bony surface in order to guarantee immediate, stable fixation.

> Cementing the tibia and femur is still considered the gold standard by many authors and has delivered excellent results and low loosening rates across all age groups in all the registries.

However, cementless implants with biological fixation and preservation of bone stock have also had some good results. Cementless TKR relies on good bone quality and is, therefore, more commonly indicated in younger patients with healthy bone stock and bone metabolism. Advantages of cementless TKR are reduced operative time, preservation of bone stock with easier revisions and no cement-associated complications like loose bodies, third body wear, and cement-related osteolysis (Aprato 2016).

Cementless TKR relies on very accurate bone cuts in order to improve host–implant contact and maximize stability whereas when using cemented implants, the cement will fill in these gaps resulting in a more forgiving situation.

> A proper cementing technique is essential to the good outcome of a cemented TKR (Cawley et al. 2013; Vanlommel et al. 2011).

The first generation of cementless implants encountered many complications leading to higher revision rates for aseptic loosening mostly on the tibial side (Hungerford et al. 1982; Dodd et al. 1990; Ebert et al. 1992). These were due to poor press-fit design leading to micromotion and lack of osteoconductive surfaces resulting in failure to gain primary fixation. The new generation of implants have improved design and utilized bioactive surfaces (e.g., porous coating, trabecular metal) offering more reliable options. However, this use of newer technology has led to modern cementless implants being significantly more expensive compared to cemented prostheses, triggering the discussion if they are worth being used since the overall performance does not differ in the registries. Looking at the literature (Nakama et al. 2012) it can be stated that cemented implants show less motion within the first 2 years on RSA studies and tend to migrate "late." This can be understood as a continuous remodeling process at the bone–cement interface. Cementless implants, on the other hand, have an initial migration phase that settles as soon as bone in-growth has been achieved and it is postulated that they guarantee a better long-term stability. Current evidence, including prospective randomized trials (Park and Kim 2011) and a meta-analysis (Gandhi et al. 2009) still cannot prove which of these two options leads to better results in terms of loosening rates with fully cemented TKR still being the mainstay in most countries (68% in the latest Australian Joint Registry) but improved uncemented implants are certainly a viable option for selected patients.

> In our practice, we currently believe that fully cemented TKR provides the most secure and consistent long-term results (Gandhi et al. 2009) and the higher costs of cementless implants do not justify the after-all minimal operative time saved during the procedure itself (11 min on average according to (Nam et al. 2019)).

26.5.2 Implant Design/Constraint/Bearing

With increasing degrees of constraint, the interface between implant and prosthesis potentially have more forces transferred to them, logically increasing the risk of component loosening (Easley et al. 2000). This becomes important mainly in the setting of complex primary TKR and revision arthroplasty where higher degrees of constraint are required to compensate for instability. It is, therefore, sensible to consider offloading the interfaces by obtaining metaphyseal and/or diaphyseal fixation with the use of stems and/or sleeves when implanting semi- or fully constrained TKR.

In primary TKR the difference in constraint between cruciate-retaining (CR) and cruciate-sacrificing, posterior-stabilized (PS) implants is minimal and has almost no influence on the revision rate for loosening (2% vs. 2.3% in the Australian NJR).

When considering bearing mobility, we should differentiate between fixed-bearing TKR, rotating platforms, and mobile-bearing implants. The original idea of a rotating platform was a more conforming tibiofemoral articular surface with lower contact stress combined with bearing rotational freedom in order to improve kinematics and increase articular congruity throughout the range of motion. In theory, this should reduce polyethylene wear through minimizing shear forces and increasing linear motion and reduce aseptic loosening by reducing strain transference to the interfaces. Also, the phenomenon of backside wear in fixed bearings should be reduced. However, there has been little good clinical evidence to back this up as yet in primary knee, although in the revision literature there is increasing evidence that rotating platforms have better results in terms of loosening (Kim et al. 2017). At the moment there is little evidence that mobile/rotating bearings are superior to fixed-bearing TKR regarding pain, range of motion, function, and failure rate (Gøthesen et al. 2013). On the contrary in some specific implant brands, the relative risk for failure due to loosening is increased (Gothesen et al. 2017).

> It is our belief that, generally associating aseptic loosening with a particular primary bearing design is not correct. It is necessary to analyze the single brands for long-time performance before drawing anticipated conclusions.

> In our practice, we rely on rotating platform, PS implants because we believe that these theoretically reduce wear, off-load the interfaces, improve patellar tracking, improve kinematics, and reduce the chance of malrotation of the tibial component.

26.5.3 Osteolysis and Wear

Periprosthetic osteolysis may be a factor in aseptic loosening. The process is very complex and still not fully understood; polyethylene, PMMA and metal wear particles initiate chronic inflammation and subsequent bone resorption by following the path of least resistance within the joint driven by hydrodynamic pressure (Gallo 2013). This is similar to that which has been observed for loosening patterns after total hip replacement. In addition to this, mechanical forces contribute to weaken the bone bed so that component alignment, the patients' bodyweight and activity must be considered when discussing osteolysis. A TKR offers a larger bearing surface compared to a prosthetic hip, so the amount of polyethylene wear particles generated will be higher but also very variable in size (Shanbhag et al. 2000). The different wear mechanisms, particle number and size as well as the fact that the volume within the joint is usually bigger in a knee than in a hip, are all reasons that limit the comparison of wear processes between hip and knee replacements.

26.5.4 Malalignment

Component malalignment is one of the major surgeon-related contributors to loosening. Malpositioning of the implants leads to pathological load transfer of the components to the interface regardless of implant design, constraint, bearing, or patient-related factors. In particular, the bone–cement interface can be degraded by excessive forces. In addition to that, malalignment increases polyethylene wear and, therefore, can trigger osteolysis. Different studies have demonstrated that tibial varus of >3° already causes accelerated wear and increases failure rate (Srivastava et al. 2012; Berend et al. 2004). Also, a valgus femoral cut of >8° increases the revision rate by five times (Ritter et al. 2011). It is, therefore, mandatory to assess a lose TKR for component malpositioning. Many studies in the last years have shown that the use of computer navigation in TKR can improve the accuracy of component positioning without clear evidence for an increased implant survival compared to conventional surgery (Jones and Jerabek 2018). Nevertheless, the trend toward computer-navigated TKR is evident with 33% of navigated joints in Australia in 2017 according to the registry.

> At this state, we currently limit the use of navigation to cases where conventional alignment cannot be reliably achieved because of extra-articular deformities, intramedullary implants, etc. We perform intramedullary alignment of the tibia in nearly all cases.

In particular for overweight patients with abundant soft tissues it can be difficult to correctly assess the anatomical axis of the tibial shaft. Therefore, inserting an intramedullary rod, in our opinion is the most reliable technique to correctly align the tibia. If IM-alignment of the tibia is performed, we restrict the medullary canal prior to cementing in order to prevent cement to migrate too distally down the tibia and improve cement pressurization and filling, optimizing fixation.

26.5.5 Cement and Cementing Technique

Cement type and consistency, bone quality at the interface, cement application, penetration, and thickness of the mantle are all factors contributing to an optimal primary fixation.

> In our practice, we currently use fully cemented implants, as supported by the registry data.

There has recently been an increased interest in improving the effectiveness of cementing our implants in TKR (Cawley et al. 2013; Saari et al. 2009), and quite a few papers have been written about the influence of cementing technique on the outcome after TKR (Cawley et al. 2013; Vanlommel et al. 2011; Bannister and Miles 1988). It appears that a poor cementing technique results in insufficient initial fixation which automatically increases micromotion at the interface. Poor cementing may also impair the mechanical properties of the cement through fat, air, and fluid contamination.

In our opinion, evidence does not justify the use of a tourniquet for the whole length of the procedure, as it often reduces access, does not reduce blood loss, and increases postoperative pain and delays rehabilitation (Jiang et al. 2015; Tai et al. 2012; Tarwala et al. 2014). If desired, a tourniquet can be inflated before implantation to improve cementing. When IM alignment has been used, we usually restrict the medullary canal of the tibia with a bone plug, to achieve a higher cement concentration around the baseplate through increased pressurization. In addition to this the plug prevents cement to escape distally down the medullary canal which can complicate future revision surgery. Pulsatile lavage is used to clean the cut surfaces of blood, fat, and debris. The surfaces are then dried with suction and sponges. In case of areas of sclerotic bone on the medial or lateral side of the tibial plateau we drill a number of holes with the 2.5 mm drill bit to improve cement fixation. Most of our joint replacements are performed under spinal anesthesia which contributes to lower blood pressure in both arterial and venous system and therefore reduces bleeding contributing to a cleaner surgical field.

The use of antibiotic-loaded bone cement in joint replacement has steadily increased worldwide in the registries and in Australia currently stands at almost 90%. There is a good evidence out of the Australian registry that using antibiotic cement reduces the overall revision rate and in particular revision rates for infection, loosening, and lysis. Concerns about possible alteration of mechanical properties of the cement by the antibiotic with subsequent weakening of the interface have not been proven whether in hip nor in knee replacements (Chiu et al. 2002; Bohm et al. 2012; Adalberth et al. 2002; Engesæter et al. 2006). The discussion about the risk of promoting antibiotic resistance with the use of antibiotic cement has been brought up early; in vitro evidence exists about the survival, resistance, and selection of bacteria on bone cement (Hendriks et al. 2005; Van De Belt et al. 2001) but the literature is still lacking on hard facts to this topic. A recent study by Hansen et al. (Hansen et al. 2014) could not prove that routine use of antibiotic-loaded cement in primary TKR leads to increased microbial resistance but further investigations will be needed in this field.

Cementing Procedure

- The authors use Palacos® cement (Heraeus, Wertheim, Germany), medium-viscosity PMMA with gentamicin, vacuum mixed, and delivered with a gun.
- The cement is first placed on the tibial, patella, and femoral components to maximize the chemical bond to the implant (Billi et al. 2019). In particular, the posterior aspect of the femoral component should be covered with cement since this part of the bone cannot be reached with the cement gun.
- After this the cement is perpendicularly delivered to the tibial plateau and pressurized. Particular attention should be paid to have a dry cement surface free of blood and lipids before impacting the tibial component.
- The tibia is then impacted and the residual cement removed.
- Now cement is applied with the gun to the distal and anterior aspect of the femur and in the lug holes.
- The femoral component is impacted and after removal of excess cement the trial liner is inserted.
- We then reduce the knee into extension carefully avoiding hyperextension which can result in posterior lift off of the tibial tray and tension in the flexion gap.
- The patella is then cemented and compressed with the help of the specific clamp.
- The knee is kept in extension until the cement is set. In this phase any kind of stability testing or cycling the knee should be avoided.

26.5.6 Patient-Related Factors for Loosening

Obesity, activity, age, and bone quality are all factors that can play a significant role in the outcome of a TKR in terms of revision rates. The sum of the forces around the knee is proportional to the body weight and, therefore, the higher the weight the more stress results on the prosthetic components and the interface regardless of the prosthetic type and design. Already in 2004, the group of Berend et al. (2004) postulated that BMI >33.7 was associated with increased failure of the tibial component. These results were confirmed again later in particular if a higher body mass is combined with a smaller surface of the tibial component (Berend et al. 2008). Our rationale in active morbidly obese patients is to evaluate the use of tibial sleeves for primary TKR in order to extend fixation to the metaphysis. Metaphyseal sleeves have shown good results in the revision setting (Agarwal et al. 2013).

Elevated weight also influences fixation of the patellar component. Meding et al. describe a patellar loosening rate up to 5%, mostly associated with higher BMI in a retrospective series of more than 8500 cemented all-poly patellae (Meding et al. 2008). The same group found that obese patients have a 6.5 times higher risk for patellar loosening and, therefore, concluded that in some of those cases, depending on implant design, it might be an option to leave the patella un-resurfaced. Patellar loosening alone though, should not be a reason not to perform patellar resurfacing since overall secondary resurfacing rate is around 10% (Barrack et al. 1997).

Patient activity is generally considered a risk factor with young and highly active patients accumulating mechanical stresses on protheses, bone surface, interface, and soft tissue structures over the years. This has led to the observation that patients younger than 50 years have a very significantly higher revision rate for mechanical failure if compared to older age cohort (Meehan et al. 2014).

> Since most patient-related factors for loosening cannot be influenced it is essential to recognize patients at risk for TKR failure in order to be able to correctly select those amendable for surgery and choose the most appropriate technique and implant anticipating potentially severe complications.

26.6 Clinical Presentation, Diagnosis, and Treatment

In early stages loosening is frequently asymptomatic and it is, therefore, important to carefully evaluate routine follow-up radiographs in order not to miss radiologic early signs. Asymptomatic patients presenting with radiolucent lines around the components should be closely monitored. Some modern TKAs have shown an increased number of these radiolucent lines on plain radiographs, especially around the tibial component, without any clinical evidence for loosening (Staats et al. 2019). It is postulated that these findings may be related to the surgical technique or to the implant.

> Patients with loosening of a TKR usually complain of pain during startup activities which worsens on weight-bearing and is localized around the loose component.

> While septic loosening frequently causes pain at rest and night pain, aseptic loosening can be much more subtle in its clinical presentation and, therefore, challenging to diagnose.

Physical examination can variate from unremarkable with good range of motion, correct patellar tracking and stable gaps to catastrophic with extreme stiffness or laxity as well as severe deformity in the case of varus or valgus collapse. Attention should be directed toward joint effusion and erythema that are often present in late hematogenous periprosthetic infections along with other systemic symptoms.

> All patients with a painful TKR should be screened for infection with blood tests (CRP and ESR) and joint aspiration (cell count, neutrophil differential, polarizing microscopy, and prolonged culture).

Standard imaging includes weight-bearing plain radiographs of the knee (anteroposterior, lateral, and skyline) including Macquet views. In addition to that CT scans for alignment and malrotation assessment and evaluation of bone stock may be performed. Technetium bone scans can aid to confirm the diagnosis of loosening in the absence of obvious signs of failure but are only reliable after 12–18 months after the primary operation. The addition of Gallium to this scan protocol may help differentiate septic from aseptic loosening.

> Unless a revision operation is considered life-threatening for a patient, or would clearly not improve his quality of life, revision surgery is the only viable option to treat a symptomatic loose TKR.

Careful evaluation of the tibial and the femoral pattern of bone loss as well as the ligamentous situation will allow to decide the type of implant, the degree of constraint, and the options regarding augmentation and fixation.

For fixation in revision, the concept of zonal fixation as proposed by Morgan-Jones et al. is very attractive and suggests that a solid fixation should be achieved in at least two of the three anatomical zones: the epiphyseal, the metaphyseal, and the diaphyseal (Morgan-Jones et al. 2015). However, we believe that achieving isolated excellent metaphyseal, biological fixation alone with a porous sleeve or cone is both desirable and effective in most cases. This encourages loading of the metaphyseal bone, and avoidance of potential overload in the diaphysis with stems. This in turn maintains healthy metaphyseal bone stock and reduces the likelihood of stem tip pain.

> Usually we achieve metaphyseal fixation with porous-coated sleeves, and if we achieve good fixation here, then we believe that further fixation in the epiphyseal zone and diaphyseal zone, is probably unnecessary.

> This has led to a very streamlined surgical technique based around the sleeves when paired with a rotating platform tibial baseplate and greatly reduced need for both augments and long stems.

In our practice, every total knee revision case is carefully planned based on imaging and clinical findings.

Take-Home Messages

- Loosening is the most frequent cause for revision of total knee replacement (TKR) in Australia.
- Fully cemented TKR still provides the most reliable fixation option regardless of implant design and age group.
- A correct cementing technique is essential to achieve good initial fixation and significantly reduces the revision rate for loosening.
- Aseptic loosening cannot be associated with a particular primary bearing design.
- Malalignment is one of the most frequent surgeon-related factors in loosening. The authors rely on conventional, intramedullary alignment of the femur and the tibia for most primary TKRs. The use of navigation is limited to special situations such as extra-articular deformities, intramedullary implants, previous history of osteomyelitis, etc.
- Patient-related risk factors for loosening (age, activity, BMI, bone quality, etc.) often cannot be successfully influenced. It is essential to carefully select patients amendable for surgery and choose the correct implant and technique on an individual basis.
- Classical symptoms for TKR loosening are startup and activity-related pain. Routine radiological follow-up is essential, even though radiological findings are variable. Technetium bone scans on the tibial side may be negative in the presence of a loose component.
- Periprosthetic joint infection must be ruled out before performing revision surgery for a loose TKR.
- Metaphyseal fixation with porous-coated sleeves is the authors' preference in the revision setting. It is also a viable option to increase tibial fixation in morbidly obese patients requiring primary TKR.

References

Adalberth G, Nilsson KG, Kärrholm J, Hassander H (2002) Fixation of the tibial component using CMW-1 or Palacos bone cement with gentamicin: similar outcome in a randomized radiostereometric study of 51 total knee arthroplasties. Acta Orthop Scand 73:531–538. https://doi.org/10.1080/000164702321022802

Agarwal S, Azam A, Morgan-Jones R (2013) Metal metaphyseal sleeves in revision total knee replacement. Bone Joint J 95(B):1640–1644. https://doi.org/10.1302/0301-620X.95B12.31190

Aprato A (2016) Cementless total knee arthroplasty. Ann Transl Med 98B:867–873. https://doi.org/10.1302/0301-620X.98B7.37367

Australian Orthopaedic Association National Joint Replacement Registry (AOANJRR) (2018) Hip, knee & shoulder arthroplasty: 2018 annual report. AOA, Adelaide

Bannister GC, Miles AW (1988) The influence of cementing technique and blood on the strength of the bone-cement interface. Eng Med 17:131–133. https://doi.org/10.1243/EMED_JOUR_1988_017_034_02

Barrack RL, Wolfe MW, Waldman DA, Milicic M, Bertot AJ, Myers L (1997) Resurfacing of the patella in total knee arthroplasty. A prospective, randomized, double-blind study*. J Bone Joint Surg Am 79:1121–1131. https://doi.org/10.2106/00004623-199708000-00002

Berend ME, Ritter MA, Meding JB, Faris PM, Keating EM, Redelman R et al (2004) Tibial component failure mechanisms in total knee arthroplasty. Clin Orthop Relat Res (428):26–34. https://doi.org/10.1097/01.blo.0000148578.22729.0e

Berend ME, Ritter MA, Hyldahl HC, Meding JB, Redelman R (2008) Implant migration and failure in total knee arthroplasty is related to body mass index and tibial component size. J Arthroplast 23:104–109. https://doi.org/10.1016/j.arth.2008.05.020

Billi F, Kavanaugh A, Schmalzried H, Schmalzried TP (2019) Techniques for improving the initial strength of the tibial tray-cement interface bond. Bone Joint J 101B:53–58. https://doi.org/10.1302/0301-620X.101B1.BJJ-2018-0500.R1

Bohm E, Petrak M, Gascoyne T, Turgeon T (2012) The effect of adding tobramycin to Simplex P cement on femoral stem micromotion as measured by radiostereometric analysis: a 2-year randomized controlled trial. Acta Orthop 83:115–120. https://doi.org/10.3109/17453674.2011.652885

Cawley DT, Kelly N, McGarry JP, Shannon FJ (2013) Cementing techniques for the tibial component in primary total knee replacement. Bone Joint J 95-B:295–300. https://doi.org/10.1302/0301-620x.95b3.29586

Chiu FY, Chen CM, Lin CFJ, Lo WH (2002) Cefuroxime-impregnated cement in primary total knee arthroplasty: a prospective, randomized study of three hundred and forty knees. J Bone Joint Surg Am 84:759–762+Adv92

Dodd CAF, Hungerford DS, Krackow KA (1990) Total knee arthroplasty fixation: comparison of the early results of paired cemented versus uncemented porous coated anatomic knee prostheses. Clin Orthop Relat Res (260):66–70

Easley ME, Insall JN, Scuderi GR, Bullek DD (2000) Primary constrained condylar knee arthroplasty for the arthritic valgus knee. Clin Orthop Relat Res (380):58–64. https://doi.org/10.1097/00003086-200011000-00008

Ebert FR, Krackow KA, Lennox DW, Hungerford DS (1992) Minimum 4-year follow-up of the PCA total knee arthroplasty in rheumatoid patients. J Arthroplast 7:101–108. https://doi.org/10.1016/0883-5403(92)90039-S

Engesæter L, Espehaug B, Lie S, Furnes O, Havelin L (2006) Does cement increase the risk of infection in primary total hip arthroplasty? Revision rates in 56,275 cemented and uncemented primary THAs followed for 0-16 years in the Norwegian Arthroplasty register. Acta Orthop 77:351–358. https://doi.org/10.1080/17453670610046253

Gallo J (2013) Osteolysis around total knee arthoplasty: a review of pathogenetic mechanisms. Acta Biomater 9:1–7. https://doi.org/10.1038/jid.2014.371

Gandhi R, Tsvetkov D, Davey JR, Mahomed NN (2009) Survival and clinical function of cemented and uncemented prostheses in total knee replacement: a meta-analysis. J Bone Joint Surg Br 91:889–895. https://doi.org/10.1302/0301-620X.91B7.21702

Gøthesen O, Espehaug B, Havelin L, Petursson G, Lygre S, Ellison P et al (2013) Survival rates and causes of revision in cemented primary total knee replacement: a report from the Norwegian arthroplasty register 1994-2009. Bone Joint J 95 B:636–642. https://doi.org/10.1302/0301-620X.95B5.30271

Gothesen O, Lygre SHL, Lorimer M, Graves S, Furnes O (2017) Increased risk of aseptic loosening for 43,525 rotating-platform vs. fixed-bearing total knee replacements: a Norwegian–Australian registry study, 2003–2014. Acta Orthop 88:649–656. https://doi.org/10.1080/17453674.2017.1378533

Hansen EN, Adeli B, Kenyon R, Parvizi J (2014) Routine use of antibiotic laden bone cement for primary total knee arthroplasty: impact on infecting microbial patterns and resistance profiles. J Arthroplast 29:1123–1127. https://doi.org/10.1016/j.arth.2013.12.004

Hendriks JGE, Neut D, van Horn JR, van der Mei HC, Busscher HJ (2005) Bacterial survival in the interfacial gap in gentamicin-loaded acrylic bone cements. J Bone Joint Surg Br 87:272–276. https://doi.org/10.1302/0301-620X.87B2.14781

Hungerford DS, Kenna RV, Krackow KA (1982) The porous-coated anatomic total knee. Orthop Clin North Am 13:103–122

Jiang FZ, Zhong HM, Hong YC, Zhao GF (2015) Use of a tourniquet in total knee arthroplasty: a systematic review and meta-analysis of randomized controlled trials. J Orthop Sci 20:110–123. https://doi.org/10.1007/s00776-014-0664-6

Jones CW, Jerabek SA (2018) Current role of computer navigation in total knee arthroplasty. J Arthroplast 33:1989–1993. https://doi.org/10.1016/j.arth.2018.01.027

Kim RH, Martin JR, Dennis DA, Yang CC, Jennings JM, Lee GC (2017) Midterm clinical and radiographic results of mobile-bearing revision total knee arthroplasty. J Arthroplast 32:1930–1934. https://doi.org/10.1016/j.arth.2017.01.014

Meding JB, Fish MD, Berend ME, Ritter MA, Keating EM (2008) Predicting patellar failure after total knee arthroplasty. Clin Orthop Relat Res 466:2769–2774. https://doi.org/10.1007/s11999-008-0417-y

Meehan JP, Danielsen B, Kim SH, Jamali AA, White RH (2014) Younger age is associated with a higher risk of early periprosthetic joint infection and aseptic mechanical failure after total knee arthroplasty. J Bone Joint Surg Am 96:529–535. https://doi.org/10.2106/JBJS.M.00545

Morgan-Jones R, Oussedik SIS, Graichen H, Haddad FS (2015) Zonal fixation in revision total knee arthroplasty. Bone Joint J 97-B:147–149. https://doi.org/10.1302/0301-620X.97B2.34144

Nakama GY, Peccin MS, Almeida GJ, Neto ODAL, Queiroz AA, Navarro RD (2012) Cemented, cementless or hybrid fixation options in total knee arthroplasty for osteoarthritis and other non-traumatic diseases. Cochrane Database Syst Rev. https://doi.org/10.1002/14651858.cd006193.pub2

Nam D, Lawrie CM, Salih R, Nahhas CR, Barrack RL, Nunley RM (2019) Cemented versus cementless total knee arthroplasty of the same modern design. J Bone Joint Surg Am 101:1185–1192. https://doi.org/10.2106/jbjs.18.01162

National Joint Registry for England, Wales Northern Ireland and the Isle of Man. 15th Annual Report 2018

Norwegian National Advisory Unit on Arthroplasty and Hip Fractures, Report June 2018

Park JW, Kim YH (2011) Simultaneous cemented and cementless total knee replacement in the same patients: a prospective comparison of long-term outcomes using an identical design of NexGen prosthesis. J Bone Joint Surg Br 93(B):1479–1486. https://doi.org/10.1302/0301-620X.93B11.27507

Ritter MA, Davis KE, Meding JB, Pierson JL, Berend ME, Malinzak RA (2011) The effect of alignment and BMI on failure of total knee replacement. J Bone Joint Surg Am 93:1588–1596. https://doi.org/10.2106/JBJS.J.00772

Saari T, Li MG, Wood D, Nivbrant B (2009) Comparison of cementing techniques of the tibial component in total knee replacement. Int Orthop 33:1239–1242. https://doi.org/10.1007/s00264-008-0632-x

Shanbhag AS, Bailey HO, Hwang DS, Cha CW, Eror NG, Rubash HE (2000) Quantitative analysis of ultrahigh molecular weight polyethylene (UHMWPE) wear debris associated with total knee replacements. J Biomed Mater Res 53:100–110. https://doi.org/10.1002/(SICI)1097-4636(2000)53:1<100::AID-JBM14>3.0.CO;2-4

Sharkey PF, Lichstein PM, Shen C, Tokarski AT, Parvizi J (2013) Why are total knee arthroplasties failing today-has anything changed after 10 years? J Arthroplast 29:1774–1778. https://doi.org/10.1016/j.arth.2013.07.024

Srivastava A, Lee GY, Steklov N, Colwell CW, Ezzet KA, D'Lima DD (2012) Effect of tibial component varus on wear in total knee arthroplasty. Knee 19:560–563. https://doi.org/10.1016/j.knee.2011.11.003

Staats K, Wannmacher T, Weihs V, Koller U, Kubista B, Windhager R (2019) Modern cemented total knee arthroplasty design shows a higher incidence of radiolucent lines compared to its predecessor. Knee Surg Sport Traumatol Arthrosc 27:1148–1155. https://doi.org/10.1007/s00167-018-5130-0

Tai TW, Chang CW, Lai KA, Lin CJ, Yang CY (2012) Effects of tourniquet use on blood loss and soft-tissue damage in total knee arthroplasty: a randomized controlled trial. J Bone Joint Surg Am 94:2209–2215. https://doi.org/10.2106/JBJS.K.00813

Tarwala R, Dorr LD, Gilbert PK, Wan Z, Long WT (2014) Tourniquet use during cementation only during total knee arthroplasty: a randomized trial knee. Clin Orthop Relat Res 472:169–174. https://doi.org/10.1007/s11999-013-3124-2

The Swedish Knee Arthroplasty Register. Annual Report 2018

Van De Belt H, Neut D, Schenk W, Van Horn JR, Van Der Mei HC, Busscher HJ (2001) Staphylococcus aureus biofilm formation on different gentamicin-loaded polymethylmethacrylate bone cements. Biomaterials 22:1607–1611. https://doi.org/10.1016/S0142-9612(00)00313-6

Vanlommel J, Luyckx JP, Labey L, Innocenti B, De Corte R, Bellemans J (2011) Cementing the tibial component in total knee arthroplasty. Which technique is the best? J Arthroplast 26:492–496. https://doi.org/10.1016/j.arth.2010.01.107

Cemented, Cruciate-Retaining Total Knee Arthroplasty: The Evolution of a Technique

Stefano A. Bini and Giulio Santi

Contents

E. Hansen, K.-D. Kühn (eds.), *Essentials of Cemented Knee Arthroplasty*,
https://doi.org/10.1007/978-3-662-63113-3_27

27

27.1 Introduction

Over the past few decades advancements in total knee arthroplasty (TKA) surgery techniques and implant design have aimed to reproduce as closely as possible both the anatomy and biomechanics of the native knee. The posterior cruciate ligament-retaining (CR) TKA is the least constrained of the knee prostheses and in theory should have attained better postoperative knee proprioception, kinematics, and flexion due to retention of the posterior cruciate ligament (PCL) as compared to posterior-stabilized (PS) devices that sacrifice it. However, the clinical results of CR TKA have not been shown to be consistently superior to those of posterior-stabilized (PS) TKA and patient perception of both implant designs have not appreciably improved over the past 20 years.

In this chapter, we will discuss the recently introduced caliper-based kinematic alignment (KA) technique for TKA and how it favors the retention of the PCL as a means by which to more closely replicate a knee's native kinematic motion. We will also take some time to focus on the importance of cementation technique in ensuring excellent longevity of cemented TKA.

27.2 Case Example

O.C. is a 64-year-old male with a history of deep venous thrombosis, hypertension, obesity, hyperlipidemia, low-back pain, and a history of left total knee replacement and lumbar spine surgery, who presents with right knee pain with activity. He is taking ibuprofen and has failed prior cortisone injections due to limited relief. On exam, he is 210 lbs. and 5′ 5″ for a BMI of 35, with a knee range of motion of 0–110° with medial joint line tenderness and no instability. He is noted to have moderate swelling and synovitis with minimal patellofemoral crepitus, or any neuromuscular deficits. He has a negative hip exam and straight leg raise.

Presurgical imaging reveals narrowing of the medial joint space, subchondral sclerosis, and cysts (■ Fig. 27.1a) on the anteroposterior view; a moderate posterior femoral offset, approximately 3° of joint line obliquity of the tibial plateau, and 6° of posterior slope on the lateral view (■ Fig. 27.1b); and a well-centered patella on the sunrise view (■ Fig. 27.1c).

Postoperative images reveal an accurate restoration of the patient's preoperative anatomy (■ Fig. 27.2) compared to the preoperative images.

27.3 Surgical Technique

While my practice for the past 7 years has been to perform TKA using kinematic alignment (KA) principles, many if not all of the surgical technique principles outlined in this chapter are not specific to KA and can be applied to any CR TKA technique. For patients in whom the joint line is within a few degrees of neutral to the tibial axis, mechanical alignment (MA), balanced gap (BG) techniques, and KA result in similar component positioning and, therefore, the case that has been selected for presentation (▶ Sect. 27.2) has only a small amount of varus tilt on the tibia to minimize the impact

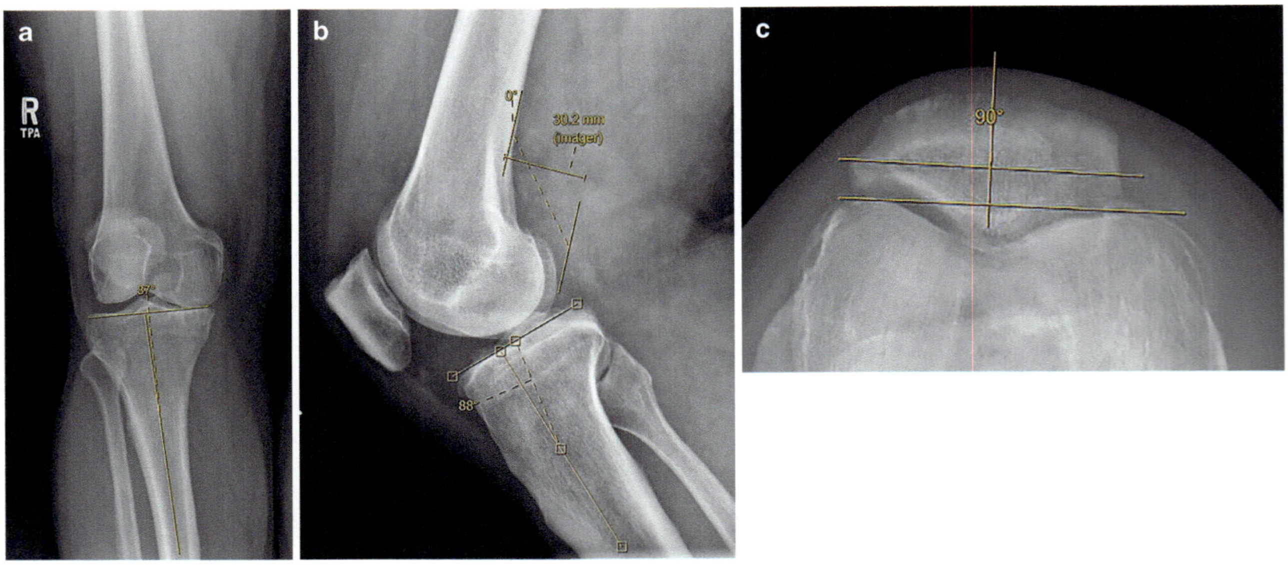

■ **Fig. 27.1** **a–c** Presurgical imaging reveals medial joint line wear with narrowing of the joint space and subchondral sclerosis, and cysts on the anteroposterior view **a**, a moderate posterior femoral offset, approximately 3° of joint line obliquity of the tibial plateau, and 2° of posterior slope on the lateral view **b**, and a well-centered patella on the sunrise view **c**

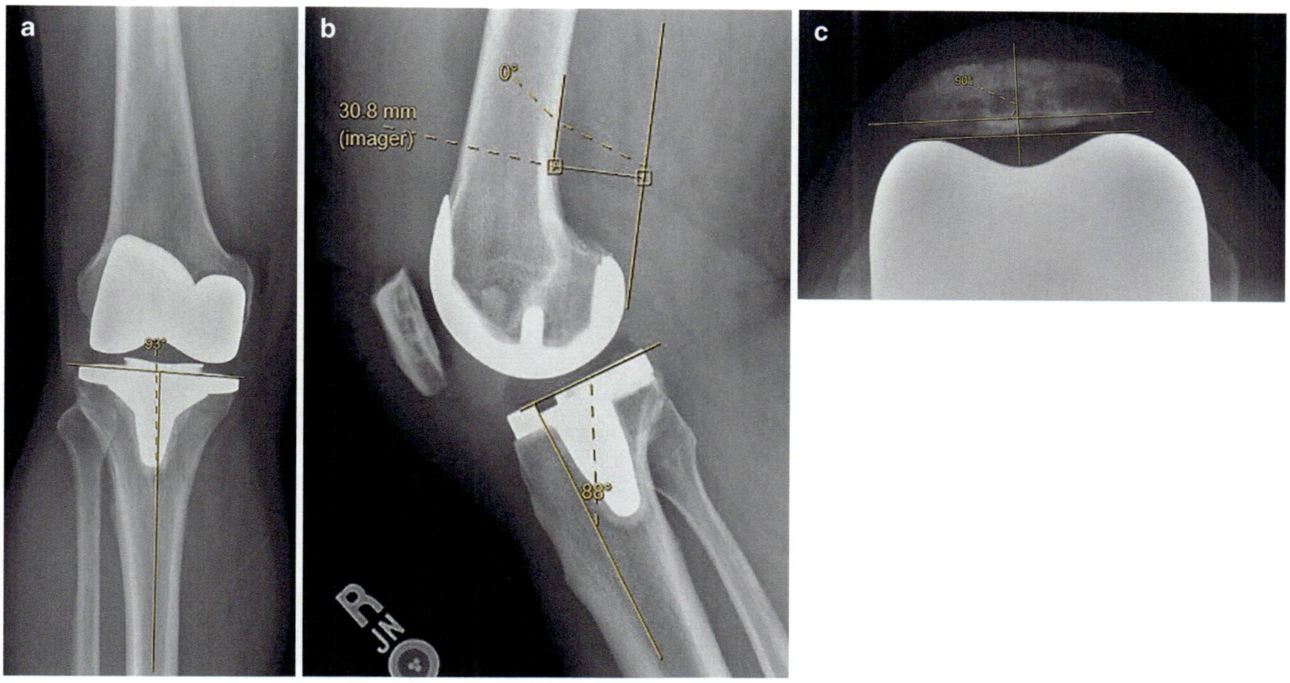

Fig. 27.2 **a–c** Postoperative imaging reveals restoration of the patient's preoperative anatomy; the femoral joint line angle

of alignment selection on the discussion of the surgical technique. However, where the methodology by which the goal of a balanced total knee is achieved using a cruciate-retaining (CR) TKA through KA principles differs from MA, the text will clearly explain how the technique varies.

27.3.1 General

There are a few general thoughts that are best addressed in the beginning:

1. The technique I use for of KA TKA uses a "femur first" approach. The femur and tibia are addressed independently, like a measured gap MA technique, but unlike a BG technique in which the posterior femoral cut, which sets rotation of the femoral component, is based on the tibial cut and, therefore, follows it.
2. I prefer to stand at the foot of the bed with the knee flexed before me and to extend the leg to the side onto a Mayo stand when extension is needed, rather than standing to the side of the knee as most surgeons do. I find that looking directly at the knee rather than obliquely allows for more accurate evaluation of the knee and better ergonomics.
3. I went back to using a tourniquet after a multiyear experience without one as I prefer a reliably dry and bloodless bony bed for cementation. As long as the tourniquet pressures are approximately 100 mmHg above systolic pressure and the tourniquet times are less than 30–40 min, I have not seen any clinical penalty to its use (Olivecrona et al. 2013).
4. After dabbling a bit with not resurfacing the patella, I have gone back to an anatomic designed resurfacing for all knees except in the very young patient or the very thin patella (<18 mm).

27.3.2 Positioning

As mentioned earlier, the patient is placed on the bed so that their leg can rest at maximum flexion against a cross bar placed just proximal to the break of the foot of the bed. A lateral post holds the thigh and, therefore, the leg in place when flexed. Once prepped and draped, the foot of the bed is folded under the table so as to allow the surgeon to stand directly in front of the knee, with one assistant to one side and the scrub tech and sterile table to the other. In this way, everyone on the team has unobstructed access to the knee. The only exception for primary knees where I will use a traditional set up is in patients who cannot flex the knee past 90°. For simplicity, the images shown in this chapter show the procedure being performed from the side of the bed.

A tourniquet is placed prior to draping as high as possible above the knee and as close as possible to the inguinal ligament. If the patient has an abductor canal catheter, the tourniquet can be applied directly over it without dislodging the catheter.

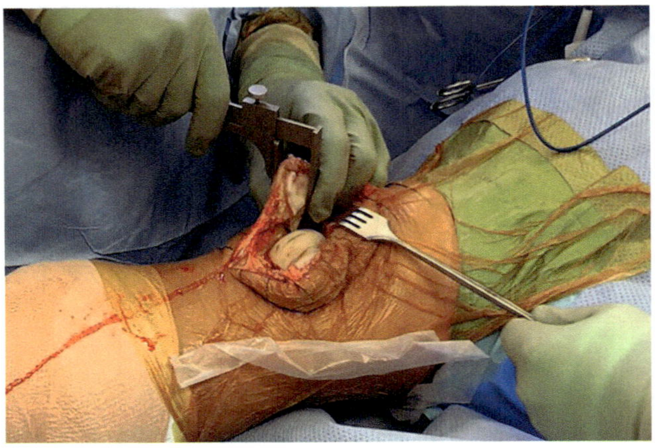

Fig. 27.3 Measuring the height of the patella

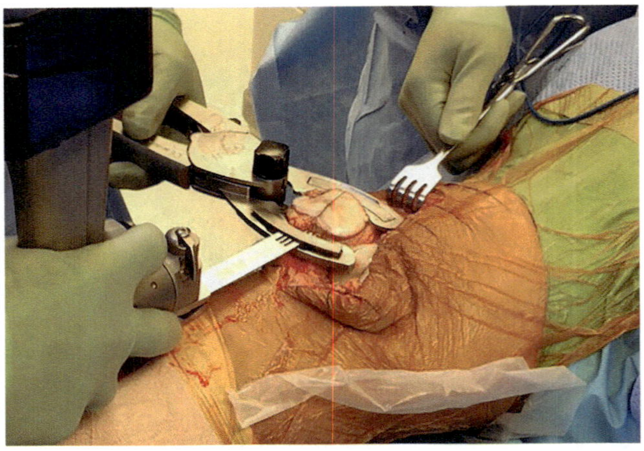

Fig. 27.4 Using a patella resection guide to make the patellar cut

27.3.3 Exposure

I use a midline incision with a traditional parapatellar arthrotomy. The arthrotomy extends along the medial aspect of the quadriceps leaving the bulk of the tendon intact and taking only 3 mm of tendon with the vastus medialis to help support the closure. A 3 mm cuff of tendon is also left along the patella to help obtain a secure closure. The knee is now brought into extension and the patella released and reflected laterally. The patellar release is performed by taking a bovie knife and finding the "nose" of the patella (anatomically named the "apex"). Any tissue deep to the apex is not part of the patellar tendon whereas any tissue dorsal to is. Once this plane is identified, the scarred fat pad is incised distally and then along the inferior lateral border of the patella, while applying an eversion force. This simple maneuver allows the patella to reflect laterally so that it can be easily accessed, measured, and cut.

27.3.4 Patella First

The patella is cut first so that it can be allowed to slide laterally without being everted. Cutting the patella also decompresses the joint space and allows better knee visualization through a smaller incision (Yang et al. 2016). The goal of resurfacing is to restore normal patellar height (Fig. 27.3) and make appropriate compensatory adjustments if there has been bone loss. The patella functions best with a normal lever arm (restored height), if it tracks orthogonally in the trochlea, and if it engages in the groove at around 15° of flexion.

To achieve these goals, I always use a cutting guide (Fig. 27.4), choose an anatomic patella design, and try to restore patellar height rather than replicate the height of the worn patella (Ali et al. 2018). In the absence of historical images or a healthy contralateral knee X-ray to evaluate the normal height of the pre-wear patella, I aim for a minimum combined patellar height of 20 mm (Fig. 27.5). A useful check to ensure the patella is cut correctly is to place the compression clamp onto the trial patellar button prior to cementation. If the clamp is not parallel to the undersurface of the patella, the cut is not orthogonal to the patella's axis and needs to be reevaluated (Fig. 27.6, checking the patellar cut).

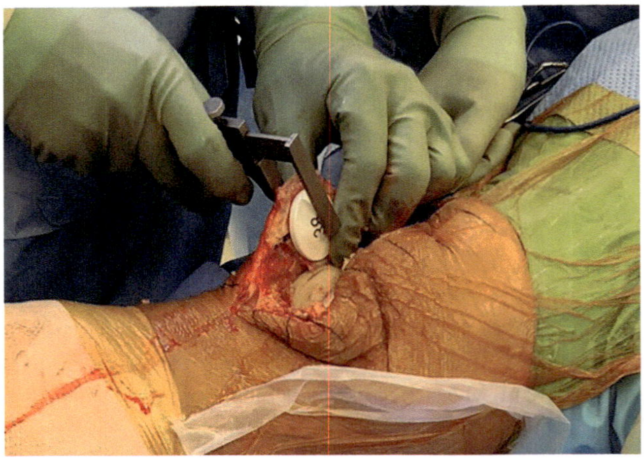

Fig. 27.5 Measuring the composite patellar height

Once cut, the patella is protected from retractors with a metal disk.

27.3.5 Femur Second

The femur is cut next. When using traditional instrumentation, the distal femoral cuts are made using a cutting block that is stabilized and aligned using an intramedullary rod (Fig. 27.7). This cut is critical and sets the joint line orientation for the knee as well as the height of the joint line. The only plane not set at this point is rotation.

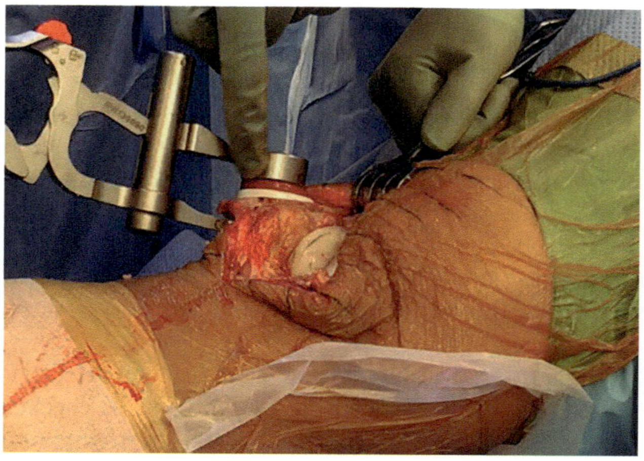

Fig. 27.6 Ensuring the patellar cuts are orthogonal to the patellar axis

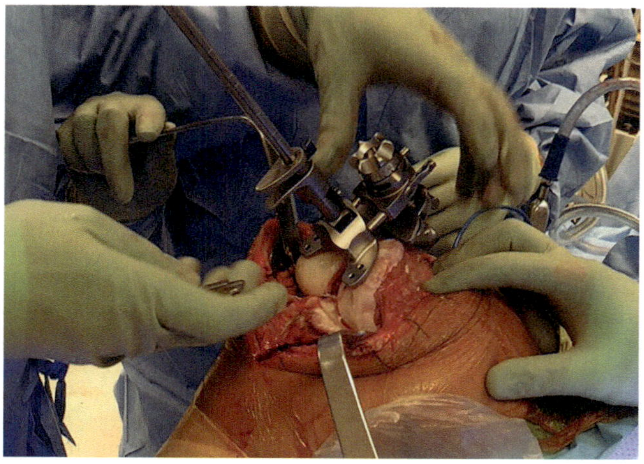

Fig. 27.7 Using an intramedullary rod to guide the distal femoral resection block

CR TKA requires careful attention to this step as the retention of the PCL requires that the joint line is maintained at exactly the same height as the native joint line, particularly on the medial side.

Measured resection techniques designed to resect an amount of bone and cartilage equal to the thickness of the femoral component are the norm in CR techniques (Sheth et al. 2017).

- If the intent is to set the joint line orthogonal to a mechanical axis that runs from the hip, through the knee and the ankle, the bone resection from the distal femur will be asymmetric in varus knees and placed in 5–7° of valgus.
- If the intent is to set the joint line equal to its native alignment and parallel to the floor when standing as in KA, the resection will be symmetric and in more valgus.

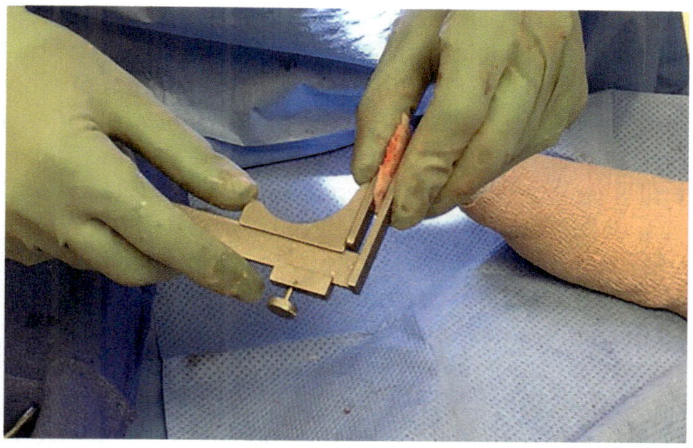

Fig. 27.8 Using a caliper to measure the amount of bone resected

The choice of MA versus KA alignment will also dictate whether the component is externally rotated 3° from the posterior condylar axis or set to match it. Regardless, the flexion and extension gaps in CR knee replacement surgery need to be meticulously matched if the PCL is to remain appropriately balanced throughout the arc of motion. We will discuss this in much greater detail later in this chapter.

In KA, the surgeon uses a caliper (Fig. 27.8) to ensure the accuracy of the cuts and adjusts them accordingly.

Prior to completing the cuts, there are several *check points that bear noting*:

Femoral component flexion beyond the native 0–3° is to be avoided (Okamoto et al. 2019).

- Flexion effectively decreases the extension gap while increasing the flexion gap and decreases the proximal extent of the trochlea potentially impacting patellar tracking. Passing a guide (alias: angel wing) through the anterior chamfer cutting slot should place the guide at the level of and parallel to the anterior femoral cortex.
- Further, the medial lateral extent of the femoral component should not extend past the bony margins, particularly medially. I personally will aim to seat the femoral component to match the lateral femoral condyle border to optimize patellar tracking.
- Lastly, osteophytes should be removed from the articular margins, the notch and the posterior knee as they can impact collateral and posterior ligament function.

Once all the cuts are complete and all the osteophytes from the femur and those from the tibial margin are removed, I will seat the trial femoral component and take the knee through a full range of motion. Generally, the previously contracted knee will come into full extension and be stable without the need for releases. How can this be the case? With the possible exception of truly deformed knees (>20° off axis) or patients with inflammatory pathologies, KA principles hold that the collateral ligaments are neither contracted nor stretched and that decompressing them as noted above, without releasing them, allows them to return to their normal length. In KA, the femoral component should be aligned exactly as the native knee was originally both in terms of its valgus alignment and its rotation.

If that was achieved, and the trial implant is essentially resurfacing the femur, the knee should be perfectly stable with a full range of motion (ROM) and any residual laxity can be assigned to bone loss on the tibial side caused by wear. If we are happy with the cuts and the component alignment, we will drill the lug holes.

We understand that there will be some ambivalence about this concept among those reading this chapter and that the MA literature is replete with articles discussing how best to "balance" contracted ligaments through selective "releases" so it is worth a deeper "dive." MA surgeons who are accustomed to releasing ligaments to balance the knee consider the ligaments on the convex side "contracted." However, KA principles hold that in such situations the ligaments appear tight not because they are contracted but because the component position does not match native anatomy. In MA the femoral components are positioned so as to "correct" native anatomy into less valgus than the native plane and in more external rotation than the native femur. This changes the relationship between the origin and the insertion of the ligaments. Doing so in a healthy knee would require soft tissue releases to balance the knee, so it is not surprising that it should be so in an arthritic knee. If the knee is not balanced in KA, the assumption is not that the ligament has contracted but rather that there has not been an accurate restoration of the native joint line.

> In essence, KA surgeons balance the knee through bony adjustments and assume the ligaments are not compromised, whereas MA surgeons will prioritize bony cuts to achieve mechanical alignment and perform soft tissue releases to balance the knee.

As in the last 7 years, I have actively needed to perform only a handful of ligamentous releases in the context of CR knee surgery, and that even in those cases the soft tissue releases were minor. I have come to agree that in the majority of KA-aligned patients no releases are necessary precisely because the position of the new component matches pre-arthritic anatomy and since the knee is perfectly balanced, the ligaments are not contracted or alternatively, lax, as a result of arthritis. The best evidence we have that this may actually be the case is from research showing reported intraoperative contact pressures are lower in KA-aligned knees (Shelton et al. 2019) without releases than in MA-aligned knees balanced through releases (MacDessi et al. 2020; Meneghini et al. 2016). That said, it is fair to suggest that more work needs to be performed on this topic and that the above arguments may not hold in severe malalignment or patients with collagen disorders and untreated inflammatory arthropathies.

Regardless of what one does once the femoral trial is seated, it is recommended that the implant be checked for medial to lateral fit (to avoid medial overhang) and anterior posterior fit (in particular we like to ensure that the femur seats easily, without going into flexion due to an insufficient anterior femoral chamfer resection). Once the fit is optimized, the lug holes are drilled. These are intended for pegs placed behind the femoral condyles of CR femoral components to provide stability to the implant in the absence of the bulky and stabilizing PCL "box." The femoral canal entry hole is then packed with bone graft, or bone wax, to prevent bleeding in the knee joint once the tourniquet is released.

27.3.6 Tibia Third

> The tibial cut is more difficult than most people give it credit for.

The tibial joint line is, on average, in 3° of varus relative to the tibial anatomic axis. However, in varus knees, it averages 4.5° of varus with a great deal of variation (Bellemans et al. 2012). To complicate matters, cartilage and bone wear can adversely impact proximal tibial geometry. Flexion contractures and rotational deformities of the tibial shaft are also common and need to be taken into account along with variations in the posterior tibial slope. Matters are further complicated by the fact that the lateral and medial tibial slope may vary by as much as 2.5° in the same knee.

> Interestingly, a shared goal for all knee alignment philosophies is that the knee should be perfectly balanced in extension.

This is because the knee should be very stable at heel strike. It is also the case that the distal femur dictates the level of the joint line, not the tibia. It is also, therefore, a fact that to be stable in extension these two cuts, the tibial cut and the distal femoral cut, need to be parallel by the end of the case. This is true for KA, BG, and MA knees. As noted above, KA achieves balance by cutting the tibia to match the distal femoral cut regardless of the varus angle this produces at the tibia and, as a result, needs no soft tissue balancing. MA and BG techniques prefer to cut the tibia in neutral to the mechanical axis and balance the resulting gap through soft tissue releases.

Things get a little more interesting in flexion.

> MA and BG techniques aim for a balanced flexion gap while KA prefers to restore the physiologic lateral flexion gap which averages 2–3 mm of laxity and, therefore, aims for a trapezoidal gap.

However, all three techniques aim for a tight medial gap throughout the arc of motion to stabilize the knee.

Having decided on coronal plane alignment, we must now consider flexion and rotation. Due to our historical preoccupation with coronal alignment, inappropriate flexion of the tibial component in the sagittal plane is an often-overlooked cause of implant failure, knee pain, and poor ROM and may be more problematic than poor coronal alignment, particularly in CR TKA (Akagi et al. 1999; Bellemans et al. 2005; Kang et al. 2018; Panni et al. 2018).

> For CR surgeons, tibial flexion must match native anatomy or risk causing a tight flexion gap (too extended) or a block to full extension (too flexed), or mid-flexion instability (correct slope, wrong rotational plane).

Native posterior slope should be measured on preoperative images so as to know the target prior to surgery, but slopes in excess of 8–9° should not be matched. Conversely, it is rare that the tibia should ever be positioned in extension. Rotation is also critical when the tibial cut is placed at an angle to the anatomic axis of the tibia as it is in CR knees. To judge rotation, one has to consider what is rotating around what. In the normal knee under physiologic loads, the medial knee joint is relatively fixed, and the lateral side translates, or better, rotates around this axis.

> The longitudinal axis of the lateral tibial plateau is thus a close approximation of the true AP axis of the tibia.

A line bisecting the lateral plateau is parallel to a line that bisects the tibial spines. Therefore, I use the electrocautery to mark a line that bisects the tibial spines and take this line over the anterior rim of the tibial plateau to make a mark distal to the tibial cut (Fig. 27.9). It will later be used to set tibial component rotation.

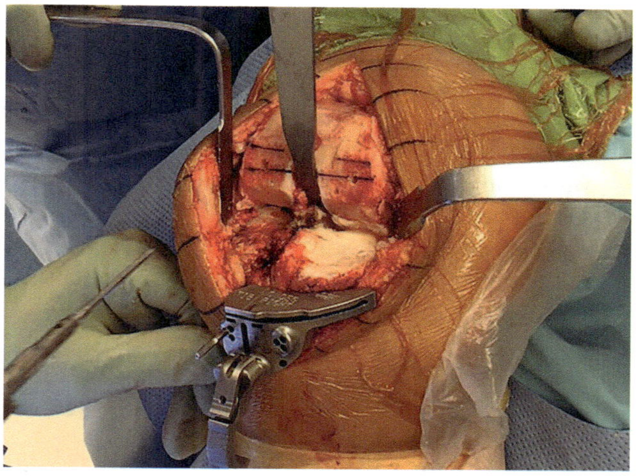

Fig. 27.9 Using the bovie to mark the tibial axis as a bisector of the interspinous ridge

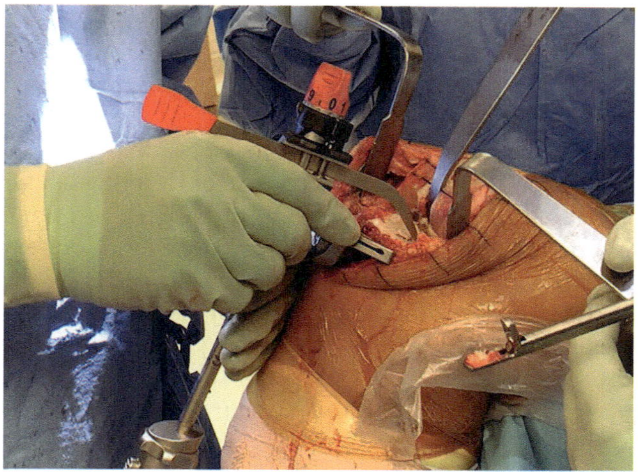

Fig. 27.10 Using the extramedullary jig to measure bone resection from the tibia and setting the varus–valgus angle of the cut

> The medial third of the tibial tubercle has, unfortunately, no more than a perfunctory relationship with the rotational axis of the tibia and cannot be relied upon as a landmark (Akagi et al. 2005; Baldini et al. 2013; Cobb et al. 2008; Eckhoff et al. 1995).

The tibial resection height is the last decision that needs to be made before the extramedullary cutting guide is pinned in place. In varus knees, the bone resection should account for the full height of the tibial tray plus the smallest tibial insert available. In knees with >15° of valgus, some surgeons recommend a more conservative tibial cut, perhaps 2 mm less, as the knee joint may open slightly in order to balance the MCL (Fig. 27.10). However, as per the discussion of ligamentous laxity above, I have not seen this as an issue with KA.

Once the alignment of the tibial cutting jig is decided, I use as many as three pins to ensure that it stays put while I pass the saw blade through it. A couple of options need to be considered at this point:

- The first is to downsize the size of the saw for patients with smaller knees to avoid unwanted collateral tissue damage.
- The second is to consider placing a small osteotome in the tibia just in front of the PCL to avoid cutting through the ligament origin inadvertently.

> Releasing the top 8–10 mm of the PCL origin from the posterior tibia, specifically that part of the tibial plateau that is being resected, will release the anterolateral bundle of the PCL.

> This can make sense in the context of a flexion contracture of long standing but should be performed carefully, taking care to not release the posterior-medial bundle of the PCL from the tibia entirely (Foge et al. 2019; Zhang et al. 2016).

Ideally, I try to retain this bone island and its PCL attachments. If there is any concern for the potential for a delayed or intraoperative PCL rupture, I will use an insert with a raised anterior polyethylene lip to prevent posterior translation of the tibia on the femur if the PCL fails (cruciate substituting [CS] inserts) (Mazzucchelli et al. 2016).

> Rotational alignment of the tibial tray onto the tibia is not trivial.

Various tibial designs exist that cover varied amounts of the exposed tibial bone. My goal is generally to ensure that whatever tibial plate I use sits on as much tibial cortex as I can arrange, while not internally rotating the tibia relative to the mark made earlier on the anterior tibial bone. Should that mark no longer be available and knowing that the tibial tubercle is not reliable, I have been happy to use the anterior tibial spine and the second metatarsal ray as secondary markers.

Several articles have documented the deleterious effects on knee pain of an internally rotated tibia, while there has not ever been an article documenting a problem associated with external tibial rotation. Of note, in CR knees that are placed in near-anatomic alignment with a well-balanced PCL, lateral rollback is accentuated, and it is important to place the tibial tray far enough posterolaterally to allow for an adequate "runway" for the lateral femoral condyle.

As mentioned above, knee stability can be restored in almost all planes. However, the plane of motion that cannot be easily addressed by modern TKA designs

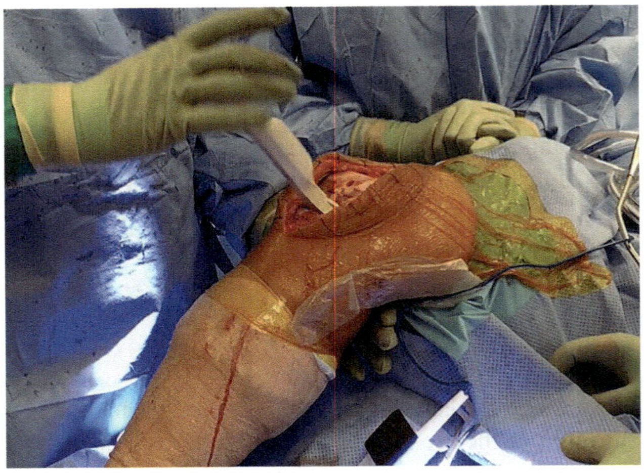

Fig. 27.11 Using a spacer block in flexion to check for stability

(both CR and PS) is anterior translation of the tibia on the femur due to ACL deficiency and an absent medial meniscus. This type of instability can cause anterior knee pain similar to chronic tendonitis and patients report an inability to perform prolonged activity due to diffused ligamentous knee pain. It is the senior author's opinion that this instability is one of the primary reasons for dissatisfaction following TKA.

The medially congruent design of "medial pivot" knees is a solution that may help provide increased AP stability to current TKA design and provide an answer to this problem.

KA principles that further restore normal kinematics to the CR knee coupled to design changes in the inserts may get us closer to a "forgotten knee." Work to create a functional bicruciate TKA continues in some quarters.

27.3.7 Balancing

Having completed all the cuts and injected the soft tissues with the PAIC, I first test the knee with spacer blocks *in flexion*, using the largest we can fit. It should be tight medially, but slightly loose laterally (2–8 mm gap). The lateral gap should match the gap seen with the femoral trial prior to performing the tibial cut (Fig. 27.11). Next we go into *extension* and the same spacer block should enable full extension. If there is any play greater than 1 mm, I will recheck the resected bone fragments to ensure that the resections are appropriate and that all osteophytes have been removed. Next, if necessary, I will recut the tibia until the knee is balanced in extension, usually from the tight side. Small resections of as little as 1 mm are often sufficient.

If working using an MA technique, balancing occurs using any sequence of soft tissue releases, usually starting with the tightest structures first. Some surgeons perform this step with the trials or even the actual components in place as they have no intention of altering the bone cuts.

Next, a laminar spreader can be used to gap the knee open in flexion and allow for the injection of the periarticular cocktail which I use to not only control perioperative hemarthroses, thanks to the epinephrine in the cocktail, but also to minimize joint pain in the immediate perioperative period.

Next, I check the TKA with trial component to ensure excellent stability, full extension, appropriate AP stability, and midline patellar tracking. If we have the appropriate instrument, we also check the femoral offset. The femoral component offset in this context is the distance that the femoral component sits back from the tibia when trialling and can be used to check if the PCL is balanced.

> It should be the same as it was at the time of the original arthrotomy. Any variance may suggest the PCL is too tight (femur too far posterior) or too lax (femur too far forward).

Another check is whether the tibial trial insert has any tendency towards "popping up" from the tray in deep flexion. Any evidence of poor PCL balance can be addressed through changing insert thickness or by changing the slope of the tibial cut.

The beauty of retaining a well-balanced PCL is that, doing so can help restore near-normal kinematics. Flexion and rotation in particular are driven by the PCL and retaining it can create a near-normal rollback and flexion. Later in this chapter, we will address why this is not always the case and why KA techniques may favor CR designs more than traditional MA techniques. Generally, as already noted, I try to avoid PCL releases.

27.3.8 Cementation

As I have previously worked at an organization that kept excellent records and lost very few patients to follow up, I was able to track all my patients from 2002 to 2015. In that time frame, I was fortunate to not have any patients revised for aseptic loosening of tibial implants. While it is possible that some patients were missed, I believe that the cementing technique I learned early on from one of my colleagues may have something to do with it. Prior to cementing, the bone is washed clean of blood and fat using pulsatile lavage and normal saline. Next it is dried with a gauze sponge. While the cement is still malleable, it is hand-packed into the tibia with as much pressure as

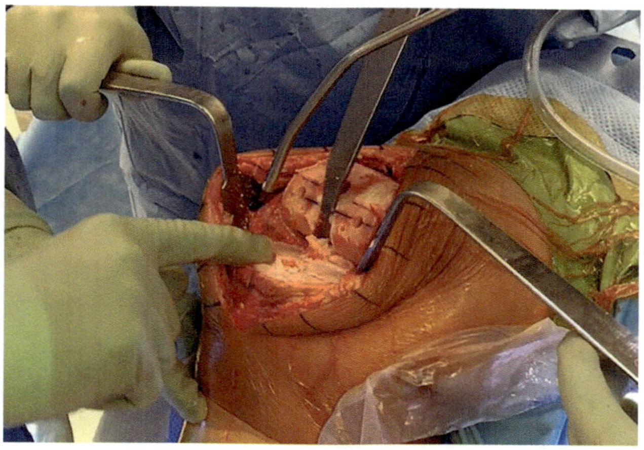

Fig. 27.12 Manually pressuring the cement into the cancellous bone to displace any fat or blood

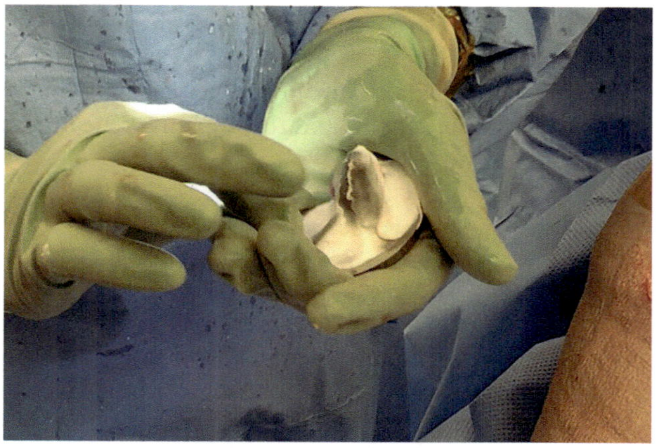

Fig. 27.13 Coating the implants and ensuring the entire surface is completely covered with cement

can be applied, first in the tibial canal, and secondly along the tibial surface.

> The goal is to pressurize the cement into the cancellous bone and displace the fat and bone marrow from the interstices of the trabecular bone (Fig. 27.12).

> The strength of the metal–cement interface is not that of a chemical bond, rather it is that of a mechanical lock between the cement and the grooves and niches of the undersurface of the tibial plate (Fig. 27.13).

Therefore, the back surfaces of the components are also manually coated with cement, and the cement is physically pushed into every nook and cranny of the device to ensure an excellent lock between the cement and the component. The same diligence is applied to the femur and patella.

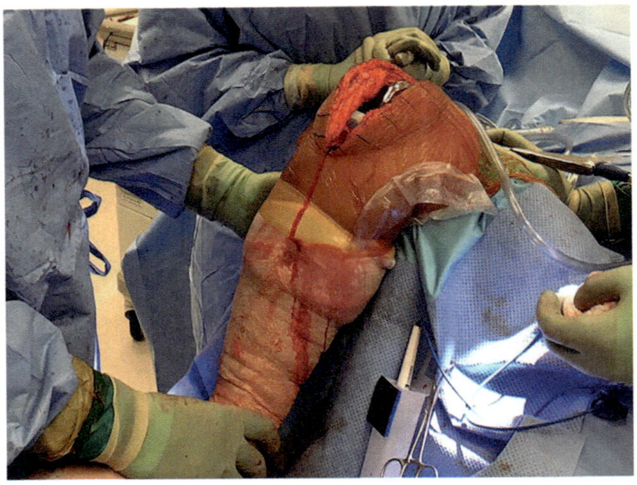

Fig. 27.14 Testing stability

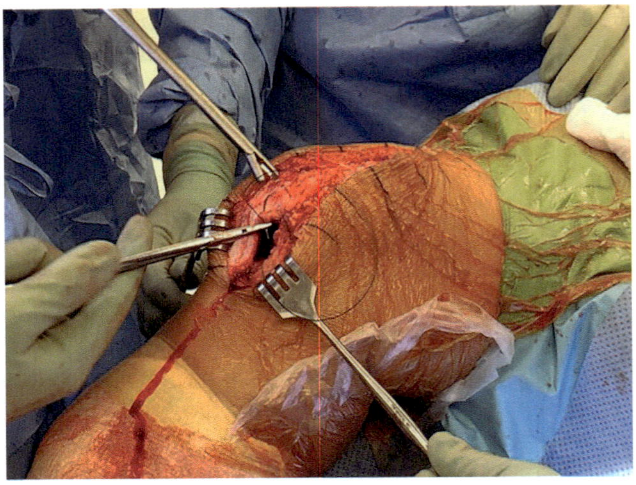

Fig. 27.15 Using running sutures

As the tibial component is being seated, any residual fat in the cancellous bone has nowhere to go to make room for the incoming metal. The only place it can go is in the space between the cement and the implant, beneath the tibial component.

> This displaced fat is the cause for the "lipid layer" occasionally seen on X-rays as a thin radiolucent line between the baseplate and the cement.

Next, a trial liner is seated, and the knee is taken through a range of motion to ensure that the components are completely seated and that full range of motion is restored to the knee. The relationship (offset) between the femur and tibia noted prior to implanting the device is reviewed. The knee is then brought into 90° and any excess cement removed. The cement is allowed to cure with the knee in extension while the joint is bathed in dilute betadine. The tourniquet is released once the implants are seated. I do not use antibiotic-loaded cement in primary knee arthroplasty.

27.3.9 Insert Trialing

Once the cement has cured, the trial liner can be exchanged if a modular base plate has been selected. The trial that provides the best balance and ROM should be selected. The PCL's tightness should be assessed for either a tight flexion gap or excessive rollback (Fig. 27.14).

There is no known published "downside" to using a CS insert in a CR knee at this time and its use is encouraged though the reader should check with the supplier if the cost of these raised rim inserts varies from the standard components. Flexion stability should also never be tested with the patella dislocated or reflected laterally as it tends to act as a checkrein and tighten the flexion gap. In obese patients, the compressive force of the thigh may also provide a false assessment of flexion stability and the assistant should be asked to apply a distracting force to the thigh while the knee joint's stability is tested.

Patellar tracking should be rechecked only once the cement has set and the tourniquet has been released. If there is any exposed lateral patellar facet it is undermined and resected to avoid painful impingement on the lateral femoral trochlear ridge. Maltracking of the patella may be caused by internal rotation of the tibia, flexion of the femoral component, a non-orthogonal cut of the tibia, or excessive patellar height. Ideally, these checks were performed at the time of trialing, but are worth repeating in case the implants seated in a different position than intended as the cement cured.

27.3.10 Closure

The deep, middle, and superficial layers are all closed with running barbed sutures that are carefully sewn with the knee in flexion using throws that are closely approximated to avoid leakage through the wounds (Fig. 27.15). If the wound is tight, we will sew in flexion but pull the sutures tight after three throws with the knee in extension. The subdermal layer in particular is closed tightly to take pressure off the superficial subcuticular layer. All three layers use running barber sutures (0, 2-0, and 3-0) and while we have had very occasional problems with skin breakdown, the incidence is not more common than with other subcuticular sutures.

The wound is then further sealed with skin glue. We recently stopped using any thin, adhesive bandages like "Steri Strips" and have been happy with the excellent results and lack of blistering. The resulting scars are usually thin, and patients love the cosmetic results and

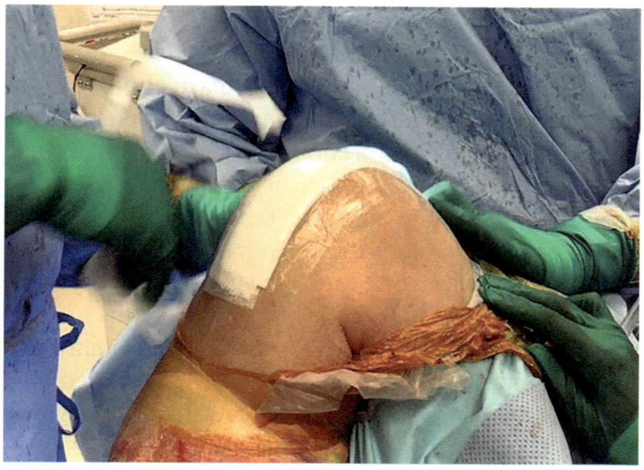

Fig. 27.16 A cost-effective, waterproof dressing that can stay on for 5 days

the lack of staples. One strip of a non-adherent bandage like Telfa is then placed on the wound followed by four layers of gauze for a very thin bandage. The dressing is covered with thin polyurethane adhesive bandage such as Tegaderm which must be placed without tension in full flexion to avoid causing traction blisters. This low-cost bandage is entirely waterproof, highly flexible, and does not impede range of motion (Fig. 27.16).

Patients are encouraged to shower immediately and at will.

> The original dressing placed in the sterile operating room environment stays on for 5 days and when it is removed at home by the patient it is not replaced.

The patient may continue to shower ad-lib but is asked to avoid baths and soaking the incision for 14 days from surgery.

27.4 Postoperative Care

Patients are encouraged to use cryotherapy several times a day for the next 1–2 months.

> Formal physical therapy is self-directed for the first 3–4 weeks after which patients who need or request formal therapy are referred for treatment while others are encouraged to walk ever increasing distances with pain as their primary guide.

Patients with weak quadriceps, however, are encouraged to work with a therapist or a trainer to regain strength. Narcotic pain medication is offered for the first 2 weeks and then tapered aggressively in patients who were previously narcotic-naive.

27.5 CR Knees: Why Retain the Cruciate?

There are several biomechanical arguments in favor of CR TKA.

> One potential advantage in conserving the PCL is to maintain proprioception of the knee after TKA.

Increased proprioception may contribute to patient satisfaction and good functional outcomes. Several studies have shown that PCL mechanoreceptors in knees with osteoarthritis are decreased but still present, and that they occupy similar areas in the PCL before and after implantation of a TKA (Çabuk et al. 2017).

> As mentioned above, PCL retention in the context of an anatomically correct trapezoidal flexion gap further promises to achieve an increased potential range of motion by restoring a more anatomic lateral femoral rollback.

This can reproduce more closely the kinematics of a normal knee, with the femur moving posterior-laterally during flexion and avoiding tibiofemoral impingement. The femoral rollback is also important for the patellofemoral joint, which functions better with a larger extensor lever arm when femoral rollback moves the tibial tubercle more anteriorly. Another advantage of CR TKA is the preservation of more bone than PS designs, which requires a box cutout to accommodate the tibial post.

> However, while the debate on CR versus PS knees in MA continues, the KA technique was designed to retain the PCL whenever it is present and little to no data exists relative to performing PS knees in KA alignment.

Indeed, the caliper-based technique would not be able to judge a priori the flexion gap induced by resecting the PCL and would tendentially create flexion and extension gap mismatches that would be difficult to adjust.

27.6 Design Features of CR Knees

CR implants are the least constrained of the knee prostheses. Traditional thinking suggests that knee stability is provided best in the presence of minimal bone loss, minimal soft tissue laxity, and an intact PCL. The lateral distal femoral condyle is sometimes larger than the medial condyle in some CR designs to facilitate translational and rotational movement, and to more closely replicate the medial pivot motion of a healthy knee.

There is no cam in the central portion of the femoral component and no post in the tibial polyethylene insert.

The insert on the tibial articular surface was historically less conforming to the femoral component in the sagittal plane to allow for femoral rollback and more normal motion of the knee.

> However, several in vivo kinematic analyses showed that these low-conforming inserts allowed a roll-forward positioning of the medial condyle during flexion akin to ACL-deficient/medial meniscal-deficient native knees.

This reduced femoral rollback, and limited ROM in flexion while exposing the tibial insert to higher risk of polyethylene wear due to elevated contact stress (Cates et al. 2008).

> Newer designs have taken a different approach with medial ultra-congruent shapes and anterior constraints to prevent the medial femoral condyle from sliding forward and constraining it as a medial pivot to restore sufficient knee stability even in cases of PCL loosening.

In contrast, the lateral tibial plateau is designed to allow the femur to move more freely with minimal congruency and, in some cases, going so far as having a convex surface. These implants are generally called Cruciate Stabilized (CS) or Medial Pivot (MP) designs based on the extent of the medial conformity of the polyethylene insert and to some extent the constrain features of the lateral compartment.

27.7 Balancing the PCL

Achieving optimal tension in the PCL throughout the arc of motion is of crucial importance if one is to balance knee flexion and extension. The PCL is composed of both anterolateral and posteromedial bundles. The anterolateral bundle becomes tight in flexion and induces posterior femoral translation, whereas the posteromedial bundle is tight in extension and mainly controls tibial rollback.

> If the PCL is normal, restoring normal kinematics such as one does with KA alignment will allow the PCL to function normally and no adjustments are required.

> If, however, the axis of rotation and overall alignment is altered, the PCL may need to be adjusted to allow the knee to be balanced throughout the arc of motion.

This is not different to the need to release the MCL or LCL in MA or BG knees. However, in patients with long-standing contractures, particularly in the varus knee, the PCL may be too tight, and a partial release will help create an optimal flexion gap and achieve coronal plane balance. A PCL which is too tight can lead to reduced flexion gap and excessive femoral rollback, which can accelerate posterior tibial polyethylene wear reducing the survivorship of the implant. In extreme cases, a very tight PCL in flexion can make the femoral condyles override the posterior edge of the tibial polyethylene, causing extremely high polyethylene contact stresses and wear. A PCL that is made too lax may lead to flexion instability, and postoperative pain.

Historically, CR TKA techniques recommended the release of the anterolateral bundle of the PCL from the bone island at the tibial attachment site, leaving only the posteromedial bundle of the PCL intact. The idea was to avoid PCL contracture-related space reduction that could interfere with knee flexion or cause conflict between the femur and the tibia.

> However, recent studies have concluded that both the anterolateral and posteromedial bundles of the PCL play an important role in maintaining knee stability. Zhang et al. showed that knee functional scores were significantly higher when the entire PCL had been retained (Foge et al. 2019).

Currently, it is my practice to release the anterolateral bundle in most knees, and to use a CS style tibial insert to not only support and protect the remaining PCL but also to help adjust for the absence of a medial meniscus.

27.8 Tibial Slope

> Reproducing an anatomic posterior tibial slope (PTS) in CR TKA is important to maintain the correct tension of the PCL throughout the arc of motion and to facilitate femoral rollback during knee flexion.

Since balancing the PCL mainly impacts anteroposterior tightness in flexion, in patients with significant deformity in the coronal plane leading to severe flexion contractures working with the PCL may not be enough. Several cadaver and computer-model studies have shown that increasing the PTS in CR TKA is more effective in reducing varus/valgus, anteroposterior, and rotational tightness in flexion than a limited PCL recessing or partial release. In an early paper, Walker and Garg reported that knees with PTS of 10° could flex 30° more than those with slope of 0° (Walker and Garg 1991). Bellemans later showed that an average gain of 1.7° of flexion could be expected for every degree of additional tibial slope acquired (Akagi et al. 1999). Conversely, Kang et al. warned that a decrease in PTS, as well as an increase in posterior condylar offset of more than 2 mm, could lead to degeneration of the PCL due to overtightening (Bellemans et al. 2005). However, an excessive PTS may induce anterior subluxation of the tibial component, increase polyethylene wear on the posterior tibial surface, and lead to aseptic loosening (Marra et al. 2017).

27.9 Indications/Contraindications

> CR TKA is mainly indicated in the arthritic knee with minimal bone loss, minimal soft tissue laxity, and an intact PCL.

Contraindications include the following:
- Posterior cruciate ligament insufficiency
- Posterolateral instability
- Significant coronal deformity
- Extensor mechanism deficiency

Other conditions which can increase the risk of conversion from a CR-type prosthesis to a PS type are as follows:
- Severe flexion contracture (>20°)
- High posterior slope
- History of previous osteotomy around the knee
- Chronic dislocation of the patella
- Small femoral component size (Bae et al. 2016; Song et al. 2019)

Rheumatoid arthritis has historically been considered a contraindication to CR TKA. However, more recent studies have suggested that CR TKA can yield results comparable to PS TKA in RA patients at a long-term follow-up.

> Intraoperatively, the status of PCL should be evaluated carefully.

The finding of PCL loosening or of poor elasticity constitutes a possible contraindication to traditional CR TKA though with newer CS inserts this is less clear. The presence of large bone defects or the need for augments are factors that do not favor the use of CR TKA. Patients who have previously undergone knee osteosynthesis, high tibial osteotomy, unicompartmental knee arthroplasty, or complex trauma leading complex deformity about the knee, may be better suited to PS TKA. In patients with an excessive (>10°) preoperative posterior tibial slope, the ability to match the slope through bone resection of the posterior aspect of the tibial plateau is limited. In such cases, the posterior aspect of the tibial component will be placed too proximal to the original joint line possibly leading to flexion–extension gap mismatch. In these patients it could be necessary to resect more tibia, decrease the PTS, release the PCL, and convert to PS TKA (Baldini et al. 2015).

Another situation which could lead to a conversion to a PS TKA is the inadvertent excessive elevation of the joint line leading to flexion–extension mismatch that can only be addressed with revision augments (generally not available for primary CR TKA femoral components) or the release of the PCL and conversion to a PS TKA. Bae et al. showed that this scenario can happen in the case of femoral component downsizing (Walker and Garg 1991).

> Finally, it should be stated that the recently introduced CS inserts are designed to be used specifically in the context to a PCL deficiency.

Several authors, ourselves included, have started to use it in all CR knees as the long-term presence of the PCL cannot be guaranteed. Others are using this insert after actively resecting the PCL in order to avoid performing the femoral resections required for the cam-and-post mechanism. Thus, accidentally transecting the ACL may not require an automatic conversion to a PCL knee if the CS inserts are available.

27.10 Clinical Results: CR Versus PS

> Many studies have compared CR TKA and PS TKA, but it is still unclear whether one design has superior clinical outcomes than the other.

Several studies have shown excellent short- and mid-term survival rates of both designs, with no differences in terms of functional and radiological outcomes, patient-reported outcomes, and complication rates.

In theory, CR TKA should attain better postoperative knee proprioception, kinematics, and flexion due to retention of the PCL and improved femoral rollback. However, many recent studies have shown that PS TKA achieved a higher postoperative ROM than CR knees due to a more uniform femoral rollback. Modern PS TKA knees that place the cam/post mechanism more posteriorly than older designs engage the tibial post sooner during flexion than older designs and thus create a more reliable rollback. CR TKA requires a near-perfect tensioning of the PCL to function like a normal knee. Indeed, CR TKAs have shown a paradoxical forward translation of the femorotibial contact point during weight-bearing flexion, probably due to a loose PCL (Jiang et al. 2016; Longo et al. 2018).

Other studies have directly compared the two prosthetic designs in bilateral total knee arthroplasties in which one knee was treated with a PS implant and the other knee with a CR implant. These studies have confirmed greater flexion in the posterior-stabilized knees, which were more stable and showed no anterior translation under weight-bearing conditions (Maruyama et al. 2004; Yoshiya et al. 2005). However, this difference was likely not clinically important, since there were no differences in functional and clinical outcomes.

Another argument promoting PCL substitution is that a significant deformity can be more reliably corrected with its use. While more relevant in MA than KA alignment, the tethering effect of a contracted PCL can make extensive collateral ligament release not effective in achieving varus–valgus balance.

> Kinematic alignment concepts may change the paradigm in favor of retaining the PCL.

It is important to note that all these prior studies have compared CR TKA versus PS TKA in the context of MA. As previously discussed, MA TKA by definition changes the rotational axis and joint kinematics of the knee to facilitate placing the knee in line with the mechanical axis. Doing so makes perfectly balancing the PCL, particularly in the context of multiple soft tissue releases to address coronal deformity, very difficult in the MA knee. In many ways, CR TKA in the context of mechanical alignment principles is a harder operation than a modern PS TKA which is why PS has become the preferred design of most arthroplasty surgeons in the US and abroad with recent increasing interest in MA CS TKA.

However, KA principles have challenged those assumptions. KA retains the PCL in order to avoid alterations of the flexion gap and further assists the normal function of the knee by maintaining the native rotational axes of the femur and the integrity of the collateral ligaments. In this context, releasing or otherwise lengthening the PCL is seldom required and the PCL is able to function normally throughout the arc of motion. While there cannot be a specific head-to-head comparison of CR versus PS in KA knees as the latter is contraindicated for KA, CR KA knees are reporting very favorable clinical outcomes suggesting that the challenges associated with retaining and balancing the PCL in MA TKA that are listed in the preceding paragraphs may not be as relevant in the KA context. The role of CS TKA in KA knees with absent or insufficient PCLs is still to be studied.

> A possible advantage of CR TKA irrespective of alignment philosophy is that it is more friendly to the patellofemoral joint.

CR designs do not allow alteration of the height of the preoperative joint line whereas PS TKAs frequently need to balance the increased flexion gap that occurs when the PCL is sacrificed with increased resection of bone from the distal femur. The resulting elevation of the joint line can lead to patella baja and increased patellofemoral joint contact forces. These effects can lead to decreased ROM and anterior knee pain. Moreover, in PS TKA, the patella and hypertrophic synovium on the undersurface of the quadriceps tendon can bind in the femoral cam, leading to a clinical entity known as “patellar clunk syndrome”. Despite the fact that current PS designs offer longer trochlear grooves to reduce hypertrophy of the synovium, cases of this complication are still reported in the literature, although less frequently (Agarwala et al. 2013; Putman et al. 2019).

Both designs have shown a low risk of revision due to wear of the polyethylene tibial insert. In CR TKA with a poorly functioning PCL and a low-conformity tibial insert, paradoxical anterior tibial translation in flexion may lead to early polyethylene wear. In PS TKA the contact point between the tibial post and the femoral component can be a site of wear and occasional breakage, particularly when the femoral component is flexed, the tibial component has an excessive posterior slope, or when the knee hyperextends.

The loosening rates in most reported studies show equal survivorships of posterior-stabilized TKA and cruciate-retaining TKA. However, some recent retrospective studies (Abdel et al. 2011; Spekenbrink-Spooren et al. 2018; Vertullo et al. 2017) have shown a higher risk of major revision in PS TKA than CR TKA, mainly due to loosening of the tibial component. It has been hypothesized that added prosthetic constraint may transfer more stress with higher shear forces to the prosthesis–bone interface on the tibial component of PS TKA designs.

▪ Conclusion

In summary, CR TKA is a well-established surgical technique that is more complex to perform than PS TKA. However, the clinical results of an appropriately indicated and well-performed TKA are comparable between the two designs. New surgical alignment theories, such as kinematic alignment, recreate the knee’s native rotational axis which aids in the retention of the PCL. Careful attention to the cementing technique is crucial to the longevity of the CR TKA.

Take-Home Messages

- Cemented TKA is reliant on excellent cement technique for long-term success and remains the standard of care against which press-fit devices will be measured.
- Mechanically aligned (MA) cemented CR TKA is a complex procedure because the retained PCL makes the gaps difficult to match, and because it is difficult to release collateral ligaments to balance the knee throughout the arc of motion in the context of an altered ("corrected") anatomical relationship between femur and tibia.
- Cemented kinematic alignment (KA) TKA principles favor retention of the PCL by closely restoring the native bony anatomy and restoring the normal biomechanics and motion of the knee without collateral ligament releases. Therefore, KA TKA is easier to balance than MA CR techniques.
- KA aims to restore pre-arthritic anatomy through caliper-based bony cuts that replicate the original position of the joint line while avoiding releases of any ligaments. MA aims to place the knee in mechanical alignment with the tibial joint line orthogonal to the mechanical axis of the limb and uses selective ligament releases to balance the knee.
- Tibial component alignment is complex and impactful. It should be carefully checked and rechecked and match the desired goal for the alignment technique selected.
- Understanding that bone cement is a grout and not an adhesive informs how we prepare both the bony and implant surfaces to avoid long-term aseptic loosening of CR TKA.
- Current implant designs create ACL and medial meniscal-deficient TKAs. Medial pivot designs that aim to address this deficiency coupled to KA may bring us closer to a more physiologic feeling TKA than we have been able to document in the past.

References

Abdel MP, Morrey ME, Jensen MR, Morrey BF (2011) Increased long-term survival of posterior cruciate-retaining versus posterior cruciate-stabilizing total knee replacements. J Bone Joint Surg Am 93(22):2072–2078. https://doi.org/10.2106/JBJS.J.01143

Agarwala SR, Mohrir GS, Patel AG (2013) Patellar clunk syndrome in a current high flexion total knee design. J Arthroplasty 28(10):1846–1850. https://doi.org/10.1016/j.arth.2013.03.019

Akagi M, Matsusue Y, Mata T, Asada Y, Horiguchi M, Iida H, Nakamura T (1999) Effect of rotational alignment on patellar tracking in total knee arthroplasty. Clin Orthop Relat Res. https://doi.org/10.1097/00003086-199909000-00019

Akagi M, Mori S, Nishimura S, Nishimura A, Asano T, Hamanishi C (2005) Variability of extraarticular tibial rotation references for total knee arthroplasty. Clin Orthop Relat Res (436):172–176. https://doi.org/10.1097/01.blo.0000160027.52481.32

Ali AA, Mannen EM, Rullkoetter PJ, Shelburne KB (2018) In vivo comparison of medialized dome and anatomic patellofemoral geometries using subject-specific computational modeling. J Orthop Res 36(7):1910–1918. https://doi.org/10.1002/jor.23865

Bae DK, Song SJ, Kim KI, Hur D, Lee HH (2016) Intraoperative factors affecting conversion from cruciate retaining to cruciate substituting in total knee arthroplasty. Knee Surg Sports Traumatol Arthrosc 24(10):3247–3253. https://doi.org/10.1007/s00167-015-3971-3

Baldini A, Indelli PF, de Luca L, Mariani PC, Marcucci M (2013) Rotational alignment of the tibial component in total knee arthroplasty: the anterior tibial cortex is a reliable landmark. Joints 1(4):155–160. https://doi.org/10.11138/jts/2013.1.4.155

Baldini A, Castellani L, Traverso F, Balatri A, Balato G, Franceschini V (2015) Instructional review the difficult primary total knee arthroplasty: a review. Bone Joint J 97-B(10 Suppl A):30–39. https://doi.org/10.1302/0301-620X.97B10.36920

Bellemans J, Robijns F, Duerinckx J, Banks S, Vandenneucker H (2005) The influence of tibial slope on maximal flexion after total knee arthroplasty. Knee Surg Sports Traumatol Arthrosc 13(3):193–196. https://doi.org/10.1007/s00167-004-0557-x

Bellemans J, Colyn W, Vandenneucker H, Victor J (2012) The Chitranjan Ranawat award: is neutral mechanical alignment normal for all patients?: the concept of constitutional varus. Clin Orthop Relat Res 470(1):45–53. https://doi.org/10.1007/s11999-011-1936-5

Çabuk H, Kuşku Çabuk F, Tekin AÇ, Dedeoğlu SS, Çakar M, Büyükkurt CD (2017) Lower numbers of mechanoreceptors in the posterior cruciate ligament and anterior capsule of the osteoarthritic knees. Knee Surg Sports Traumatol Arthrosc 25(10):3146–3154. https://doi.org/10.1007/s00167-016-4221-z

Cates HE, Komistek RD, Mahfouz MR, Schmidt MA, Anderle M (2008) In vivo comparison of knee kinematics for subjects having either a posterior stabilized or cruciate retaining high-flexion total knee arthroplasty. J Arthroplasty 23(7):1057–1067. https://doi.org/10.1016/j.arth.2007.09.019

Cobb JP, Dixon H, Dandachli W, Iranpour F (2008) The anatomical tibial axis: reliable rotational orientation in knee replacement. J Bone Joint Surg Br 90(8):1032–1038. https://doi.org/10.1302/0301-620X.90B8.19905

Eckhoff DG, Metzger RG, Vandewalle MV (1995) Malrotation associated with implant alignment technique in total knee arthroplasty. Clin Orthop Relat Res (321):28–31. https://doi.org/10.1097/00003086-199512000-00005

Foge DA, Baldini TH, Hellwinkel JE, Hogan CA, Dayton MR (2019) The role of complete posterior cruciate ligament release in flexion gap balancing for total knee arthroplasty. J Arthroplasty 34(7S):S361–S365. https://doi.org/10.1016/j.arth.2019.03.017

Jiang C, Liu Z, Wang Y, Bian Y, Feng B, Weng X (2016) Posterior cruciate ligament retention versus posterior stabilization for total knee arthroplasty: a meta-analysis. PLoS One 11(1):e0147865. https://doi.org/10.1371/journal.pone.0147865

Kang KT, Koh YG, Son J, Kwon OR, Lee JS, Kwon SK (2018) A computational simulation study to determine the biomechanical influence of posterior condylar offset and tibial slope in cruciate retaining total knee arthroplasty. Bone Joint Res 7(1):69–78. https://doi.org/10.1302/2046-3758.71.BJR-2017-0143.R1

Longo UG, Ciuffreda M, Mannering N, D'Andrea V, Locher J, Salvatore G, Denaro V (2018) Outcomes of posterior-stabilized compared with cruciate-retaining total knee arthroplasty. J Knee Surg 31(4):321–340. https://doi.org/10.1055/s-0037-1603902

MacDessi SJ, Griffiths-Jones W, Chen DB, Griffiths-Jones S, Wood JA, Diwan AD, Harris IA (2020) Restoring the constitutional alignment with a restrictive kinematic protocol improves quantitative soft-tissue balance in total knee arthroplasty: a randomized controlled trial. Bone Joint J 102-B(1):117–124

Marra MA, Strzelczak M, Heesterbeek PJ, van de Groes S, Janssen DW, Koopman BF, Wymenga AB, Verdonschot NJ (2017) The effect of tibial slope on the biomechanics of cruciate-retaining TKA: a musculoskeletal simulation study. J Orthop Res 11(5): page 2423

Maruyama S, Yoshiya S, Matsui N, Kuroda R, Kurosaka M (2004) Functional comparison of posterior cruciate-retaining versus posterior stabilized total knee arthroplasty. J Arthroplasty 19(3):349–353. https://doi.org/10.1016/j.arth.2003.09.010

Mazzucchelli L, Deledda D, Rosso F, Ratto N, Bruzzone M, Bonasia DE, Rossi R (2016) Cruciate retaining and cruciate substituting ultra-congruent insert. Ann Transl Med 4(1):2. https://doi.org/10.3978/j.issn.2305-5839.2015.12.52

Meneghini RM, Ziemba-Davis MM, Lovro LR, Ireland PH, Damer BM (2016) Can intraoperative sensors determine the "target" ligament balance? Early outcomes in total knee arthroplasty. J Arthroplasty 31(10):2181–2187

Okamoto Y, Otsuki S, Nakajima M, Jotoku T, Wakama H, Neo M (2019) Sagittal alignment of the femoral component and patient height are associated with persisting flexion contracture after primary total knee arthroplasty. J Arthroplasty 34(7):1476–1482. https://doi.org/10.1016/j.arth.2019.02.051

Olivecrona C, Lapidus LJ, Benson L, Blomfeldt R (2013) Tourniquet time affects postoperative complications after knee arthroplasty. Int Orthop 37(5):827–832. https://doi.org/10.1007/s00264-013-1826-4

Panni AS, Ascione F, Rossini M, Braile A, Corona K, Vasso M, Hirschmann MT (2018) Tibial internal rotation negatively affects clinical outcomes in total knee arthroplasty: a systematic review. Knee Surg Sports Traumatol Arthrosc 26(6):1636–1644. https://doi.org/10.1007/s00167-017-4823-0

Putman S, Boureau F, Girard J, Migaud H, Pasquier G (2019) Patellar complications after total knee arthroplasty. Orthop Traumatol Surg Res 105(1S):S43–S51. https://doi.org/10.1016/j.otsr.2018.04.028

Shelton TJ, Howell SM, Hull ML (2019) Is there a force target that predicts early patient-reported outcomes after kinematically aligned TKA? Clin Orthop Relat Res 477(5):1200

Sheth NP, Husain A, Nelson CL (2017) Surgical techniques for total knee arthroplasty: measured resection, gap balancing, and hybrid. J Am Acad Orthop Surg 25(7):499–508. https://doi.org/10.5435/JAAOS-D-14-00320

Song SJ, Park CH, Bae DK (2019) What to know for selecting cruciate-retaining or posterior-stabilized total knee arthroplasty. CiOS Clin Orthop Surg 11(2):142–150. https://doi.org/10.4055/cios.2019.11.2.142

Spekenbrink-Spooren A, Van Steenbergen LN, Denissen GAW, Swierstra BA, Poolman RW, Nelissen RGHH (2018) Higher mid-term revision rates of posterior stabilized compared with cruciate retaining total knee arthroplasties: 133,841 cemented arthroplasties for osteoarthritis in the Netherlands in 2007–v2016. Acta Orthop 89(6):640–645. https://doi.org/10.1080/17453674.2018.1518570

Vertullo CJ, Lewis PL, Lorimer M, Graves SE (2017) The effect on long-term survivorship of surgeon preference for posterior-stabilized or minimally stabilized total knee replacement an analysis of 63,416 prostheses from the Australian Orthopaedic Association national joint replacement registry. J Bone Joint Surg Am 99(13):1129–1139. https://doi.org/10.2106/JBJS.16.01083

Walker PS, Garg A (1991) Range of motion in total knee arthroplasty: a computer analysis. Clin Orthop Relat Res (262):227–235. https://doi.org/10.1097/00003086-199101000-00031

Yang G, Huang W, Xie W, Liu Z, Zheng M, Hu Y, Tian J (2016) Patellar non-eversion in primary TKA reduces the complication rate. Knee Surg Sports Traumatol Arthrosc 24(3):921–930. https://doi.org/10.1007/s00167-015-3528-5

Yoshiya S, Matsui N, Komistek RD, Dennis DA, Mahfouz M, Kurosaka M (2005) In vivo kinematic comparison of posterior cruciate-retaining and posterior stabilized total knee arthroplasties under passive and weight-bearing conditions. J Arthroplasty 20(6):777–783. https://doi.org/10.1016/j.arth.2004.11.012

Zhang B, Cheng CK, Qu TB, Hai Y, Lin Y, Pan J, Wang ZW, Wen L (2016) Partial versus intact posterior cruciate ligament-retaining total knee arthroplasty: a comparative study of early clinical outcomes. Orthop Surg 8(3):331–337. https://doi.org/10.1111/os.12269

Posterior Stabilized Total Knee Arthroplasty

Musa B. Zaid and Thomas P. Vail

Contents

E. Hansen, K.-D. Kühn (eds.), *Essentials of Cemented Knee Arthroplasty*,
https://doi.org/10.1007/978-3-662-63113-3_28

28

28.1 Introduction

The decision to utilize a cruciate-retaining versus a posterior stabilized total knee arthroplasty continues to be an area of debate as one technique has not separated itself from the other in achieving optimized pain relief and functional outcome. While current literature suggests that posterior stabilized knee arthroplasty may provide increased postoperative range of motion, there is minimal difference in rates of aseptic loosening or patient-reported outcomes when compared to cruciate-retaining total knee arthroplasty. The purpose of this chapter is to highlight the surgical technique of performing a cemented posterior stabilized total knee arthroplasty as well as to briefly discuss the kinematic considerations of a posterior stabilized knee arthroplasty and explore some of the recent literature examining functional and patient-related outcomes between cruciate-retaining and posterior stabilized implant designs.

28.2 Case Example

A 75-year-old female with a past medical history of hypertension has been followed in the arthroplasty clinic with bilateral, left greater than right, knee pain that has progressively worsened over the last year. She describes activity-related, dull-aching pain located in her anterior knees that gets worse with using stairs, prolonged standing, and walking. Additionally, she has noticed increased bowing of her knees. The patient currently can ambulate greater than six blocks and does not use any assistive devices. She has previously attempted oral anti-inflammatories and intra-articular cortisone injections experiencing mild relief of her symptoms. Her review of systems is notable for joint pain; she denies back pain or other significant joint symptoms.

On examination, her body mass index is 26 kg/m^3. She walks with an antalgic gait, valgus thrust. She has full painless passive and active range of motion of her bilateral hips with no pain on active straight leg raise. Examination of her knees is significant for mild medial and lateral joint line tenderness and no effusion. The patient has bilateral, left greater than right, valgus knee alignment with a symmetrical range of motion of 0–130°. She is stable to anterior–posterior stress exam and her valgus deformity is passively correctable with solid endpoints on collateral ligament testing. She is neurovascularly intact.

Anterior–posterior, sunrise, lateral, and Rosenberg view radiographs of the bilateral knees demonstrate valgus alignment with bone-on-bone lateral joint space narrowing and associated subchondral sclerosis (Fig. 28.1).

Given the severity of the patient's symptoms, the associated limitation of her activities, and impact on her quality of life, staged bilateral total knee arthroplasty is recommended. As her left knee is more symptomatic, the patient elects to have a left total knee arthroplasty first. Postoperative results are shown in Fig. 28.2.

28.3 Surgical Technique

28.3.1 Positioning

The patient is placed supine on a standard operating room Table. A well-padded, high-thigh tourniquet is placed on the operative extremity and is only inflated during final component cementation. The operative extremity is prepped and draped in the usual sterile fashion and then placed in a knee positioning device and secured. The ankle is left free to allow for visualization of the malleoli during placement of the extramedullary tibial alignment guide.

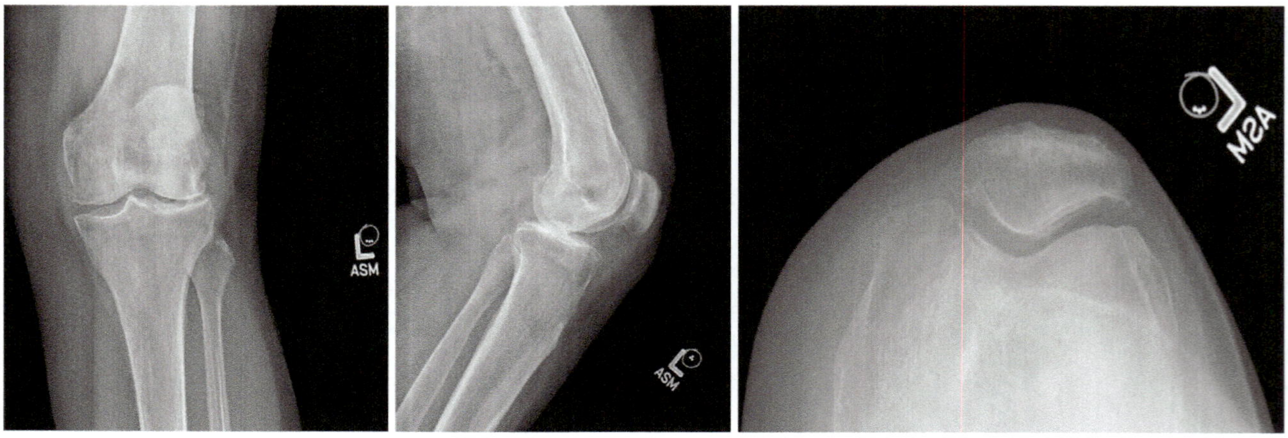

Fig. 28.1 Preoperative radiographs demonstrating valgus alignment with medial-sided bone-on-bone arthritis and osteophyte formation

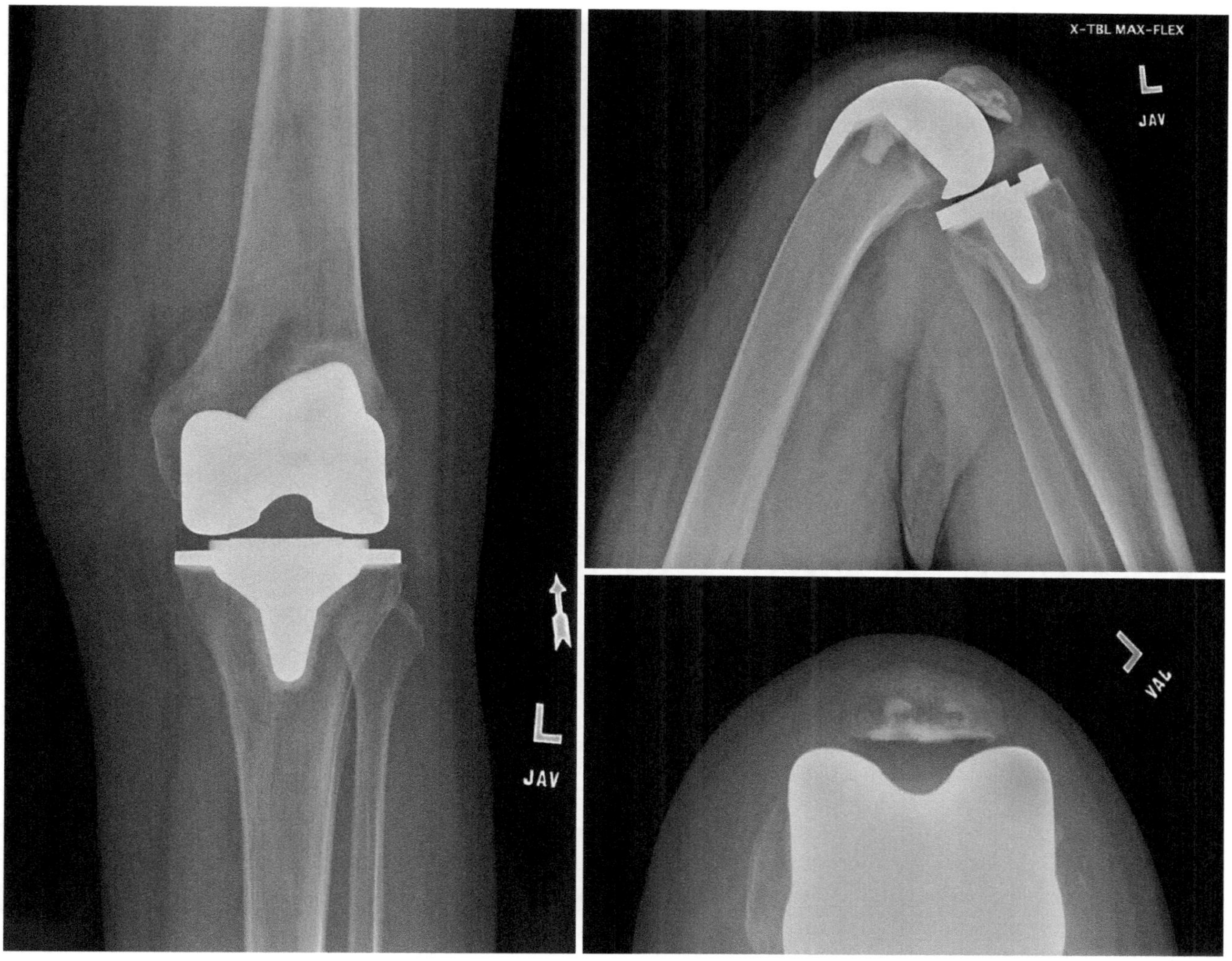

Fig. 28.2 Postoperative radiographs demonstrating a well-sized, well-fixed, cemented posterior stabilized total knee arthroplasty

28.3.2 Exposure

With the knee in a 40–45° flexed position, a curved medial peripatellar skin incision, avoiding the tibial tubercle and other bony prominences, is used. A capsular incision is then performed starting distally using a knife, proceeding from the medial one-third of the tibial tubercle, incorporating the medial 6–8 mm of the infrapatellar ligament, creating a cuff of tissue around the medial aspect of the patella, and then proceeding proximally in the medial 6–8 mm of the quadriceps tendon to a distance of about one patella diameter above the superior pole of the patella. The patella is then reflected laterally and the fat pad is excised.

An "internal release of the patella" is performed by elevating the capsular attachment to the patella along the lateral patellar border at the osteochondral junction. The lateral patellofemoral ligament is divided sharply. A limited synovectomy is performed (this can be more extensive if there is extensive synovitis or synovial thickening). Exposure in standard varus or valgus knee with a correctable deformity (as opposed to a more severe, fixed deformity required a greater release of contracture) includes minimal elevation of the deep MCL to allow visualization of the proximal tibia sufficient to perform a proximal tibial resection.

Once this standard exposure is completed, the knee is flexed with the patella subluxated to the lateral gutter. This allows sufficient visualization of the distal femur and proximal tibia to begin the bone resection and assessment of the flexion and extension gaps.

28.3.3 Distal Femoral Preparation

The knee is brought into flexion and a rongeur is used to remove any osteophytes that may be present along the articular cartilage edges sufficiently large to interfere with the assessment of the joint line using the distal femoral resection guide. For intramedullary guidance of the distal femoral cut, the diaphysis of the distal femur is then opened above the notch toward its medial border at

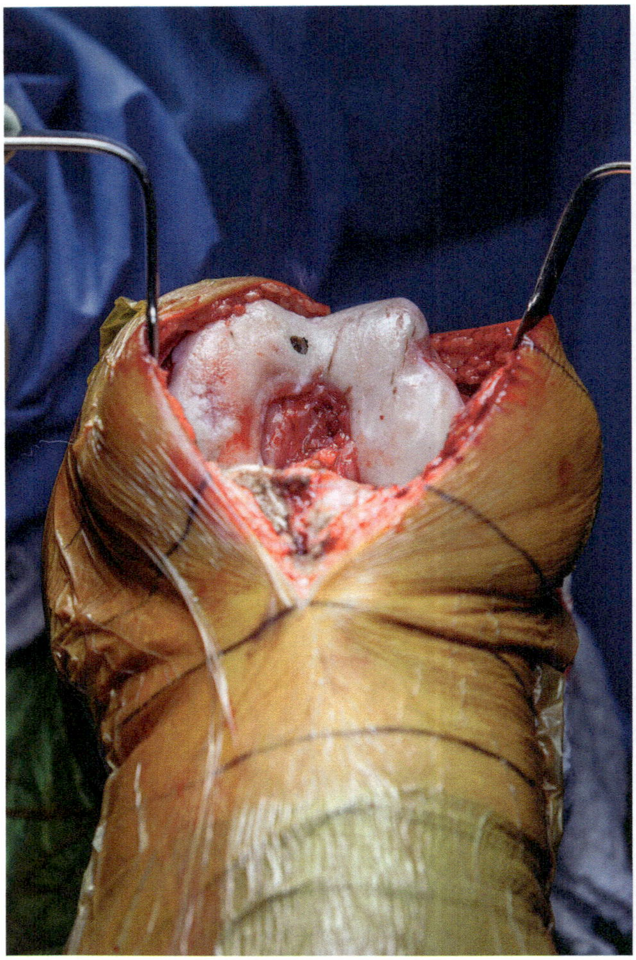

Fig. 28.3 Intraoperative photograph demonstrating exposure of the distal femur as well as marking the start site for the intramedullary alignment guide located 7–10 mm anterior and just medial to the femoral origin of the posterior cruciate ligament

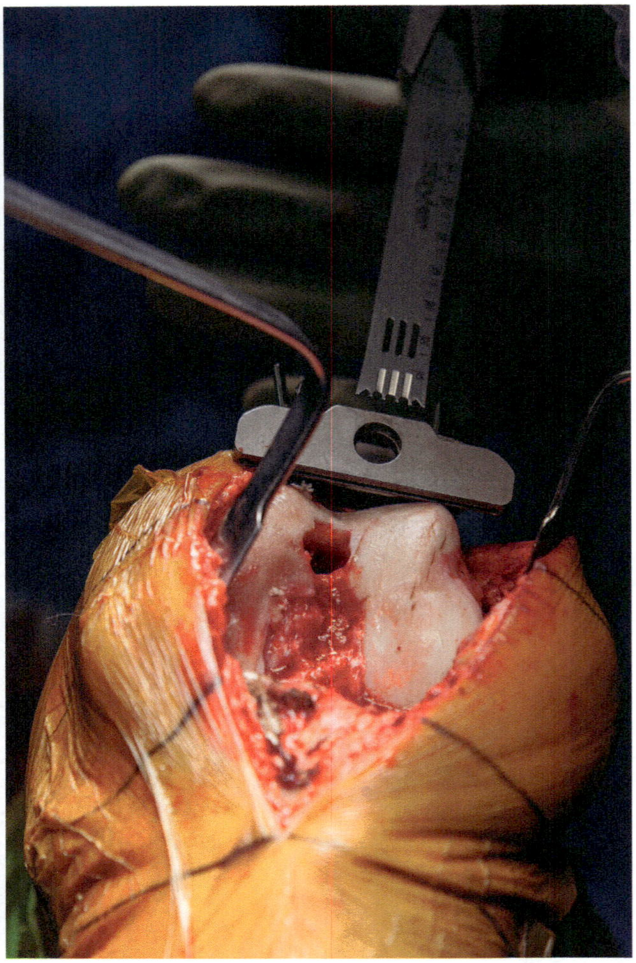

Fig. 28.4 Intraoperative photograph demonstrating placement of the distal femoral cutting guide followed by removal of the intramedullary alignment guide. Note the entry position of the intramedullary guide just above the notch and slightly medial to the mid-line. An oscillating saw is used to make this cut through the guide

a location 7–10 mm anterior and just medial to the femoral origin of the posterior cruciate ligament (Fig. 28.3). The intramedullary alignment rod is inserted into the distal femur with the attached distal femoral cutting block preset at the desired valgus angle relative to the anatomic axis. This desired angle can be determined with preoperative imaging. The resection level is set such that the resected bone matches the thickness of the prosthesis, thereby preserving the joint line. Once positioned, the cutting jig is secured with pins allowing removal of the alignment rod and creation of the distal femoral using an oscillating saw through the jig (Fig. 28.4).

> Care should be taken to assure that the cutting instrument does not deviate off of sclerotic bone thereby moving the cut off of the desired angle.

28.3.4 Tibial Preparation

Following distal femur preparation, the knee is brought into 90° of flexion to prepare the proximal tibia. While it is possible to create both the distal femoral and proximal tibial cuts with navigation or custom blocks, most often an extramedullary tibial guide is used. Likewise, it is also acceptable to make the proximal tibial cut first, and the distal femoral cut next, using the proximal tibia to guide the femoral cut. In either workflow, the extramedullary guide is secured to the leg via pins at the joint line and clamps that reach around the tibial at or above the lateral and medial malleoli. The position of the jig proximally sets the relationship of the proximal tibial cut to the mechanical and anatomic axes. Some surgeons prefer a predetermined proximal tibial angle, others use

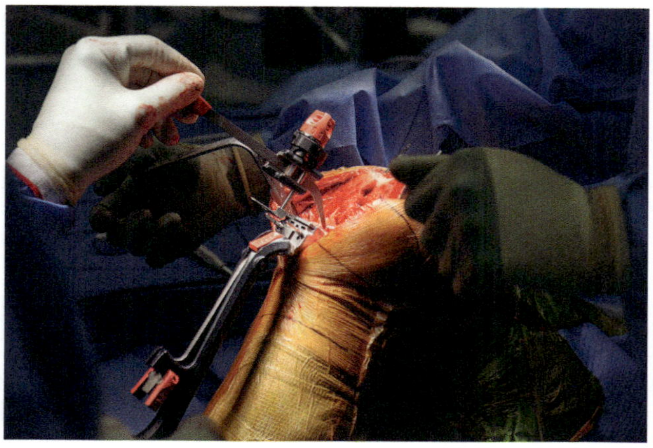

Fig. 28.5 Intraoperative photograph demonstrating placement of the extramedullary tibial alignment guide. The resection stylus is placed on the tibial plateau to set the proper level of proximal tibial bone resection. The amount of resection correlates with the combined thickness of the metal prosthetic tray and tibial insert

surface anatomy such as the intermalleolar position distally and the medial third of the tibial tubercle proximally, and others choose to make the proximal tibial cut perpendicular to the mechanical axis.

> With any of those choices, it is assumed that the surgeon accounts for the variability in individual anatomy and preexisting deformity to achieve the desired outcome.

When performing a posterior stabilized knee replacement, to accommodate the articular design of the prosthesis, the posterior slope is typically set to 5° or less. The desired varus and valgus alignment of the extramedullary tibial guide can be checked using a drop rod from anterior portion of the alignment guide and adjusted relative to surface landmarks on the tibia such as the tibial crest or the malleoli. While not critical at this stage, rotation of the proximal tibial cutting block is set by aligning the central mark on the cutting block with the medial third of the tibial tubercle. To the extent that any slope is incorporated into the cut, the rotation does become important as rotation of the cutting block that has a greater anterior than posterior resection can translate into varus or valgus if rotation is off of the midline.

Finally, the resection stylus is placed on the tibial plateau to set the proper level of bone resection (Fig. 28.5). Depending upon the point of reference, the resection level can vary, with less bone being removed if the point of reference is from a deficient area, and bone resection commensurate with the implant thickness if the point of reference is taken from the healthy joint line. The proximal tibia cut is then made using an oscillating saw.

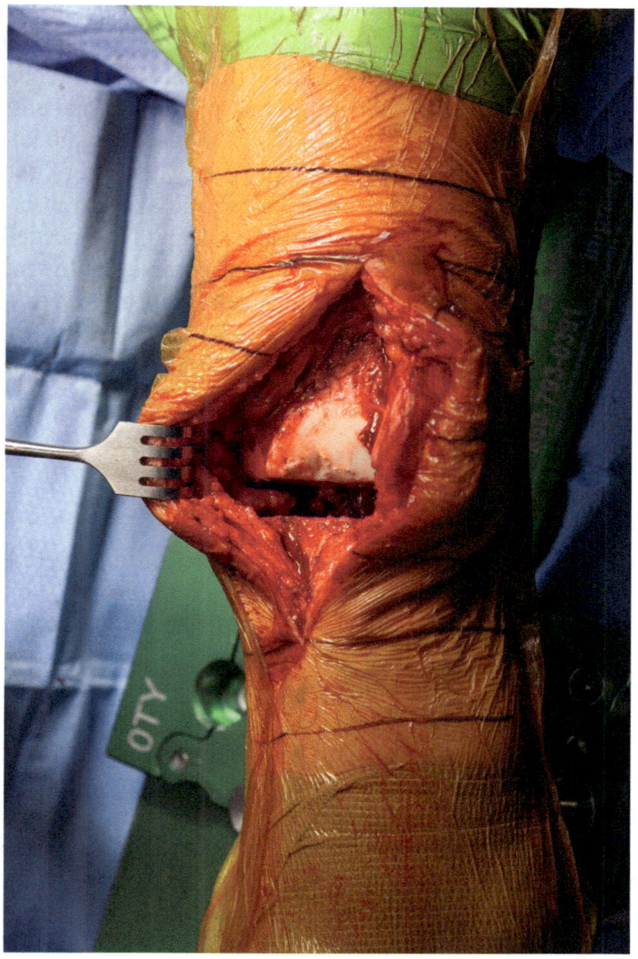

Fig. 28.6 Intraoperative photograph demonstrating a balanced or rectangular extension gap

> Great care should be taken to protect the collaterals, and to feel the posterior cortex, moving slowly with the saw as the posterior vascular structures, collaterals, and capsule are at particular risk when making the tibial cut.

28.3.5 Extension Gap Balancing

After the distal femur and proximal tibia cuts have been made, the extension gap is checked. The leg is brought into a full extension and a spacer block is inserted to evaluate the balance of the extension gap. Ideally, the extension gap is close to being rectangular rather than trapezoidal (Fig. 28.6). There should be no significant medial to lateral laxity, or differences of >2 mm, when the spacer block is placed and ligament balance is assessed.

> This is a very subjective step in the procedure, as there is no defined magnitude of varus or valgus stress that should be applied when assessing the extension gap balance.

However, if the surgeon determines that the extension gap is not acceptably balanced, then some soft tissue releases may be needed (assuming that the desired resection angle of the distal femoral and proximal tibial cuts has been achieved). Typically for a valgus knee, the lateral capsule at the joint line can be elevated off of the tibia, followed by elevation of the iliotibial band insertion just above Gerdy's tubercle, and finally if needed the popliteofibular ligament (capsule complex below the popliteus). For a varus knee, the medial capsule, the posteromedial corner, and the superficial medial collateral can be released in sequence to achieve balance in the extension gap.

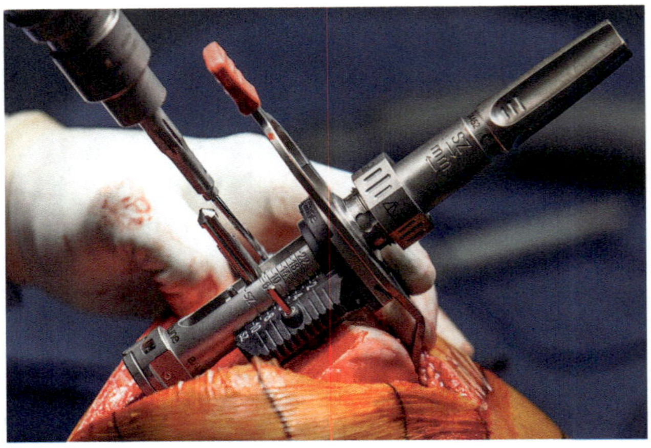

Fig. 28.7 Intraoperative photograph demonstrating distal femoral sizing. Subsequent to sizing, the rotational position of the distal femoral component is established using a ligament-tensioning device in a gap-balancing workflow. This can be accomplished with a lamina spreader, an electronic tensiometer, or a specially designed instrument. In this example, the intramedullary rod serves as the pivot point, allowing balancing of the medial and lateral flexion gaps as the ligaments are tensioned by the instrument. Once the optimal rotation and size are established, the femoral cutting guide is pinned in place and removed

28.3.6 Femoral Sizing and Rotation

Once optimal extension gap balance has been achieved, one can proceed with femoral sizing and finishing. This step can be done either using a measured resection method or a gap balance method. Some surgeons using a measured resection technique prefer to start with the distal femoral cut and then finish the femoral preparation using the epicondylar axis or Whiteside's line to set rotation, balancing ligaments at the end after all of the desired femoral and tibial cuts are made. In the gap-balancing workflow, the releases are performed at the outset once the extension gap cuts have been made.

The femoral finishing, which included the anterior, posterior, and chamfer cuts, is then made using the tibial cut and the ligament tension to set the rotation. For the gap-balancing workflow, the knee is brought into 90° of flexion and the femur size is determined. The femoral component rotation is then set using a ligament-tensioning device or a spacer block that sits on the tibia and is used as a reference for setting femoral component rotation (Fig. 28.7). At this step, a varus and valgus force can be applied to check for symmetry and lift off of the jig from the proximal tibia to assess the flexion gap balance. Adjustments can be made in the size of the femoral component, the thickness of the polyethylene insert, or the rotation of the femoral component before the cuts are made to set the rotation.

> Ideally, the extension and flexion gaps should be close to equal; if the flexion space is too large, upsizing the femoral component should be considered. If the flexion space is too small, the femoral component can be downsized.

Once the optimal rotation and size are established, the femoral cutting guide is pinned in place and removed (Fig. 28.7). Retractors are placed to protect soft tissues, and an oscillating saw is then used to cut the anterior, anterior chamfer, posterior, and posterior chamfer cuts at the distal femur. The notch cut is then completed (Fig. 28.8). The medial–lateral position of the notch cut determines the ultimate medial–lateral position of the implant. It should be placed as far lateral as possible without lateral overhang to facilitate patella tracking. Next, a lamina spreader can be used to distract the flexion gap to gain visualization of the posterior femoral condyles to remove residual osteophytes. Trial implants can now be inserted and overall balance, fit, and range of motion rechecked.

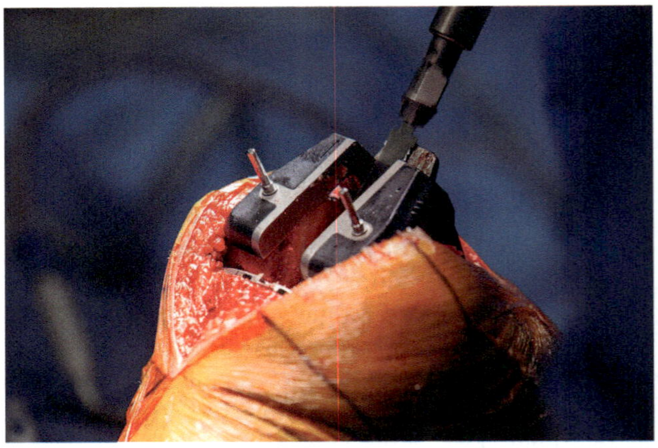

Fig. 28.8 Intraoperative photograph of the notch cut being performed. The medial–lateral position of the notch cut determines the ultimate medial–lateral position of the implant. It should be placed as far lateral as possible without lateral overhang to facilitate patella tracking

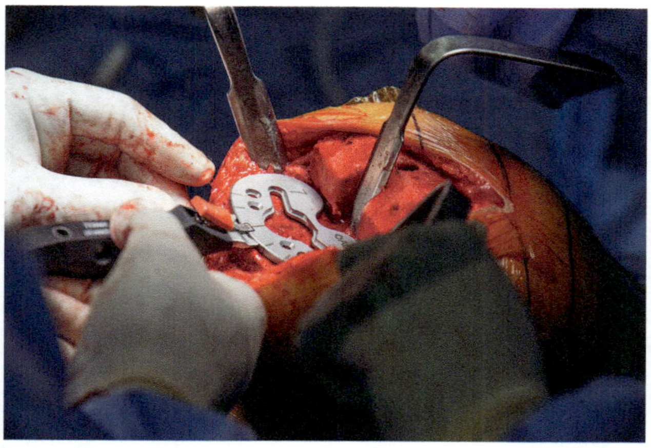

Fig. 28.9 Intraoperative photograph showing tibial sizing. The tibia is sized by selecting a tibial baseplate that maximizes tibial coverage without overhang. Rotation of the implant is set using anatomic landmarks such as the tibial tubercle and ankle joint

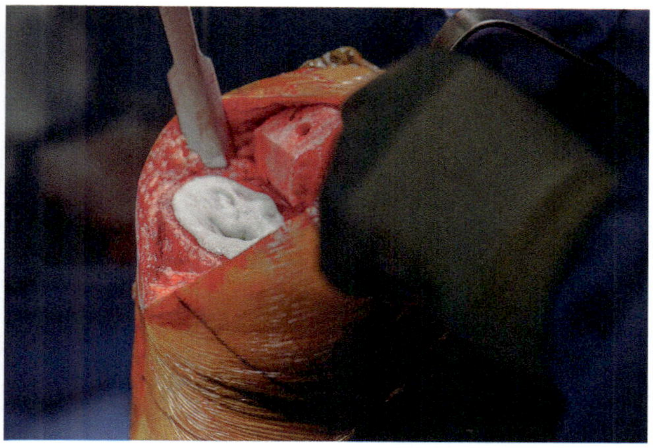

Fig. 28.10 Intraoperative photograph demonstrating finger-packed cement along the proximal tibial surface. Cement is also placed along the distal femur prior to placement of the femoral component (not shown). Keeping blood and fat out of the interface between the implant and the cement is important for optimal implant fixation

28.3.7 Patellar Preparation

The patella is sized and the cutting guide is set according to the available patellar bone. Generally, the patella is cut at its osteochondral border, noting that the lateral facet is generally longer, thinner, and less steep than the medial facet of the patella.

28.3.8 Trialing and Tibial Sizing

With the trial femoral component impacted onto the femur and the tibial trial in place, a visual check should be performed to ensure that the distal femur cuts are appropriate, fitting into the femoral trial. The tibia is sized by selecting a tibial baseplate that maximizes tibial coverage without overhang (Fig. 28.9). Tibial component rotation can be assessed before finalizing the preparation by putting the trial construct through a range of motion and marking the tibial component rotation at the joint line. If the knee is stable and well balanced, and the desired tibial component rotation is established, then the final tibial preparation is performed using the drill and punch method.

28.3.9 Cementation and Final Component Placement

The tourniquet is inflated and a pulse lavage is used to prepare all the bony surfaces which are subsequently patted dry. First, the tibial component is cemented into place. Cement is placed and finger-packed (some surgeons use a cement gun) along the proximal tibial surface and the keel hole as well as on the tibial baseplate (Figs. 28.10 and 28.11). Cement is placed onto the

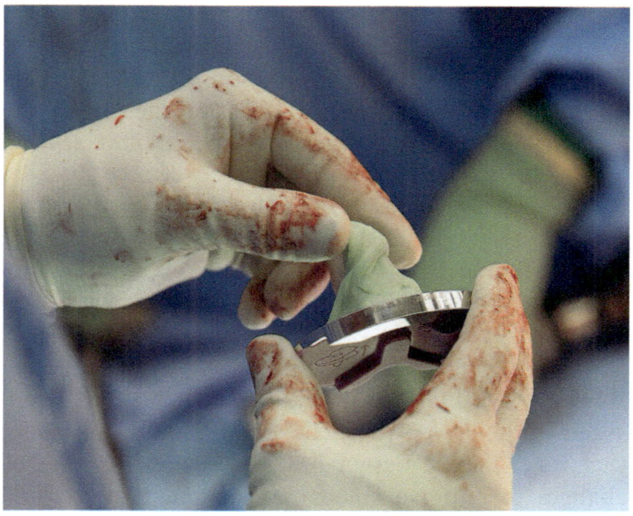

Fig. 28.11 Cement is placed onto the dry implant coating the cement-facing surface of the tibia (shown) and femur

dry implant coating the cement-facing surface of the tibia and femur. Similarly, cement is placed on the anterior and distal femoral cuts, and a small amount of cement is placed on the posterior flanges of the implant. The components are then placed and impacted. Excess cement is removed. A trial liner is placed and the knee is brought into extension.

> It is important to keep the knee very still and properly aligned while the cement cures. Movement of the knee while the cement is in a plastic phase can lead to bone–cement or implant–cement radiolucency and suboptimal cement mantle.

The patellar component is cemented in place after the tibia and femur. The knee is once again checked for a stable range of motion once the cement is allowed to fully harden. The tourniquet is deflated and the polyethylene liner is placed.

28.3.10 Closure

The knee capsule is closed anatomically using monofilament absorbable suture on the deep layers, and either nylon suture, stables, or a running subcuticular closure on the skin. The wound is dressed with a sterile dressing.

28.4 Literature Review

- **Introduction**

For the primary total knee arthroplasty, numerous prosthesis designs exist with the two most common being the cruciate-retaining (CR) and posterior stabilized (PS). While the cruciate-retaining implant design relies on the patient's native posterior cruciate ligament to allow for femoral rollback during deep flexion, the posterior stabilized design utilizes a central post on the tibial polyethylene insert which engages with a transverse cam located on the femoral component between the condyles (Fig. 28.12). In the PS design, during deep flexion, the cam and post engage, which in theory limits the degree of anterior femoral translation and leads to subsequent femoral rollback allowing increased knee flexion (Insall et al. 1982).

The first iteration of the posterior stabilized design was introduced in 1978 by Insall and Burstein and consisted of an all-polyethylene tibial component. Since that time, the PS design has undergone a variety of changes to improve kinematics and durability (Insall and Clarke 1993).

> The posterior stabilized total knee arthroplasty is a popular implant design with numerous studies demonstrating excellent range of motion, survivorship, and functional outcomes.

- **Range of Motion**

It has been hypothesized that replacing the native posterior cruciate ligament with a cam and post can improve the range of motion through mechanical enforcement of femoral rollback (Pagnano et al. 1998; Bercik et al. 2013). Numerous studies have demonstrated the ability to obtain excellent range of motion with a posterior stabilized knee. In a prospective cohort of over 240 knees, Hirsch et al. compared range of motion between posterior-stabilized, cruciate-retaining, and cruciate-sacrificing knees and found that posterior stabilized knees obtained significantly increased range of motion as compared to cruciate-retaining knees (112° vs. 104°) (Hirsch et al. 1994). This finding of improved range of motion compared to cruciate-retaining implants has been reproduced in numerous studies (Maruyama et al. 2004; Yoshiya et al. 2005; Catani et al. 2004) including a recent meta-analysis by Bercik et al. which concluded that PS knees had on average an increase of 3.33° of range of motion as compared to CR knees (Bercik et al. 2013). In addition to improved overall range of motion, numerous studies have found that posterior stabilized knees may provide increase flexion as compared to cruciate-retaining knees. Similar to range of motion, the recent meta-analysis by Bercik et al. showed that patients were able to obtain significantly more flexion in posterior stabilized knees as compared to cruciate-retaining knees (Bercik et al. 2013).

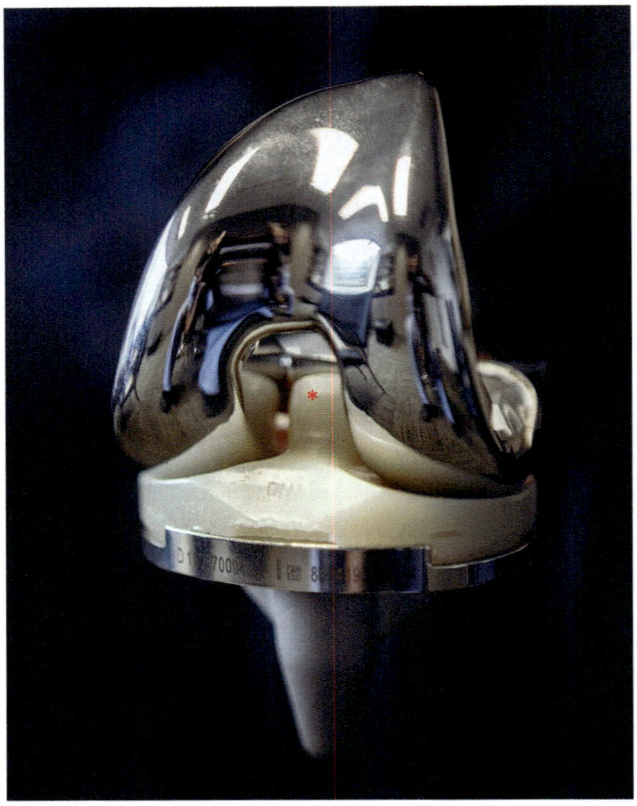

Fig. 28.12 The posterior stabilized total knee implant utilizes a central post (*) on the tibial polyethylene insert which engages with a transverse cam located on the femoral component between the condyles

- **Loosening and Survivorship**

Although early on it was hypothesized that retaining the native posterior cruciate ligament could mitigate aseptic loosening by resisting shear forces at the bone–implant interface (Pagnano et al. 1998), early biomechanical testing of posterior stabilized knees demonstrated that articulation of the post-and-cam mechanism on a PS knee led to compressive rather than shear forces at the proximal tibia (Insall et al. 1982). These biomechanical findings support today's clinical results.

In a long-term prospective cohort study of 55 young patients (<60 years at index surgery) undergoing a posterior stabilized knee arthroplasty, Meftah et al. experienced no cases of aseptic loosening at an average follow-up of 12.3 years (range 11–13) (Meftah et al. 2015). Additionally, the posterior stabilized implants had excellent survivorship of 98% at final follow-up (Meftah et al. 2015). Even at 15-year follow-up, Lachiewicz et al. experienced an aseptic loosening rate of <1% and survivorship of 96.8% for a cohort of patients who underwent a modular posterior stabilized knee arthroplasty.

> These results suggest that posterior stabilized knees may not be at an increased risk for aseptic loosening and have excellent survivorship.

Functional Outcomes

Patient-reported outcomes following posterior stabilized knee arthroplasty are similar to those of cruciate-retaining knee replacements as demonstrated by numerous randomized trials. In a recent randomized controlled trial comparing PS to CR knees, Scott et al. found no significant difference in Knee Society pain, function, and motion scores at a minimum follow-up of 2 years in a cohort of 111 patients (Scott and Smith 2014). Similarly, Maruyama et al. found no significant difference in postoperative knee scores at an average follow-up of 31.7 months in a prospective randomized comparison of patients undergoing posterior stabilized versus cruciate-retaining total knee arthroplasty (Maruyama et al. 2004). Additionally, a meta-analysis of randomized trials comparing posterior stabilized and cruciate-retaining implants failed to demonstrate a significant difference in functional outcomes and postoperative Knee Society pain scores at 2- and 5-year average follow-up (Li et al. 2014).

Kinematics and Gait

As previously discussed, it is theorized that the cam-and-post mechanism on a posterior stabilized knee recreates native femoral rollback and allows for increased knee flexion. Numerous studies have compared the kinematics of cruciate-retaining and posterior stabilized implants. While initially it was thought that retaining the PCL would allow for predictable femoral rollback that mimicked native knee kinematics, this has failed to be proven. Dennis et al. demonstrated the concept of "paradoxical anterior femoral translation" where abnormal anterior femoral translation upon the tibia can occur in cruciate-retaining implants (Dennis et al. 1996). This abnormal femoral motion can theoretically lead to increased tibial polyethylene wear and shear forces. Unlike CR implant designs, posterior stabilized total knee implants have been shown to restore physiological femoral rollback. Using in vivo fluoroscopy, Fantozzi et al. have demonstrated that posterior stabilized implants successfully recreate physiological femoral rollback during activities of daily living such as walking, going from sitting to standing posture, and during stair climbing (Fantozzi et al. 2006).

Take-Home Messages

- Posterior stabilized total knee implants utilize a cam-and-post mechanism to recreate native femoral rollback.
- Posterior stabilized total knee implants have demonstrated excellent 10- and 15-year survivorship with low rates of aseptic loosening.
- Posterior stabilized implants may offer slightly more increased flexion as compared to cruciate-retaining implants.
- Functional outcomes following posterior stabilized knee replacement are comparable to cruciate-retaining implants.
- Joint kinematics may be more closely restored with a posterior stabilized implant as compared to a cruciate-retaining implant.
- Keeping blood and fat out of the interface between the implant and the cement is important for optimal implant fixation.

References

Bercik MJ, Joshi A, Parvizi J (2013) Posterior cruciate-retaining versus posterior-stabilized total knee arthroplasty: a meta-analysis. J Arthroplasty 28:439–444

Catani F, Leardini A, Ensini A et al (2004) The stability of the cemented tibial component of total knee arthroplasty. J Arthroplasty 19:775–782

Dennis DA, Komistek RD, Hoff WA, Gabriel SM (1996) In vivo knee kinematics derived using an inverse perspective technique. Clin Orthop Relat Res 331:107–117

Fantozzi S, Catani F, Ensini A, Leardini A, Giannini S (2006) Femoral rollback of cruciate-retaining and posterior-stabilized total knee replacements: in vivo fluoroscopic analysis during activities of daily living. J Orthop Res 24:2222–2229

Hirsch HS, Lotke PA, Morrison LD (1994) The posterior cruciate ligament in total knee surgery. Save, sacrifice, or substitute? Clin Orthop Relat Res 309:64–68

Insall JN, Clarke HD (1993) Historic development, classification, and characteristics of knee prostheses. In: Insall & Scott surgery of the knee, 6th edn, pp 1375–1404.e6

Insall J, Lachiewicz P, Burstein A (1982) The posterior stabilized condylar prosthesis: a modification of the total condylar design. Two to four-year clinical experience. J Bone Joint Surg Am 64:1317–1323

Li N, Tan Y, Deng Y, Chen L (2014) Posterior cruciate-retaining versus posterior stabilized total knee arthroplasty: a meta-analysis of randomized controlled trials. Knee Surg Sports Traumatol Arthrosc 22:556–564

Maruyama S, Yoshiya S, Matsui N, Kuroda R, Kurosaka M (2004) Functional comparison of posterior cruciate-retaining versus posterior stabilized total knee arthroplasty. J Arthroplasty 19:349–353

Meftah M, White PB, Ranawat AS, Ranawat CS (2015) Long-term results of total knee arthroplasty in young and active patients with posterior stabilized design. Knee 23:318–321

Pagnano MW, Cushner FD, Scott WN (1998) Role of the posterior cruciate ligament in total knee arthroplasty. J Am Acad Orthop Surg 6:176–187

Scott D, Smith R (2014) A prospective, randomized comparison of posterior stabilized versus cruciate-substituting total knee arthroplasty: a preliminary report with minimum 2-year results. J Arthroplasty 29:179–181

Yoshiya S, Matsui N, Komistek RD, Dennis DA, Mahfouz M, Kurosaka M (2005) In vivo kinematic comparison of posterior cruciate-retaining and posterior stabilized total knee arthroplasties under passive and weight-bearing conditions. J Arthroplasty 20:777–783

Bicruciate-Retaining Total Knee Arthroplasty

Michael D. Ries

Contents

E. Hansen, K.-D. Kühn (eds.), *Essentials of Cemented Knee Arthroplasty*,
https://doi.org/10.1007/978-3-662-63113-3_29

29

29.1 Introduction

Bicruciate-retaining total knee arthroplasty was performed regularly in the 1970s, but the procedure was largely abandoned in the United States in the 1980s. Early bicruciate-retaining knee replacements essentially consisted of two unicondylar knee replacements in which the tibial components were connected by an anterior bar or bridge which allowed retention of the anterior cruciate ligament. However, unacceptable failure rates were reported with these early designs, usually as a result of tibial failure due to loosening, implant breakage, wear, and baseplate–insert dissociation (▫ Fig. 29.1). Other complications included stiffness and fracture of the eminence or tibial bone island containing the ACL insertion (Ries et al. 2018; Coventry et al. 1973; Gunston and MacKenzie 1976). Results with ACL-sacrificing, posterior cruciate-retaining (CR), or posterior cruciate-substituting (PS) designs have consistently provided reproducible pain relief and implant survivorship. However, approximately 20% of TKA patients are unsatisfied with the functional results of the procedure (Noble et al. 2006). This has been attributed to many factors including altered kinematics and flexion instability that likely results from loss of ACL function in CR and PS designs (Pagnano et al. 1998; Dennis et al. 2003).

Newer bicruciate-retaining TKA designs have been developed with the expectation that modern implant materials, surgical techniques, and instrumentation would allow retention of both cruciate ligaments in TKA, but avoid the problems that occurred historically with older bicruciate-retaining TKAs (Ries et al. 2018).

> Bicruciate-retaining TKA is generally considered appropriate for younger more active patients with an intact ACL, minimal knee deformity, and relatively good bone stock.

29.2 Illustrative Cases

29.2.1 Case 1

An active 65-year-old female developed lateral and anterior knee pain, which impaired routine and recreational activities. Treatment with NSAIDs did provide satisfactory relief and injections with cortisone were ineffective. Her knee range of motion is 0–130°, and the knee is stable to varus-valgus and anteroposterior stress. Radiographs demonstrate osteoarthritis primarily involving the lateral tibiofemoral compartment (▫ Fig. 29.2).

The patient is treated with bicruciate-retaining TKA. Exposure is performed through a medial parapatellar approach and standard femoral bone cuts made for a CR femoral component, which allows exposure of the medial tibial plateau (▫ Fig. 29.3a). Extramedullary alignment is used to orient depth, coronal, and sagittal alignment of the medial tibial plateau resection (▫ Fig. 29.3b). The medial tibial plateau is resected preserving the tibial eminence and cruciate ligaments (▫ Fig. 29.3c). A trial reduction is performed for the femoral component and medial tibial insert to ensure adequate bone has been removed from the medial tibial plateau. A lateral cutting guide is then attached to the extramedullary alignment jig which allows making a lateral plateau resection parallel to the medial plateau resection (▫ Fig. 29.3d).

A trial reduction is performed with various medial and lateral insert thicknesses and slopes to balance the soft tissues (▫ Fig. 29.3e).

> In order to optimize cement fixation of the tibial component, cancellous bone is curetted around the tibial keel (▫ Fig. 29.3f). Cement is applied in a relatively liquid state to allow optimal penetration into the bone (▫ Fig 29.3g).

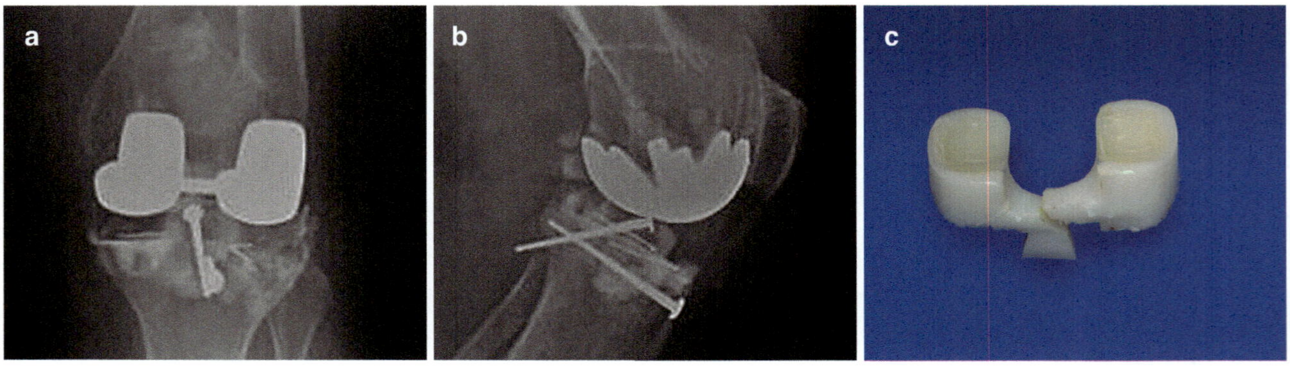

▫ **Fig. 29.1** **a** Anteroposterior radiograph of a 68-year-old female with rheumatoid arthritis 28 years after bicruciate-retaining TKA with a Geometric (Stryker, Mahwah, NJ) prosthesis including an all-poly tibial component and patellar non-resurfacing. **b** Lateral radiograph demonstrates screws that had been placed in the tibial eminence during the original surgery. **c** Revision TKA was performed. The tibial component was found to be loose and fractured at the anterior bridge between the two plateaus

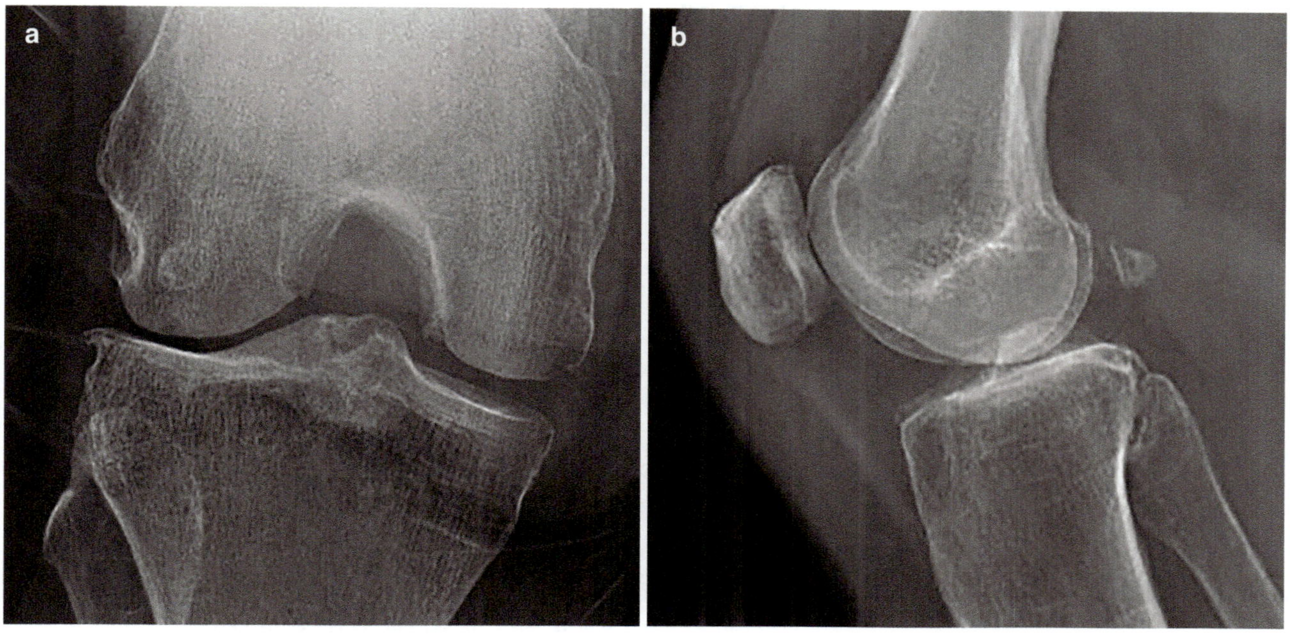

■ **Fig. 29.2** **a** AP and **b** lateral radiographs demonstrate osteoarthritis

The anterior part of the tibial eminence is removed and final components are cemented in place (■ Fig 29.3h).

29.2.2 Case 2

An active 38-year-old woman presented with complaints of left knee pain limiting routine activities of daily living. She had sustained a knee injury as a result of a fall which caused loss of cartilage on both the medial and lateral femoral condyles. Her knee was subsequently treated with three arthroscopic procedures in an effort to restore the integrity of the articular cartilage. However, she developed severe debilitating pain with all weight-bearing activity. Her range of motion is 0–125°, and the knee is well-aligned clinically. Radiographs demonstrate mild medial joint space narrowing (■ Fig. 29.4a) and relative preservation of the patellofemoral joint (■ Fig. 29.4b). She is treated with bicruciate-retaining TKA and patellar non-resurfacing (■ Fig. 29.4c–e).

About 3 years after surgery, she had no knee pain and carries out all routine activities as well as hiking and cycling long distances. Range of motion is 0–135°, and strength and knee stability are normal.

29.3 Results

Steihl et al. assessed kinematics in bicruciate-retaining TKA patients compared to CR TKA patients using in vivo fluoroscopy (Stiehl et al. 2000) (■ Table 29.1). Bicruciate TKA demonstrated gradual posterior femoral rollback during knee flexion. CR TKA demonstrated paradoxical motion and femorotibial contact began significantly posterior in extension with progressive anterior translation during knee flexion. Moro-oka et al. similarly compared the kinematics of bicruciate-retaining and CR TKAs using in vivo fluoroscopy (Moro-oka et al. 2007). Posterior translation of the lateral condyle was significantly greater for the bicruciate-retaining than CR TKAs during stair climbing and maximum flexion activities. Kono et al. studied 17 bicruciate-retaining TKA patients during squatting and cross-legged sitting activity using in vivo fluoroscopy (Kono et al. 2019). During cross-legged sitting, a medial pivot was observed beyond 60° of flexion. From 80–110° of flexion, femoral external rotation during squatting was significantly larger than that during cross-legged sitting.

> These studies suggest that bicruciate-retaining TKAs roll back and externally rotates in a pattern that is similar to the normal knee.

ACL retention in TKA has been advocated to preserve more normal proprioception, kinematics, and joint function than conventional CR or PS TKA. Baumann et al. assessed proprioception by balance testing during single-leg stance with eyes closed compared to eyes open in patients with bicruciate TKA, UKA, and PS TKA (Baumann et al. 2017). The authors found a lower difference in the area of sway between eyes closed and eyes open for the BCR and UKA patients compared to the PS TKA group. Pritchett reported on functional out-

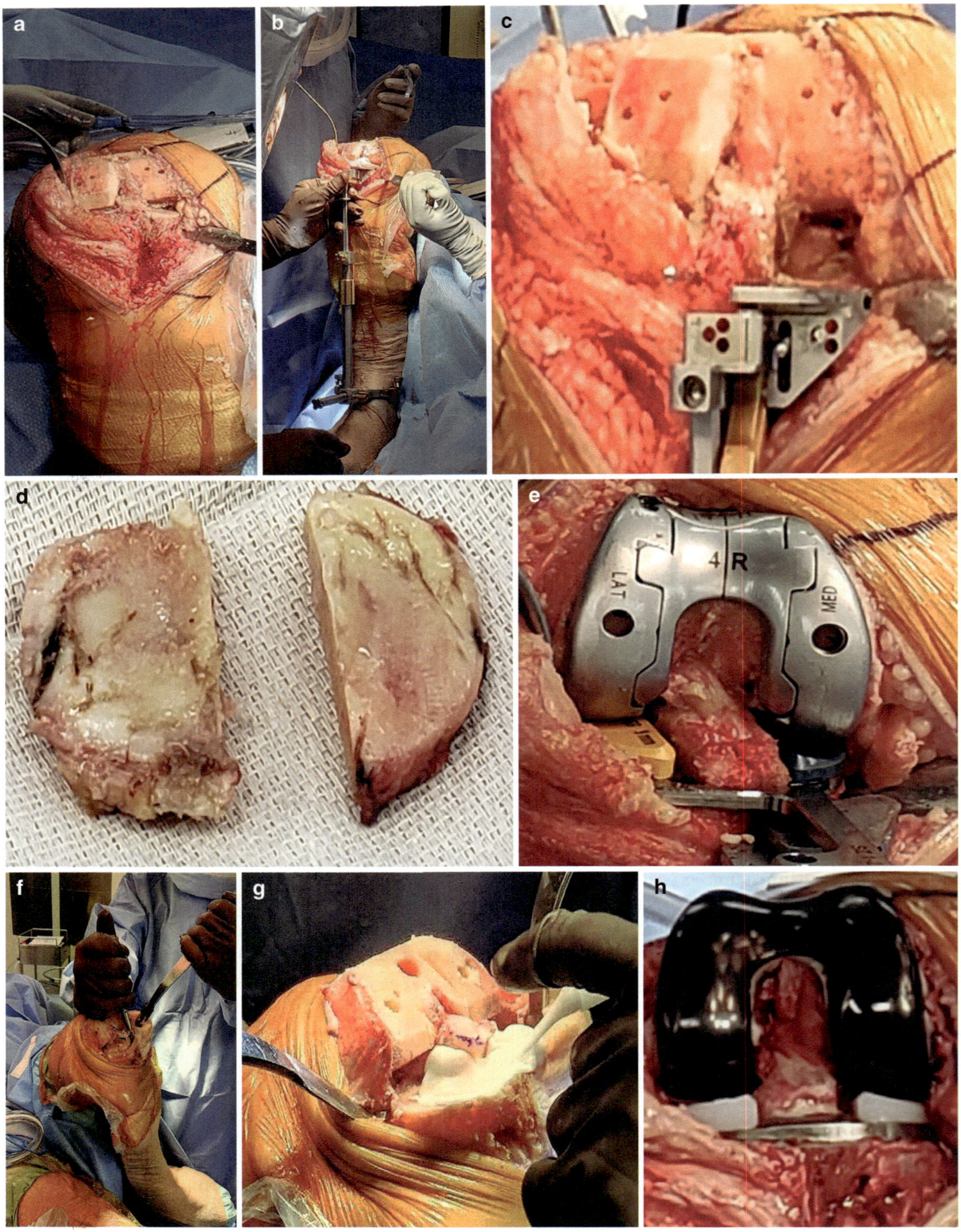

Fig. 29.3 **a** The femoral bone cuts are prepared for a CR femoral component. After removal of resected femoral bone, the medial tibial plateau is exposed. A trial reduction is then performed for the femoral component and medial tibial insert to ensure adequate bone has been removed from the medial tibial plateau. **b** Extramedullary tibial alignment is used to orient depth, coronal, and sagittal orientation of the medial tibial plateau resection. **c** The medial tibial plateau is resected similar to that of medial unicompartmental knee arthroplasty. **d** A lateral tibial plateau bone cut is made parallel to the medial plateau bone cut. The resected bone surfaces can be used to assess tibial component size. **e** Trial reduction is performed with various medial and lateral tibial insert thicknesses and posterior slopes to determine the optimal soft tissue tension. **f** In order to optimize cement fixation of the tibial component, cancellous bone is curetted around the tibial keel. **g** Cement is applied in a low to medium viscosity state to penetrate into the tibial bone. **h** The anterior part of the tibial eminence is removed and the final components are cemented in place

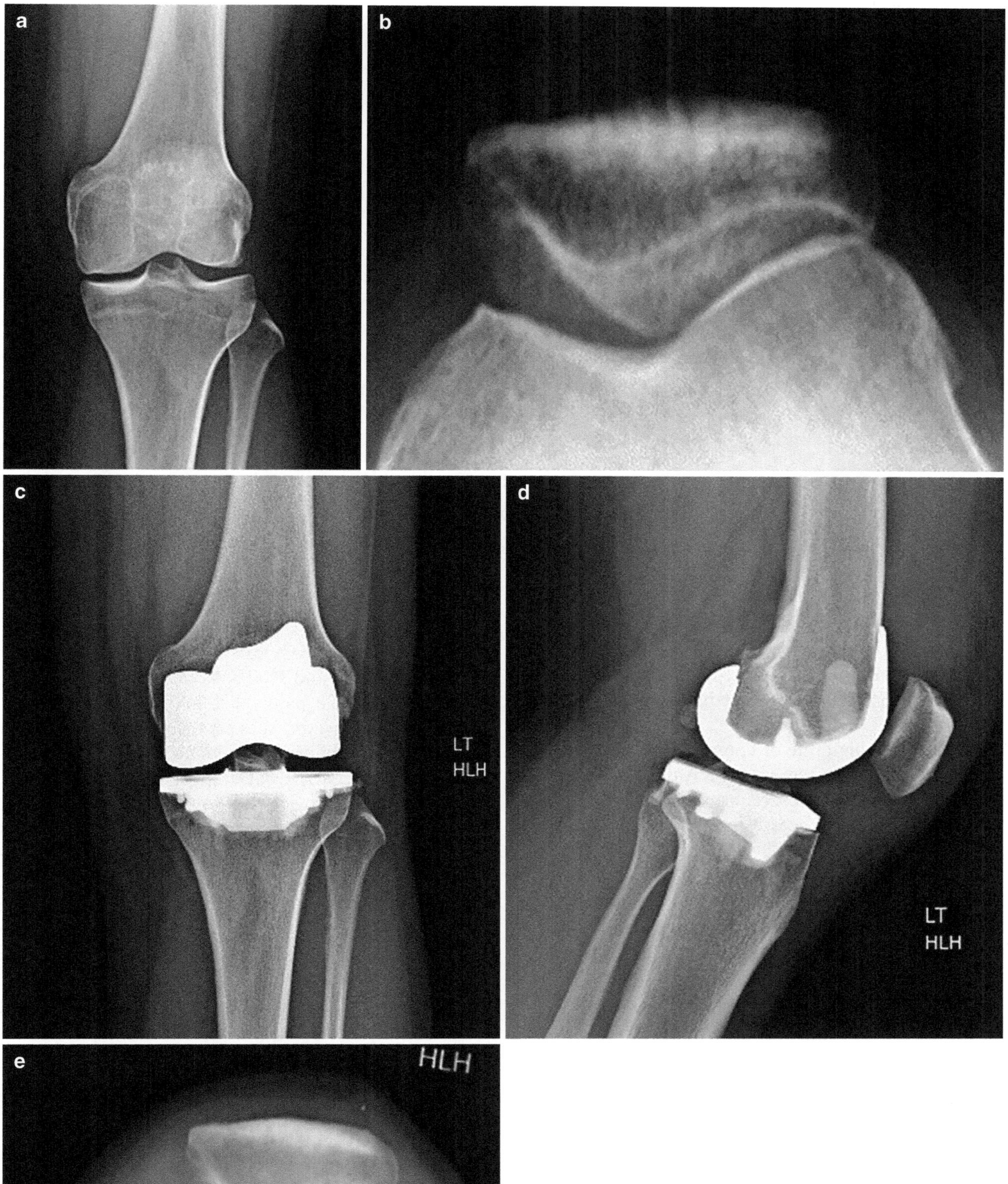

Fig. 29.4 **a** Preoperative AP radiograph demonstrates mild medial compartment joint space narrowing and minimal bony deformity. **b** Axial patellar radiograph shows mild patellofemoral arthritic changes. **c** 3 years after surgery, AP radiograph demonstrates stable position of the prosthetic components. **d** Lateral radiograph demonstrates cement penetration below the tibial keel and absence of any radiolucencies. **e** Patellar radiograph demonstrates central tracking of the unresurfaced patella

Table 29.1 Recent studies evaluating modern bicruciate-retaining TKA

Publication	Methods	Number of Patients	Results
Steihl et al. (2000)	Kinematic fluoroscopic	16 BCR, 6 CR	BCR had gradual posterior femoral rollback, CR most abnormal kinematics
Moro-oka et al. (2007)	Kinematic fluoroscopic	9 BCR, 5 CR	BCR showed greater posterior translation than CR
Kono et al. (2019)	Kinematic fluoroscopic	17 BCR	Relatively normal kinematics after BCR
Baumann et al. (2017)	Balance testing – single-leg stance with eyes closed compared to eyes open	20 BCR, 20 UKA, 20 PS	Superior balance ability after preservation of both cruciate ligaments
Pritchett (2011)	Comparative cohort study	440 bilateral TKA	89.1% preferred bicruciate TKA to PS TKA and 76.2% preferred medial pivot TKA to PS TKA
Pritchett (2015)	Retrospective review	489 BCR	89% survivorship at 23 years
Sabouret et al. (2013)	Retrospective review	163 BCR	82% survivorship at 22.4 years
Pelt et al. (2019)	Retrospective review	141 BCR	88% survivorship at 3 years
Boese et al. (2019)	Prospective multicenter study	149 BCR	Clinically significant improvements in both functional and quality of life outcomes

29

comes of 440 patients who underwent staged bilateral TKA using a different type of prosthesis on each side (Pritchett 2011). 89.1% preferred bicruciate TKA to PS TKA and 76.2% preferred medial pivot TKA to PS TKA.

A relatively high rate of complications was reported with early bicruciate-retaining TKA designs (Ries et al. 2018). However, Pritchett reported favorable long-term survivorship in 489 knees using a bicruciate-retaining, minimally constrained device (Pritchett 2015). The Kaplan–Meier survivorship was 89% at 23 years with revision for any reason as the endpoint. Sabouret et al. reported on 163 bicruciate-retaining Hermes 2C total knee replacements in 130 patients at a mean follow-up of 22.4 years (Sabouret et al. 2013). The survival rate using revision for any reason as the endpoint was 82%. However, Pelt et al. reported on 141 bicruciate-retaining TKAs with a more modern design (Pelt et al. 2019). At 3 years, survivorship was 88% which is lower than that expected for conventional CR and PS designs. Failures occurred as a result of isolated tibial loosening, anterior cruciate ligament (ACL) impingement, pain, unknown reasons, femoral and tibial loosening, ACL deficiency, and arthrofibrosis.

> More favorable early results have been reported in 156 patients (165 knees) with a newer implant design having a large keel and a more anatomically oriented joint line (Boese et al. 2019).

29.4 Discussion

Conventional CR and PS TKAs that sacrifice the ACL provide predictable pain relief and favorable implant survivorship. However, these implants have also been associated with abnormal kinematics and flexion instability (Pagnano et al. 1998; Dennis et al. 2003). Retention of the ACL can provide more normal proprioception, kinematics, and joint function. Partial knee replacements (UKA, patellofemoral replacement, and bicompartmental knee arthroplasty) can provide more favorable functional results than TKA as a result of preservation of the ACL. However, the durability and implant survivorship of partial knee replacements has generally been less favorable than TKA (Wilson et al. 2019).

Bicruciate-retaining TKAs have also demonstrated kinematics and function closer to the normal knee than after CR or PS TKA. Early patient satisfaction after bicruciate-retaining TKA has been high. However, variable implant survivorship results have been reported after bicruciate-retraining TKA. Early designs used in the 1970s and 1980s were associated with a relatively high rate of implant failure usually on the tibial side due to wear, loosening, fracture, baseplate–insert dissociation, and implant breakage (Ries et al. 2018). However, some of these designs demonstrated survivorship at 20 years of over 80%, which is similar to conventional CR and PS TKAs implanted during the same time period (Pritchett 2015; Sabouret et al. 2013).

Newer designs using modern implant materials and surgical techniques could mitigate the problems associated with early bicruciate-retaining TKA. However, results of one design with a cobalt-chrome tibial component and mechanically aligned joint line demonstrate survivorship of only 88% at 3 years, which is lower than conventional CR and PS TKA (Pelt et al. 2019). Early results with a newer design having a tibial keel and kinematically oriented joint line appear more favorable and suggest that bicruciate-retaining TKA may be a feasible option for relatively active patients with minimal deformity, an intact ACL, and good bone stock (Boese et al. 2019). However, the long-term durability and implant survivorship in comparison to currently available CR and PS TKA has not been established.

Take-Home Messages

- Retention of both cruciate ligaments is possible in TKA.
- BCR TKA can result in more normal kinematics and favorable joint function in comparison to conventional TKA.
- Early BCR TKAs used in the 1970s and 1980s were associated with a high failure rate in comparison to conventional CR or PS TKA.
- Early clinical results with a modern implant design and surgical method which emphasizes cement technique have been favorable.
- In order to optimize cement fixation of the tibial component, cancellous bone is curetted around the tibial keel. Cement is applied in a relatively liquid state to allow optimal penetration into the bone.
- Long-term durability of currently available new BCR designs has not been established.

References

Baumann F, Bahadin Ö, Krutsch W, Zellner J, Nerlich M, Angele P, Tibesku CO (2017) Proprioception after bicruciate-retaining total knee arthroplasty is comparable to unicompartmental knee arthroplasty. Knee Surg Sports Traumatol Arthrosc 25: 1697–1704

Boese K, MacDonald J, Huang W, Schwarzkopf R, Gerlinger T, Swank M, Huff T, Schinsky M, Amin N, Ast M, Ries M, Roche M, Jones J, Cooper H. Early clinical and patient-reported results of a bi-cruciate retaining total knee implant: six-month results of a prospective multicenter study of 149 primary TKAs. European Orthopaedic Research Society, October 2–5, 2019

Coventry MB, Upshaw JE, Riley LH, Finerman GA, Turner RH (1973) Geometric total knee arthroplasty.II Patient data and complications. Clin Orthop Relat Res 94:177–184

Dennis DA, Komistek RD, Mahfouz MR, Haas BD, Stiehl JB (2003) Multicenter determination of in vivo kinematics after total knee arthroplasty. Clin Orthop Relat Res 416:37–57

Gunston FH, MacKenzie RI (1976) Complications of polycentric knee arthroplasty. Clin Orthop Relat Res 120:11–17

Kono K, Inui H, Tomita T, Yamazaki T, Taketomi S, Tanaka S (2019) In vivo kinematics of bicruciate-retaining total knee arthroplasty with anatomical articular surface under high-flexion conditions. J Knee Surg. https://doi.org/10.1055/s-0039-1696959. [Epub ahead of print]

Moro-oka TA, Muenchinger M, Canciani JP, Banks SA (2007) Comparing in vivo kinematics of anterior cruciate-retaining and posterior cruciate-retaining total knee arthroplasty. Knee Surg Sports Traumatol Arthrosc 15:93–99

Noble PC, Conditt MA, Cook KF, Mathis KB (2006) Patients expectations affect satisfaction with total knee arthroplasty. Clin Orthop Relat Res 452:35–43

Pagnano MW, Hanssen AD, Lewallen DG, Stuart MJ (1998) Flexion instability after primary posterior cruciate retaining total knee arthroplasty. Clin Orthop Relat Res 356:39–46

Pelt CE, Sandifer PA, Gililland JM, Anderson MB, Peters CL (2019) Mean three-year survivorship of a new bicruciate-retaining total knee arthroplasty: are revisions still higher than expected? J Arthroplasty 34:1957–1962

Pritchett JW (2011) Patients prefer a bicruciate-retaining or the medial pivot total knee prosthesis. J Arthroplasty 26: 224–228

Pritchett JW (2015) Bicruciate-retaining total knee replacement provides satisfactory function and implant survivorship at 23 years. Clin Orthop Relat Res 473:2327–2333

Ries MD, Lenz N, Jerry G, Salehi A, Haddock S (2018) Is modern bicruciate retaining TKA feasible? Semin Arthroplasty 29:55–57

Sabouret P, Lavoie F, Cloutier JM (2013) Total knee replacement with retention of both cruciate ligaments: a 22-year follow-up study. Bone Joint J 95-B:917–922

Stiehl JB, Komistek RD, Cloutier JM, Dennis DA (2000) The cruciate ligaments in total knee arthroplasty: a kinematic analysis of 2 total knee arthroplasties. J Arthroplasty 15:545–550

Wilson HA, Middleton R, Abram SGF, Smith S, Alvand A, Jackson WF, Bottomley N, Hopewell S, Price AJ (2019) Patient relevant outcomes of unicompartmental versus total knee replacement: systematic review and meta-analysis. BMJ 364:l352

Fixed- Versus Mobile-Bearing Total Knee Arthroplasty

Daniel N. Bracey and Douglas A. Dennis

Contents

E. Hansen, K.-D. Kühn (eds.), *Essentials of Cemented Knee Arthroplasty*,
https://doi.org/10.1007/978-3-662-63113-3_30

30.1 Introduction

The first widely used mobile-bearing implant was the Oxford knee, a unicompartmental knee arthroplasty introduced in 1976 (Capella et al. 2016). Following FDA approval in 1984, the Low Contact Stress TKA (LCS, formerly the New Jersey Knee; Depuy, Warsaw, IN) was released (Hamelynck 2006). It introduced a second articulating surface under the polyethylene bearing, in contrast to fixed-bearing designs where the polyethylene bearing is locked into a metal-backed tibial tray which was designed to prevent inferior surface motion (◘ Fig. 30.1) (Post et al. 2010). Utilization of mobile-bearing TKA (MB TKA) has varied (Heckmann et al. 2019; Nguyen et al. 2015). Recent analysis from the American Joint Replacement Registry showed that mobile-bearing use was 9.4% in 2016 versus the New Zealand Joint Registry in which mobile-bearing utilization approaches 30% in the 2018 report. Mobile-bearing technology offers potential advantages over fixed-

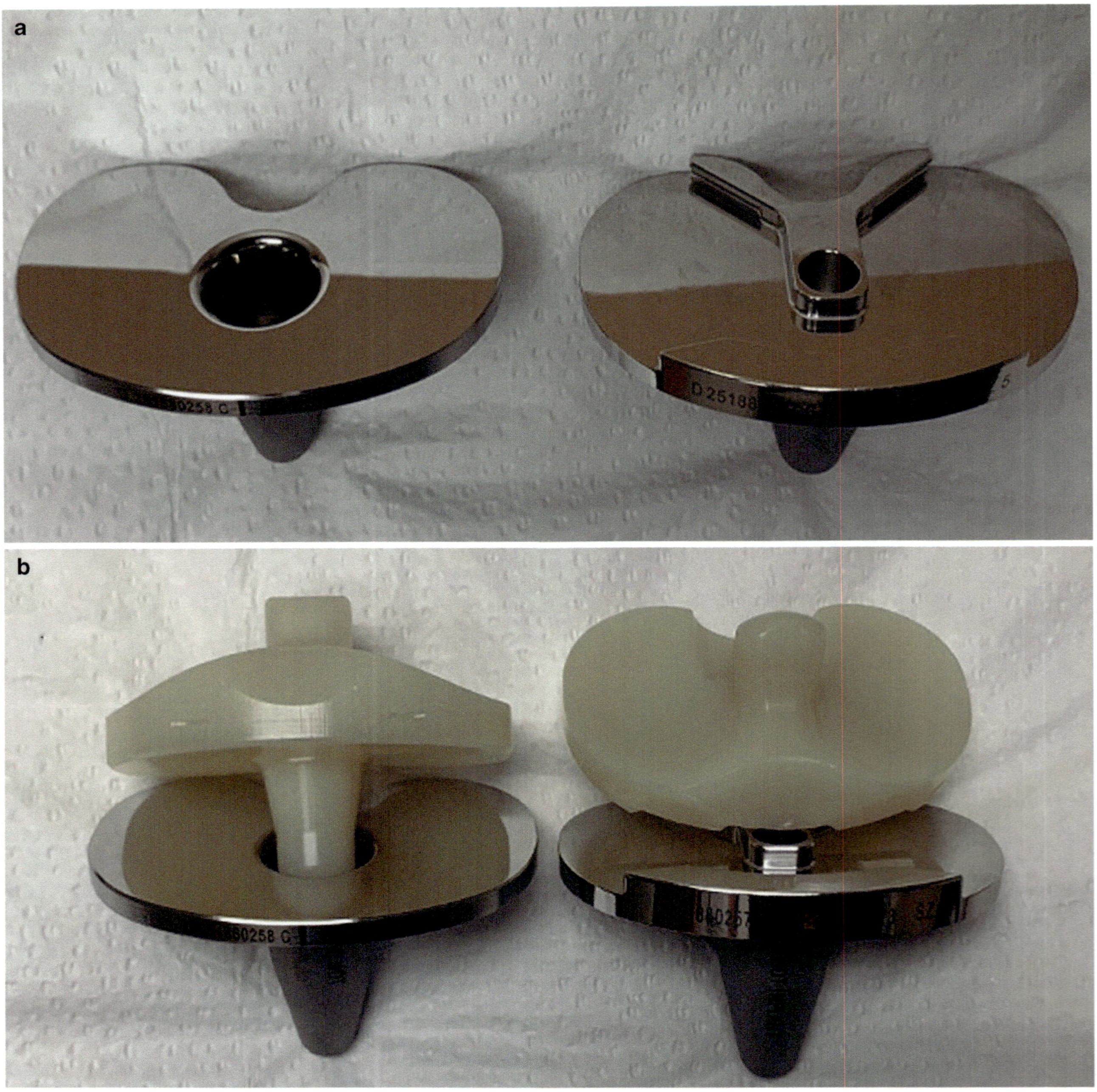

◘ **Fig. 30.1** Conventional fixed-bearing (*right*) and rotating platform TKA design (*left*). **a** The fixed-bearing tray has a locking mechanism no longer required with RP design. **b** The tray accepts the RP bearing (*left*) which rotates around a central post while the fixed-bearing tray (*right*) engages the polyethylene with its locking mechanism (Post et al. (2010), with permission from Elsevier)

bearing designs with regard to knee kinematics, implant fixation, wear, and longevity which are discussed in this chapter.

30.2 Case Example

A 62-year-old female with advanced right knee medial and patellofemoral compartment osteoarthritis failed extensive conservative treatment and is indicated for surgical intervention (Fig. 30.2). We elect to proceed with total knee arthroplasty (TKA) using a posterior stabilized, mobile-bearing design.

Extension Gap Preparation

> A thigh tourniquet is no longer used at our institution except for cementation based on our randomized trial which demonstrated that tourniquet use is associated with quadriceps strength deficits up to 3 months after TKA (Dennis et al. 2016).

Following a standard midline incision, a medial parapatellar arthrotomy is performed (Fig. 30.3a). A distal femur osteotomy is made with an intramedullary guide typically set at 4–6° valgus depending on the severity of

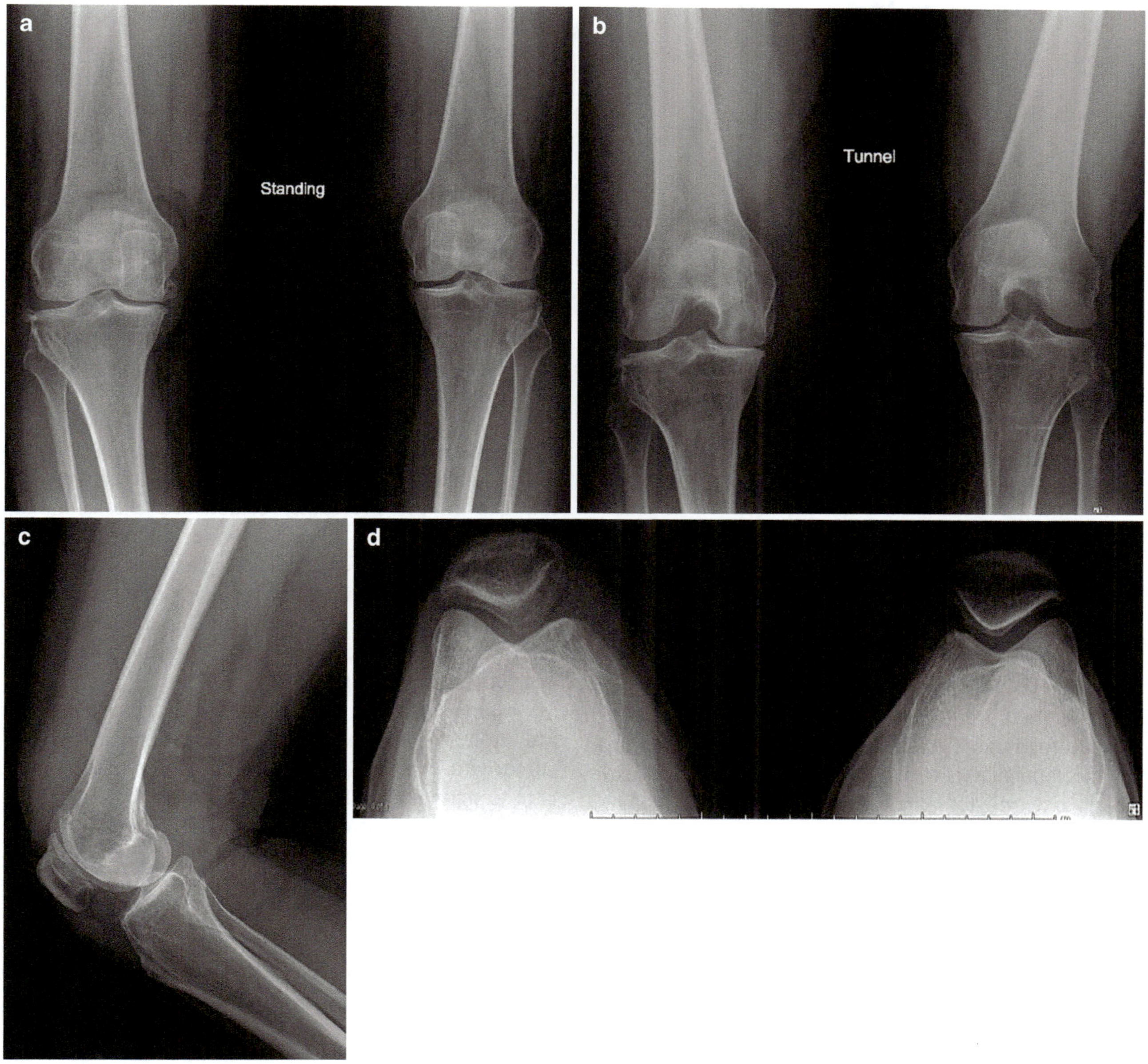

Fig. 30.2 Preoperative radiographs routinely obtained in our clinic include standing AP **a**, tunnel **b**, lateral **c**, Merchant **d**, and full-length standing **e** views. These images confirm the patient's diagnosis of degenerative osteoarthritis with the collapse of the medial and patellofemoral joint spaces, subchondral sclerosis, and medial joint line osteophyte formation

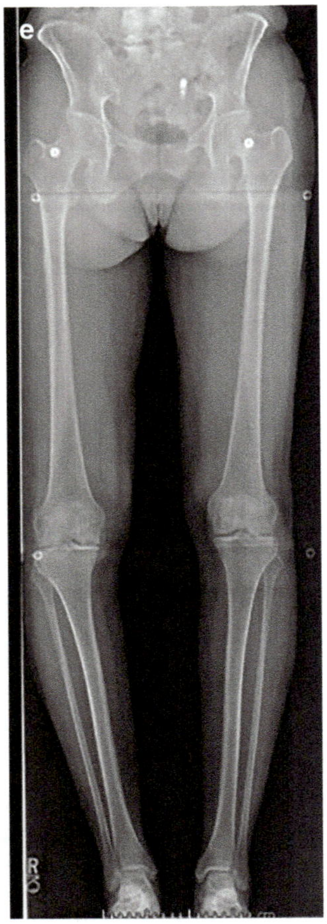

Fig. 30.2 (continued)

coronal plane deformity present and restoration of mechanical alignment.

> Distal femoral osteophytes tenting the collateral ligaments are identified (Fig. 30.3b) and removed with an osteotome (Fig. 30.3c) to initiate obtaining soft tissue balance.

The knee is then dislocated, menisci and cruciate ligaments are removed, and a tibial osteotomy is made with an extramedullary guide seeking a cut perpendicular to the mechanical axis with 0–3° of posterior slope. Medial tibial osteophytes are removed with a rongeur (Fig. 30.3d) and both the femoral and tibial components are sized at this time. As part of *an extension gap first balancing technique*, a spacer block is inserted to assess the stability of the extension gap (Fig. 30.4e). We accept 1–2 mm of balanced coronal plane laxity at this stage.

> If coronal imbalance is present, appropriate soft tissue releasing procedures are executed to ensure adequate extension gap balance.

An electrocautery cord is extended from a point two finger widths medial to the anterior superior iliac spine to the middle of the tibial plafond to assess alignment versus the mechanical axis (Fig. 30.3e).

Flexion Gap Preparation

Gap balancing is performed with the knee at 90° flexion.

The transepicondylar (TEA) and anteroposterior (AP) axes are marked, and laminar spreaders are used to equally tension the collateral ligaments (Fig. 30.4a).

> Care is taken to avoid over-tensioning the medial laminar spreader as this results in femoral component internal rotation as well as excessive medial collateral ligament tension and subsequent loss of knee flexion using the technique described.

If the tibial resection and outlined axes are accurately executed, and the primary flexion gap stabilizing structures are intact (superficial MCL medially; lateral collateral ligament and popliteus laterally), the TEA should typically parallel the tibial osteotomy and be perpendicular to the AP axis.

> To match the flexion gap to our previously defined extension gap, the extension gap block is placed on the anterior aspect of the proximal tibia, and the AP distal femoral cutting guide is positioned on top of the block (Fig. 30.4b).

This ensures the posterior femoral condylar bone resections are made at a level that matches the tensioned flexion gap to the previously established extension gap (Fig. 30.4c). The block is pinned in place, lamina spreaders are removed, and the spacer block is left in place at which time we assess the medial and lateral stability of our flexion gap to ensure it is stable and symmetrically balanced before posterior condylar resections are performed (Fig. 30.4d).

After completing all femoral cuts, trial components are implanted and examined. Patellar thickness is measured with a caliper, and an osteotomy is made taking care to maintain uniform facet thickness. The patella is sized and trialed to ensure central patellar tracking. If necessary, a lateral release is performed but in our experience, this is relatively uncommon with a rotating platform (RP) design (Yang et al. 2008).

> The lateral margin of the patellar component is traced and excess bone and osteophytes are removed with a rongeur to ensure no impingement exists between patellar bone and the femoral component (Fig. 30.4e).

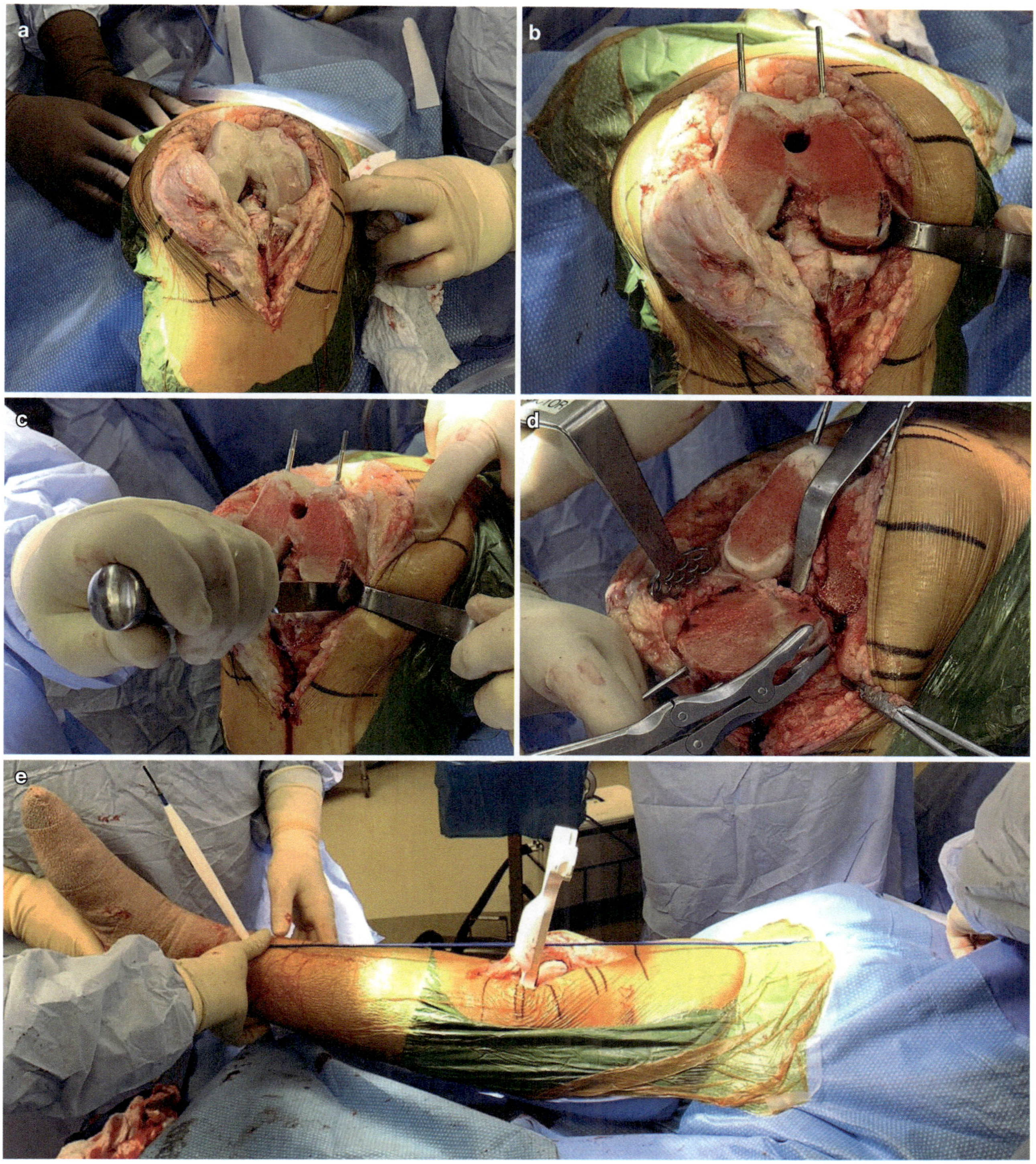

Fig. 30.3 **a–c** Intraoperative photographs demonstrating exposure and extension gap preparation. **a** Exposure is obtained using a medial parapatellar arthrotomy. **b** Medial distal femoral osteophytes which tent the medial collateral ligament (*MCL*) are outlined (*blue marking*) for removal. **c** An osteotome is used to remove osteophytes under the collateral ligament. **d** Osteophytes along the medial tibia are removed to facilitate extension gap balance. **e** Extension gap balance is first assessed with a spacer block. Mechanical alignment is roughly evaluated with a *drop line* (bovie cord)

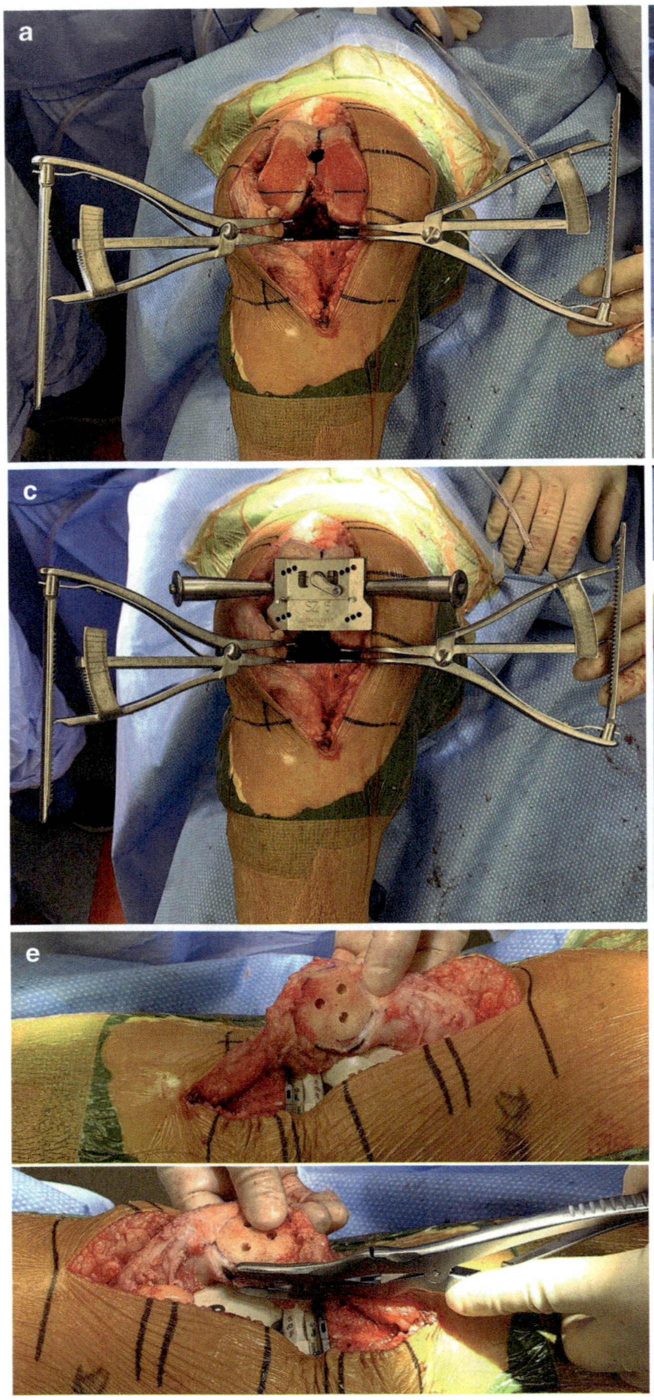

Fig. 30.4 **a–e** Intraoperative photographs demonstrating a gap balancing technique. **a** Lamina spreaders are used to tension the collateral ligaments taking care to never excessively tighten medially. The transepicondylar axis (horizontal femoral line) should be parallel to the resected tibial surface and be perpendicular to the AP axis (vertical femur line). **b** The femoral cutting block is placed on the extension gap block to set femoral component rotation. **c** The pinned cutting block should parallel the tibial osteotomy. Planned posterior femoral resection will match our flexion and extension gaps. **d** Medial and lateral flexion gap stabilities are assessed with the extension gap spacer block in place after laminar spreader removal to ensure gaps are balanced. **e** Following the patella osteotomy, the patellar button margin is traced (*blue line*) and excess lateral facet is resected to ensure there is no bony impingement on the femoral component

At this time, the limb is exsanguinated, and a pneumatic tourniquet is inflated to begin preparing bony surfaces for cementation.

- **Cementation and Component Implantation**

The sclerotic bone surfaces are penetrated multiple times with a 1.5 mm drill bit to improve cement penetration. All bone surfaces are then washed with pulsatile lavage and dried with a lap sponge (◘ Fig. 30.5a).

> Pulsatile lavage is crucial to remove intra-osseous lipid and debris which enhances cement penetration and cannot be compensated for with cement pressurization alone without pre-washing (Schlegel et al. 2014; Maistrelli et al. 1995).

We utilize a *tibial component with under-surface cement pockets* (◘ Fig. 30.5b) to improve peripheral cement penetration by reducing cement escape (Vertullo and Davey 2001).

Currently, we use a low-viscosity cement to improve implant adherence and prevent lipid penetration into the cement mantle, recognizing that conflicting data exist regarding appropriate cement viscocity (Silverman et al. 2014; Buller et al. 2020). The tibial and femoral components (◘ Fig. 30.5c) are precoated with cement. Precoating ensures a clean, dry interface between the component and cement which has been shown to improve fixation strength (Billi et al. 2019). The bone surface is similarly coated with cement knowing that precoating the tibial component alone has been shown to be insufficient for proper cement penetration (Vanlommel et al. 2011).

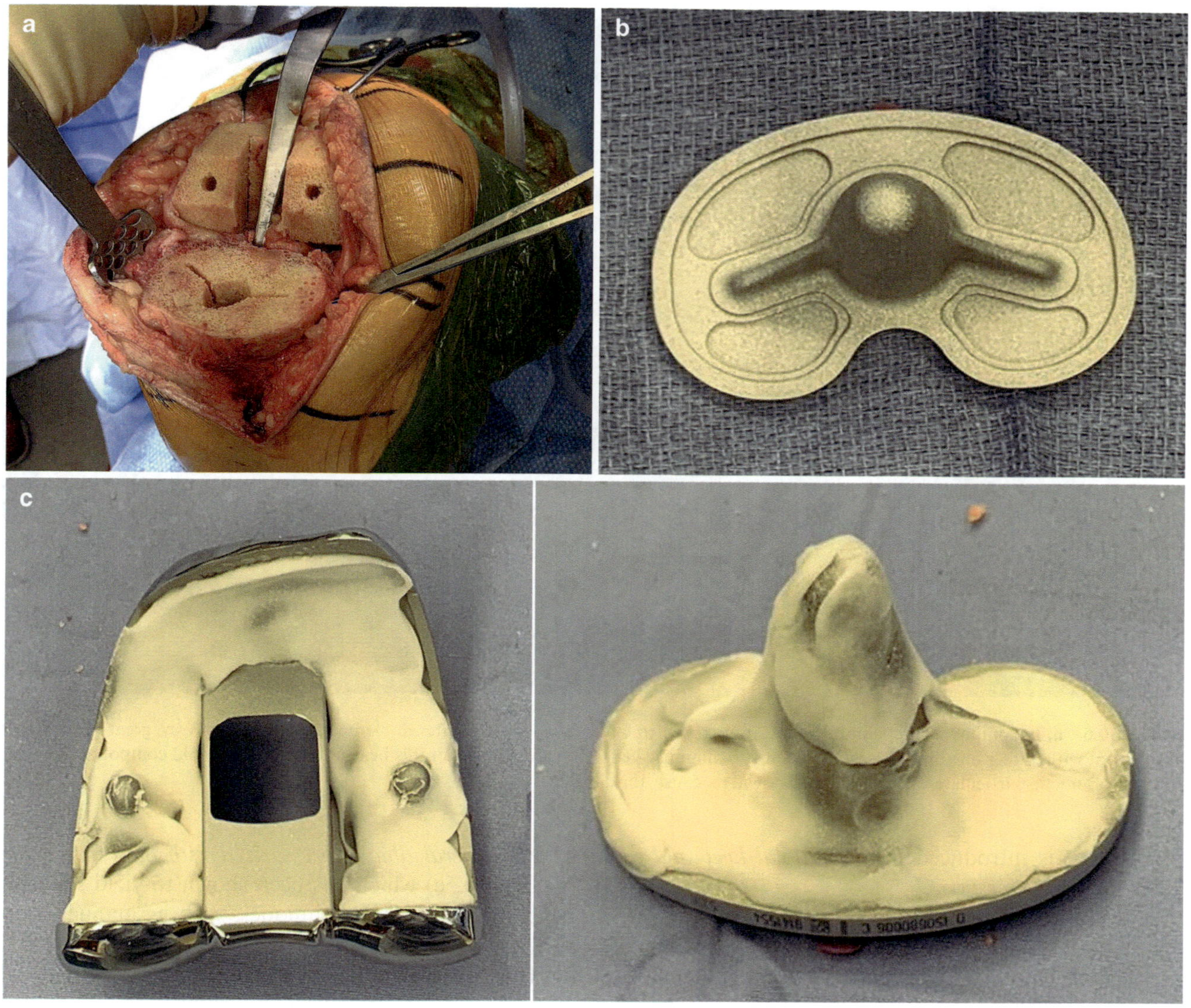

◘ **Fig. 30.5** **a–e** The bone surfaces are prepared for cementation. **a** The cancellous bone surfaces are pulse-lavaged and dried with sponges to prepare a dry surface devoid of blood/lipid contamination. **b** A tibial component with cement pockets is utilized to improve peripheral pressurization and penetration. **c** The tibial and femoral components are precoated with cement to improve fixation stress by avoiding fluid contamination at the cement–prosthesis interface. **d** Cement injected into the central keel is manually pressurized which expels lipid-rich fluid (*arrow*) which is suctioned to lessen lipid contamination of the fixation interface. **e** The cement gun is used to pressurize the peripheral bone bed

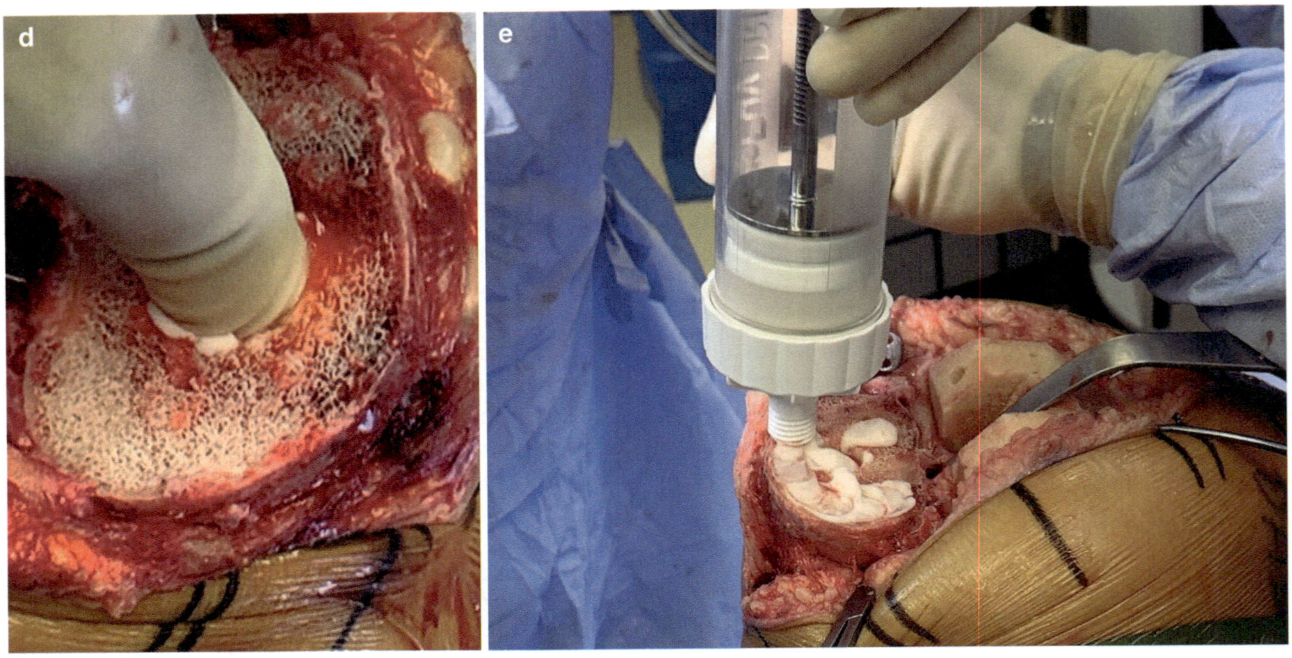

Fig. 30.5 (continued)

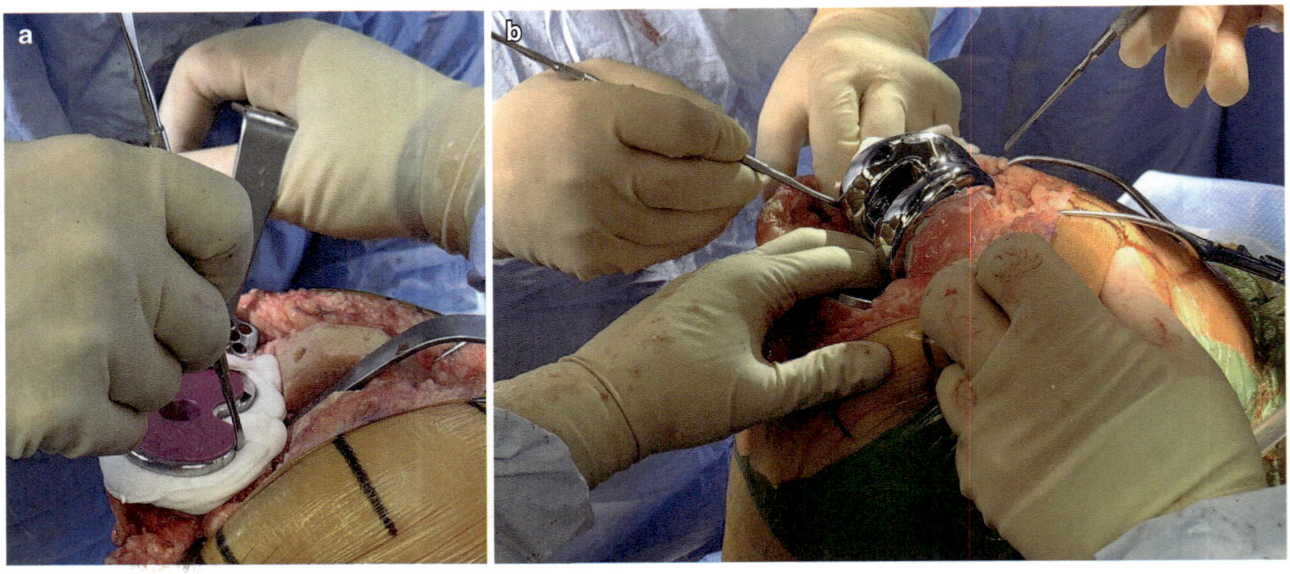

Fig. 30.6 **a, b** Component implantation. **a** Care is taken to cut the cement with a freer one time in large fragments to minimize generation of micro-particulate cement debris known to cause third body wear. **b** After implantation of the tibial tray, great care is taken to always protect this bearing surface and avoid component scratching

Cement is introduced into the *tibial keel void* and then *manually pressurized.*

> This typically expels a notable amount of lipid-rich fluid (Fig. 30.5d), which is removed with suction and lap sponges. Removing this fluid is critical to lessen lipid contamination of the cement mantle which has been associated with tibia debonding (Billi et al. 2019).

The *peripheral tibia* is *pressurized with the cement gun* (Fig. 30.5e) which has been shown to yield superior penetration to other techniques, such as manual pressurization (Lutz et al. 2009; Ritter et al. 1994).

The tibial component is now inserted with equal manual pressure followed by impaction. Extruded cement is cut at the component edge with a freer elevator and removed in large fragments (Fig. 30.6a), ideally only once.

> We avoid multiple passes with the freer and avoid scraping cement with curettes, which generates more particulate debris that could contribute to later third body wear.

We now re-dry the femoral bone surface before implanting the precoated femoral component.

> Given that the mobile-bearing surface of the tibial component is exposed at this stage, great care is taken to protect it during femoral component implantation (◘ Fig. 30.6b).

Following impaction of the femoral component and removal of the excess cement, a trial polyethylene is inserted, and the knee is brought into extension. The patella is then washed, dried and its component is cemented into place. The knee is kept in full extension until the cement is fully cured. Previous lab data has shown that component motion and final polyethylene bearing insertion during cement curation can significantly reduce fixation strength (Mason 2018).

▪ **Closure and Rehabilitation**

After the cement has cured, the knee is brought into flexion, and stability is assessed a final time before the final polyethylene insert is selected and inserted. The joint is irrigated, and then thoroughly examined to ensure all particulate debris has been evacuated. The wound is then closed in a layered fashion. Rehabilitation is initiated on the day of operation with hospital discharge typically within 24 h of admission. A supervised outpatient physical therapy program is continued for 4–6 weeks postoperatively. Postoperative radiographs are obtained at 6 weeks and every 2–3 years thereafter (◘ Fig. 30.7).

30.3 Kinematics of the Native Knee and Total Knee Arthroplasty

Native knee kinematics are driven by the geometry of the femur–tibia articulation and the soft tissue constraints provided by the surrounding ligaments, joint capsule, andmyotendinous structures. Kinematic analyses have proven that knee motion is certainly more complex than a simple hinge. The medial femoral condyle is stabilized by the relatively immobile medial meniscus and medial ligamentous structures. Subsequently, the medial femoral condyle experiences less sagittal anterior–posterior (AP) motion compared to the lateral femoral condyle which is stabilized by a relatively mobile lateral meniscus and dynamic tendinous structures. With flexion, the lateral femoral condyle translates posteriorly on the tibia ("posterior femoral rollback"), and pivots around the relatively immobile medial femoral condyle ("screw-home mechanism"). This internally rotates the tibia relative to the femur with knee flexion and externally rotates the tibia during knee extension. In vivo fluoroscopic analyses of native human knees undergoing deep knee bend maneuver (DKB; 0° to 120°) have shown 14.1–21.07 mm of posterior translation of the lateral condyle, in contrast to 1.5–1.94 mm of posterior translation medially (◘ Fig. 30.8) (Mahfouz et al. 2004; Komistek et al. 2003). During this same range of motion, the tibia internally rotates 16.8–23.67° (Mahfouz et al. 2004; Komistek et al. 2003).

> Native knee kinematics are difficult to reproduce after TKA and multiple kinematic variances from normal knee kinematics have been observed such as paradoxical anterior femoral translation, reverse axial rotation, decreased posterior femoral rollback, and femoral condylar liftoff (Dennis et al. 1998a, 2003a).

Posterior-stabilized (PS) TKA components rely on cam–post engagement during knee flexion to reproduce posterior femoral translation on the tibia and typically provide a greater amount of rollback when compared to cruciate-retaining (CR) TKA designs in deep knee flexion (Dennis et al. 2003a). Posterior femoral translation is desirable because it minimizes impingement between the posterior femur and tibia and improves knee flexion (Dennis et al. 1998b). Paradoxical anterior translation of the femur has been reported with less constrained designs, such as the CR TKA, and increases shear forces across the polyethylene surface, accelerates polyethylene wear, and weakens the moment arm of the quadriceps tendon (Banks et al. 2003; Stiehl et al. 1999; Dennis et al. 2003b; Greenwald and Heim 2005; Blunn et al. 1991). Reverse axial rotation lateralizes the tibial tubercle, and increases the Q-angle in deep flexion, which leads to patellar maltracking, risk of patella subluxation, and decreased knee flexion as posterior femoral rollback is reduced (Dennis et al. 2004).

TKA component design has evolved to mitigate these undesirable kinematic patterns. Congruity of the articulation between the femur and polyethylene as well as the amount of constraint provided by components have been utilized to balance the forces transmitted through the TKA components and implant–host fixation interfaces against the forces experienced by the surrounding soft tissue stabilizers. While implant constraint and congruity afford greater stability to the TKA articulation, they also transfer forces previously shared by the

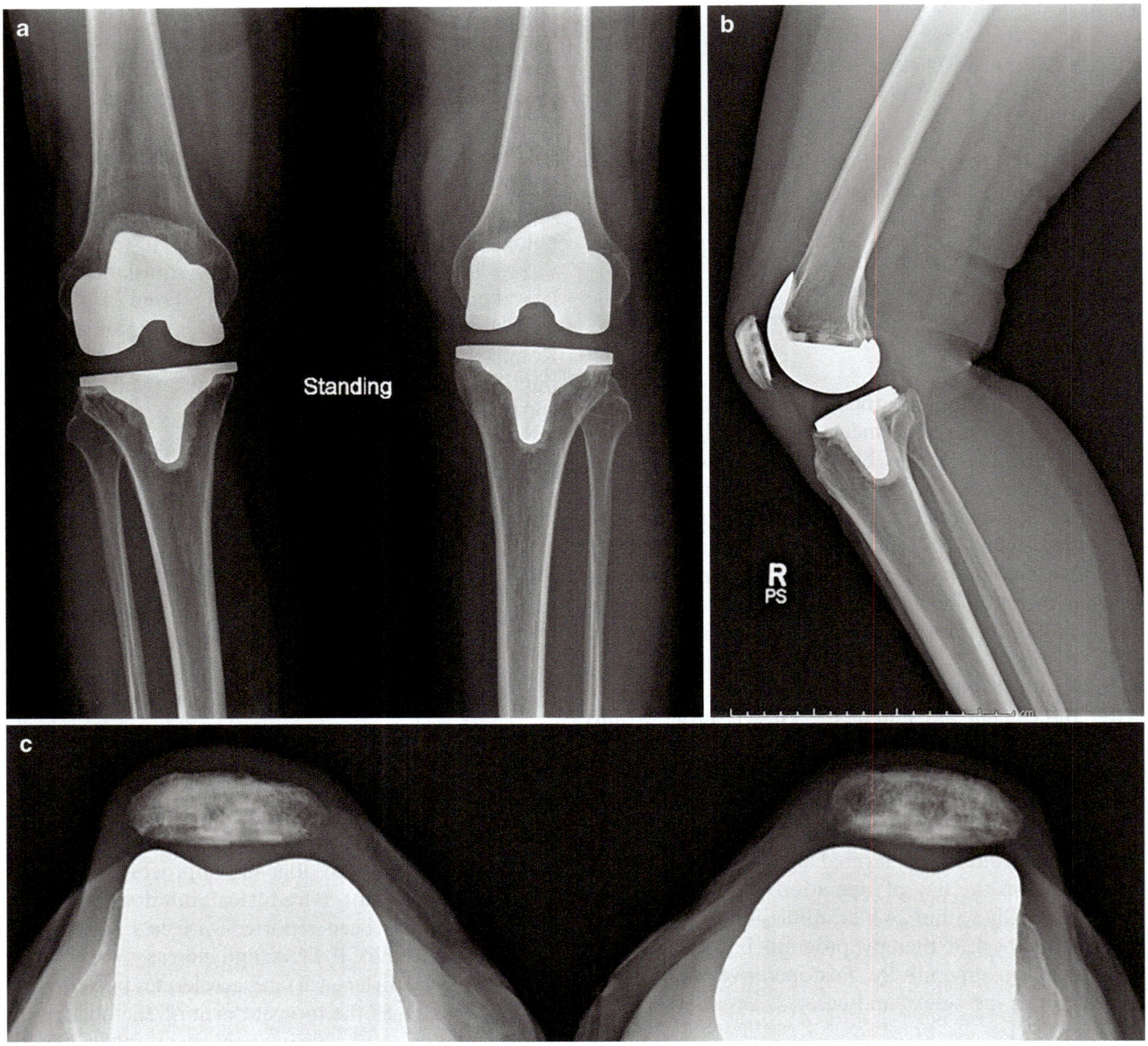

Fig. 30.7 a–c Radiographs obtained at 5 years postoperatively. AP **a**, lateral **b**, and Merchant **c** views are obtained which demonstrate excellent cement mantle around the tibial and femoral components with a symmetric depth of penetration. The patellar resection yielded symmetric thickness along the superior and inferior poles with a component centered in the trochlear groove

surrounding soft tissue structures to the implant–bone interface, which ultimately puts these components at risk for aseptic loosening (D'Lima et al. 2001; Bartel et al. 1986). TKA components with less constraint offload forces seen at the bone–implant interface, but these round-on-flat or flat-on-flat articulation designs have lower contact areas which increase polyethylene contact pressure and accelerate wear leading to premature TKA failure (Stiehl et al. 1999; Sharkey et al. 2002; Lonner et al. 1999). Increasing component contact area by increasing congruity in the coronal and sagittal planes can reduce contact pressures and polyethylene wear. A contact area of 300–350 mm^2 dramatically reduces contact stresses (Greenwald and Heim 2005). With knee flexion, the contact area moves posterior with femoral translation and tibial axial rotation, which reduces the contact area and increases stresses (Sharma et al. 2007).

> Mobile-bearing designs increase the contact area relative to fixed-bearing designs, which effectively reduces contact stresses, polyethylene wear, and aseptic loosening rates (Jones et al. 1999; Ranawat et al. 2004; Walker et al. 2002).

Contact area may exceed 800 mm^2 with mobile-bearing designs, compared to fixed-bearing designs which fail to exceed 300 mm^2 (Fig. 30.9) (Greenwald and Heim 2005).

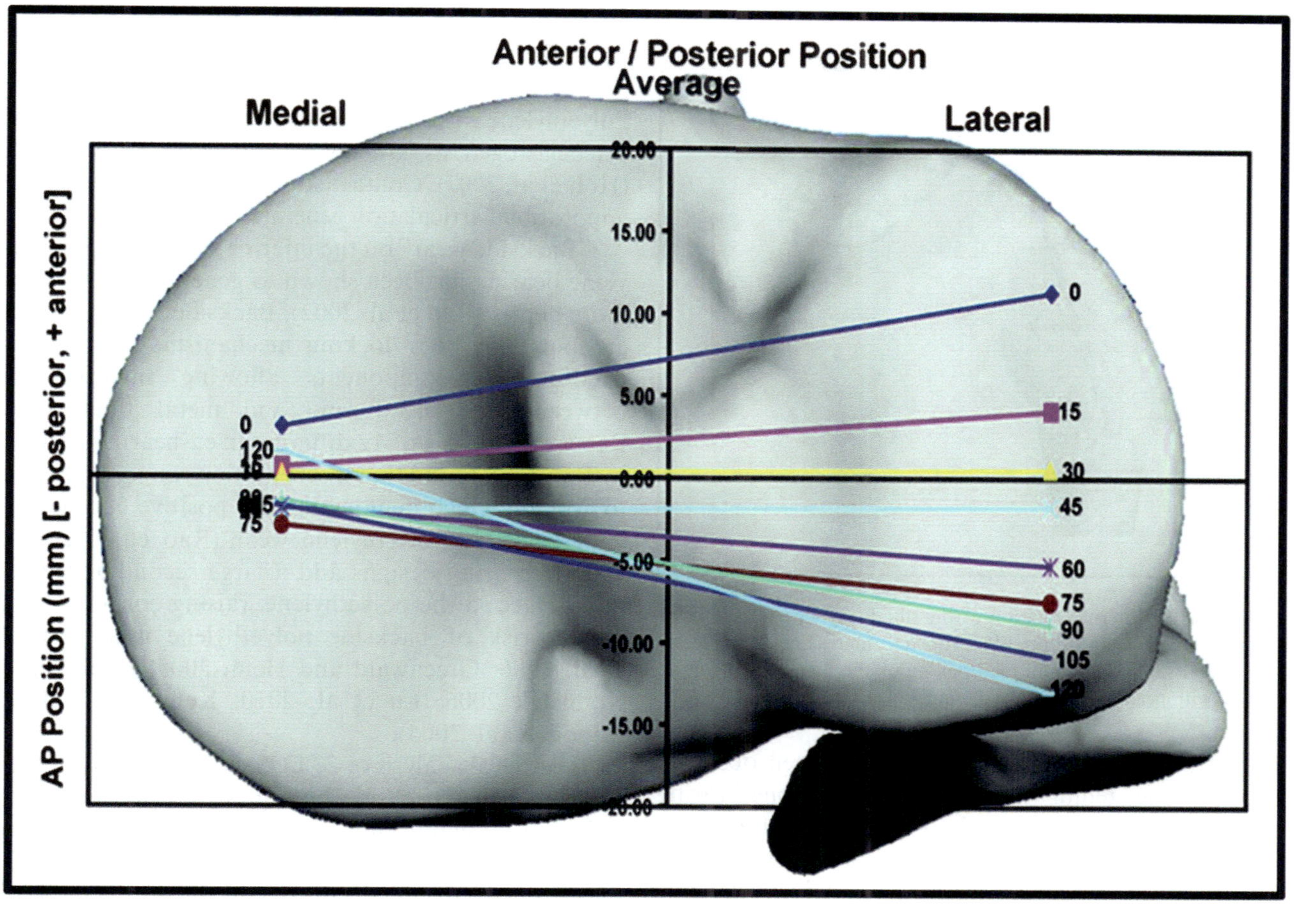

■ Fig. 30.8 Posterior femoral rollback of the lateral femoral condyle on the tibial plateau during various degrees of knee flexion exceeds that of the relatively immobile medial femoral condyle (Mahfouz et al. (2004), with permission from Wolters Kluwer Health, Inc.)

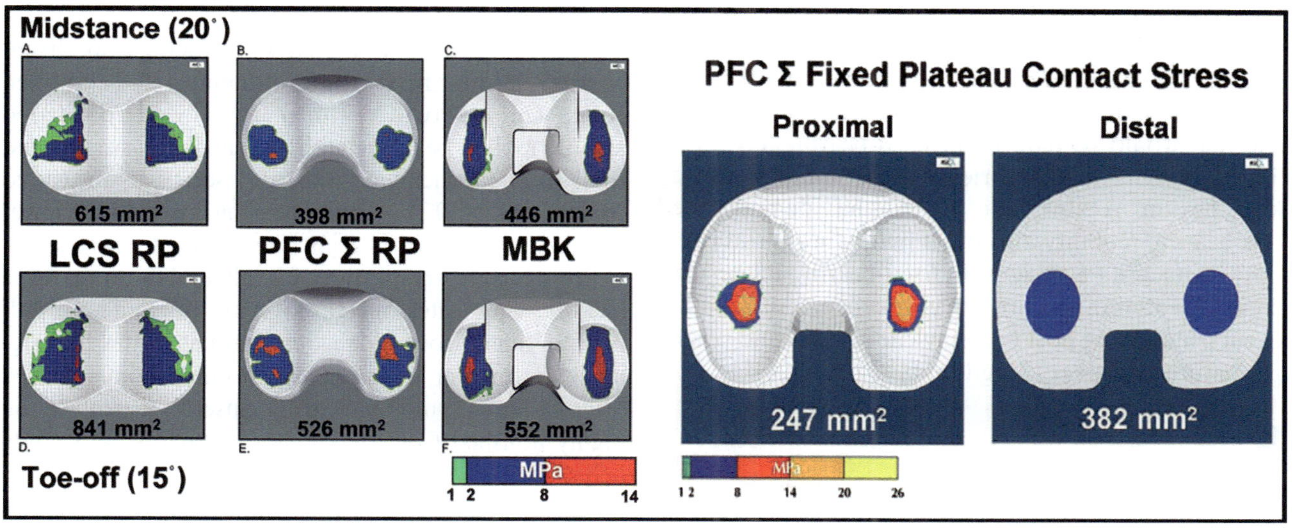

■ Fig. 30.9 Contact areas seen in mobile rotating platform (RP) designs exceed those seen with fixed-bearing (FB) designs which effectively reduces the contact pressures seen on the polyethylene surface (Greenwald and Heim (2005), courtesy of the U.S. National Library of Medicine)

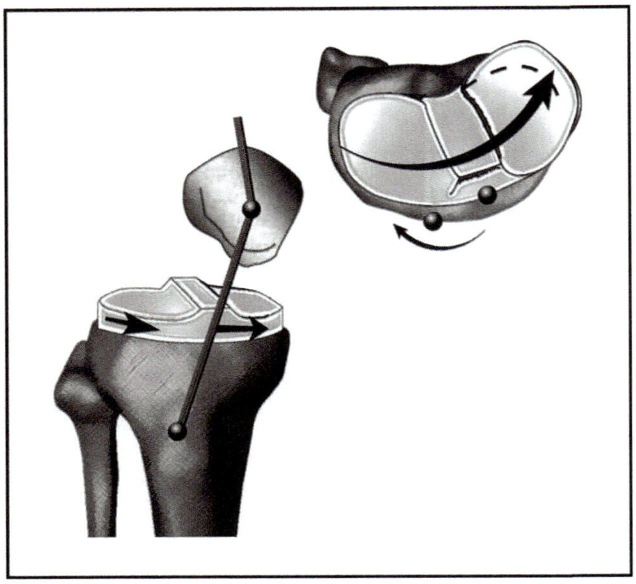

Fig. 30.10 Internal rotation of the tibial tray with a fixed-bearing design will lateralize the tibial tubercle, increasing Q-angle and risk lateral subluxation and maltracking of the patella (Yang et al. (2008), with permission from Wolters Kluwer Health, Inc.)

Larger amounts of axial rotation have been observed between the femur and tibia with mobile-bearing designs. A fluoroscopic study of patients performing a DKB after TKA showed that mean axial rotation was 4.1° for a fixed-bearing prosthesis and 7.3° for patients with a mobile-bearing prosthesis (Ranawat et al. 2004). Numerous studies have shown that the majority of this rotation with mobile-bearing designs occurs between the polyethylene under-surface and the highly polished tibial tray as the polyethylene "follows" the femur (Dennis et al. 2004, 2005; D'Lima et al. 2001; Komistek et al. 2004). Axial rotation of the bearing maintains congruity and contact area between the femur and polyethylene that would be reduced in fixed-bearing TKA (FB TKA) designs that experience axial rotation during knee flexion. A kinematic analysis has demonstrated this bearing mobility also helps maintain central cam–post-contact in PS designs. In fixed-bearing PS designs, if axial rotation occurs, eccentric cam–post-contact occurs, increasing post polyethylene stresses and risk of premature post wear (Zingde et al. 2014).

Bearing design also affects patellar kinematics.

In FBTKA, tibial tray rotation relative to the tibial tubercle will alter the Q-angle and patellar tracking. If the tray is internally rotated, the tubercle is lateralized, which disrupts patellar tracking and risks lateral subluxation (Fig. 30.10) (Yang et al. 2008). Regardless of tibial tray rotation, MB TKAs allow the tubercle to self-correct to the appropriate rotation when dynamically loaded.

30.4 Fears Associated with Mobile-Bearing TKA

Polyethylene wear debris leads to macrophage-activated osteoclastogenesis, osteolysis, and early TKA failure (Holt et al. 2007). Contact stress and shear forces at the femorotibial articulation generate wear debris.

"Backside wear" on the inferior surface of polyethylene bearing has been shown to generate 2–100 times more debris (Rao et al. 2002). Backside wear has been attributed to poor locking mechanisms in modular fixed-bearing components allowing micromotion between the polyethylene and metal tibial tray. Retrieval analysis of 12 different fixed-bearing designs by Rao et al. found that insert motion ranged from 104 to 760 μm which demonstrated a positive correlation with backside polyethylene wear (Rao et al. 2002). Mobile-bearing designs add a large second articulating surface to the polyethylene, raising concerns of a greater risk of backside polyethylene wear (Bartel et al. 1986; Greenwald and Heim 2005; Dennis and Komistek 2006; Lu et al. 2010; Kelly et al. 2011; Minoda et al. 2004).

A retrieval analysis of 23 LCS mobile-bearing inserts confirmed that backside pitting, scratching, and burnishing were significantly greater than that observed on the 31 fixed-bearing inserts retrieved (Engh et al. 2009). The authors attributed pitting and scratching to third body debris, but the scratching was specific to implant design given it was concentric and aligned with rotational movement of the polyethylene. Interestingly, linear wear rates were similar for fixed-bearing and mobile-bearing designs.

In a separate retrieval analysis by Berry et al., fixed-bearing inserts from rough titanium and polished cobalt–chrome (CoCr) tibial trays were compared against mobile bearings with polished CoCr trays, and total through-thickness wear of inserts was measured (Berry et al. 2012). Mobile-bearing inserts had lower wear rates than fixed-bearing inserts and mobile-bearing wear rates were irrespective of implanted duration while fixed-bearing rates increased with time. The fixed-bearing liners from rough titanium baseplates had significantly greater wear rates than liners from polished trays. Because mobile-bearing inserts articulate on highly polished CoCr baseplates, data from this study helps explain the bearing surface's contribution to reduced wear rates. Knee simulator studies presented by McEwen et al. compared mobile-bearing and fixed-bearing designs and found a three- to four-fold reduction in wear per millions of cycles with mobile-bearing designs (McEwen et al. 2001, 2005). More recently, Delport et al. presented comparative TKA simulator data that also showed four-fold reductions in wear rates with mobile-bearing designs (Delport et al. 2010).

Atwood et al. reported on 100 retrieved LCS mobile-bearing components after >2 years and calculated volumetric wear rates at 54 mm^3/year (Atwood et al. 2008). Wear rates decreased with time and the damaged appearance did not correlate with actual wear (loss of material). This volumetric wear rate is lower than the 120 mm^3/year rates reported with fixed-bearing designs (Atwood et al. 2008).

> Despite the theoretical concerns presented, backside polyethylene wear has not emerged as a clinically relevant concern with MB TKA designs.

Osteolysis has also been proposed as a risk associated with the use of mobile-bearing technology. Studies have again cited increased polyethylene wear rates with mobile-bearing designs contributing to the greater risk of osteolysis (Greenwald and Heim 2005; Kim et al. 2010). Polyethylene wear particle size and biologic reactivity present different risks of developing osteolytic pathology (Utzschneider et al. 2009; Fisher et al. 2004). Minoda et al. aspirated fluid from both mobile-bearing and FB TKAs and found no difference in polyethylene wear particle size (Minoda et al. 2004). In a follow-up report, the same authors followed patients who underwent bilateral TKAs using both mobile-bearing and fixed-bearing designs and aspirated their knees 3.5 years after surgery (Minoda et al. 2017). They found no difference in polyethylene wear particle size, shape, or number. Knee simulator data has supported these in vivo studies and shown no difference in wear debris characterization (Fisher et al. 2004, 2006). Clinical outcome studies have found no difference in the rates of osteolysis with fixed- or mobile-bearing designs. Kim et al. published 10-year outcomes on 444 patients who underwent simultaneous bilateral TKA using mobile-bearing and fixed-bearing in the same patient and found no difference in radiographic rates of osteolysis (Kim et al. 2014).

> With the advent of highly cross-linked polyethylene and improved sterilization techniques, the rates of polyethylene wear and osteolysis continue to decline with both FB and MB TKA designs.

A concern unique to mobile-bearing design is the risk of the polyethylene bearing dislocation or "spin-out." This has typically been reported in deep knee flexion where the bearing rotates 90° around its central axis, with the posterolateral lip of the polyethylene slipping posterior behind the lateral femoral condyle (◘ Fig. 30.11). This is typically caused by a mismatch between the flexion and extension gaps and is usually reduced in a closed fashion although revision may be required in cases of substantial gap inequality. Use of gap balancing techniques with attention to ligament-balancing has greatly reduced the incidence of spin-out (Ulivi et al. 2015). Diamond et al. highlighted the association between ligament-balancing and mobile-bearing spin-out in their review of 8373 consecutive primary MBTKAs (Diamond et al. 2018). The incidence of spin-out was low (0.58%) but after adopting a gap balancing technique, the incidence was reduced to 0.2% ($p < 0.01$). Chiavetta et al. reported a series of 426 MBTKAs using a gap balancing technique where there were no reported cases of bearing spin-out (Chiavetta et al. 2006). Consistent with these results, the senior author has yet to experience a bearing dislocation following a primary TKA using a gap balancing method in a 20-year experience with MBTKA.

30.5 Benefits of a Mobile-Bearing Design

> MB TKA balances implant conformity, constraint, and contact area without significantly increasing stresses seen at the polyethylene bearing or bone–implant fixation interface.

Bearing mobility allows increased implant conformity and constraint in both the sagittal and coronal planes without dramatically increasing fixation stresses (Jones et al. 1999). By increasing sagittal plane conformity in MBTKA, in vivo fluoroscopic analyses have demonstrated improved control of anteroposterior translation with reduced paradoxical anterior femoral translation, particularly when tested during gait (Dennis et al. 2003a). The increased coronal plane conformity typically present in MBTKAs increases the contact area and lessens the increased contact stresses which are present if femoral condylar liftoff occurs (Dennis and Komistek 2006).Compared to fixed-bearing designs, mobile-bearing designs maintain greater contact area throughout knee flexion as the bearing rotates on the tibial tray and follows the femur, maintaining ideal congruency in both the sagittal and coronal planes in addition to optimizing cam–post mechanics (◘ Fig. 30.11).

Puloski et al. performed a retrieval analysis of FB PS TKA polyethylene bearings showing that 40% of the post-surface area was worn or deformed at the time of retrieval, drawing attention to this as a potential source of polyethylene wear and implant failure (Puloski et al. 2001). Nakayama et al. measured cam–post-contact area and stress in four different TKA designs and found cam–post-contact stress increased significantly with internal rotation of the tibial tray because contact area decreased and the posterolateral edge of the post impinged on the medial edge of the lateral femoral condyle (◘ Fig. 30.12) (Nakayama et al. 2005). Peak con-

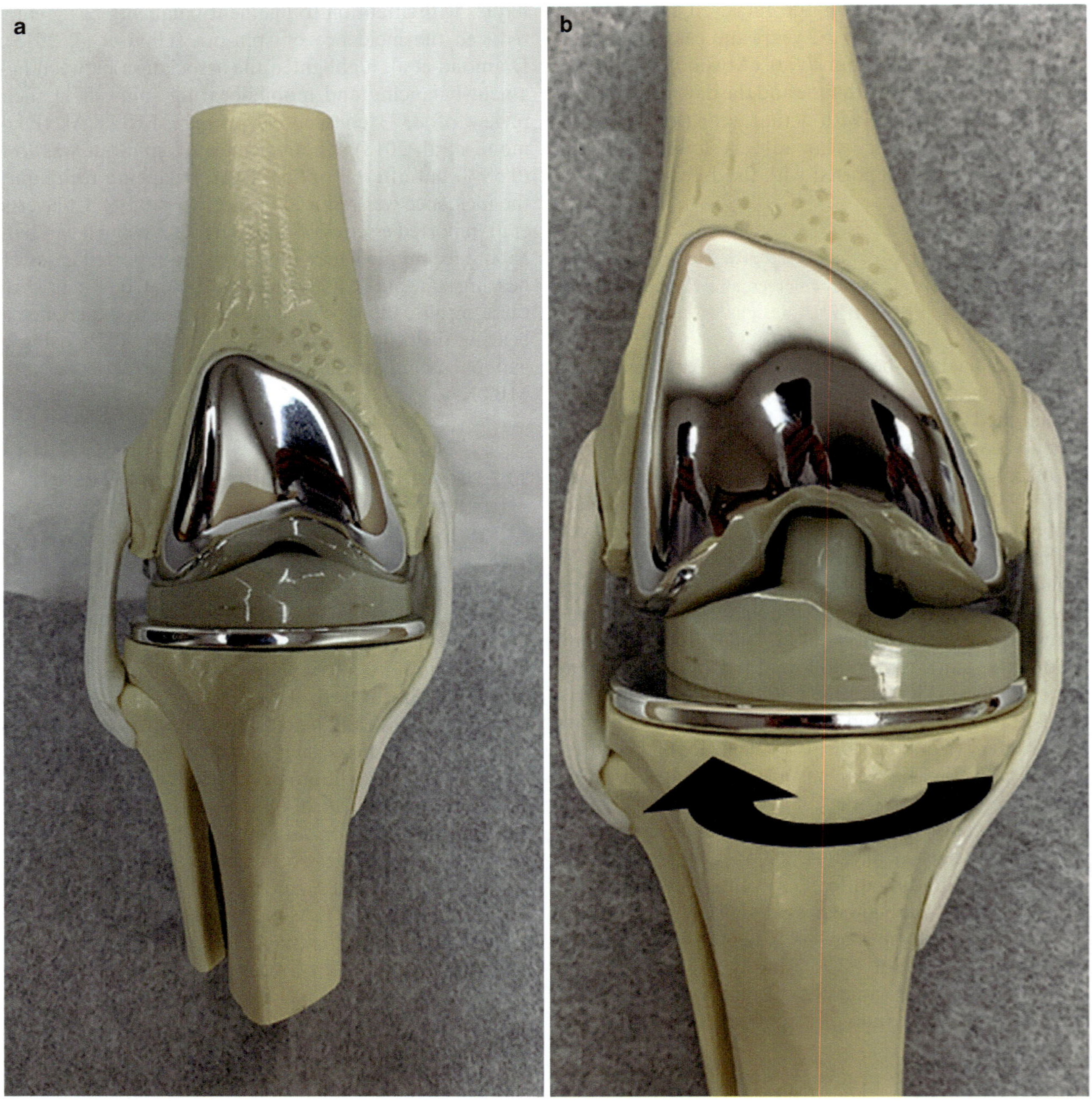

Fig. 30.11 **a, b** Rotating platform bearing "spin-out." **a** The RP bearing maintains articular congruity with the femoral component. **b** A RP knee can experience bearing dislocation or "spin-out" with axial rotation during knee flexion, most commonly where the posterolateral aspect of the polyethylene goes posterior to the lateral femoral condyle

tact stresses were not increased with internal rotation of the one mobile-bearing design tested (NexGen LPS Flex Mobile TKA; Zimmer Biomet, Warsaw, IN) suggesting that mobile bearings are protective against this cam–post wear pattern. Zingde et al. studied cam–post mechanics by performing an in vivo fluoroscopic analysis of fixed-bearing and MBPS TKA (Zingde et al. 2014). The authors found that cam–post engagement was located more centrally in rotating platform designs versus more eccentric cam–post contact in fixed-bearing designs (Fig. 30.13).

Self-alignment of the polyethylene bearing with the femoral component reduces cross shear stresses on the bearing by decoupling the multidirectional motion patterns (rotational, translational, and flexion–extension) present in FB TKA to unidirectional motion in MB TKA which occurs at two different interfaces (flexion–extension on the superior aspect of the bearing and rota-

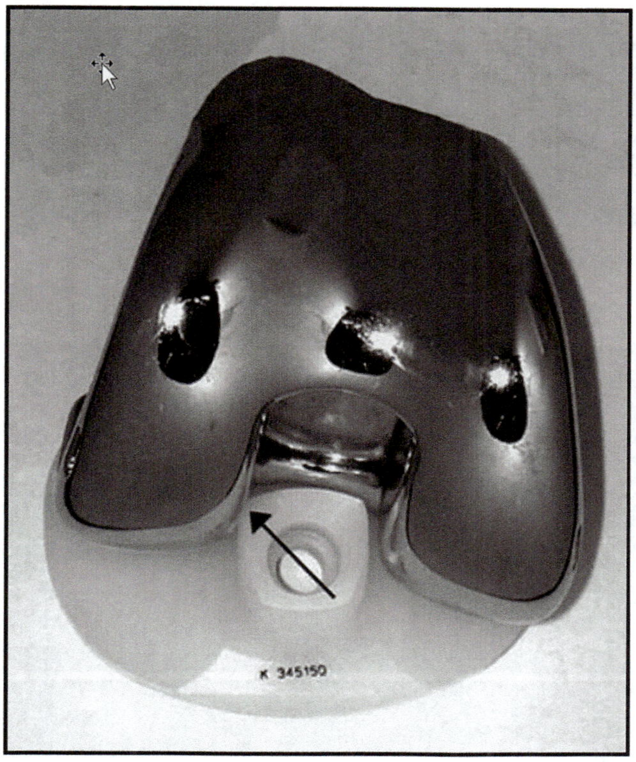

Fig. 30.12 Internal rotation of the tibial tray alters the cam–post-contact area, effectively decreasing contact area which was found to significantly increase contact stresses. Additionally, this leads to post impingement (*arrow*), accelerated wear, and risk of failure (From Nakayama et al. (2005). © The British Editorial Society of Bone and Joint Surgery, with permission)

tion occurring on the inferior surface). Multidirectional motion increases shear forces and accelerates wear as compared with unidirectional motion (Jones et al. 1999; Bragdon et al. 1996). More specifically, simulator data has shown polyethylene to have a lower coefficient of friction when loaded with unidirectional motion which results in lower wear rates (Pooley and Tabor 1972; Abdelgaied et al. 2013). This likely explains why mobile-bearing inserts have been shown to have equivalent or lower wear rates compared to fixed-bearing inserts despite having an additional bearing surface (Jones et al. 1999; Lu et al. 2010; Engh et al. 2009; McEwen et al. 2001, 2005; Delport et al. 2010; Fisher et al. 2004, 2006, 2010; Bragdon et al. 1996).

> The uncoupling of rotational strain transmission from the implant to fixation interface has been shown to lessen fixation stresses.

Bottlang et al. compared strains transmitted to the proximal tibia in cadavers implanted with fixed and MB TKA designs and found 33% less compressive strain and 68–73% less torsional strain with MB TKA (Bottlang et al. 2006). Malinzak et al. compared the mechanical response of the tibia to femoral component rotation in composite tibia specimens implanted with primary and revision fixed-bearing or mobile-bearing components in an effort to study the relationship between constraint and force transmission to proximal tibia (Malinzak et al. 2014). Using digital image correlation mapping, the authors found that fixed-bearing designs exerted 13.8x greater torque and 69% greater cortical strain on the proximal tibia than RP designs (Fig. 30.14).

Reducing stress at the fixation interface should lower the risk of fixation failure and component loosening. Despite these theoretical advantages with mobile-bearing design, registry data has not proven mobile-bearing design to have lower aseptic loosening rates compared to fixed-bearing design in primary TKA (Gothesen et al. 2017). Differences in bearing design may be more relevant in settings that require the use of highly constrained constructs, such as revision TKA where significant bone loss may be encountered in addition to disrupted ligaments or unbalanced soft tissues.

Increasing constraint helps address ligament imbalance at the price of increasing stress on component fixation to bone that may already be compromised from osteolysis or implant removal in the revision setting (Mow and Wiedel 1998; Peters et al. 1997; Rand 1991). Failure after revision TKA is most frequently caused by infection, but aseptic loosening is commonly cited as the second most common mode of failure, accounting for 4.9–42% of failures (Rosso et al. 2019; Suarez et al. 2008; Siqueira et al. 2014; Mortazavi et al. 2011; Agarwal et al. 2019). A mobile-bearing interface can decrease implant fixation stress and reduce the risk of aseptic loosening after revision TKA.

We previously reported our own midterm clinical and radiographic results of 280 revision TKAs performed with a mobile-bearing revision TKA system (Kim et al. 2017). At a mean follow-up duration of 59.9 months, 4 cases failed due to aseptic loosening (1.4%). More recently, Reina et al. reported on 367 revision TKAs with a mean 4-year follow-up duration using a varus–valgus constrained implant (Sigma TC3 Rotating-Platform) (Reina et al. 2019). The incidence of failure due to aseptic loosening was 3%. The same institution also published long-term results after revision TKA with rotating-hinge prostheses, an implant design that has historically, resulted in high failure rates in fixed-bearing hinge designs secondary to aseptic loosening (Cottino et al. 2017). Cumulative incidence of revision for aseptic loosening at 10 years was surprisingly low at 4.5%.

> The authors attributed this low incidence largely to the mobile-bearing design reducing fixation interface stress but also to the benefits of enhanced metaphyseal fixation associated with the use of metaphyseal sleeves.

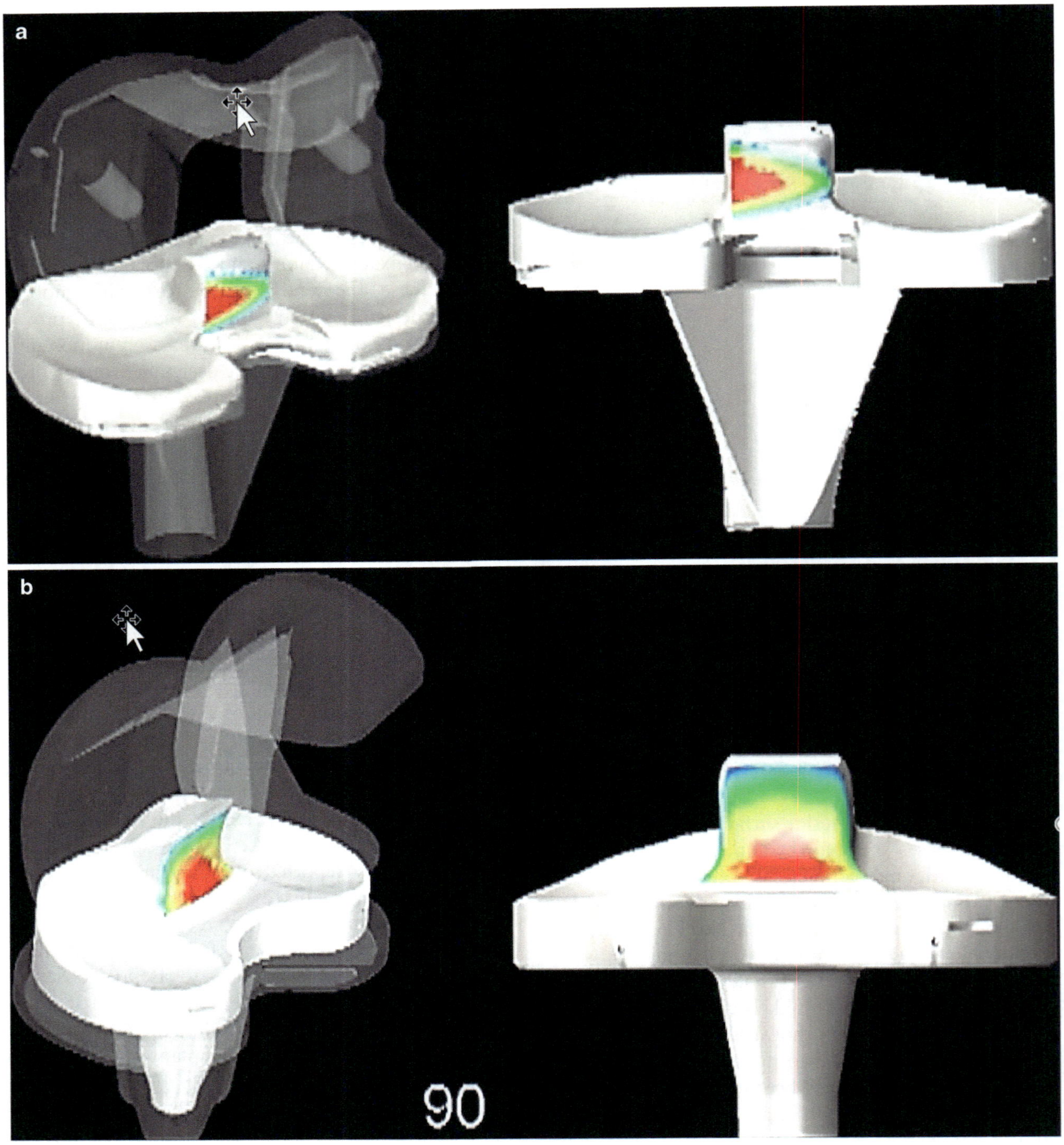

Fig. 30.13 In vivo kinematic study of cam–post engagement patterns with fixed-bearing **a** and mobile-bearing **b** PS TKA designs identified where the cam engages on the posterior aspect of the polyethylene post. Axial rotation of the rotating platform polyethylene bearing keeps the cam and post nearly parallel throughout range of motion to allow more central engagement on the post, while fixed-bearing knees engaged the medial aspect of the post. (Zingde et al. 2014; Greenwald and Heim 2005, with permission from Wolters Kluwer Health, Inc.)

Patellar tracking is also improved in MB TKA as axial rotation of the polyethylene helps centralize the extensor mechanism. With FB TKA, any internal rotation of the tibial tray will lateralize the tubercle and extensor mechanism which can lead to maltracking or even lateral subluxation of the patella (Fig. 30.10) (Yang et al. 2008).

RP designs can accommodate mismatches in rotation of the tibial tray through self-alignment of the bearing. At our institution, we retrospectively reviewed

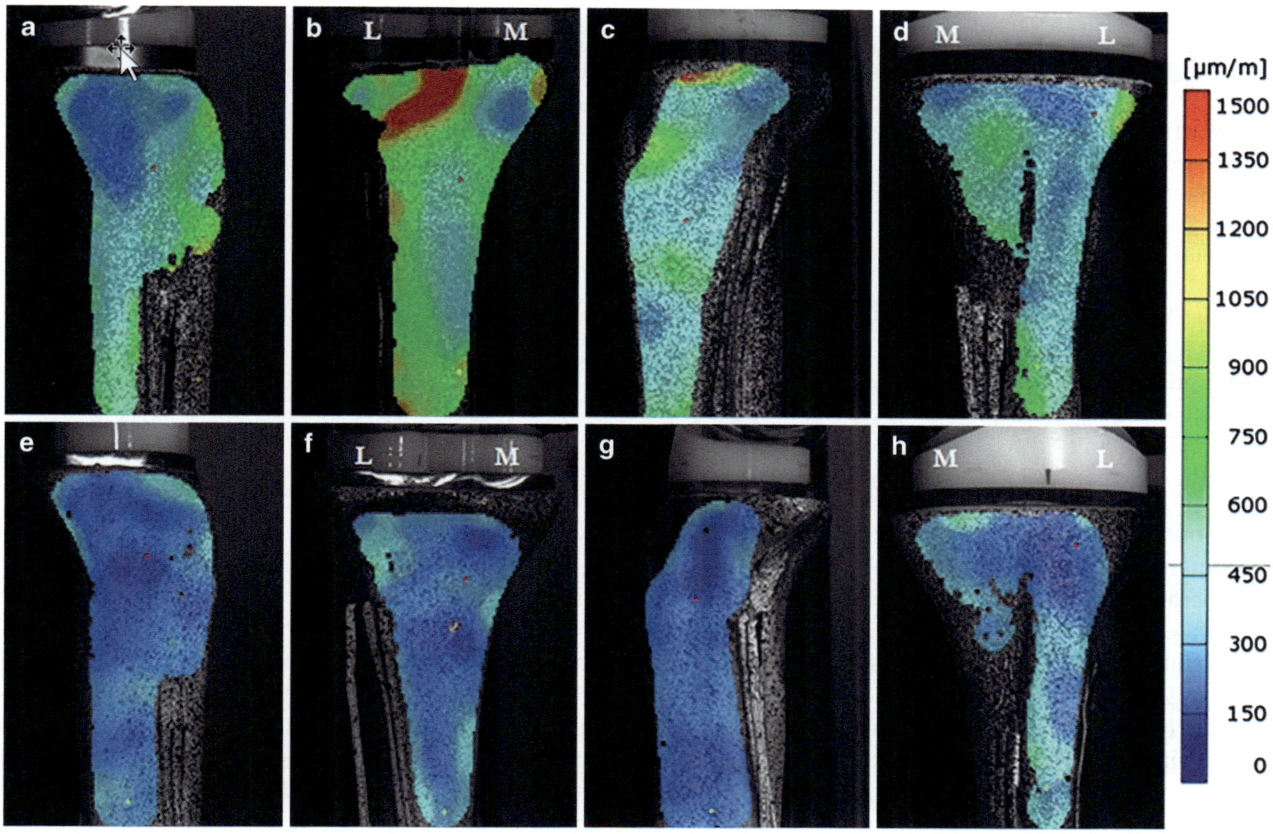

Fig. 30.14 Digital image correlation mapping of the torsion-induced von Mises strain response in the proximal tibia following 10° femoral external rotation in specimens implanted with fixed-bearing **a–d** or rotating platform components **e–h** (Malinzak et al. 2014 (2014), with permission from Elsevier)

1318 consecutive primary TKAs performed with PFC Sigma PS implants (Depuy Synthes; Warsaw, IN) using mobile (n = 940) or fixed-bearing (n = 378) inserts, to assess the incidence of lateral retinacular release (LRR) required to achieve perfect patellar tracking assessed using the rule of "no thumb" (Yang et al. 2008). LRR FB TKAs was 14.3% compared to 5.3% with MB TKA ($p < 0.0001$) lending further evidence to improved patellar kinematics with mobile-bearing design. Sawaguchi et al. performed an in vivo evaluation of 66 PS TKAs using computer navigation, analyzing patellar tracking and contact stresses with both fixed- and mobile-bearing inserts (Sawaguchi et al. 2010). They observed superior patellar tracking and lower contact stresses in the MB cohort. Despite other studies finding similar results supporting improved patellar kinematics with MB TKA (Rees et al. 2005), Pagnano et al. (2004) did not find differences in LRR or clinical outcome measures at both 3 months and 1 year in a comparative study of FB versus MB TKAs.

Previous kinematic studies have documented axial rotation on the under-surface of the mobile-bearing against the tibial tray, but the question remained if this rotational freedom was preserved over time as the soft tissues may encapsulate the bearing. Assessment of long-term bearing mobility has been done during in vivo fluoroscopic studies in which tantalum beads were embedded within the bearing to determine if bearing mobility is present. Analyses at 3 and 15 months, 5 years, and finally at 10 years demonstrated bearing mobility was maintained over a 10-year period (Dennis et al. 2005; LaCour et al. 2014).

30.6 Clinical Outcomes After Mobile Versus Fixed-Bearing TKA

TKA is a reliable surgery for the treatment of advanced osteoarthritis, and pooled registry data indicate that 82% of TKAs last 25 years (Evans et al. 2019).

> Despite the theoretical advantages of mobile-bearing design that we present, comparative outcomes studies against fixed-bearing design have produced similar clinical results in registries and trials with up to 15-year follow-up duration (Capella et al. 2016; Post et al. 2010; Heckmann et al. 2019; Namba et al. 2011).

Table 30.1 Cumulative percent revision of primary total knee replacement by bearing mobility (Primary Diagnosis OA) (Australian Orthopaedic Association National Joint Replacement Registry (AOANJRR)) (2019)

Bearing mobility	*N* revised	*N* total	1 year	3 years	5 years	10 years	15 years	18 years
Fixed	18,044	515,200	1.0 (1.0, 1.0)	2.5 (2.4, 2.5)	3.3 (3.2, 3.3)	5.0 (4.9, 5.1)	7.1 (6.9, 7.2)	8.3 (7.9, 8.6)
Mobile	6671	127,815	1.2 (1.1, 1.3)	3.4 (3.2, 3.5)	4.5 (4.4, 4.6)	6.3 (6.2, 6.5)	8.3 (8.0, 8.5)	9.6 (9.1, 10.2)
Total	**24,715**	**643,015**						

OA osteoarthritis
Note: Excludes 186 procedures with unknown bearing mobility

Mobile-bearing implants have good survivorship in meta-analyses with reliable clinical outcomes. Carothers et al. performed a meta-analysis of 3506 MB TKAs at an average follow-up duration of 8.6 years (Carothers et al. 2011). 15-year survivorship of rotating platform designs (96.4%) was greater than meniscal bearing implants (86.5%). Mean component loosening (0.33%) and bearing instability (<1%) for all subgroups were uncommon. Implants placed prior to 1995 exhibited higher rates of bearing complications (1.6% vs. 0.1%), believed due to improvements in gap balancing techniques in later years of the analysis. A recent prospective 20-year analysis of a single surgeon's mobile-bearing experience produced similar results (Milligan et al. 2019). In a cohort of 487 RP TKAs (DePuy LCS), 139 patients had a 20-year follow-up with cumulative survivorship of 98%.

However, other authors have cited that most clinical studies supporting mobile-bearing technology have been smaller-scale single-center reports (Namba et al. 2011), while the majority of registry studies have failed to identify any difference in clinical outcomes with MB versus FB TKA. Registry-based comparative data has shown cumulative revision rates to be higher with use of MB TKA (Table 30.1) (Gøthesen et al. 2013, 2017; Namba et al. 2013; Jorgensen et al. 2019). These reports typically include all different designs of MB TKA analyzed collectively. In vivo fluoroscopic studies have demonstrated variable kinematic patterns based on the design of the MB TKA (Dennis et al. 1998a, 2003a). Similarly, clinical survivorship has varied based on implant design. For example, rotating platform designs have exhibited superior results when compared with meniscal bearing implants (Carothers et al. 2011). The senior author believes improved gap balancing surgical technique development over the last two decades will improve long-term results of MB TKA since these designs are less forgiving (than FB TKA) of imperfect gap balance due to the risk of bearing instability.

Conclusion

TKA-bearing design significantly influences knee kinematics and polyethylene wear properties. Registry studies reflect the limited use of mobile-bearing designs both in the United States and abroad, but critical advantages are seen with mobile-bearing use compared to fixed-bearing design. With axial rotation in knee flexion, the mobile-bearing design increases contact area between the femur and tibia, and effectively reduces contact stress on the polyethylene bearing. Axial rotation of the mobile-bearing on the tibial tray uncouples rotational strain between the implant and fixation interface at the bone which is critical to reducing aseptic loosening with use of highly constrained TKA constructs. The rotating bearing also allows the extensor mechanism to auto-centralize into the trochlear groove of the femoral component which improves patellar tracking and leads to improved kinematic indices, reduced patellofemoral contact stresses, and in our experience, significantly lower lateral retinacular release rates.

Proposed risks with mobile-bearing design use have historically included increased polyethylene wear associated with the second articulating surface on the backside of the polyethylene, and also mobile-bearing dislocation, termed "spin-out." Retrieval analyses have shown decreased volumetric polyethylene wear with mobile-bearing designs over time, and bearing spin-out has rarely been reported in TKAs done with appropriate gap balancing techniques.

Despite the reported advantages with mobile-bearing design, registry data has shown equivalent clinical outcomes and survivorship with fixed- and mobile-bearing designs. While it is possible that subgroup analysis of the mobile-bearing design (rotating platform, meniscal bearing, specific implant system) may show differences, that data has been limited to smaller single-center studies. The senior author has seen improved clinical outcomes in his practice with use of a mobile-bearing design. Surgeons should be aware of the advantages associated with mobile-bearing design use, but ultimately should implant the bearing design they feel most comfortable with.

Take-Home Messages

- Key elements to effective cementation technique include the following:
  - Preparing a dry bony surface devoid of marrow/blood lipid contamination
  - Pressurization of the tibial surface periphery due to cement escape
  - Repeated evacuation of lipid-rich liquid expelled by pressurization
  - Removing cement in large fragments to minimize generation of third body debris particles
  - Avoidance of micromotion during cement curation to preserve fixation strength
- MB TKA designs increase the femoral–tibial contact area relative to FB TKA which lowers contact pressures and reduces polyethylene wear.
- Axial freedom of the polyethylene bearing allows the component to self-align with the femoral component which centralizes the extensor mechanism and improves patellar tracking.
- Concerns of mobile-bearing spin-out/dislocation have been minimized by precise gap balancing surgical techniques.
- MB TKA designs uncouple force transmission to the component fixation interface. This should be considered in settings with impaired bone stock, such as revision TKA where highly constrained components with high fixation stresses are utilized.
- Registry data have failed to demonstrate superior implant survivorship associated with mobile-bearing use. Ultimately, surgeon preference and judgment are required to pick the best bearing design for their patients.

References

Abdelgaied A, Brockett CL, Liu F, Jennings LM, Fisher J, Jin Z (2013) Quantification of the effect of cross-shear and applied nominal contact pressure on the wear of moderately cross-linked polyethylene. Proc Inst Mech Eng H 227(1):18–26. https://doi.org/10.1177/0954411912459423

Agarwal S, Kabariti R, Kakar R, Lopez DJ, Morgan-Jones R (2019) Why are revision knee replacements failing? Knee 26(3):774–778. https://doi.org/10.1016/j.knee.2019.04.012

Atwood SA, Currier JH, Mayor MB, Collier JP, Van Citters DW, Kennedy FE (2008) Clinical wear measurement on low contact stress rotating platform knee bearings. J Arthroplasty 23(3):431–440. https://doi.org/10.1016/j.arth.2007.06.005

Australian Orthopaedic Association National Joint Replacement Registry (AOANJRR) (2019) 20th Annual Report. p 230 (Table KT17). https://aoanjrr.sahmri.com/annual-reports-2019

Banks S, Bellemans J, Nozaki H, Whiteside LA, Harman M, Hodge WA (2003) Knee motions during maximum flexion in fixed and mobile-bearing arthroplasties. Clin Orthop Relat Res 410:131–138. https://doi.org/10.1097/01.blo.0000063121.39522.19

Bartel DL, Bicknell VL, Wright TM (1986) The effect of conformity, thickness, and material on stresses in ultra-high molecular weight components for total joint replacement. J Bone Joint Surg Am 68(7):1041–1051. https://doi.org/10.2106/00004623--198668070-00010

Berry DJ, Currier JH, Mayor MB, Collier JP (2012) Knee wear measured in retrievals: a polished tray reduces insert wear. Clin Orthop Relat Res 470(7):1860–1868. https://doi.org/10.1007/s11999-012-2248-0

Billi F, Kavanaugh A, Schmalzried H, Schmalzried TP (2019) Techniques for improving the initial strength of the tibial tray-cement interface bond. Bone Joint J 101-B(1_Supple_A):53–58. https://doi.org/10.1302/0301-620X.101B1.BJJ-2018-0500.R1

Blunn GW, Walker PS, Joshi A, Hardinge K (1991) The dominance of cyclic sliding in producing wear in total knee replacements. Clin Orthop Relat Res (273):253–260. https://doi.org/10.1097/00003086-199112000-00036

Bottlang M, Erne OK, Lacatusu E, Sommers MB, Kessler O (2006) A mobile-bearing knee prosthesis can reduce strain at the proximal tibia. Clin Orthop Relat Res 447:105–111. https://doi.org/10.1097/01.blo.0000203463.27937.97

Bragdon CR, O'Connor DO, Lowenstein JD, Jasty M, Syniuta WD (1996) The importance of multidirectional motion on the wear of polyethylene. Proc Inst Mech Eng H 210(3):157–165. https://doi.org/10.1243/PIME_PROC_1996_210_408_02

Buller LT, Rao V, Chiu Y-F, Nam D, McLawhorn AS (2020) Primary total knee arthroplasty performed using high-viscosity cement is associated with higher odds of revision for aseptic loosening. J Arthroplasty 35(6):S182–S189. https://doi.org/10.1016/j.arth.2019.08.023

Capella M, Dolfin M, Saccia F (2016) Mobile bearing and fixed bearing total knee arthroplasty. Ann Transl Med 4(7):1–9. https://doi.org/10.21037/atm.2015.12.64

Carothers JT, Kim RH, Dennis DA, Southworth C (2011) Mobile-bearing total knee arthroplasty. A meta-analysis. J Arthroplasty 26(4):537–542. https://doi.org/10.1016/j.arth.2010.05.015

Chiavetta J, Fehring TK, Odum S, Griffin W, Mason JB (2006) Importance of a balanced-gap technique in rotating-platform knees. Orthopedics 29(9 Suppl):S45–S48. http://www.ncbi.nlm.nih.gov/pubmed/17002148

Cottino U, Abdel MP, Perry KI, Mara KC, Lewallen DG, Hanssen AD (2017) Long-term results after total knee arthroplasty with contemporary rotating-hinge prostheses. J Bone Joint Surg Am 99(4):324–330. https://doi.org/10.2106/JBJS.16.00307

D'Lima DD, Trice M, Urquhart AG, Colwell CW (2001) Tibiofemoral conformity and kinematics of rotating-bearing knee prostheses. Clin Orthop Relat Res 386:235–242. https://doi.org/10.1097/00003086-200105000-00031

Delport HP, Sloten JV, Bellemans J (2010) Comparative gravimetric wear analysis in mobile versus fixed-bearing posterior stabilized total knee prostheses. Acta Orthop Belg 76(3):367–373. http://www.ncbi.nlm.nih.gov/pubmed/20698459

Dennis DA, Komistek RD (2006) Mobile-bearing total knee arthroplasty. Clin Orthop Relat Res 452:70–77. https://doi.org/10.1097/01.blo.0000238776.27316.d6

Dennis DA, Komistek RD, Colwell CE et al (1998a) In vivo anteroposterior femorotibial translation of total knee arthroplasty: a multicenter analysis. Clin Orthop Relat Res 356:47–57. https://doi.org/10.1097/00003086-199811000-00009

Dennis DA, Komistek RD, Stiehl JB, Walker SA, Dennis KN (1998b) Range of motion after total knee arthroplasty: the effect of implant design and weight-bearing conditions. J Arthroplasty 13(7):748–752. https://doi.org/10.1016/s0883-5403(98)90025-0

Dennis DA, Komistek RD, Mahfouz MR, Haas BD, Stiehl JB (2003a) Conventry award paper: multicenter determination of in vivo kinematics after total knee arthroplasty. Clin Orthop Relat Res 416(416):37–57. https://doi.org/10.1097/01.blo.0000092986.12414.b5

Dennis DA, Komistek RD, Mahfouz MR (2003b) In vivo fluoroscopic analysis of fixed-bearing total knee replacements. Clin Orthop Relat Res 410:114–130. https://doi.org/10.1097/01.blo.0000062385.79828.72

Dennis DA, Komistek RD, Mahfouz MR, Walker SA, Tucker A (2004) A multicenter analysis of axial femorotibial rotation after total knee arthroplasty. Clin Orthop Relat Res 428:180–189. https://doi.org/10.1097/01.blo.0000148777.98244.84

Dennis DA, Komistek RD, Mahfouz MR, Outten JT, Sharma A (2005) Mobile-bearing total knee arthroplasty: do the polyethylene bearings rotate? Clin Orthop Relat Res 440:88–95. https://doi.org/10.1097/01.blo.0000185464.23505.6e

Dennis DA, Kittelson AJ, Yang CC, Miner TM, Kim RH, Stevens-Lapsley JE (2016) Does tourniquet use in TKA affect recovery of lower extremity strength and function? A randomized trial. Clin Orthop Relat Res 474(1):69–77. https://doi.org/10.1007/s11999-015-4393-8

Diamond OJ, Doran E, Beverland DE (2018) Spinout/dislocation in mobile-bearing total knee arthroplasty: a report of 26 cases. J Arthroplasty 33(2):537–543. https://doi.org/10.1016/j.arth.2017.09.016

Engh GA, Zimmerman RL, Parks NL, Engh CA (2009) Analysis of wear in retrieved mobile and fixed bearing knee inserts. J Arthroplasty 24(6 SUPPL):28–32. https://doi.org/10.1016/j.arth.2009.03.010

Evans JT, Walker RW, Evans JP, Blom AW, Sayers A, Whitehouse MR (2019) How long does a knee replacement last? A systematic review and meta-analysis of case series and national registry reports with more than 15 years of follow-up. Lancet 393(10172):655–663. https://doi.org/10.1016/s0140--6736(18)32531-5

Fisher J, McEwen HMJ, Tipper JL et al (2004) Wear, debris, and biologic activity of cross-linked polyethylene in the knee. Clin Orthop Relat Res 428:114–119. https://doi.org/10.1097/01.blo.0000148783.20469.4c

Fisher J, McEwen H, Tipper J et al (2006) Wear-simulation analysis of rotating-platform mobile-bearing knees. Orthopedics 29(9 Suppl):S36–S41. http://www.ncbi.nlm.nih.gov/pubmed/17002146

Fisher J, Jennings LM, Galvin AL, Jin ZM, Stone MH, Ingham E (2010) 2009 Knee Society presidential guest lecture: polyethylene wear in total knees. Clin Orthop Relat Res 468(1):12–18. https://doi.org/10.1007/s11999-009-1033-1

Gøthesen EB, Havelin L et al (2013) Survival rates and causes of revision in cemented primary total knee replacement: a report from the Norwegian arthroplasty register 1994–2009. Bone Joint J 95 B(5):636–642. https://doi.org/10.1302/0301-620X.95B5.30271

Gothesen O, Lygre SHL, Lorimer M, Graves S, Furnes O (2017) Increased risk of aseptic loosening for 43,525 rotating-platform vs. fixed-bearing total knee replacements. Acta Orthop 88(6):649–656. https://doi.org/10.1080/17453674.2017.1378533

Greenwald AS, Heim CS (2005) Mobile-bearing knee systems: ultra-high molecular weight polyethylene wear and design issues. Instr Course Lect 54:195–205. https://doi.org/10.1054/arth.2002.33550

Hamelynck KJ (2006) The history of mobile-bearing total knee replacement systems. Orthopedics 29(9 Suppl):S7–S12. http://www.ncbi.nlm.nih.gov/pubmed/17002140

Heckmann N, Ihn H, Stefl M et al (2019) Early results from the American Joint Replacement Registry: a comparison with other national registries. J Arthroplasty 34(7):S125–S134.e1. https://doi.org/10.1016/j.arth.2018.12.027

Holt G, Murnaghan C, Reilly J, Meek RMD (2007) The biology of aseptic osteolysis. Clin Orthop Relat Res 460:240–252. https://doi.org/10.1097/BLO.0b013e31804b4147

Jones VC, Barton DC, Fitzpatrick DP, Auger DD, Stone MH, Fisher J (1999) An experimental model of tibial counterface polyethylene wear in mobile bearing knees: the influence of design and kinematics. Biomed Mater Eng 9(3):189–196. http://www.ncbi.nlm.nih.gov/pubmed/10572623

Jorgensen NB, McAuliffe M, Orschulok T, Lorimer MF, de Steiger R (2019) Major aseptic revision following Total knee replacement. J Bone Joint Surg Am 101(4):302–310. https://doi.org/10.2106/JBJS.17.01528

Kelly NH, Fu RH, Wright TM, Padgett DE (2011) Wear damage in mobile-bearing TKA is as severe as that in fixed-bearing TKA. Clin Orthop Relat Res 469(1):123–130. https://doi.org/10.1007/s11999-010-1557-4

Kim YH, Choi Y, Kim JS (2010) Osteolysis in well-functioning fixed- and mobile-bearing TKAs in younger patients. Clin Orthop Relat Res 468(11):3084–3093. https://doi.org/10.1007/s11999--010-1336-2

Kim Y-H, Park J-W, Kim J-S, Kulkarni SS, Kim Y-H (2014) Long-term clinical outcomes and survivorship of press-fit condylar sigma fixed-bearing and mobile-bearing total knee prostheses in the same patients. J Bone Joint Surg Am 96(19):e168. https://doi.org/10.2106/JBJS.M.01130

Kim RH, Martin JR, Dennis DA, Yang CC, Jennings JM, Lee GC (2017) Midterm clinical and radiographic results of mobile-bearing revision total knee arthroplasty. J Arthroplasty 32(6):1930–1934. https://doi.org/10.1016/j.arth.2017.01.014

Komistek RD, Dennis DA, Mahfouz M (2003) In vivo fluoroscopic analysis of the normal human knee. Clin Orthop Relat Res 410(410):69–81. https://doi.org/10.1097/01.blo.0000062384.79828.3b

Komistek RD, Dennis DA, Mahfouz MR, Walker S, Outten J (2004) In vivo polyethylene bearing mobility is maintained in posterior stabilized total knee arthroplasty. Clin Orthop Relat Res 428(428):207–213. https://doi.org/10.1097/01.blo.0000147135.60185.39

LaCour MT, Sharma A, Carr CB, Komistek RD, Dennis DA (2014) Confirmation of long-term in vivo bearing mobility in eight rotating-platform TKAs. Clin Orthop Relat Res 472(9):2766–2773. https://doi.org/10.1007/s11999-014-3642-6

Lonner JH, Siliski JM, Scott RD (1999) Prodromes of failure in total knee arthroplasty. J Arthroplasty 14(4):488–492. https://doi.org/10.1016/S0883-5403(99)90106-7

Lu Y-C, Huang C-H, Chang T-K, Ho F-Y, Cheng C-K, Huang C-H (2010) Wear-pattern analysis in retrieved tibial inserts of mobile-bearing and fixed-bearing total knee prostheses. J Bone Joint Surg Br 92-B(4):500–507. https://doi.org/10.1302/0301--620X.92B4.22560

Lutz MJ, Pincus PF, Whitehouse SL, Halliday BR (2009) The effect of cement gun and cement syringe use on the tibial cement mantle in total knee arthroplasty. J Arthroplasty 24(3):461–467. https://doi.org/10.1016/j.arth.2007.10.028

Mahfouz MR, Komistek RD, Dennis DA, Hoff WA (2004) In vivo assessment of the kinematics in normal and anterior cruciate

30

ligament-deficient knees. J Bone Joint Surg Am 86(SUPPL. 2):56–61. https://doi.org/10.2106/00004623-200412002-00009
Maistrelli GL, Antonelli L, Fornasier V, Mahomed N (1995) Cement penetration with pulsed lavage versus syringe irrigation in total knee arthroplasty. Clin Orthop Relat Res 312:261–265. http://www.ncbi.nlm.nih.gov/pubmed/7634612
Malinzak RA, Small SR, Rogge RD et al (2014) The effect of rotating platform TKA on strain distribution and torque transmission on the proximal tibia. J Arthroplasty 29(3):541–547. https://doi.org/10.1016/j.arth.2013.08.024
Mason JB (2018) Simultaneous femoral and tibial cementation negatively effects tibial fixation in total knee arthroplasty. Am Acad Orthop Surg 2018 Annu Meet Sci Exhib 15
McEwen HMJ, Fisher J, Goldsmith AAJ, Auger DD, Hardaker C, Stone MH (2001) Wear of fixed bearing and rotating platform mobile bearing knees subjected to high levels of internal and external tibial rotation. J Mater Sci Mater Med 12(10–12):1049–1052. https://doi.org/10.1023/a:1012850224565
McEwen HMJ, Barnett PI, Bell CJ et al (2005) The influence of design, materials and kinematics on the in vitro wear of total knee replacements. J Biomech 38(2):357–365. https://doi.org/10.1016/j.jbiomech.2004.02.015
Milligan DJ, O'Brien S, Doran E, Gallagher NE, Beverland DE (2019) Twenty-year survivorship of a cemented mobile bearing total knee arthroplasty. Knee 26(4):933–940. https://doi.org/10.1016/j.knee.2019.06.004
Minoda Y, Kobayashi A, Iwaki H et al (2004) Characteristics of polyethylene wear particles isolated from synovial fluid after mobile-bearing and posterior-stabilized total knee arthroplasties. J Biomed Mater Res 71B(1):1–6. https://doi.org/10.1002/jbm.b.30005
Minoda Y, Hata K, Ikebuchi M, Mizokawa S, Ohta Y, Nakamura H (2017) Comparison of in vivo polyethylene wear particles between mobile- and fixed-bearing TKA in the same patients. Knee Surg Sport Traumatol Arthrosc 25(9):2887–2893. https://doi.org/10.1007/s00167-016-4027-z
Mortazavi JSM, Molligan J, Austin MS, Purtill JJ, Hozack WJ, Parvizi J (2011) Failure following revision total knee arthroplasty: infection is the major cause. Int Orthop 35(8):1157–1164. https://doi.org/10.1007/s00264-010-1134-1
Mow CS, Wiedel JD (1998) Revision total knee arthroplasty using the porous-coated anatomic revision prosthesis: six- to twelve-year results. J Arthroplasty 13(6):681–686. https://doi.org/10.1016/S0883-5403(98)80013-2
Nakayama K, Matsuda S, Miura H, Higaki H, Otsuka K, Iwamoto Y (2005) Contact stress at the post-cam mechanism in posterior-stabilised total knee arthroplasty. J Bone Joint Surg Br 87-B(4):483–488. https://doi.org/10.1302/0301-620X.87B4.15684
Namba RS, Inacio MCS, Paxton EW, Robertsson O, Graves SE (2011) The role of registry data in the evaluation of mobile-bearing total knee arthroplasty. J Bone Joint Surg Am 93(Suppl 3):48–50. https://doi.org/10.2106/JBJS.K.00982
Namba RS, Cafri G, Khatod M, Inacio MCS, Brox TW, Paxton EW (2013) Risk factors for total knee arthroplasty aseptic revision. J Arthroplasty 28(8 SUPPL):122–127. https://doi.org/10.1016/j.arth.2013.04.050
Nguyen LCL, Lehil MS, Bozic KJ (2015) Trends in total knee arthroplasty implant utilization. J Arthroplasty 30(5):739–742. https://doi.org/10.1016/j.arth.2014.12.009
Pagnano MW, Trousdale RT, Stuart MJ, Hanssen AD, Jacofsky DJ (2004) Rotating platform knees did not improve patellar tracking: a prospective, randomized study of 240 primary total knee arthroplasties. Clin Orthop Relat Res 428:221–227. https://doi.org/10.1097/01.blo.0000148892.31464.81
Peters CL, Hennessey R, Barden RM, Galante JO, Rosenberg AG (1997) Revision total knee arthroplasty with a cemented posterior-stabilized or constrained condylar prosthesis: a minimum 3-year and average 5-year follow- up study. J Arthroplasty 12(8):896–903. https://doi.org/10.1016/S0883-5403(97)90159-5
Pooley CM, Tabor D (1972) Friction and molecular structure: the behaviour of some thermoplastics. Proc R Soc A Math Phys Eng Sci 329(1578):251–274. https://doi.org/10.1098/rspa.1972.0112
Post ZD, Matar WY, van de Leur T, Grossman EL, Austin MS (2010) Mobile-bearing total knee arthroplasty: better than a fixed-bearing? J Arthroplasty 25(6):998–1003. https://doi.org/10.1016/j.arth.2009.07.014
Puloski SKT, McCalden RW, MacDonald SJ, Rorabeck CH, Bourne RB (2001) Tibial post wear in posterior stabilized total knee arthroplasty. An unrecognized source of polyethylene debris. J Bone Joint Surg Am 83(3):390–397. https://doi.org/10.2106/00004623-200103000-00011
Ranawat CS, Komistek RD, Rodriguez JA, Dennis DA, Anderle M (2004) In vivo kinematics for fixed and mobile-bearing posterior stabilized knee prostheses. Clin Orthop Relat Res 80222(418):184–190. https://doi.org/10.1097/00003086-200401000-00030
Rand JA (1991) Revision total knee arthroplasty using the total condylar III prosthesis. J Arthroplasty 6(3):279–284. https://doi.org/10.1016/S0883-5403(06)80175-0
Rao AR, Engh GA, Collier MB, Lounici S (2002) Tibial interface wear in retrieved total knee components and correlations with modular insert motion. J Bone Joint Surg Am 84(10):1849–1855. https://doi.org/10.2106/00004623-200210000-00017
Rees JL, Beard DJ, Price AJ et al (2005) Real in vivo kinematic differences between mobile-bearing and fixed-bearing total knee arthroplasties. Clin Orthop Relat Res (432):204–209. https://doi.org/10.1097/01.blo.0000150372.92398.ba
Reina N, Salib CG, Pagnano MW, Trousdale RT, Abdel MP, Berry DJ (2019) Varus-valgus constrained implants with a mobile-bearing articulation: results of 367 revision total knee arthroplasties. J Arthroplasty 35(4):1060–1063. https://doi.org/10.1016/j.arth.2019.11.023
Ritter MA, Herbst SA, Keating EM, Faris PM (1994) Radiolucency at the bone-cement interface in total knee replacement. The effects of bone-surface preparation and cement technique. J Bone Joint Surg Am 76(1):60–65. https://doi.org/10.2106/00004623-199401000-00008
Rosso F, Cottino U, Dettoni F, Bruzzone M, Bonasia DE, Rossi R (2019) Revision total knee arthroplasty (TKA): mid-term outcomes and bone loss/quality evaluation and treatment. J Orthop Surg Res 14(1):1–9. https://doi.org/10.1186/s13018-019-1328-1
Sawaguchi N, Majima T, Ishigaki T, Mori N, Terashima T, Minami A (2010) Mobile-bearing total knee arthroplasty improves patellar tracking and patellofemoral contact stress. In vivo measurements in the same patients. J Arthroplasty 25(6):920–925. https://doi.org/10.1016/j.arth.2009.07.024
Schlegel UJ, Püschel K, Morlock MM, Nagel K (2014) An in vitro comparison of tibial tray cementation using gun pressurization or pulsed lavage. Int Orthop 38(5):967–971. https://doi.org/10.1007/s00264-014-2303-4
Sharkey PF, Hozack WJ, Rothman RH, Shastri S, Jacoby SM (2002) Insall award paper. Why are total knee arthroplasties failing today? Clin Orthop Relat Res 404(404):7–13. https://doi.org/10.1097/00003086-200211000-00003
Sharma A, Komistek RD, Ranawat CS, Dennis DA, Mahfouz MR (2007) In vivo contact pressures in total knee arthroplasty. J Arthroplasty 22(3):404–416. https://doi.org/10.1016/j.arth.2006.07.008

Silverman EJ, Landy DC, Massel DH, Kaimrajh DN, Latta LL, Robinson RP (2014) The effect of viscosity on cement penetration in total knee arthroplasty, an application of the squeeze film effect. J Arthroplasty 29(10):2039–2042. https://doi.org/10.1016/j.arth.2014.05.010

Siqueira M, Klika A, Higuera C, Barsoum W (2014) Modes of failure of total knee arthroplasty: registries and realities. J Knee Surg 28(02):127–138. https://doi.org/10.1055/s-0034-1396014

Stiehl JB, Komistek RD, Dennis DA (1999) Detrimental kinematics of a flat on flat total condylar knee arthroplasty. Clin Orthop Relat Res 365:139–148. https://doi.org/10.1097/00003086--199908000-00019

Suarez J, Griffin W, Springer B, Fehring T, Mason JB, Odum S (2008) Why do revision knee arthroplasties fail? J Arthroplasty 23(6):99–103. https://doi.org/10.1016/j.arth.2008.04.020

Ulivi M, Orlandini L, Meroni V, Consonni O, Sansone V (2015) Survivorship at minimum 10-year follow-up of a rotating-platform, mobile-bearing, posterior-stabilised total knee arthroplasty. Knee Surg Sport Traumatol Arthrosc 23(6):1669–1675. https://doi.org/10.1007/s00167-014-3118-y

Utzschneider S, Paulus A, Datz J-C et al (2009) Influence of design and bearing material on polyethylene wear particle generation in total knee replacement. Acta Biomater 5(7):2495–2502. https://doi.org/10.1016/j.actbio.2009.03.016

Vanlommel J, Luyckx JP, Labey L, Innocenti B, De Corte R, Bellemans J (2011) Cementing the tibial component in total knee arthroplasty: which technique is the best? J Arthroplasty 26(3):492–496. https://doi.org/10.1016/j.arth.2010.01.107

Vertullo CJ, Davey JR (2001) The effect of a tibial baseplate undersurface peripheral lip on cement penetration in total knee arthroplasty. J Arthroplasty 16(4):487–492. https://doi.org/10.1054/arth.2001.22270

Walker PS, Komistek RD, Barrett DS, Anderson D, Dennis DA, Sampson M (2002) Motion of a mobile bearing knee allowing translation and rotation. J Arthroplasty 17(1):11–19. https://doi.org/10.1054/arth.2002.28731

Yang CC, McFadden LA, Dennis DA, Kim RH, Sharma A (2008) Lateral retinacular release rates in mobile- versus fixed-bearing TKA. Clin Orthop Relat Res 466(11):2656–2661. https://doi.org/10.1007/s11999-008-0425-y

Zingde SM, Leszko F, Sharma A, Mahfouz MR, Komistek RD, Dennis DA (2014) In vivo determination of cam-post engagement in fixed and mobile-bearing TKA knee. Clin Orthop Relat Res 472(1):254–262. https://doi.org/10.1007/s11999-013-3257-3

All-Polyethylene Tibial Components in Primary Total Knee Arthroplasty: Why It Works and Why I Do Not Use It Anymore?

Ahmed Siddiqi, Abdullah Aftab, and Amar S. Ranawat

Contents

E. Hansen, K.-D. Kühn (eds.), *Essentials of Cemented Knee Arthroplasty*,
https://doi.org/10.1007/978-3-662-63113-3_31

31

31.1 Introduction

The utilization of all-polyethylene tibial (APT) components in TKA has clear advantages, especially in patients with correctable deformity with minimal tibial bone loss. As indicated by the study conducted at our institution, the survivorship of APT TKAs in young and active patients is comparable to that of MBT TKAs and excellent clinical results were observed after 10–18 years. The cost advantage of APT components is substantial per case and even greater cumulatively at long-term. Although APT components lack modularity and do not allow for the usage of stems and augments in complex primary TKAs, they completely eliminate the concerns surrounding the issue of backside wear. APT components are a viable and excellent cost-saving option in contemporary TKA.

31.2 Case Example

An 80-year-old female with past medical history of hypertension, coronary artery disease, and a body mass index of 35 kg/m^2 presents to the clinic with debilitating left knee pain for a few years from primary end-stage osteoarthritis. Over the past 6 months, the patient's symptoms did not improve with activity modifications, corticosteroid, and hyaluronic acid injections. Her radiographs demonstrate several medial compartment and patellofemoral joint space narrowings with osteophyte formation and subchondral cysts and sclerosis (Fig. 31.1). On physical examination, the patient has a correctable varus deformity without a thrust during ambulation. After discussing risks, benefits, and alternatives, the patient elects to undergo primary left total knee arthroplasty. During the surgical procedure, after all bony cuts and soft-tissue releases are performed to have equal medial–lateral, flexion–extension balanced gaps, a posterior stabilized femoral component and all-polyethylene tibial (APT) component is cemented into place (Fig. 31.2). During a long-term follow-up of 10 years, patient continues to have full range of motion (0–120°) and is pain-free.

31.3 Background

> "Modularity is like an addiction. You know it is bad for you, but you do it anyway." (Chitranjan S. Ranawat, MD)

All-polyethylene tibial (APT) components and metal-backed tibias represent the original total condylar tibial component design with long-term survivorship over 90% (Ranawat et al. 1993; Gill et al. 1999). Despite excellent outcomes, biomechanical studies in the early

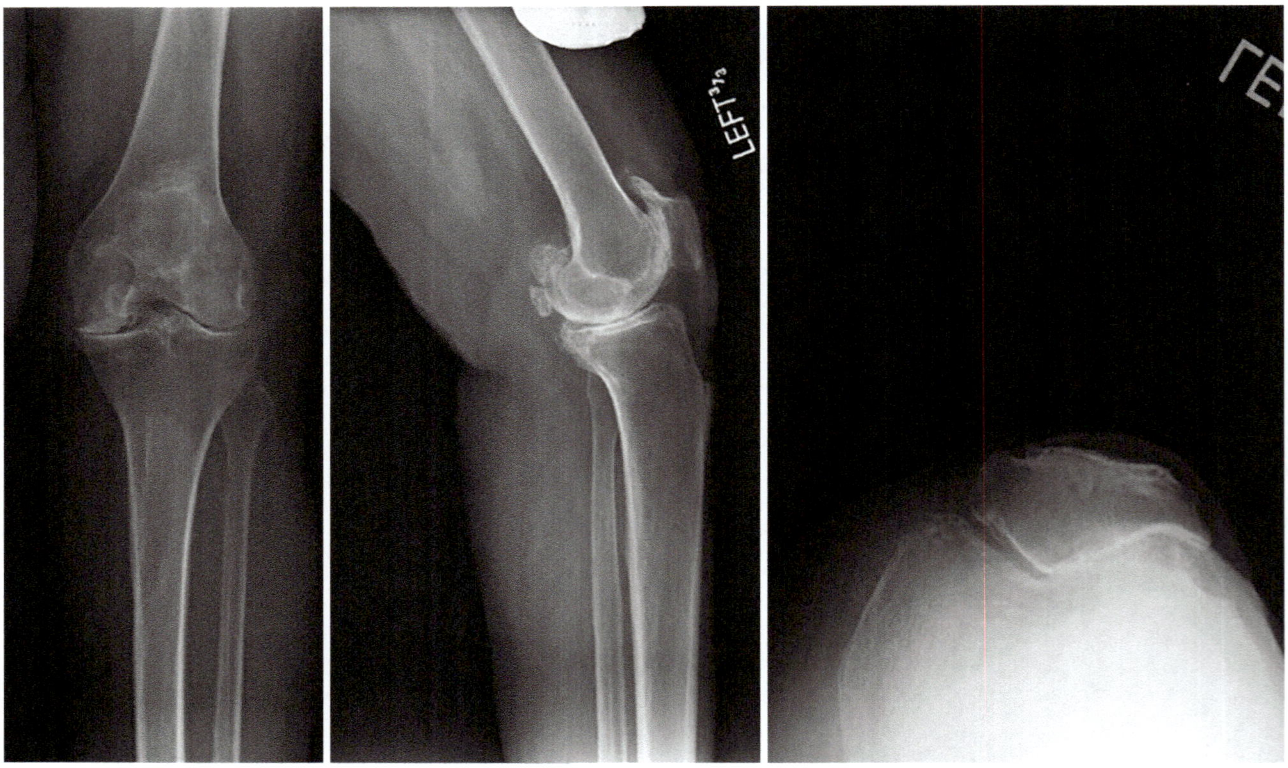

Fig. 31.1 Anteroposterior, lateral, and Merchant radiographs demonstrating severe tricompartmental degenerative joint disease

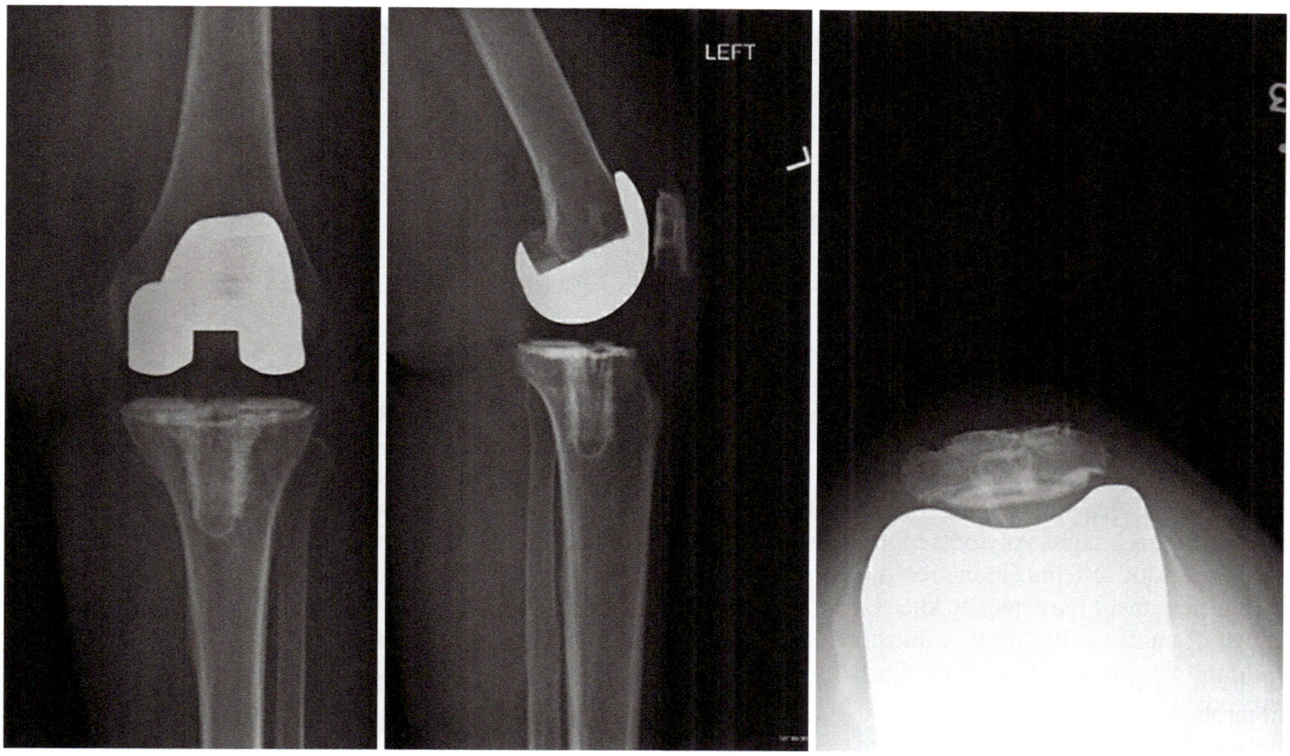

Fig. 31.2 Anteroposterior, lateral, and Merchant radiographs demonstrating posterior-stabilized primary TKA with an all-polyethylene tibial component

1980s described modularity advances that led to widespread adoption of cemented metal-backed modular (MBT) tibial components globally (Lewis et al. 1982; Fipp 1983; Bartel et al. 1986). The Annual Report of the National Joint Registry for England and Wales in 2007 showed that only 3.9% of primary TKAs utilized APT components (Bettinson et al. 2009). Proponents of MBT components cite greater intraoperative flexibility with modularity and the ability to apply a porous coating for cementless fixation (Small et al. 2010; Gioe et al. 2007a). However, many studies comparing APT to MBT have not been able to demonstrate significant difference in outcomes and implant survivorship (Bettinson et al. 2009; Gioe et al. 2007b; Blumenfeld and Scott 2010; Robinson and Green 2011).

In a finite element analysis, Fipp et al. (1983) found that compressive stress on cancellous bone was substantially increased when the load was applied to a single tibial plateau but when the load was equally distributed to both plateaus, the cancellous bone stress under APT components was nearly equal to the cancellous bone under metal-backed tibial (MBT) components. Therefore, when utilizing APT, it is essential to make a flat tibial cut that is perpendicular to the mechanical axis to ensure equal load distribution and implant longevity. In a study of 536 flat non-conforming coronal design APT in 405 patients, Faris et al. (2003) reported a failure rate of 68% at 10 years. Fifty-seven (73%) of 79 failures occurred in association with loosening or medial tibial plateau collapse likely attributed to a varus or valgus tibia cut. The authors found the implant–bone stresses were the highest with extreme edge-loading with varus or valgus tilt of the implants with a flat articular geometric coronal plane design.

> Although APT-conforming geometric designs have substantially improved over the past decade to minimize liftoff and edge-loading, the basic tenet of a flat perpendicular tibial cut and overall limb mechanical alignment is of utmost importance (Stiehl et al. 1999).

31.4 Surgical Technique

Proper preparation and implantation of APT components require adequate exposure. Ran-Sall maneuver (Meftah et al. 2012a) is important to properly expose the tibial surface to ensure an even flat cut without soft-tissue interposition. It is also critical to preserve medial subchondral bone that will bear the shear stresses across the APT component during cyclical loading. Since the APT implants are non-modular, the surgeon must be satisfied with intraoperative stability and soft-tissue balance during trialing prior to final cementation.

> We recommend cementing the femoral component first as cementing the tibia initially is likely to obscure visualization and not allow for proper removal of excess cement from the posterior portion of the femoral component.

> This is especially important when using posterior-stabilized implants since the post of the APT may prevent femoral component seating.

> Surgeons newer to this technique may consider using separate bags of cement for the femur and tibia to ensure appropriate component alignment without liftoff.

Implants are cemented using the conventional third-generation technique. Any posterior extruded cement is removed prior to femur reduction on the APT implant. After the cement hardens, the knee is put through a full range of motion (ROM) to confirm proper balancing followed by standard closure of the arthrotomy, subcutaneous tissue, and skin.

Advantages

From a technical viewpoint, the tibial resection is generally more conservative to accommodate the minimum thickness of polyethylene. The lack of modularity eliminates the issue of backside wear from modularity. The absence of a metal base plate allows the use of thicker polyethylene inserts, thus reducing the amount of wear and reducing shear stresses occurring at the cement–prosthesis and cement–bone interfaces.

Disadvantages

Unlike MBT, APT implants may be reserved for individuals with minimal coronal deformity, adequate tibial bone stock, and normal proximal tibial anatomy. The lack of modularity significantly limits intraoperative options if instability is noted after final implant cementation (Doran et al. 2015). Furthermore, there are no options for liner removal in procedures involving irrigation and debridement for acute periprosthetic joint infection or late TKA revision for instability that requires a thicker or varus–valgus constrained polyethylene insert (Blumenfeld and Scott 2010; Doran et al. 2015). Finally, as cementless TKA is garnering increasing interest, there are limited APT press-fit options.

31.5 Implant Cost

In the current cost-conscious healthcare environment, there is increased attention to improving the quality of care while curtailing expenditure. Limiting implant cost has been an area of focus in an effort to decrease overall spend per episode of care provided.

> APT implants have been shown to have substantial cost-saving implications with some studies demonstrating 20% to 50% lower costs versus MBT (Gioe et al. 2006, 2007a, b; Muller et al. 2006; Gioe and Bowman 2000; Healy et al. 2002; Najibi et al. 2003; Pomeroy et al. 2000).

Although some authors have suggested that keeping both APT and MBT on the shelf increases inventory costs (Pagnano et al. 1999), the cost appears to be minimal compared with potential savings. In a randomized controlled trial of 111 APT and 102 MBT TKA, Gioe et al. (Gioe and Bowman 2000) reported contemporary congruent APT components with equivalent function to MBT at mean 49-month follow-up with an average of $675 (USD) cost-saving per procedure for APT. In another registry study, Gioe et al. (2007a) reported 99.4% survival at 14.3 years with all-cause revision as the primary endpoint. The estimated cost savings for the APT was $729 (USD) per case compared to MBT. The authors further reported that if all patients older than 75 years old in the registry received APT, the projected implant cost savings would be greater than $1.2 million (USD) (Gioe et al. 2007a).

Browne et al. (2018) constructed a Markov model analysis to examine cost-effectiveness of APT and determine what difference in revision rates would make MBT implants a more cost-saving choice. Cost data from the authors' institution was used in conjunction with published United States implant list prices and modeled with a 3% discount rate. The study found that over a 20-year period, a failure rate greater than 27% for APT would be needed to achieve equivalent cost compared with the proposed failure rate of 18% for MBT. The authors concluded that APT implants are cost-effective if the excess total revision rate increases by less than 9% in 20 years compared with MBT TKA (Browne et al. 2018).

31.6 Clinical Outcomes

In a study conducted at the Hospital for Special Surgery, a 10–18-year follow-up study for 44 APT TKAs in 32 patients (12 bilateral TKA) that were 60 years and younger demonstrated good to excellent outcome in 96% of patients with implant survivorship greater than 95%. (Meftah et al. 2012b) The implants were either posterior stabilized Pressed Fit Condylar (PFC) Modular or Sigma designs (DePuy Orthopaedics, Inc., Warsaw, Ind). Clinical analysis included pre- and postoperative validated Knee Society Score (KSS), Knee Society Function Score (KSFS), Western Ontario and McMaster Universities Osteoarthritis Index (WOMAC), UCLA activity score and a detailed Patient Administered Questionnaire (ROC-PAQ) containing separate sections for pain, daily living activities, sport participation, and satisfaction (Rasquinha et al. 2006; Cooper et al. 2010; Ranawat et al. 2004). The KSS improved from 38.3 ± 9.7 to 94 ± 7 and KSFS improved from 51.5 ± 14.1 to 89 ± 20 at an average of 12.4 ± 2.7 years of follow-up. None of the patients in the study indicated that they were dissatisfied (satisfaction score less than 5 on the ROC-PAQ) and the mean satisfaction score was 9.2 ± 1.4. 62% of patients were participating in sporting activities such as running, gym exercises, and playing tennis or golf.

The survivorship of MBT TKAs is widely reported in the literature and ranges from 88.9% to 97.2% at 8–13 years (Gioe et al. 2007b; Bozic et al. 2005; Ehrhardt et al. 2011; Parsch et al. 2009; Stern and Insall 1992). A number of good-quality studies have also compared survivorship and function of APT and MBT TKAs (Bettinson et al. 2009; Gioe et al. 2007b).

> The general conclusion has been that the results are similar at 10 years with regard to function, survivorship, patient satisfaction, and radiological parameters.

One prospective study followed APT TKA patients over 14 years and found 99% cumulative survival as compared to 95.1% for MBT patients. The cumulative revision rate for the APT group was 1%, which was significantly lower than the 4.9% CRR in the MBT group ($p = 0.02$).

Houdek et al. (2016) reviewed 31,939 patients undergoing primary TKA (28,224 (88%) MBT and 3715 (12%) APT) over a 43-year period and found APT components to have significantly improved survivorship ($p < 0.0001$) compared to MBT. Interestingly, APT TKA had improved survival for all body mass index (BMI) groups except in the morbidly obese subgroup (BMI ≥ 40) where there was no statistical difference ($p > 0.05$). Additionally, APT implants were found to have significantly lower rates of periprosthetic joint infections, instability, aseptic loosening, periprosthetic fractures, and fewer radiolucent lines. Herschmiller et al. (2019) also found statistically fewer radiolucent lines ($p < 0.001$) around APT on plain radiographs compared to MBT. However, the authors appropriately concluded that the clinical implications of fewer radiolucencies are unknown. Through radiostereometric analysis (RSA) testing, however, Nouta et al. (Nouta et al., 2012) found that APT had better fixation compared with MBT as the maximum total point motion for APT was 0.6 (± 0.2) versus 0.89 (± 1.3) for the MBT.

A recent meta-analysis of 32 articles evaluating 58,942 TKA patients demonstrated no significant differences in patient-reported outcome measures (PROMs) and functional outcome scores. However, APT had statistically higher revision rates compared with MBT (2.02% vs. 1.85%, $p < 0.00001$, respectively). The authors concluded that this finding demonstrates a negative impact on APT cost-effectiveness and that MBT should remain the implant of choice. However, the findings from the study should be taken with caution since the quality of evidence of the studies included was low according to GRADE scoring. Conversely, another recent meta-analysis of 30 studies from 2000 to 2016 reported level 1 evidence comparing APT and MBT with no statistically significant survivorship difference (Kumar et al. 2019).

In a registry study, Mohan et al. (2013) evaluated the risk of revision in younger patients (<65 years old) and in older patients (≥65 years old) with APT TKA. 27,657 TKAs were evaluated with 2306 (8%) patients having APT TKA and 25,351 (92%) with MBT components. In adjusted models, the risk of early all-cause revision (hazard ratio [HR] = 0.5) and aseptic revision (HR = 0.6) was lower for the APT cohort than for the MBT cohort. In older patients, the early risk of all-cause revision was 0.6 for the APT patients compared to the MBT cohort. In younger patients, the adjusted risk of all-cause revision (HR = 0.3) and the adjusted risk of aseptic revision (HR = 0.3) were lower for the APT cohort than for the MBT group. Overall, APT TKA patients had a 49% lower risk of early all-cause revision and a 41% lower risk of aseptic revision compared to MBT (Mohan et al. 2013). Furthermore, the risk of early revision for any causes was even lower in younger patients ($p < 0.01$).

Why I Do Not Use It Anymore

Despite the widespread literature on APT longevity and survivorship, the senior author is no longer a routine utilizer of APT components. As implant MBT design has improved polyethylene manufacturing and tibial locking mechanism over the past decade, MBT disadvantages have been significantly mitigated. Although APT is significantly more cost-effective, this cost may be offset by overall improved workflow efficiency with decreased number of implant trays, especially at higher volume centers. Additionally, in most communities APT does not represent a standard of care. The comfort of modularity is here to stay and has similarly demonstrated long-term viability and success.

31

Take-Home Messages

- The utilization of APT components in TKA has clear advantages, especially in patients with correctable deformity with minimal tibial bone loss.
- APT avoids locking mechanism problems and backside wear unique with MBT implants.
- Although APT-conforming geometric designs have substantially improved over the past decade to minimize liftoff and edge-loading, the basic tenet of a flat perpendicular tibial cut and overall limb mechanical alignment is of utmost importance.
- We recommend cementing the femoral component first as cementing the tibia initially is likely to obscure visualization and does not allow for proper removal of excess cement from the posterior portion of the femoral component. This is especially important when using posterior stabilized implants since the post of the APT may prevent femoral component seating. Surgeons newer to this technique may consider using separate bags of cement for the femur and tibia to ensure appropriate component alignment without liftoff.
- APT implants have been shown to have substantial cost-saving implications with some studies demonstrating 20–50% lower costs versus MBT. APT offers significant cost reduction of up to $725 USD per case and even greater savings cumulatively.
- The lack of modularity for APT limits intraoperative and postoperative options that require simple polyethylene insert exchange or increased constraint.
- APT is shown to have excellent functional clinical outcomes and long-term survivorship among varying age groups and BMI compared to MBT.

References

Bartel DL, Bicknell VL, Wright TM (1986) The effect of conformity, thickness, and material on stresses in ultra-high molecular weight components for total joint replacement. J Bone Joint Surg Am 68(7):1041–1045. https://doi.org/10.2106/00004623-198668070-00010

Bettinson KA, Pinder IM, Moran CG, Weir DJ, Lingard EA (2009) All-polyethylene compared with metal-backed tibial components in total knee arthroplasty at ten years: a prospective, randomized controlled trial. J Bone Joint Surg Am 91(7):1587–1594. https://doi.org/10.2106/JBJS.G.01427

Blumenfeld TJ, Scott RD (2010) The role of the cemented all-polyethylene tibial component in total knee replacement. A 30-year patient follow-up and review of the literature. Knee 17(6):412–416. https://doi.org/10.1016/j.knee.2009.11.008

Bozic KJ, Kinder J, Menegini M, Zurakowski D, Rosenberg AG, Galante JO (2005) Implant survivorship and complication rates after total knee arthroplasty with a third-generation cemented system: 5 to 8 years followup. Clin Orthop Relat Res (430):117–124. https://doi.org/10.1097/01.blo.0000146539.23869.14

Browne JA, Dempsey IJ, Novicoff W, Wanchek T (2018) When would a metal-backed component become cost-effective over an all-polyethylene tibia in total knee arthroplasty? Am J Orthop (Belle Mead NJ). https://doi.org/10.12788/ajo.2018.0039

Cooper HJ, Ranawat AS, Potter HG, Foo LF, Koob TW, Ranawat CS (2010) Early reactive synovitis and osteolysis after total hip arthroplasty. Clin Orthop Relat Res 468(12):3278–3285. https://doi.org/10.1007/s11999-010-1361-1

Doran J, Yu S, Smith D, Iorio R (2015) The role of all-polyethylene tibial components in modern TKA. J Knee Surg 28(5):382–389. https://doi.org/10.1055/s-0035-1551832

Ehrhardt J, Gadinsky N, Lyman S, Markowicz D, Westrich G (2011) Average 7-year survivorship and clinical results of a newer primary posterior stabilized total knee arthroplasty. HSS J 7(2):120–124. https://doi.org/10.1007/s11420-011-9196-1

Faris PM, Ritter MA, Keating EM, Meding JB, Harty LD (2003) The AGC all-polyethylene tibial component: a ten-year clinical evaluation. J Bone Joint Surg Am 85(3):489–493. https://doi.org/10.2106/00004623-200303000-00014

Fipp GJ (1983) Performance of the tibial component in total knee replacement. J Bone Joint Surg Am 64(7):1026–1033. https://doi.org/10.2106/00004623-198365030-00031

Gill GS, Joshi AB, Mills DM (1999) Total condylar knee arthroplasty: 16- to 21-year results. Clin Orthop Relat Res (367):210–215. https://doi.org/10.1097/00003086-199910000-00026

Gioe TJ, Bowman KR (2000) A randomized comparison of all-polyethylene and metal-backed tibial components. Clin Orthop Relat Res (380):108–115. https://doi.org/10.1097/00003086-200011000-00015

Gioe TJ, Killeen KK, Mehle S, Grimm K (2006) Implementation and application of a community total joint registry: a twelve-year history. J Bone Joint Surg Am 88(6):1399–1404. https://doi.org/10.2106/JBJS.E.01198

Gioe TJ, Sinner P, Mehle S, Ma W, Killeen KK (2007a) Excellent survival of all-polyethylene tibial components in a community joint registry. Clin Orthop Relat Res 464:88–92. https://doi.org/10.1097/BLO.0b013e31812f7879

Gioe TJ, Stroemer ES, Santos ERG (2007b) All-polyethylene and metal-backed tibias have similar outcomes at 10 years: a randomized level II evidence study. Clin Orthop Relat Res 455:212–218. https://doi.org/10.1097/01.blo.0000238863.69486.97

Healy WL, Iorio R, Ko J, Appleby D, Lemos DW (2002) Impact of cost reduction programs on short-term patient outcome and hospital cost of total knee arthroplasty. J Bone Joint Surg Am 84(3):348–353. https://doi.org/10.2106/00004623-200203000-00003

Herschmiller T, Bradley KE, Wellman SS, Attarian DE (2019) Early to midterm clinical and radiographic survivorship of the all polyethylene versus modular metal backed tibia component in primary total knee replacement. J Surg Orthop Adv 28(2):108–114. https://doi.org/10.3113/jsoa.2019.0108

Houdek MT, Wagner ER, Wyles CC, Watts CD, Cass JR, Trousdale RT (2016) All-polyethylene tibial components: an analysis of long-term outcomes and infection. J Arthroplasty 31(7):1476–1482. https://doi.org/10.1016/j.arth.2015.12.048

Kumar V, Hasan O, Umer M, Baloch N (2019) Cemented all-poly tibia in resource constrained country, affordable and cost-effective care. Is it applicable at this era? Review article. Ann Med Surg 47:36–40. https://doi.org/10.1016/j.amsu.2019.09.010

Lewis JL, Askew MJ, Jaycox DP (1982) A comparative evaluation of tibial component designs of total knee prostheses. J Bone Joint Surg Am. https://doi.org/10.2106/00004623-198264010-00018

Meftah M, Blum YC, Raja D, Ranawat AS, Ranawat CS (2012a) Correcting fixed varus deformity with flexion contracture during total knee arthroplasty: the "inside-out" technique. AAOS exhibit selection. J Bone Joint Surg Am 94(10):e66. https://doi.org/10.2106/JBJS.K.01444

Meftah M, Ranawat AS, Sood AB, Rodriguez JA, Ranawat CS (2012b) All-polyethylene tibial implant in young, active patients. A concise follow-up, 10 to 18 years. J Arthroplasty 27(1):10–14. https://doi.org/10.1016/j.arth.2011.05.013

Mohan V, Inacio MCS, Namba RS, Sheth D, Paxton EW (2013) Monoblock all-polyethylene tibial components have a lower risk of early revision than metal-backed modular components. Acta Orthop 84(6):530–536. https://doi.org/10.3109/17453674.2013.862459

Muller SD, Deehan DJ, Holland JP et al (2006) Should we reconsider all-polyethylene tibial implants in total knee replacement? J Bone Joint Surg Br 88(12):1596–1602. https://doi.org/10.1302/0301-620X.88B12.17695

Najibi S, Iorio R, Surdam JW, Whang W, Appleby D, Healy WL (2003) All-polyethylene and metal-backed tibial components in total knee arthroplasty: a matched pair analysis of functional outcome. J Arthroplasty 18(7 Suppl 1):9–15. https://doi.org/10.1016/S0883-5403(03)00304-8

Nouta KA, Verra WC, Pijls BG, Schoones JW, Nelissen RGHH (2012) All-polyethylene tibial components are equal to metal-backed components: systematic review and meta-regression. Clin Orthop Relat Res 470(12):3549–3559. https://doi.org/10.1007/s11999-012-2582-2

Pagnano MW, Levy BA, Berry DJ (1999) Cemented all polyethylene tibial components in patients age 75 years and older. Clin Orthop Relat Res (367):73–80. https://doi.org/10.1097/00003086-199910000-00009

Parsch D, Krüger M, Moser MT, Geiger F (2009) Follow-up of 11-16 years after modular fixed-bearing TKA. Int Orthop 33(2):431–435. https://doi.org/10.1007/s00264-008-0543-x

Pomeroy DL, Schaper LA, Badenhausen WE et al (2000) Results of all-polyethylene tibial components as a cost-saving technique. Clin Orthop Relat Res (380):140–143. https://doi.org/10.1097/00003086-200011000-00018

Ranawat CS, Flynn WF, Saddler S, Hansraj KK, Maynard MJ (1993) Long-term results of the total condylar knee arthroplasty: a 15-year survivorship study. Clin Orthop Relat Res (286):94–102. https://doi.org/10.1097/00003086-199301000-00015

Ranawat AS, Rossi R, Loreti I, Rasquinha VJ, Rodriguez JA, Ranawat CS (2004) Comparison of the PFC sigma fixed-bearing and rotating-platform total knee arthroplasty in the same patient: short-term results. J Arthroplasty 19(1):35–39. https://doi.org/10.1016/j.arth.2003.08.010

Rasquinha VJ, Ranawat CS, Cervieri CL, Rodriguez JA (2006) The press-fit condylar modular total knee system with a posterior cruciate-substituting design: a concise follow-up of a previous report. J Bone Joint Surg Am 88(5):1006–1010. https://doi.org/10.2106/JBJS.C.01104

Robinson RP, Green TM (2011) Eleven-year implant survival rates of the all-polyethylene and metal-backed modular Optetrak posterior stabilized knee in bilateral simultaneous cases. J Arthroplasty 26(8):1165–1169. https://doi.org/10.1016/j.arth.2011.01.009

Small SR, Berend ME, Ritter MA, Buckley CA (2010) A comparison in proximal tibial strain between metal-backed and all-polyethylene anatomic graduated component total knee arthroplasty tibial components. J Arthroplasty 25(5):820–825. https://doi.org/10.1016/j.arth.2009.06.018

Stern SH, Insall JN (1992) Posterior stabilized prosthesis. Results after follow-up of nine to twelve years. J Bone Joint Surg Am 74(7):980–986. https://doi.org/10.2106/00004623-199274070-00004

Stiehl JB, Komistek RD, Dennis DA (1999) Detrimental kinematics of a flat on flat total condylar knee arthroplasty. Clin Orthop Relat Res (365):139–148. https://doi.org/10.1097/00003086-199908000-00019

Cementless Total Knee Arthroplasty

Bradley A. King and Arthur L. Malkani

Contents

E. Hansen, K.-D. Kühn (eds.), *Essentials of Cemented Knee Arthroplasty*,
https://doi.org/10.1007/978-3-662-63113-3_32

32.1 Introduction

Cemented fixation for total knee arthroplasty (TKA) remains the gold standard for primary TKA worldwide with a record of excellent clinical outcomes and implant survivorship for up to 20 years (Scuderi and Insall 1992; Attar et al. 2008; Falatyn et al. 1995). Cementless TKA designs have been present since the 1980s with variable outcomes (Meneghini and Hanssen 2008). Early cementless implants contained flaws and never gained traction due to multiple factors such as patch porous coating, poor polyethylene locking mechanisms, tibial screw augmentation leading to screw track osteolysis, femoral component fracture, and patella failures. Corrections of these design flaws, together with advances in biomaterials, have led to a new generation of cementless TKA implants. As demonstrated in total hip arthroplasty (THA), cementless fixation is advantageous because of intimate biologic fixation, leading to long-term durable survivorship.

32

Joint arthroplasty, previously performed in a more sedentary and elderly population with end-stage osteoarthritis, continues to experience a changing demographic to include younger, more active, and obese patients (Kurtz et al. 2007, 2009; Dalury 2016). The proportion of younger patients undergoing TKA increased between 1993 and 2006. The demand for primary TKA in patients ages 45–54 years is projected to increase by 17 times from 2006 to 2030. Patients younger than 65 years are expected to make up the majority of demand for primary or revision TKA by 2030 (Kurtz et al. 2009). The prevalence of TKA has increased across all age groups in the past two decades. In 2015, the estimated prevalence of patients living with a TKA in the United States was 0.68% at 50 years, 2.92% at 60 years, 7.29% at 70 years, 10.38% at 80 years, and 8.48% at 90 years (Maradit Kremers et al. 2015). Increased life expectancy, together with this increasing prevalence of TKA, means more patients are living longer with knee implants, therefore placing increased stress at the bone–cement–implant interface.

Obesity continues to be a major problem in the United States. The combined number of patients undergoing TKA categorized as obese or morbidly obese (BMI ≥30) increased significantly from 1990 to 2005 from 42% to 60%. Obese patients make up a disproportionately large proportion of TKA patients, as the nationwide prevalence of obesity in 2005 was 32% (compared to 60% of TKA population) (Fehring et al. 2007). By 2030, it is estimated that 87% of adults in the United States will be either overweight or obese (Wang et al. 2008).

Aseptic loosening is the one of the most common reasons for revision TKA. The cement–bone interface has been shown to attenuate over time (Miller et al. 2014). Studying a series of postmortem retrieved knee implants, it was found that implants with greater time in service had less interlock at the cement–bone interface, demonstrated by resorption of the trabeculae in the cement interlock region (Miller et al. 2014; Sharkey et al. 2014).

> Younger patients with active lifestyles and obese patients pose a challenge to cemented TKA due to greater amounts of stress on the cement–bone interface.

Cement has poor resistance to shear and tension forces that are present in greater amounts at this interface in larger or active patients (Lewis 1997; Harrysson et al. 2004). Abdel et al. (2015) demonstrated that patients with a BMI > 35 experienced a two times greater risk of revision with cemented implants due to aseptic tibial loosening compared to patients with a BMI < 35, regardless of age or coronal alignment. Patients experiencing aseptic loosening of the tibia in their study were statistically younger. Meehan et al. (2014) demonstrated that the risk of revision surgery due to aseptic loosening in cemented primary TKA at 1 year postoperatively in patients <50 years old was 4.7 times greater than that of a >65-year-old cohort.

> Long-term component fixation remains a concern in the obese and younger population.

32.2 Cementless TKA Designs

Given the current and anticipated demand for TKA by younger and heavier patients, there is an emphasis on improving the reliability and survivorship of joint replacements. With the past success of cementless THA, there has been an increased interest in the use of cementless TKA to provide biologic fixation over mechanical cement fixation for long-term durability. However, given the failure rates of first-generation cementless TKA, a cautious approach is needed in proceeding with newer- or second-generation cementless TKA designs.

32.2.1 Early Cementless TKA Designs

> The first generation of cementless TKA designs in the 1980s had limited acceptance due to fixation and design flaws leading to high failure and poor clinical outcomes.

Early cementless implants had multiple design flaws including the following

- Patch porous coating
- Poor polyethylene locking mechanisms
- Tibial screw augmentation leading to screw track osteolysis
- Femoral component fracture
- Patella failures

Additionally, these first-generation design implants did not provide adequate mechanical fixation for immediate implant stability (Meneghini and Hanssen 2008; Cherian et al. 2014; Berger et al. 2001).

Tibial component fixation in early designs was inconsistent and had issues with initial fixation. Dunbar et al. (2009) used radiostereometric analysis to demonstrate that immediate rigid implant stability is essential for long-term biological fixation in cementless TKA. Early designs did not attain adequate initial mechanical fixation to allow for bony ingrowth due to multiple reasons, in addition to issues with liftoff and subsidence (Matassi et al. 2014). These first-generation designs had an increased incidence of progressive radiolucent lines at the implant–bone interface leading to aseptic loosening (Rand 1991; Rosenberg et al. 1990). Stems or screws were added to enhance initial fixation to allow for osseointegration. These screw tracks created an access channel into the tibial metaphysis for debris. Together with first-generation polyethylene and a poor polyethylene liner locking mechanism, particulate debris caused osteolysis along the screw track (◘ Fig. 32.1). The incidence of screw track osteolysis was reported to be greater than 30% in some cementless tibial component designs (Lewis et al. 1995; Peters Jr et al. 1992). Holloway et al. (2010) showed reliable fixation with screwless cementless tibial baseplates at an average of 7.6 years follow-up. Other studies have also demonstrated no advantage to using tibial baseplate with or without screws (Ferguson et al. 2008; Schepers et al. 2012; Ritter and Meneghini 2010). Another cause of metaphyseal osteolysis and loosening was baseplates with a patch porous coating, which created access channels that allowed particulate debris to spread into the metaphysis (Whiteside 1995). Subsequent designs had a circumferential and fully porous-coated surface to prevent this problem.

Early patellar failures were due to both flawed design and surgical technique. Femoral components had a nonanatomic trochlea (Varadarajan et al. 2011). Less atten-

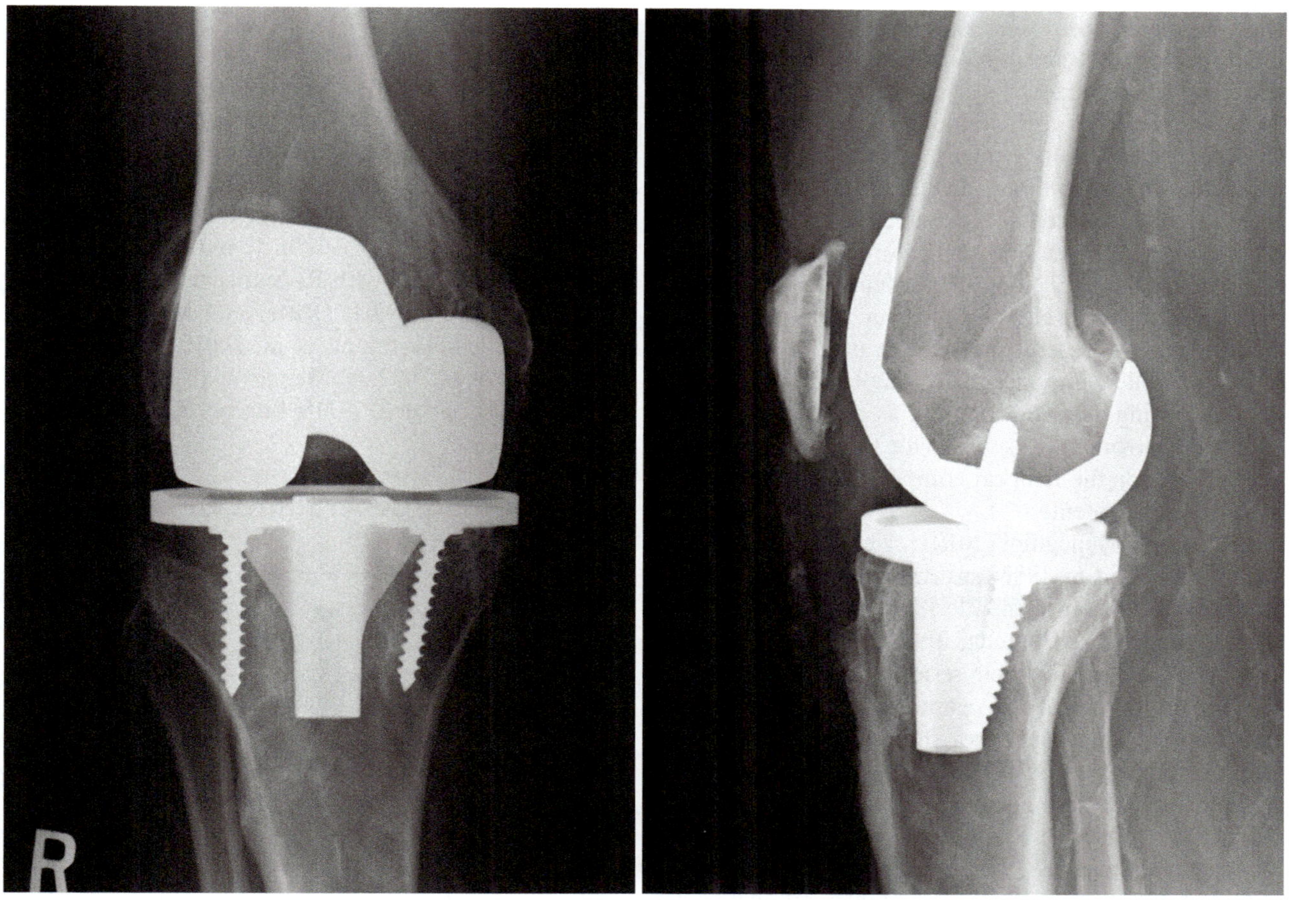

◘ **Fig. 32.1** AP and lateral radiographs of first-generation cementless TKA with polyethylene wear and osteolysis along the screw track in the tibial metaphysis tion was given to femoral component rotation leading to malalignment and wear (Ritter and Meneghini 2010). The use of first-generation polyethylene along with a metal-backed patella also accelerated polyethylene wear leading to metal-on-metal articulation with the femoral component and eventual metallosis (Berger et al. 2001; Ritter and Meneghini 2010). Failure of the metal-backed patella was the most common mode of failure of early cementless TKA designs due to polyethylene wear, failure of ingrowth, and dissociation of the metal and polyethylene components (Rosenberg et al. 1988; Lombardi Jr et al. 1988).

While early designs of cementless tibial and patellar implants had concerns, early design cementless femoral components fared well. The femoral implant attains its initial mechanical stability through the multiplanar bone cut providing initial stability for bony ingrowth. Some early design cementless femoral components did fail due to fatigue fracture at weak points along the implant (Whiteside et al. 1993). Early femoral components, both cemented and cementless, were not designed to optimize patellar tracking, which contributed to patella polyethylene wear and metal-backed patellar component failure.

Despite design flaws and problems with the metal-backed patella, there were successes with femoral and tibial fixation. In a review of primary cementless TKA with the Miller-Galante 1 system (Zimmer, Warsaw, IN) at an average of 11 years follow-up, Berger et al. (2001) reported mixed results: cementless femoral fixation was excellent, whereas 48% of metal-backed patellar components were revised. These patellar component failures led to a 12% femoral revision rate due to femoral component damage. None of the femoral components were loose and none had radiolucency. Cementless tibial fixation had a 9% aseptic loosening rate and 12% of the well-fixed tibial components had small osteolytic lesions develop. Using aseptic loosening as the end point, the 10-year survivorship was 90.7% for the patellar component, 100% for the femoral component, and 94.3% for the tibial component.

Ritter and Meneghini (2010) reviewed 73 cementless knees from 1984 to 1986 and demonstrated that many of the early cases of cementless TKA failures were due to the metal-backed patella. Twelve of the 15 failures leading to revision in their series were due to patellar component failure with an overall 76.4% survivorship at 20 years. The survivorship of the cementless tibial and femoral components was 96.8%.

Bassett (1998) reviewed 1000 consecutive primary TKA using the Performance prosthesis (Biomet/Kirschner, Warsaw, IN) from 1988–1993. Of these, 584 cases had cementless femoral and tibial components. All had a cemented all-polyethylene patella. At an average of 5.2-year follow-up, the implant survival rate in the cementless group was 99%, with slightly higher subjective and functional knee scores for cementless knees compared to knees with cemented components. There were a number of early cementless TKA designs that were able to achieve successful long-term results similar to cemented TKA with 10-year survival rates greater than 94% (Table 32.1) (Ritter and Meneghini 2010; Whiteside 1994; Hofmann et al. 2001; Schroder et al. 2001; Khaw et al. 2002; Hardeman et al. 2006; Watanabe et al. 2004; Tarkin et al. 2005; Buechel Sr et al. 2001).

Table 32.1 First-generation cementless TKA survivorship studies

Research group	Length of follow-up (years)	Survivorship (%)	Design
Whiteside (1994)	10	94.1	Ortholoc
Hofmann et al. (2001)	10	95.1	Natural
Schroder et al. (2001)	10	97.1	AGC-2000
Khaw et al. (2002)	10	95.6	PFC
Hardeman et al. (2006)	10	97.1	Profix
Watanabe et al. (2004)	13	96.7	Osteonics
Tarkin et al. (2005)	17	97.9	LCS-RP
Buechel Sr et al. (2001)	18	98.3	LCS-RP
Ritter and Meneghini (2010)	20	98.6	AGC

32.2.2 Second-Generation Cementless TKA Designs

> Lessons learned from early cementless TKA design flaws, together with advances in biomaterials and manufacturing processes, have led to the creation of a second generation of cementless TKA implants.

The emergence of new biomaterials, such as hydroxyapatite (Soballe et al. 1991a, b, 1992), porous tantalum (Bobyn et al. 1999; Cohen 2002; Zhang et al. 1999), and highly porous titanium (Frenkel et al. 2004), and advanced manufacturing techniques have led to implants with improved ability to achieve early mechanical stability to allow for long-term biologic ingrowth. The initial fixation strength can be achieved without screw fixation eliminating the risk of screw track osteolysis. Improved wear characteristics of highly cross-linked polyethylene along with improved polyethylene tibial baseplate locking mechanisms have minimized the risk of polyethylene wear and osteolysis.

Modern-design cementless TKA implants are composed of highly porous metals, such as tantalum or titanium with increased porosity leading to improved capacity for osseointegration compared to first-generation implants (Levine et al. 2006). The greatest potential for biologic fixation exists with a pore size range of 100–700 μm, an average pore size of 400–500 μm, and 55–65% overall porosity (Bobyn et al. 1999; Levine et al. 2006). In the absence of screw fixation, the initial fixation and immediate stability comes from interference fit and frictional resistance to motion. A high-friction surface is desirable in order to improve initial fixation (Dimaano et al. 2010). Highly porous tantalum has been used in the manufacturing of cementless TKA (Trabecular Metal™, Zimmer-Biomet, Warsaw, IN) (◘ Fig. 32.2). Porous tantalum has improved material elasticity and increased surface friction compared to first-generation designs. The coefficient of friction of porous tantalum (0.88–0.98) is greater than prior cementless designs that included porous coating or sintered beads (0.66). The modulus of elasticity of tantalum is between cortical and cancellous bone, creating a more physiologic stress transfer to the periprosthetic bone interface (Lombardi Jr et al. 2007; Karageorgiou and Kaplan 2005).

Highly porous titanium, formed using laser sintering technology through an additive manufacturing process, has also been used in modern-design cementless TKA (Tritanium®, Stryker, Mahwah, NJ) (◘ Fig. 32.3). This porous titanium tibial baseplate has a porosity of 65–70%, which is greater than that of traditional titanium or cobalt–chrome beads. Highly porous titanium has a coefficient of friction of 1.01 ± 0.18 (Dimaano et al. 2010). The manufacturing process consists of laser rapid manufacturing wherein commercially pure titanium or a titanium alloy powder is deposited layer by layer using computer-based designs and laser sintering technology. Advantages of additive manufacturing include the creation of either solid, porous, or fenestrated features on an implant of any form that cannot be attained through conventional manufacturing. This technology can optimize porosity for ingrowth and has the ability to manufacture complex geometries including the solid keel with porous tibial fixation at the baseplate or porous pegs designed at specific locations.

Initial implant stability is crucial to allow for osseointegration, which had been an issue with first-generation cementless tibial component designs. Bhimji and Meneghini (2014) studied two cementless baseplate designs:

- One with two hexagonal pegs made of porous tantalum without a keel.
- The other with four cruciform pegs of porous titanium which also included a keel.

Their findings demonstrated that a baseplate with dual-hex peg fixation without a keel experienced more rocking motions, making it susceptible to larger amounts of liftoff than the baseplate with a keel and four surrounding pegs.

Hydroxyapatite (HA) coatings are osteoconductive, facilitating the formation of bone structure and potentially contributing to more stable fixation over the years. HA coatings can enhance the stability of implants by promoting early bone ingrowth even in the presence of small gaps or initial instability (Dumbleton and Manley 2004). In a review of HA-coated cementless tibia components, Voigt and Mosier (2011) found that longer term durability may be enhanced with HA-coated implants, particularly in patients who are younger than 70 years of age.

32.3 Surgical Technique

Adequate bone quality is needed for mechanical stability and osseointegration. When compared to normal controls, cementless tibial components show decreased mechanical stability in osteoporotic bone (Meneghini et al. 2011).

> However, at present, definite objective preoperative studies from which to base a selection criteria for cementless TKA are lacking. The author's indications include young, active patients, and morbidly obese patients with good bone quality.

Preoperative radiographs can be used initially as a tool to determine bone quality, but intraoperative evaluation of the patient's bone quality is needed.

> Contraindications may include patients with osteoporotic bone, the elderly, posttraumatic arthritis where the bone vascularity is compromised, and in cases with bone loss requiring grafts or augments.

Whereas cemented fixation allows for slightly imperfect bony cuts, bony defects, and variable bone porosity, cementless TKA requires a rim fit with maximum coverage of the available host proximal tibia bone surface for coverage with the tibial implant. The preparation

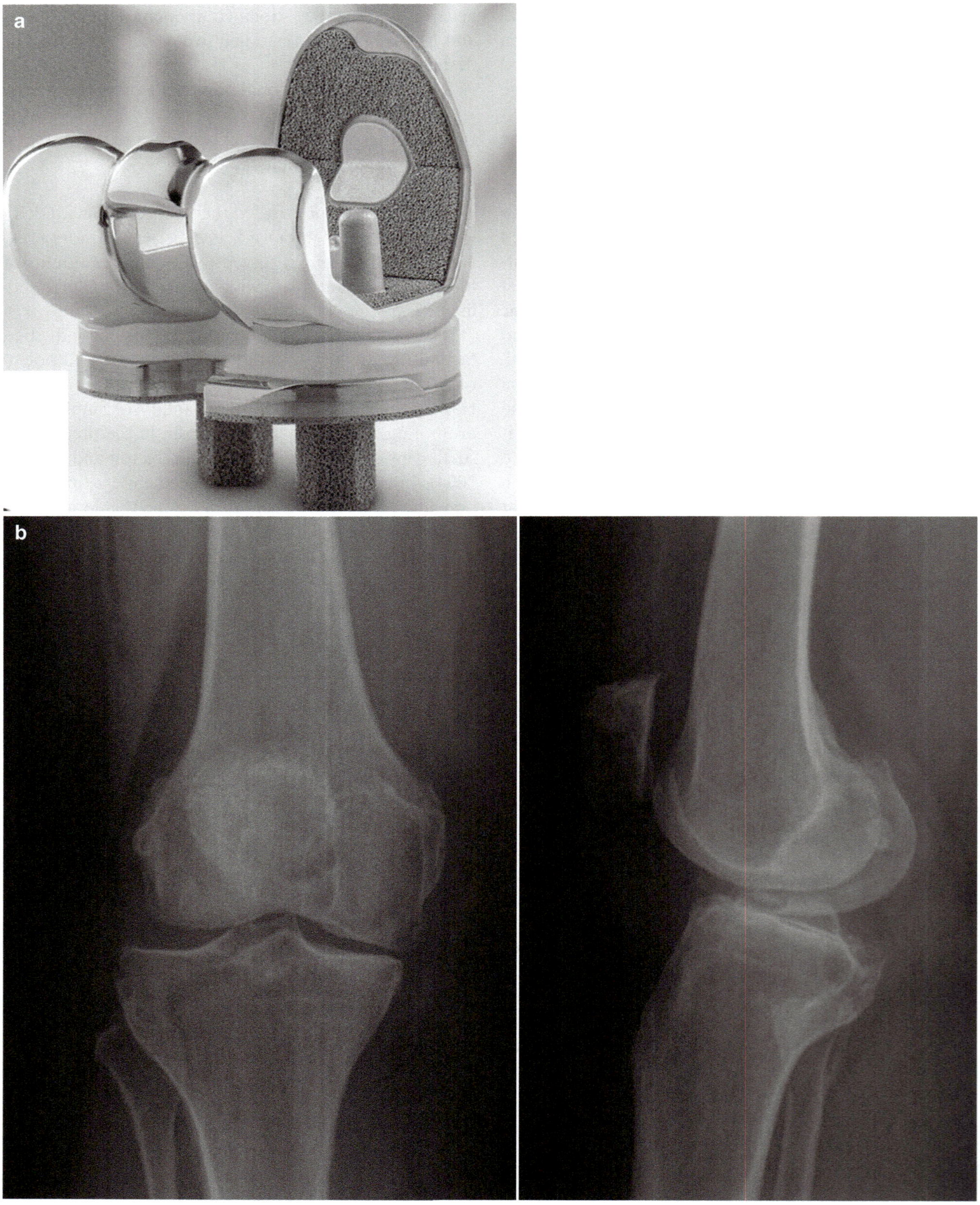

■ **Fig. 32.2** **a** Zimmer Persona® cementless TKA design. **b** Preoperative AP and lateral radiographs of a 67-year-old female with right knee osteoarthritis. **c** Postoperative AP and lateral knee radiographs using the Persona® design

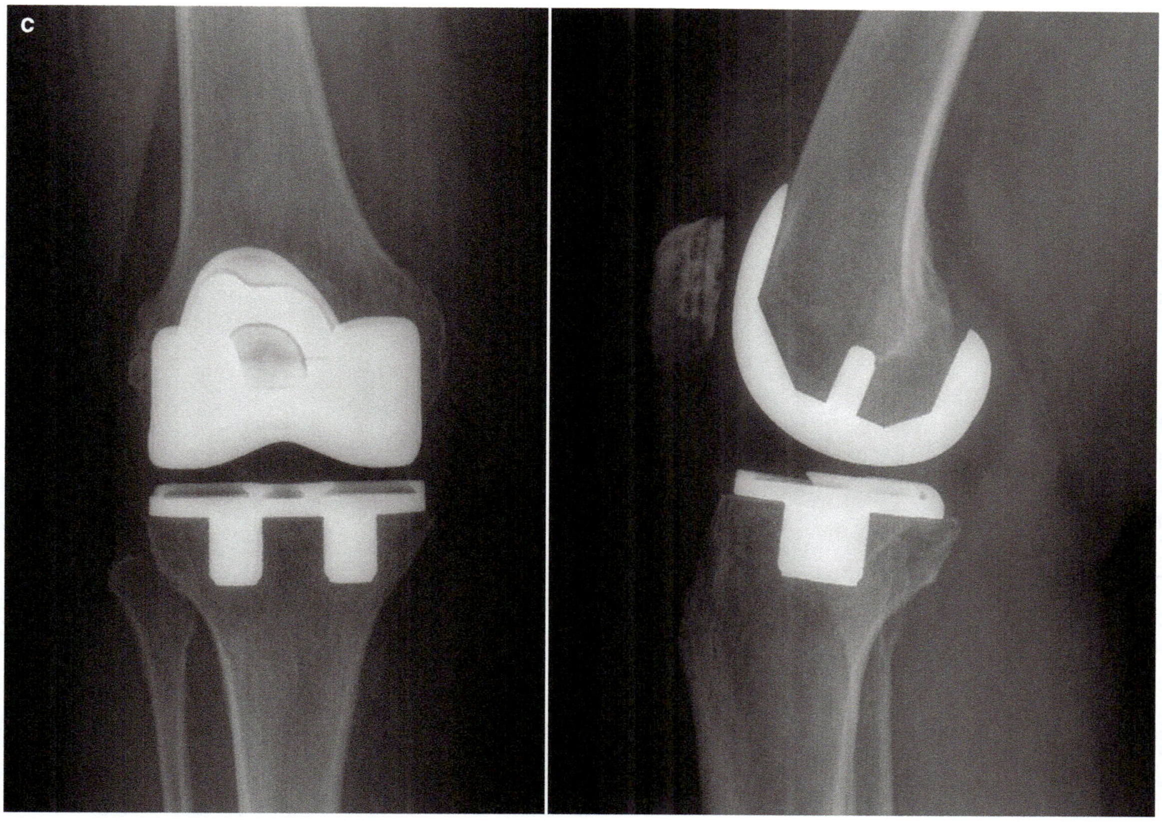

Fig. 32.2 (continued)

of the tibial plateau can result in an uneven surface in cases of very sclerotic bone as the saw blade can skive off the dense sclerotic bone. Togsvig-Larsen and Ryd (1991) reported the potential of a 1–2 mm gap between the uppermost and lowermost points of a cut tibial surface. An uneven cut may contribute to implant instability with weight-bearing and possible subsequent loss of fixation. The tibial cut can be evaluated intraoperatively with the "four corners" technique described by Whiteside, that being digital impaction of each corner of a flat tibial baseplate trial to ensure no liftoff. Cementless posteriorly stabilized (PS) TKA carried additional concerns about micromotion at the tibial fixation interface caused by cam–post engagement potentially leading to aseptic loosening (Mikulak et al. 2001). These early concerns have not endured. Harwin et al. (2018) reviewed cementless PS TKA at minimum 7-year follow-up, and at a mean of approximately 8 years excellent survivorship of 98% was maintained.

32.4 Results

> Several recent studies have compared the survivorship of cemented versus cementless TKA with promising results for modern cementless TKA designs.

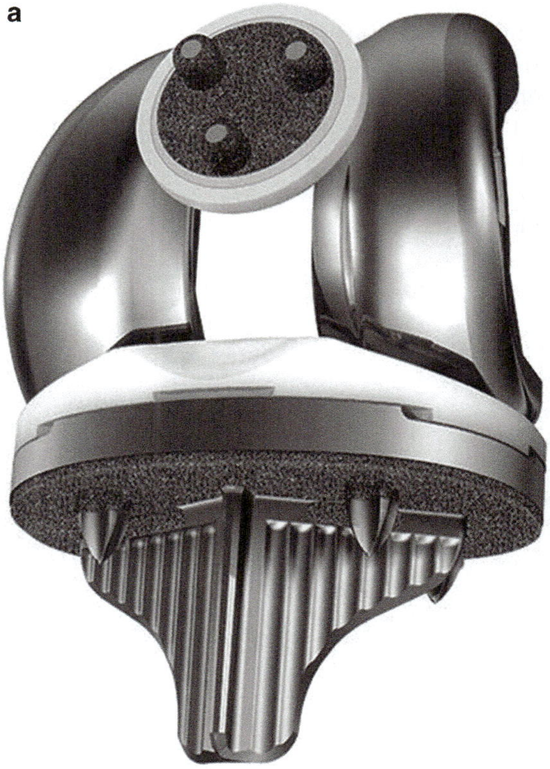

Fig. 32.3 **a** Stryker Triathlon® cementless TKA design. **b** Preoperative AP and lateral radiographs of a 63-year old female with left knee osteoarthritis. **c** Postoperative AP and lateral knee radiographs using the cementless Triathlon®

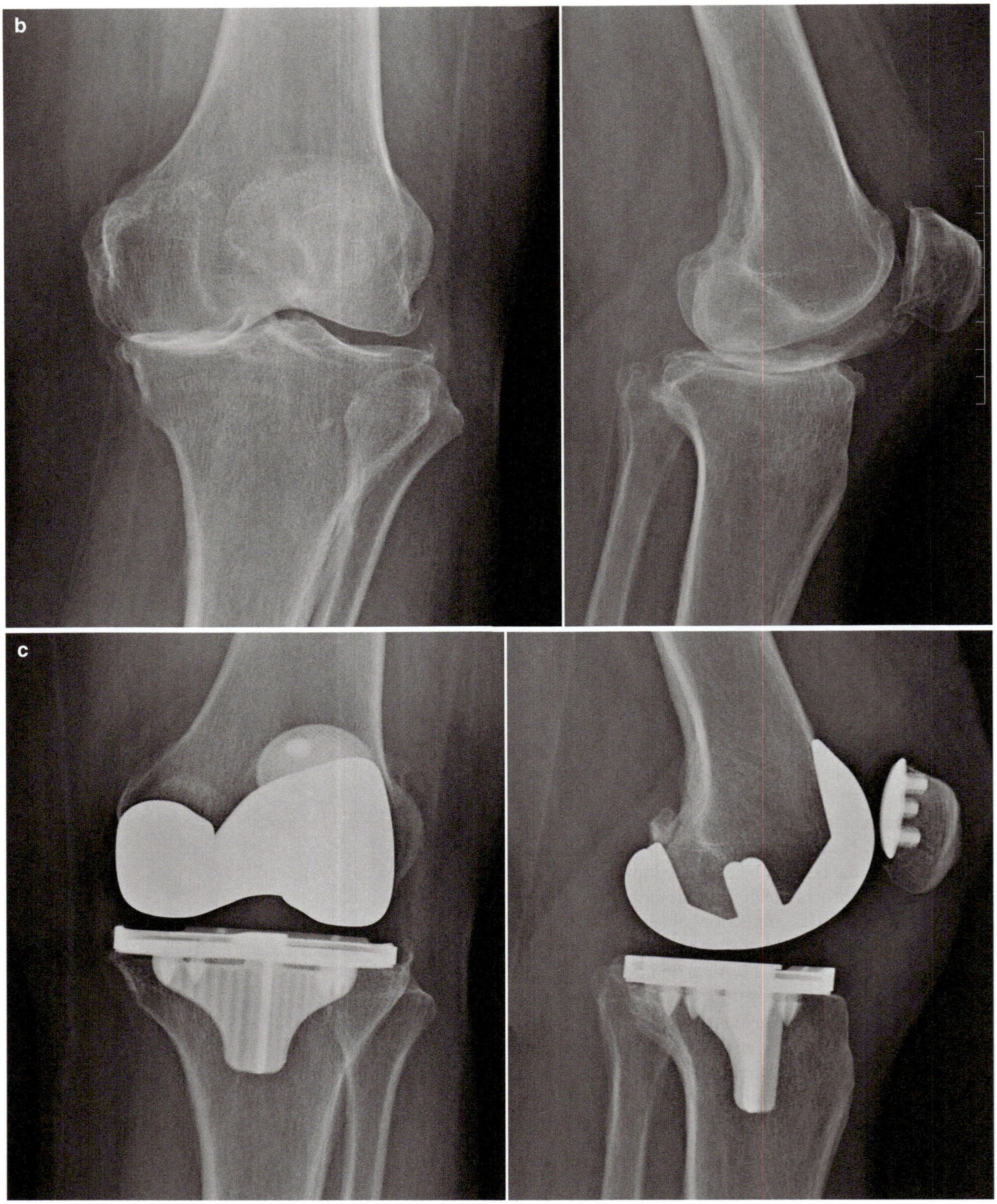

■ **Fig. 32.3** (continued)

In a retrospective study comparing cemented versus cementless fixation for primary TKA using the same implant design, Miller et al. (2018) demonstrated a failure rate due to aseptic loosening of 0.5% at an average follow-up of 2.4 years following TKA using a cementless highly porous tibial baseplate. The matched cemented cohort with the same implant design had an aseptic failure rate of 2.5%. Boyle et al. (2018) performed a similar retrospective review using a single CR system in cemented versus cementless TKA in patients with BMI > 30 with a mean follow-up of 5.7 years. In their study, 154 uncemented patients and 171 cemented patients were found to have a 99.3% and 99.4% survivorship for tibial aseptic loosening, respectively.

In a retrospective study of cemented versus cementless PS TKA in morbidly obese patients with a mean BMI of 45 and 5-year follow-up, there was an overall revision rate of 5.4% with a revision rate of 0.9% for aseptic loosening in the cementless group versus a 25.9% overall revision rate and 11.8% aseptic loosening failure in the cemented cohort. Survivorship with aseptic loosening as the end point was 92.9% at 5 years for the cementless group and 88.2% at 8 years for the cemented group (Sinicrope et al. 2019). In a similar earlier study at the same institution, Bagsby et al. (2016) demonstrated improved survivorship of the cementless TKA prosthesis over the cemented TKA for all causes of revision and for aseptic loosening. Their study demonstrated that morbidly obese patients undergoing cementless TKA had a lower rate of aseptic revision, greater improvement in functional scores, and comparable postoperative range-of-motion to patients who underwent cemented TKA.

They concluded that cementless fixation may provide biologic bony ingrowth leading to a more durable implant–bone interface, which may better tolerate the added mechanical stress generated in this challenging patient population.

Cementless TKA has also been effective in a younger population. In a review of 29 young patients (mean age 45 years) undergoing cementless TKA, at average of 4-year follow-up, the overall implant survivorship was 100%. There were no failures or revision surgeries performed and no evidence of radiographic loosening (Mont et al. 2017). In a separate study, a Kaplan–Meier survivorship analysis showed primary cemented TKA patients <55 years old had significantly higher rates of revision due to aseptic loosening at both 5 and 10 years postoperatively compared with cementless TKA (McCalden et al. 2013).

There are multiple studies demonstrating excellent survivorship for modern cementless TKA designs

Table 32.2 Modern design cementless TKA survivorship studies

Research group	Length of follow-up (years)	Survivorship (%)	Design
Harwin et al. (2015)	4	99.5	Triathlon®
Boyle et al. (2018)	5	99.3	Triathlon®
Kwong et al. (2014)	7	95.7	NexGen®
Cross and Parish (2005)	10	99.6	Active
Tai and Cross (2006)	12	97.5	Active
Kim et al. (2014)	17	98.9	NexGen®

(Table 32.2) (Boyle et al. 2018; Harwin et al. 2015; Kwong et al. 2014; Cross and Parish 2005; Tai and Cross 2006; Kim et al. 2014).

Cementless components experience a period of initial migration before osseointegration. In a study investigating the press-fit fixation of Stryker Triathlon® cementless tibial baseplate and metal-backed patella to the underlying bone, most component migration was observed over the first 6 postoperative weeks, after which no significant migration between the 12- and 24-month timepoints was observed. This demonstrates the biphasic migration pattern in cementless components, characterized by a high initial migration followed by stabilization. This suggests osseointegration of the components at about 6 weeks (Nevelos et al. 2019). The micromotion experienced by cementless tibial components may indicate a lower initial mechanical stability than cemented components. However, this difference in initial stability may be subclinical, as the differences between average cemented and cementless micromotion were <150 μm in one study (Crook et al. 2017). In a study by Dunbar et al. (2009), 70 patients were randomized to a cemented or cementless tantalum tibial baseplate (NexGen®, Zimmer-Biomet, Warsaw, IN). A radiosteroemetric analysis was performed at 6, 12, and 24 months. Cementless components experienced migration, with 9/28 components migrating >1 mm at 1 year. These components then stabilized and none were considered be at risk for early aseptic loosening, whereas 4/21 cemented components were at risk for early aseptic loosening.

Radiolucent lines (RLL) following TKA are concerning for osteolysis and loosening. In a study by

Aebli et al. (2004), the radiographic results from 91 cementless TKA over a 7.5-year follow-up showed that RLL appeared most frequently near the tibial plateau and that most RLL were present immediately postoperatively or appeared within the first year (96%). RLL were largely non-progressive (99%). In a review of a primary cementless TKA using a CR RP TKA system, there were femoral and/or tibial radiolucencies at almost all time points including 6 weeks, 1 year, and final follow-up with an average final follow-up of 9.6 years. These were found to be non-progressive partial and stable lines at final follow-up. In addition, the presence of these stable RLLs did not seem to affect the functional outcome of these patients at final follow-up (Costales et al. 2020). These results suggest that if RLLs are visible within the first year postoperatively, but do not increase further, observation or conservative treatment can be pursued.

Nam et al. (2017) compared cementless versus cemented total knee implants and demonstrated no difference in blood loss or change in hemoglobin but did show decreased operative time in the cementless group. There have been concerns of increased bleeding due to lack of tamponade by cement that have not been substantiated. Given the ongoing transition to alternative payment models by insurance providers, the value of healthcare continues to be evaluated. Cementless components are more expensive than their cemented counterparts. However, savings in the non-implant costs of decreased surgical time and not using cement negate these higher implant costs (Yayac et al. 2020). There are several modern design implants available for cementless TKA fixation at present (Table 32.3).

Table 32.3 Modern design cementless TKA implants available in the United States

Company	System
DePuy	Attune®
Donjoy	EMPOWR™
Exactech	Truliant®
Medacta	GMK
MicroPort	Evolution®
Stryker	Triathlon®
Zimmer	NexGen®
Zimmer	Persona®

Take-Home Messages

- Younger patients with active lifestyles and obese patients pose a challenge to cemented components due to greater amounts of stress on the cement–bone interface. Long-term component fixation remains a concern in this population.
- First-generation cementless knee components contained design flaws. Lessons learned from these flaws, together with advances in materials and manufacturing techniques, have given rise to the modern generation of cementless components with excellent mid-term results.
- Modern-design cementless TKA components have demonstrated equivalent and even improved survivorship in certain patient populations, including the young and the morbidly obese. Cementless fixation may provide biologic bony ingrowth leading to a more durable implant–bone interface, which may better tolerate the added mechanical stress generated inthesepatient populations.
- Objective preoperative studies from which to base a selection criteria for cementless TKA are lacking. The author's indications include young, active patients, and morbidly obese patients with good bone quality. Contraindications may include patients with osteoporotic bone, the elderly, post-traumatic arthritis where the bone vascularity is compromised, and in cases with bone loss requiring grafts or augments.

References

Abdel MP, Bonadurer GF, Jennings MT, Hanssen AD (2015) Increasedaseptic tibial failures in patients with a BMI ≥ 35 and well-aligned total knee arthroplasties. J Arthroplasty 30(12):2181–2184

Aebli N, Krebs J, Schwenke D, Hii T, Wehrli U (2004) Progression of radiolucent lines in cementless twin-bearing low-contact-stress knee prostheses: a retrospective study. J Arthroplasty 19(6):783–789

Attar FG, Khaw FM, Kirk LM, Gregg PJ (2008) Survivorship analysis at 15 years of cemented press-fit condylar total knee arthroplasty. J Arthroplasty 23(3):344–349

Bagsby DT, Issa K, Smith LS, Elmallah RK, Mast LE, Harwin SF, Mont MA, Bhimani SJ, Malkani AL (2016) Cemented vs cementless total kneearthroplasty in morbidly obese patients. J Arthroplasty 31(8):1727–1731

Bassett RW (1998) Results of 1,000 performance knees: cementless versus cemented fixation. J Arthroplasty 13(4):409–413

Berger RA, Lyon JH, Jacobs JJ, Barden RM, Berkson EM, Sheinkop MB, Rosenberg AG, Galante JO (2001) Problems with cementless total knee arthroplasty at 11 years followup. Clin Orthop Relat Res 392(392):196–207

Bhimji S, Meneghini RM (2014) Micromotion of cementless tibial baseplates: keels with adjuvant pegs offer more stability than pegs alone. J Arthroplasty 29(7):1503–1506
Bobyn JD, Stackpool GJ, Hacking SA, Tanzer M, Krygier JJ (1999) Characteristics of boneingrowth and interface mechanics of a new poroustantalumbiomaterial. J Bone Joint Surg Br 81(5):907–914
Boyle KK, Nodzo SR, Ferraro JT, Augenblick DJ, Pavlesen S, Phillips MJ (2018) Uncemented vs cemented cruciate retaining total knee arthroplasty in patients with body mass index greater than 30. J Arthroplasty 33(4):1082–1088
Buechel FF Sr, Buechel FF Jr, Pappas MJ, D'Alessio J (2001) Twenty-year evaluation of meniscal bearing and rotating platform knee replacements. Clin Orthop Relat Res (388):41–50
Cherian JJ, Banerjee S, Kapadia BH, Jauregui JJ, Harwin SF, Mont MA (2014) Cementless total knee arthroplasty: a review. J Knee Surg 27(3):193–197
Cohen R (2002) A porous tantalum trabecular metal: basic science. Am J Orthop 31(4):216–217
Costales TG, Chapman DM, Dalury DF (2020) The natural history of radiolucencies following uncemented total knee arthroplasty at 9 years. J Arthroplasty 35(1):127–131
Crook PD, Owen JR, Hess SR, Al-Humadi S, Wayne JS, Jiranek WA (2017) Initial stability of cemented vs cementless tibial components under cyclicload. J Arthroplasty 32(8):2556–2562
Cross MJ, Parish EN (2005) A hydroxyapatite-coated total knee replacement: prospective analysis of 1000 patients. J Bone Joint Surg Br 87(8):1073–1076
Dalury DF (2016) Cementless total knee arthroplasty: current concepts review. Bone Joint J 98-B(7):867–873
Dimaano F, Hermida J, D'Lima D, Cowell CW, Kulesha G (2010) Comparison of the coefficient of friction of porous ingrowth surfaces. 56th annual meeting of the Orthopaedic Research Society
Dumbleton J, Manley MT (2004) Hydroxyapatite-coated prostheses in total hip and knee arthroplasty. J Bone Joint Surg Am 86(11):2526–2540
Dunbar MJ, Wilson DA, Hennigar AW, Amirault JD, Gross M, Reardon GP (2009) Fixation of a trabecular metal knee arthroplasty component. A prospective randomized study. J Bone Joint Surg Am 91(7):1578–1586
Falatyn S, Lachiewicz PF, Wilson FC (1995) Survivorship analysis of cemented total condylar knee arthroplasty. Clin Orthop Relat Res (317):178–184
Fehring TK, Odum SM, Griffin WL, Mason JB, McCoy TH (2007) The obesityepidemic: its effect on total joint arthroplasty. J Arthroplasty 22(6):71–76
Ferguson RP, Friederichs MG, Hofmann AA (2008) Comparison of screw and screwless fixation in cementless total knee arthroplasty. Orthopedics 31(2):127–110
Frenkel SR, Jaffe WL, Dimaano F, Iesaka K, Hua T (2004) Bone response to a novel highly porous surface in a canine implantable chamber. J Biomed Mater Res B Appl Biomater 71(2):387–391
Hardeman F, Vandenneucker H, Van Lauwe J, Bellemans J (2006) Cementless total knee arthroplasty with Profix: a 8- to 10-year follow-up study. Knee 13(6):419–421
Harrysson OLA, Robertsson O, Nayfeh JF (2004) Higher cumulative revision rate of knee arthroplasties in younger patients with osteoarthritis. Clin Orthop Relat Res 421:162–168
Harwin SF, Elmallah RK, Jauregui JJ, Cherian JJ, Mont MA (2015) Outcomes of a newer-generation cementless total knee arthroplasty design. Orthopedics 38(10):620–624
Harwin SF, Levin JM, Khlopas A, Ramkumar PN, Piuzzi NS, Roche M, Mont MA (2018) Cementless posteriorly stabilized total knee arthroplasty: seven-year minimum follow-up report. J Arthroplasty 33(5):1399–1403
Hofmann AA, Evanich JD, Ferguson RP, Camargo MP (2001) Ten- to 14-year clinical followup of the cementless natural knee system. Clin Orthop Relat Res 388:85–94
Holloway IP, Lusty PJ, Walter WL, Walter WK, Zicat BA (2010) Tibial fixation without screws in cementless knee arthroplasty. J Arthroplasty 25(1):46–51
Karageorgiou V, Kaplan D (2005) Porosity of 3D biomaterial scaffolds and osteogenesis. Biomaterials 26(27):5474–5491
Khaw FM, Kirk LM, Morris RW, Gregg PJ (2002) A randomised, controlled trial of cemented versus cementless press-fit condylar total knee replacement. Ten-year survival analysis. J Bone Joint Surg Br 84(5):658–666
Kim YH, Park JW, Lim HM, Park ES (2014) Cementless and cemented total knee arthroplasty in patients younger than fifty five years. Which is better? Int Orthop 38(2):297–303
Kurtz S, Ong K, Lau E, Mowat F, Halpern M (2007) Projections of primary and revision hip and knee arthroplasty in the United States from 2005 to 2030. J Bone Joint Surg Am 89(4):780–785
Kurtz SM, Lau E, Ong K, Zhao K, Kelly M, Bozic KJ (2009) Future young patient demand for primary and revision joint replacement: national projections from 2010 to 2030. Clin Orthop Relat Res 467(10):2606–2612
Kwong LM, Nielsen ES, Ruiz DR, Hsu AH, Dines MD, Mellano CM (2014) Cementless total knee replacement fixation: a contemporary durable solution--affirms. Bone Joint J 96-B(11 Supple A):87–92
Levine BR, Sporer S, Poggie RA, Della Valle CJ, Jacobs JJ (2006) Experimental and clinical performance of porous tantalum in orthopedic surgery. Biomaterials 27(27):4671–4681
Lewis G (1997) Properties of acrylicbonecement: state of the art review. J Biomed Mater Res 38(2):155–182
Lewis PL, Rorabeck CH, Bourne RB (1995) Screw osteolysis after cementless total knee replacement. Clin Orthop Relat Res (321):173–177
Lombardi AV Jr, Engh GA, Volz RG, Albrigo JL, Brainard BJ (1988) Fracture/dissociation of the polyethylene in metal-backed patellar components in total knee arthroplasty. J Bone Joint Surg Am 70(5):675–679
Lombardi AV Jr, Berasi CC, Berend KR (2007) Evolution of tibial fixation in total kneearthroplasty. J Arthroplasty 22(4):25–29
Maradit Kremers H, Larson DR, Kremers WK, Crowson CS, Berry DJ, Washington RE, Steiner CA, Jiranek WA (2015) Prevalence of total hip and knee replacement in the United States. J Bone Joint Surg Am 97(17):1386–1397
Matassi F, Carulli C, Civinini R, Innocenti M (2014) Cemented versus cementless fixation in total knee arthroplasty. Joints 1(3):121–125
McCalden RW, Robert CE, Howard JL, Naudie DD, McAuley JP, MacDonald SJ (2013) Comparison of outcomes and survivorship between patients of different age groups following TKA. J Arthroplasty 28(8):83–86
Meehan JP, Danielsen B, Kim SH, Jamali AA, White RH (2014) Younger age is associated with a higher risk of early periprosthetic joint infection and aseptic mechanical failure after total knee arthroplasty. J Bone Joint Surg Am 96(7):529–535
Meneghini RM, Hanssen AD (2008) Cementless fixation in total kneearthroplasty: past, present, and future. J Knee Surg 21(4):307–314

Meneghini RM, Daluga A, Soliman M (2011) Mechanicalstability of cementless tibial components in normal and osteoporotic-bone. J Knee Surg 24(03):191–196
Mikulak SA, Mahoney OM, dela Rosa MA, Schmalzried TP (2001) Loosening and osteolysis with the press-fit condylar posterior-cruciate-substituting total knee replacement. J Bone Joint Surg Am 83(3):398
Miller M, Goodheart J, Izant T, Rimnac C, Cleary R, Mann K (2014) Loss of cement-bone interlock in retrieved tibial components from total knee arthroplasties. Clin Orthop Relat Res 472(1):304–313
Miller AJ, Stimac JD, Smith LS, Feher AW, Yakkanti MR, Malkani AL (2018) Results of cemented vs cementless primary total knee arthroplasty using the same implant design. J Arthroplasty 33(4):1089–1093
Mont MA, Gwam C, Newman JM, Chughtai M, Khlopas A, Ramkumar PN, Harwin SF (2017) Outcomes of a newer-generation cementless total knee arthroplasty design in patients less than 50 years of age. Ann Transl Med 5(Suppl 3):S24
Nam D, Kopinski JE, Meyer Z, Rames RD, Nunley RM, Barrack RL (2017) Perioperative and early postoperative comparison of a modern cemented and cementless total knee arthroplasty of the same design. J Arthroplasty 32(7):2151–2155
Nevelos J, Maclean L, Sporer S, Harwin S, Nam D, Nunley R, Malkani A (2019) Design, migration and earlyclinicalresults of the first mass produced 3D printedcementless total knee implants. Scientific Exhibit Presented at AAOS. Las Vegas, NV, 12–16 Mar 2019
Peters PC Jr, Engh GA, Dwyer KA, Vinh TN (1992) Osteolysis after total knee arthroplasty without cement. J Bone Joint Surg Am 74(6):864–876
Rand JA (1991) Cement or cementless fixation in total knee arthroplasty? Clin Orthop Relat Res (273):52–62
Ritter MA, Meneghini RM (2010) Twenty-year survivorship of cementless anatomic graduated component total knee arthroplasty. J Arthroplasty 25(4):507–513
Rosenberg AG, Andriacchi TP, Barden R, Galante JO (1988) Patellar component failure in cementless total knee arthroplasty. Clin Orthop Relat Res (236):106–114
Rosenberg AG, Barden RM, Galante JO (1990) Cemented and ingrowth fixation of the miller-galante prosthesis. clinical and roentgenographic comparison after three- to six-year follow-up studies. Clin Orthop Relat Res (260):71–79
Schepers A, Cullingworth L, van der Jagt DR (2012) A prospective randomized clinical trial comparing tibial baseplate fixation with or without screws in total knee arthroplasty: a radiographic evaluation. J Arthroplasty 27(3):454–460
Schroder HM, Berthelsen A, Hassani G, Hansen EB, Solgaard S (2001) Cementless porous-coated total knee arthroplasty: 10-year results in a consecutive series. J Arthroplasty 16(5): 559–567
Scuderi GR, Insall JN (1992) Total knee arthroplasty. current clinical perspectives. Clin Orthop Relat Res (276):26–32
Sharkey PF, Lichstein PM, Shen C, Tokarski AT, Parvizi J (2014) Why are total knee arthroplasties failing today – has anything changed after 10 years? J Arthroplasty 29(9):1774–1778
Sinicrope BJ, Feher AW, Bhimani SJ, Smith LS, Harwin SF, Yakkanti MR, Malkani AL (2019) Increased survivorship of cementless versus cemented TKA in the morbidly obese. A minimum 5-year follow-up. J Arthroplasty 34(2):309–314
Soballe K, Hansen ES, Brockstedt-Rasmussen H, Hjortdal VE, Juhl GI, Pedersen CM, Hvid I, Bunger C (1991a) Fixation of titanium and hydroxyapatite-coated implants in arthriticosteopenic-bone. J Arthroplasty 6(4):307–316
Soballe K, Hansen ES, Brockstedt-Rasmussen H, Hjortdal VE, Juhl GI, Pedersen CM, Hvid I, Bunger C (1991b) Gap healing enhanced by hydroxyapatite coating in dogs. Clin Orthop Relat Res (272):300–307
Soballe K, Hansen ES, Brockstedt-Rasmussen H, Pedersen CM, Bunger C (1992) Bone graft incorporation around titanium-alloy- and hydroxyapatite-coated implants in dogs. Clin Orthop Relat Res (274):282–293
Tai CC, Cross MJ (2006) Five- to 12-year follow-up of a hydroxyapatite-coated, cementless total knee replacement in young, active patients. J Bone Joint Surg Br 88(9):1158–1163
Tarkin IS, Bridgeman JT, Jardon OM, Garvin KL (2005) Successful biologic fixation with mobile-bearing total knee arthroplasty. J Arthroplasty 20(4):481–486
Toksvig-Larsen S, Ryd L (1991) Surface flatness after bone cutting. A cadaver study of tibial condyles. Acta Orthop Scand 62(1):15–18
Varadarajan KM, Rubash HE, Li G (2011) Are current total knee arthroplasty implants designed to restore normal trochlear groove anatomy? J Arthroplasty 26(2):274–281
Voigt JD, Mosier M (2011) Hydroxyapatite (HA) coating appears to be of benefit for implant durability of tibial components in primary total knee arthroplasty. Acta Orthop 82(4):448–459
Wang Y, Beydoun MA, Liang L, Caballero B, Kumanyika SK (2008) Will all Americans become overweight or obese? Estimating the progression and cost of the US obesity epidemic. Obesity 16(10):2323–2330
Watanabe H, Akizuki S, Takizawa T (2004) Survival analysis of a cementless, cruciate-retaining total knee arthroplasty. Clinical and radiographic assessment 10 to 13 years after surgery. J Bone Joint Surg Br 86(6):824–829
Whiteside LA (1994) Cementless total knee replacement. nine- to 11-year results and 10-year survivorship analysis. Clin Orthop Relat Res (309):185–192
Whiteside LA (1995) Effect of porous-coating configuration on tibial osteolysis after total knee arthroplasty. Clin Orthop Relat Res (321):92–97
Whiteside LA, Fosco DR, Brooks JG Jr (1993) Fracture of the femoral component in cementless total knee arthroplasty. Clin Orthop Relat Res (286):71–77
Yayac M, Harrer S, Hozack WJ, Parvizi J, Courtney PM (2020) The use of cementless components does not significantly increase procedural costs in total knee arthroplasty. J Arthroplasty 35(2):407–412
Zhang Y, Ahn PB, Fitzpatrick DC, Heiner AD, Poggie RA, Brown TD (1999) Interfacial frictional behavior: cancellous bone, cortical bone, and a novel porous tantalum biomaterial. J Musculoskelet Res 03(04):245–251

Custom/Patient-Specific Total Knee Arthroplasty

Nana O. Sarpong, Darwin Chen, and H. John Cooper

Contents

E. Hansen, K.-D. Kühn (eds.), *Essentials of Cemented Knee Arthroplasty*,
https://doi.org/10.1007/978-3-662-63113-3_33

33.1 Introduction

With the growing demand for TKA and with procedures being performed in younger and more active patients, there is an increasing need to achieve longer survivorship, better clinical outcomes, and improved patient satisfaction after TKA. While most patients report reasonable satisfaction after TKA, up to 30% of patients remain dissatisfied with their procedure (Bourne et al. 2010). Dissatisfaction following TKA is multifactorial, and may be attributable to improper implant sizing, positioning of the components, or instability (Meier et al. 2019; Patil et al. 2015).

Anatomic studies of the knee have demonstrated distinct geometrical differences in gender and race, which may result in imperfect positioning and bony coverage of traditional (i.e., off-the-shelf) components during TKA (Patil et al. 2015). As such, implant manufacturers have developed newer implants that are, at times, marketed as ethnic- and gender-specific (i.e., available in more sizes in both mediolateral and anteroposterior planes) to address some of these challenges (Hirschmann and Behrend 2018). However, even with the newer gender-specific implants, studies have demonstrated asymmetrical variations between medial and lateral femoral condyles that are not accounted for (Patil et al. 2015; Mahoney and Kinsey 2010). These challenges have led to the development of custom, patient-specific TKA designs, with the goals of improving the implant fit, restoring each patient's native anatomy, and recreating normal knee kinematics, the end-result being regarded as the holy grail in TKA (Leyvraz and Rakotomanana 2000).

Custom TKA aims to restore knee anatomy and kinematics using anatomical data obtained primarily from advanced preoperative imaging such as computed tomography (CT), from which both patient-specific cutting jigs and custom implants unique to the patient are developed for the procedure (Arbab et al. 2018). We describe this unique approach to knee arthroplasty below using the iTotal CR TKA system (ConforMIS, Bellerica, MA) as a case study.

33.2 Case Study

History and Physical Examination

A 70-year-old man with medical comorbidities including hypertension, hyperlipidemia, and well-controlled diabetes presents with worsening left knee pain for the previous 9 months. He has exhausted conservative treatment modalities including non-steroidal anti-inflammatory medications, acetaminophen, tramadol, aerobic exercises, corticosteroid, and gel injections.

On examination, he ambulates with a left-sided antalgic gait and has no previous incisions about his left knee. His left knee exhibits varus alignment that is partially correctable on examination. He is mostly tender to palpation on the medial joint line with minimal effusion and crepitation appreciated. His left knee range of motion is 5–120° of flexion, stable to varus and valgus stress, and has a normal neurovascular examination.

Preoperative Imaging

Preoperative plain radiography including a standing three-joint-radiograph and a left knee anteroposterior and lateral radiograph demonstrate left knee tricompartmental arthritis with varus alignment of his right lower extremity (▫ Fig. 33.1).

The patient undergoespreoperative CT imaging of his lower extremity in preparation for a left TKA using the iTotal CR ConforMIS system. iView (ConforMIS, Bellerica, MA) patient-specific planning images are obtained and available preoperatively from the manufacturer. These images provide patient-specific tibial and femoral resection values, jig placement, and final implant positioning information (▫ Fig. 33.2).

Surgical Technique

The patient is given regional anesthesia with an adductor canal block and hypotensive spinal anesthesia. No tourniquet is used. An anterior midline incision is made followed by a standard medial parapatellar arthrotomy, a medial release, patellar fat pad resection, and release of the anterior horns of both menisci. Operative findings include significant sclerosis and osteophytes, all of which are preserved as they were captured in the preoperative CT scan and are built into the custom jigs.

Tip

Do not remove osteophytes at this point, as they are necessary landmarks for placement of the custom cutting jigs.

The distal femur is prepared by placing the initial positioning jig onto the femur so it finds its natural conforming location (designed to reference osteophytes), which is then used as a guide to remove any remaining cartilage above the subchondral bone from the medial and lateral condyles (▫ Fig. 33.3, left). A second jig is then placed which can reference both the peripheral osteophytes as well as the subchondral bone of both distal condyles (▫ Fig. 33.3, right). This second jig is used to set both the distal resection level as well as femoral rotation. The distal femoral resection is carried out after placement of the custom distal cutting guide, which has a patient-specific surface that extends over the trochlea and may or may not have a step cut.

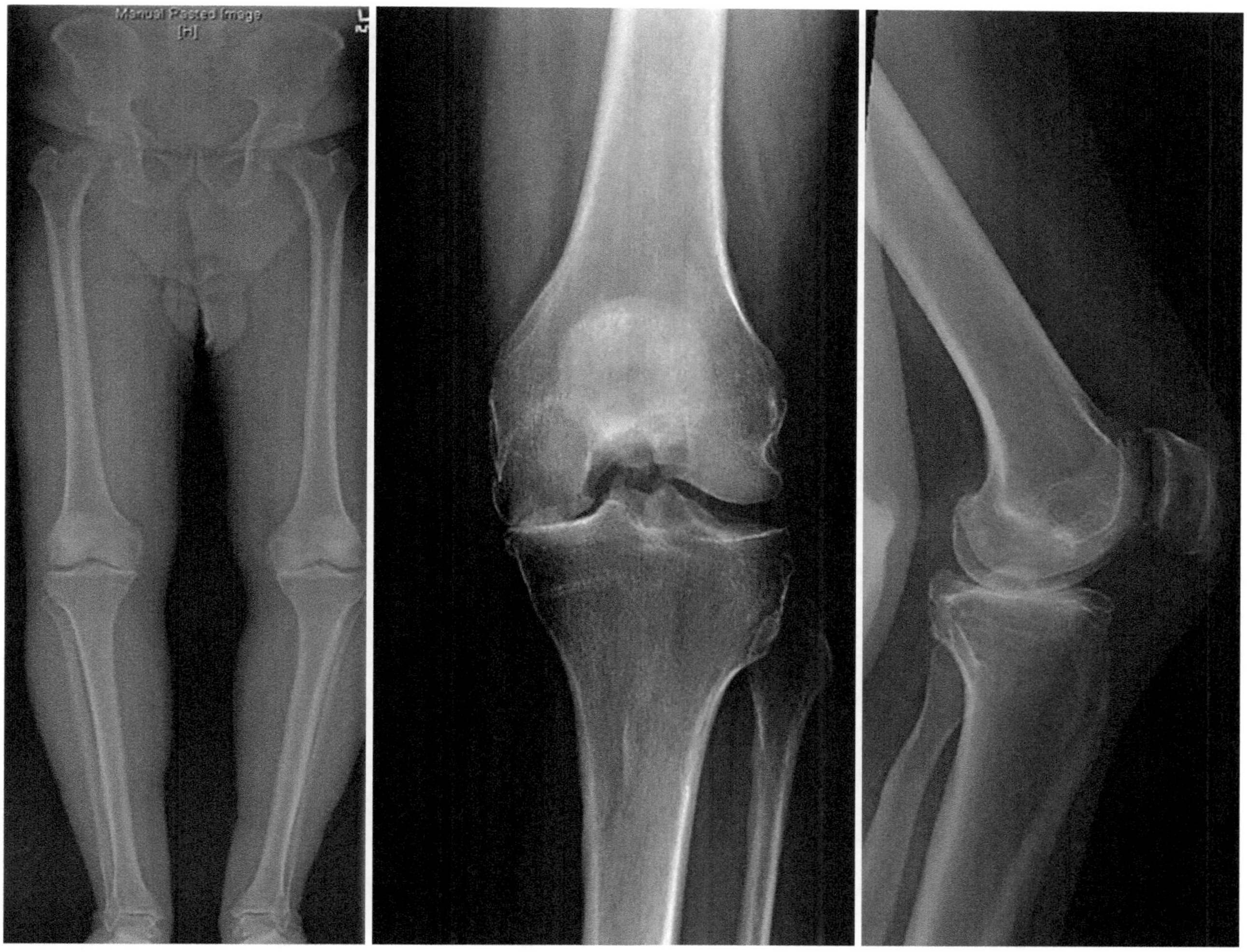

Fig. 33.1 Preoperative plain radiography

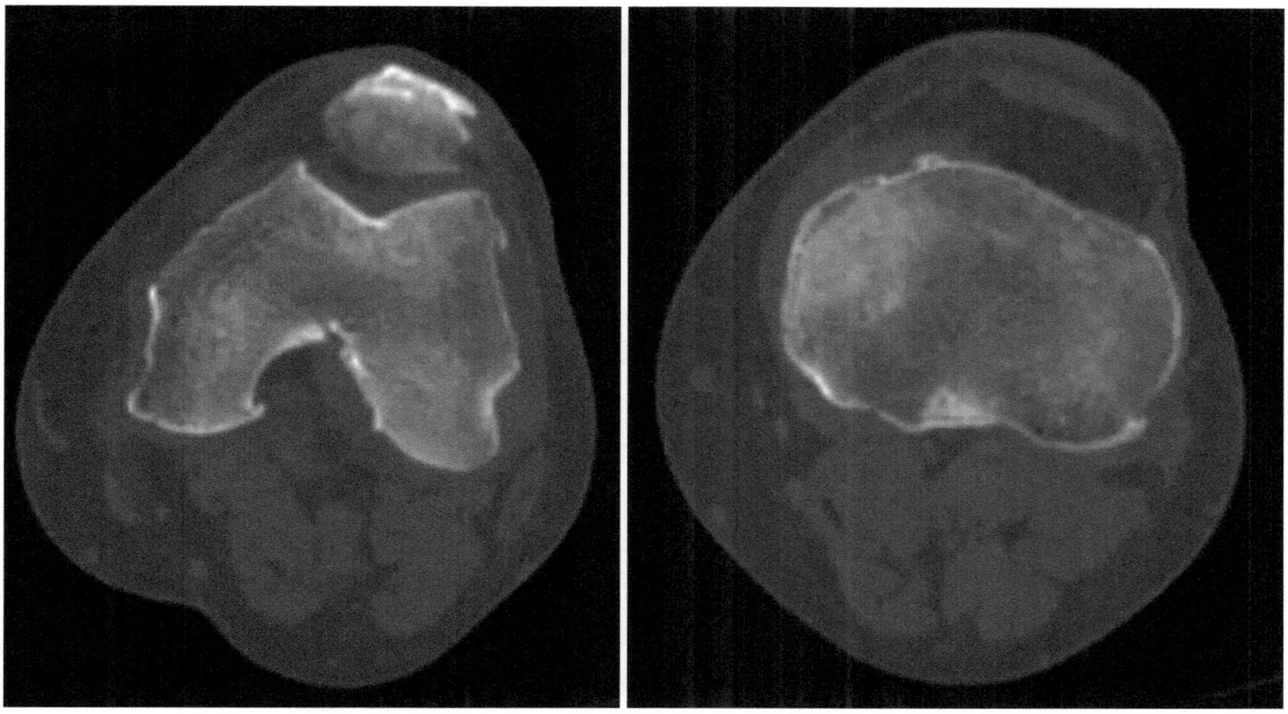

Fig. 33.2 Preoperative axial CT imaging (representative cuts of distal femur and proximal tibia)

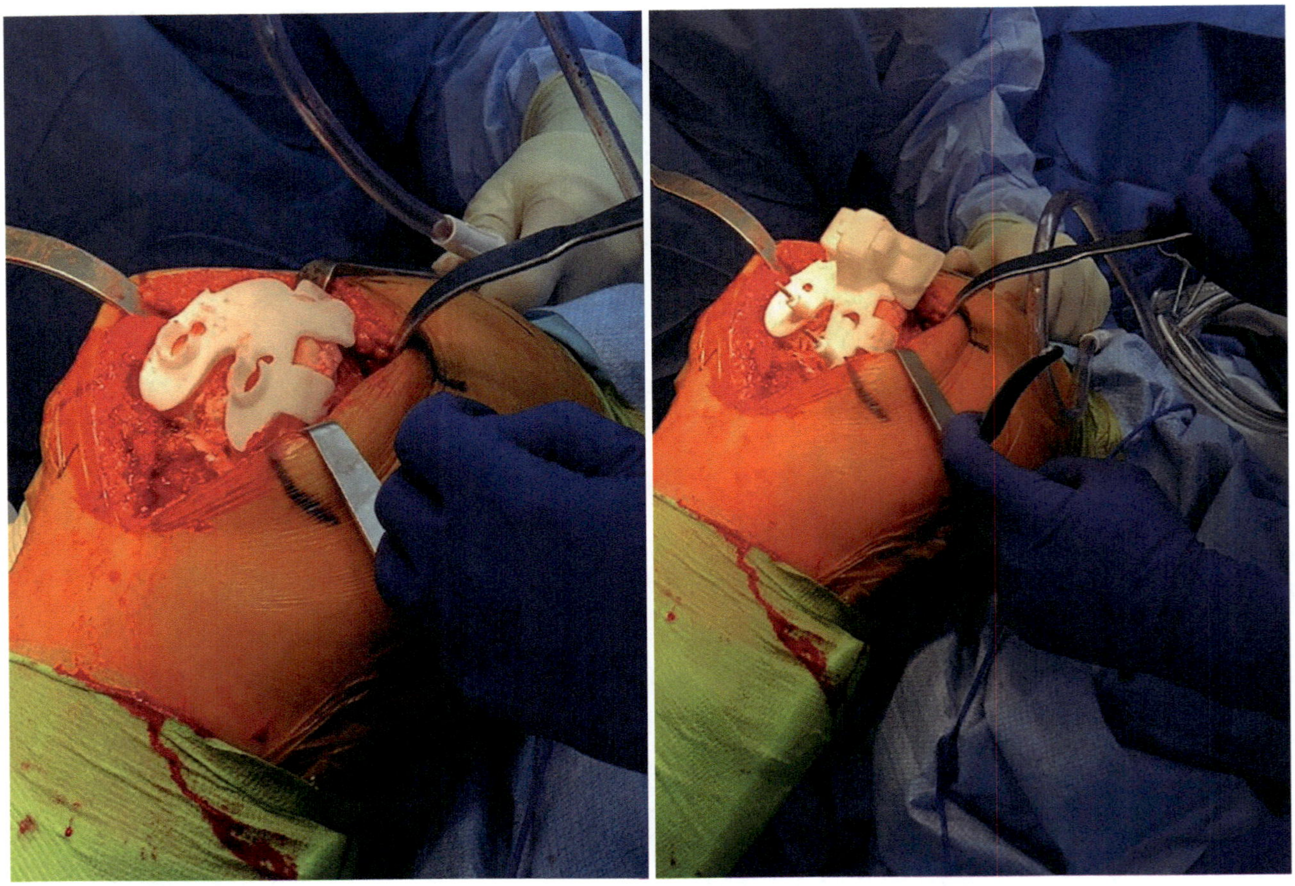

Fig. 33.3 Intraoperative clinical images demonstrating ConforMIS iJigs utilized for femoral preparation

Tip

In rare instances, the initial jig may not secure firmly onto the femur due to uncaptured osteophytes on CT imaging. In such cases, it is helpful to reference the iView planning images for proper jig placement.

> The distal femoral cuts should be checked carefully to confirm planar resections.

Using the previously referenced rotational pin holes from the initial custom guides, anterior, posterior, and chamfer cuts are carried out using additional cutting guides.

> Care should be taken that these guides sit flush along the cut surfaces of bone.

Tibial preparation is also carried out using a custom cutting guide that matches the patient's native tibial slope, within certain manufacturer specifications. The custom tibial guide is used, and sagittal and coronal alignment can be confirmed prior to the cut using an attached alignment rod. Proximal tibial resection is performed, followed by the removal of all peripheral tibial and femoral osteophytes. Femoral and tibial trials can then be placed to test the knee for stability throughout a range of motion. With the iTotal CR system, there is no custom jig for the patella and as such, the patella is prepared using conventional methods.

Once all cuts are made, the bony surfaces are copiously irrigated with pulse lavage.

> Final components are cemented into place using standard modern cementing technique polymethylmethacrylate (PMMA) bone cement. The authors' standard practice is not to inflate tourniquet for this step.

Tip

Ensure exposed bony surfaces are completely dry prior to cementation to achieve optimal osteointegration to cancellous bone.

Trial liners are placed while the PMMA is allowed to polymerize, and is exchanged for the real liner(s) after any remaining cement particles are removed. Of note, current custom cruciate-retaining designs feature medial and lateral components with separate polyethylene inserts, while posterior-stabilized designs feature a single polyethylene insert.

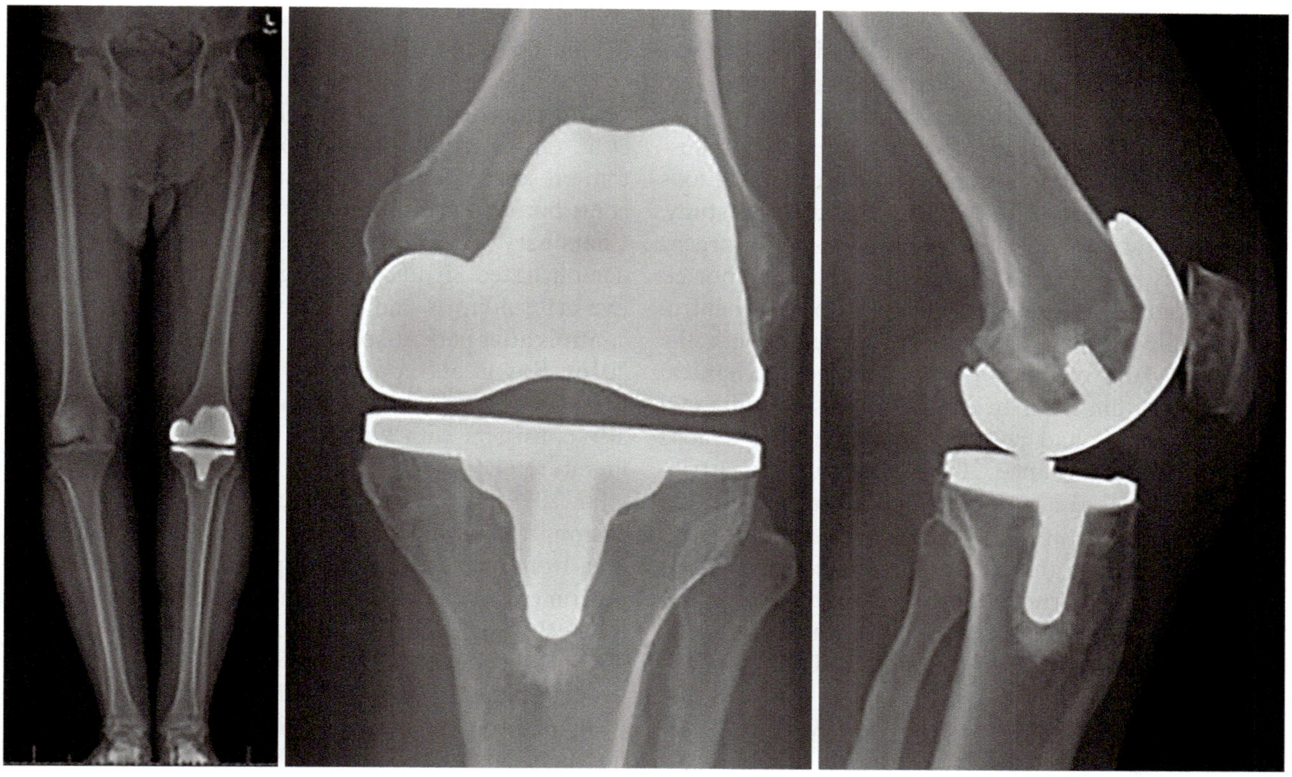

Fig. 33.4 Postoperative plain radiography

Postoperative Course

The patient undergoes an uneventful postoperative course and is discharged to his home on the first postoperative day after ambulating 600 feet with the physical therapist and navigating stairs. His mechanical alignment is restored to neutral (Fig. 33.4).

33.3 Discussion

As the number of patients undergoing TKA continues to rise, so will the number of patients dissatisfied with their outcomes from the procedure. The arthroplasty literature suggests that residual pain is the leading cause of patient dissatisfaction following TKA, with approximately 30% of clinically significant knee pain attributable to implant malalignment (Mahoney and Kinsey 2010). Furthermore, about half of early revision TKA is related to malalignment, instability, and failure of fixation (Sharkey et al. 2014). Previous studies have demonstrated that postoperative alignment within 0–3° of the mechanical axis is recommended (Jeffery et al. 1991). Many attempts have been made by implant companies to improve the accuracy of traditional (i.e., off-the-shelf) TKA implants, however, significant variations in bony anatomy, limitations of conventional jigs, and surgeon error can result in component malpositioning (Bäthis et al. 2004).

Custom, patient-specific TKA represents a different approach to the conventional surgical technique for knee arthroplasty. Given the substantial variation in anatomical geometry between patients, some surgeons theorize that custom implants may be advantageous when compared with ethnic- or gender-specific TKA (van den Heever et al. 2012). These techniques aim to improve postoperative alignment using the patient's unique anatomical data from preoperative axial CT or MRI to create TKA components that are unique to the patient's anatomy, which can be implanted using custom disposable cutting jigs. The iTotal CR and PS systems available through ConforMIS are examples of modern custom TKA systems.

Several recent reports have compared this technology to the traditional TKA systems. It has been hypothesized that refining implant component design using a custom TKA philosophy allows for more normal kinematics than patients undergoing traditional TKA (Zeller et al. 2017). Using state-of-the-art mobile fluoroscopy, Zeller et al. analyzed in vivo tibiofemoral kinematics during deep knee bend and rising from a seated position for patients who had undergone custom TKA, compared to patients with traditional off-the-shelf implants. They reported that the patients undergoing custom TKA exhibited greater weight-bearing knee flexion, greater posterior femoral rollback, greater axial rotation, and minimal liftoff (hence better stability in early to mid-flexion) when compared with patients who underwent traditional TKA. The authors concluded that the custom TKA implant demonstrated kinematics that were more similar to a normal knee (Zeller et al. 2017).

Another study investigated the accuracy of custom TKA in restoring coronal plane mechanical axis alignment (Levengood and Dupee 2018). In this study, Levengood et al. utilized computer-assisted surgery to objectify the mechanical alignment and reported that custom TKA implants resulted in perfect neutral coronal alignment (0°) in 84% of patients, with the remaining 16% exhibiting postoperative mechanical alignment within 2° of neutral. They also highlighted that no patients had postoperative extension deficits (Levengood and Dupee 2018). The authors attributed the increased accuracy to the use of the full-set of patient-specific jigs with the custom implants, with each jig custom to the patient, compared to previous patient-specific instrumentation techniques which utilized a starter jig on the femur and a single starter jig on the tibia, but all subsequent steps utilized standard instrumentation.

Another study by Arbab et al. also evaluated postoperative alignment in a retrospective study of patients undergoing custom (ConforMIS iTotal) compared to conventional (Triathlon; Stryker, Mahwah, NJ) TKA (Arbab et al. 2018). They reported that the rate of outliers within 3° of neutral limb alignment was 16% in the custom TKA cohort and 26% in the conventional TKA group. They concluded that the custom TKA technique may offer an advantage over conventional TKA in terms of restoration of the mechanical axis (Arbab et al. 2018).

> While the aforementioned reports have highlighted improved overall alignment with custom TKA, there is a dearth of high-quality evidence on the benefits of custom TKA on clinical functional outcomes and survivorship.

Tait et al. conducted a multicenter prospective trial of patients undergoing custom TKA and evaluated patient-reported outcome measures and adverse events at midterm (Tait et al. n.d.). They reported that there were statistically significant improvements in the average range of motion, KOOS, and three out of four domains of the KSS (objective, function, satisfaction), when compared to preoperative measures. Moreover, they observed a 3.1% manipulation under anesthesia (MUA) rate and a 92% and 90% overall satisfaction rate at 1 and 2 years, respectively (Tait et al. n.d.). They highlighted that at 2 years, the observed MUA rate was consistent with previously published reports of MUA after TKA (Rubinstein and DeHaan 2010).

The rate of MUA for newer generation custom TKA was investigated in another prospective study by Kay et al. (2018), given that previous iterations of the custom prosthesis design had been implicated as a possible contributor to arthrofibrosis (Cates and Schmidt 2009; Chaudhary et al. 2008). These previous reports had demonstrated significantly higher rates of postoperative arthrofibrosis and need for MUA versus matched controls after patient-specific TKA (White and Ranawat 2016). Kay et al. reported a 3.05% rate of MUA with the second-generation ConforMIS iTotal TKA, which is also consistent with typical MUA rates reported in the literature (1.5–6%), regardless of implant design (Kay et al. 2018). A few more clinical outcome studies after custom TKA are under way. More recently, internal data from our institution compared short-term clinical outcomes of custom versus traditional TKA in a retrospective study (Frederick et al. n.d.). We found that at 3 months, patients with a custom TKA experienced statistically betterSF-12 PCS and Knee Society scores when compared to patients undergoing traditional TKA, but no significant difference in SF-12 MCS or WOMAC scores. Furthermore, at 1 year, we observed that custom TKA patients exhibited superior KSS scores (Frederick et al. n.d.).

> Although the majority of published studies to date have highlighted the potential benefits of custom TKA, reports of complications also exist, notably in earlier generations of custom TKA designs.

In a retrospective study, Meheux et al. compared traditional TKA to an older (ConforMIS iTotal G2) and newer (ConforMIS iTotal G2 Plus) generation custom TKA designs (Meheux et al. 2019). The authors highlighted that the use of the older generation design was discontinued after reports of early failure. They reported no difference in mechanical axis alignment between the three cohorts, but did observe that the newer generation custom TKA system had superior KSS scores compared to the traditional and older generation TKA systems at all time points. Furthermore, they reported shorter hospital length of stay and blood loss with the newer generation compared to the older generation and traditional TKA systems. The principal finding of their study, however, was the significant failure rate in the older generation (23%) compared to the newer generation (0%) and traditional (3%) TKA designs. The most common mode of failures in the older generation system were tibial component subsidence and polyethylene locking mechanism failure, which were eliminated when the manufacturer modified the design to the newer generation system (Meheux et al. 2019).

> Later generation custom TKA designs have greatly reduced the reported early failures, but knee arthroplasty surgeons must still recognize that even these refined systems are not without limitations and certain patients may not be ideal candidates for this technology.

As these custom TKA systems rely on advanced three-dimensional imaging for preoperative planning, the accuracy of custom jig fabrication may be significantly affected in patients with flexion contractures greater than 20° or with previous knee instrumentation, as these may prevent accurate anatomic knee landmarking planning studies (Nam et al. 2016). Furthermore, manufacturers recommend against the use of their custom TKA systems in situations of severe (>15°) coronal alignment, severe instability due to significant bone loss and/or the absence of collateral ligament instability, and metal insensitivity, particularly to nickel (ConforMIS iTotal G2 Surgical Technique Guide 2015). Additionally, as in traditional TKA systems, careful attention to the cruciate ligaments is recommended during the preoperative examination to prevent inadvertent implantation of a cruciate-retaining custom implant when a cruciate-sacrificing implant is actually warranted.

> In conclusion, custom TKA has been demonstrated to improve postoperative lower extremity alignment and some clinical outcome measures in the few studies that exist to date, and these benefits may impact postoperative resource utilization for patients undergoing TKA.

A recent study by O'Connor et al. compared TKA episode expenditure among Medicare fee-for-service beneficiaries who underwent custom versus traditional TKA (O'Connor and Blau 2019). They reported that the average total episode spending was $1695 less for patients who underwent custom TKA compared to traditional TKA, and this was attributable to lower average spending on in-patient, skilled nursing facility, and home health services. Thus, they concluded that the use of custom TKA may reduce healthcare spending for those undergoing TKA (O'Connor and Blau 2019). However, these results may not necessarily be applicable to the wider Medicare population undergoing TKA, as it is possible that new technologies (i.e., custom TKA) are more likely to be used in the healthier population.

Take-Home Messages

- Restoration of patient anatomy and normal knee kinematics is the holy grail in TKA.
- Custom TKA systems have been shown to improve lower extremity mechanical alignment when compared to traditional TKA systems.
- Several studies have demonstrated improved clinical outcomes with custom compared to traditional TKA systems.
- Osteophytes should be preserved prior to bony preparation as they are captured in the preoperative CT scan and accounted for in the patient-specific jigs.
- In rare instances, custom jigs may not secure firmly onto the bone due to uncaptured osteophytes on CT imaging. In such cases, it is helpful to reference the iView planning images for proper jig placement.
- The authors' standard practice is not to inflate tourniquet during cementation of the custom TKA components.
- A recent study demonstrated potential economic savings with the use of custom TKA implants in the Medicare population.

References

Arbab D, Reimann P, Brucker M, Bouillon B, Lüring C (2018) Alignment in total knee arthroplasty - A comparison of patient-specific implants with the conventional technique. Knee 25:882–887. https://doi.org/10.1016/j.knee.2018.05.017

Bäthis H, Perlick L, Tingart M, Lüring C, Zurakowski D, Grifka J (2004) Alignment in total knee arthroplasty. A comparison of computer-assisted surgery with the conventional technique. J Bone Joint Surg Br 86:682–687. https://doi.org/10.1302/0301--620x.86b5.14927

Bourne RB, Chesworth BM, Davis AM, Mahomed NN, Charron KDJ (2010) Patient satisfaction after total knee arthroplasty: who is satisfied and who is not? Clin Orthop Relat Res 468:57–63. https://doi.org/10.1007/s11999-009-1119-9

Cates HE, Schmidt JM (2009) Closed manipulation after total knee arthroplasty: outcome and affecting variables. Orthopedics 32:398. https://doi.org/10.3928/01477447-20090511-10

Chaudhary R, Beaupré LA, Johnston DWC (2008) Knee range of motion during the first two years after use of posterior cruciate-stabilizing or posterior cruciate-retaining total knee prostheses. A randomized clinical trial. J Bone Joint Surg Am 90:2579–2586. https://doi.org/10.2106/JBJS.G.00995

ConforMIS iTotal G2 Surgical Technique Guide 2015

Frederick J, Jennings E, Geller J, Shah R, Cooper H (n.d.) Custom individually-made total knee implants are associated with slightly better improvements in early patient-reported outcomes

Hirschmann MT, Behrend H (2018) Functional knee phenotypes: a call for a more personalised and individualised approach to

total knee arthroplasty? Knee Surg Sports Traumatol Arthrosc 26:2873–2874. https://doi.org/10.1007/s00167-018-4973-8
Jeffery RS, Morris RW, Denham RA (1991) Coronal alignment after total knee replacement. J Bone Joint Surg Br 73:709–714
Kay A, Kurtz W, Martin G, Huber B, Tait R, Clyburn T (2018) Manipulation rate is not increased after custom total knee arthroplasty. Reconstr Rev 8:1–48
Levengood GA, Dupee J (2018) Accuracy of coronal plane mechanical alignment in a custom, individually made total knee replacement with patient-specific instrumentation. J Knee Surg 31:792–796. https://doi.org/10.1055/s-0037-1608946
Leyvraz PF, Rakotomanana L (2000) The anatomy and function of the knee – the quest for the holy grail? J Bone Joint Surg Br 82:1093–1094. https://doi.org/10.1302/0301-620x.82b8.11656
Mahoney OM, Kinsey T (2010) Overhang of the femoral component in total knee arthroplasty: risk factors and clinical consequences. J Bone Joint Surg Am 92:1115–1121. https://doi.org/10.2106/JBJS.H.00434
Meheux CJ, Park KJ, Clyburn TA (2019) A retrospective study comparing a patient-specific design total knee arthroplasty with an off-the-shelf design: unexpected catastrophic failure seen in the early patient-specific design. J Am Acad Orthop Surg Glob Res Rev 3:e10.5435. https://doi.org/10.5435/JAAOSGlobal-D--19-00143
Meier M, Zingde S, Steinert A, Kurtz W, Koeck F, Beckmann J (2019) What is the possible impact of high variability of distal femoral geometry on TKA? A CT data analysis of 24,042 knees. Clin Orthop Relat Res 477:561–570. https://doi.org/10.1097/CORR.0000000000000611
Nam D, Park A, Stambough JB, Johnson SR, Nunley RM, Barrack RL (2016) The Mark Coventry Award: custom cutting guides do not improve total knee arthroplasty clinical outcomes at 2 years followup. Clin Orthop Relat Res 474:40–46. https://doi.org/10.1007/s11999-015-4216-y
O'Connor MI, Blau BE (2019) The economic value of custom versus off-the-shelf knee implants in medicare fee-for-service beneficiaries. Am Health Drug Benefits 12:66–73
Patil S, Bunn A, Bugbee WD, Colwell CW, D'Lima DD (2015) Patient-specific implants with custom cutting blocks better approximate natural knee kinematics than standard TKA without custom cutting blocks. Knee 22:624–629. https://doi.org/10.1016/j.knee.2015.08.002
Rubinstein RA, DeHaan A (2010) The incidence and results of manipulation after primary total knee arthroplasty. Knee 17:29–32. https://doi.org/10.1016/j.knee.2009.07.001
Sharkey PF, Lichstein PM, Shen C, Tokarski AT, Parvizi J (2014) Why are total knee arthroplasties failing today – has anything changed after 10 years? J Arthroplasty 29:1774–1778. https://doi.org/10.1016/j.arth.2013.07.024
Tait H, Kurtz W, Clyburn T (n.d.) Outcomes after custom individually made total knee arthroplasty. ICJR Pan Pacific Congress 2016 Presentation 1632
van den Heever DJ, Scheffer C, Erasmus P, Dillon E (2012) Classification of gender and race in the distal femur using self organising maps. Knee 19:488–492. https://doi.org/10.1016/j.knee.2011.06.009
White PB, Ranawat AS (2016) Patient-specific total knees demonstrate a higher manipulation rate compared to "off-the-shelf implants". J Arthroplasty 31:107–111. https://doi.org/10.1016/j.arth.2015.07.041
Zeller IM, Sharma A, Kurtz WB, Anderle MR, Komistek RD (2017) Custom versus patient-sized cruciate-retaining total knee arthroplasty: an in vivo kinematics study using mobile fluoroscopy. J Arthroplasty 32:1344–1350. https://doi.org/10.1016/j.arth.2016.09.034

Alternative Bearings in Total Knee Arthroplasty

Brian P. Chalmers and Steve B. Haas

Contents

E. Hansen, K.-D. Kühn (eds.), *Essentials of Cemented Knee Arthroplasty*,
https://doi.org/10.1007/978-3-662-63113-3_34

34.1 Introduction

While there have been a number of technological and philosophical evolutions in primary total knee arthroplasty (TKA) over the last several decades, the principles remain the same: achieve a well-balanced and well-aligned TKA with durable fixation (Mercuri and Schwarzkopf 2019; Dennis 1991; Donaldson et al. 2015; Nikolaou et al. 2014).

> While cementless TKA is becoming more common, cemented TKA remains the gold standard (Nugent et al. 2019). Proper and meticulous surgical technique is essential for achieving these principles, including proper cementation technique.

The goal of this chapter is to outline the senior author's (SBH) surgical technique in achieving a well-aligned and well-balanced TKA with proper cement technique with an illustrative case example. Finally, the current literature on alternative bearing surfaces in primary TKA will be reviewed.

34.2 Case Example

Our case example is a 62-year-old male with end-stage right knee varus degenerative arthritis that has failed a comprehensive conservative management program and has been indicated for primary TKA (Fig. 34.1). Prior to surgery, we obtain long leg standing radio-

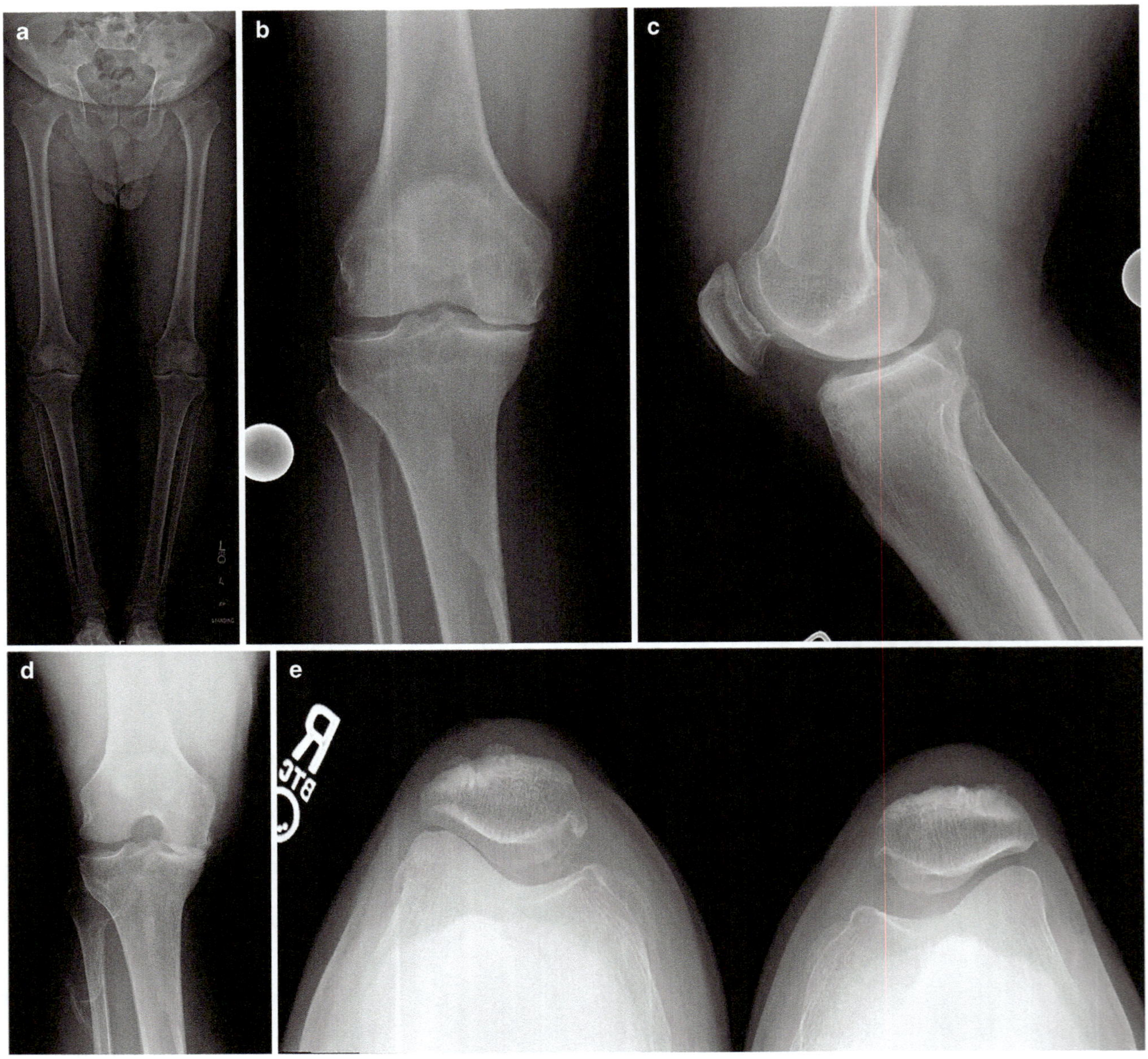

Fig. 34.1 Full-length standing **a**, standing AP **b** and lateral **c**, PA flexion **d**, and Merchant view **e** patellar radiographs of the right knee obtained routinely for preoperative assessment

graphs to assess overall alignment and any pathology of the contralateral limb or hips (◘ Fig. 34.1a). We also obtain an AP, lateral, PA flexion, and Merchant view of the knee as we routinely note significant posteromedial degenerative, bone-on-bone changes on the PA flexion view (◘ Fig. 34.1d), more so than the AP view (◘ Fig. 34.1b). We template our femoral and tibial cuts on the full-length standing view to better plan our bony resections. We also template sizes for a posterior stabilized, oxidized zirconium TKA with calibrated radiographs in order to better prepare for surgery (◘ Fig. 34.2).

34.3 Surgical Technique

The senior author has utilized a minimally invasive, modified mini-midvastus surgical approach that has been previously reported with excellent results for the past several decades (Haas et al. 2004, 2006). A medial release is performed, the extent of which is determined by the preoperative deformity, and the anterior cruciate ligament (ACL), posterior cruciate ligament (PCL), and anterior horn of the lateral meniscus are incised.

After measuring the patellar thickness, a preliminary flush cut is made to gain exposure and make a flat surface for a thin bent Homan to retract upon; in patients with softer bone or thinner patellae, this step is skipped. The femoral canal is then accessed with an opening reamer, starting typically just superior to the origin of the PCL. After irrigating, an intramedullary guide is inserted in the femoral canal with a 5° valgus cut angle planned, variable depending on the patient's anatomy on the preoperative long-standing radiograph, and a 9 mm resection planned. The angular guide is pinned to the distal medial femoral condyle (MFC) (and should be proud on the distal lateral femoral condyle [LFC]) and the cutting guide is pinned in place with two headless pins. The distal femoral resection is adjusted with the guide in order to achieve a bony resection to the trochlear groove. Patients with remaining cartilage may require a "+2" distal femoral cut, while patients with distal MFC bone loss, which may be evident as the guide sitting flush with the LFC, may require an initial "–2"

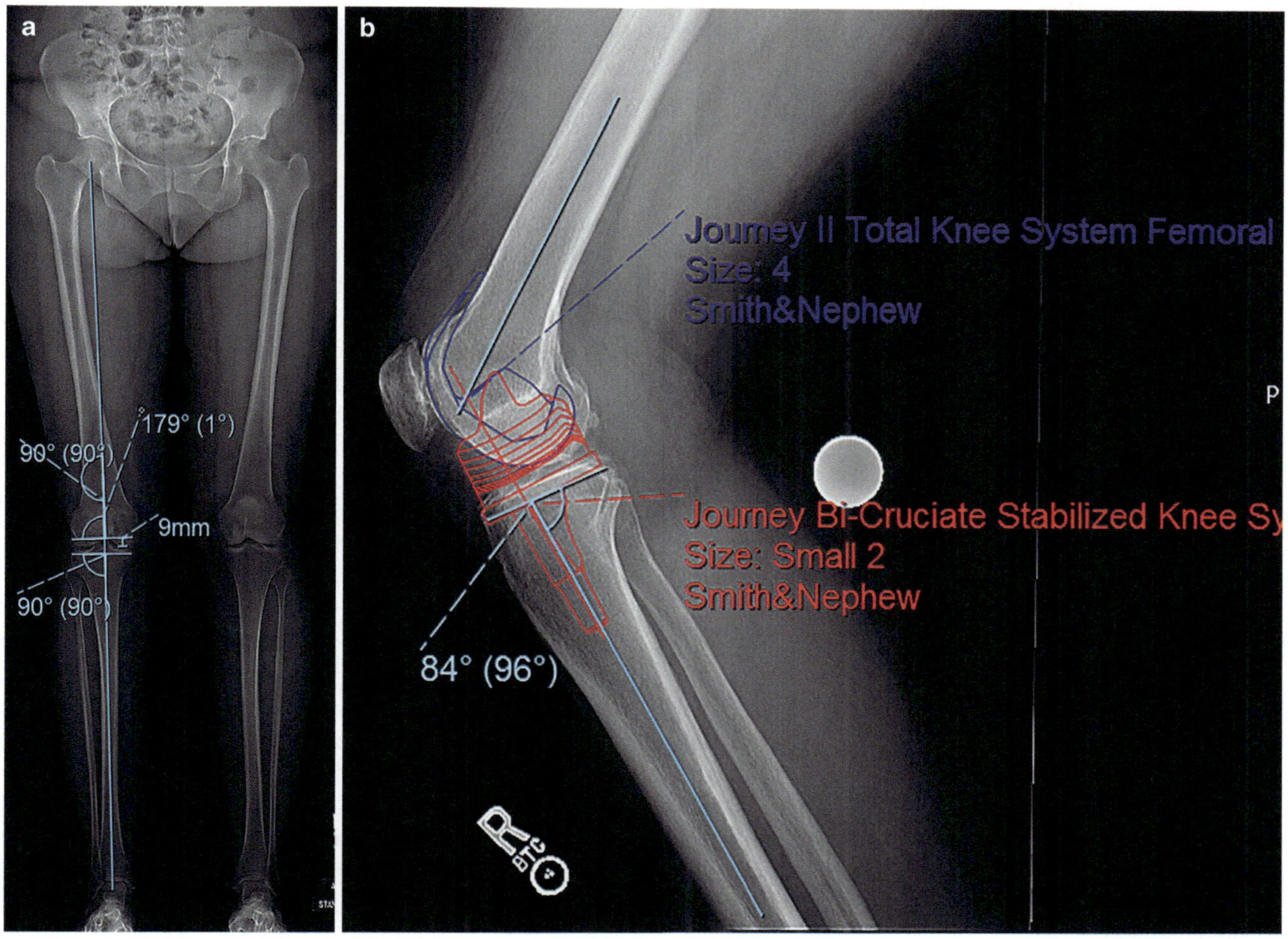

◘ **Fig. 34.2** Full-length standing **a** radiograph with the femoral and tibial cuts templated. The component sizes can be accurately templated on the lateral radiograph **b**

cut. After the bony resection, the intramedullary guide is re-inserted to check the quality of the resection; the resection is re-visited until the distal angular guide is flush with the distal femoral resection.

The tibiais then exposed in the normal fashion with the knee subluxated forward. An extramedullary tibial cutting guide or accelerometer-based navigation guide is utilized to cut the tibia at 3° of posterior slope and 90° to the mechanical axis, referencing the preoperative long leg template to approximate the depth of the tibial resection medially and laterally. A spacer block with a drop rod is utilized to ensure that the cut runs along the tibial crest, in patients with neutral tibial anatomy, and points to the second ray. The spacer block is then utilized to balance the knee in extension and check the overall limb alignment. A drop rod is placed caudad and cephalad in the spacer block to ensure that the tibial alignment is neutral and the femoral alignment rod points toward the femoral head which lies roughly two fingerbreadths medial to the anterior superior iliac spine (ASIS).

Once satisfied with the overall alignment and balance in extension, attention is turned to the femur. One of the most crucial steps in the operation is setting femoral rotation in order to properly balance the knee as well as ensure proper patellofemoral tracking and mechanics. The senior author utilizes a medially pivoting sizing guide that allows variable rotation in order to customize femoral external rotation to a patient's anatomy. The medial pivot maintains the posterior medial resection and augments the posterior lateral resection, rather than a central pivoting guide which would over-resect posterior medial bone in order to add femoral external rotation (Coyle et al. 2019). Whiteside's line and the posterior condyles are utilized as a reference to set femoral external rotation (Poilvache et al. 1996; Arima et al. 1995; Anouchi et al. 1993). Once rotation is set, the guide is drilled, the appropriate size is selected with the sizing guide. The four-in-one cutting block is placed and the anterior, posterior, anterior chamfer, and posterior chamfer resections are made.

> Care is taken on the anterior femoral resection in order to avoid notching the femoral cortex but also to ensure that the proper size has been selected.

The resection should be close to or right in line with the cortex in order to avoid overstuffing the patellofemoral joint and ensuring proper posterior offset is restored for a balanced flexion space. With the knee at 90° of flexion and with a laminar spreader, the medial and lateral menisci are removed as well as any posterior osteophytes that may tension the posterior capsule and affect soft tissue balancing.

The tibia is then exposed with the knee subluxated and various sized tibial trays are trialed in proper external rotation, in line with the medial one-third of the tibial tubercle, to select the appropriately sized tibial tray. The senior author utilizes an asymmetric tibial tray that fits the anatomy of the tibial plateau, optimizes tibial plateau implant coverage, and allows proper external rotation of the component without posterolateral uncoverage (Minoda et al. 2018; Stulberg and Goyal 2015). Once the size and rotation are set, the tibial tray is pinned in place and the tibia is prepared. We utilize the drill initially on forward but then drill on reverse at the last one-third to compact the bone distally as a plug for later cementation. In sclerotic bone, a small saw is utilized prior to impaction of the keel to avoid fracture of the tibial plateau or shifting of the component position. The keel is then punched.

The femoral trial is then inserted and the box is prepared. A PS polyethylene trial is inserted and the range of motion, balance, and alignment are trialed with various polyethylene thicknesses. Alignment rods are again utilized to check the femoral, tibial, and overall limb alignment. If required for proper balance or alignment, additional tibial or distal femoral resections are performed and the TKA is re-trialed. Finally, the patella is recut to a straight surface to a level in which the overall thickness, taking into account the thickness of the planned polyethylene implant, is similar to the pre-resection thickness of the native patella as measured previously. The patella is sized with appropriate medialization of the component to lateralize the patella and ensure proper patellar tracking. The knee is taken through range of motion to confirm that the patella tracks centrally without any lateral tilt or subluxation.

Once satisfied with the overall TKA balance, alignment, and patellar tracking, the knee is copiously irrigated and the femoral, tibial, and patellar surfaces are thoroughly dried. Meticulous cement technique is essential for the durability of cemented TKA implants. Drill holes are made in any sclerotic bone in order to enhance cement interdigitation. The senior author cements the tibia, femur, and patella in that order. Cement is mixed manually in a bowl. Antibiotic cement is not routinely utilized but reserved for patients at potentially higher risk of developing a periprosthetic joint infection (PJI) (obesity, diabetes mellitus, etc.).The tibia is subluxated and circumferentially exposed. Utilizing high-viscosity (HV) cement in the early stages, the keel is finger-pressurized (◘ Fig. 34.3a) until fat and marrow contents are seen from the tibia guide pins and the tibial plateau; the prior bone plug created by reverse reaming assists in creating a plug for pressurization into the tibia. The tibial plateau is then fully coated with cement, interdigitating the cement with finger pressure into the plateau (◘ Fig. 34.3b).

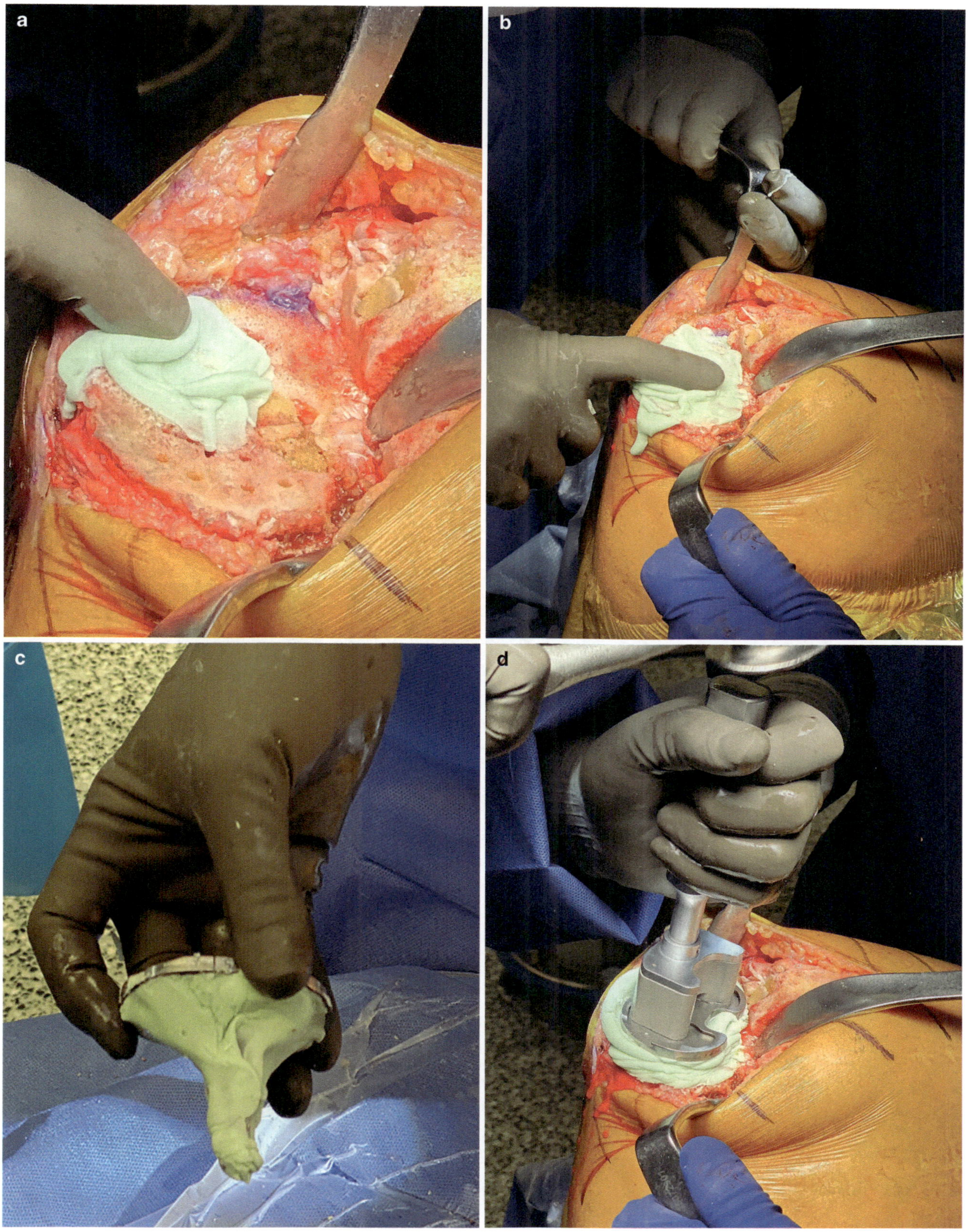

Fig. 34.3 **a–h** Meticulous cementation techniques of the tibia and the femur are important for a successful TKA. The keel **a** and the tibial cut surface **b** are manually pressurized to assure cement interdigitation. The entire tibial component cemented surface is coated with cement **c** and impacted into place **d**, removing all excess cement. The femur is then coated with cement **e**, similarly interdigitating the cement into the bone. The femur-cemented surface is coated **f** and the component is impacted into place **g**, taking care to remove all excess cement **h**

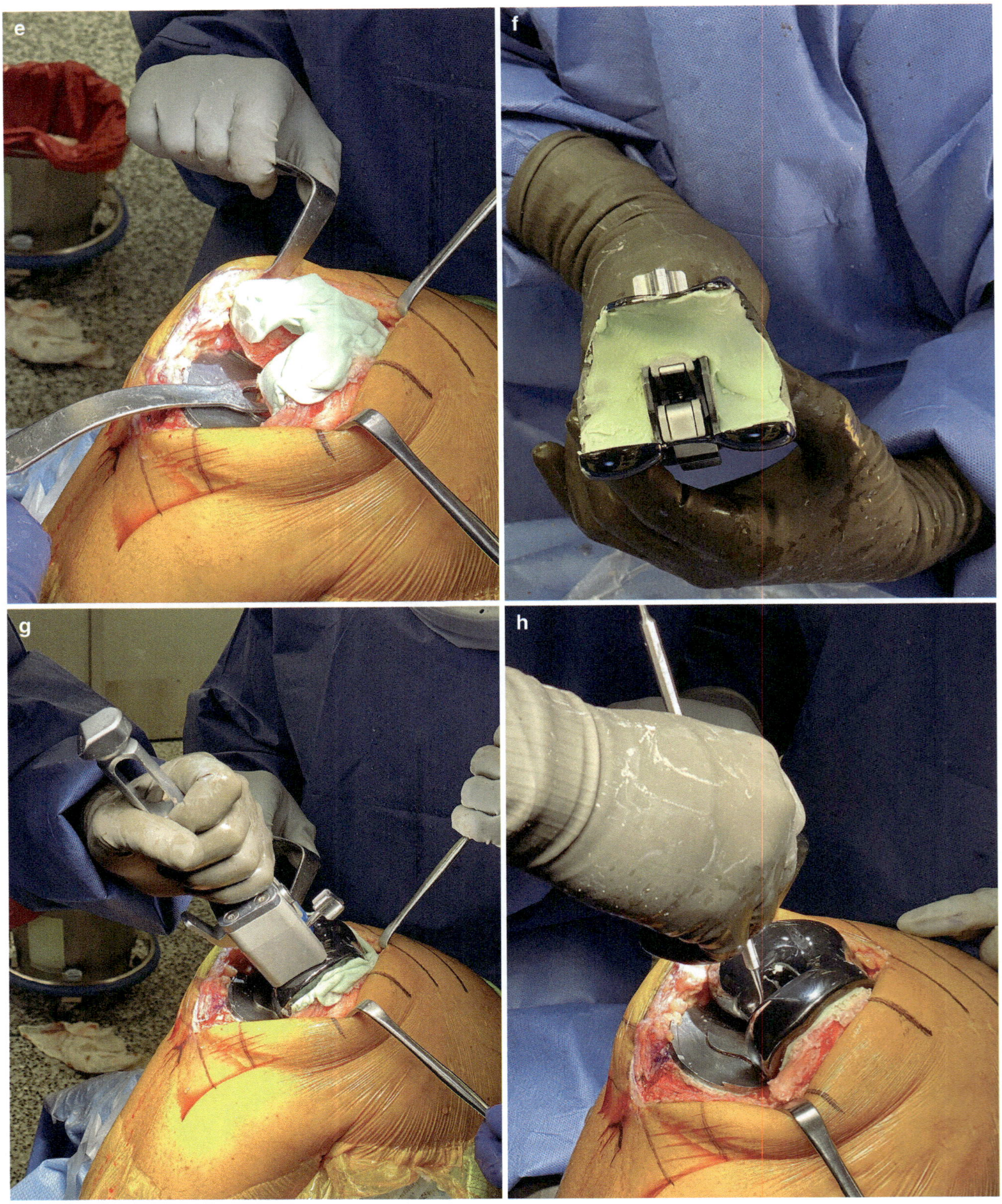

Fig. 34.3 (continued)

> The entirety of the cemented surface of the tibial implant is coated with cement prior to implantation (Fig. 34.3c). Recent biomechanical data has shown that cementing early in a runnier phase rather than a doughier phase improves initial tibial fixation by 48–72% (Billi et al. 2019).

> Furthermore, cementing the keel increases initial tibial fixation strength by roughly 150% (Billi et al. 2019).

The real tibial component is then impacted into place fully and the cement is methodically cleaned (Fig. 34.3d). The femur is then exposed; a PCL retractor under the femur can help elevate the femur for easier cementation but also places pressure on the tibial component, ensuring that it does not lift off (Fig. 34.3e).Cement is placed on the femur and interdigitated with the cancellous bone with finger pressurization (Fig. 34.3e). The entirety of the cemented surface of the femoral component is coated with cement (Fig. 34.3f) and the oxidized zirconium femoral component is impacted into place (Fig. 34.3g). The oxidized zirconium femoral component is black, as seen in Fig. 34.3g and h, and has an excellent undersurface for cement bonding. Cement is cleaned methodically from the knee (Fig. 34.3h).

> We coat the implant as biomechanical data that has shown that contamination of the implant interface by fat reduces mean fixation strength by roughly 90% and that adding cement to the tray prior to implantation increases fixation strength by 50% (Billi et al. 2019).

This technique produces reliable cement penetration and interdigitation of both components, but especially the tibial component, as seen in Fig. 34.4. To achieve optimal patella cement penetration, the senior author prepares a separate batch of cement for the patella to assure that the cement is in the early stage (Billi et al. 2019).

34.4 Ceramic Bearings

The senior author has been utilizing oxidized zirconium, a ceramicized metal, as a bearing surface in primary and revision TKA for two decades with excellent results. Oxidized zirconium implants were introduced in 1997 for knee arthroplasty as an alternative bearing surface to cobalt–chromium (CoCr) in an attempt to reduce polyethylene wear and improve long-term implant survival (Patel and Spector 1997).

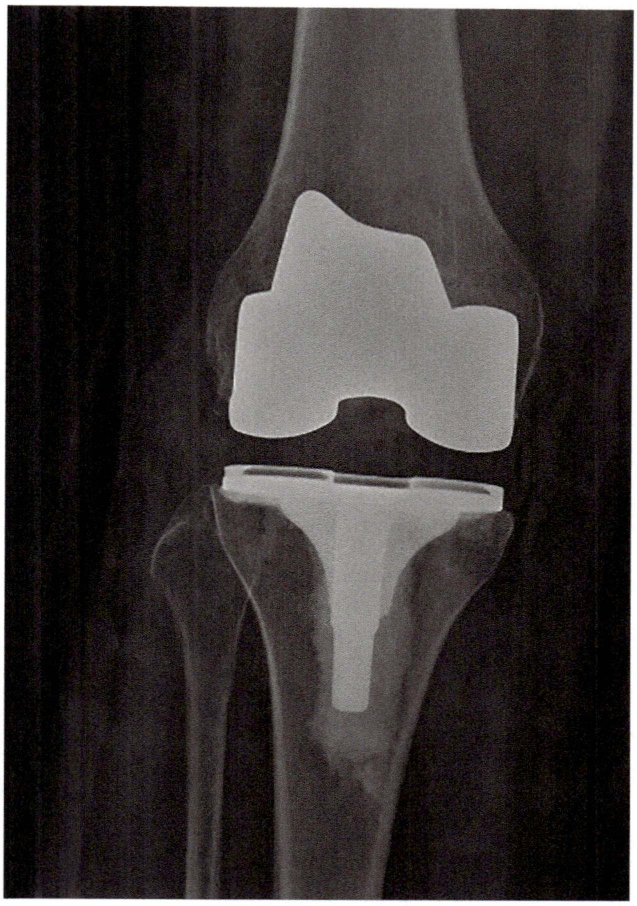

Fig. 34.4 Postoperative AP radiograph of a right TKA with excellent cement mantle and penetration in the tibia

> Oxidized zirconium is a ceramicized metal, which allows it to have the potential advantages of a ceramic bearing surface without the fragility of ceramics (Bal et al. 2007).

While other ceramic or ceramicized total knee implants have been developed, most have shown overall poor results and high failure rates compared to CoCr or oxidized zirconium implants (Song et al. 2020; Lionberger et al. 2019).

34.5 Metal Allergy

There is continued debate on the impact of patients' metal and nickel allergies on the incidence of true metal hypersensitivity to total knee implants (Saccomanno et al. 2019; Innocenti et al. 2017; Schmidt et al. 2019; Bravo et al. 2016; Faschingbauer et al. 2017; Hofer and Ezzet 2014).While some studies have shown that metal allergy is associated with inferior outcomes after primary TKA, other studies have shown that metal allergy or patching testing does not affect clinical outcomes (Saccomanno et al. 2019; Innocenti et al. 2017; Schmidt et al. 2019; Bravo et al. 2016; Faschingbauer et al. 2017; Hofer and Ezzet 2014).

> However, ceramicized metals, such as oxidized zirconium, are an alternative bearing surface that are "hypoallergenic" (Hofer and Ezzet 2014). As such, in patients that are highly concerned about metal allergy affecting their total knee outcomes, ceramicized components are an attractive option (Hofer and Ezzet 2014).

34.6 Wear Properties

A number of biomechanical studies have shown decreased wear of oxidized zirconium compared to CoCr-bearing surfaces (White et al. 1994; Ezzet et al. 2004, 2012; Tsukamoto et al. 2006; Ries et al. 2002).Several in vitro studies report between 42% and 85% reduced wear of oxidized zirconium implants compared to CoCr with ultra-high molecular weight polyethylene (UHMWPE) after five million or more cycles on a knee simulator (White et al. 1994; Ezzet et al. 2004, 2012; Tsukamoto et al. 2006; Ries et al. 2002).

34

> Oxidized zirconium's improved wear characteristics are attributed to its surface lubricity (Bal et al. 2007) that results in a decreased coefficient of friction, its increased hardness compared to CoCr, and reduced in vivo surface roughening compared to CoCr (Bal et al. 2007).

In order to simulate the degree that roughening of components contributes to wear, Ries et al. (2002) intentionally roughened CoCr and oxidized zirconium components and tested their wear characteristics after five million cycles on a knee simulator. They reported that roughened oxidized zirconium produced 85% less wear than roughened CoCr (Ries et al. 2002). Therefore, it appears that all of these factors play a role in the reduction of polyethylene wear seen in oxidized zirconium compared to CoCr-bearing surfaces.

> Reassuringly, oxidized zirconium does not produce different polyethylene wear particulate debris compared to CoCr-induced polyethylene wear particles (Minoda et al. 2014; Kim et al. 2010).

Kim et al. (2010) analyzed synovial fluid of 100 patients with an oxidized zirconium implant in one TKA and a CoCr implant in the contralateral TKA. They did not find any significant difference in polyethylene particle size or shape (Kim et al. 2010).

Furthermore, retrieval analyses have supported the decreased in vitro damage, surface roughness, and polyethylene wear of oxidized zirconium compared to CoCr-bearing surfaces (Heyse et al. 2011a, b, 2014). Heyse et al. (2011a) reported in a matched-pair retrieval analysis of 11 oxidized zirconium and 11 CoCr femoral components at a mean of 20 months of implantation that there were significantly lower damage scores of the femoral components and polyethylene inserts in the oxidized zirconium compared to the CoCr-bearing surfaces. Further, in a different matched-pair retrieval analysis, profilometry of 10 oxidized zirconium and 10 CoCr femoral components showed significantly greater surface roughness of the CoCr femoral components compared to the oxidized zirconium implants (Heyse et al. 2014). This building evidence shows that enhanced in vivo performance of oxidized zirconium compared to CoCr-bearing surfaces in TKA.

34.7 Clinical Outcomes

Oxidized zirconium-bearing surfaces also produce reliable patient clinical outcomes and durable implant survivorship (Innocenti et al. 2010, 2014; Laskin 2003; Hui et al. 2011; Hofer and Ezzet 2014). Innocenti et al. (2014) reported a 98% implant survival at 10 years and a mean Knee Society score (KSS) of 84 and a mean Knee Society function score (KFS) of 83 in 98 patients with oxidized zirconium-bearing surfaces at a mean 11 years of follow-up. Similarly, Hofer and Ezzet (2014) reported excellent sustained clinical outcomes with mean KSSs of 92 and KFS of 81 in 109 TKAs with oxidized zirconium-bearing surfaces.

Conclusion

In conclusion, cemented primary TKA remains the gold standard knee arthroplasty option. Meticulous surgical and cementation technique and avoiding common surgical pitfalls, as outlined in this chapter, is essential to achieving well-aligned, well-balanced, and durable TKAs. Furthermore, oxidized zirconium-bearing articulations show significant promise in reducing polyethylene wear and may further enhance implant durability and longevity.

Take-Home Messages

- Preoperative planning and intraoperative assessment of bony cuts and alignment help ensure that one achieves a well-aligned TKA.
- Achieving proper femoral component rotation for an individual patient's anatomy while not over-resecting the posterior medial femoral condyle is essential in properly balancing a TKA.
- Meticulous cement techniques, including pressurization and cementation of the tibial keel and coating of the tibial and femoral implants, are crucial for fixation strength and implant durability.
- Oxidized zirconium-bearing surfaces in primary TKA have reduced polyethylene wear compared to CoCr-bearing surfaces in in vitro knee simulator studies.
- Oxidized zirconium-bearing surfaces can result in up to 98% implant survival at 10 years with reliable and sustained improvement in clinical outcome measures.
- Retrieval analyses show that oxidized zirconium has decreased damage, wear properties, and surface roughness compared to CoCr femoral components.

References

Anouchi YS, Whiteside LA, Kaiser AD, Milliano MT (1993) The effects of axial rotational alignment of the femoral component on knee stability and patellar tracking in total knee arthroplasty demonstrated on autopsy specimens. Clin Orthop Relat Res (287):170–177

Arima J, Whiteside LA, McCarthy DS, White SE (1995) Femoral rotational alignment, based on the anteroposterior axis, in total knee arthroplasty in a valgus knee. A technical note. J Bone Joint Surg Am 77(9):1331–1334

Bal BS, Garino J, Ries M, Rahaman MN (2007) A review of ceramic-bearingmaterials in total joint arthroplasty. Hip Int 17(1):21–30

Billi F, Kavanaugh A, Schmalzried H, Schmalzried TP (2019) Techniques for improving the initial strength of the tibial tray-cement interface bond. Bone Joint J 101-B(1_Supple_A): 53–58

Bravo D, Wagner ER, Larson DR, Davis MP, Pagnano MW, Sierra RJ (2016) No increased risk of knee arthroplasty failure in patients with positive skin patch testing for metal hypersensitivity: a matched cohort study. J Arthroplasty 31(8):1717–1721

Coyle RM, Bas MA, Rodriguez JA, Hepinstall MS (2019) The effect of femoral cutting jig design on restoration of femoral offset in posterior-referenced total knee arthroplasty. Orthopedics 42(6):316–322

Dennis DA (1991) Principles of total knee arthroplasty. Semin Arthroplasty 2(1):2–11

Donaldson J, Joyner J, Tudor F (2015) Current controversies of alignment in total knee replacements. Open Orthop J 9:489–494

Ezzet KA, Hermida JC, Colwell CW Jr, D'Lima DD (2004) Oxidized zirconium femoral components reducepolyethylene wear in a knee wear simulator. Clin Orthop Relat Res 428:120–124

Ezzet KA, Hermida JC, Steklov N, D'Lima DD (2012) Wear of polyethylene against oxidized zirconium femoral components effect of aggressive kinematic conditions and malalignment in total knee arthroplasty. J Arthroplasty 27(1):116–121

Faschingbauer M, Renner L, Boettner F (2017) Allergy in total knee replacement. Does it exist?: review article. HSS J 13(1):12–19

Haas SB, Cook S, Beksac B (2004) Minimally invasive total knee replacement through a mini midvastus approach: a comparative study. Clin Orthop Relat Res (428):68–73

Haas SB, Manitta MA, Burdick P (2006) Minimally invasive total knee arthroplasty: the mini midvastus approach. Clin Orthop Relat Res 452:112–116

Heyse TJ, Chen DX, Kelly N, Boettner F, Wright TM, Haas SB (2011a) Matched-pair total knee arthroplasty retrieval analysis: oxidized zirconium vs. CoCrMo. Knee 18(6):448–452

Heyse TJ, Davis J, Haas SB, Chen DX, Wright TM, Laskin RS (2011b) Retrieval analysis of femoral zirconium components in total knee arthroplasty: preliminary results. J Arthroplasty 26(3):445–450

Heyse TJ, Elpers ME, Nawabi DH, Wright TM, Haas SB (2014) Oxidized zirconium versus cobalt-chromium in TKA: profilometry of retrieved femoral components. Clin Orthop Relat Res 472(1):277–283

Hofer JK, Ezzet KA (2014) A minimum 5-year follow-up of an oxidized zirconium femoral prosthesis used for total knee arthroplasty. Knee 21(1):168–171

Hui C, Salmon L, Maeno S, Roe J, Walsh W, Pinczewski L (2011) Five-year comparison of oxidized zirconium and cobalt-chromium femoral components in total knee arthroplasty: a randomized controlled trial. J Bone Joint Surg Am 93(7):624–630

Innocenti M, Civinini R, Carulli C, Matassi F, Villano M (2010) The 5-year results of an oxidized zirconium femoral component for TKA. Clin Orthop Relat Res 468(5):1258–1263

Innocenti M, Matassi F, Carulli C, Nistri L, Civinini R (2014) Oxidized zirconium femoral component for TKA: a follow-up note of a previous report at a minimum of 10 years. Knee 21(4):858–861

Innocenti M, Vieri B, Melani T, Paoli T, Carulli C (2017) Metal hypersensitivity after knee arthroplasty: fact or fiction? Acta Biomed 88(2S):78–83

Kim YH, Kim JS, Huh W, Lee KH (2010) Weight of polyethylene wear particles is similar in TKAs with oxidized zirconium and cobalt chrome prostheses. Clin Orthop Relat Res 468(5): 1296–1304

Laskin RS (2003) An oxidized Zr ceramic surfaced femoral component for total knee arthroplasty. Clin Orthop Relat Res 416: 191–196

Lionberger D, Conlon C, Wattenbarger L, Walker TJ (2019) Unacceptable failure rate of a ceramic-coated posterior cruciate-substituting total knee arthroplasty. Arthroplast Today 5(2):187–192

Mercuri JJ, Schwarzkopf R (2019) Coronal and sagittal balancing of total knee arthroplasty old principles and new technologies. Bull Hosp Jt Dis (2013) 77(1):45–52

Minoda Y, Hata K, Iwaki H et al (2014) No difference in in vivo polyethylene wear particles between oxidized zirconium and cobalt-chromium femoral component in total knee arthroplasty. Knee Surg Sports Traumatol Arthrosc 22(3):680–686

Minoda Y, Ikebuchi M, Mizokawa S, Ohta Y, Nakamura H (2018) Asymmetric tibial component improved the coverage and rotation of the tibial component in a medial pivot total knee prosthesis. J Knee Surg 31(5):416–421

Nikolaou VS, Chytas D, Babis GC (2014) Common controversies in total knee replacement surgery: Current evidence. World J Orthop 5(4):460–468

Nugent M, Wyatt MC, Frampton CM, Hooper GJ (2019) Despite improved survivorship of uncemented fixation in total knee arthroplasty for osteoarthritis, cemented fixation remains the gold standard: an analysis of a national joint registry. J Arthroplasty 34(8):1626–1633

Patel AM, Spector M (1997) Tribological evaluation of oxidized zirconium using an articular cartilage counterface: anovelmaterial for potential use in hemi arthroplasty. Biomaterials 18(5):441–447

Poilvache PL, Insall JN, Scuderi GR, Font-Rodriguez DE (1996) Rotation all and marks and sizing of the distal femur in total knee arthroplasty. Clin Orthop Relat Res (331):35–46

Ries MD, Salehi A, Widding K, Hunter G (2002) Polyethylene wear performance of oxidized zirconium and cobalt-chromium knee components under abrasive conditions. J Bone Joint Surg Am 84-A(Suppl 2):129–135

Saccomanno MF, Sircana G, Masci G et al (2019) Allergy in total knee replacement surgery: is it a real problem? World J Orthop 10(2):63–70. Published 2019 Feb 18

Schmidt KJ, Huang PS, Colwell CW Jr, McCauley JC, Pulido PA, Bugbee WD (2019) Self-reported metal allergy and early outcomes after total knee arthroplasty. Orthopedics 42(6):330–334

Song SJ, Lee HW, Bae DK, Park CH (2020) High incidence of tibial component loosening after total knee arthroplasty using ceramic titanium-nitride-coated mobile bearing prosthesis in moderate to severe varus deformity: a matched-pair study between ceramic-coated mobile bearing and fixed bearing prostheses. J Arthroplasty 35(4):1003–1008

Stulberg SD, Goyal N (2015) Which tibial tray design achieves maximum coverage and ideal rotation: anatomic, symmetric, or asymmetric? An MRI-based study. J Arthroplasty 30(10):1839–1841

Tsukamoto R, Chen S, Asano T et al (2006) Improved wear performance with cross linked UHMWPE and zirconia implants in knee simulation. Acta Orthop 77(3):505–511

White SE, Whiteside LA, McCarthy DS, Anthony M, Poggie RA (1994) Simulated knee wear with cobalt chromium and oxidized zirconium knee femoral components. Clin Orthop Relat Res 309:176–184

Contemporary Rotating Hinged Prostheses in Primary Total Knee Arthroplasty

Benjamin M. Wooster and Matthew P. Abdel

Contents

E. Hansen, K.-D. Kühn (eds.), *Essentials of Cemented Knee Arthroplasty*,
https://doi.org/10.1007/978-3-662-63113-3_35

35.1 Introduction

The utilization of fixed hinged prostheses in TKAs has been traditionally reserved for complex revision scenarios where issues such as extensive bone loss, ligament incompetence, and extensor mechanism dysfunction prevented the use of implants with lesser constraint (Sculco 2006; Dauwe and Vandenneucker 2018). While the initial stability afforded by these devices can be beneficial in these difficult revision situations, the historically high failure rate of early fixed hinged designs moderated their widespread adoption. The etiology of failure of older hinged prostheses was likely multifactorial in nature, but largely related to flaws in the biomechanical design and poor kinematics of these implants (Dauwe and Vandenneucker 2018; Chelman et al. 1975).

The first-generation of fixed hinged prostheses were introduced in the early 1950s and consisted of linked, monobloc components of various metal alloys that only allowed uniaxial motion in the sagittal plane (Jones 1973; Shiers 1954; Lettin et al. 1978; Mazas 1973). This degree of constraint resulted in significantly increased force transmission to the bone–cement interface yielding unacceptable early failure rates due to aseptic loosening (Dauwe and Vandenneucker 2018; Jackson and Elson 1973). Second-generation hinged prostheses were introduced nearly two decades later featuring design modifications that permitted some additional motion in the axial and coronal planes (Sheehan 1978; Herbert and Herbert 1973; Matthews et al. 1973; Hoogland and Bosma 1981; Flynn 1979). However, early failure and high complication rates persisted despite these modifications (Kester et al. 1988; Knutson et al. 1986).

Contemporary, third-generation rotating-hinge (RH) constructs first appeared in the market in the early 1990s and incorporated modularity and mobile bearings into the design (Jones 2006; Barrack 2001). The reduced prosthetic constraint afforded by these modern implants functioned to mitigate the forces transmitted to the bone–cement interface and resulted in increased survival rates compared to earlier designs.

> Consequently, the indications for RHs have expanded in both primary and revision TKA scenarios.

35.2 Case Example

A 90-year-old female with a history of right total hip arthroplasty for primary osteoarthritis presents to clinic with a chief complaint of progressively worsening left knee pain, instability, and deformity refractory to conservative management strategies. Physical examination demonstrates a severe, fixed, valgus deformity of the left knee measuring approximately 75° (Fig. 35.1). Passive and active range of motion is limited from 10° shy of full extension to 100° of flexion. Ligamentous testing demonstrates complete incompetence of the medial collateral ligament (MCL) with valgus stress (Fig. 35.2). Radiographs of the left knee demonstrate severe genu valgus with advanced degenerative changes of the lateral and patellofemoral compartments, lateral subluxation of the patella with erosion of the lateral patellar facet, and gapping of the medial joint space consistent with MCL insufficiency (Fig. 35.3). Standing hip–knee–ankle (HKA) radiographs demonstrate a windswept deformity with moderate varus alignment of the right lower extremity and significant valgus alignment of the left lower extremity (Fig. 35.4).

Given the severe coronal deformity and lack of a competent MCL, the plan is for a TKA with an RH prosthesis. Intraoperative evaluation demonstrates severe tricompartmental arthritis with substantial erosion of the posterolateral tibia and lateral facet of the patella (Fig. 35.5). The patient receives a cemented Modular Rotating Hinge (MRH) construct (Stryker; Mahwah, NJ) with cemented tibial and femoral stems. The postoperative course is uneventful and the patient has an excellent recovery.

At the most recent follow-up (3 years postoperative), the patient reports significant improvement in her pain and function. She is ambulating without the use of gait aids. Physical examination demonstrates a neutral mechanical axis of her left lower extremity. Range of motion of the left knee is from 0° to 130°. Radiographs of the left knee demonstrate a well-fixed and well-aligned RH TKA (Fig. 35.6). The postoperative HKA radiograph demonstrates neutral mechanical alignment of the left lower extremity (Fig. 35.7).

35.3 Surgical Technique

Typical anesthesia includes spinal anesthesia, single-shot adductor canal block, and periarticular injection. Patients are placed on the operative table in the supine position. An examination of the knee is performed under anesthesia. Thereafter, a non-sterile pneumatic tourniquet is placed on the thigh followed by sterile preparation and draping of the operative extremity. Prophylactic antibiotics consisting of a weight-based dose of a second-generation cephalosporin (e.g., cefazolin) and 1 g of tranexamic acid are administered intravenously (IV). The limb is then exsanguinated and the tourniquet is inflated.

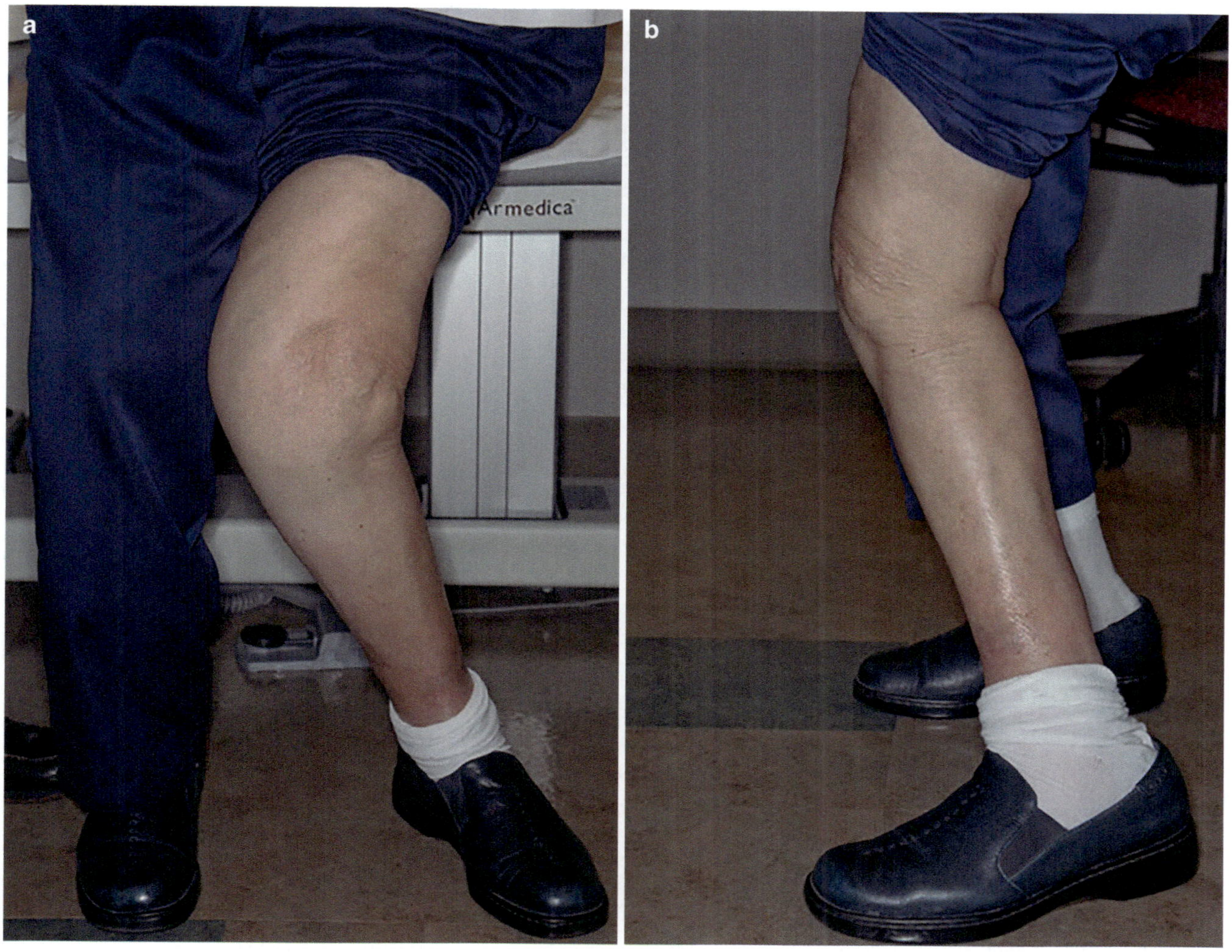

Fig. 35.1 Clinical photographs of patient's bilateral lower extremities including an anteroposterior view **a** demonstrating a fixed valgus deformity of the left knee and a lateral view **b** demonstrating an approximate 10° flexion contracture of the left knee

35.3.1 Exposure

A straight midline anterior longitudinal incision is performed with the knee in approximately 90° of flexion. Sharp dissection is carried through the subcutaneous tissue to the level of the fascia. A standard medial parapatellar arthrotomy is performed to expose the knee joint. If difficulty exposing the knee joint is encountered, a quadriceps snip and/or complete takedown of the collateral ligaments from their femoral insertions are performed to facilitate exposure of the joint (Fig. 35.8). A medial release is performed around the proximal tibia. The patella is subluxed or everted laterally and the knee joint is evaluated. Osteophytes, menisci, and the cruciate ligaments are excised.

35.3.2 Tibial Preparation

An external alignment guide is used to align the tibial resection guide perpendicular to its axis in the frontal plane.

> Of important note, when completing an RH TKA in the primary setting, additional tibial and femoral bony resections must be completed to accommodate the prosthesis, including the hinge mechanism.

Typically, the tibial resection required is 10–12 mm from the involved side, but varies based upon the preoperative radiographs and intraoperative pathology. The guide is secured to the tibia with pins and the tib-

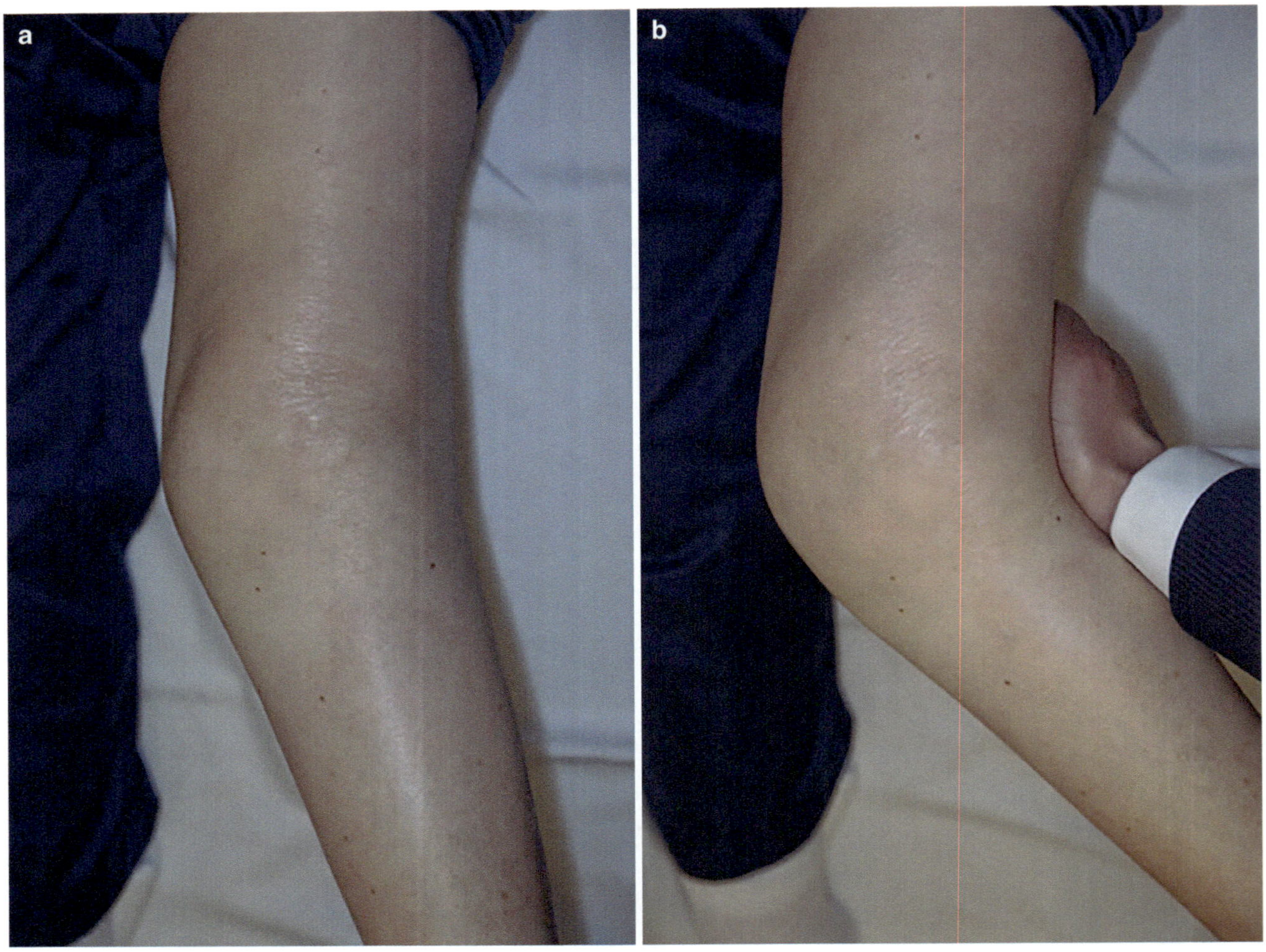

Fig. 35.2 Clinical photographs of the patient's left knee demonstrating fixed valgus deformity **a** and medial gapping with valgus stress testing, indicating complete incompetence of the medial collateral ligament **b**

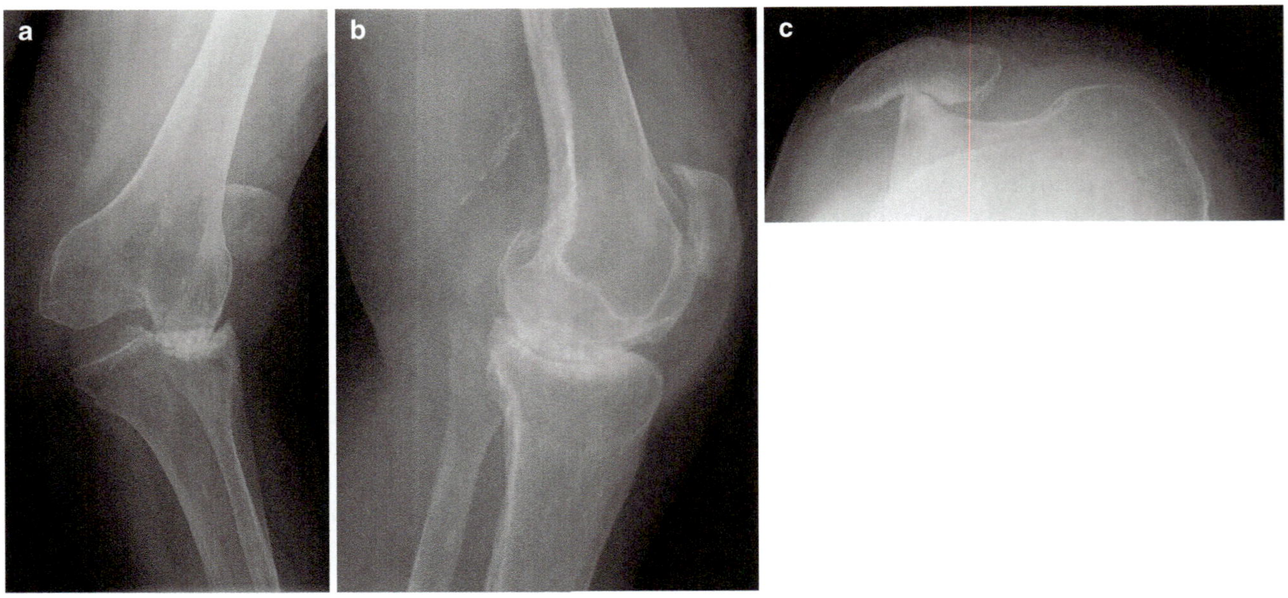

Fig. 35.3 Preoperative radiographs including anteroposterior **a**, lateral **b**, and sunrise **c** views of the patient's left knee demonstrating marked valgus deformity, advanced degenerative changes of the lateral and patellofemoral compartments, gapping of the medial joint space consistent with ligamentous insufficiency, and lateral subluxation of the patella

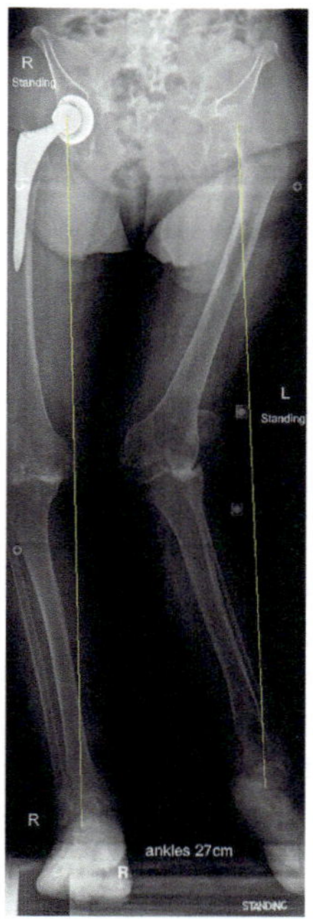

■ **Fig. 35.4** Preoperative standing hip–knee–ankle radiograph of the patient demonstrating windswept deformity of the bilateral lower extremities with moderate varus alignment of the right lower extremity and severe valgus alignment of the left lower extremity

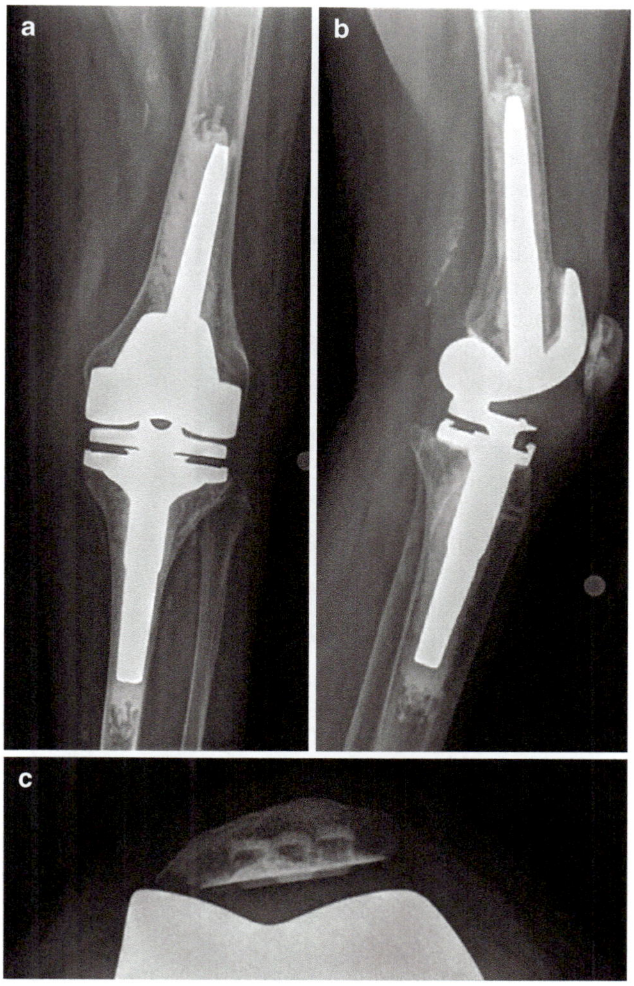

■ **Fig. 35.6** Postoperative radiographs including anteroposterior **a**, lateral **b**, and sunrise **c** views of the patient's left knee demonstrating a well-fixed and well-aligned cemented contemporary rotating-hinge TKA

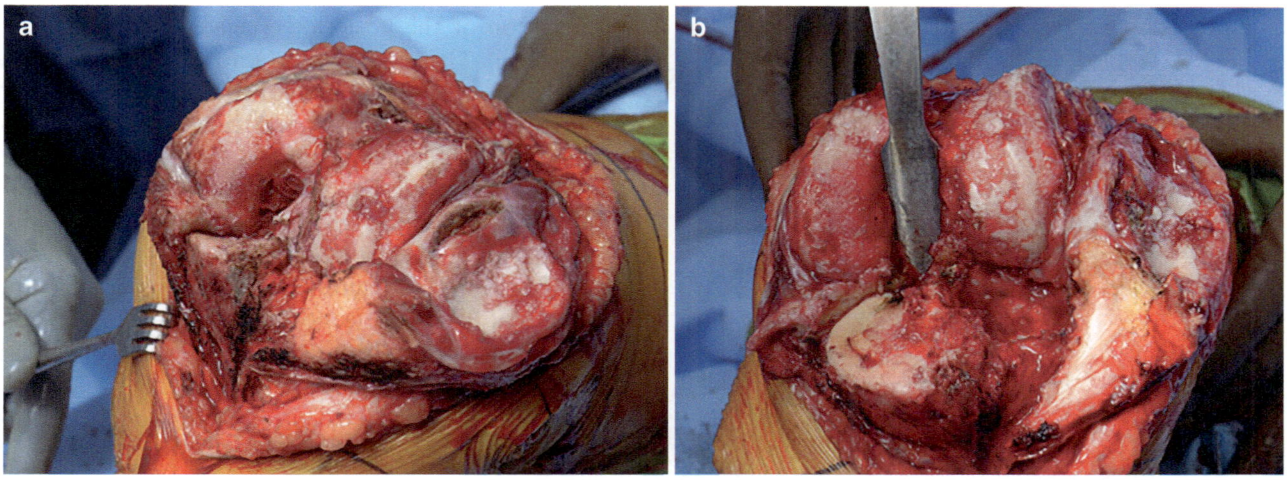

■ **Fig. 35.5** **a**, **b** Intraoperative clinical photographs of the patient's left knee demonstrating severe tricompartmental degenerative changes with substantial erosion of the posterolateral tibia and lateral facet of the patella

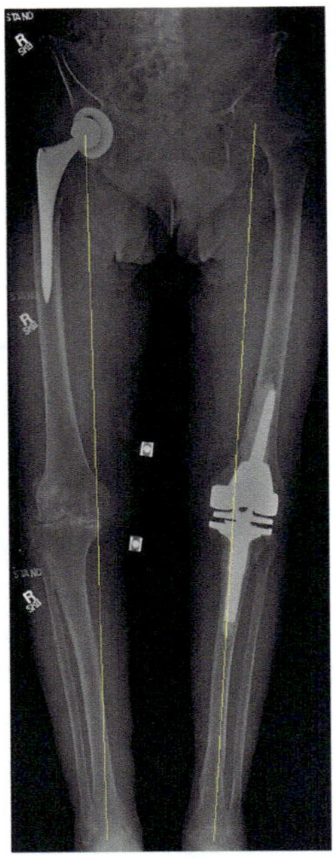

Fig. 35.7 Postoperative standing hip–knee–ankle radiograph of the patient demonstrating improvement in mechanical alignment of left lower extremity following left total knee arthroplasty with a rotating-hinge TKA

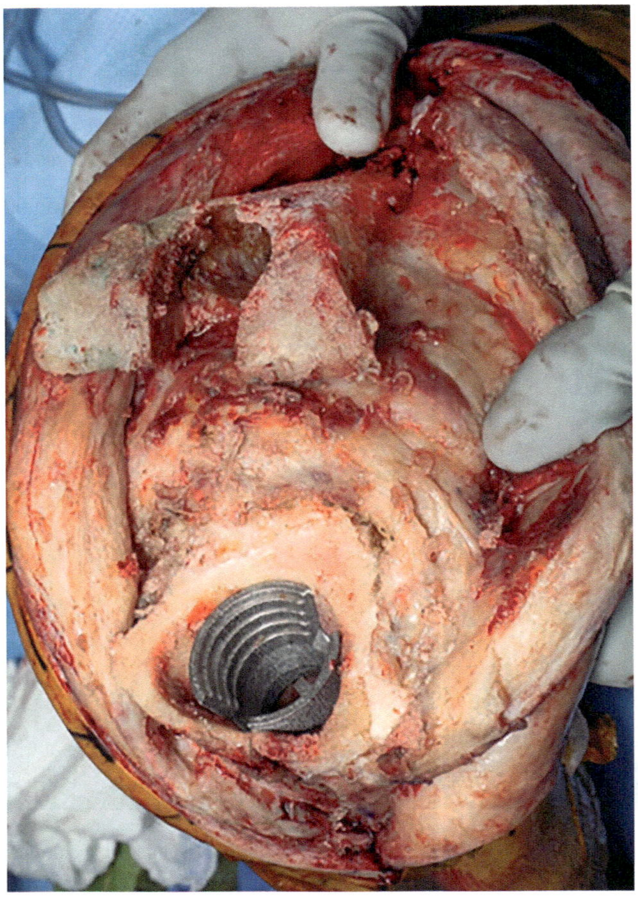

Fig. 35.8 Intraoperative clinical photograph demonstrating excellent exposure of the knee joint facilitated by complete takedown of the collateral ligaments from their femoral insertions

ial resection is performed with an oscillating saw. The tibia is sized and the alignment of the tibial resection is assessed with a drop rod to the second ray of the foot with the ankle in neutral flexion. The tibial finishing template is secured to the proximal tibia with pins utilizing the middle of the tibial tubercle and tibial crest as anatomic landmarks for appropriate rotation. The tibial stem keel punch guide is then applied to the tibial finishing template and the keel is punched in the proximal tibia. Thereafter, the intramedullary canal of the tibia is opened with a stepped drill and the canal is reamed with fluted reamers until there is appropriate chatter in the diaphysis. Typically, that is 14 mm in diameter at a depth of 175 mm. In most scenarios, this allows for a 12 mm stem with a 2 mm cement mantle. A 50–75 mm stem extender is usually more than adequate in the primary setting.

> Of note, the reamer should be pulsed proximally rather than being utilized in a continuous fashion to prevent complete denudation of cancellous bone (and thus inhibition of interdigitation of the bone cement in the intramedullary canal).

It has become the preference of the senior author (MPA) to utilize a tibial cone (Fig. 35.9) when performing an RH TKA given the increased loads at the bone–cement interface. Preparation for the tibial cone is performed with a milling reamer over the intramedullary reamer and is typically sized large enough to accept the revision tibial component for the RH TKA.

35.3.3 Femoral Preparation

A pilot hole is drilled slightly anterior to the femoral insertion of the posterior cruciate ligament with a stepped drill. Thereafter, an intramedullary guide rod is introduced with a distal femoral cutting guide set to 6° of valgus (as that is what is mandated by most manufacturers). The distal femoral cutting block is secured to the femur with pins and the distal femoral resection is performed with an oscillating saw. At a minimum, 10–12 mm of distal femoral bone should be removed from the distal aspect of the medial femoral condyle. After completion of the distal femoral resection, spacer blocks specific to the RH construct are utilized to assess the mechanical alignment of the limb and ensure the knee comes out to full extension. If full extension is not possible, additional distal femoral bone must be removed. The femur is then sized with femoral sizing templates and the corresponding three-in-one cutting block is secured to the distal femur with pins. Rotation of the cutting block is set in line with the transepicondylar axis of the femur to make a rectangle with the in situ tibial trial, which should be cut perpendicular to the coronal and sagittal

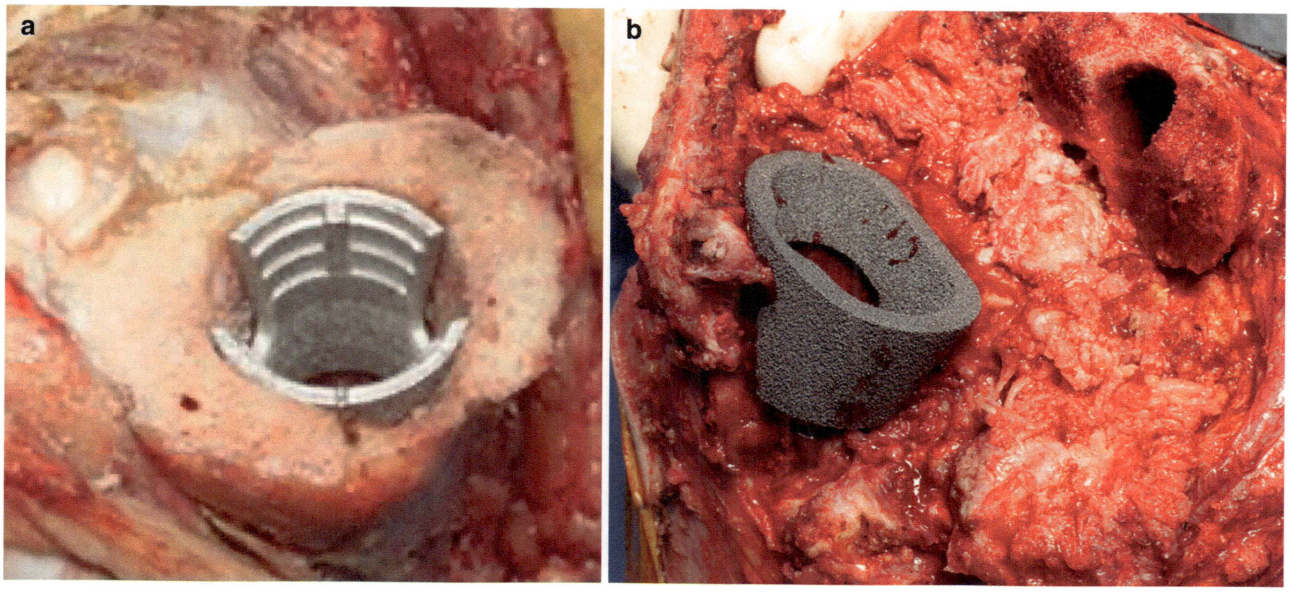

Fig. 35.9 Intraoperative clinical photographs demonstrating two types of highly porous metaphyseal tibial cone augments including Stryker Triathlon® Tritanium tibial cone **a** and Zimmer Trabecular Metal™ tibial cone **b**

axes of the tibia. If anything, additional external rotation is placed to assist with patellofemoral tracking. The anterior femoral, anterior chamfer, and posterior condylar resections are carefully performed with an oscillating saw after the soft tissues on the posterior aspect of the femur are taken directly off the bone to protect the neurovascular bundle from injury by the saw blade. Fluted reamers are then sequentially advanced into the femoral canal until there is appropriate chatter in the diaphysis. Typically, the diameter is 15 mm for a 13 mm stem with a 2 mm cement mantle. Moreover, the length of the stem in the primary setting is usually 50–75 mm. As with preparing the tibial canal, the femoral reamer should be utilized in a pulsatile fashion to avoid reaming away all of the cancellous bone.

Similar to the tibial side, it has become the preference of the senior author (MPA) to utilize femoral cones (Fig. 35.10) when performing an RH TKA given the increased loads at the bone–cement interface. Preparation for the femoral cone is performed with a milling reamer over the intramedullary reamer and is typically sized large enough to accept the revision femoral component for the RH TKA.

35.3.4 Patellar Preparation

The patella is everted with the knee in extension and stabilized with a pair of pointed towel clamps. Excessive osteophytes are removed with a rongeur and the patella is circumferentially denervated with electrocautery. The thickness of the patella is measured with a caliper and the patella resection is performed free-hand with an oscillating saw to restore the patellar height. However, the patella is never resected below 12 mm. The patellar thickness is reassessed in four quadrants to ensure an even resection. The patella is sized and anchor holes are preferentially drilled on the superomedial aspect of the patella. The trial patellar component is then placed and a partial lateral facetectomy is performed with a high-speed burr or rongeur.

35.3.5 Trialing

Trial femoral and tibial components are assembled on the back table and impacted onto the prepared bony surfaces. Knee stability (in the form of obtaining full extension without recurvatum) and patellar tracking are tested with trial spacer inserts of various thicknesses. Intraoperative radiographs (anteroposterior and lateral) are obtained to confirm appropriate sizing, positioning, and alignment of all the components. If patellar maltracking is encountered, the tourniquet is deflated and patellar tracking is reassessed. If maltracking persists with the tourniquet deflated, then a lateral release is performed with care taken to preserve the superior lateral geniculate artery. After sizing, positioning, alignment, stability, and patellar tracking are deemed satisfactory, the trial components are removed, the wound is copiously irrigated with sterile saline via pulsatile lavage, and the exposed bony surfaces are thoroughly dried.

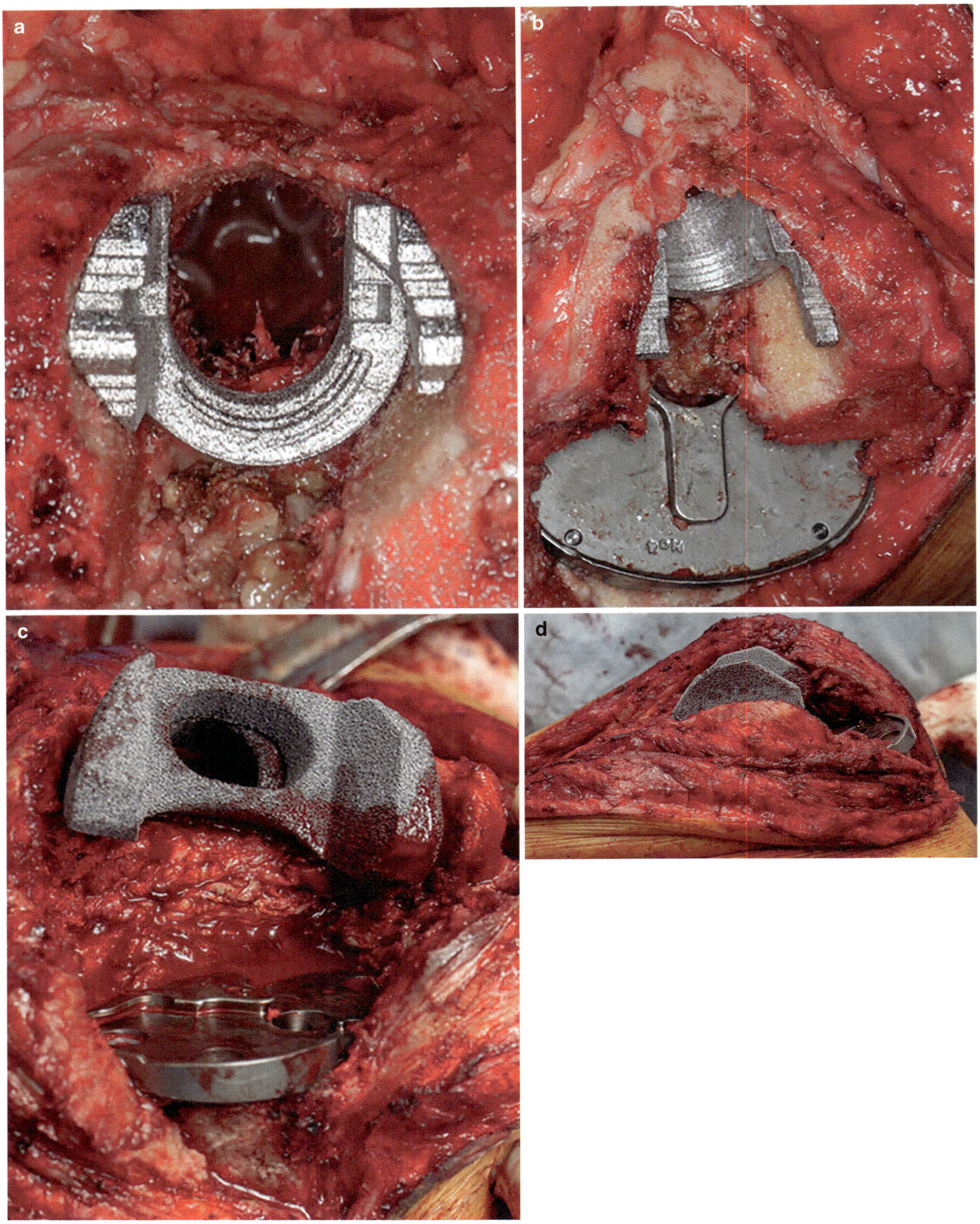

Fig. 35.10 Intraoperative clinical photographs demonstrating two types of highly porous metaphyseal femoral cone augments including Stryker Triathlon® Tritanium femoral cone **a** and **b** and Zimmer Trabecular Metal™ femoral cone **c** and **d**

35.3.6 Final Implant Placement

Final implants are opened and assembled according to manufacturer guidelines on the back table. Cement restrictors are placed in the tibia and femur at depths only a few millimeters past the end of the stems. This allows for excellent pressurization of the cement into the cancellous bone. Thereafter, the uncemented tibial and femoral cones are impacted.

> Cementation of the final tibial and femoral components are completed separately with the tibia performed first.

Two batches of 40 mg low-viscosity polymethylmethacrylate bone cement are mixed by hand on the back table with a combination of 2 g of vancomycin and 2.4 g of gentamicin powder. After achieving a doughy consistency, liberal amounts of cement are applied to the back of the final tibial component baseplate and the exposed bony surfaces of the tibia with a cement gun. The final tibial component is impacted into place through the uncemented cone, ensuring rotation is kept in line with the middle of the tibial tubercle and tibial crest. Excess cement is meticulously removed with a freer and the cement is allowed to completely cure. Attention is then turned to cementation of the final femoral and patellar components. Cementation of the final femoral component is performed in a similar fashion as previously described for the tibial component with care taken to ensure that rotation remains in line with the transepicondylar axis of the femur. Finally, cement is applied to the patellar surface by hand and the final patellar component is clamped into place until the cement has completely cured.

After all the cement has cured, the knee is then brought to approximately 45° of flexion to facilitate final assembly of the hinge. A tibial sleeve is first inserted into the tibial baseplate and the final polyethylene insert is secured into place. The rotating tibial platform is then placed into the polyethylene insert. The femoral bushings are inserted into the femoral component with care to ensure that the flanges are inside the intercondylar cutout. The rotating tibial platform is then aligned with the femoral component bushings and the axle is slid through the assembly housing with care to ensure that the axle recess is aligned inferiorly. The bumper (typically neutral) is then aligned with the axle recess and gently impacted into place.

The wound is copiously irrigated with a dilute betadine solution followed by sterile saline via pulse lavage. The tourniquet is deflated and meticulous hemostasis is achieved with electrocautery. The wound is then closed in sequential layers and sterile dressings are applied.

35.4 Indications for Rotating Hinges in Primary TKA

The utilization of RHs in complex primary TKA has been steadily increasing since the turn of the twenty-first century. According to the National Joint Registry for England and Wales, the use of RHs in primary TKA experienced a fourfold increase between 2003 and 2010 (National Joint Registry for England and Wales 2010). Similarly, the use of these implants in primary TKA has nearly doubled from 2010 to 2018 according to the Norwegian Arthroplasty Register (Norwegian National Advisory Unit on Arthroplasty and Hip Fractures 2019).

Despite the increasing utilization of RHs in primary TKA, specific non-oncologic indications for their use remain controversial in the literature. Some authors suggest imposing strict limitations on the use of these devices in primary TKA. Gehrke et al. (2014) recommend that the use of RHs in primary TKA be restricted to patients older than 75 years who possess either of the following:

- Collateral ligament insufficiency
- Bony destruction of the distal femur or proximal tibia
- Hyperlaxity
- Fixed varus or valgus deformity greater than 20°
- Severe rheumatoid arthritis

These selected indications were established by the authors after finding age- and deformity-related discrepancies in the mid-term revision-free survival rates of the Endo-Model® prosthesis (Waldemar Link; Hamburg, Germany). In their study, the authors retrospectively reviewed the mid-term outcomes and survival of this specific type of RH in a cohort of 238 patients with a mean age of 67 years. The overall survivorship free of all-cause revision for the entire cohort was 90% at 13 years. However, after adjusting survival by age at implantation, the 13-year survivorship free of all-cause revision was 94% for patients older than 60 years compared to only 77% for patients younger than 60 years old. Similarly, after adjusting for preoperative deformity, the 13-year survivorship free of all-cause revision for patients with a preoperative varus deformity was 97% while survivorship was only 79% in patients with a preoperative valgus deformity.

> Based on these results, the authors concluded that RHs can be safely and effectively utilized in primary TKA for selected indications. However, they emphasized that the need for these devices in primary TKA is exceedingly rare with <2% of the primary TKAs performed at their institution in 1 year.

There are other non-oncologic indications beyond the criteria suggested by Gehrke et al. (2014) where the use of RHs in the primary TKA may be warranted. Specifically, patients with neuropathic (Charcot) arthropathy or neuromuscular conditions. Patients with neuropathic arthropathy can develop rapid and progressive joint destruction, deformity, and instability resulting from loss of nociception attributable to various etiologies (◘ Fig. 35.11) (Bae et al. 2009; Tibbo et al. 2018). Consequently, many surgeons recommend utilizing implants with increased levels of constraint when performing TKA in these patients, regardless of age. Tibbo et al. (2018) recently investigated implant utilization and contemporary mid-term results of primary TKA in patients with neuropathic arthropathy attributed to multiple underlying conditions. Their study included 27 patients (37 knees) with a mean age of 60 years. Posterior stabilized implants were used in 19% of cases (7 knees), varus-valgus constrained (VVC) devices were used in 46% of cases (18 knees), and RHs were utilized in 35% of cases (13 knees). Supplemental fixation with highly porous metaphyseal cones was used in 16% of the cases (5 knees). Kaplan–Meier estimated survivorship free of all-cause revision was 91% at 5 years and 70% at 10 years. However, estimated survivorship free of all-cause re-operation was much lower at 83% at 5 years and 65% at 10 years. The majority of revisions and re-operations in this cohort were related to postoperative wound issues and periprosthetic joint infection (PJI). Conversely, revisions due to aseptic loosening or mechanical failure of the implants were rare. In fact, the survivorship free of aseptic loosening was 100% at 5 years and 88% at 10 years. The authors attributed these findings to poor host characteristics and the selective use of highly porous metaphyseal cones in these patients.

Although the incidence of poliomyelitis has significantly decreased since the introduction of its vaccine, patients afflicted by this condition develop varying degrees of generalized hypotonia (Tigani et al. 2009). Muscle weakness often leads to compensated gait patterns that result in characteristic deformities of the knee joint. Specifically, patients with poliomyelitis often present with significant knee flexion contractures and recurvatum deformities related to imbalances in quadriceps and hamstring function (Tigani et al. 2009). Consequently, the utilization of devices with increased constraint is similarly advocated when performing primary TKA in patients with this condition. There are few studies in the literature reporting on the outcomes of primary TKA in patients with poliomyelitis. In a systematic review of six retrospective case series, Prasad et al. (2018) explored implant utilization trends and mid-term outcomes of primary TKA in 82 patients with poliomyelitis. The mean age of the patients was 63 years. Thirty-six patients (44%) possessed preoperative recurvatum deformities ranging from 5° to 30°. Cruciate-retaining (CR) implants were used in 24% of patients, PS devices were used in 35% of patients, VVC implants were used in 14% of patients, and RHs were used in 27% of patients. At a mean follow-up of 6 years, there were only 6 patients (7%) who required revision TKA. Indications for revision included PJI (2 patients), instability (2 patients), periprosthetic fracture (1 patient), and aseptic loosening (1 patient). Ten (28%) of the 36 patients with a preoperative recurvatum deformity developed recurrent deformity after surgery. Although this complication was observed most commonly in patients who received CR devices (5 patients), deformity recurrence was also observed in 4 patients who received VVC devices and 1 patient who received an RH. Only 2 patients with post-

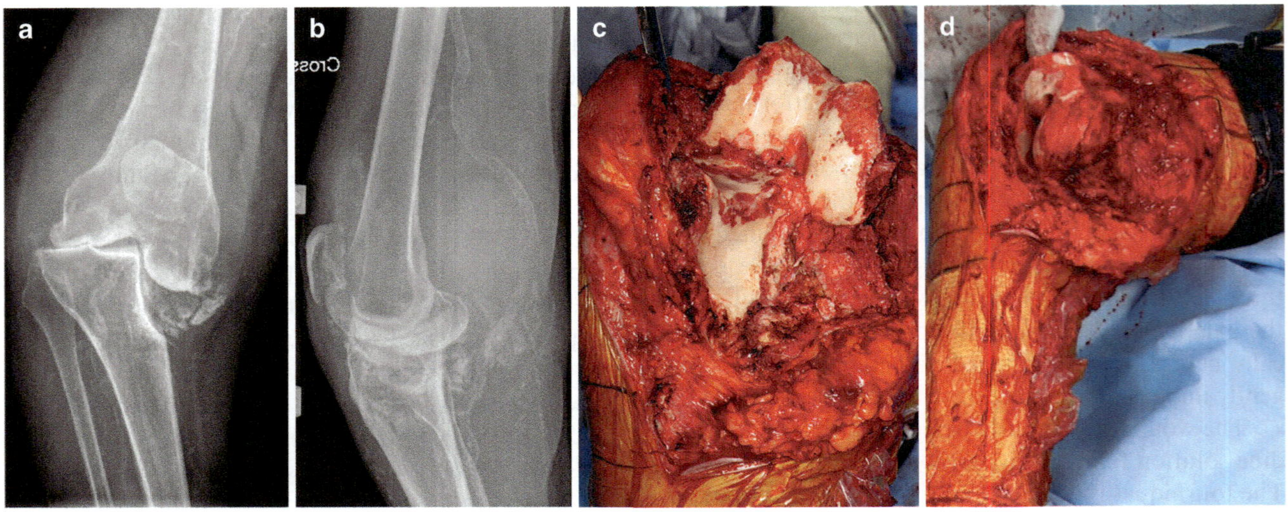

◘ **Fig. 35.11** Preoperative radiographs including anteroposterior **a** and lateral **b** views of a patient with neuropathic arthropathy of the right knee demonstrating extensive bony destruction of the distal femur and proximal tibia. Images **c** and **d** demonstrate intraoperative photographs of the left knee of the same patient

35

operative deformity recurrence required revision TKA and were successfully treated by increasing the level of implant constraint.

35.5 Clinical Outcomes

35.5.1 Short- and Mid-Term Outcomes

The increased utilization of RHs in primary TKA has been supported in the literature by a number of studies demonstrating that the early outcomes of these devices are comparable to implants with lesser constraint. In a retrospective analysis of the National Joint Registry for England and Wales, Baker et al. (2014) found that the mid-term survival of RHs in primary TKA was similar to unconstrained implants irrespective of the indication for surgery. Their study included 964 patients with a mean age of 73 years who underwent primary TKA with several types of RHs. Indications for surgery included osteoarthritis (71%), inflammatory arthritis (10%), and post-traumatic arthritis (8%). The survivorship free of all-cause revision for the entire cohort at 5 years was 97% and was not dependent on the primary indication for surgery. Specifically, the 5-year survivorship free of all-cause revision was 97% for patients with osteoarthritis, 96% for patients with inflammatory arthritis, and 100% for patients with post-traumatic arthritis (p = not significant). The authors noted that these survival rates were comparable to the 5-year survivorship free of all-cause revision of cemented, unconstrained primary TKAs reported in the same National Registry database (96%) and the Australian National Registry database (95%). Multiple studies have similarly demonstrated promising short- and mid-term survivorship of RHs in primary TKA for multiple indications (Zhang et al. 2014; Bistolfi et al. 2013; Bohler et al. 2017; Sanguineti et al. 2014; Badawy et al. 2019; Efe et al. 2012; Neri et al. 2019; Kowalczewski et al. 2014).

> Based on these results, many authors consider RHs as not only necessary but also safe and effective options for complex primary TKA in elderly patient populations.

35.5.2 Long-Term Outcomes

Currently, there is a paucity of studies in the literature that have investigated the long-term outcomes of RHs in primary TKA. To our knowledge, Martin et al. (2016) has published the only study reporting on the long-term survival of these implants in primary arthroplasty setting. Their study included 246 patients with a mean age of 52 years who underwent primary TKA with several types of RHs at a single tertiary referral center between 1979 to 2013. Indications included degenerative joint disease (19%), congenital or pediatric conditions (13%), post-traumatic arthritis (12%), inflammatory arthritis (2%), and other (53%). Kaplan–Meier estimated survivorship free of all-cause revision was 75% at 10 years but decreased to 40% at 20 years. The estimated survivorship free of all-cause re-operation for this cohort was even lower at both 10 years (49%) and 20 years (17%).

In the same study, the authors subsequently compared the survivorship of RHs to VVC (n = 427) and unconstrained (n = 27,994) devices in patients who underwent primary TKA for similar indications. After adjusting for potential confounding factors, the estimated survivorship free of all-cause revision was not significantly different between the RH and unconstrained cohorts at 10 and 20 years (Hazard Ratio [HR] = 1.5; p = 0.05). However, the adjusted survivorship free of all-cause re-operation was significantly lower in patients with RHs compared to the unconstrained cohort at 10 and 20 years (HR = 2.07; $p < 0.001$). The increased rate of re-operation in the RH cohort was primarily attributed to higher risk of infection (HR = 4; $p < 0.001$) and wound complications (HR = 2; $p < 0.001$).

> It is important to note that the mean age of patients who received RHs in this study was significantly lower than the studies demonstrating favorable short- and mid-term outcomes of these devices.

Further, congenital and pediatric conditions or "other" diagnoses were cited as the primary indication for RH in more than half of the patients in this study. These characteristics likely contributed to the considerably lower survivorship reported in this cohort at a longer follow-up.

> Nevertheless, these results suggest that the early comparable outcomes of RHs to devices with lesser constraint may not persist with longer follow-up and caution should, therefore, be exercised when utilizing RHs in younger patient populations.

35.6 Complications

35.6.1 Early Perioperative Complications

Although the utilization of RHs in primary TKA is often reserved for complex pathology in patients who often have multiple co-morbid conditions, the early perioperative complications do not appear different to patients undergoing TKA with implants of lesser constraint. Sodhi et al. (2018) recently used the American College of Surgeons National Surgical Quality Improvement

Program database to investigate the differences in the 30-day perioperative outcomes of over 151,000 TKAs performed in the United States between 2011 and 2015. In their study, the authors identified 99 patients with a mean age of 67 years who underwent primary TKA with several types of RHs. Indications for RH were not specified beyond excluding patients who underwent conversion or revision TKA or who received an RH for malignancy. These patients were subsequently propensity score-matched to a group of patients who underwent primary TKA with unconstrained devices in a 1:3 ratio based on patient demographics and medical co-morbidities. Although the adjusted mean operative times in the RH cohort were significantly higher than the unconstrained cohort (116 vs. 94 min, $p < 0.001$), no differences were observed in 30-day readmission rates (6% vs. 2%, $p = 0.1$) or complication rates (13% vs. 12%, $p = 0.86$) between groups.

35.6.2 Delayed Complications

The comparable early perioperative complications between patients undergoing primary TKA with RHs and unconstrained devices may not persist with longer follow-up. In a retrospective analysis of the Norwegian Arthroplasty Register, Badawy et al. (2019) found that the risk of revision of RHs at a mid-term follow-up was significantly higher than implants with lesser constraint. In their study, the authors identified 197 patients with a mean age of 67 years who underwent primary TKA with several types of RHs between 1994 and 2017. Indications for surgery included osteoarthritis (33%), inflammatory arthritis (8%), post-fracture arthritis (14%), post-ligament injury (19%), post-infection (5%), instability (6%), neurologic sequelae (5%), and other (10%). The authors compared the mid-term risk of revision of RHs to patients who underwent primary TKA with VVC ($n = 204$) and unconstrained ($n = 71,515$) implants for similar indications during the same timeframe. Kaplan–Meier estimated survivorship free of all-cause revision at 5 years was 95% for unconstrained devices, 94% for VVC devices, and 86% for RHs. After adjusting for potential confounding factors, patients who underwent primary TKA with RHs demonstrated a significantly higher risk of revision compared to the unconstrained cohort (HR = 2.4; $p < 0.001$). Infection was the major complication necessitating revision TKA in all of the groups; however, this complication contributed to a higher percentage of revisions in the RH cohort (73%), compared to the VVC (4%) and unconstrained (22%) cohorts. Interestingly, when revision for infection was excluded from the analysis, Kaplan–Meier estimated survivorship at 5 years was 96% for all three groups.

> Infection has been persistently demonstrated to be the most common complication requiring revision of contemporary RH devices in multiple studies (Bistolfi et al. 2013; Neri et al. 2019; Yang et al. 2012; Guenoun et al. 2009).

While the increased risk of infection associated with RHs is multifactorial, poor host characteristics, deformity complexity, and the increased operative time required to perform these procedures likely play predominant roles. Managing PJI in patients with RHs can be particularly challenging. Successful removal of the long stems and robust cement mantles often seen with these devices can predispose patients to other complications, particularly intraoperative fractures (Gehrke et al. 2014). Furthermore, the resultant bony defects and ligamentous instability that remain after explanation limit options for staged re-implantation. Consequently, Gehrke et al. (2014) recommend the use of shorter stems and modular versions of hinged implants during the index procedure to help mitigate the future risk of complications should revision TKA be required for any reason.

> It is our recommendation that shorter cemented stems with metaphyseal cones be utilized for this reason.

The incidence of failure of RHs attributable to aseptic loosening has significantly decreased with modern designs, but it remains a relatively common mode of failure of these implants at mid-term follow-up. Neri et al. (2019) investigated the survival rate and complication profile of several types of RHs in a cohort of 112 patients with a mean age of 68 years who underwent primary TKA at 14 centers between 2006 and 2011. Indications for surgery were severe deformity (55%), arthritis and arthropathy (35%), and ligamentous deficiency/instability (10%). The overall complication rate in this cohort was 25% at a mean follow-up of 7 years. While the most common complication observed in these patients was infection (11%), aseptic loosening occurred in 4% of patients at this mid-term follow-up. Other complications requiring revision cited in this study included stiffness (5%) and patellofemoral instability (4%). Multiple studies have demonstrated similar rates of aseptic loosening of contemporary RHs at mid-term follow-up (Baker et al. 2014; Bistolfi et al. 2013; Badawy et al. 2019).

The utilization of uncemented highly porous metaphyseal cones may be a successful technique to mitigate the risk of aseptic loosening in primary TKA with contemporary RHs. Highly porous metaphyseal cones have been demonstrated in the literature to successfully reduce the risk of aseptic loosening in revision TKA by decreasing stress at the bone–cement interface (Meneghini et al. 2009; Kamath et al. 2015). The role of these augments in primary TKA has been less studied. Cottino et al. (2017) recently reported on the mid-term outcomes of 392 patients (408 knees) who received several types of RHs at a single academic institution between 2002 and 2012 for various non-oncologic indications including complex primary (18%) and revision (82%) TKA (Cottino et al. 2017). Mean age of patients was 69 years. Highly porous metaphyseal cones (Trabecular Metal; Zimmer, Warsaw, IN) were utilized in 28% of the patients. Although the authors reported that the cumulative incidence of any revision in this cohort was 10% at 2 years and 23% at 10 years, the cumulative incidence of revision for aseptic loosening was only 2% at 2 years and 5% at 10 years. Kaplan–Meier survivorship analysis demonstrated a trend toward a lower risk of revision in the cohort of patients with highly porous metaphyseal cones, but this was not statistically significant (HR = 0.69; $p = 0.20$).

These results suggest that the utilization of highly porous metaphyseal cone augments may reduce the risk of failure of contemporary RHs attributed to aseptic loosening at mid-term follow-up, but further studies investigating these augments in complex primary TKA at longer follow-up are needed.

Conclusion

There has been a wave of enthusiasm for the use of RHs in complex primary TKAs. While the specific non-oncologic indications for the use of these devices in primary TKA remain controversial, many authors agree that RHs may be safely and effectively utilized in elderly patient populations with knee pathology that precludes the use of implants with lower levels of constraint. Specifically, patients with gross knee instability, excessive femoral or tibial bone loss, severe coronal or sagittal deformity, or incompetent extensor mechanisms may benefit from an RH TKA. The mid-term outcomes and survivorship of RHs in primary TKAs support their use in elderly patients as they appear comparable to implants with lesser constraint. However, the high failure rates of RHs demonstrated with longer follow-up warrants surgeons to exercise caution when selecting these implants, especially in younger patient populations. Infection remains the most common complication requiring revision in RHs and this risk appears to be multifactorial in nature. Consequently, it is imperative that patients with modifiable risk factors for infection be effectively optimized prior to undergoing surgery. While the incidence of aseptic loosening has significantly improved with modern implant designs, it remains a common mode of failure at mid-term follow-up. The concomitant utilization of highly porous metaphyseal cones with RHs may further decrease the risk of aseptic loosening in contemporary RHs, but further studies are required.

Take-Home Messages

- The primary non-oncologic indications for contemporary RHs in primary TKAs include elderly patient populations with gross knee instability, excessive femoral or tibial bone loss, severe coronal or sagittal deformity, or incompetent extensor mechanisms.
- The mid-term outcomes and implant survivorship of RHs in primary TKAs appear comparable to implants with lesser constraint in large registry databases, but these comparable outcomes may not persist with longer follow-up.
- PJI remains the most common complication requiring revision in primary TKAs with RHs and patients with modifiable risk factors should undergo optimization prior to proceeding with surgical intervention.
- Failure of RHs attributable to aseptic loosening has decreased with improvements in implant design, but remains a common mode of failure at mid-term follow-up.
- The risk of aseptic loosening with RHs in primary TKA may be further mitigated by the concomitant utilization of highly porous metaphyseal cones, but additional studies are needed.

References

Badawy M, Fenstad AM, Furnes O (2019) Primary constrained and hinged total knee arthroplasty: 2- and 5-year revision risk compared with unconstrained total knee arthroplasty: a report on 401 cases from the Norwegian Arthroplasty Register 1994-2017. Acta Orthop 5:467–472

Bae DK, Song SJ, Yoon KH, Noh JH (2009) Long-term outcome of total knee arthroplasty in Charcot joint: a 10- to 22-year follow-up. J Arthroplasty 8:1152–1156

Baker P, Critchley R, Gray A, Jameson S, Gregg P, Port A, Deehan D (2014) Mid-term survival following primary hinged total knee replacement is good irrespective of the indication for surgery. Knee Surg Sports Traumatol Arthrosc 3:599–608

Barrack RL (2001) Evolution of the rotating hinge for complex total knee arthroplasty. Clin Orthop Relat Res 392:292–299

Bistolfi A, Lustig S, Rosso F, Dalmasso P, Crova M, Massazza G (2013) Results with 98 Endo-Modell rotating hinge prostheses for primary knee arthroplasty. Orthopedics 6:e746–e752

Bohler C, Kolbitsch P, Schuh R, Lass R, Kubista B, Giurea A (2017) Midterm results of a new rotating hinge knee implant: a 5-year follow-up. Biomed Res Int 2017:7532745

Chelman B, Walker PS, Shoji H, Erkman MJ (1975) Kinematics of the knee after prosthetic replacements. Clin Orthop Relat Res 108:149–157

Cottino U, Abdel MP, Perry KI, Mara KC, Lewallen DG, Hanssen AD (2017) Long-term results after total knee arthroplasty with contemporary rotating-hinge prostheses. J Bone Joint Surg Am 4:324–330

Dauwe J, Vandenneucker H (2018) Indications for primary rotating-hinge total knee arthroplasty. Is there consensus? Acta Orthop Belg 3:245–250

Efe T, Roessler PP, Heyse TJ, Hauk C, Pahrmann C, Getgood A, Schmitt J (2012) Mid-term results after implantation of rotating-hinge knee prostheses: primary versus revision. Orthop Rev (Pavia) 4:e35
Flynn LM (1979) The noiles hinge knee prosthesis with axial rotation. Orthopedics 6:602–605
Gehrke T, Kendoff D, Haasper C (2014) The role of hinges in primary total knee replacement. Bone Joint J 11(Supple A): 93–95
Guenoun B, Latargez L, Freslon M, Defossez G, Salas N, Gayet LE (2009) Complications following rotating hinge Endo-Modell (Link) knee arthroplasty. Orthop Traumatol Surg Res 7:529–536
Herbert JJ, Herbert A (1973) A new total knee prosthesis. Clin Orthop Relat Res 94:202–210
Hoogland T, Bosma G (1981) The Attenborough total knee arthroplasty. Neth J Surg 5:237–242
Jackson JP, Elson RA (1973) Evaluation of the Walldius and other prostheses for knee arthroplasty. Clin Orthop Relat Res 94: 104–114
Jones GB (1973) Total knee replacement-the Walldius hinge. Clin Orthop Relat Res 94:50–57
Jones RE (2006) Total knee arthroplasty with modular rotating-platform hinge. Orthopedics 9(Suppl):S80–S82
Kamath AF, Lewallen DG, Hanssen AD (2015) Porous tantalum metaphyseal cones for severe tibial bone loss in revision knee arthroplasty: a five to nine-year follow-up. J Bone Joint Surg Am 3:216–223
Kester MA, Cook SD, Harding AF, Rodriguez RP, Pipkin CS (1988) An evaluation of the mechanical failure modalities of a rotating hinge knee prosthesis. Clin Orthop Relat Res 228:156–163
Knutson K, Lindstrand A, Lidgren L (1986) Survival of knee arthroplasties. A nation-wide multicentre investigation of 8000 cases. J Bone Joint Surg Br 5:795–803
Kowalczewski J, Marczak D, Synder M, Sibinski M (2014) Primary rotating-hinge total knee arthroplasty: good outcomes at mid-term follow-up. J Arthroplasty 6:1202–1206
Lettin AW, Deliss LJ, Blackburne JS, Scales JT (1978) The Stanmore hinged knee arthroplasty. J Bone Joint Surg Br 3:327–332
Martin JR, Beahrs TR, Stuhlman CR, Trousdale RT (2016) Complex primary Total knee arthroplasty: long-term outcomes. J Bone Joint Surg Am 17:1459–1470
Matthews LS, Sonstegard DA, Kaufer H (1973) The spherocentric knee. Clin Orthop Relat Res 94:234–241
Mazas FB (1973) Guepar total knee prosthesis. Clin Orthop Relat Res 94:211–221
Meneghini RM, Lewallen DG, Hanssen AD (2009) Use of porous tantalum metaphyseal cones for severe tibial bone loss during revision total knee replacement. Surgical technique. J Bone Joint Surg Am 91:131–138
National Joint Registry for England and Wales (2010) 8th Annual Report. https://www.njrcentre.org.uk/njrcentre/Portals/0/Documents/NJR%208th%20Annual%20Report%202011pdf
Neri T, Boyer B, Papin PE, Martz P, Vaz G, Eichler D, Ehlinger M, Pasquier G (2019) Contemporary rotating hinge arthroplasty can safely be recommended in complex primary surgery. Knee Surg Sports Traumatol Arthrosc
Norwegian National Advisory Unit on Arthroplasty and Hip Fractures; Report June 2019 (2019). http://nrlweb.ihelse.net/eng/Rapporter/Report2019_english.pdf
Prasad A, Donovan R, Ramachandran M, Dawson-Bowling S, Millington S, Bhumbra R, Achan P, Hanna SA (2018) Outcome of total knee arthroplasty in patients with poliomyelitis: a systematic review. EFORT Open Rev 6:358–362
Sanguineti F, Mangano T, Formica M, Franchin F (2014) Total knee arthroplasty with rotating-hinge Endo-Model prosthesis: clinical results in complex primary and revision surgery. Arch Orthop Trauma Surg 11:1601–1607
Sculco TP (2006) The role of constraint in total knee arthoplasty. J Arthroplasty 4(Suppl 1):54–56
Sheehan JM (1978) Arthroplasty of the knee. J Bone Joint Surg Br 3:333–338
Shiers LG (1954) Arthroplasty of the knee; preliminary report of new method. J Bone Joint Surg Br 4:553–560
Sodhi N, Patel YH, George J, Sultan AA, Anis HK, Newman JM, Kryzak TJ, Khlopas A, Moskal JT, Mont MA (2018) Operative time, length of stay, short-term readmission, and complications after hinged primary total knee arthroplasty: a propensity score matched analysis. J Knee Surg 10:940–945
Tibbo ME, Chalmers BP, Berry DJ, Pagnano MW, Lewallen DG, Abdel MP (2018) Primary total knee arthroplasty in patients with neuropathic (Charcot) arthropathy: contemporary results. J Arthroplasty 9:2815–2820
Tigani D, Fosco M, Amendola L, Boriani L (2009) Total knee arthroplasty in patients with poliomyelitis. Knee 6:501–506
Yang JH, Yoon JR, Oh CH, Kim TS (2012) Primary total knee arthroplasty using rotating-hinge prosthesis in severely affected knees. Knee Surg Sports Traumatol Arthrosc 3:517–523
Zhang F, Liu Y, Xiao Y, Liu W (2014) Clinical outcomes of primary rotating-hinge knee arthroplasty for knees with severe deformity. Chin Med J 9:1791–1793

Patellar Component

Yoav S. Zvi and Eli Kamara

Contents

E. Hansen, K.-D. Kühn (eds.), *Essentials of Cemented Knee Arthroplasty*,
https://doi.org/10.1007/978-3-662-63113-3_36

36.1 Introduction

In this chapter, we review the patellar component in cemented knee arthroplasty. The authors' preferred surgical technique for patellar resurfacing is the onlay method using an all-polyethylene cemented implant. Surgical technique for patellar resurfacing is discussed, including tips to avoid pitfalls and minimize potential complications postoperatively. When resurfacing the patella, specific considerations regarding bony resection and implant positioning should be kept in mind to optimize fixation, patellofemoral tracking, and quadriceps muscle efficiency. It is important to restore the combined thickness of the resected patella and implant to the thickness of the native patellar bone. Surgeons should also select patellar implants that will maximize bony coverage. Furthermore, implants should be positioned such that the patellar component lies along the anatomic medial ridge.

Patellofemoral complications including loosening, fracture, and maltracking are a primary reason for revision knee arthroplasty, highlighting the importance of these concepts.

36.2 Case Example

A 62-year-old female presents to the orthopedic surgery clinic with complaints of 2 years of atraumatic, progressively worsening left knee pain. The patient describes a sharp, grinding pain that is aggravated with weight bearing, specifically while climbing stairs. On exam, her pain localizes to the medial and lateral joint line, as well as the anterior aspect of the knee. A moderate, partially correctable valgus deformity is noted, with a range of motion of 5–110°. The patient is otherwise neurovascularly intact. Radiographic imaging of the knee demonstrates significant valgus angular deformity, osteophytes, subchondral sclerosis, and joint space narrowing affecting the medial, lateral, and patellofemoral joint spaces (▫ Fig. 36.1).

A trial of conservative management is started – this includes physical therapy, activity modifications, nonsteroidal anti-inflammatory medications (NSAIDs), as well as multiple corticosteroid injections to the knee. Her symptoms are alleviated for 2 years, at which point conservative treatment is no longer effective. At that time, she is indicated for a total knee arthroplasty for definitive treatment. Postoperatively, the patient reports complete alleviation of her pain; her valgus deformity and joint alignment are restored (▫ Fig. 36.2). She remains well at her most recent postoperative visit, with no evidence of component loosening or functional deficits.

36.3 Surgical Technique

The authors' preferred surgical technique is an onlay patellar resurfacing. After joint exposure through a medial parapatellar approach, femoral and tibial bony

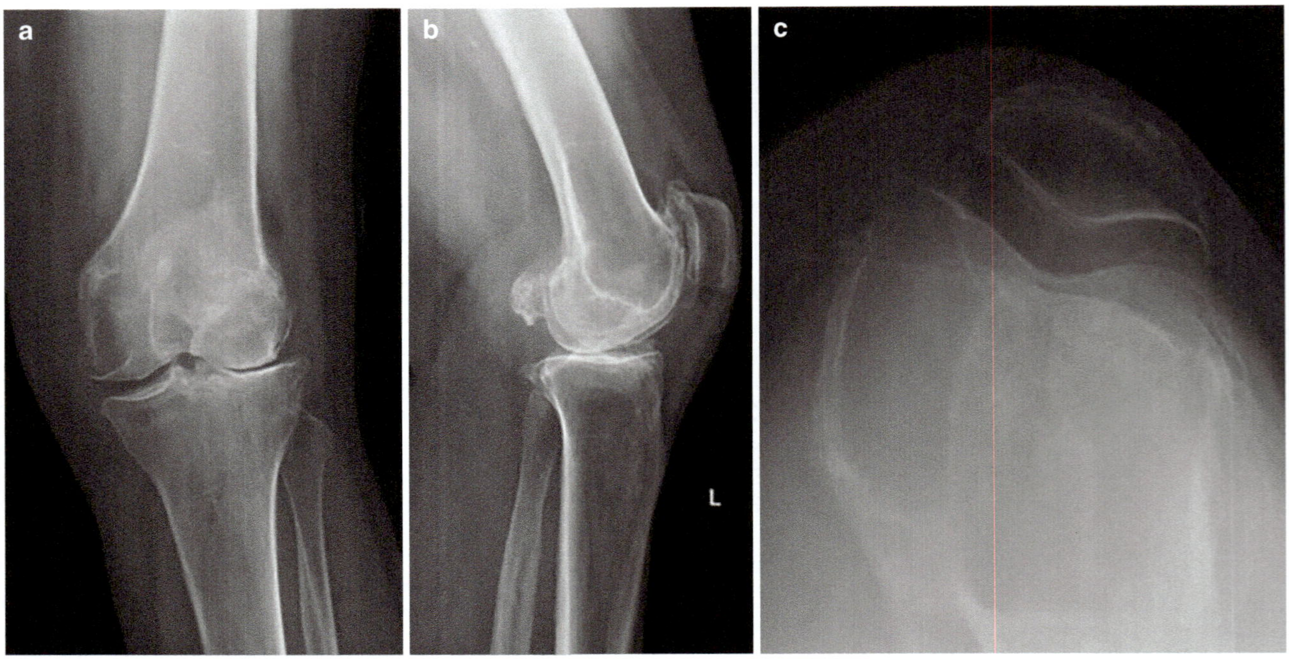

▫ **Fig. 36.1** **a–c** Preoperative left knee radiographs. Anteroposterior **a**, lateral **b**, and sunrise **c** radiographic views demonstrating significant tricompartmental disease. A valgus angular deformity is seen with diffuse osteophytes, subchondral sclerosis, and joint-space narrowing

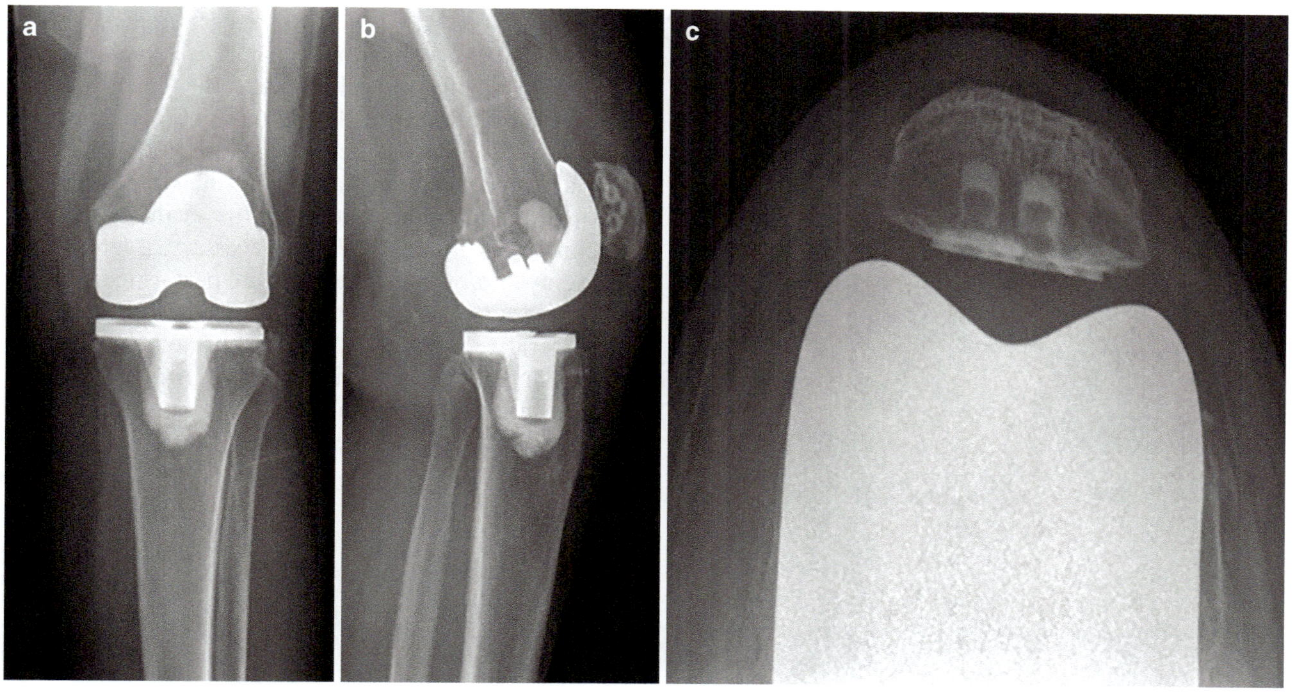

■ **Fig. 36.2** a–c Postoperative left knee radiographs. Anteroposterior **a**, lateral **b**, and sunrise **c** radiographic views demonstrating total knee arthroplasty with restoration of joint space and mechanical alignment

cuts are made. Using a gap-balancing technique, the joint is balanced in both flexion and extension, ensuring an adequate mechanical alignment is maintained throughout range of motion. Attention is then shifted to patellar preparation.

> The goals of resurfacing are
> - to restore the combined thickness of the resected patella and implant to the native patella thickness,
> - to ensure proper patella tracking of the implant without bony impingement on the prosthesis.

The borders of the patella are carefully defined using electrocautery. If present, osteophytes surrounding the rim of the patella are removed with a rongeur. The native thickness of the patella is measured with a hand-held caliper (■ Fig. 36.3). A minimum of 10 mm thickness is required for this technique to prevent the onlay implant peg from protruding through the native patella, but 12–14 mm is preferred to decrease the risk of patella fracture. Using the patellar cutting guide, the patella is cut with an oscillating saw to a goal of 10–12 mm thickness depending on the implant used (■ Fig. 36.4).

> Care should be taken to ensure that a level surface with even thickness throughout the patella is maintained – this will help avoid patellar tilt.

The cut patella is then re-measured, and if necessary, additional cuts are made (■ Fig. 36.5). This prevents under- or over-resecting the native patella, which can lead to either over- or under-stuffing, respectively, when the final component is placed. Over-stuffing may lead to postoperative anterior knee pain, loss of flexion, patellar fracture, maltracking, and/or early patellar component loosening, while under-stuffing may cause patellar maltracking, patella fracture, osteonecrosis, and loss of extensor mechanism efficiency.

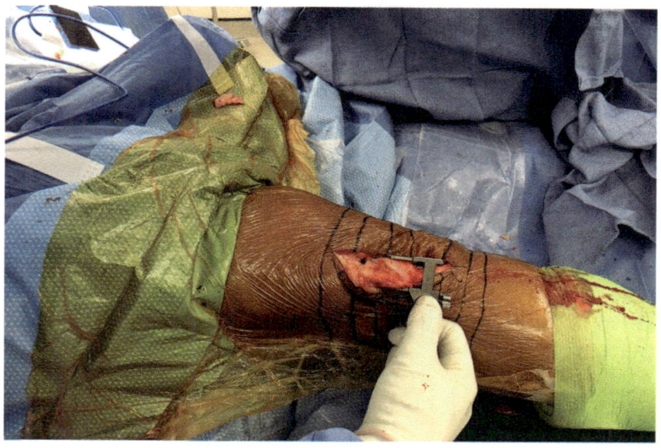

■ **Fig. 36.3** Measuring native patella bone thickness using hand-held caliper

The patella is sized with a measuring plate with consideration for positioning (■ Fig. 36.6). In general, the apex position of the patellar component should be along the median ridge of the native patella while maximizing the osseous coverage that is provided by the

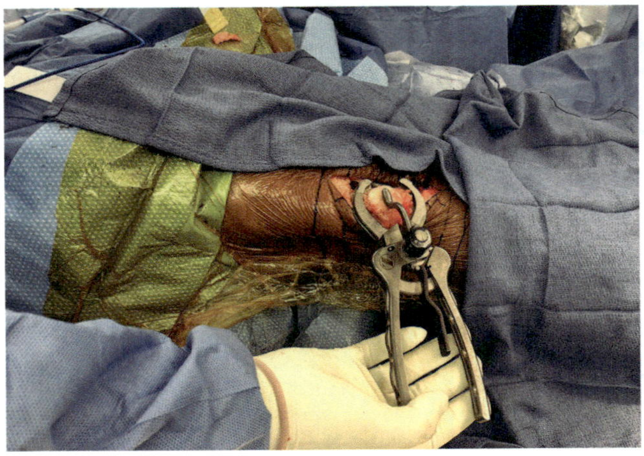

■ **Fig. 36.4** Patella cutting guide positioned for bony cut using oscillating saw

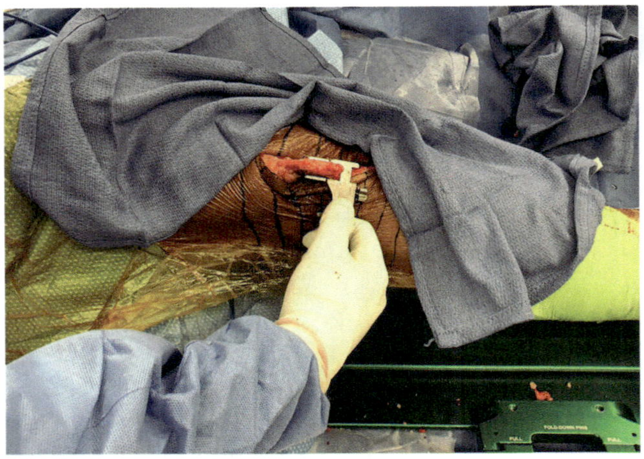

■ **Fig. 36.5** Resected patella thickness measured using handheld caliper

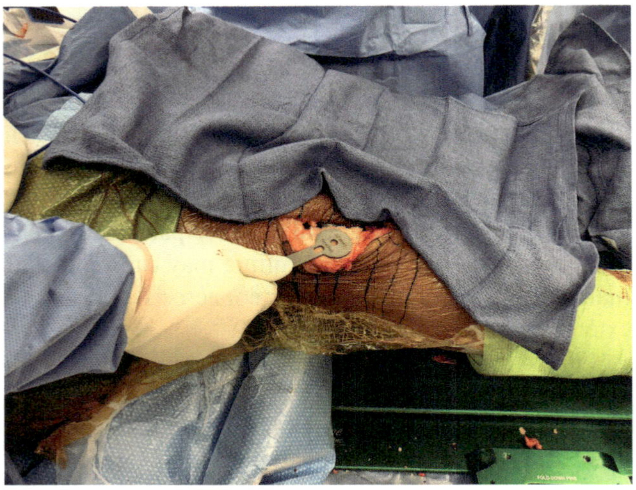

■ **Fig. 36.6** Patella is sized using a measuring plate

patellar implant. If between sizes, use of a smaller size with medialization may be appropriate to achieve this. Following sizing and placement, the corresponding drill-guide is used to drill one or three holes into the patella depending on the implant used (■ Fig. 36.7). A trial dome patella is placed, and the knee is brought through flexion and extension to evaluate patellar tracking (■ Fig. 36.8). When necessary, a lateral facetectomy and/or lateral releases are performed in order to relieve tension forces that may lead to maltracking postoperatively. Lastly, the thickness of the resected patella and trial implant is measured using a handheld caliper, in order to ensure that the native patellar thickness was restored as closely as possible (■ Fig. 36.9).

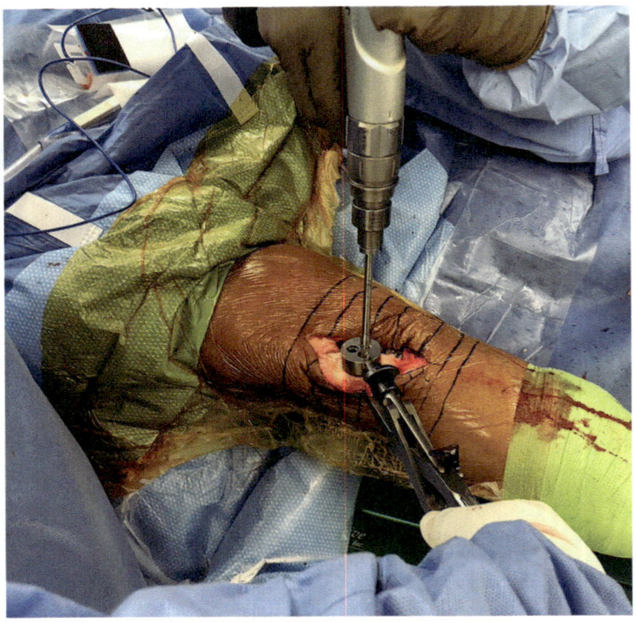

■ **Fig. 36.7** Corresponding drill guide used to drill 3 holes into resected patella

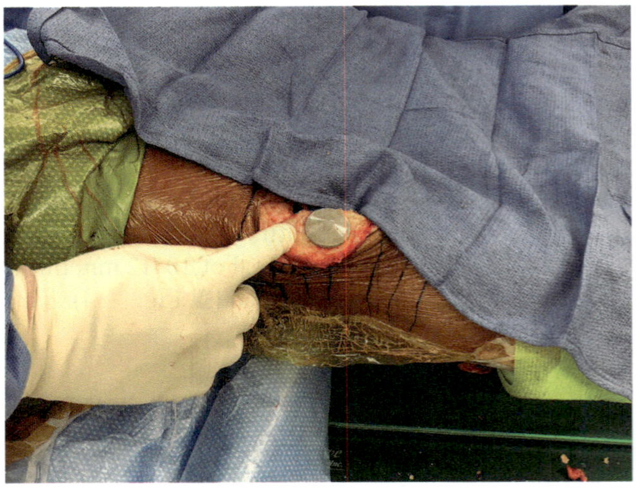

■ **Fig. 36.8** Trial implant placed and tested for adequacy of patellar tracking in flexion and extension

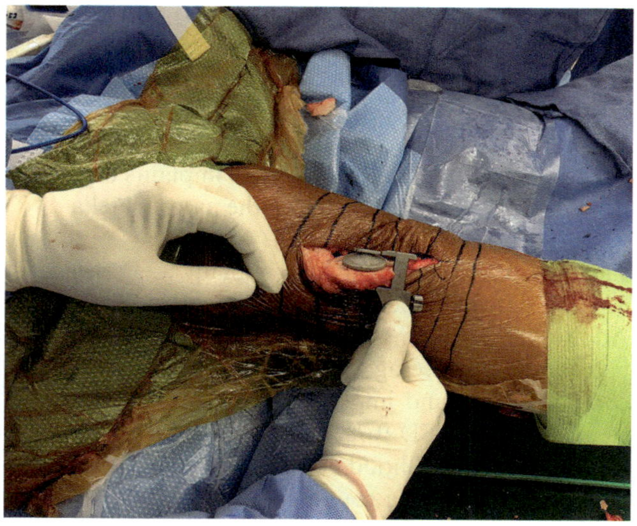

■ **Fig. 36.9** Thickness of resected patella and trial implant measured using handheld caliper

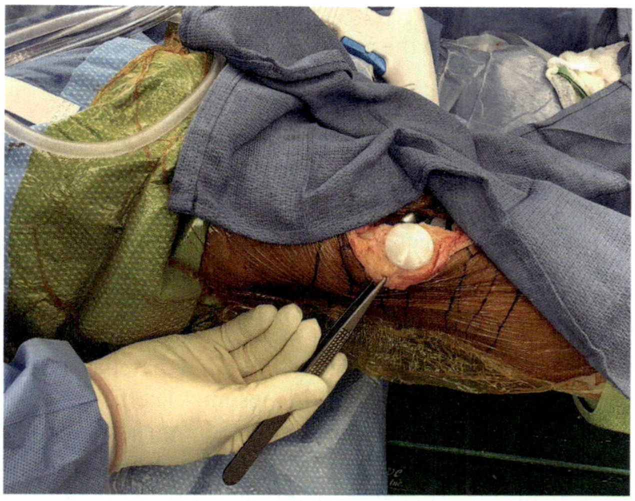

■ **Fig. 36.10** Final patella implant after cementing of all components

> After finalizing femoral, tibial, and patellar trial components and achieving acceptable soft-tissue balancing and patellar tracking, final components are cemented (■ Fig. 36.10). Cement is used for all 3 components, the order of insertion of implants being tibia, femur, trial liner, and patella.

The authors prefer using an all-polyethylene, three-pegged, dome-shaped patellar component, but anatomic patellar components may also be used when deemed appropriate.

36.4 Relevant Literature

When resurfacing the patella, for either a total knee or patellofemoral arthroplasty, two surgical techniques are generally used. The onlay method involves cutting the patella to resect a pre-measured thickness of bone, while the inset method uses a reamer to create a circular dome within the native patella in which the component will be placed.

> Regardless of technique that is used, careful attention to component design, size, and positioning is paramount to optimize postoperative patellar tracking and extensor mechanism efficiency.

Patellofemoral complications including anterior knee pain, maltracking, clunk syndrome, implant loosening, and patella fracture continue to be a primary reason for revision knee arthroplasty (Schiavone Panni et al. 2014; Abdel et al. 2014), highlighting the importance of surgical technique. Review of the literature can offer insight into certain surgical and component principles that may yield improved outcomes and minimize these potential complications.

The role of cemented implant fixation when resurfacing the patella has been demonstrated in a study conducted by Healy et al. (1995). They reported on implant design and patient risk factors on postoperative complications in total knee arthroplasty. In their series of 211 patients treated with total knee arthroplasty, 160 patients treated with cemented patella implants were compared with 37 patients treated with cementless patella implants. In the total cohort, 5 patients (2.4%) were found to have patellar fractures; of these patients, 4 were treated with cementless fixation. Additionally, they found the rate of *patellar loosening* in *cementless* implant fixation to be *significantly higher* than cemented implant fixation (13.5% vs. 1.2%; $p < 0.01$).

> Patient outcomes were best with a cemented, all-polyethylene domed patellar component demonstrating lower rates of overall complications when compared with cementless implant fixation.

> The study concludes that cement contributes significantly to patella implant stability. While this study was conducted a number of years ago, most surgeons today still prefer to use cemented patella implant fixation for this reason.

Onlay and inset patellar fixation techniques are both widely reported in the literature. It is debated which surgical technique will yield superior outcomes while minimizing complications, though both are still in use with reasonable results. Greenwald et al. sought to compare the fixation strength of onlay and inset implants through a biomechanical study (Rosenstein et al. 2007). Synthetic solid foam patellae were prepared with identical dimensions of 29 mm diameter and 12.5 mm height; 3-pegged onlay or inset components were then cemented in place. Mounting blocks were then used to load the components onto an Instron Testing Machine that recreated a chair rise motion by applying a compressive joint force perpendicular to the anterior patella. A shearing force was then introduced, and the maximal load to failure was recorded. Their study found the inset component group to have significantly higher maximal shear force than the onlay component group (mean: 715 lbf, SD: 41.8 vs. mean: 571 lbf, SD 52.7; $p < 0.01$).

> The authors conclude that although this was a small sample-sized biomechanical study, the increased resistance to shear forces demonstrated by the inset components may offer improved durability of patellar fixation in vivo.

The patella experiences significant anterior forces as the knee is flexed. This has certain implications when deciding not only on surgical technique, but also on prosthesis selection, amount of bone to resect, and composite thickness of resected patella and implant.

> Increased surface strains across an overly resected patella can lead to patella fracture, which is why conservative patella cuts should be considered.

Incavo et al. investigated these concepts in a biomechanical cadaver study (Wulff and Incavo 2000). Using a cadaveric patella with the quadriceps and patellar tendons attached, onlay and inset implants were used to resurface the patella. Specimens were then mounted to a loading fixture in 50° of flexion, previously reported to show maximum anterior surface strain, and a strain gauge was placed along the anterior cortical surface of the patella. Flexion angle, load rate, and maximum load (1000 N) were all kept constant. The study showed that both implants increased anterior strain on the patella; however, when the native patellar height was reproduced the inset implant had significantly higher strain than the onlay implant (28% vs. 22%; $p < 0.05$). They also demonstrated that increasing patella resection at 2 mm increments is directly related to increased patellar strain. The onlay implant was able to tolerate more resection than the inset prosthesis. Lastly, they showed that with an over-resected patella, restoring the native height by using a thicker prosthesis significantly increased the anterior patellar strain, regardless of implant type. Increased anterior forces along the patella suggest that loosening and fracture are more likely; however, this study did not specifically report on these complications.

Patellar design is another aspect that can affect both the size and positioning of the component. A study conducted by Laz et al. sought to determine how round and oval designs of the patella affected size selection and coverage (Yang et al. 2017). Their study involved 100 patients undergoing primary total knee arthroplasty, and analyzed 3 parameters:

- Intraoperative assessment of component size
- Digitally measured bony coverage
- Apex positioning of the patellar implants compared to the medial-lateral ridge of the native patella

They found that a larger oval implant was selected in 82% of patients when compared to a round implant. Additionally, oval implants were found to have a greater percent bony coverage of the resected patella when compared to round implants (mean 82.7%, SD 10.7% vs. mean 80.9%, SD 9.7%; $p = 0.02$). The authors also report that the likelihood of upsizing was higher with an oval component vs. a round component, and was generally preferred by the operating surgeon. Lastly, they demonstrated improvement in apex positioning with respect to the native medial ridge with oval components than round components (mean 0.25 mm lateral to anatomic median ridge, SD 2.45 mm vs. mean 1.16 mm, SD 2.54 mm medial to the anatomic median ridge; $p < 0.01$).

> Admittedly, while these findings are statistically significant and theoretically should correspond to better outcomes based on component principles, it is difficult to determine whether these marginal differences translate into long-term clinically relevant improvements.

With patellar resurfacing, it is crucial to restore native patellofemoral biomechanics such that patellar tracking, contact forces, and quadriceps muscle efficiency are optimized. Shelburne et al. conducted an in vivo biomechanical study comparing medialized dome vs. medialized anatomic patellar implants in 20 patients (10 per group), to investigate these parameters (Ali et al. 2018). Anatomic patellar implants differ from dome patellar implants in that they possess a medialized peak that more closely mimics the geometry of native medial and lateral facets of the patella. In their study, patients were asked to perform seated knee extension and weight-bearing lunge exercises. Using high-speed stereo radiography (HSSR) they collected patient-specific parameters while performing these activities. Marker-based motion capture and force plate data were used for musculoskeletal simulations, and data analysis of each patient's patellofemoral mechanics was done through finite element modeling (◘ Fig. 36.11).

The authors note that kinematic differences between knee extension and lunge activities were not significant. When comparing medialized dome and medialized anatomic subjects, noticeable differences were seen during the lunge. Anatomic patients demonstrated larger patellofemoral flexion–extension angles with an average dif-

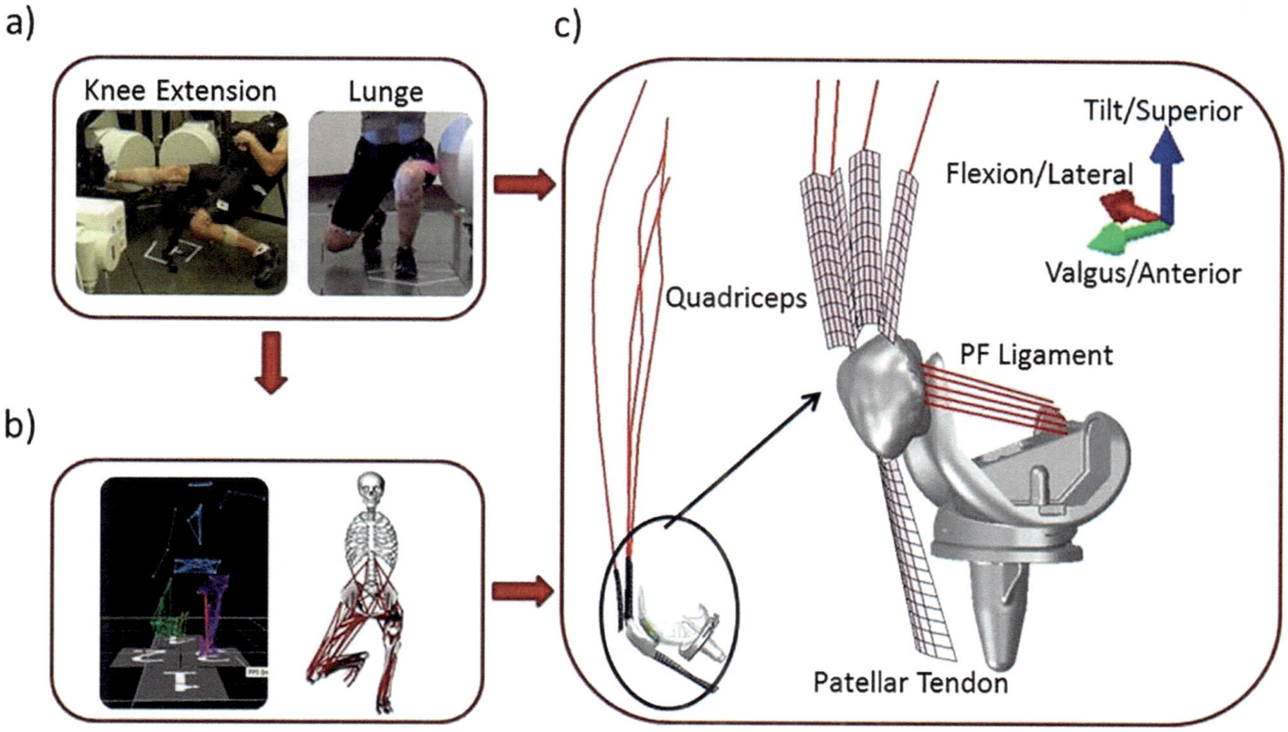

Fig. 36.11 Workflow of study. **a** HSSR data collection. **b** Musculoskeletal modeling. **c** Finite element modeling. (Courtesy of John Wiley & Sons)

ference of 11° ± 3°; dome patients were also found to have an increase in patellar tilt by an average of 6° ± 5°. When comparing quadriceps force, little difference was found during knee extension between groups, though during lunge, dome patients exhibited higher forces at mid-flexion (60°) while anatomic patients exhibited higher forces at deep flexion (90°).

Contact forces were, as expected, shown to decrease during knee extension and increase during lunge – forces were translated superiorly on the patellar component with flexion. Contact force ratios, defined as the ratio between total force due to patellar contact and total quadriceps force, were shown to be larger in dome patients compared to anatomic patients during lunge activity. Patellar force ratio, defined as the ratio of patellar tendon force divided by total quadriceps force, decreased as knee flexion increased. In knee extension, similar patellar force ratios were measured between dome and anatomic patients; however, during lunge, anatomic patients showed larger patellar force ratios in deep flexion (>75°).

> Taken together, the authors conclude that their findings imply that anatomic patellar implants more closely replicate native patellofemoral mechanics.

In summary, there are multiple factors that can affect postoperative complications when resurfacing the patella. Patellar implants have a variety of different designs that play a critical role in optimizing patellar tracking, quadriceps efficiency, and implant stability.

> Surgeons should pay close attention to surgical technique with regard to bony resection and implant positioning, and be aware of the added stability with cemented implant fixation when choosing implants.

With consideration of these concepts when performing patellar resection, patient outcomes can be optimized.

Take-Home Messages

- After finalizing femoral, tibial, and patellar trial components and achieving acceptable soft-tissue balancing and patellar tracking, final components are cemented. The order of insertion of implants being the tibia, femur, trial liner, and patella.
- When resurfacing the patella it is important to restore the native anatomy as best as possible to optimize patellar tracking and quadriceps muscle efficiency.
- The combined thickness of the resected patella and final implant should be the same as the native patellar bone to avoid over- or under-stuffing the patellofemoral joint.

- Under-stuffing (i.e., over-resecting) can decrease quadriceps muscle efficiency, lead to patellar osteonecrosis or fracture, while over-stuffing (i.e., under-resecting) can lead to anterior knee pain, decreased ROM, patellar component loosening, or fracture of the patella.
- A minimum of 10 mm thickness is required for this technique to prevent the onlay implant peg from protruding through the native patella, but 12–14 mm is preferred to decrease the risk of patella fracture.
- The apex position of the patellar component should be along the median ridge of the native patella.
- Implant size should maximize the osseous coverage of the resected patella. If between sizes, the use of a smaller size with medialization may be appropriate.
- A lateral facetectomy and/or lateral releases are performed in order to relieve tension forces that may lead to maltracking postoperatively.
- Cement has been shown to minimize patellar fracture and implant loosening.
- Both onlay and inset techniques demonstrate successful clinical outcomes when performed appropriately.
- Inset implants have demonstrated higher maximal shear force to failure, suggesting improved durability over onlay implants.
- Oval implants were shown to enable maximal osseous coverage and medial ridge positioning when compared to round implants.
- Medialized anatomic patella implants more closely replicate native patellofemoral biomechanics when compared to medialized dome patella implants.

References

Abdel MP, Parratte S, Budhiparama NC (2014) The patella in total knee arthroplasty: to resurface or not is the question. Curr Rev Musculoskelet Med 7(2):117–124

Ali AA et al (2018) In vivo comparison of medialized dome and anatomic patellofemoral geometries using subject-specific computational modeling. J Orthop Res 36(7):1910–1918

Healy WL et al (1995) Patellofemoral complications following total knee arthroplasty. Correlation with implant design and patient risk factors. J Arthroplasty 10(2):197–201

Rosenstein AD, Postak PD, Greenwald AS (2007) Fixation strength comparison of onlay and inset patellar implants. Knee 14(3): 194–197

Schiavone Panni A et al (2014) Patellar resurfacing complications in total knee arthroplasty. Int Orthop 38(2):313–317

Wulff W, Incavo SJ (2000) The effect of patella preparation for total knee arthroplasty on patellar strain: a comparison of resurfacing versus inset implants. J Arthroplasty 15(6):778–782

Yang CC et al (2017) Patellar component design influences size selection and coverage. Knee 24(2):460–467

Databases Afterwards Database

Contents

International Registries – A Comparison of Outcomes

Kevin A. Lawson, Spencer J. Montgomery, and James I. Huddleston

Contents

E. Hansen, K.-D. Kühn (eds.), *Essentials of Cemented Knee Arthroplasty*,
https://doi.org/10.1007/978-3-662-63113-3_37

37.1 Introduction

Along with the numerous successes of total knee arthroplasty (TKA), there have been many major failures during the course of implant development and our refinement in surgical technique (Maloney 2001). With the ever-increasing number of TKAs performed (Kurtz et al. 2007; Sloan et al. 2018; Losina et al. 2012) and the large financial cost to society, it is incumbent on the joint surgery community to track outcomes and treatment trends (Delaunay 2015). As orthopedic surgeons realized that it would be impossible for an individual surgeon to base his choice of optimal operative methods and/or implants on his/her own experience, it became apparent that aggregation of data was essential (Swedish Knee Arthroplasty Register 2018). However, examples set by early arthroplasty pioneers such as Charnley, Insall, and many others to insist on close, detailed follow-up and to develop systems for tracking their patients and documenting outcomes led to the early development of the large international registries we have today (Malchau et al. 2018). Here, we report on the outcomes of many large national registries as they pertain to TKA. We included those registries which deliver English language annual reports. We focus on outcomes based on indications and patient factors. We also report on some notable trends in care.

37.2 Registries

The purpose of a registry is to collect institutional, regional, or national data in order to analyze and draw statistically significant conclusions regarding patient, surgical technique, and implant-associated factors that lead to good or poor outcomes. The goal is to have enough data to allow adequate statistical analysis, mechanisms to track long-term results, assessment of quality, and recurring analysis to identify trends in care. With a significant cross section of the treatment community, registries possibly avoid performance bias, and reflect care provided in the wider community (Hughes et al. 2017). Registries also provide for post-market surveillance of implants, with numerous examples of registry-derived recalls (Furnes et al. 1997; Craviotto 2001). Additionally, registries also allow for the generation of scientific evidence, as well as assessment of large-scale cost-saving effects (Maloney 2001). Large clinical trials, which may answer some of these same questions, are independently time-consuming and costly for surgeons, groups, and health systems to perform.

37.2.1 History

The Mayo Clinic total joint registry is an institutionally based registry initiated by Dr. Mark Coventry in 1965 (Berry et al. 1997). This registry is commonly cited as being the first institutional arthroplasty registry (Delaunay 2015). The level of detail, including referencing radiographs and patient-reported outcome measures, allows a diversity and depth of study of questions that is different from, and complimentary to, large national registries. Because additional clinical information is archived, as compared to current national registries, institutional registries have the ability to identify the performance of specific implants in specific settings (Howard et al. 2011; Joglekar et al. 2012). William H. Harris, MD, DSc followed the Mayo Registry to create the second institutional joint registry in the United States at Mass General (Malchau et al. 2018). Similar to the Mayo, this registry began with the archiving of pre- and postoperative radiographs following the advent of digital radiography. Major contributions from this registry include evaluation of developments from the Harris Orthopedic Laboratory, including the creation and long-term follow-up of highly crosslinked polyethylene (Harris 1995). The first federally funded institutional hip and knee arthroplasty registry was created by David Schurman, MD at Stanford University in 1972.

Registries moved from an institutional and regional concept to one of analysis of a whole country's outcomes with the initiation of the Swedish Knee Arthroplasty Register in 1974 (Robertsson et al. 2000a; Knutson and Robertsson 2010). This allows for much larger patient numbers and more generalizable data secondary to the differences of practice settings represented (Herberts et al. 1989). It is estimated that this register currently captures 98% of all arthroplasty admissions in Sweden (Swedish Knee Arthroplasty Register 2018). Some early pioneering work from this registry includes risk factors and epidemiology of periprosthetic joint infection as well as early analysis of techniques or implants with high failure rates (Bengston et al. 1989; Knutson et al. 1981). These reports demonstrated the power of aggregated data of a national registry to the wider arthroplasty community.

> Following the Swedish example, multiple other national registries have been created (see overview of National Arthroplasty Registries below).

National Arthroplasty Registries – Developed between 1975–2007

- *Swedish Knee Arthroplasty Register*
  - Established in 1975
  - First National Total Knee Registry ever
  - >275,000 procedures
- *Swedish Hip Arthroplasty Register*
  - Established in 1979
  - First National Total Hip Registry ever
  - >450,000 procedures
- *Finnish National Arthroplasty Register*
  - Established in 1980
  - >400,000 procedures
- *Norwegian Arthroplasty Register*
  - Established in 1987
  - >200,000 procedures
- *Danish Hip Arthroplasty Register*
  - Established in 1995
  - >150,000 procedures
- *Danish Knee Arthroplasty Register*
  - Established in 1997
  - >100,000 procedures
- *New Zealand National Joint Register*
  - Established in 1998
  - >130,000 procedures
- *Australian National Joint Registry*
  - Established in 1999
  - >1,200,000 procedures
- *UK National Joint Registry*
  - Established in 2003
  - The world's largest joint registry
  - >2,350,000 procedures
- *Slovak National Arthroplasty Register*
  - Established in 2003
  - >40,000 procedures
- *Dutch Arthroplasty Register*
  - Established in 2007
  - >250,000 procedures

The majority of these registries have been established by professional societies (Swedish Knee Arthroplasty Register 2018; Finnish Arthroplasty Register 2017; American Joint Replacement Registry (AJRR) 2019) or as directed by national healthcare authorities (Canadian Institute for Health Information 2020; National Joint Registry 2018).

The Functional Outcomes Research for Comparative Effectiveness in Total Joint Replacement and Quality Improvement (FORCE-TJR) Registry was developed with the support from the Agency for Healthcare Quality and Research that was started in 2010 and was funded for 5 years (Franklin et al. 2013). This was one of the first attempts at a national American registry. The American Joint Replacement Registry (AJRR) followed the same year and was established by the American Academy of Orthopedic Surgeons (AAOS) to capture hip and knee arthroplasty data to conduct implant-specific survivorship analyses, produce risk-adjusted patient outcome data, and provide hospitals with quality benchmarks (Etkin and Springer 2017). The registry has rapidly spread throughout the United States, but is still capturing less than 50% of the nearly one million arthroplasties performed annually in the United States each year (AJRR report). With over two million hip and knee replacement procedures, it is currently the largest registry in the world based on procedure volume.

37.2.2 Collaboration

The International Society of Arthroplasty Registries (ISAR) was created in 2004 (▶ https://www.isarhome.org/). ISAR was established as a voluntary international organization with Professor Stephen Graves as inaugural president. Some of the goals of ISAR are to foster registry development, maintenance, cooperation, and the free reporting of outcomes. Encouraging uniformity of data collection in national registries allows for worldwide comparison of outcomes. Membership requires participation of over 80% of national hospitals and reporting of a minimum of 90% of procedures from each unit. Data collected must be validated. Associate members include registries with less than 80% coverage. There are currently 13 full-time members throughout the world (▶ https://www.isarhome.org/members). These include Australian, New Zealand, Romanian, UK NJR, Dutch, Danish, Swiss, Slovak, Swedish, Norwegian, Finish, and Lithuanian registries. The only US-based registry included as a full ISAR member is the Kaiser Permanente National Total Joint Registry (▶ https://national-implantregistries.kaiserpermanente.org/).

Further examples of international cooperation have been shown by the Nordic registries with the creation of The Nordic Arthroplasty Register Association (Havelin et al. 2009). This created a common Nordic database to compare results and further pool data.

37.2.3 Data Collected

International total joint replacement registries have traditionally focused on implant revision rates and tracked the length of time between the initial total joint replacement and implant removal. In this model, national registries incorporate large numbers of arthroplasties to identify device longevity. While the implant revision rate remains an important outcome, implant materials and technology have matured and patients and insurers want to understand the quality of care of the vast majority of patients who do not have a revision each year. Recently many registries have begun to add more data, including the capture and reporting on patient-reported outcome measures.

37.2.4 Weaknesses

> With all the success of national registries, there is a danger of using large observational data sets to make erroneous conclusions.

Correlations can be identified but causation cannot be concluded from these national registries (Lübbeke et al. 2017). Many types of bias can affect such associations including selection bias, performance bias, and in some cases, reporting bias. Interactions among variables may be difficult to tease apart. Risk stratification has often not been performed or may be rudimentary when reporting outcomes. Finally, as stated earlier, registries typically use revision as an endpoint and other outcome measures such as pain relief and function are equally as important to many patients.

37.3 Registries and Their Respective Sizes

37

The longest running national arthroplasty registry is the Swedish Joint Registry (Swedish Knee Arthroplasty Register 2018), which was started in 1974 as the Swedish Knee Arthroplasty Register and began reporting results in the early 1980s. Other international registries followed, including the Finnish (Finnish Arthroplasty Register 2017), Norwegian (Norwegian Arthroplasty Register 2019), Danish, New Zealand (New Zealand Orthopaedic Association 2018), Australian (Australian Orthopaedic Association National Joint Replacement Registry 2018), and UK Registries (National Joint Registry 2018) in that order. Other registries described in this chapter include the Canadian (Canadian Institute for Health Information 2020), Belgian (Orthopride Belgian Hip and Knee Arthroplasty Registry Annual Report 2018), Dutch (Dutch Arthroplasty Register (LROI) 2018), and the American Joint Replacement Registry (AJRR) (2019).

Registry basic information is included in Table 37.1. One of the largest databases is the National Joint Registry from the UK. The data in that registry spans 15 years (2003–2018), with the current total number of patients listed at 1,193,830. Over the most recent 3-year period they reported 274,495 procedures performed. This is secondary to the UK's large population size and capture rate. The AJRR's most recent report lists 828,999 total knee replacements captured over 6 years (2002–2018). With the large US population and number of procedures performed each year, it is likely that the AJRR will soon grow to be one of the largest national knee registries, even with a relatively low inclusion rate when compared to other national registries (Sloan et al. 2018). Another large database is the Australian registry with 658, 596 total knee patients. The Canadian Joint Replacement Registry (CJRR), which is relatively new, reported 202,319 total cases between 2012 and 2018, and likely will grow to be one of the larger registries as well. The Swedish registry, being the longest collecting TKA data (1974–2017), includes 270,159 patients. The most recent year lists 14,957 TKAs per-

Table 37.1 Registry sizes and reported participation

Registry	American	Australian	Belgian	Canadian	Dutch	Finnish	New Zealand	Norwegian	Swedish	UK/Wales
Years included	2012–2018	1999–2018	2009–2018	2012–2018	2010–2017	1980–2019	1999–2018	1994–2018	1974–2017	2003–2018
Participation	Unknown	95.9%	Est. 100%[a]	72.1%	>95% (+)	95.0%	>95.0%	97.1%	98.1%	95.2%
Registry case volumes										
TKA (No.)	828,999	782,600	–	202,319	220,499	230,529	110,678	97,022	270,159	1,193,830
Primary TKA in most recent year (No.)	139,582	56,259	25,915	70,502	32,258	12,679	8392	7567	14,957	105,278

TKA total knee arthroplasty
(+) van Steenbergen et al. (2015)
[a]Prosthesis reimbursement in Belgium is coupled to prosthesis entry into the registry as of September 1, 2015

formed. The majority of these databases demonstrated an increase in the number of cases performed over time.

Reported capture rates of patients in the included European registries range from approximately 95% in the Dutch, Finnish, and UK registries to 98.1% in the Swedish registry.

> Of note, the highest trajectory for capture comes from the Belgium registry where prosthesis reimbursement is dependent on its entry into the database as of September 1, 2015, resulting in an estimated 100% capture rate moving forward (Orthopride Belgian Hip and Knee Arthroplasty Registry Annual Report 2018).

The capture rate in North America is considerably lower, and given the impressive estimated annual procedural rates of total knee replacements in the United States ranging from 400,000 to −680,000 (Sloan et al. 2018; Losina et al. 2012; Singh et al. 2019) the AJRR current capture rate is approaching 50% of this annual volume in 2020.

Patient demographics can be seen in ◘ Table 37.2. The range of mean ages reported is 67–68.5 years. Age at which TKA prevalence peaks differs between the registries, with a high of 80–85 years old in the Swedish Registry to peaking in the 60–65 years old cohort in the AJRR. The majority of surgeries performed are on female patients. This is from a low of 51.8% of all patients in the New Zealand registry to 68.3% of patients in the Finnish registry.

ASA class is also commonly reported in these registries, with the majority of patients following into ASA II class (52–72%) depending on the registry. Body mass index (BMI) is reported in fewer than half of the included registries, although many intend on including these data moving forward. In the registries that include this data, only 10.6–17% are considered to fall into a healthy weight category with a BMI <25 while 31.1–69.4% of patients are classified as overweight with a BMI 25–30 and 16.1–56.1% of patients categorized as obese with BMI 30 or greater. The Dutch and Finnish registries are the only registries in which the majority of the patients have a BMI of <30 (58% and 83.95% of patients, respectively). The Australian registry included 58.3% of patients with a BMI >30.

Across registries, the majority of the surgeries included were for primary or idiopathic osteoarthritis (88–98.8%). The second and third most common diagnoses are post-traumatic arthritis and rheumatoid arthritis, respectively.

37.4 Outcomes Reporting

Reported outcomes in the registries vary but generally encompass the notion of cumulative revision rate or revision-free survival at multiple given time points reported by age, sex, fixation type, implant design, and by individual implants among other categories. Some registries include the measured revision rate as a portion of observed component years to standardize the differences in patient numbers seen at the various time points in follow-up (New Zealand Orthopaedic Association 2018). It has further been suggested that annual revision burden, the percentage of total cases that are revision arthroplasties, may also be a viable surrogate measure for comparative procedural success and quality improvement initiatives (American Joint Replacement Registry (AJRR) 2019).

▪ Osteoarthritis

As a vast majority of cases in the registries are due to osteoarthritis as a primary cited etiology, it is, therefore, generalized that the overall reported results pertain to this diagnosis. When overall cumulative revision rates are reported by years of follow-up, they have been recorded here in 5-year increments (◘ Table 37.3). At the earliest time point of 5 years post-procedure, reported cumulative revision rate ranges from 2.0% to 3.5% while at the longest reported time points (18–20 years) revision rates vary from 5.5% in Belgium to 14.4% in Finnish males and 12.5% in Finnish females. Younger registries such as the Dutch LROI report outcomes at 5 and 9 years, respectively. Overall revision burden of the most recently reported year of the respective registry is also presented in ◘ Table 37.3. The Dutch registry reports the greatest revision burden of 9.4% while the Swedish registry claims the lowest revision burden of 5.2%.

> Pooled analysis of registries with greater than 15-year follow-up lists the 25-year survival of TKA at 82% (Evans et al. 2019).

▪ Rheumatoid Arthritis

Outcomes for rheumatoid arthritis are discussed specifically in the Australian and Swedish registries. As a diagnosis, rheumatoid arthritis is responsible for as little as 1.3% of cases in Australia and as many as 4.9% of cases in Norway. The overall trend in etiologic burden is decreasing with improvements in the medical management for rheumatoid arthritis resulting in the prevention of articular erosion (Swedish Knee Arthroplasty

Table 37.2 Incidence of patient characteristics, fixation methods, and diagnoses by registry

Registry	American	Australian	Belgian	Canadian	Dutch	Finnish	New Zealand	Norwegian	Swedish	UK/Wales
Mean age										
Overall	67.0	68.5	67.6	–	68.6	–	–	68.5	68.9	69.0
Female	–	–	68.8	68.5	–	–	68.5	69.1	–	70.0
Male	–	–	68.1	68.1	–	–	67.9	67.5	–	69.0
Sex distribution										
Female (%)	61.1	56.6	61.3	61.3	64.0	68.3	51.6	62.5	56.0	56.7
Male (%)	38.9	43.4	38.7	38.7	36.0	31.7	48.4	37.5	44.0 (2017)	43.3
ASA class										
I (%)	–	6.0	–	–	12.0	8.0	11.0	14.6	–	11.9
II (%)	–	55.5	–	–	68.0	52.0	64.0	66.0	–	72.0
III (%)	–	37.4	–	–	20.0	39.9	24.0	19.3	–	15.8
IV (%)	–	1.1	–	–	–	–	1.0	0.1	–	0.3
BMI										
<25 (%)	–	10.6	–	–	17.0	14.5	11.3	–	–	–
25–30 (%)	–	31.1	–	–	41.0	69.4	32.7	–	–	–
30–40 (%)	–	47.7	–	–	38.0	16.1 (BMI >30)	46.7	–	–	–
>40 (%)	–	10.6	–	–	4.0		9.4	–	–	–
Diagnosis										
Osteoarthritis (%)	–	97.7	94.8	98.8	96.0	93.8	94.9	88[a]	>96[b]	97.4
Post-traumatic (%) (incl. ligament injury)	–	–	2.2	–	2.0	2.6	1.9	10.2[a]	<2[b]	–
Rheumatoid arthritis (%)	–	1.3	–	–	1.0	2.1	2.1	4.2[a]	<2[b]	–
Other inflammatory (%)	–	0.5	0.7	–	–	0.1	0.8	0.5[a]	–	–
Avascular necrosis (%)	–	0.3	1.3	–	1.0	0.5	0.3	0.2[a]	–	–
Neoplastic (%)	–	–	–	–	–	–	0.1	–	–	–

[a]Diagnoses are not mutually exclusive in the Norwegian registry
[b]Estimate from most recent time point in a line graph (1975–2017)

Register 2018; Australian Orthopaedic Association National Joint Replacement Registry 2018). Outcomes for rheumatoid arthritis appear non-contributory to implant survival. The Australian registry states that although the early revision rate (within 3 months) is higher in rheumatoid patients, by 9 months post-op the cumulative survival of the prosthesis is in fact better than their osteoarthritic cohort (Fig. 37.1). Likewise, the Swedish registry showcases a survival curve in rheumatoid arthritis patients that demonstrates no significant difference compared to patients with osteoarthritis as a primary diagnosis at 10-year follow-up (Fig. 37.2).

Table 37.3 Revision rate data by registry

Registry	American	Australian	Belgian		Canadian	Dutch	Finnish		New Zealand	Norwegian	Swedish	UK/Wales
Revision burden												
7.5	8.7	8.0	6.9		9.4	6.9	7.5		8.6	5.2	6.0	
Cumulative revision rate												
At 5 yrs (%)	–	3.5	–		2.0	–	3.9 female 4.3 male		2.4	–	3.0[a]	2.7
At 10 yrs (%)	–	5.3	–		–	5.6 (9 yrs)	6.3 female 6.8 male		4.3	–	3.9[a]	4.4
At 15 yrs (%)	–	7.3	–		–	–	9.3 female 10.1 male		6.3	–	–	6.4
At 20 yrs (%)	–	8.6 (18 yrs)	5.5		–	–	12.5 female 14.4 male		7.9 (19 yrs)	10.5	7.0[b]	–
Revision rate by sex												
Time point	**–**	**18 yrs**	**–**		**–**	**9 yrs**	**10 yrs**	**25 yrs**	**Overall cohort**	**–**	**–**	**5 yrs**
Female (%)	–	7.9	–		–	5.8	6.3	15.9	3.1	–	–	6.0
Male (%)	–	9.5	–		–	5.5	6.8	17.9	3.6	–	–	6.3
Revision rate by age group												
Time point	–	**5 yrs**	**18 yrs**		–	–	**5 yrs**		**Overall cohort**	–	**5 yrs**	**5 yrs**
<55 yrs old (%)	–	6.6	17.8		–	–	5.0 female 6.5 male		6.7	–	4.0[a] (age <65)	4.4 female 5.0 male
55–64 yrs old (%)	–	4.5	11.7		–	–	2.9 female 3.8 male		4.4	–		2.8 female 3.3 male
65–74 yrs old (%)	–	3.3	7		–	–	1.9 female 2.7 male		2.9	–	2.7[a]	1.9 female 2.2 male
>75 yrs old (%)	–	2.2	3.6		–	–	1.7 female 2.1 male		1.6	–	2.5[a]	1.8 female 1.4 male
Time point	**3 months**	–	**5 yrs**	**10 yrs**	–	**9 yrs**	–		–	**5 yrs**	–	–

(continued)

Table 37.3 (continued)

Registry	American	Australian		Belgian		Cana-dian	Dutch	Finnish		New Zealand	Norwe-gian	Swedish	UK/ Wales
<50 yrs old (%)	0.69	–		13[b]	17.5[b]	–	13.3	–		–	9.0 female 10.0 male	–	–
50–59 yrs old (%)	0.49	–		7[b]	14[b]	–	9.2	–		–		–	–
60–69 yrs old (%)	0.41	–		3.5[b]	4.5[b]	–	5.9	–		–		–	–
70–79 yrs old (%)	0.38	–		2.5[b]	3[b]	–	4.3	–		–	5.0 female 4.5 male	–	–
80–89 yrs old (%)	0.42	–		2[b]	2[b]	–	2.3 (age >80)	–		–		–	–
>89 yrs old (%)	0.49	–		(age >80)	–	–	–	–		–		–	–
Revision rate by fixation type													
Time point	**5 yrs**	**5 yrs**	**15 yrs**	–		–	–	**10 yrs**	**20 yrs**	**Overall cohort**	–	–	**15 yrs**
Cemented (%)	1.6[b]	2.9 (MS) 3.9 (PS) 3.3 (MP)	6.5 (MS) 7.0 (PS) 6.8 (MP)	–		–	–	6.0	11.3	3.2	–	–	4.7
Uncemented (%)	2.1[b]	4.2 (MS) 4.9 (PS) 5.8 (MP)	8.3 (MS) 7.0 (PS) 7.2 (MP)	–		–	–	12.8	27.1	5.2	–	–	6.2
Hybrid (%)	–	3.0 (MS) 5.4 (PS) 3.8 (MP)	6.5 (MS) 9.6 (PS)	–		–	–	–		4.5	–	–	4.4

Reasons for revision										
Aseptic loosening (%)	25	25	27.7	26.7	29.8	8.7	35.9	23.3	25[a]	27.5
Instability (%)	12.6	8.1	19.2	15.8	27.7	21.9	–	16.6	14[a]	16.5
Infection (%)	20.5	23.3	20.5	21.2	20.3	34.5	26.6	18.2	30[a]	25.4
Pain (%)	–	18	20.2	–	–	10.1	29.5	26.8	–	14.4
Other notable (%)	22.5 Other mechanical complications	–	11.8 Due to progressive OA	–	–	Non-exclusive diagnoses	Non-exclusive diagnoses	–	–	–

MS minimally stabilized (includes cruciate-retaining and ultra-congruent polyethylene prosthesis designs), *PS* posteriorly stabilized prostheses, *MP* medial pivot prosthesis

[a]Denotes estimate from 2007 to 2016 data set

[b]Denotes estimated of percentage from survival curve diagram

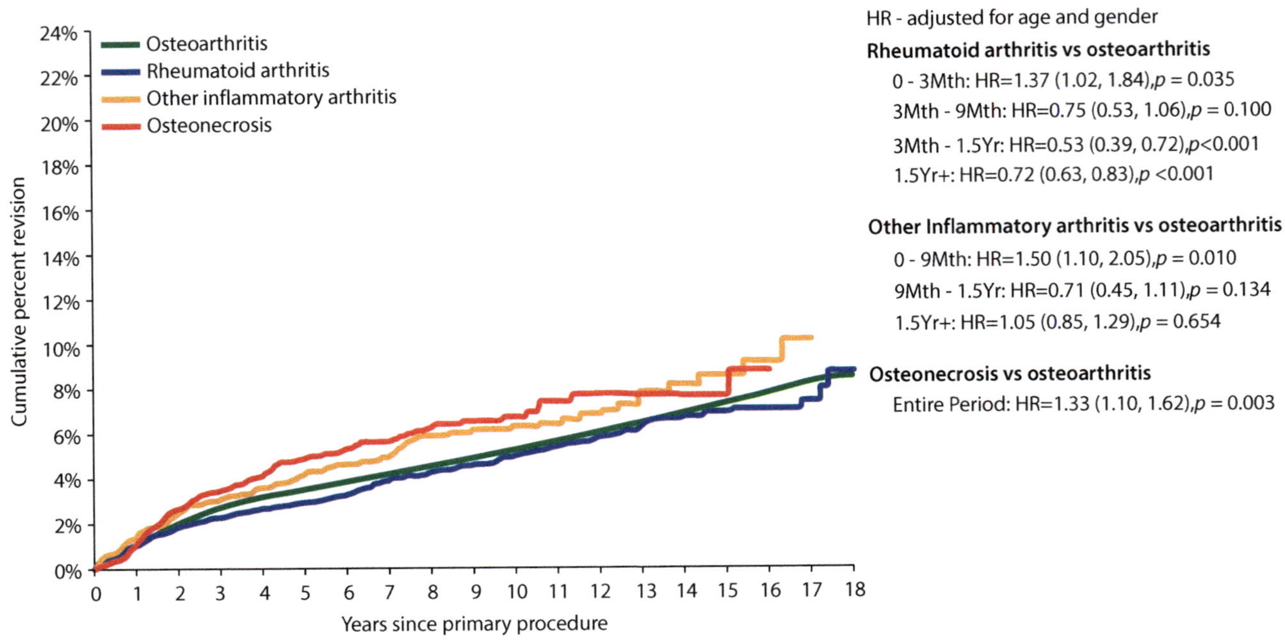

Fig. 37.1 Cumulative percent revision of primary total knee replacement by primary diagnosis

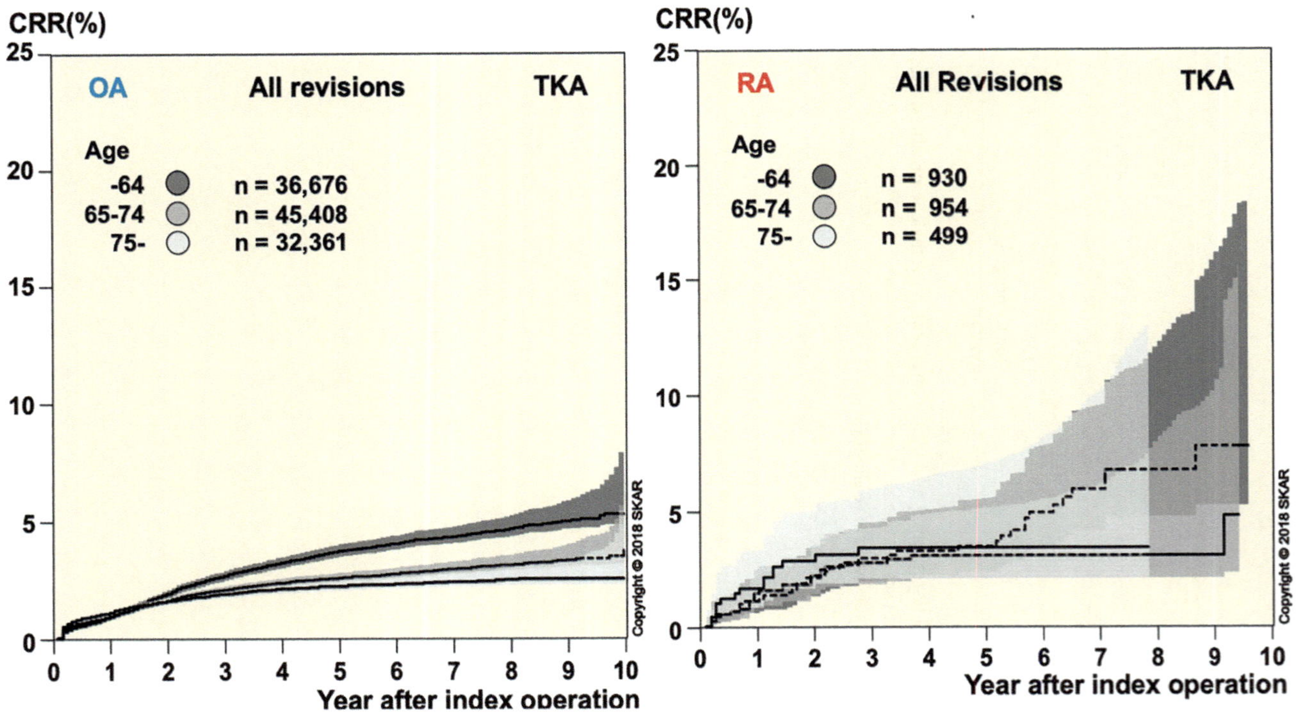

Fig. 37.2 Survival curve in rheumatoid arthritis (*RA*) patients compared to patients with osteoarthritis (*OA*) as a primary diagnosis at 10-year follow-up. *CRR* cumulative recurrence rate, *TKA* total knee arthroplasty (© Swedish Knee Arthroplasty Register [SKAR] 2018, with permission)

37.4.1 Outcomes Based on Patient Characteristics

37.4.1.1 Effect of Age

Assessment of implant survival based on patient age at the time of procedure is generally well-reported across registries (◘ Table 37.3). Reported age categories vary from commonly reported groupings such as <55, 55–64, 65–74, and 75+ years to groupings by decade of life. Timing varies from reports of early failure (within 3 months) reported in AJRR to 18-year data in the Australian registry and 20-year data in the Finnish registry, with most registries able to report outcomes at the 5-year mark. Some registries provided survival curve diagrams but not actual values, which require an estimation when extracting data. Consistent across all registries is a trend to lower revision rates with increasing age. In patients aged less than 55 years at the time of surgery the 5-year revision rates range from a low of 4.4% in female patients in the UK to a high of 9% in males in the Norwegian registry (in the age under 60 years category). At longer follow-up this age group sees the highest rates of revision documented at 17.8% at 18 years in the Australian registry and a remarkable 26.9% revision rate at 20 years in the Finnish registry. Revision rate in the 55–64-year age group at 5 years follow-up ranges from 2.8% in females in the UK to 4.8% in all sexes in the Finnish registry with long-term revision rates approaching 18.6%. The 65–74-year age group has documented revision rates at the 5-year time point ranging from 1.9% to 3.7% with long-range revision rates from 7% to 10.2%. The older age groups being 75 years or greater at the time of surgery have the lowest revision rates ranging from 1.4% to 5.0% at 5 years and comparatively very low revision rates at long-term follow-up, granted the longevity of the implant may outlast the remainder of the patients' years at this stage, with reported revision rates for those who survive to the 18- and 20-year time points of 3.6–5.0%, respectively.

> Younger age at implantation, specifically in males, has been shown to significantly increase revision rates, presumably from higher demand and heavier stress placed on the implants (Bayliss et al. 2017).

- **Effect of Sex**

Overall cumulative survival reported by sex was provided in 5 registries (◘ Table 37.3). The overall revision rate for males is higher than that for females in all registries other than the Dutch registry, albeit by never more than 2%. The Dutch registry reports revision rates of 5.8% and 5.5% for female and male patients, respectively, at 9-year follow-up. From the registries that report on sex differences in outcomes at multiple time points the difference between male and female revision rates becomes more apparent with time as the greatest differences are seen at final follow-up. The largest difference between the sexes at final follow-up is 2% seen in the Finnish registry at 25 years (revision rates of 15.9% for females and 17.9% for males) and in the UK registry at 15 years (15.5% for females and 17.5% for males). The Australian registry reports revision rates of 7.9% for females and 9.5% for males at 18-year follow-up. Patient-reported outcomes based on sex have not been currently reported. Previous studies have demonstrated worse postoperative patient-reported outcomes in females, but this may be secondary to worse preoperative function and pain (Barrack et al. 2014).

> However, as seen in this registry data, aggregation of large clinical studies has shown a trend toward higher revision rates in males following TKAs (O'Connor 2011).

- **Effect of BMI**

The effect of BMI is increasingly becoming a focus of registries moving forward; however, only the Australian and New Zealand registries have reported data available in their annual reports. Data on BMI has been collected since 2015 in the Australian registry. While no difference has been detected in revision rates between patients of normal weight and those classified as overweight or obesity class 1, early revision rates (within the first 6 months) are increased in patients in the obesity class 2 or greater categories (◘ Fig. 37.3).

> Of note, the Australian registry further showcases that BMI class experiences more revisions due to infection.

The New Zealand registry has collected BMI data since 2010 and reports revision rate of BMI categories by rate of revision per 100 component years. There have only been 89 revisions in patients with BMI <19 providing 331.6 observed component years with a reported observed rate of revision of 0.00 (95% CI 0.00–1.11). Patients with BMI 19–24 demonstrate a revision rate per 100 component years of 0.66 (95% CI 0.54–0.80), while patients within BMI ranges 25–29 and 30–39 have demonstrated rates of 0.57 (95% CI 0.50–0.64) and 0.59 (95% CI 0.53–0.65), respectively. Patients with BMI scores of 40 and higher demonstrate the highest rate of revision at 0.83 revisions per 100 component years (95% CI 0.26–1.08). The New Zealand registry also provides data on patient-reported outcomes by way of an Oxford knee score compared to BMI status at 5 years follow-up. Oxford knee scores range from a low of 36.11 seen in patients with BMI 40+ to a high of 39.81 seen with

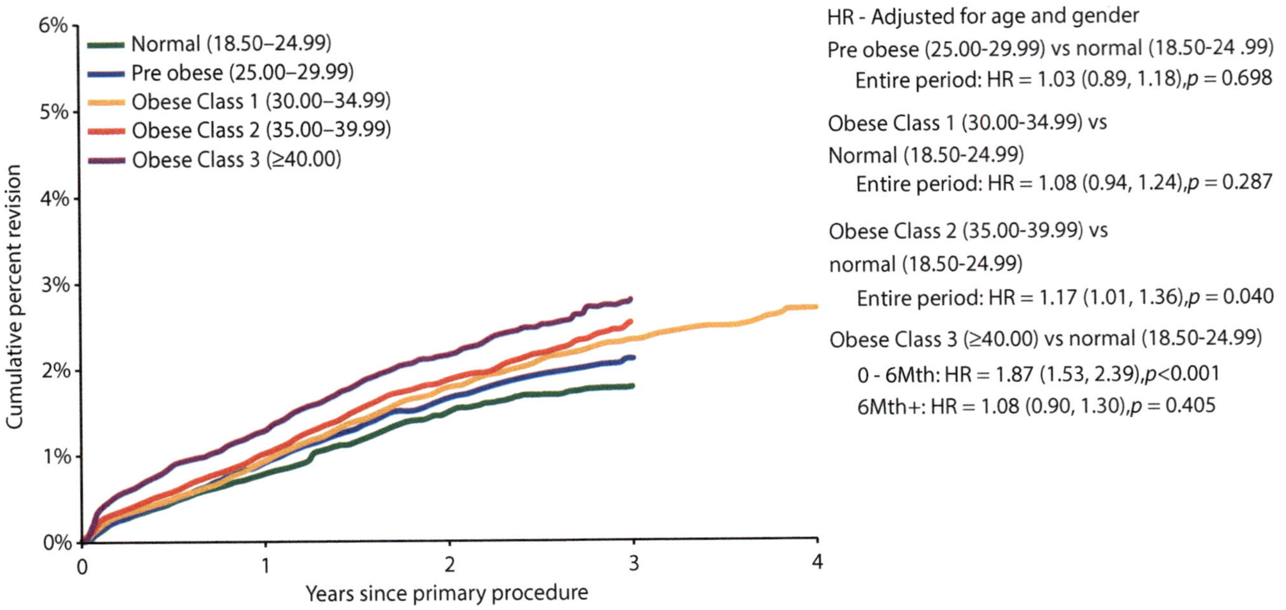

Fig. 37.3 Cumulative percent revision of primary total knee replacement by BMI category (primary diagnosis OA)

patients with a BMI 19–24. The outcomes of morbidly obese patients (>40 BMI), compared to simply obese patients, have shown to have worse outcomes in multiple other previous studies (George et al. 2018).

Effect of ASA Status

37

Data on outcomes based on ASA status are available in the Australian, Dutch, and New Zealand registries. The Australian registry has reported data on ASA status in 285,168 patients with up to 4 years follow-up for ASA class V patients, 5 years follow-up for ASA class I and IV patients, and 6 years follow-up for ASA class II and III patients. At these respective time points, revision rates are reported as

- 2.9% for class I,
- 3.2% for class II,
- 3.6% for class III,
- 4.4% for class IV, and
- 0% for the 16 patients registered in ASA class V.

In addition to cumulative revision rates, the Australian registry also provides a chart that highlights the reasons for revision within ASA classes I–IV which shows an increasing risk of infection in ASA class III and IV and potentially an increasing risk of loosening in ASA class IV, though exact values and confidence intervals are not provided (Fig. 37.4).

The Dutch registry provides a cumulative revision graph on survival based on competing risk assessment by ASA class showing a small but significant increase in revision rates at 9 years for patients with ASA class I compared to all others with a rate of

- 6.2% (95% CI 5.9–6.5%) for ASA class I
- 5.2% (95% CI 5.0–5.4%) for class II
- 5.1% (95% CI 4.7–5.5%) for a combined cohort of ASA class III and IV patients (Fig. 37.5)

However, in their Kaplan-Meier assessment, only the ASA class I and class II cohorts have non-overlapping 95% confidence intervals.

The New Zealand registry began collecting ASA classification data in 2005 and provides revision rates per 100 component years of

- 0.53 (95% CI 0.47–0.59) for ASA class I
- 0.48 (95% CI 0.48–0.51) for class II
- 0.56 (95% CI 0.52–0.60) for class III
- 0.57 (95% CI 0.26–1.08) for ASA class IV

37.4.2 Outcomes Based on Method of Fixation

Many registries report objective values for incidence of cemented, uncemented, and hybrid total knee arthroplasties (Table 37.4).

> The most notable outlier is Australia as the only registry reporting rates of fully cemented total knee arthroplasty below 90% (68.6%).

Outcomes by fixation method are reported in the American, Australian, Finnish, New Zealand, and UK registries at various time points ranging from 5 to 20 years (Table 37.3). The American registry provides a sur-

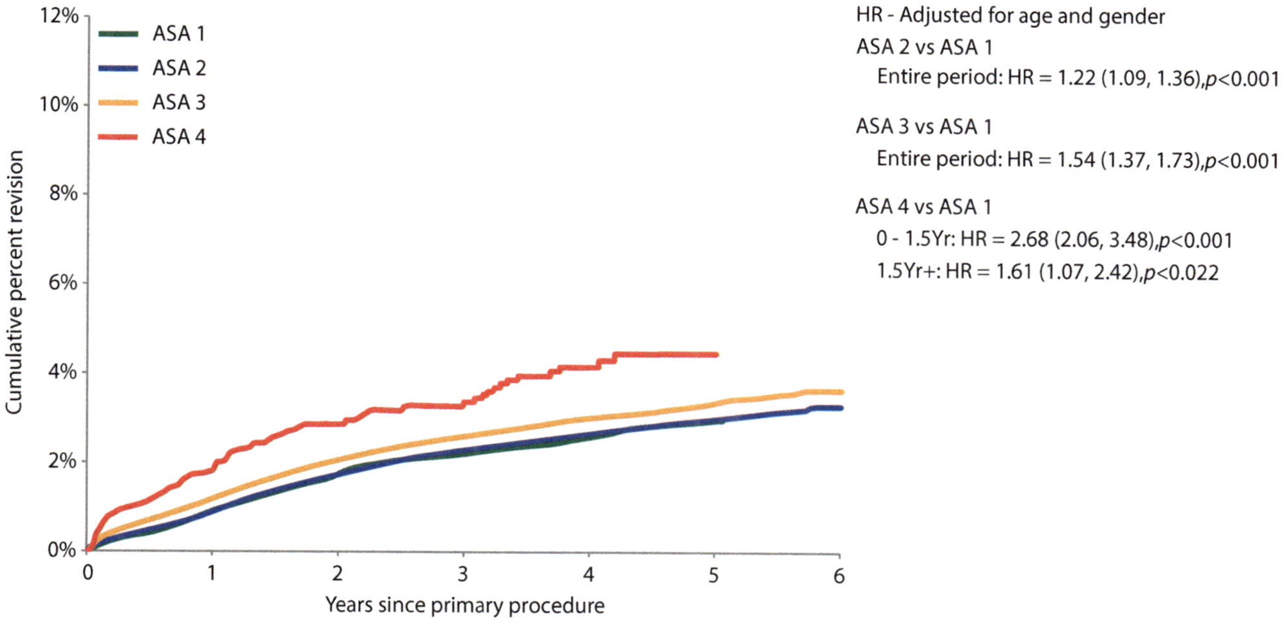

Fig. 37.4 Cumulative percent revision of primary total knee replacement by ASA score (primary diagnosis OA)

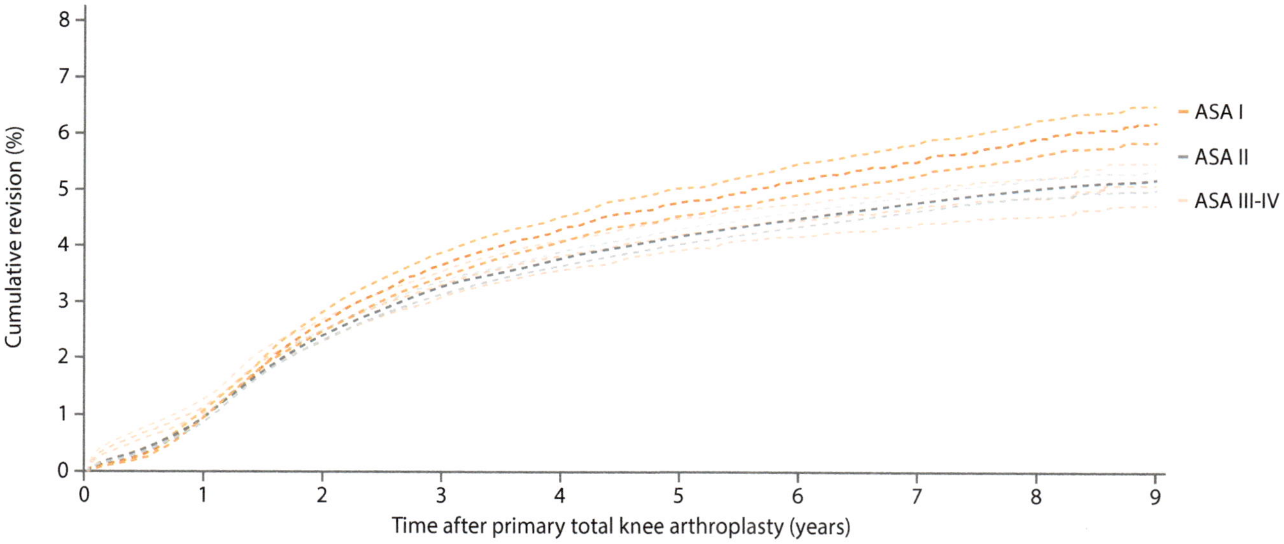

Fig. 37.5 Cumulative percent revision of primary total knee arthroplasties by ASA score in The Netherlands in 2007–2017 ($N = 206{,}162$). *Dotted lines* represent upper and lower limits of the 95% confidence interval (© Dutch Arthroplasty Register [LROI], with permission)

vival curve diagram which permits estimation of revision rate at 5 years of approximately 1.6% and 2.1% for cemented and uncemented/hybrid fixation methods, respectively. The Australian registry separates survival analysis by both fixation method and implant type. For minimally stabilized prostheses, uncemented fixation techniques are reported to have the highest cumulative revision rates while no difference is seen between cemented and hybrid cemented techniques. In posteriorly stabilized prostheses there is a time-dependent difference in survival based on technique with cemented fixation demonstrating lower revision rates for the first 2.5 years while after 4.5 years cementless fixation techniques demonstrate a lower revision rate, with hybrid fixation of posteriorly stabilized prostheses having the highest revision rate at all time points. When analyzing the medial pivot prosthesis design, the Australian registry demonstrates higher revision rates in cementless techniques compared to cemented techniques with no difference detected between either technique and hybrid fixation. The Finnish registry demonstrates a substantially higher cumulative revision rate in uncemented techniques which are double that of cemented at 10 years (6.0% cemented vs. 12.8% uncemented) with the gap

Table 37.4 Implantation technique, use of navigation and Rate of patellar resurfacing by registry

Registry	American	Australian	Belgian	Canadian	Dutch	Finnish	New Zealand	Norwegian	Swedish	UK/Wales
Fixation method (TKA)										
Cemented (%)	93.8	68.6	91.1	–	93.2	93.5	92.0	–	92.6	94.9
Uncemented (%)	6.2	9.9	4.8	–	4.1	5.8	5.0	–	7.0	4.2
Hybrid (%)	–	21.5	3.9	–	2.7	0.7	3.0	–	0.1 (2017 data)	0.9
Use of navigation										
(%)	–	33.2	–	–	–	–	13.1[a]	–	–	–
Patellar resurfacing										
(%)	90.6	66.6	–	–	92.8	–	37.0	8.6	2.4	–

TKA total knee arthroplasty
[a]Includes approaches classified as image-guided and robot navigation

widening with time such that at 20 years follow-up cemented fixation results in a revision rate of 11.3% while uncemented fixation techniques display a 27.1% cumulative revision rate. Cementless fixation technique is associated with higher mean cumulative revision rates in the New Zealand and UK registries as well, to a lesser degree however (Table 37.3).

37

37.4.3 Reasons for Revision

All registries provided a method for reporting the reasons for revisions in TKA and at minimum the 3 most common reasons are reported in Table 3. The majority of registries list aseptic loosening as the number one cause of revision. An outlier in this area is the Finnish registry reporting a rate of revision for aseptic loosening of only 8.7% yet a rate of revision for infection of 34.5%. Whereas the New Zealand registry reports non-exclusive diagnoses with 35.9% of revisions carrying at least one diagnosis of a loose component. The Canadian and Swedish registries list infection as the number one reason for revision. In Norway, pain is the most commonly provided reason listed at the time of revision, although in the Norwegian database revision reasons are non-exclusive.

As some registries have all reported diagnostic reasons compiled such that rates are non-exclusive and total percentages add up to greater than 100%, the level of detail provided in revision cases varies considerably. Furthermore, it has been demonstrated that the most common causes of revision differ depending on if you look at acute vs. late causes (Sharkey et al. 2014) and this is not specified in the registries. Overall, in registries with exclusive diagnoses, the rate of instability ranges from 8.1% to 19.2%, rate of infection ranges from 18.2% to 34.5% and where reported the revision rate for a primary diagnosis of pain ranges from 10.1% to 26.8%.

Other notable reported reasons for revision include the Belgian registry reporting an 11.8% rate of revision due to progressive OA in unaddressed compartments and the American registry reporting 22.5% of revisions being performed for mechanical complications other than aseptic loosening and instability.

37.4.4 Notable Trends

Some trends have been shown in these international registries, one of which is the trend in number of cases performed yearly has increased in all the registries we included.

> This increase in TKA utilization cannot be explained by simply an increase in the population and may indicate expanded indications and patient demand (Losina et al. 2012).

The use of navigation has begun to be tracked by several registries and is now being reported on. Australia has reported an increase from 2.4% of TKA cases performed in 2003 using navigation to 33.2% in 2018 (Fig. 37.6). Some registries have begun to capture the use of robotics but currently this has not been reported in annual reports. In the Australian registry, patients aged <65 years have a

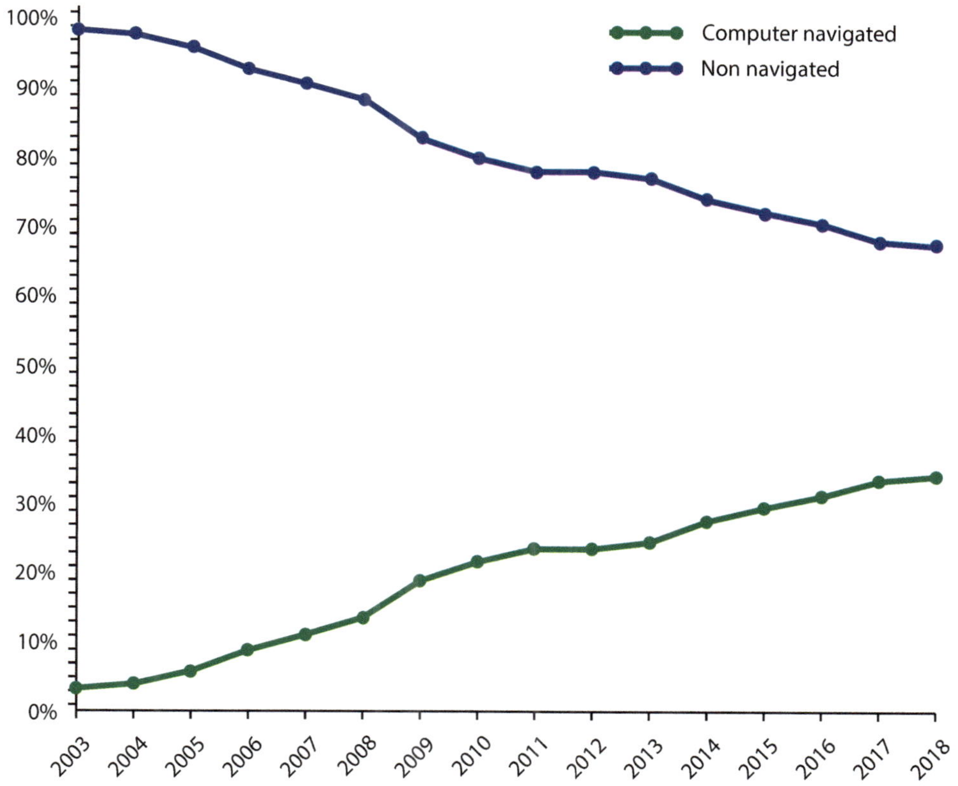

Fig. 37.6 Primary total knee replacement by computer navigation

lower rate of revision when computer navigation is used compared to when it is not used.

Resurfacing vs. non-resurfacing of the patella is also reported on and some notable trends can be seen. In the Australian registry the rate of patella resurfacing was as low as 41.5% in 2003 and has now increased to 69.1% in 2018 (Fig. 37.7). Norway has also demonstrated an increase in percentage of patella resurfacings, currently at 8.6% of TKAs from 2.2% in 2010. The Norwegian registry cited a report on their own data demonstrating higher KOOS scores in resurfaced TKAs as driving this trend (Aunan et al. 2016). The highest reported amount of patella resurfacing is seen in the AJRR at 90.6%. This is down from a high of 93.6% reported in 2012. The lowest reported percentage of resurfacing was reported in Sweden at 2.4%, which have been decreasing since the 1980s. Their recent high was 15% in 2005. In New Zealand 63% of the TKAs had no patella resurfacing, with 37% having a patella resurfaced.

The use of highly cross-linked polyethylene continues to increase. The use of highly cross-linked polyethylene has continued to increase from a low of 7.1% to 64.2% of TKAs in the Australian registry. The use of antioxidant polyethylene has increased from 2.5% in 2012 to 23.2% of TKAs in the current AJRR report. Unicondylar knee arthroplasty (UKA) use in the Swedish registry has decreased over time compared to TKA (Fig. 37.8) but has increased in utilization in the past 5 years.

In the Australian registry, the use of partial knee replacements has decreased from a high of 12.3% of all procedures to a 5.8% in 2018. The 2018 value is, however, slightly increased from a low of 4.2% in 2014. In the UK, NJR UKAs have remained relatively steady since they began recording data in 2003 with a rate around 10% of the procedures.

Norway has demonstrated a decreasing trend in the use of a surgical drain, from a high of 49% in 2011 to a low of 15% in 2018.

When examining the mean length of stay as reported to AJRR, there has been a significant decrease of 0.9 days for TKAs comparing 2012–2018. A significant decrease in mean length of stay for partial knee arthroplasties of 1.2 days was also seen.

37.4.5 Patient-Reported Outcome Measures

Traditional TJA registries were designed to collect data useful to monitoring implant survival and failure as defined by revision rates (Franklin et al. 2013). While the implant revision rate remains an important outcome, registries are currently utilizing patient-reported outcome measures (PROMs) to contextualize patient function prior to a revision.

Fig. 37.7 Primary total knee replacement by patella usage

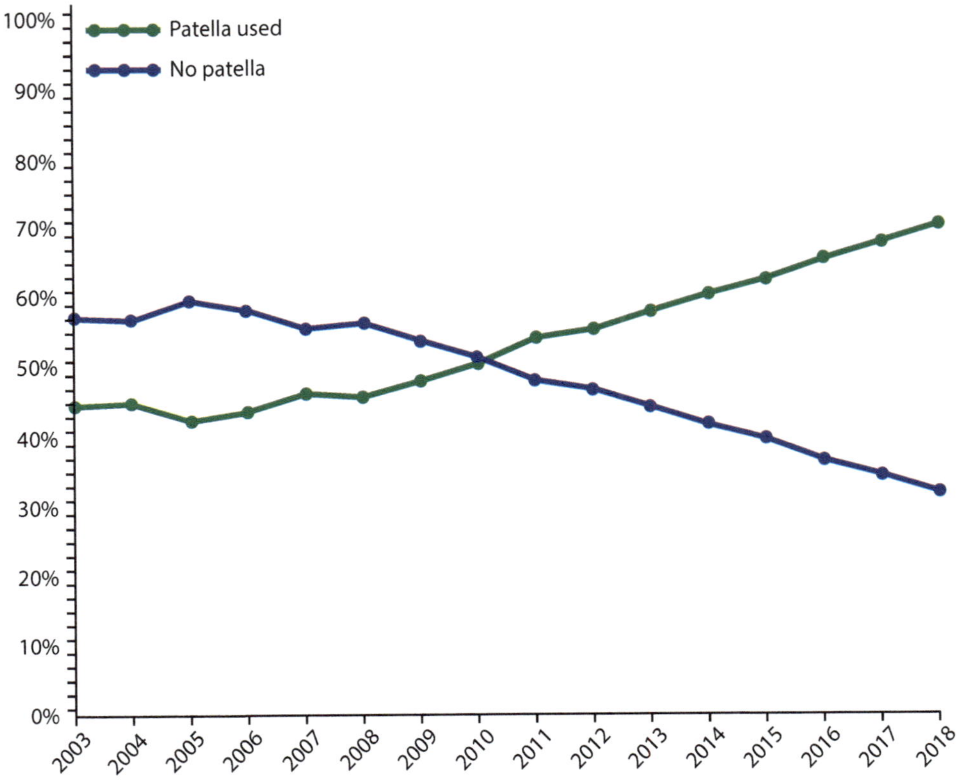

Fig. 37.8 Relative yearly distribution of implant types used for primary surgery (© Swedish Knee Arthroplasty Register [SKAR] 2018, with permission)

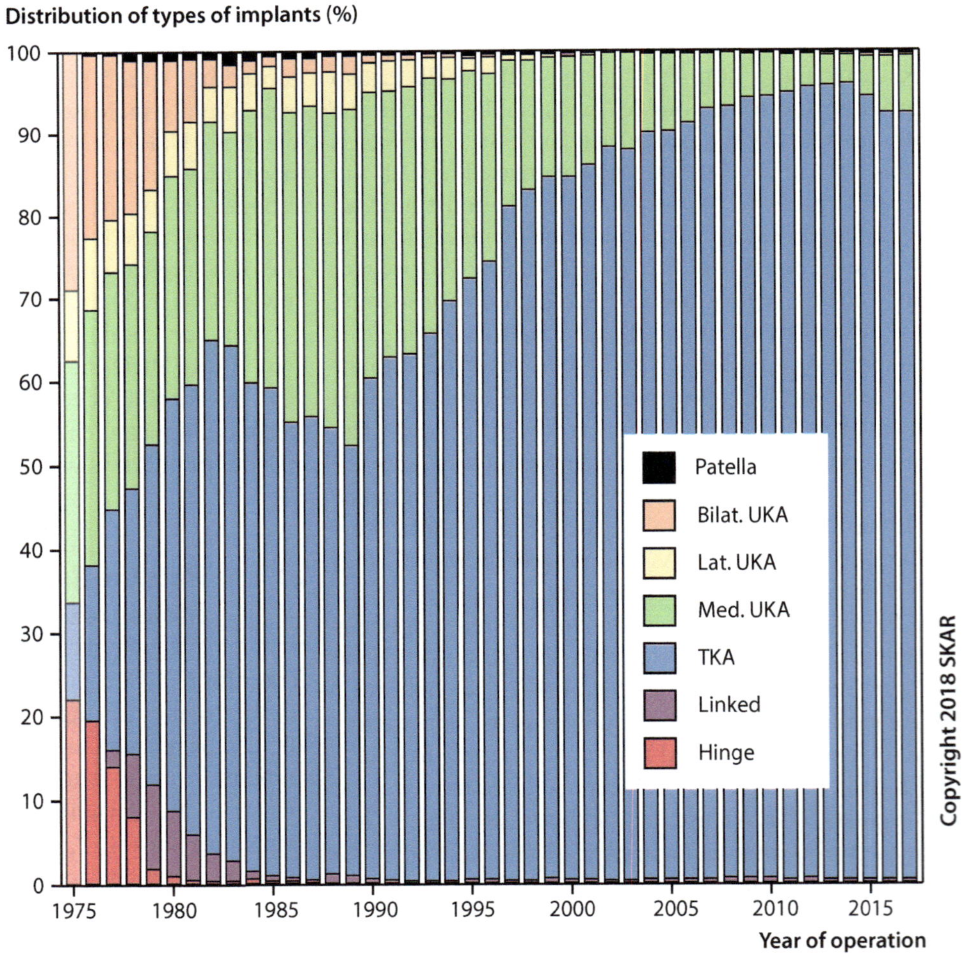

Total joint arthroplasty is performed to decrease pain as well as to restore function and quality of life. It is, therefore, important to measure these same outcomes when assessing the registry results of TKA (Wilson et al. 2019).

Revision itself as an endpoint is rather straightforward, but it is likely insufficient as a measure of success given the fact that 1-year TKA survivorship is almost 100%, while only 80% of the patients are satisfied (Robertsson et al. 2000b). However, numerous barriers exist to the implementation of PROM collection for national registries including, but not limited to, cost, time, and response rate. Given this difficulty, ISAR PROMs Working Group proposes a 60% threshold for an acceptable frequency of collection based on these external difficulties in collection (ISAR Website 2020). The New Zealand registry was an early adopter of postoperative PROMs for hip and knee procedures, beginning at its inception in 1998. Other European registries followed with the Swedish hip registry in 2002, the UK NJR in 2009, and the Norwegian hip fracture registry in 2005 (Rolfson et al. 2011). The current national knee registries'annual reports that include PROMs include AJRR, Canada, Dutch, New Zealand, and Swedish Joint Registry (■ Table 37.5). The UK NJR registry reports annual PROMs separately on the NHS website (NHS Digital 2020).

Not all registries collect the same PROMs, which differ in the type of data collected. The Canadian, Dutch, UK NKR, and New Zealand registries collect the Oxford knee score. The Canadian, Dutch, UK NJR Wales, and Swedish registries all collect the EQ-5D. The Swedish, Dutch, and American registries collect the knee injury and osteoarthritis outcome score (KOOS). AJRR also collects PROMIS and VR-12. The Dutch collect the numeric rating scale (NRS). The Swedish and UK NJR also collect the visual analog scale (VAS). The Swedish registry collects the OMERACT-OARSI.

At this stage, the vast majority of these registries' PROMs are currently reported as overall outcomes from preoperative to postoperative and are not broken down into comparisons based on patient demographics, surgical techniques, or specific implants.

As an exception, the New Zealand joint registry has reported Oxford knee scores by BMI class at 6 months postoperatively in a cohort of 8663 patients.

Conclusion

Here, we reported on the current status of the international registries. We included national registries which report annual English language analyses. We attempted to give an overall picture of the status of the registries and the outcomes that can be learned from them. The quality of data obtained from these registries continues to improve, as the number of national registries and their capture rates has grown. As collaboration progresses as well, we will continue to learn more about our total knee arthroplasty outcomes from a global perspective.

Table 37.5 Patient-reported outcome details by registry

Registry	American	Australian	Belgian	Canadian	Dutch	Finnish	New Zealand	Norwegian	Swedish	UK/Wales
Patient-reported outcome measures										
Oxford knee	–	–	–	Oxford knee	Oxford knee	–	Oxford knee	–	–	Oxford knee
KOOS	KOOS JR	KOOS-12	–	–	KOOS PS	–	–	–	KOOS	
EQ-5D	–	–	–	EQ-5D-5L	EQ-5D index EQ-5D thermometer	–	–	–	EQ-5D	EQ-5D
PROMIS	PROMIS-10	–	–	–	–	–	–	–	–	–
VR-12	VR-12	–	–	–	–	–	–	–	–	–
NRS	–	–	–	–	NRS rest NRS activity	–	–	–	–	–
OMERACT-OARSI	–	–	–	–	–	–	–	–	OMERACT-OARSI	–
VAS	–	–	–	–	–	–	–	–	VAS	EQ VAS
Time points being collected										
Time point	Pre-op 1 yr post-op	–	–	–	Pre-op 6 mos post-op 1 yr post-op	–	6 mos post-op 5 yrs post-op 10 yrs post-op 15 yrs post-op 20 yrs post-op	–	Pre-op 1 yr post-op	Pre-op post-op

KOOS knee injury and osteoarthritis outcome score, *EQ-5D* EuroQol-5D, *PROMIS* patient-reported outcomes measurement information system, *VR-12* veterans RAND 12, *NRS* numeric rating scale, *OMERACT–OARSI* outcome measures in arthritis clinical trials – Osteoarthritis research society international, *VAS* visual analogue scale

Take-Home Messages

- The aggregation of data via registries is essential to allow for adequate statistical analysis, the ability to track long-term results, and recurring analysis to identify trends in care.
- The first institutional-based registry began at the Mayo Clinic, Rochester, Minnesota in 1965.
- Registries have now grown to the national scale, with the first national registry formed in Sweden in 1974.
- The American Joint Replacement Registry (AJRR) is a national registry in the United States, established and managed by the American Association of Orthopedic Surgeons (AAOS) in 2011.
- With all the success of national registries, there is a danger of using large observational data sets to make erroneous conclusions. Correlations can be identified but causation cannot be concluded.
- Pooled data from international registries demonstrates 82% TKA survivorship at 25-year follow-up.
- Traditional TJA registries were designed to collect data useful to monitoring implant survival and failure as defined by revision rates. While the implant revision rate remains an important outcome, registries are currently utilizing patient-reported outcome measures (PROMs) to contextualize patient function prior to a revision

References

American Joint Replacement Registry (AJRR) (2019) 6th annual report on hip and knee arthroplasty data. http://connect.ajrr.net/2019-ajrr-annual-report. Accessed April 19, 2020

Aunan E, Næss G, Clarke-Jenssen J, Sandvik L, Kibsgård TJ (2016) Patellar resurfacing in total knee arthroplasty: functional outcome differs with different outcome scores: a randomized, double-blind study of 129 knees with 3 years of follow-up. Acta Orthop 87(2):158–164. https://doi.org/10.3109/17453674.2015.1111075

Australian Orthopaedic Association National Joint Replacement Registry (2018) Hip, knee & shoulder annual report 2018. https://aoanjrr.sahmri.com/annual-reports-2018. Accessed April 20, 2020

Barrack RL, Ruh EL, Chen J et al (2014) Impact of socioeconomic factors on outcome of total knee arthroplasty. Clin Orthop Relat Res 472(1):86–97. https://doi.org/10.1007/s11999-013-3002-y

Bayliss LE, Culliford D, Monk AP et al (2017) The effect of patient age at intervention on risk of implant revision after total replacement of the hip or knee: a population-based cohort study. Lancet 389(10077):1424–1430. https://doi.org/10.1016/S0140-6736(17)30059-4

Bengston S, Knutson K, Lidgren L (1989) Treatment of infected knee arthroplasty. Clin Orthop Relat Res 245:173–178

Berry DJ, Kessler M, Morrey BF (1997) Maintaining a hip registry for 25 years. Mayo Clinic experience. *Clin Orthop Relat Res* 344:61–68. https://doi.org/10.1097/00003086-199711000-00007

Canadian Institute for Health Information. Hip and Knee Replacements in Canada, 2017–2018: Canadian joint replacement registry annual report. CIHI, Ottawa. https://www.cihi.ca/sites/default/files/document/cjrr-annual-report-2019-en-web_0.pdf. Accessed April 20, 2020

Craviotto DF (2001) Dissemination of information, among orthopaedic surgeons, regarding early failure of total joint implants. J Bone Joint Surg Am 83(10):1580–1581. https://doi.org/10.2106/00004623-200110000-00019

Delaunay C (2015) Registries in orthopaedics. Orthop Traumatol Surg Res 101(1 Suppl):S69–S75. https://doi.org/10.1016/j.otsr.2014.06.029

Dutch Arthroplasty Register (LROI) (2018) Online LROI annual report 2018. https://www.lroirapportage.nl/media/pdf/PDF%20Online%20LROI%20annual%20report%202019.pdf. Accessed April 20, 2020

Etkin CD, Springer BD (2017) The American joint replacement registry-the first 5 years. Arthroplast Today 3(2):67–69. https://doi.org/10.1016/j.artd.2017.02.002

Evans JT, Walker RW, Evans JP, Blom AW, Sayers A, Whitehouse MR (2019) How long does a knee replacement last? A systematic review and meta-analysis of case series and national registry reports with more than 15 years of follow-up. Lancet 393(10172):655–663. https://doi.org/10.1016/S0140-6736(18)32531-5

Finnish Arthroplasty Register (2017) Total hip and knee arthroplasty report 2017. https://www2.thl.fi/endo/report/#html/opendata. Accessed April 21, 2020

Franklin PD, Harrold L, Ayers DC (2013) Incorporating patient-reported outcomes in total joint arthroplasty registries: challenges and opportunities. Clin Orthop Relat Res 471(11):3482–3488. https://doi.org/10.1007/s11999-013-3193-2

Furnes O, Lie SA, Havelin LI, Vollset SE, Engesaeter LB (1997) Exeter and Charnley arthroplasties with Boneloc or high viscosity cement: comparison of 1, 127 arthroplasties followed for 5 years in the Norwegian Arthroplasty Register. Acta Orthop Scand 68(6):515–520. https://doi.org/10.3109/17453679708999017

George J, Piuzzi NS, Ng M, Sodhi N, Khlopas AA, Mont MA (2018) Association between body mass index and thirty-day complications after total knee arthroplasty. J Arthroplast 33(3):865–871. https://doi.org/10.1016/j.arth.2017.09.038

Harris WH (1995) The problem is osteolysis. Clin Orthop Relat Res 311:46–53

Havelin LI, Fenstad AM, Salomonsson R et al (2009) The Nordic Arthroplasty Register Association: a unique collaboration between 3 national hip arthroplasty registries with 280,201 THRs. Acta Orthop 80(4):393–401. https://doi.org/10.3109/17453670903039544

Herberts P, Ahnfelt L, Malchau H, Strömberg C, Andersson GB (1989) Multicenter clinical trials and their value in assessing total joint arthroplasty. Clin Orthop Relat Res 249:48–55

Howard JL, Kudera J, Lewallen DG, Hanssen AD (2011) Early results of the use of tantalum femoral cones for revision total knee arthroplasty. J Bone Joint Surg Am 93(5):478–484. https://doi.org/10.2106/JBJS.I.01322

Hughes RE, Batra A, Hallstrom BR (2017) Arthroplasty registries around the world: valuable sources of hip implant revision risk data. Curr Rev Musculoskelet Med 10(2):240–252. https://doi.org/10.1007/s12178-017-9408-5

ISAR Website. https://sites.google.com/view/isaropen. Accessed April 25, 2020

Joglekar SB, Rose PS, Lewallen DG, Sim FH (2012) Tantalum acetabular cups provide secure fixation in THA after pelvic irradiation at minimum 5-year followup. Clin Orthop Relat Res 470(11):3041–3047. https://doi.org/10.1007/s11999-012-2382-8

Knutson K, Robertsson O (2010) The Swedish Knee Arthroplasty Register (www.knee.se): the inside story. Acta Orthop 81(1):5–7. https://doi.org/10.3109/17453671003667267

Knutson K, JóSnsson G, Andersen JL, Lárusdóttir H, Lidgren L (1981) Deformation and loosening of the tibial component in knee arthroplasty with unicompartmental endoprostheses. Acta Orthop Scand 52(6):667–673. https://doi.org/10.3109/17453678108992165

Kurtz S, Ong K, Lau E, Mowat F, Halpern M (2007) Projections of primary and revision hip and knee arthroplasty in the United States from 2005 to 2030. JBJS 89(4):780–785. https://doi.org/10.2106/JBJS.F.00222

Losina E, Thornhill TS, Rome BN, Wright J, Katz JN (2012) The dramatic increase in total knee replacement utilization rates in the United States cannot be fully explained by growth in population size and the obesity epidemic. J Bone Joint Surg Am 94(3):201–207. https://doi.org/10.2106/JBJS.J.01958

Lübbeke A, Silman AJ, Prieto-Alhambra D, Adler AI, Barea C, Carr AJ (2017) The role of national registries in improving patient safety for hip and knee replacements. BMC Musculoskelet Disord 18(1):414. https://doi.org/10.1186/s12891-017-1773-0

Malchau H, Garellick G, Berry D et al (2018) Arthroplasty implant registries over the past five decades: development, current, and future impact. J Orthop Res 36(9):2319–2330. https://doi.org/10.1002/jor.24014

Maloney WJ (2001) National Joint Replacement Registries: has the time come? J Bone Joint Surg Am 83(10):1582–1585. https://doi.org/10.2106/00004623-200110000-00020

National Joint Registry (2018) 16th annual report 2018 National Joint Registry for England, Wales, Northern Ireland and the Isle of Man. https://reports.njrcentre.org.uk/Portals/0/PDFdownloads/NJR%2016th%20Annual%20Report%202019.pdf. Accessed April 19, 2020

New Zealand Orthopaedic Association (2018) The New Zealand Joint Registry. The New Zealand Joint Registry 19 Year Report. https://nzoa.org.nz/system/files/DH8152_NZJR_2018_Report_v6_4Decv18.pdf. Accessed April 20, 2020

NHS Digital. Patient reported outcome measures. https://digital.nhs.uk/data-and-information/data-tools-and-services/dataservices/patient-reported-outcome-measures-proms. Accessed April 22, 2020

Norwegian Arthroplasty Register (2019) Norwegian national advisory unit on arthroplasty and hip fractures. http://nrlweb.ihelse.net/eng/Rapporter/Report2019_english.pdf. Accessed April 20, 2020

O'Connor MI (2011) Implant survival, knee function, and pain relief after TKA: are there differences between men and women? Clin Orthop Relat Res 469(7):1846–1851. https://doi.org/10.1007/s11999-011-1782-5

Orthopride Belgian Hip and Knee Arthroplasty Registry Annual Report (2018). https://www.ehealth.fgov.be/file/view/AXDOTDE0mTlaOSp4Nmeq?filename=Orthopride_Annual_Report_2018.pdf. Accessed April 25, 2020

Robertsson O, Lewold S, Knutson K, Lidgren L (2000a) The Swedish knee arthroplasty project. Acta Orthop Scand 71(1):7–18. https://doi.org/10.1080/00016470052943829

Robertsson O, Dunbar M, Pehrsson T, Knutson K, Lidgren L (2000b) Patient satisfaction after knee arthroplasty: a report on 27,372 knees operated on between 1981 and 1995 in Sweden. Acta Orthop Scand 71(3):262–267. https://doi.org/10.1080/000164700317411852

Rolfson O, Rothwell A, Sedrakyan A et al (2011) Use of patient-reported outcomes in the context of different levels of data. J Bone Joint Surg Am 93(Suppl 3):66–71. https://doi.org/10.2106/JBJS.K.01021

Sharkey PF, Lichstein PM, Shen C, Tokarski AT, Parvizi J (2014) Why are total knee arthroplasties failing today--has anything changed after 10 years? J Arthroplast 29(9):1774–1778. https://doi.org/10.1016/j.arth.2013.07.024

Singh JA, Yu S, Chen L, Cleveland JD (2019) Rates of total joint replacement in the United States: future projections to 2020–2040 using the national inpatient sample. J Rheumatol. https://doi.org/10.3899/jrheum.170990

Sloan M, Premkumar A, Sheth NP (2018) Projected volume of primary total joint arthroplasty in the U.S., 2014 to 2030. J Bone Joint Surg Am 100(17):1455–1460. https://doi.org/10.2106/JBJS.17.01617

Swedish Knee Arthroplasty Register (2018) Swedish Knee Arthroplasty Register 2018 Annual Report. http://www.myknee.se/pdf/SVK_2018_Eng_1.0.pdf. Accessed April 21, 2020

van Steenbergen LN, Denissen GAW, Spooren A et al (2015) More than 95% completeness of reported procedures in the population-based Dutch Arthroplasty Register. Acta Orthop 86(4):498–505

Wilson I, Bohm E, Lübbeke A et al (2019) Orthopaedic registries with patient-reported outcome measures. EFORT Open Rev 4(6):357–367. https://doi.org/10.1302/2058-5241.4.180080

USA AJRR – Total Knee Arthroplasty: Lessons Learned

Paul Hoogervorst and Patrick K. Horst

Contents

E. Hansen, K.-D. Kühn (eds.), *Essentials of Cemented Knee Arthroplasty*,
https://doi.org/10.1007/978-3-662-63113-3_38

38.1 Introduction

The first nationwide orthopedic implant registries were implemented between 1975 and 1995 in the three Scandinavian countries and Finland with the aim to collect data on total knee arthroplasty (TKA) and total hip arthroplasty (THA) (Delaunay 2015; Malchau et al. 2018) (◘ Fig. 38.1).

❯ The American Joint Replacement Registry (AJRR) is considerably newer since it was established in 2010 by the American Academy of Orthopedic Surgeons. Its

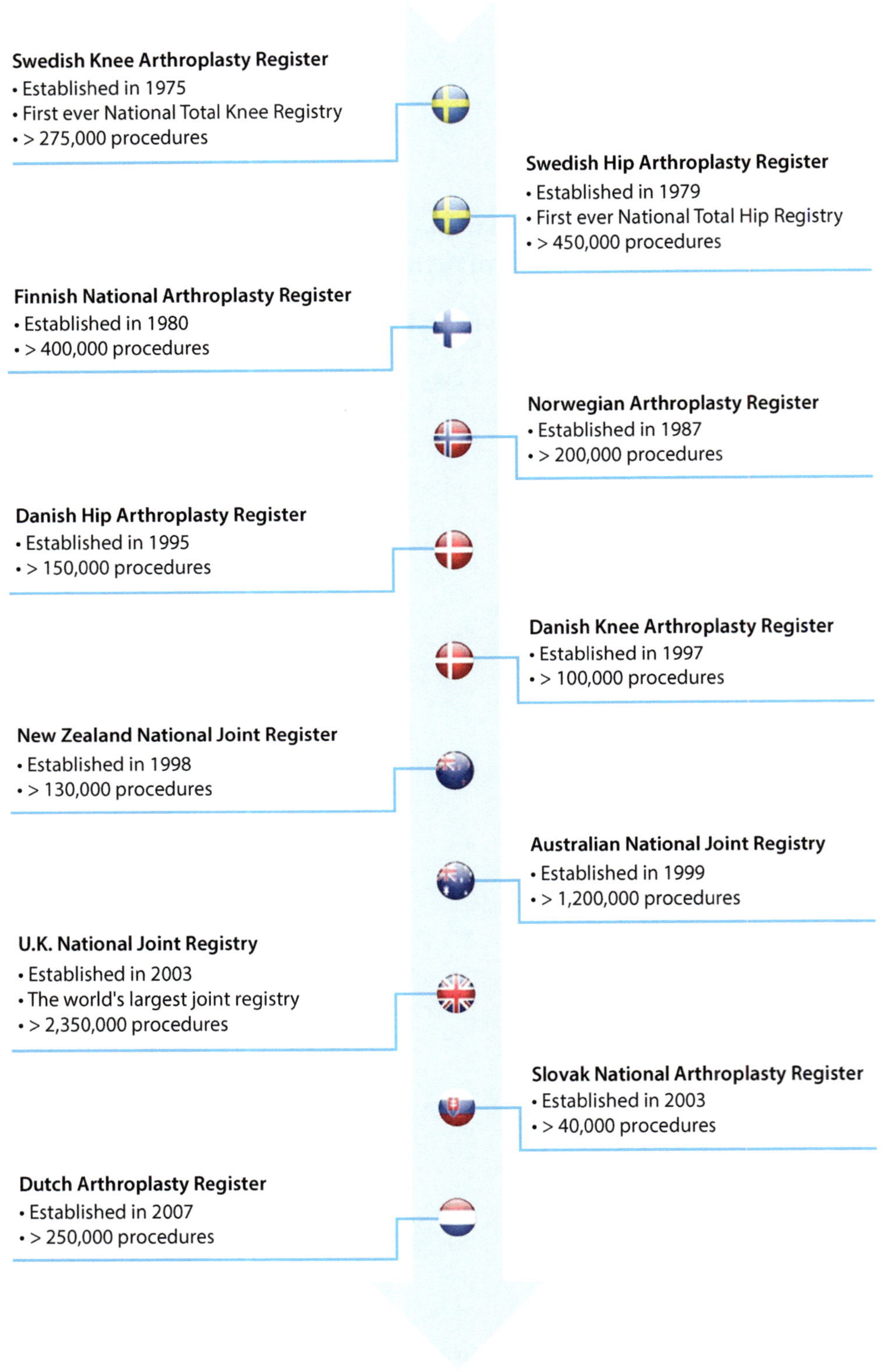

◘ **Fig. 38.1** Earliest registry development. (Adapted from Malchau et al. (2018); by courtesy of John Wiley & Sons)

goals are to capture hip and knee arthroplasty data to conduct implant-specific survivorship analyses, produce risk-adjusted patient outcome data, and provide hospitals with quality benchmarks (Etkin and Springer 2017).

Currently, the AJRR contains data on over 1.5 million procedures from 1133 hospitals, 104 ambulatory surgery centers (ASCs), and 65 private practice groups in all 50 states and the District of Columbia.

> It covers approximately 32% of all arthroplasties performed nationwide.

This number is significantly lower than the Swedish, Finnish, Norwegian, and UK registries which report a coverage of 93.8–98.1% (Swedish Knee Arthroplasty Register 2019; National Joint Registry 2019; Norwegian National Advisory Unit on Arthroplasty and Hip Fractures: Annual Report 2019; Finnish Arthroplasty Registry 2019). The AJRR collects hip and knee arthroplasty procedures in 3 data types:

- Procedural
- Postoperative
- Patient-reported outcome measures (PROMs) data (Table 38.1) (American Joint Replacement Registry (AJRR) 2019)

Table 38.1 Data captured by AJRR

Procedural	Patient	Name (last, first) Date of birth Social Security Number Diagnosis (ICD-9/10, CPT) Gender Race/ethnicity Height + weight/Body Mass Index Payer status
	Site of Service	Name and address (TIN, NPI)
	Surgeon	Name (NPI) Trainee
	Procedure	Type (ICD-9/10, CPT) Date of surgery Length of stay Surgical approach Surgical technique Laterality Implants (maufacturer, lot #) Anesthesia
Postoperative		Comorbidities CJR risk variables Height + weight/body mass index Length of stay American Society of Anaesthesiologists score Charlson index Operative and postoperative complications
PROMs		HOOS Jr. KOOS Jr. PROMIS-10 Global VR-12

38.2 Primary TKA

In 2018, the total number of primary TKAs registered in the American Joint Replacement Registry (AJRR) was 828,999 which amounts to 55.1% of all procedures collected.

The mean per surgeon volume of TKAs in 2018 was 44.8 with an interquartile range (IQR) of 7–56. The average age for patients undergoing TKA was 66.7 years (SD 9.6). This is in line with other national registries which report a mean age at surgery of approximately 68 years (National Joint Registry 2019; Norwegian National Advisory Unit on Arthroplasty and Hip Fractures: Annual Report 2019; Australian Orthopaedic Association National Joint Replacement Registry 2019; The New Zealand Joint Registry 20 Year Report 2019; Hip and Knee Replacements in Canada, 2017–2018 2019; Grimberg et al. 2019; Dutch Arthroplasty Register (LROI) 2019). The mean length of stay recorded in 2018 was 2.0 days (95% CI, 1.9–2.0). Approximately 60–65% of all patients undergoing TKA were female. This is consistent throughout the different age groups.

> Posterior stabilized (PS) designs were most commonly used (51.6%) as compared to cruciate-retaining (CR) designs (43.8%) (Fig. 38.2).

The use of these different designs varies throughout the world. Registries from The Netherlands (49.6%) (Dutch Arthroplasty Register (LROI) 2019) and Canada (62.5%) (Hip and Knee Replacements in Canada, 2017–2018 2019) report a more common use of PS designs, while countries like Norway (68.2%) (Norwegian National Advisory Unit on Arthroplasty and Hip Fractures: Annual Report 2019), UK (69.0%) (National Joint Registry 2019), and Sweden (90.8%) (Swedish Knee Arthroplasty Register 2019) report a more common use of CR designs. Although the AJRR reports an improved implant survival of the CR designs compared to the PS designs in those over 65 years of age

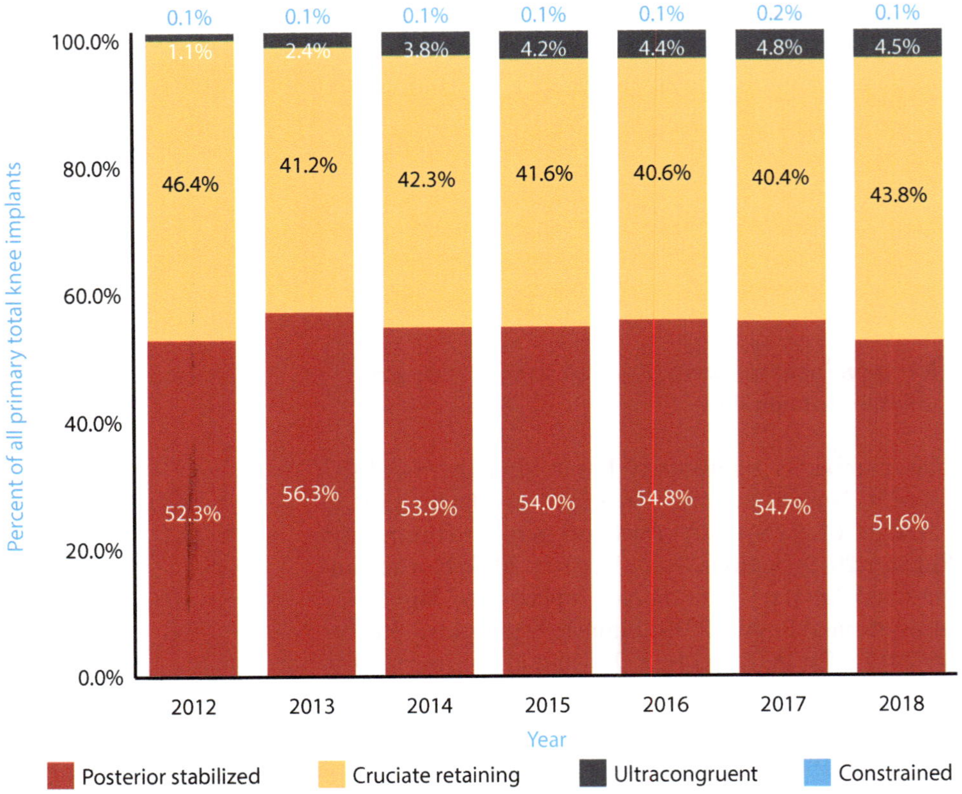

Fig. 38.2 Primary TKA implant design, 2012–2018 ($N = 591{,}773$). (Reprinted with permission from American Joint Replacement Registry [AJRR]: 2019 Annual Report. Rosemont, IL: American Academy of Orthopaedic Surgeons [AAOS], 2019 (American Joint Replacement Registry (AJRR) 2019))

(HR = 0.712, 95% CI, 0.658–0.770, $p < 0.0001$), the difference was small (<1%) and the analysis does not account for multiple confounders. To further put this finding in perspective, multiple systematic reviews and meta-analyses comparing the outcomes and complications of both designs have not shown any differences besides a possible increase of postoperative range of motion in the PS group (Bercik et al. 2013; Jiang et al. 2016; Li et al. 2014; Longo et al. 2018a; Migliorini et al. 2019).

38

The use of mobile-bearing primary TKA designs in the United States was reported in 7% of the cases which is more than those reported in Canada (1.9%) (Hip and Knee Replacements in Canada, 2017–2018 2019) and less than reported in Germany (15.9%) (Grimberg et al. 2019). Antioxidant polyethylene liners in the United States were used in 23.2% of cases while either conventional polyethylene (UHMWPE) and highly cross-linked polyethylene liners were used in the other cases.

> Patellar resurfacing is common practice in the United States in 90.8% of patients (Heckmann et al. 2019).

This is in contrast to other international registries such as Australia (66.6%) (Australian Orthopaedic Association National Joint Replacement Registry 2019), New Zealand (37.0%) (The New Zealand Joint Registry 20 Year Report 2019), The Netherlands (20.9%) (Dutch Arthroplasty Register (LROI) 2019), Germany (11.2%), Norway (9.5%) (Norwegian National Advisory Unit on Arthroplasty and Hip Fractures: Annual Report 2019), and Sweden (2.4%) (Swedish Knee Arthroplasty Register 2019) that report substantially lower rates. Multiple systematic reviews evaluating the potential benefit of patellar resurfacing have not resulted in unequivocal recommendations (Arirachakaran et al. 2015; Cheng et al. 2014; Grassi et al. 2018; Longo et al. 2018b) and could explain the disparities between countries.

> Comparable to other registries, in the large majority of TKAs (91.6%) in 2018 polymethylmetacrylate (PMMA) was used for fixation (Swedish Knee Arthroplasty Register 2019; National Joint Registry 2019; Finnish Arthroplasty Registry 2019; American Joint Replacement Registry (AJRR) 2019; The New Zealand Joint Registry 20 Year Report 2019; Grimberg et al. 2019; Dutch Arthroplasty Register (LROI) 2019).

The AJRR also contains data on the type of PMMA used (high viscosity vs. low viscosity). In 2012 both high-viscosity and low-viscosity cement was used equally at 46.0% and 47.9%, respectively.

> However, Kelly et al. reported that by 2017 high-viscosity cement gained in popularity and was used in 61.3% of TKAs (Kelly et al. 2018).

The difference between the two types of PMMA is that high-viscosity PMMA mixes faster and has a prolonged working phases as compared to the low-viscosity PMMA (Hazelwood et al. 2015). In animal and cadaveric models, it has been shown that high-viscosity cement results in inferior trabecular cement interdigitation, weaker cement–implant shear strengths and is, therefore, thought to be one of the factors involved in the occurrence of aseptic loosening (Rey Jr. et al. 1987; Reading et al. 2000). An increase in the use of high-viscosity PMMA in TKAs between 2012 (46.0%) and 2017 (61.3%) has been identified (Kelly et al. 2018). The AJRR can be an important tool in evaluating whether the use of different types of PMMA is indeed influential in the long-term survival of TKAs.

> Compared to 2017 the use of cementless fixation increased from 5.7% to 8.4%.

According to the data in the AJRR there was no difference identified in survivorship between cemented and cementless TKAs for those diagnosed with primary osteoarthritis and revision as an endpoint (HR = 0.92 [0.83–1.01], $p = 0.0917$).

38.3 Primary Unicompartmental Knee Arthroplasty (UKA) and Patellofemoral Arthroplasty (PFA)

> According to the AJRR, unicompartmental knee arthroplasties (UKA) accounted for only 2.2% of all primary knee arthroplasties 2018.

This is far less than those numbers reported in Norway (14.5%) (Norwegian National Advisory Unit on Arthroplasty and Hip Fractures: Annual Report 2019), Germany (12.6%) (Grimberg et al. 2019), The Netherlands (12.3%) (Dutch Arthroplasty Register (LROI) 2019), UK (9.1%) (National Joint Registry 2019), and Australia (7.8)% (Australian Orthopaedic Association National Joint Replacement Registry 2019).

The use of PFAs in 2018 was even more limited accounting to less than 0.1% of all arthroplasties performed which is consistent with those reported in the national registries of New Zealand, England and Wales, and Sweden (Swedish Knee Arthroplasty Register 2019; National Joint Registry 2019; The New Zealand Joint Registry 20 Year Report 2019).

Like the registry from England (National Joint Registry 2019), the AJRR demonstrated better survivorship for TKAs compared to UKAs constructs in patients >65 years of age between 2012 and 2018 (HR = 6.71 (5.58–8.07), $p < 0.001$).

38.4 Epidemiology Revision TKA from AJRR

> The AJRR has collected data on 58,409 revision TKAs up to 2018. In 2018, the revision burden for all TKA procedures documented in the AJRR was of 7.5% (Heckmann et al. 2019).

This proportion has been stable over the last 5 years. Other registries have reported stable and similar revision burdens between 6.9% and 10.3% (Norwegian National Advisory Unit on Arthroplasty and Hip Fractures: Annual Report 2019; Australian Orthopaedic Association National Joint Replacement Registry 2019; The New Zealand Joint Registry 20 Year Report 2019; Hip and Knee Replacements in Canada, 2017–2018 2019; Dutch Arthroplasty Register (LROI) 2019; McGrory et al. 2016).

To identify reasons for revision surgery ICD-9 or ICD-10 codes were used. The numbers reported may be difficult to adequately interpret because of categories such as "other" and "other mechanical complications". Mechanical loosening was reported to be the most common reason for all knee revision surgery at 25.0% (Fig. 38.3). When focusing on early revision, defined as revision <3 months after index surgery, the most common reason for revision was infection (63.2%). Loosening, infection, patellofemoral pain, and instability are consistently reported throughout the other national registries as the most common causes for revision (National Joint Registry 2019; Australian Orthopaedic Association National Joint Replacement Registry 2019; Grimberg et al. 2019; Dutch Arthroplasty Register (LROI) 2019). The infection burden for TKA reported in the AJRR between 2010 and 2015 varied from 0.80% to 1.08% (Springer et al. 2019).

The use of antioxidant liners in revision TKA has increased to 12.8%. The use of mobile-bearing designs in the revision setting has continued to hover around 18% for the past 6 years.

38.5 Future Directions

Large databases and national registries have the potential of being powerful instruments to not only improve the outcomes of joint replacement surgery, but also to be used as a health economic instrument. This is especially true if the registries include patient-reported outcomes and can be linked to reimbursement in health care and other insurance and societal costs (Malchau et al. 2018). However, when conducting research utilizing these instruments it is important to realize each type of database can vary in its methodology of data acquisition which could potentially influence results (Bedard et al. 2018).

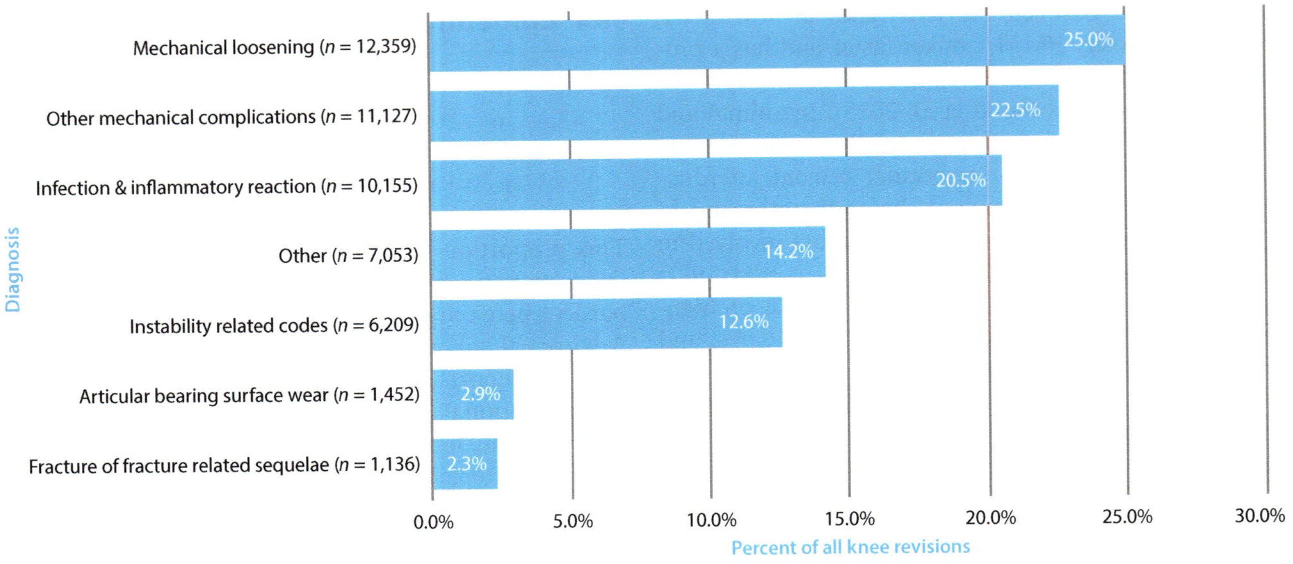

Fig. 38.3 Primary diagnosis for all knee revisions, 2012–2018 (N = 49,491). (Reprinted with permission from American Joint Replacement Registry [AJRR]: 2019 Annual Report. Rosemont, IL: American Academy of Orthopaedic Surgeons [AAOS], 2019 (American Joint Replacement Registry (AJRR) 2019))

> One of the prerequisites for being useful is a coverage and completeness of >80% of joint replacement procedures performed.

Since the AJRR is currently capturing only 32% of all procedures performed, it is important to improve upon this.

In an attempt to make the various national registries more uniform so results can be compared, the International Society of Arthroplasty Registries (ISAR) was established in 2004. In spite of this, it is notable that differences and disparities in the data reported, terminology used, and statistical analysis used remain. To utilize the trove of potential knowledge available from these registries, it is important to continue and support the effort of ISAR to make the data captured and reported more interchangeable.

38

Take-Home Messages

- It is imperative to increase the coverage/completeness of the AJRR from only 32% to >80% to make it more reliable and representative.
- Similar to countries like Canada and The Netherlands the use of posterior stabilized TKA designs is more common in the USA.
- Contrary to other national registries patellar resurfacing is almost standard practice in the USA.
- UKAs accounted for only 2.2% of all primary knee arthroplasties in 2018.
- The revision burden for all TKA procedures documented in the AJRR was of 7.5% and has been stable over the past 5 years.

References

American Joint Replacement Registry (AJRR) (2019) 2019 Annual report. American Academy of Orthopaedic Surgeons (AAOS), Rosemont. Available from: http://connect.ajrr.net/2019-ajrr-annual-report

Arirachakaran A, Sangkaew C, Kongtharvonskul J (2015) Patellofemoral resurfacing and patellar denervation in primary total knee arthroplasty. Knee Surg Sports Traumatol Arthrosc 23(6):1770–1781. Epub 2014/09/15

Australian Orthopaedic Association National Joint Replacement Registry (2019) Hip, knee & shoulder annual report 2018. [cited 2020 04/24/2020]. Available from: https://aoanjrr.sahmri.com/annual-reports-2018

Bedard NA, Pugely AJ, McHugh M, Lux N, Otero JE, Bozic KJ et al (2018) Analysis of outcomes after TKA: do all databases produce similar findings? Clin Orthop Relat Res 476(1):52–63. Epub 2018/03/13

Bercik MJ, Joshi A, Parvizi J (2013) Posterior cruciate-retaining versus posterior-stabilized total knee arthroplasty: a meta-analysis. J Arthroplasty 28(3):439–444. Epub 2013/02/26

Cheng T, Zhu C, Guo Y, Shi S, Chen D, Zhang X (2014) Patellar denervation with electrocautery in total knee arthroplasty without patellar resurfacing: a meta-analysis. Knee Surg Sports Traumatol Arthrosc 22(11):2648–2654. Epub 2013/06/08

Delaunay C (2015) Registries in orthopaedics. Orthop Traumatol Surg Res 101(1 Suppl):S69–S75. Epub 2015/01/03

Dutch Arthroplasty Register (LROI) (2019) Online LROI annual report 2019

Etkin CD, Springer BD (2017) The American Joint Replacement Registry-the first 5 years. Arthroplast Today 3(2):67–69. Epub 2017/07/12

Finnish Arthroplasty Registry (2019). Available from: https://www.thl.fi/far/#index

Grassi A, Compagnoni R, Ferrua P, Zaffagnini S, Berruto M, Samuelsson K et al (2018) Patellar resurfacing versus patellar retention in primary total knee arthroplasty: a systematic review of overlapping meta-analyses. Knee Surg Sports Traumatol Arthrosc 26(11):3206–3218. Epub 2018/01/18

Grimberg A JV, Melsheimer O, Steinbrück A (2019) Endoprothesenregister Deutschland (EPRD). Mit Sicherheit mehr Qualität
Hazelwood KJ, O'Rourke M, Stamos VP, McMillan RD, Beigler D, Robb WJ 3rd. (2015) Case series report: early cement-implant interface fixation failure in total knee replacement. Knee 22(5):424–428. Epub 2015/03/22
Heckmann N, Ihn H, Stefl M, Etkin CD, Springer BD, Berry DJ et al (2019) Early results from the American Joint Replacement Registry: a comparison with other national registries. J Arthroplasty 34(7S):S125–S34 e1. Epub 2019/02/04
Hip and Knee Replacements in Canada, 2017–2018 (2019) Canadian Joint Replacement Registry Annual Report
Jiang C, Liu Z, Wang Y, Bian Y, Feng B, Weng X (2016) Posterior cruciate ligament retention versus posterior stabilization for total knee arthroplasty: a meta-analysis. PLoS One 11(1):e0147865. Epub 2016/01/30
Kelly MP, Illgen RL, Chen AF, Nam D (2018) Trends in the use of high-viscosity cement in patients undergoing primary total knee arthroplasty in the United States. J Arthroplasty 33(11):3460–3464. Epub 2018/07/31
Li N, Tan Y, Deng Y, Chen L (2014) Posterior cruciate-retaining versus posterior stabilized total knee arthroplasty: a meta-analysis of randomized controlled trials. Knee Surg Sports Traumatol Arthrosc 22(3):556–564. Epub 2012/11/03
Longo UG, Ciuffreda M, Mannering N, D'Andrea V, Locher J, Salvatore G et al (2018a) Outcomes of posterior-stabilized compared with cruciate-retaining total knee arthroplasty. J Knee Surg 31(4):321–340. Epub 2017/07/01
Longo UG, Ciuffreda M, Mannering N, D'Andrea V, Cimmino M, Denaro V (2018b) Patellar resurfacing in total knee arthroplasty: systematic review and meta-analysis. J Arthroplasty 33(2):620–632. Epub 2017/10/17
Malchau H, Garellick G, Berry D, Harris WH, Robertson O, Karrlholm J et al (2018) Arthroplasty implant registries over the past five decades: development, current, and future impact. J Orthop Res 36(9):2319–2330. Epub 2018/04/18
McGrory BJ, Etkin CD, Lewallen DG (2016) Comparing contemporary revision burden among hip and knee joint replacement registries. Arthroplast Today 2(2):83–86. Epub 2016/01/01
Migliorini F, Eschweiler J, Tingart M, Rath B (2019) Posterior-stabilized versus cruciate-retained implants for total knee arthroplasty: a meta-analysis of clinical trials. Eur J Orthop Surg Traumatol 29(4):937–946. Epub 2019/01/17
National Joint Registry (2019) 16th annual report National Joint Registry for England, Wales, Northern Ireland and the Isle of Man 2019; Available from: https://reports.njrcentre.org.uk/Portals/0/PDFdownloads/NJR%2016th%20Annual%20Report%202019.pdf
Norwegian National Advisory Unit on Arthroplasty and Hip Fractures: Annual Report 2019 (2019)
Reading AD, McCaskie AW, Barnes MR, Gregg PJ (2000) A comparison of 2 modern femoral cementing techniques: analysis by cement-bone interface pressure measurements, computerized image analysis, and static mechanical testing. J Arthroplasty 15(4):479–487. Epub 2000/07/07
Rey RM Jr, Paiement GD, McGann WM, Jasty M, Harrigan TP, Burke DW et al (1987) A study of intrusion characteristics of low viscosity cement Simplex-P and Palacos cements in a bovine cancellous bone model. Clin Orthop Relat Res 215:272–278. Epub 1987/02/01
Springer BD, Etkin CD, Shores PB, Gioe TJ, Lewallen DG, Bozic KJ (2019) Perioperative periprosthetic femur fractures are strongly correlated with fixation method: an analysis from the American Joint Replacement Registry. J Arthroplasty 34(7S):S352–S3S4. Epub 2019/03/11
Swedish Knee Arthroplasty Register (2019) Swedish Knee Arthroplasty Register 2018 Annual Report. 2019 [cited 2020 04/24/2020]; Available from: http://www.myknee.se/pdf/SVK_2018_Eng_1.0.pdf
The New Zealand Joint Registry 20 Year Report (2019). Available from: https://nzoa.org.nz/system/files/DH8328_NZJR_2019_Report_v4_7Nov19.pdf

US National Databases – Total Knee Arthroplasty: Lessons Learned

Christie Bergerson, Derek Holyoak, and Kevin Ong

Contents

E. Hansen, K.-D. Kühn (eds.), *Essentials of Cemented Knee Arthroplasty*,
https://doi.org/10.1007/978-3-662-63113-3_39

39.1 Introduction

Motivated by the goal of improving the longevity of implants as well as reducing the incidence of complications and the need for implant removal, national orthopedic registries were developed in Scandinavia in the 1970s to track revisions as a function of surgeon, patient, and implant characteristics (Malchau et al. 2002). Over the past few decades, orthopedic registries have expanded across Europe, Canada, Australia, and New Zealand. In the United States, it was not until early 2011 that a national orthopedic registry, the American Joint Replacement Registry (AJRR), was initiated with 15 pilot sites, and now has grown substantially to 1312 sites in 50 states as of early 2020 (American Joint Replacement Registry 2020).

However, the absence of a national-based registry in the United States before then led researchers to leverage other regional or national administrative claims data sets or large clinical registries to study the epidemiology, utilization, and outcomes following various orthopedic procedures. Even though the AJRR is gaining maturity, the administrative claims data sets and large clinical registries are still heavily relied upon to help evaluate less common risk factors, which may be more difficult to study in other data sets with smaller sample sizes.

Moreover, public accessibility to AJRR data is also limited. Thus, these claims data sets and large clinical registries still have their place in research (Pugely et al. 2015a, b), to help further drive the development of hypotheses that can then be further examined in clinical studies.

39.2 Available Databases

A multitude of national or regional administrative claims databases and clinical registries are available for studying trends in total knee arthroplasty (TKA), each with its own unique data structure, collection method, sampling scheme, and geographic scope within the United States. A few of these are briefly described below.

National Hospital Discharge Survey/National Hospital Care Survey The National Hospital Discharge Survey (NHDS) was an annual survey conducted by the National Center for Health Statistics (NCHS) from 1965 to 2010 (National Center for Health Statistics 2020). This has since evolved to the National Hospital Care Survey (NHCS). The NHCS is a relatively new survey that integrates inpatient data formerly collected by the NHDS with the emergency department (ED), outpatient department (OPD), and ambulatory surgery center (ASC) data collected by the National Hospital Ambulatory Medical Care Survey (NHAMCS). The integration of these two surveys along with the collection of personal identifiers (protected health information) allows the linking of care provided to the same patient in the ED, OPD, ASC, and inpatient departments. The 2013–2016 unweighted inpatient and ambulatory NHCS data sets are now accessible through the NCHS Research Data Center. Collected information includes patient demographics, disease diagnosis, type of procedure performed, institutional characteristics, and resource utilization.

National/Nationwide Inpatient Sample The National/Nationwide Inpatient Sample (NIS) is a larger and more recent database of inpatient discharge data compared to the NHDS. The NIS was established in 1988 by the Healthcare Cost and Utilization Project (HCUP) of the Agency of Healthcare Quality and Research. Compared to the NHDS, the NIS has 25 times more records with five to eight million records per year and also includes twice the number of hospitals. In 2012, the NIS was redesigned to capture a sample of discharges from all hospitals participating in HCUP, instead of all discharges in a 20% sample of hospitals. The NIS captures patient, payer, hospitalization factors, as well as information about the charges and cost for the hospitalization.

Medicare The Medicare data set is available from the Center for Medicare and Medicaid Services (CMS) in 5% or 100% formats. The 5% data set consists of 7 components: hospital inpatient, hospital outpatient, home health agency, skilled nursing facility, hospice care, physician carrier (Part B), and durable medical equipment. The 100% data set includes all Medicare beneficiaries but does not include data from the durable medical equipment or physician carrier components. A denominator file is also available to track the date of death and enrollment information for Medicare beneficiaries. Patients are uniquely identified by an encrypted Medicare beneficiary identification number that remains consistent across all parts of the database, as well as over time, which allows follow-up of the patient. In 2017, this included data for approximately 58 million enrollees, of whom 85% were over 65 years old, while the remaining enrollees who were under 65 were insured by Medicare due to their physical disabilities or end-stage renal disease (Medicare Interactive 2020).

State Inpatient Database The State Inpatient Database (SID) comprises state discharge databases that are consolidated into a uniform format for comparison and incorporation into the NIS. These databases operate under the HCUP umbrella, but participation may vary by state. State inpatient databases are available for >90% of the states from HCUP. Although the data collection is similar to the NIS, some states collect additional information.

PearlDiver PearlDiver is a health data analytics company with one of the largest healthcare databases, incorporating over one billion US records. The data set includes private insurance claims (Humana and United Healthcare), government claims (Medicare), and other databases in a simplified, de-identified format. The PearlDiver database contains information pertaining to procedure volumes, patient demographics, charges, and reimbursements.

ACS NSQIP The American College of Surgeons (ACS) National Surgical Quality Improvement Program (NSQIP) is a surgical quality improvement program that prospectively collects 30-day morbidity and mortality data. The NSQIP originated from a 1990s Veterans Affairs (VA) System pilot program to collect risk-adjusted outcomes. The NSQIP received funding from the Agency for Healthcare Research and Quality in 1998, and then was adopted by the ACS at the end of 2004. Since the creation of the ACS NSQIP in 2005, more than 500 institutions have participated in the program. Each site has a surgical clinical reviewer who is independently trained and audited. A systematic (8-day) sampling process is used to collect a subset of cases. The NSQIP collects data on more than 250 patient, operative, and outcomes variables. In terms of postoperative data, NSQIP reports on 30-day, predefined complications that contribute to morbidity and mortality.

ABOS The American Board of Orthopaedic Surgery (ABOS) was established in 1934 to standardize orthopedic surgical competency through the board certification process. The ABOS maintains a database of cases from board-eligible candidates (Part II certification), generally within 22 months after residency completion. The case information is self-reported by each candidate and is entered into an Internet-based system. The candidates must submit the information for all of their cases during the time period of interest. The database contains cases reported by candidates during their Part-II 6-month board collection period. Information pertaining to patient demographics, comorbidities, procedures performed, length of follow-up, and complications has been captured electronically since 1999. Complications are separated into medical (stroke, myocardial infarction, etc.) and surgical procedure-related (hemorrhage, implant failure, etc.) groups.

Strengths and Weaknesses

These data have given researchers powerful tools to evaluate a wide variety of clinical questions, such as those related to orthopedic disease and its treatment, volume, resource utilization, costs, and complications.

> Despite an impressive sample size, large-scale databases have notable limitations. Understanding the nuances of these data is critical for surgeons, patients, hospitals, and policy makers.

Many of these differences relate to trends over time, geographic variation, patient comorbidities, inpatient complications, short-term complications, long-term complications, financial analysis, and accessibility. For example, although Medicare claims comprise one of the most robust data sets used to perform orthopedic research, the data are limited primarily to those 65 years and older. On the other hand, private claims data often comprise more heterogeneous patient demographic samples, while still allowing longitudinal analysis similar to that offered by Medicare claims, but employers and beneficiaries may switch insurance carriers, thus potentially limiting accessibility to continuous coverage data.

Many of these data sets are expensive to purchase, as well as complicated and labor-intensive to use. Furthermore, some data sets provide only limited follow-up. The NIS is not as well suited for investigating postoperative adverse outcomes because it only includes inpatient events and the NSQIP is limited due to its short 30-day follow-up.

Some disadvantages of the administrative claims data sets include lack of precision of ICD-9 (International Classification of Diseases, Ninth Revision) coding schemes. Although clinical registries typically have a more robust list of variables, with relatively precise prospective data input, management infrastructure, and reporting systems, they tend to have a smaller number of patients, inconsistent follow-up duration, and their findings may not be generalizable to the rest of the patient population. The ABOS has limitations in terms of its narrow source of input data from a select, novice group of surgeons as well as the fact that the self-reported complication follow-up is limited and variable, ranging from a few weeks to 6 months. The ABOS database also does not contain non-operative cases or clinical information such as certain patient demographics, medications, and comorbidity severity.

> It is important to understand the source of the data and whether an appropriate data set is being used for drawing the types of conclusions investigated by a study.

An understanding of the fundamentals is necessary when interpreting conclusions or considering the use of data sets for further research.

39.3 Unicompartmental Knee Arthroplasty (UKA)

39.3.1 Prevalence

The prevalence of UKA in both the elderly (>65 years) and younger (<65 years) populations has been studied using the 2002 to 2011 5% sample of the Medicare Part B data set, as well as the 2004 to June 2012 MarketScan Commercial and Medicare Supplemental Databases, respectively (Hansen et al. 2018). The rates of UKA increased until 2008, after which they declined. However, the data showed that males age 55 to 74 were the only group whose UKA rates appeared to be trending upwards consistently. The highest proportion of UKA procedures was observed in the South and Midwest United States. Over 95% of the recipients were white, with only 5.1% of recipients having lower socioeconomic status.

39.3.2 Outcomes and Risk Factors

UKA outcomes have also been widely examined for various patient subgroups and risk factors using various national and regional data sets. Sundaram 2019 examined the influence of BMI on 30-day postoperative complications after UKA for 8209 patients in the NSQIP data set (Sundaram et al. 2019). They found that overweight and obese individuals who undergo UKA may not have an increased risk of 30-day postoperative complications compared to normal-weight individuals. Morbidly obese patients had a greater risk of superficial skin infection after UKA. Bovonratwet 2017 compared the outcomes between 568 outpatient and 5312 inpatient UKA in the NSQIP database (Bovonratwet et al. 2017). No significant differences were found in any perioperative complications or any post-discharge complications, including 30-day re-admissions, between the outpatient and inpatient cohorts. UKA outpatient procedures were also found to be biased toward lower American Society of Anesthesiologists (ASA) classes.

39

> The authors suggested that outpatient UKA is equivalent regarding complication risks, thus more patients can likely be considered safe for an outpatient UKA if appropriate clinical support is in place during the immediate postoperative period.

39.3.3 Surgical Technique

Robotic-assisted UKA (RAUKA) is a field of growing interest, because of its radiographic and patient-specific advantages. Vakharia et al. compared the primary and revision utilization rates, revision surgery risk factors, and survivorship between RAUKA and manual UKA techniques (Vakharia et al. 2019). A total of 13,617 RAUKA and 21,444 UKA patients between 2005 and 2014 were identified in the Medicare database. Compared with manual UKA techniques, RAUKA had a significantly lower revision incidence (0.99% vs. 4.24%). In addition, survivorship 3 years after index procedures was over 99% for RAUKA patients and 97.5% for manual UKA patients.

39.3.4 UKA vs. TKA

National databases have also been used to compare outcomes for UKA patients and TKA patients. For example, after matching 32,379 UKA patients with 250,377 TKA patients from the IBM MarketScan Commercial Database, the IBM MarketScan Medicare Supplemental Database, the Optum Clinformatics Datamart, and a United Kingdom-based primary care electronic medical record database (THIN), the following was shown:

> UKA was found to be associated with a higher risk for long-term revision, but lower risks for persistent pain and acute venous thromboembolism after surgery (Prieto-Alhambra et al. 2019).

The authors speculated that the higher revision rate came from the surgeons being more willing to revise the UKAs. Opioid use was also found to be reduced by up to 30% in UKA patients in the 3 to 12 months following surgery.

Courtney et al. studied whether Medicare should remove TKA from its inpatient-only list, similar to the policy that exists for UKA. To answer this, they compared the surgical outcomes of patients aged 65 years or older who underwent TKA vs. UKA. Using the ACS-NSQIP database, they investigated factors such as comorbidities, 30-day complications, and length of stay (LOS). Based on a total of 49,136 TKA and 1351 UKA patients, TKA patients had longer LOS (2.97 vs. 1.57 days) and a higher complication rate (9% vs. 3%) than UKA patients.

> The authors concluded that caution should be used when applying UKA data to TKA patients and that a clear difference in risk exists between the two procedures in the Medicare population.

Hansen et al. sought to compare the risk of complications, risk of revisions, hospital re-admission, and mortality of TKA and UKA patients. The study population consisted of patients from the 2002–2011 5% sample of Medicare data and the 2004–2012 MarketScan Commercial and Medicare Supplemental Databases to further compare the procedures in patients younger vs. older

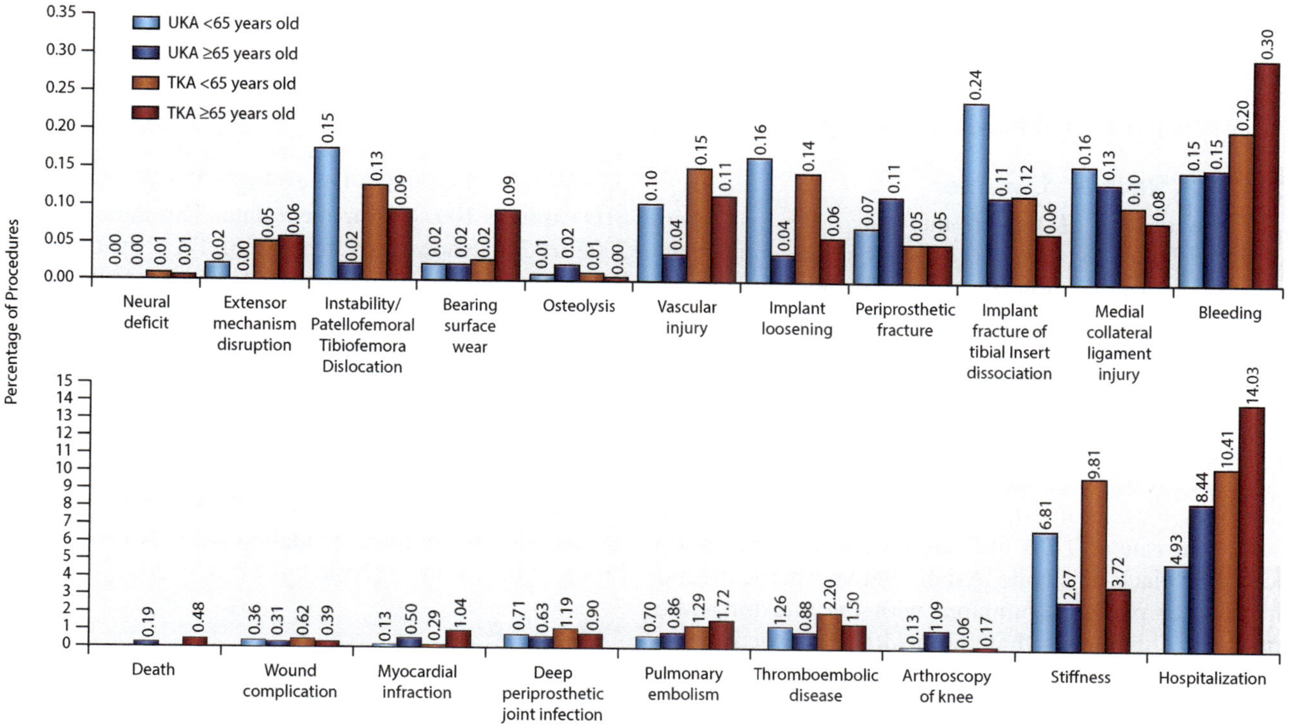

Fig. 39.1 Outcomes following UKA and TKA within 90 days of follow-up for patients younger and older than 65 years of age. (Adapted from Hansen et al. (2018); courtesy of the U.S. National Library of Medicine)

than 65 years of age. A total of 25,135 UKA and 362,589 TKA matched patients were analyzed in the study. UKA patients had significantly lower rates of wound complications, pulmonary embolism, periprosthetic joint infection, re-admission, and death, compared to TKA patients (Fig. 39.1). However, UKA had lower survivorship compared to TKA, regardless of age. Specifically, at the 7-year postoperative time point, survivorship for the younger population was 74.4% for UKA and 91.9% for TKA, and survivorship for the elderly population was 80.9% for UKA and 95.7% for TKA.

The study determined that although UKA has fewer complications and hospital re-admissions compared to TKA, the survivorship of UKA was lower than TKA within 10 years follow-up.

39.4 Primary and Revision Total Knee Arthroplasty

39.4.1 General Outcomes

TKAs are a popular surgical option for patients in the United States, and their utilization has been increasing. Survey of the NIS and Census Bureau data sets between 1993 and 2012 showed a total of 7.8 million primary TKAs were performed in the United States and the number of surgeries increased by 224% over that time (Kurtz et al. 2016). This annual TKA volume increase was more pronounced after the year 2000. Prior to 2000, the average increase was 10,520 procedures per year. This accelerated to an average increase of 32,730 procedures/year after 2000, nearly tripling the rate of increase. As evidence of the increasing trend in popularity, TKAs in Massachusetts from the SID data set experienced a similar 80% increase from 10.8 procedures/10,000 in 2002 to 19.4 procedures/10,000 in 2011. The trends in Massachusetts were similar to the trends seen across the nation as a whole for that time period, which experienced a 69% increase. National utilization was 12.2 procedures per 10,000 in 2002 and rose to 20.65 in 2011, as seen from the NIS data set. This is an interesting contrast with the Medicare population examined over a similar time period. Analysis of the Medicare database within the PearlDiver 2005 to 2011 data set showed a modest increase in annual utilization from a minimum of 287,006 in 2006 to a maximum of 301,956 in 2010 (Nwachukwu et al. 2015).

Databases allow for objective measures of utilization of services across racial, gender, and regional lines and show that there are geographic, racial, gender, and patient-age-dependent variations in the utilization, complication rates, and reimbursement for TKAs. Differences exist between the region with the most procedures performed and the region with the highest annual increase. The utilization of TKAs was found to be less from many minority groups as compared to white patients. The complication types and rates are different between males and females following TKA, and reimbursements and outcomes vary significantly by age. More detail on each of these variables is provided below.

39.4.1.1 Race and Gender

The use of the SID from multiple states has been explored by Zhang et al. to examine racial and ethnic disparities in utilization of primary TKA (Zhang et al. 2016). The SID data from Arizona, Colorado, Iowa, North Carolina, New Jersey, Rhode Island, Wisconsin, and Florida demonstrated an increase in TKA utilization over 2002 to 2008 for all racial groups. However, lower rates of TKA utilization were observed for minorities. After adjusting for co-variables such as differing patient demographics, health conditions, and socioeconomic status, the rate of TKA utilization was still significantly lower for black, Hispanic, Asian, Native American, and mixed-race patients compared with the rate for white patients. This means that the healthcare system characteristics explained only some of the racial disparities in utilization of and outcomes after TKA. Using NIS data, Gwam and coworkers found significant racial differences in age of presentation, health, and income status of TKA patients (Gwam et al. 2019a).

> The authors found that black patients underwent TKA at a younger age, lower median household income, and decreased age-adjusted Charlson comorbidity index.

Racial and ethnicity effects on primary TKA outcomes have also been studied. Zhang used 8 years of SID data from 8 racially diverse states, studying Arizona, Colorado, Iowa, North Carolina, New Jersey, Rhode Island, Wisconsin, and Florida from 2001 to 2008 (Zhang et al. 2016).

39

> Racial disparities were found with respect to mortality and complications after adjusting for patient-related and healthcare system characteristics.

The risk of perioperative mortality was significantly higher for black, Native American, and mixed-race patients than for white patients. In addition, the rates of in-hospital complications were significantly higher for black and mixed-race patients than for white patients in these specific states. On the other hand, using ACS-NSQIP data for 62,075 primary elective TKAs, Cram found similar 30-day complication rates after TKA for white and black patients (Cram et al. 2018).

Regarding gender, Cram et al. examined the same ACS-NSQIP database for 62,075 primary, elective TKAs and found that while women had markedly higher complication rates than men, the differences were driven almost entirely by higher rates of blood transfusion in women.

> Gender should further be explored in future publications.

39.4.1.2 Region

State-based data have also been used to assess utilization for individual states. For example, the Massachusetts SID captures 100% of inpatient data. This data set from 2002 to 2011 showed an increase in TKA incidence by 80% from 10.8 procedures per 10,000 population in 2002 to 19.4 in 2011 (Kurtz et al. 2016). Gwam et al. (2019a) identified the Midwest region with the fastest growth per capita, as compared to the Northeast, South, and West regions (Gwam et al. 2019a). Regarding regions with largest current patient populations, the Medicare database within the PearlDiver data set indicated that the highest volumes of TKA procedures are in the South but the average reimbursement rates are highest in the Northeast and lowest in the Midwest (Nwachukwu et al. 2015).

39.4.1.3 Age

Nwachukwu et al. examined 2,040,667 TKAs in the 2005 to 2011 Medicare database of PearlDiver and showed that TKAs were performed most frequently on patient ages 65–69, which was also the age group with the lowest reimbursement cost per procedure ($10,956) (Nwachukwu et al. 2015). TKAs were performed least frequently in patients 84+ years old and surgeries in this group had the highest amount reimbursed per procedure ($11,838).

In-hospital complication rates in octogenarians and nonagenarians undergoing revision TKA have been examined using NIS data (Smith et al. 2019). Based on 30,471 revision TKAs between 2010 and 2014, nonagenarians were found to have significantly longer lengths of stay (5.88 vs. 4.88 days) and higher total charges ($98,828 vs. $86,203) than octogenarians. Nonagenarians also had a significantly higher inpatient mortality rate (2.73% vs. 0.81%) than octogenarians. They tended to develop pneumonia or pneumonitis (1.28% vs. 0.44%), urinary tract infection (14.06% vs. 7.20%), acute kidney injury (15.28% vs. 8.73%), and cardiogenic shock (0.26% vs. 0.02%) at a significantly higher rate than octogenarians. Orthopedic surgeons can expect increased rates of some complications in nonagenarians undergoing revision TKA.

> As such, orthopedic surgeons need to be alert to inpatient postoperative management of nonagenarians to help mitigate some of the increased risk of select postoperative complications, and to thereby help to reduce length of stay and total charges.

39.4.2 Comorbidities

39.4.2.1 Smoking and Malnutrition

The ACS-NSQIP database was used to identify patients who underwent revision TKA between 2006 and 2014 (Bedard et al. 2018). Of the 8776 revision TKA patients,

11.6% were current smokers. Multivariate analysis identified current smokers as being at a significantly increased risk of any wound complication and deep infection after revision TKA. There was also a strong, albeit insignificant ($p = 0.051$) trend toward re-operation in smokers compared to non-smokers.

Malnutrition as measured by low serum albumin has been shown to increase the rate of perioperative complications in primary total joint arthroplasties including TKAs. An ACS-NSQIP study by Kamath et al. further showed that patients with low serum albumin (<3.5 mg/dL) were more likely to develop deep surgical site infection, organ space surgical site infection, pneumonia, urinary tract infection, and sepsis (Kamath et al. 2017).

Modifiable risk factors, such as smoking and malnutrition, can have an impact on postoperative complications.

> Therefore, greater attention needs to be placed on better understanding of whether smoking cessation programs could help reduce these postoperative complication risks, and whether hypoalbuminemia may be used to help identify higher risk patients.

39.4.2.2 Opioid Use Disorder and Associated Adverse Events

Opioid use disorder (OUD) is associated with adverse health events and increased odds of developing venous thromboembolism (VTE) (Vakharia et al. 2019). To determine whether opioids affect the outcome of primary TKA, Vakharia et al. evaluated patients with OUD after TKA for the presence of VTEs, re-admissions, and costs of care (Vakharia et al. 2019). The study compared 10,929 patients with OUD vs. 43,551 patients without OUD who underwent TKA between 2005 and 2014 using the Medicare Standard Analytical Files from the PearlDiver database.

> Compared to patients without OUD, patients with OUD had higher incidence of VTE in the 90 days following primary TKA surgery (2.48% vs. 1.10%). In addition, re-admission rates and costs of care were both higher in patients with OUD (◘ Fig. 39.2).

Jones et al. sought to characterize the impact of the opioid-based analgesia after TKA. Specifically, they focused on the incidence and clinical/economic impact of opioid-related adverse drug events (ORADEs) (Jones

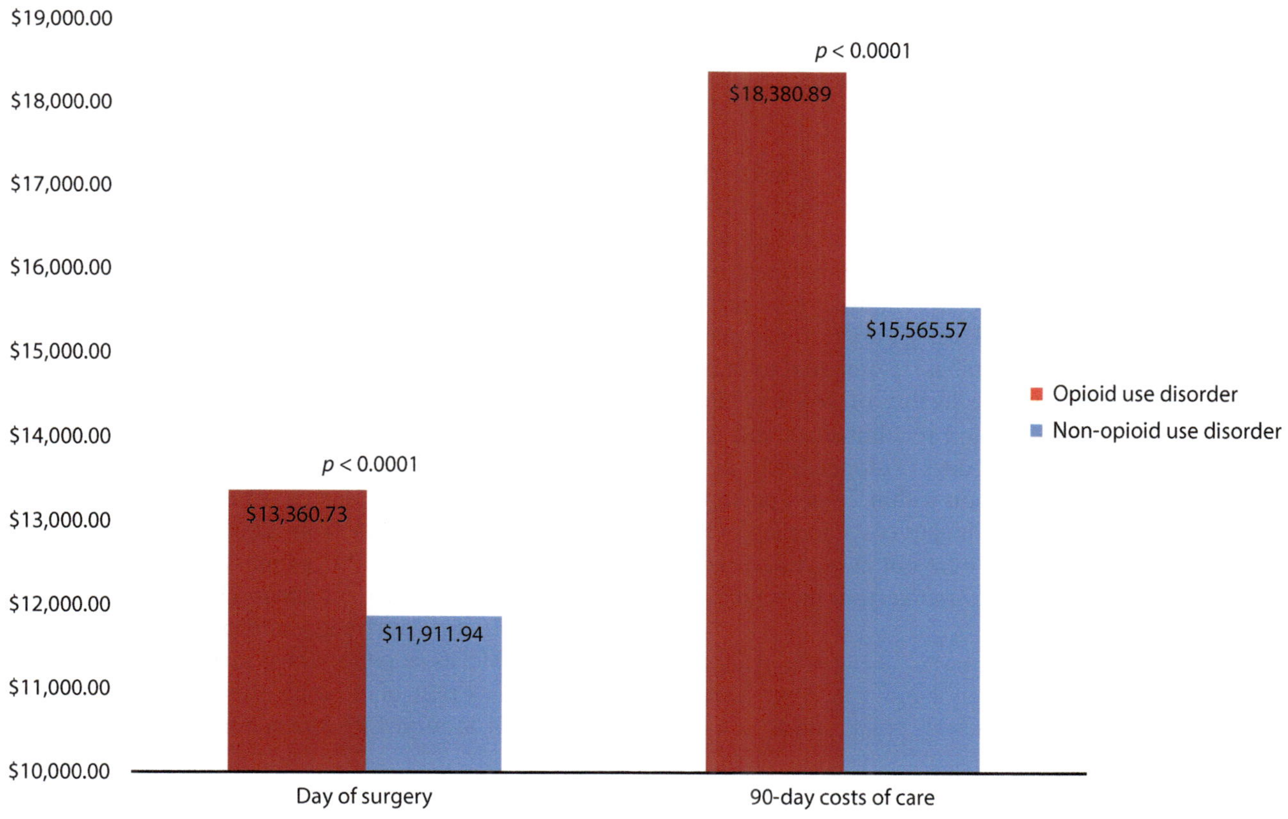

◘ **Fig. 39.2** Day of surgery and total global 90-day episode of care costs among opioid use disorder and non-opioid use disorder patients following primary TKA. (Adapted from Vakharia et al. 2019, with permission from Elsevier) (Vakharia et al. 2019)

et al. 2019). The study population consisted of 316,858 patients who underwent TKA between 2016 and 2017 from the Medicare Limited Data Set, which represents approximately 35% of all inpatient hospital discharges in the United States. Potential ORADE occurrence was determined using a series of ICD-10 codes that included codes for events including drug-induced constipation, altered mental status, different types of acute respiratory failure, and others. The incidence of potential ORADE in these patients was determined to be 8%. Patients who experienced at least one ORADE had longer hospital stays compared to patients without an ORADE (3.42 vs. 2.38 days). In addition, ORADEs resulted in lower daily hospital revenue per day in discharges ($4680 vs. $6014). Lastly, ORADEs were associated with increased risk of clinical conditions such as pneumonia, shock, septicemia, gastrointestinal hemorrhage, and acute myocardial infarction.

Gonzales et al. also evaluated the risk, incidence, and expense associated with potential opioid-related adverse events after primary and revision TKA (Gonzales et al. 2018). Using the Medicare 5% Limited Data Set, 41,702 TKA patients and 3817 revision TKA patients were analyzed. At 90 days after surgery, respiratory complications, postoperative nausea and vomiting, and urinary retention were the most common ORADEs after primary and revision TKA. Suffering an ORADE increased medical costs by 39% for primary TKA patients and 26% for revision TKA patients.

39.4.2.3 Disease

Quinlan et al. evaluated whether multiple sclerosis (MS) was a potential risk factor for complications following TKA (Quinlan et al. 2019). The study included 6437 patients with a history of MS and 64,370 patients from a matched control cohort, all of whom underwent primary TKA between 2005 and 2014, using the PearlDiver patient records from a Medicare database. Compared to patients without MS, patients with a history of MS had significantly higher rates of hospital re-admissions and emergency room visits within 30 days postoperatively, as well as periprosthetic joint infection within 2 years postoperatively and longer stays with higher costs accrued overall. However, patients with MS were not at increased risk of postoperative stiffness, revision surgery, or mortality.

> This research indicates that MS patients who require TKA should be provided appropriate counseling regarding the increased risks of complications.

Vakharia et al. sought to determine the influence of schizophrenia on primary TKA outcomes (Vakharia et al. 2019). Specifically, they investigated the hospital length of stay, re-admission rates, complications, and costs of care. The study evaluated 8196 patients with schizophrenia and 40,980 matched patients without schizophrenia within the Medicare claims database. Schizophrenia resulted in significantly longer hospital stays (3.73. vs. 3.22 days) and higher re-admission rates (18.3% vs. 12.1%). In addition, medical and implant-related complications were both higher in patients with schizophrenia compared to controls. Generally, schizophrenia patients had higher costs of total care.

> Ultimately, schizophrenia may be a risk factor following TKA and patients should be informed of the elevated levels of risks if suffering from schizophrenia.

39.4.2.4 Immunosuppression

Curtis evaluated perioperative and 30-day outcomes in 3466 chronically immunosuppressed patients who undergo primary TKA for osteoarthritis from 2008-2014 ACS-NSQIP data, with 108,158 patients in a control group (Curtis et al. 2018). The chronically immunosuppressed group patients were more likely to be younger and female with a lower BMI. Immunosuppressed patients were defined as those with the need for oral/IV corticosteroids or immunosuppressant drugs, such as Prednisone, Decadron, or Cyclosporine. Immunosuppressed patients were at higher risks of developing organ/surgical site infection, wound dehiscence, deep venous thrombosis (DVT), pneumonia, urinary tract infection, systemic sepsis, and re-admission.

> Immunosuppression is a risk factor for surgery and surgeons should be aware of the complications involved with operating on an immunosuppressed patient.

39.4.2.5 Obesity

Discharge records from the NIS data set showed that the proportion of morbid obesity increased almost 3 times in TKA patients from 2006 to 2014 (Wang et al. 2019). The effects of obesity on VTE has been examined using ACS-NSQIP data from 2008 to 2016 by Sloan et al. (2019). From 218,997 primary TKAs, they found the risk of pulmonary embolism (PE) being elevated, but not DVT, for overweight and obese primary TKA patients. BMI as a continuous variable, meaning the value exists as part of a range, was associated with an odds ratio of around 1.03 for each increase in kg/m^2.

> A suggested optimal cut point for BMI among patients undergoing primary TKA to maximize sensitivity and specificity of risk for PE was 33.0 kg/m^2.

Combined VTE (DVT or PE resulting in treatment) within 30 days of surgery was not associated with BMI as a continuous variable for patients undergoing primary TKA.

The NIS data set has been used to evaluate obesity trends in revision TKAs as well. Based on 451,982 revision TKA patients using 2002-2012 NIS data set, the obesity rate among revision TKA patients more than doubled during this 10-year period, increasing significantly from 9.74% in 2002 to 24.57% in 2012 (Odum et al. 2016). After adjusting for all factors, revision patients treated in 2011 or 2012 were over 4 times as likely to be obese, compared to revision patients treated in 2002. Female revision patients and revision patients between the ages of 45 and 64 years were independently associated with higher obesity rates. This means that no matter the year studied, female revision patients and revision patients between the ages of 45 and 64 were more likely to be obese than other revision TKA patients. The effects of obesity on the potential for experiencing a VTE have also been examined using ACS-NSQIP data from 2008 to 2016 by Sloan et al. (2019). They found no association between obesity and increased risk of PE, DVT, or combined VTE for 15,286 revision TKA patients.

In 2014, approximately 10% of morbidly obese TKA patients were also undergoing bariatric surgery as shown in the 2006-2014 discharge records from the NIS data set (Wang et al. 2019). This data set also showed that TKA patients with prior bariatric surgery had a lower risk of pulmonary embolism, respiratory complications, death, and shorter length of stay, but also had a higher risk of blood transfusion and anemia.

With the evident trend toward patients with higher BMIs, particularly in the revision TKA category, surgeons will benefit from this research into the optimal BMI cutoff point for primary TKA surgery and the increased risk of PE for obese primary TKA patients, as well as the potential benefits of bariatric surgery and general knowledge of the associated risk factors.

39.4.3 Surgical Technique

39.4.3.1 Computer Navigation

Computer navigation and robotic assistance surgeries have been introduced in total joint replacement to provide improved accuracy in component positioning. From the 2005–2014 NIS data set, 6,060,901 TKA surgeries were examined, including 273,922 (4.5%) who used computer navigation and 24,084 (0.4%) who used robotic assistance (Antonios et al. 2019). The proportion of robotic-assisted or computer navigation in TKAs steadily increased over the study period from 1.2% in 2005 to 7.0% in 2014. However, the use of these technologies was associated with increased hospital charges, averaging $53,740 per procedure compared to $47,639 for conventional TKA, but the elevated charges appeared to be driven by computer navigation rather than robotic assistance. Most technology-assisted TKAs were performed in urban hospitals, on Caucasian patients who were Medicare beneficiaries. Though the prevalence of advanced techniques in TKA surgeries is limited thus far, it is increasing steadily. More research into the revision rates with advanced surgeries versus traditional techniques would benefit this field.

39.4.3.2 Bilateral TKAs, Staged TKAs, Combined THA/TKA, and Inpatient vs. Outpatient Surgery

Rarer procedures such as combined THA and TKA have also been evaluated using national healthcare databases. Using the 2005–2014 NIS data set, Almaguer 2019 compared in-hospital outcomes of combined total joint arthroplasty (TJA), as defined as total hip arthroplasty (THA) and total knee arthroplasty (TKA) performed during the same admission, vs. bilateral THA, bilateral TKA, single THA, and single TKA (Almaguer et al. 2019). During that period, a total of 1690 (0.0002%) patients underwent combined TJA during the same hospital stay, while 32,763 (0.3%) underwent bilateral THA and 388,812 (3.6%) underwent bilateral TKA during the same hospital admission. Single THA was performed in 3,524,055 (32.7%) patients, while 6,835,843 (63.4%) underwent single TKA.

> Combined TJA was associated with increased risk of deep vein thrombosis, prosthetic joint infection, irrigation and debridement procedures, revision arthroplasty, extended length of stay (LOS), and increased in-hospital costs compared with bilateral THA, bilateral TKA, single THA, and single TKA.

A study of the Humana subset of the PearlDiver database showed that as compared with simultaneous bilateral TKA, staged TKAs occurring within 12 months of each other had higher odds of mechanical complications and infection but lower odds of transfusion and re-admission within 90 days for any reason (Richardson et al. 2019). Those patients with staged surgeries much less than 3 months apart had significantly higher odds of undergoing manipulation under anesthesia. The study included 7747 patients, with 1637 of those undergoing simultaneous bilateral TKA.

With regard to the concern surrounding the healthcare expenditures in the United States, studies into the national trends and complication rates for inpatient vs. outpatient TKAs have been performed. Outpatient surgeries were more likely to necessitate revision for non-infectious reasons, removal, irrigation and debride-

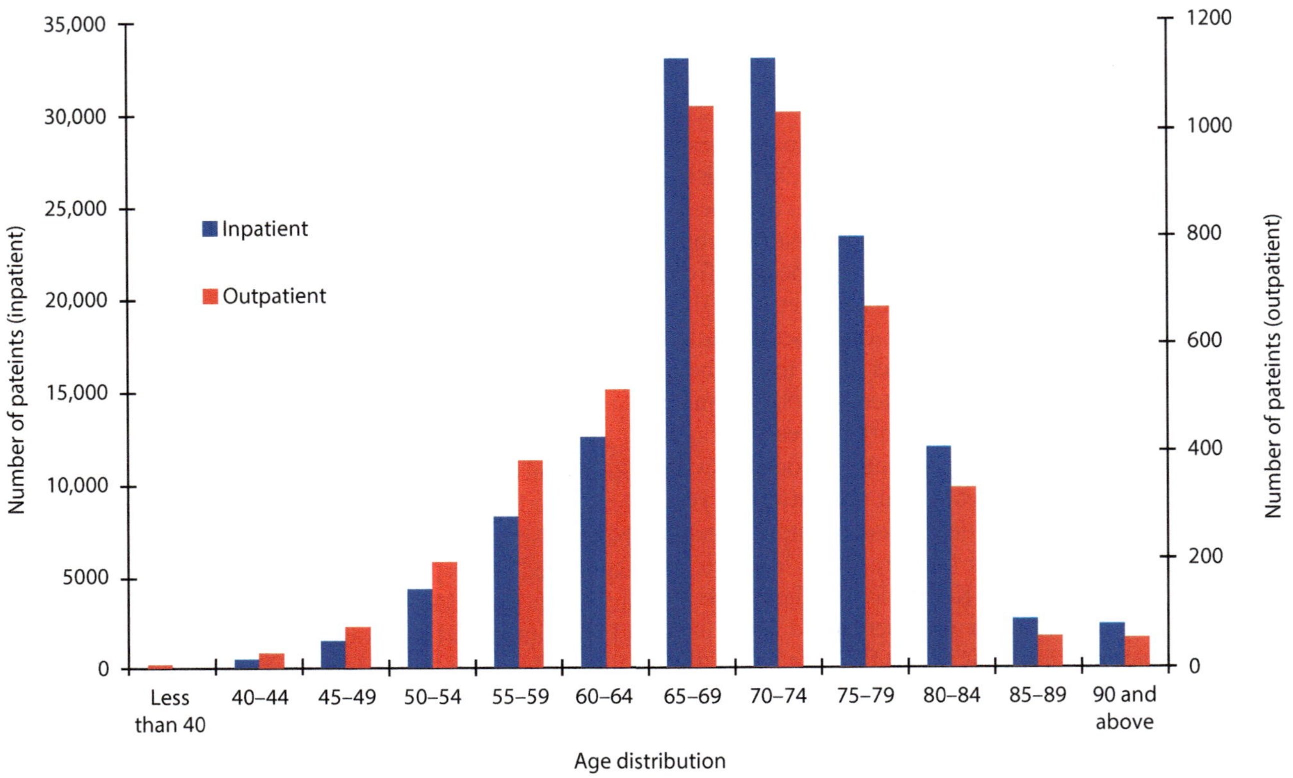

Fig. 39.3 Age distributions of patients undergoing TKA as either inpatient (*blue*) or outpatient (*red*) with Humana insurance. The age distributions were statistically comparable between the 2 groups, with median age in the 70- to 74-year age group. (From Arshi et al. 2017, by courtesy of Wolters Kluwer Health, Inc.) (Arshi et al. 2017)

ment, stiffness requiring manipulation under anesthesia, postoperative deep vein thrombosis, and acute renal failure than inpatient surgeries (Arshi et al. 2017). The Humana subset of the PearlDiver database from 2007 to 2015 was used and tracked patients for up to 1 year after surgery. A total of 4391 outpatient surgery recipients and 128,951 inpatient surgery recipients were included in the study (Fig. 39.3).

39

Combined TJA is associated with additional risks compared to any other operations involving combinations of knee or hip arthroplasties. In addition, the complication rates for outpatient TKAs are higher than inpatient procedures.

> Surgeons will benefit from this information when considering the appropriate operative approach, and patients considering TJA or outpatient procedures should be warned of the associated risks.

39.4.3.3 Cemented vs. Cementless

Selective use of cementless TKA has been demonstrated in several studies. Gwam 2019 studied the epidemiology of cemented and cementless TKA based on ICD-10 codes in the NIS data set from October 1 to December 31, 2015 (Gwam et al. 2019b). From 167,930 TKAs, only 2.9% (n = 4870) were identified as cementless TKA. Cemented TKA patients were found to be older, mostly women, residing outside of the Northeast, and being insured by Medicare.

> Cementless TKA procedures had significantly higher total inpatient mean costs ($16,010) compared to cemented TKA procedures ($15,394).

But they also had significantly higher odds of being discharged to home, with other options including inpatient rehabilitation, discharge to a skilled nursing facility, or under home health care.

No association was identified between type of fixation and acute renal failure, urinary tract infection, pulmonary embolism, superficial surgical site infection, postoperative pneumonia, or deep vein thrombosis, which encompasses all of the complications in scope for this study. The field would benefit from more data set-based research into the revision rates of cemented vs. cementless fixation.

39.4.4 Infection

Use of antibiotic-loaded bone cement in TKAs is common practice, despite the controversy surrounding it. The concern comes from the multiple adverse events associated with its use as compared to the potential reduction in infection risk.

> The data included from 1,184,270 surgeries in the Premier Healthcare claims database from 2006 to 2016 showed that antibiotic-loaded bone cement was used in 17.3% of TKA surgeries in 2006 and grew to 30.2% in 2010, when use plateaued (Chan et al. 2019).

Utilization was lower in rural hospitals (21.4% of surgeries), but higher in hospitals with over 500 beds (29.4%). Use of antibiotic-loaded bone cement was associated with a reduced incidence of early postoperative infections, but also with increased odds for acute kidney injury.

Slifka et al. investigated the effects of prosthetic joint infection (PJI) after TKA on mortality rates using claims data from the 2004 to 2012 Medicare 5% sample Standard Analytic Files (Slifka et al. 2018). A total of 80,429 TKAs were included in the study, and 1% were diagnosed with PJI. The crude mortality rate was 3.7 times greater in patients with PJI than without PJI following TKA. After accounting for comorbid conditions and additional dependent factors, the risk of death with PJI vs. non-PJI was still 2.6 times higher following TKA. The study results supported the importance of better understanding risk factors for PJI following TKA.

Cancienne et al. investigated the clinical outcomes of patients who experienced PJI following primary TKA, had their prostheses removed, and received an antibiotic spacer (Cancienne et al. 2018). A total of 18,533 patients were included in the study using Medicare data from PearlDiver. Complications within 1 year of antibiotic spacer placement included death in a hospital setting (3.7%), joint fusion (4.5%), amputation (3.1%), and repeat debridement procedures (14.5%). 12.5% of the patients retained their spacers without re-implantation, and 61.6% underwent spacer removal and re-implantation within 1 year. The study also found that multiple risk factors were associated with complications following antibiotic spacer placement, including, but not limited to, obesity, peripheral vascular disease, and tobacco/alcohol use/abuse.

> Ultimately, the study provided sobering data on the fate of patients who experience PJI and need antibiotic spacers, and further investigation is necessary to eradicate infection while minimizing morbidity and mortality of these patients.

39.4.5 Postoperative Care

Database information can also lend insight into the tendencies for postoperative care in different regions of the United States, different insurance types, and different fixation methods. Gwam et al. found that implantation with a cementless TKA was associated with higher probability of being discharged home vs. implantation with a cemented TKA (Gwam et al. 2019b). Soley-Bori et al. found that patients in the Northeast were 2.5 times more likely to be discharged to an extended care facility as compared with patients in the South who tended to be discharged home (Soley-Bori et al. 2017). Similarly, those enrolled in private insurance HMO/PPOs were more likely to use extended care facilities vs. those in non-capitated plans such as fee-for-service or exclusive provider organizations, though this did not hold true for the Northeast. The Truven Health Analytics MarketScan inpatient database from 2009 and 2010 was used for this study, and 110,643 patients met the inclusion criteria. Only 10% of these patients were discharged to an extended care facility, and large variation was observed across the states. The average patient age was 45 years, 51% were women, 30% had between two and four comorbidities, and 15% had diagnosed obesity. Those discharged to an extended care facility tended to be older, female, more obese, diagnosed with more comorbidities, and wealthier.

Furthermore, a study using the Truven Health MarketScan databases from 2009 to 2013 showed that primary and revision TKA patients were discharged to home under self-care at approximately the same rate (40.2% for primary, 40.6% for revision) (Nichols and Vose 2016). Home health organizations cared for 36.6% and 37.3% of primary and revision TKA patients, respectively, and 14.0% of primary TKA and 13.4% of revision TKA patients were discharged to skilled nursing facilities. Complications, transfusions, and a length of stay greater than 3 days were associated with greater odds of discharge to home with home health services support or to a skilled nursing facility as opposed to home under self-care. Discharge to a skilled nursing facility or home with home health services was then associated with a greater risk for re-admission. Re-admission occurred in 14.8% and 23.1% of primary and revision TKA patients, respectively, and 76.8% of primary patients stayed over 3 days for their index hospitalization as compared to 75.7% of revision patients. A total of 323,803 primary TKAs and 25,354 revision TKAs met the inclusion criteria and were followed for 90 days.

Home health care and physical therapy (PT) utilization following TKA procedures is increasing. Falvey et al. sought to determine a relationship between home health care PT utilization and functional recovery, as well as investigate any factors that may influence PT utilization after TKA (Falvey et al. 2018). A total of 5967 Medicare patients who received home health care services in 2012 were analyzed. After adjusting for factors such as age, sex, and baseline physical function, patients who received 6 PT visits or more reported significantly improved functional scores in activities of daily living compared to patients who received 5 or less PT visits. Living in a rural location, dyspnea, and depressive symptoms were all associated with lower PT utilization. These results suggest that more than 6 home health care PT visits promote functional recovery, and that certain patient populations should be monitored to ensure appropriate PT utilization.

> These data revealed that region within the nation and insurance type are more influential to the postoperative care plan of a patient compared to whether that patient is undergoing a primary or revision surgery.

> These studies also show the importance of routine PT postoperatively and provide information that can be used to screen for patients at risk for under-utilization.

39.4.6 Preventing Venous Thromboembolic Events

The ideal agents for prevention of venous thromboembolic events (VTEs) after TKA is a topic of debate. Bala et al. compared VTE incidence after TKA with the use of four agents: aspirin, enoxaparin, warfarin, or factor Xa inhibitors (Bala et al. 2017), and Runner et al. have compared the outcomes of less aggressive (i.e., aspirin) vs. more aggressive (e.g., enoxaparin and warfarin among others) prophylactic treatment strategies (Runner et al. 2019). Specifically, the occurrences of deep venous thrombosis (DVT) and pulmonary embolism (PE) were investigated by Bala by looking at a total of 18,288 patients from Medicare and Humana databases between 2007 and 2016, and a total of 22,072 cases of primary joint arthroplasty (combined TKA and THA) between 2014 and 2016 using the ABOS case list database were assessed by Runner. The use of less aggressive treatments was associated with a lower rate of DVT and PE events at 90 days post-surgery (Bala et al. 2017). Furthermore, less aggressive treatments had a lower likelihood of mild (0.2% vs. 0.9%) and moderate (0.4% vs. 1.2%) thrombotic events, as well as mild, moderate, and severe bleeding events. Less aggressive strategies also were less likely to lead to infection or death within 90 days post-surgery (Runner et al. 2019). Only 3% or less of patients using aspirin or Factor Xa inhibitors had DVT events within 90 days following TKA, while 3.5% of patients using enoxaparin and 4.8% of patients using warfarin had DVT events within 90 days. These differences were statistically significant. Similarly, PE events occurred in between 0.9% and 1.2% of patients using aspirin, Factor Xa inhibitors, or enoxaparin with 90 days, while PE occurred in 1.6% of patients using warfarin, which was again a statistically significant difference. Patients with aspirin demonstrated the lowest risk of bleeding, though the differences in occurrence between the therapies were not statistically significant.

The utilization of aspirin and factor Xa inhibitors after TKA grew 30% and 43% respectively from 2007 to 2015, while utilization of enoxaparin and warfarin remained relatively constant over the timespan (Bala et al. 2017). However, less aggressive strategies were used less frequently compared to more aggressive strategies in the study population (45.4% vs. 54.6%).

> Patients receiving less aggressive prophylactic treatment strategies were significantly more likely to have fewer or no complications with the TKA or THA compared to more aggressive strategies (95.5% vs. 93.0%).

Further research into this topic is being undertaken in the Comparative Effectiveness of Pulmonary Embolism Prevention after Hip and Knee Replacement (PEPPER) trial (Bala et al. 2017).

39.4.7 Future Trends in TKA

The use of large national-based databases provides an excellent resource for estimating the future use of TKA (Inacio et al. 2017). Projections based on logistic regression modeling of NIS data from 1993 to 2012 estimated TKA incidence to increase 69% by 2050 compared to 2012, from 429 procedures per 100,000 persons in 2012 to 725 in 2050, which corresponds with a 143% projected increase in total number of TKA procedures performed (Fig. 39.4). Taking a less conservative approach using Poisson modeling, the TKA incidence has been projected

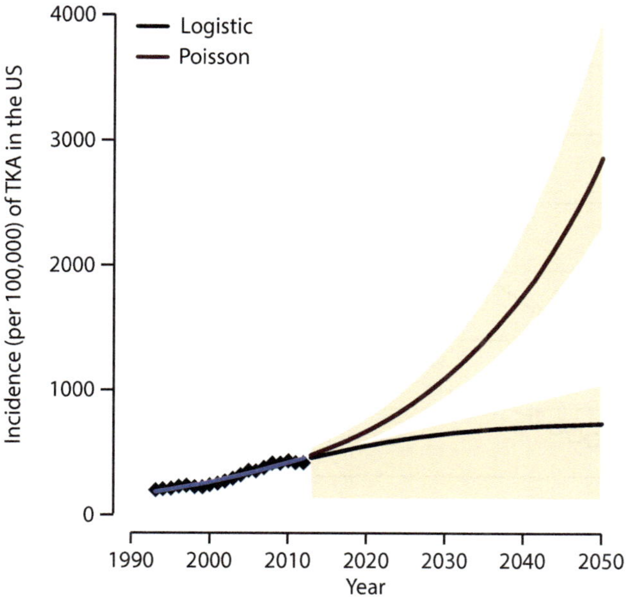

Fig. 39.4 Historical (1993–2012) and projected (2015–2050) incidence rates per 100,000 procedures of primary TKA procedures in citizens 40 years old and older from Logistic and Poisson models. (From Inacio 2017, with permission from Elsevier) (Inacio et al. 2017)

to increase 565% over the same time frame, to 2854 procedures/100,000 persons by 2050, representing an 855% projected increase in the total number of TKA procedures compared to 2012. Sloan et al. also offered an estimation using Poisson modeling, and predicted the increase by 2030 to be 147% (to 1.68 million), on the basis of the 2000 to 2014 NIS data (Fig. 39.5) (Sloan et al. 2018).

Others have also used different modeling methods, such as polynomial regression and linear projection, to account for the non-linearity and interactions between variables (Singh et al. 2019). Compared to 2014, the total annual primary TKA surgeries in the United States are projected to increase by 56% in 2020, 110% in 2025, 182% in 2030, and 401% in 2040. Sloan et al. sampled the NIS data set and used linear projection to predict that by 2030, TKA volume would increase by 84.9% (to 1.26 million) (Fig. 39.6) (Sloan et al. 2018).

> All models have indicated an increase in the annual volume of TKA procedures in the coming years. Further research is necessary to understand and predict TKA utilization, and database information provides the appropriate sample sizes and distributions from which to make these estimations.

Fig. 39.5 Data predicting the utilization from 2000 to 2030 based on the NIS data set with a Poisson Model (Sloan et al. 2018)

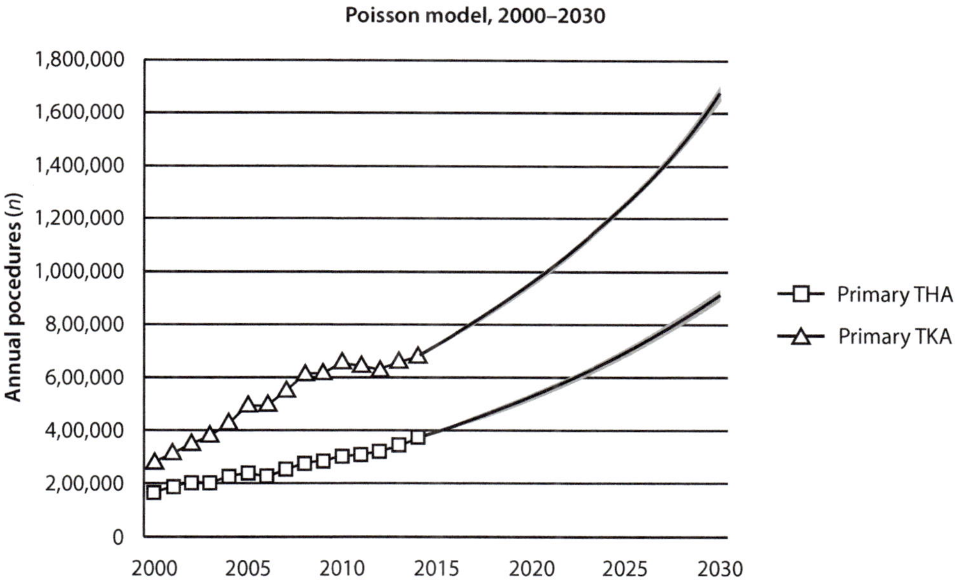

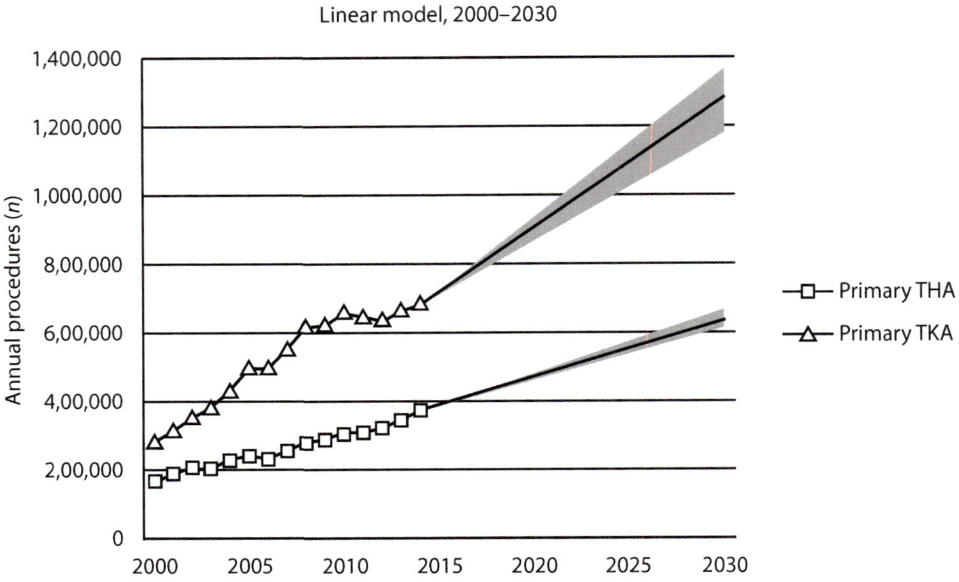

Fig. 39.6 Data predicting the utilization from 2000 to 2030 based on the NIS data set with a Linear Model (Sloan et al. 2018)

Conclusion

Administrative claims data and large-scale databases have taken on an influential role within the orthopedic surgery literature. The large sample sizes over many years and excellent capture of billable procedures or complications such as mortality remain the major advantages of their use.

Take-Home Messages

- Administrative claims data sets and large clinical registries offer powerful insight into how practices vary depending on region, insurance type and race, even after accounting for differences in the healthcare system. This type of objective insight is necessary to identify and address problems facing American surgeons and patients.
- To date, the study of cementless TKAs using administrative claims data sets and large clinical registries has been limited. However, current studies indicate that cementless TKAs were associated with increased costs with similar complication rates compared to cemented TKAs.
- Various diseases and comorbidities can have surprising correlations to complications after TKA, such as patients with opioid use disorder being more prone to experiencing VTE than a control population.
- More work in the areas of gender dynamics, influence of robotic surgeries on TKA revision rates, and the influence of cementless vs. cemented fixation on revision rates would benefit the field.
- And importantly, the lack of standardization between these databases often makes data difficult to compare. Care and attention are necessary when drawing conclusions from these immensely useful data sets.
- Cementless TKA procedures had significantly higher total inpatient mean costs ($16,010) compared to cemented TKA procedures ($15,394).
- From 1,184,270 surgeries in the Premier Healthcare claims from 2006 to 2016, antibiotic-loaded bone cement was used in 17.3% of TKA surgeries in 2006 and grew to 30.2% in 2010, but plateaued thereafter.

References

Almaguer AM, Cichos KH, McGwin G Jr, Pearson JM, Wilson B, Ghanem ES (2019) Combined total hip and knee arthroplasty during the same hospital admission: is it safe? Bone Joint J 101-B(5):573–581. https://doi.org/10.1302/0301-620X.101B5.BJJ-2018-1438

American Joint Replacement Registry. http://www.ajrr.net/. Accessed February 11, 2020

Antonios JK, Korber S, Sivasundaram L, Mayfield C, Kang HP, Oakes DA et al (2019) Trends in computer navigation and robotic assistance for total knee arthroplasty in the United States: an analysis of patient and hospital factors. Arthroplast Today 5(1):88–95. https://doi.org/10.1016/j.artd.2019.01.002

Arshi A, Leong NL, D'Oro A, Wang C, Buser Z, Wang JC et al (2017) Outpatient total knee arthroplasty is associated with higher risk of perioperative complications. JBJS 99(23):1978–1986. https://www.jbjs.org

Bala A, Huddleston JI 3rd, Goodman SB, Maloney WJ, Amanatullah DF (2017) Venous thromboembolism prophylaxis after TKA: aspirin, warfarin, enoxaparin, or factor Xa inhibitors? Clin Orthop Relat Res 475(9):2205–2213. https://doi.org/10.1007/s11999-017-5394-6

Bedard NA, Dowdle SB, Wilkinson BG, Duchman KR, Gao Y, Callaghan JJ (2018) What is the impact of smoking on revision total knee arthroplasty? J Arthroplasty 33(7S):S172–S1S6. https://doi.org/10.1016/j.arth.2018.03.024

Bovonratwet P, Ondeck NT, Tyagi V, Nelson SJ, Rubin LE, Grauer JN (2017) Outpatient and inpatient unicompartmental knee arthroplasty procedures have similar short-term complication profiles. J Arthroplasty 32(10):2935–2940. https://doi.org/10.1016/j.arth.2017.05.018

Cancienne JM, Granadillo VA, Patel KJ, Werner BC, Browne JA (2018) Risk factors for repeat debridement, spacer retention, amputation, arthrodesis, and mortality after removal of an infected total knee arthroplasty with spacer placement. J Arthroplasty 33(2):515–520. https://doi.org/10.1016/j.arth.2017.08.037

Chan JJ, Robinson J, Poeran J, Huang H-H, Moucha CS, Chen DD (2019) Antibiotic-loaded bone cement in primary total knee arthroplasty: utilization patterns and impact on complications using a national database. J Arthroplasty 34(7):S188–S94. e1

Cram P, Hawker G, Matelski J, Ravi B, Pugely A, Gandhi R et al (2018) Disparities in knee and hip arthroplasty outcomes: an observational analysis of the ACS-NSQIP clinical registry. J Racial Ethn Health Disparities 5(1):151–161. https://doi.org/10.1007/s40615-017-0352-2

Curtis GL, Chughtai M, Khlopas A, Newman JM, Sultan AA, Sodhi N et al (2018) Perioperative outcomes and short-term complications following total knee arthroplasty in chronically, immunosuppressed patients. Surg Technol Int 32:263–269

Falvey JR, Bade MJ, Forster JE, Burke RE, Jennings JM, Nuccio E et al (2018) Home-health-care physical therapy improves early functional recovery of medicare beneficiaries after total knee arthroplasty. J Bone Joint Surg Am 100(20):1728–1734. https://doi.org/10.2106/JBJS.17.01667

Gonzales J, Lovald ST, Lau EC, Ong KL (2018) Risk of opioid-related adverse events after primary and revision total knee arthroplasty. J Surg Orthop Adv 27(2):148–154

Gwam C, Rosas S, Sullivan R, Luo TD, Emory CL, Plate JF (2019a) The who, what, and where of primary TKAs: an analysis of HCUP data from 2009 to 2015. J Knee Surg. https://doi.org/10.1055/s-0039-1677857

Gwam CU, George NE, Etcheson JI, Rosas S, Plate JF, Delanois RE (2019b) Cementless versus cemented fixation in total knee arthroplasty: usage, costs, and complications during the inpatient period. J Knee Surg 32(11):1081–1087. https://doi.org/10.1055/s-0038-1675413

Hansen E, Ong K, Lau E, Kurtz S, Lonner J (2018) Unicondylar knee arthroplasty in the US patient population: prevalence and epidemiology. Am J Orthop (Belle Mead, NJ) 47(12). https://doi.org/10.12788/ajo.2018.0113

Inacio MCS, Paxton EW, Graves SE, Namba RS, Nemes S (2017) Projected increase in total knee arthroplasty in the United States – an alternative projection model. Osteoarthr Cartil 25(11):1797–1803. https://doi.org/10.1016/j.joca.2017.07.022

Jones MR, Kramer ME, Beutler SS, Kaye AD, Rao N, Brovman EY et al (2019) The association between potential opioid-related adverse drug events and outcomes in total knee arthroplasty: a retrospective study. Adv Ther. https://doi.org/10.1007/s12325-019-01122-1

Kamath AF, Nelson CL, Elkassabany N, Guo Z, Liu J (2017) Low albumin is a risk factor for complications after revision total knee arthroplasty. J Knee Surg 30(3):269–275. https://doi.org/10.1055/s-0036-1584575

Kurtz SM, Lau E, Ong KL, Katz JN, Bozic KJ (2016) Universal health insurance coverage in Massachusetts did not change the trajectory of arthroplasty use or costs. Clin Orthop Relat Res 474(5):1090–1098. https://doi.org/10.1007/s11999-015-4643-9

Malchau H, Herberts P, Eisler T, Garellick G, Soderman P (2002) The Swedish total hip replacement register. J Bone Joint Surg Am 84-A(Suppl 2):2–20. https://doi.org/10.2106/00004623-200200002-00002

Medicare Interactive. https://www.medicareinteractive.org/get-answers/medicare-basics/medicare-eligibility-overview/medicareeligibility-for-those-under-65. Accessed February 11, 2020

National Center for Health Statistics. https://www.cdc.gov/nchs/nhds/index.htm. Accessed February 11, 2020

Nichols CI, Vose JG (2016) Clinical outcomes and costs within 90 days of primary or revision total joint arthroplasty. J Arthroplasty 31(7):1400–1406. e3. https://doi.org/10.1016/j.arth.2016.01.022

Nwachukwu BU, McCormick F, Provencher MT, Roche M, Rubash HE (2015) A comprehensive analysis of Medicare trends in utilization and hospital economics for total knee and hip arthroplasty from 2005 to 2011. J Arthroplasty 30(1):15–18. https://doi.org/10.1016/j.arth.2014.08.025

Odum SM, Van Doren BA, Springer BD (2016) National obesity trends in revision total knee arthroplasty. J Arthroplasty 31(9 Suppl):136–139. https://doi.org/10.1016/j.arth.2015.12.055

Prieto-Alhambra D, Burn E, Weaver J, Sena AG, Stewart HM, Ryan P (2019) OP0174 partial knee replacement is associated with a lower risk of venous thromboembolism and OPIOID use than total knee replacement but increased risk of long-term revision: a multinational, multi-database, propensity score-matched, cohort analysis including over 280,000 patients. BMJ Publishing Group Ltd

Pugely AJ, Martin CT, Harwood J, Ong KL, Bozic KJ, Callaghan JJ (2015a) Database and registry research in orthopaedic surgery: part 2: clinical registry data. J Bone Joint Surg Am 97(21):1799–1808. https://doi.org/10.2106/JBJS.O.00134

Pugely AJ, Martin CT, Harwood J, Ong KL, Bozic KJ, Callaghan JJ (2015b) Database and registry research in orthopaedic surgery: part I: claims-based data. J Bone Joint Surg Am 97(15):1278–1287. https://doi.org/10.2106/JBJS.N.01260

Quinlan ND, Chen DQ, Werner BC, Barnes CL, Browne JA (2019) Patients with multiple sclerosis are at increased risk for postoperative complications following total hip and knee arthroplasty. J Arthroplasty 34(8):1606–1610. https://doi.org/10.1016/j.arth.2019.04.022

Richardson SS, Kahlenberg CA, Blevins JL, Goodman SM, Sculco TP, Figgie MP et al (2019) Complications associated with staged versus simultaneous bilateral total knee arthroplasty: an analysis of 7747 patients. Knee 26(5):1096–1101

Runner RP, Gottschalk MB, Staley CA, Pour AE, Roberson JR (2019) Utilization patterns, efficacy, and complications of venous thromboembolism prophylaxis strategies in primary hip and knee arthroplasty as reported by American Board of Orthopedic Surgery Part II candidates. J Arthroplasty 34(4):729–734. https://doi.org/10.1016/j.arth.2018.12.015

Singh JA, Yu S, Chen L, Cleveland JD (2019) Rates of total joint replacement in the United States: future projections to 2020-2040 using the National Inpatient Sample. J Rheumatol 46(9):1134–1140. https://doi.org/10.3899/jrheum.170990

Slifka KJ, Yi SH, Reddy SC, Baggs J, Jernigan JA (2018) The attributable mortality of prosthetic joint infection after primary hip and knee arthroplasty among medicare beneficiaries, 2005–2012. Open Forum Infect Dis 5(Suppl 1):S118. https://doi.org/10.1093/ofid/ofy210.298

Sloan M, Premkumar A, Sheth NP (2018) Projected volume of primary total joint arthroplasty in the U.S., 2014 to 2030. J Bone Joint Surg Am 100(17):1455–1460. https://doi.org/10.2106/JBJS.17.01617

Sloan M, Sheth N, Lee GC (2019) Is obesity associated with increased risk of deep vein thrombosis or pulmonary embolism after hip and knee arthroplasty? A large database study. Clin Orthop Relat Res 477(3):523–532. https://doi.org/10.1097/CORR.0000000000000615

Smith EL, Dugdale EM, Tybor D, Kain M (2019) Comparing inpatient complication rates between octogenarians and nonagenarians following primary and revision total hip arthroplasty in a nationally representative sample 2010-2014. Geriatrics (Basel) 4(4). https://doi.org/10.3390/geriatrics4040055

Soley-Bori M, Soria-Saucedo R, Youn B, Haynes AB, Macht R, Ryan CM et al (2017) Region and insurance plan type influence discharge disposition after hip and knee arthroplasty: evidence from the privately insured US population. J Arthroplasty 32(11):3286–91 e4. https://doi.org/10.1016/j.arth.2017.06.007

Sundaram K, Warren J, Anis H, George J, Murray T, Higuera CA et al (2019) An increased body mass index was not associated with higher rates of 30-day postoperative complications after unicompartmental knee arthroplasty. Knee 26(3):720–728. https://doi.org/10.1016/j.knee.2019.02.009

Vakharia RM, Sabeh KG, Cohen-Levy WB, Sodhi N, Mont MA, Roche MW (2019) Opioid disorders are associated with thromboemboli following primary total knee arthroplasty. J Arthroplasty 34(12):2957–2961. https://doi.org/10.1016/j.arth.2019.07.042

Wang Y, Deng Z, Meng J, Dai Q, Chen T, Bao N (2019) Impact of bariatric surgery on inpatient complication, cost, and length of stay following total hip or knee arthroplasty. J Arthroplasty 34(12):2884–2889. e4. https://doi.org/10.1016/j.arth.2019.07.012

Zhang W, Lyman S, Boutin-Foster C, Parks ML, Pan TJ, Lan A et al (2016) Racial and ethnic disparities in utilization rate, hospital volume, and perioperative outcomes after total knee arthroplasty. J Bone Joint Surg Am 98(15):1243–1252. https://doi.org/10.2106/JBJS.15.01009

Arthroplasty Register Data: Outcomes of Knee Arthroplasty in Younger Patients

Nils P. Hailer and Annette W-Dahl

Contents

E. Hansen, K.-D. Kühn (eds.), *Essentials of Cemented Knee Arthroplasty*,
https://doi.org/10.1007/978-3-662-63113-3_40

40.1 Introduction

The number of knee arthroplasties performed in younger patients is increasing in most countries that report arthroplasty register data, and the proportion of younger age groups among all knee arthroplasty patients is also on the rise. Within the context of knee arthroplasty surgery, "young" is mostly defined as an age below 55 years, but the definition sometimes includes persons of working age, i.e., up to 65 years.

> Compared to the mostly good or even excellent results obtained in the elderly, patients who receive a unicompartmental (UKA) or total knee arthroplasty (TKA) before the age of 55 are at higher risk of implant revision.

As in the elderly, revision rates in younger patients are considerably higher after UKA than after TKA, a finding that is consistent over all established registers. However, the threshold to revise a UKA may be lower than to revise a TKA, and this has to be considered when comparing revision rates between these two fundamentally different principles. There is no register-based evidence that uncemented knee arthroplasty gives better outcomes than cemented TKA, neither in terms of implant survival nor with respect to patient-reported outcomes. Younger patients have higher expectations on their artificial joint.

> After knee arthroplasty younger patients gain function just as the elderly do after this procedure. However, young patients are – at least in some aspects – more often dissatisfied with the outcome of their procedure.

40

In conclusion, the young patient is at increased risk of inferior outcome after both total and partial knee arthroplasty, and the cemented knee arthroplasty can still be considered a gold standard that other methods have to be measured against.

40.2 Trends in the Demography of Knee Arthroplasty Patients

Historically, the use of total knee arthroplasty was established in the group of elderly patients, and due to excellent or at least good results in many patients the method rapidly gained wide acceptance (◘ Fig. 40.1). However, since the 1990s, epidemiological studies and arthroplasty register data indicate a robust increase in the number and proportion of younger patients treated with either a total or a unicompartmental knee arthroplasty (Swedish Knee Arthroplasty Register 2019). The average age of patients treated with a total knee arthroplasty in Sweden was 71 years in 1994, and it has only slightly declined to 69 years in 2018.

> However, the proportion of patients younger than 55 at the time of index surgery has grown from 1.8% to 7% (W-Dahl et al. 2010).

In absolute numbers, the increase in the proportion of younger patients is more easily visible, and in Sweden the number of patients operated with TKA has risen almost 8-fold from 1994 to 2018 (Swedish Knee Arthroplasty Register 2019). This observation of an increasing incidence of knee arthroplasty in younger patients is consistent over the Nordic countries, where the increase in the incidence of knee arthroplasty is highest in the younger patients (Niemelainen et al. 2017).

> Generally speaking, UKA is an implant that is more frequently chosen in younger patients, such that the average age of patients at the time of insertion of this type of implant is about 5 years below that of patients receiving TKA.

The National Joint Registry of England and Wales (NJR) does not reach quite as far back in time as the Nordic arthroplasty registers, but it supports Nordic data on the demographics of patients who received total vs. unicompartmental knee arthroplasty. According to NJR data, patients receiving UKA were typically around the age of 64, whereas those operated with TKA were aged 70 years at the time of the index procedure. Moreover, females dominate in the group of patients operated with TKA, whereas 53% of all patients in the NJR who receive UKA are males (National Joint Registry 2019).

The "young knee arthroplasty patient" differs from the average knee arthroplasty patient not only in terms of age, but also in terms of the indications underlying surgery.

> While osteoarthritis of the knee dominates as the underlying diagnosis in both older and younger knee arthroplasty patients, the proportion of patients operated due to rheumatoid arthritis or previous fracture is higher in knee arthroplasty patients under the age of 55.

The proportion of patients who have undergone prior surgery in the index knee is also much higher in younger than in elderly patients. This observation reflects the fact that both soft-tissue injuries to the knee and tibial condylar fractures frequently occur in patients in their

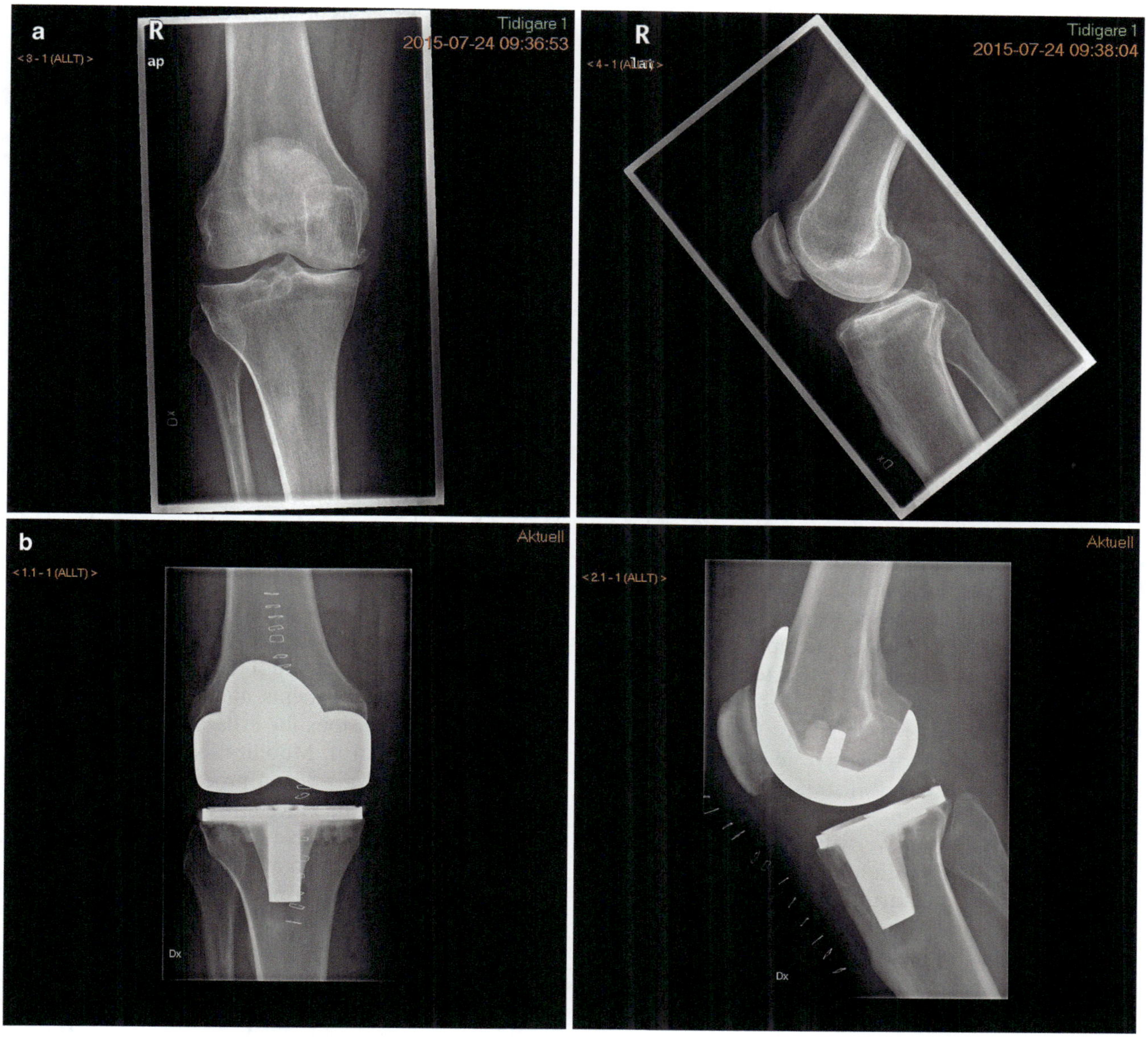

Fig. 40.1 Cemented total knee arthroplasty in a 49-year-old male with primary osteoarthritis. (**a**) Preoperative frontal and lateral views, and (**b**) postoperative frontal and lateral views

20s or 30s, and that early-onset rheumatoid arthritis can lead to severe joint destruction at a relatively young age (Wennergren et al. 2018; Innala et al. 2014). This difference in the indications underlying knee arthroplasty surgery is important to remember, since most registers consistently report that results after TKA performed for other reasons than osteoarthritis are inferior to those found after surgery due to osteoarthritis, and thus, the group of younger patients is at higher risk of implant failure than the average elderly patient.

> However, even if only patients with osteoarthritis are analyzed, younger patients who receive TKA remain at higher risk of revision than older patients, indicating that not only the underlying indication but younger age per se is a risk factor for earlier failure (Harrysson et al. 2004).

40.3 What Is "Outcome"?

The issue of implant revision leads to the next important question: What parameters contribute to the term "outcome after knee arthroplasty"? Obviously, the *occurrence of revision surgery*, performed due to implant loosening or for other reasons such as infection or instability, is an important measure of outcome, and it is the main outcome reported by all national arthroplasty registers. However, since the turn of the millennium, much well-deserved focus has been directed toward patient-reported outcomes. These are produced by patients directly reporting on their own health status without interpretation by a surgeon or other medical professionals, and a *patient-reported outcome measure (PROM)* is a specific tool, often a questionnaire, that measures different aspects of patient-reported outcomes (Wilson et al. 2019). PROMs have been used for more than 20 years and are increasing in studies as well as national arthroplasty register analyses as an integral part of the evaluation after knee arthroplasty surgery. PROMs evaluating knee arthroplasty surgery include both generic general health instruments such as the well-established EQ-5D and SF-36 as well as disease-specific instruments such as the Oxford Knee Score (OKS), Knee Injury and Osteoarthritis Outcome Score (KOOS), and The Western Ontario and McMaster Universities Arthritis Index (WOMAC). Expectations before and satisfaction after surgery are other measures that are commonly used in the evaluation of subjective outcomes.

And, as for the outcome revision surgery, we shall see that young patients differ from the average elderly patients in several facets that PROMs attempt to capture, be it pain, function, or the ability to return to work or sports.

> An important factor that affects PROMs is the preoperative level of expectation, and this also differs between young and elderly patients.

Thus, in the following we will analyze both implant survival and PROMs with a focus on younger patients operated with a knee arthroplasty. We will compare outcomes after total with those after unicompartmental arthroplasty, and evaluate whether cemented or cementless fixation gives better results.

40.4 Implant Survival

40.4.1 TKA and UKA in the Young Patient

> As a rule of thumb, most established arthroplasty registers report overall 10-year implant survival rates of more than 95% after cemented TKA.

When implant survival is stratified by age groups, the *unadjusted survival is lower in the youngest age groups*, with 10-year survival rates dropping to just above 90% in Swedish patients younger than 55 years at the time of primary arthroplasty surgery (Swedish Knee Arthroplasty Register 2019), a result that at first glance may appear quite satisfactory (Fig. 40.2a).

> However, when transformed into a relative risk of revision, it becomes apparent that younger patients have an approximately 2.1-fold higher adjusted risk of implant revision when compared to patients aged 65 to 74, the dominating age group in the Swedish Knee Arthroplasty Register.

Again, this observation is fairly *consistent throughout the Nordic arthroplasty registers*, including Norway, Denmark, and Finland. In the Danish Knee Arthroplasty Register, the risk of revision after TKA in patients younger than 40 years is about 4.6-fold higher compared to those aged 70–79 years (Dansk Knaealloplastikregister 2019). The notion that younger patients are at much higher risk of revision is also *confirmed by numbers from the NJR* where the group of patients under the age of 55 runs by far the highest risk of revision after total knee arthroplasty, both in females and in males. Average 10-year implant survival in the NJR is estimated at around 89% in this age group.

Reasons for revision after TKA differ between younger and elderly patients. In a Finnish register study, younger patients with TKA were at higher risk of revision than older patients, and the risk increase was pronounced for revisions for other reasons than infection (Julin et al. 2010). Mobilization under anesthesia is not registered as a revision procedure in most joint registries, and since the procedure can be performed on an out-patient basis, reliable numbers on this topic are often lacking. However, an analysis of the incidence of this procedure in Swedish patients after primary knee arthroplasty indicates that younger, female patients are at considerably higher risk of developing postoperative knee stiffness that requires treatment (Thorsteinsson et al. 2019).

When compared with TKA, *results after UKA are inferior in terms of implant survival*, an observation that we will discuss in more detail. The 10-year survival rate of all UKAs in the Swedish Knee Arthroplasty Register is around 86% (Swedish Knee Arthroplasty Register 2019), and the NJR reports 10-year survival rates of around 89% after UKA, compared to above 96% after cemented TKA (National Joint Registry 2019). This is consistent with findings from Norway and Denmark, with the Danish register reporting that UKA has about double the risk of revision than TKA (Dansk Knaealloplastikregister 2019).

When we take a closer look at Swedish patients younger than 55 years at the time of insertion of a unicompartmental knee arthroplasty (Fig. 40.2b), these are at 1.6-fold higher risk of conversion to a

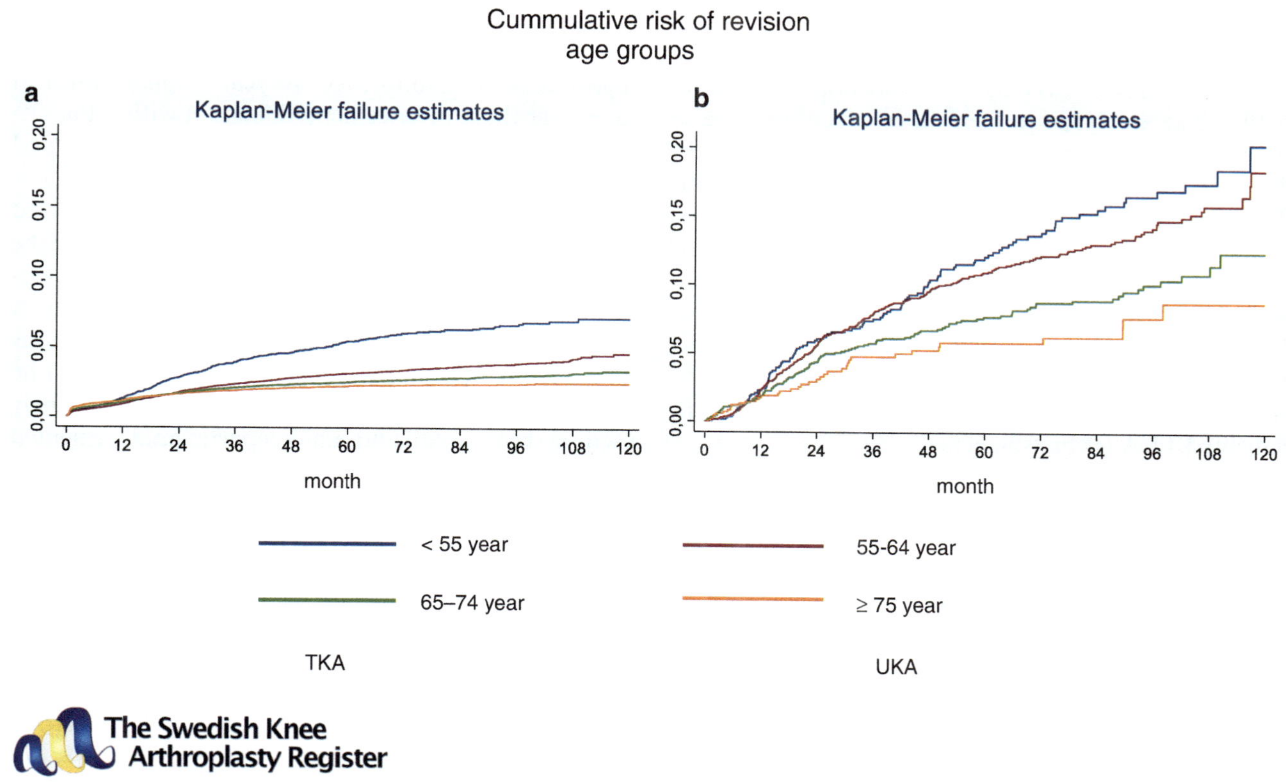

Fig. 40.2 Cumulative revision rates after total knee arthroplasty (**a**) and unicompartmental knee arthroplasty (**b**), divided by age groups

total knee arthroplasty than those in the age group between 65 and 74 (Swedish Knee Arthroplasty Register 2019).

> The NJR confirms that younger patients receiving UKA suffer from higher implant failure rates than elderly patients.

The 10-year-survival rate of the UKA inserted into patients <55 years at the time of primary surgery is 84%, compared with 91% after cemented TKA in the same age group (National Joint Registry 2019).

The discussion about revision rates after UKA vs. TKA has sometimes been heated. It has been suggested that the dissatisfied patient with UKA may more readily be considered for revision surgery. In patients with UKA and progression of disease in the contralateral compartment, insertion of a contralateral UKA or conversion to a TKA may seem an appealing solution. In contrast, the surgical option for patients who are dissatisfied after a TKA is more complex revision surgery, a decision that may be less easily taken. In addition, the average patient with UKA is younger and potentially less comorbid.

> Therefore, the threshold to revise a patient with UKA may be lower, thus giving rise to higher cumulative revision rates and lower implant survival when compared to patients with TKA.

40.4.2 Cemented Compared with Cementless Fixation

Historically, both components in TKA were fixed using bone cement, but cementless fixation of the tibial component in TKA was popularized in the late 1980s, a concept later termed "inverse hybrid" fixation (Rosenberg et al. 1989). Long-term follow-up of such cohorts in the Swedish Knee Arthroplasty Register indicates *inferior results after cementless tibial fixation*, with a relative risk of revision of 1.6 when compared with cemented implants. However, during the latest 10-year period, implant survival does not differ statistically significantly between cemented and cementless fixation of tibial components in Sweden, but the proportion of cementless fixation remains well below 10% of all Swedish knee arthroplasty procedures (Swedish Knee Arthroplasty Register 2019).

In Denmark, the risk of revision after cementless TKA is about 1.4 times higher when compared to cemented TKA (Dansk Knaealloplastikregister 2019), and in Norway, cementless fixation is also associated with slightly higher failure rates after more than 10 years, although not statistically significantly (Nasjonalt Register For Leddproteser 2019). In contrast to the "inverse hybrid" fixation described above, the combination of cementless femoral components with a cemented tibial tray in TKA has been termed "hybrid" fixation. According to a Norwegian register analysis, some hybrid designs are associated with slightly improved implant survival when compared with totally cemented TKA (Petursson et al. 2015).

> A recent Nordic register collaboration study indicates that both hybrid and inverse hybrid fixation techniques can offer 10-year survival rates of 93% or above in patients younger than 65 years.

However, the entirely cementless fixation of both femoral and tibial components is associated with a higher revision risk (Niemelainen et al. 2020). Nonetheless, in the Nordic countries cemented fixation of both components dominates by far.

In accordance with praxis in the Nordic countries, the NJR reports that entirely cementless or hybrid fixation is used in less than 4% of all knee arthroplasties, and the mean age of patients receiving hybrid or cementless knee arthroplasties is about the same as that of patients receiving cemented knee arthroplasty. Again, as in most Nordic countries, cementless fixation is by the NJR reported to be associated with slightly lower implant survival after 10 years (National Joint Registry 2019). Lower implant survivorship in cementless compared with both cemented and hybrid TKA is also described in a register study from New Zealand (Nugent et al. 2019).

> Although less popular today, the use of cemented monoblock polyethylene tibial components has proven to be fairly successful, both in Sweden and in England & Wales (Gudnason et al. 2014; National Joint Registry 2019).

In parallel with the development of cementless fixation of TKA, this type of fixation has also gained popularity in UKA.

> A recent Finnish register-based comparison of cementless with cemented fixation of a specific UKA indicates a slightly lower revision risk for uncemented components after 5 years.

However, in that study, implant survival of both cementless and cemented UKA is clearly inferior to that of cemented TKA (Knifsund et al. 2019). Cementless fixation of the same specific UKA device is also reported to have improved 10-year implant survival rates over those after cemented fixation within the setting of a register study from the NJR (Mohammad et al. 2020).

Numerous observational studies, both register-based and smaller cohort studies, support the notion that the addition of antibiotics to bone cement improves long-term implant survival after total joint arthroplasty, a finding that has been related to a reduced risk of revisions for infections (Engesaeter et al. 2003). In the Nordic countries, antibiotic-loaded bone cement is routinely used in both total and unicompartmental cemented knee arthroplasty. However, there are indications that the use of antibiotic-loaded bone cement is not as clearly associated with a reduced risk of revision for infections after TKA as after total hip arthroplasty. According to a recent study on a large cohort from the NJR, the risk of being revised due to PJI seems higher in patients receiving cemented when compared with cementless TKA fixation (Lenguerrand et al. 2019), and in a Canadian register study, the addition of antibiotics to polymethacrylate bone cement in TKA seems not as clearly associated with a reduced risk of revision due to infection as is the case after cemented total hip arthroplasty (Bohm et al. 2014).

40.5 Patient-Reported Outcomes

Patients younger than 55 years of age do not only have a longer life expectancy than older patients but the average younger patient will also have to return to work for around 10 years before retirement. Workload, leisure time, family, and economic situations of the younger patients are thus quite different compared to patients close to retirement or to those who are already retired. Younger patients expect to perform higher in many activities of daily life, both during work and leisure time, and sometimes at a challenging level (Witjes et al. 2017). The fundamentally different life situation and increased expectations among younger patients are reflected not only in their increased risk of revision but also in their patient-reported outcomes.

Patient-reported outcomes after knee arthroplasty in younger patients are not as extensively investigated when compared to those of the elderly population, and findings derived from younger knee arthroplasty cohorts are not consistent. The inconsistencies may be explained by selection bias, smaller sample sizes, lower response rates when it comes to answering questionnaires, the type of PROM used, and investigated time frames. Further, the interpretation of what a difference in PROMs between groups really means from a clinical perspective is debated since statistically significant differences in large register cohorts may not be clinically relevant.

While *some studies on younger patients report more pain and inferior function* after TKA, others report similar outcomes as in the elderly (Wood et al. 2013; Williams et al. 2013; Haynes et al. 2017; Townsend et al. 2018; Clement et al. 2018). On the other hand, even if younger patients preoperatively report more preoperative pain and lower function than older age groups (Nyvang et al. 2019) *other studies indicate that they can experience similar or even better improvements in PROMs* after arthroplasty surgery (Williams et al. 2013; Street et al. 2013).

However, there are no definitions of what a successful outcome after knee arthroplasty surgery in terms of PROMs is, mostly because the surgical goals vary with age, sex, underlying diagnosis, health status, and so forth. PROMs are commonly reported as mean values that fail to illustrate the outliers, and – when presented as an arithmetic mean – they also give no hint of the proportion of patients that have improved after surgery. This proportion may oftentimes be of greater interest than a statistical mean difference, and the "Outcome Measures in Rheumatology–The Osteoarthritis Research Society International" (OMERACT–OARSI) responder criteria can be used to evaluate this (Pham et al. 2004). The responder criteria are based on a combination of absolute and relative changes in pain, function, and total WOMAC score 1 year after surgery. These criteria have not been frequently used to compare younger with older patients, however, there seems to be no clear correlation of outcome with age (Weber et al. 2018).

> The proportion of younger patients reporting that they are satisfied with TKA surgery is lower compared to older patients: 83–86% in the young vs. 91–92% in the older patients (Williams et al. 2013; Scott et al. 2016; Lange et al. 2018; Clement et al. 2018).

The question whether UKA confers better patient-reported outcome when compared with TKA is debated. A recently published systematic review and meta-analysis of patient-reported outcomes after total vs. unicompartmental knee arthroplasty describes no relevant differences in pain – but better function in patients with UKA (Wilson et al. 2019). In contrast, a 5-year follow-up of a randomized controlled trial (RCT) indicates no statistically or clinically significant difference in Oxford Knee Score between patients operated with a total compared to a unicompartmental knee arthroplasty (Beard et al. 2019). In that study, 82% of patients receiving UKA and 77% of patients with TKA were satisfied with the surgery, without a statistically significant difference.

Several national arthroplasty registers collect patient-reported outcomes as part of the evaluation after surgery (Wilson et al. 2019). However, few registers report patient-reported outcomes in their annual reports. The SKAR has collected and reported patient-reported outcomes since 2012 from an increasing number of participating units (Swedish Knee Arthroplasty Register 2019). An analysis of almost 15,000 TKA patients, whereof 800 patients were younger than 55 years, indicates similar pain and activities of daily living in patients younger than 55 years when compared with older patients. However, younger patients reported more other symptoms, more problems in sports and recreation function, and lower knee-related quality of life compared to the older age groups 1 year after surgery when measured by the KOOS. 88% of patients younger than 55 years were considered as OMERACT–OARSI responders, a very similar proportion as among older patients (89–90%). The SKAR has an anchor question on patients' expectations since these may influence satisfaction as well as pain and function postoperatively.

> 12% of patients younger than 55 years report high expectations but were not satisfied with the surgery, compared to 7% in patients 65–74 years of age.

Independently of age-group, patients with higher expectations report considerable inferior outcomes in all five dimensions of the KOOS instrument.

Conclusion

From a register perspective, TKA and UKA result in good implant survival even in younger patients, but the risk of revision is consistently higher in younger than in older patients, irrespective of whether total or partial arthroplasty is performed. UKA confers a higher risk of revision when compared to TKA, also in younger age groups. Cemented fixation of total knee arthroplasty gives the most reliable long-term results in terms of implant survival, but some hybrid and inverse hybrid techniques seem to achieve similar results. Patient-reported outcome is not extensively studied in patients younger than 55 years of age, but younger patients seem to attain similar gains in terms of reduced pain and increased function as elderly patients. However, when compared with the elderly population, a lower proportion of young patients is satisfied with the outcome after surgery, possibly because younger patients have higher demands and expectations on their knee function when compared to the elderly knee arthroplasty population. In conclusion, register data support that despite mostly good results after total and unicompartmental knee arthroplasty, younger patients are at higher risk of both implant failure, inferior function, and dissatisfaction, findings that should be weighed in when counseling younger patients prior to knee arthroplasty.

Take-Home Messages

- An increasing number of younger patients is operated with partial or total knee arthroplasty.
- The proportion of patients who have undergone prior surgery in the index knee is higher in younger patients, and the proportion of primary osteoarthritis is lower than in the elderly, both of which can contribute to an inferior outcome.
- Knee arthroplasty patients younger than 55 at the time of surgery are at higher risk of implant revision.
- Revision rates are higher after unicompartmental than after total knee arthroplasty, even in younger patients.
- Younger patients gain knee function just as the elderly do.
- Young patients are, however, more often dissatisfied with the outcome of their procedure than elderly patients.

References

Beard DJ, Davies LJ, Cook JA, et al for the TOPKAT Study Group (2019) The clinical and cost-effectiveness of total versus partial knee replacement in patients with medial compartment osteoarthritis (TOPKAT): 5-year outcomes of a randomized controlled trial. Lancet 394:746–756

Bohm E, Zhu N, Gu J et al (2014) Does adding antibiotics to cement reduce the need for early revision in total knee arthroplasty? Clin Orthop Relat Res 472(1):162–168. https://doi.org/10.1007/s11999-013-3186-1

Clement ND, Walker LC, Bardgett M et al (2018) Patient age of less than 55 years is not an independent predictor of functional improvement or satisfaction after total knee arthroplasty. Arch Orthop Trauma Surg 138(12):1755–1763

Dansk Knaealloplastikregister (2019) Årsrapport. 2019. https://www.sundhed.dk/

Engesaeter LB, Lie SA, Espehaug B et al (2003) Antibiotic prophylaxis in total hip arthroplasty: effects of antibiotic prophylaxis systemically and in bone cement on the revision rate of 22,170 primary hip replacements followed 0–14 years in the Norwegian Arthroplasty Register. Acta Orthop Scand 74(6):644–651. https://doi.org/10.1080/00016470310018135

Gudnason A, Hailer NP, W-Dahl A et al (2014) All-polyethylene versus metal-backed tibial components – an analysis of 27,733 cruciate-retaining total knee replacements from the Swedish Knee Arthroplasty Register. J Bone Joint Surg Am 96(12):994–999. https://doi.org/10.2106/jbjs.m.00373

Harrysson OL, Robertsson O, Nayfeh JF (2004) Higher cumulative revision rate of knee arthroplasties in younger patients with osteoarthritis. Clin Orthop Relat Res 421:162–168. https://doi.org/10.1097/01.blo.0000127115.05754.ce

Haynes J, Sassoon A, Nam D et al (2017) Younger patients have less severe radiographic disease and lower reported outcome scores than older patients undergoing total knee arthroplasty. Knee 24(3):663–669

Innala L, Berglin E, Möller B et al (2014) Age at onset determines severity and choice of treatment in early rheumatoid arthritis: a prospective study. Arthritis Res Ther 16(2):R94

Julin J, Jamsen E, Puolakka T et al (2010) Younger age increases the risk of early prosthesis failure following primary total knee replacement for osteoarthritis. A follow-up study of 32,019 total knee replacements in the Finnish Arthroplasty Register. Acta Orthop 81(4):413–419. https://doi.org/10.3109/17453674.2010.501747

Knifsund J, Reito A, Haapakoski J et al (2019) Short-term survival of cementless Oxford unicondylar knee arthroplasty based on the Finnish Arthroplasty Register. Knee 26(3):768–773. https://doi.org/10.1016/j.knee.2019.03.004

Lange JK, Lee YY, Spiro SK, Haas SB (2018) Satisfaction rates and quality of life changes following total knee arthroplasty in age-differentiated cohorts. J Arthroplast 33(5):1373–1378

Lenguerrand E, Whitehouse MR, Beswick AD et al (2019) Risk factors associated with revision for prosthetic joint infection following knee replacement: an observational cohort study from England and Wales. Lancet Infect Dis 19(6):589–600. https://doi.org/10.1016/s1473-3099(18)30755-2

Mohammad HR, Matharu GS, Judge A, Murray DW (2020) Comparison of the 10-year outcomes of cemented and cementless unicompartmental knee replacements: data from the National Joint Registry for England, Wales, Northern Ireland and the Isle of Man. Acta Orthop 91(1):76–81. https://doi.org/10.1080/17453674.2019.1680924

Nasjonalt Register For Leddproteser (2019) Rapport. 2019. https://www.kvalitetsregistre.no

National Joint Registry (2019) 16th Annual Report. 2019. https://reports.njrcentre.org.uk/Portals/0/PDFdownloads/NJR%2016th%20Annual%20Report%202019.pdf

Niemelainen MJ, Makela KT, Robertsson O et al (2017) Different incidences of knee arthroplasty in the Nordic countries. Acta Orthop 88(2):173–178. https://doi.org/10.1080/17453674.2016.1275200

Niemelainen MJ, Makela KT, Robertsson O et al (2020) The effect of fixation type on the survivorship of contemporary total knee arthroplasty in patients younger than 65 years of age: a register-based study of 115,177 knees in the Nordic Arthroplasty Register Association (NARA) 2000–2016. Acta Orthop:1–7. https://doi.org/10.1080/17453674.2019.1710373

Nugent M, Wyatt MC, Frampton CM, Hooper GJ (2019) Despite improved survivorship of uncemented fixation in total knee arthroplasty for osteoarthritis, cemented fixation remains the gold standard: an analysis of a National Joint Registry. J Arthroplast 34(8):1626–1633. https://doi.org/10.1016/j.arth.2019.03.047

Nyvang JS, Naili JE, Iversen MD et al (2019) Younger age is associated with greater pain expression among patients with knee or hip osteoarthritis scheduled for a joint arthroplasty. BMC Musculoskelet Disord 20:365

Petursson G, Fenstad AM, Havelin LI et al (2015) Better survival of hybrid total knee arthroplasty compared to cemented arthroplasty. Acta Orthop 86(6):714–720. https://doi.org/10.3109/17453674.2015.1073539

Pham T, van der Heijde D, Altman RD et al (2004) OMERACT–OARSI initiative: osteoarthritis Research Society International set of responder criteria for osteoarthritis clinical trials revisited. Osteoarthr Cartil 12(5):389–399

Rosenberg AG, Barden R, Galante JO (1989) A comparison of cemented and cementless fixation with the Miller-Galante total knee arthroplasty. Orthop Clin North Am 20(1):97–111

Scott CEH, Bugler KE, Clement ND et al (2016) Patient expectations of arthroplasty of the hip and knee. Bone Joint J 98-B(12): 1625–1634

Street BD, Wong W, Rotondi M, Gage W (2013) Younger patients report greater improvement in self-reported function after knee joint replacement. J Orthop Sports Phys Ther 43(9): 666–672

Swedish Knee Arthroplasty Register (2019) Annual Report. 2019. researchgate.net

Thorsteinsson H, Hedstrom M, Robertsson O et al (2019) Manipulation under anesthesia after primary knee arthroplasty in Sweden: incidence, patient characteristics and risk of revision. Acta Orthop 90(5):484–488. https://doi.org/10.1080/17453674.2019.1637177

Townsend LA, Roubion RC, Bourgeois DM et al (2018) Impact of age on patient-reported outcome measures in total knee arthroplasty. J Knee Surg 31(6):580–584

W-Dahl A, Robertsson O, Lidgren L (2010) Surgery for knee osteoarthritis in younger patients. Acta Orthop 81(2):161–164. https://doi.org/10.3109/17453670903413186

Weber M, Craiovan B, Woerner ML et al (2018) Predictors of outcome after primary total joint replacement. J Arthroplast 33:431–435

Wennergren D, Bergdahl C, Ekelund J et al (2018) Epidemiology and incidence of tibia fractures in the Swedish Fracture Register. Injury 49(11):2068–2074. https://doi.org/10.1016/j.injury.2018.09.008

Williams DP, Price AJ, Beard DJ et al (2013) The effects of age on patient-reported outcome measures in total knee replacements. Bone Joint J 95-B(1):38–44

Wilson I, Bohm E, Lübbeke A et al (2019) Orthopaedic registries with patient-reported outcome measures. EFORT Open Rev 4(6):357–367

Witjes S, van Geenen RCI, Koenraadt KLM et al (2017) Expectations of younger patients concerning activities after knee arthroplasty: are we asking the right questions? Qual Life Res 26(2):403–417

Wood AM, Keenan ACM, Arthur CHC et al (2013) The functional outcome of total knee replacement in young patients: a 10-year matched case control study. Open J Orthop 3(2):128–132

Economics

Contents

Economics of Surgical Treatment of Knee Arthritis – A US Perspective

J. Parker Chapman, David P. Hagan, and Chancellor F. Gray

Contents

E. Hansen, K.-D. Kühn (eds.), *Essentials of Cemented Knee Arthroplasty*,
https://doi.org/10.1007/978-3-662-63113-3_41

41.1 Introduction

Symptomatic osteoarthritis of the knee is a common condition for which patients seek treatment. A Swedish study from 2012 reported a prevalence of 13.8% among persons >45 years of age of a large sample population with symptomatic osteoarthritis of the knee with a predicted increase to 15.2% by the year 2032 (Turkiewicz et al. 2014). The most complete current literature for prevalence of symptomatic radiographic osteoarthritis of the knee in the United States (US) is from the NHANES III cohort. Within the cohort of 2394 patients greater than age 60 surveyed between 1991 and 1994, 12.1% reported symptoms in addition to having radiographic evidence of osteoarthritis (Dillon et al. 2006). This data is antiquated, includes only patients >60 years of age and the percentage of affected persons is likely under-reported as radiographic evaluation only included an anterior-posterior (AP) view. It can be assumed that the prevalence of symptomatic osteoarthritis of the knee in the United States exceeds the 12.1% observed in 1991–1994 including persons younger than 60 with symptomatic osteoarthritis, population growth over the last 25 years, and the current obesity epidemic. While conservative management has a role and a financial impact on the treatment of symptomatic knee osteoarthritis, the majority of the economic impact and utilization of healthcare resources involves surgical treatment (Bedard et al. 2017).

41.2 Economic Burden of Knee Arthritis

There are multiple surgical options, but the most efficacious procedure for the treatment of global advanced (tricompartmental) osteoarthritis of the knee is total knee arthroplasty (TKA). TKA is one of the most common elective surgeries in the developed world, owing to multiple factors: an aging population with expectations of preserved activity, and increasingly safe and effective knee arthroplasty procedures. The United States boasts the highest utilization rate of TKA implants among industrialized countries with projections for exponential growth over the next decade in the number of TKA cases performed (Pabinger et al. 2015).

41

> The economic impact from a cost perspective will be significant. It is projected that the rate of primary TKA will increase as much as 673% and revision TKA by 601% by the year 2030 (Kurtz et al. 2007).

Orthopedic implants, operating room utilization, as well as postoperative hospital stay and follow-up are all significant contributors to the joint replacement expense. With the projected exponential increases the amount of total joint replacement surgeries to be performed over the next decade, the cost and quality of delivery of this modality will become increasingly important. In order to address this financial burden, changes to reimbursement in the US healthcare system have already developed (via bundled payments and other alternative payment models), and are likely to continue to grow in prevalence (Kurtz et al. 2007).

A goal of all parties involved is to create a sustainable model that decreases cost, increases quality, and does not limit access to TKA for those with comorbidities leading to higher operative risks or for those without private insurance. Creating a system that accomplishes these things will require delicate balancing of these factors.

> Although there is potential for difficulty through this transition, if done properly, benefit could be seen by each player via improved quality, streamlined payment models for hospitals and surgeons, and increased value to the population.

41.2.1 Non-TKA Treatments

Depending on the stage of knee OA, there are alternatives available prior to TKA (Fig. 41.1). Typically, TKA is reserved for moderate to severe arthritis (Kellgren and Lawrence stage III or IV) with heavy burden of symptoms, significantly impacting quality of life. The onus of proper patient selection falls on the treating surgeon, and there are no absolute guidelines for operative vs. non-operative management outside of an individual surgeon's clinical judgment. Part of a surgeon's responsibility to the patient and healthcare as a whole is the value a modality provides for the patient – whether surgical or non-surgical – and its overall cost-effectiveness.

Historically, prior to any surgical intervention, it has been important to have adequate trials and documentation of a step-wise progression through the available non-operative management options. While there are a multitude of non-operative modalities, it is important to discuss the efficacy of a modality and its role within current practice guidelines. The AAOS clinical practice guidelines are a culmination of evidence-based treatment recommendations for orthopedic pathologies. Regarding non-operative modalities, only physical therapy (low-impact aerobic activity, strengthening exercises, neuromuscular education, etc.) and the use of NSAIDs and tramadol received a recommendation strength of strong (American Academy of Orthopaedic Surgeons 2013). Few studies report on the cost-effectiveness of non-oper-

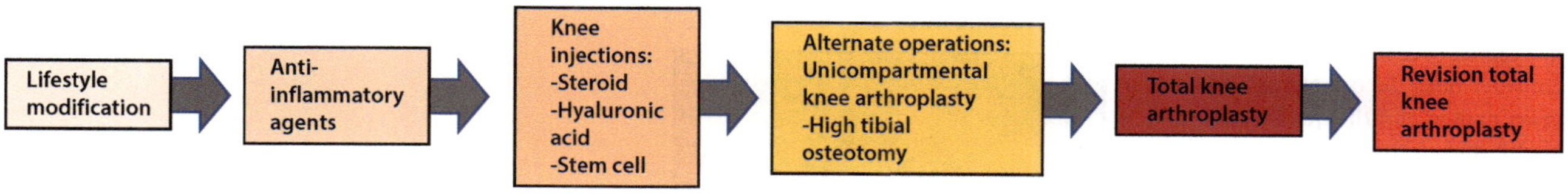

Fig. 41.1 Stage-dependent treatment of knee OA

ative management before surgical intervention. A meta-analysis from 2012 queried the available literature investigating the cost-effectiveness of non-surgical and non-pharmacologic modalities as interventions for hip and knee osteoarthritis. Their conclusion was that exercise-based programs appear to offer the best value for money when quality-adjusted life years (QALY) are used as the outcome of interest (Pinto et al. 2012). Using this measure, 0.022–0.045 additional QALY are added for $769–$796 of cost to the healthcare system, a number which is considered cost-effective.

> It is important to note that the evidence included in the analysis is limited, not standardized regarding outcome measures, and at high risk of bias.

For moderate arthritis (stage II, III), therapy typically progresses through the ever-increasing array of knee injection options. Corticosteroid, hyaluronic acid, platelet-rich plasma, and, most recently, stem cell injections have all been utilized in non-operative management of knee OA. The AAOS clinical practice guidelines consensus is inconclusive regarding steroid injections and platelet-rich plasma and cannot make a recommendation for or against the use of these modalities. While there is no consensus regarding the use of steroid injections, they continue to be used as a treatment modality and can offer temporary pain relief that in some cases may delay TKA. A recommendation of strong was given against the use of hyaluronic injections for symptomatic arthritis based on a meta-analysis of 14 studies (3 high strength and 11 moderate strength) that demonstrated no appreciable number of patients achieving a clinically relevant benefit in outcome scores.

Biologics remain a source of confusion. Though the AAOS has formally created a committee to investigate the science behind biologic therapies for musculoskeletal care, the American Academy of Hip and Knee Surgeons (AAHKS) has stated: "It is our position that biologic therapies, including stem cell and PRP injections, cannot currently be recommended for the treatment of advanced … knee arthritis."(American Academy of Hip and Knee Surgeons 2019)

> At this time, the authors cannot advocate for the use of biologics in the spectrum of knee arthritis treatment from a cost or efficacy standpoint.

The limited use of arthroscopy has been found to provide benefit for mechanical symptoms in OA; otherwise, there is limited evidence that arthroscopy provides a clinically significant improvement in symptoms or outcome measures (Hutt et al. 2015). Although each of these forms of conservative management has been used with varying efficacy in mild to moderate arthritis, it has been shown that in end-stage knee OA (stage IV), a decision for TKA is of greatest benefit in most cases.

In addition, the surgical alternatives to TKA should be noted (Fig. 41.1). High tibial osteotomy (HTO) as well as unicompartmental knee arthroplasty (UKA) have been utilized in select scenarios. HTO is beneficial in younger patients (<50 years, typically) with isolated medial compartment disease, varus deformity, and intact ligamentous stability (Smith et al. 2017). UKA is also beneficial under these circumstances but additionally can be appropriate in patients of more advanced age (Fabre-Aubrespy et al. 2016).

> Though these interventions are able to preserve more of the native anatomy, the index costs are similar and the potential need for conversion to a TKA exists, along with the associated costs.

41.2.2 Health-Related Quality of Life and Societal Benefits of TKA

As mentioned above, TKA has been targeted for cost reduction because it represents a significant expense in the budget of any health insurer – this situation reflects both its high utilization rate and high cost. The intervention continues to be highly utilized because it is effective, and it continues to be reimbursed for the same reason.

By any standard, TKA adds cost-effective value to a patient's life. QALYs are currently the standard for determination of an intervention's value to the patient within a population. QALYs effectively reflect both the quantity of time added to a patient's life as well as the quality of that time. For example, 1 year lived in perfect health is represented by one QALY. Otherwise, the QALY is calculated using a utility value based on the patient's state of health along with the time spent in that state of health (Wu et al. 2014). Utility values are based on factors such as pain, functional level, and ability to perform activities of daily living (ADLs). Governing

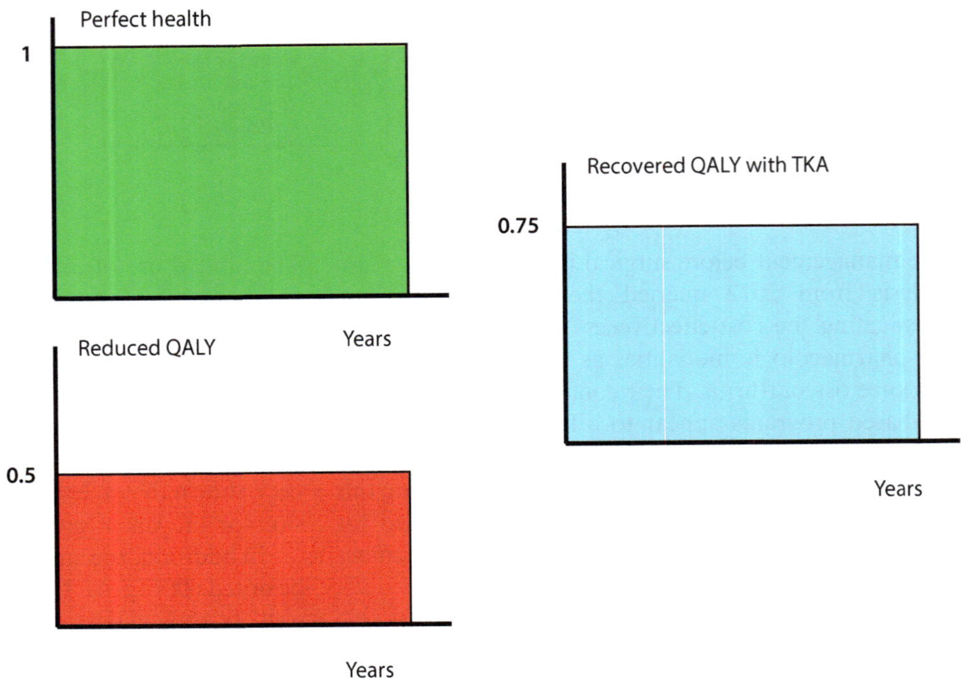

Fig. 41.2 Quality-adjusted life years (QALY). QALYs consider both the quantity of life years gained and the quality of health during those years, and assigns an associated cost to recoup the additional time and quality of life. Perfect health is assigned a value of 1, while death has a value of 0

bodies navigate this ethically and economically challenging area to set the value for a QALY. In the United States, the addition of each QALY has been valued anywhere between $50,000 and $150,000.

> Although TKA raises the lifetime cost of treatment for knee OA (average cost of TKA approximately $50,000 with wide range), the associated increase in QALYs outweighs this cost and is well within the currently accepted range of cost per QALY (Fig. 41.2).

More specifically, with TKA, lifetime costs rose from $37,100 (no TKA) to $57,900 after TKA. Nonetheless cost-effectiveness ratios remained favorable at $18,300 per QALY for low-risk patients and $28,100 per QALY for high-risk patients (Losina et al. 2009).

41

Additionally, there are economic advantages in returning patients to the workforce. For instance, for a 50-year old with symptomatic knee OA, TKA would be expected to save society nearly $70,000 over a lifetime compared to non-operative management. These cost benefits are realized quickly and are preserved throughout a lifetime (Bedair et al. 2014).

> Due to such favorable economics, TKA will continue to be the standard of care in end-stage knee OA for the foreseeable future.

41.3 Economic Considerations of TKA

Economic considerations of TKA must account for factors from before the patient with knee osteoarthritis enters the clinic door to when the patient exits the 90-day postoperative period and beyond. Each stage carries intricacies that play into the economic viability of TKA in a population.

41.3.1 Preoperative Considerations and Patient Selection

When selecting patients for primary TKA, the surgeon must consider each patient's medical comorbidities along with other factors in determining who can safely undergo surgery and experience the greatest benefit. It is well known that certain diseases such as obesity and diabetes mellitus (DM) increase the risk for postoperative infection and other postoperative complications. A personal or family history of thromboembolic disease or other prothrombotic states increases the risk of postoperative pulmonary embolism (PE) or deep venous thrombosis (DVT), and often requires more aggressive anticoagulation therapy, though acetyl salicylic acid (ASA) has been shown to be cost-effective for the majority of patients undergoing TKA (Parvizi et al. 2017).

> It is also important to account for lifestyle factors such as smoking status, alcohol consumption, and the use of any recreational drugs which can lead to any number of adverse effects.

Complications lead to increased cost to orthopedic practices, the hospital, the healthcare system, patients, and society as a whole; potentially avoidable complications must be minimized through optimization wherever possible. Preoperatively, a thorough medical history should be gathered for each patient along with identification and characterization of all comorbidities (Santaguida et al. 2008). Once identified, each risk factor should be optimized with assistance from the appropriate providers (i.e., anesthesia, cardiology) prior to operative intervention. The Charlson comorbidity index (CCI), which accounts for age, heart disease, vascular disease, endocrine disease (DM), lung disease (COPD), renal disease, etc., is a commonly used tool in preoperative evaluation and in studies evaluating outcomes in the total joint replacement literature (Baumgartner et al. 2018). Patient screening and selection techniques among surgeons display a wide range of variability. In general, despite increased risks with advanced age and multiple comorbidities, it has been shown that the benefit of TKA outweighs these risks for much of the population even when considering the increased cost. Patient-specific care will need to be addressed in payment models to prevent access limitations for patients with increased risk factors.

An innovative use of big data and machine learning could provide a solution for creating patient-specific reimbursement models through a tiered system – when more complex patients are encountered, the reimbursement would reflect this complexity (Navarro et al. 2018). At present, CMS makes a minimal distinction between the vast majority of patients and those with "major medical comorbidities", which make up very few total knee replacement episodes (around 6% nationally) (Vizient Inc 2020). This lack of granularity in risk creates disincentive to manage complex cases.

> Future work in this area will help to ensure that surgeons are able to provide TKA to patients despite increased comorbidities and the associated increase in financial burden due to an increased rate of postoperative complications.

When a TKA patient requires inpatient management postoperatively, costs begin to increase and frequently exceed the reimbursement in standard bundled payment models and Center for Medicare and Medicaid Services (CMS) standards. This is especially true for patients with postoperative PE or DVT, intensive care unit (ICU) admission, and other medical/psychiatric consultations (Baumgartner et al. 2018).

41.3.2 Postoperative and Discharge Considerations

Since the adoption of bundled payment models, the goal of the arthroplasty surgeon has been to manage the whole episode of care associated with the arthroplasty, and to minimize low value but expensive care practices (Gray et al. 2018). One such opportunity is in post-discharge planning. Discharge home, in most cases, either with or without home-care is an increasingly favored option, improving outcomes and cost (Keswani et al. 2016). The alternatives including discharge to skilled nursing or subacute rehab quickly increase episode costs for TKA and generally lead to worse outcomes.

The "risk assessment and prediction tool" (RAPT) is a frequently used assessment tool shown to be useful in predicting length of stay (LOS) requirements for patients undergoing TKA. RAPT accounts for

- Age
- Gender
- Ambulatory distance capability
- Level of assistance required for ambulation
- Level of community support
- Level of home support (Dibra et al. 2019)

It predicts whether patients will be appropriate for home discharge vs. requiring extended rehabilitation. Certain patients are unable to effectively discharge home due to their social support and functional status, and future reimbursement models will need to take this into account.

For TKA, there is emerging evidence that, for most patients, there is little difference in complications or readmission rates for patients undergoing outpatient surgery vs. those who have a short-stay surgery (Courtney et al. 2015; Bovonratwet et al. 2019; Gogineni et al. 2019). With similar outcomes, and substantially decreased costs, outpatient surgery has become a favorable pathway for optimizing value with TKA care for many patients. An increasing number of patients and surgeons are electing to proceed with outpatient surgery with promising outlook.

> Of note, hospitals and surgeons with a clearly defined care pathway postoperatively are associated with reduced costs and utilization compared to those without clearly defined pathways (Tessier et al. 2016).

Re-admission post-discharge after TKA has been shown to occur at a rate of approximately 4–10% (Gray et al. 2018; Keswani et al. 2016; Iorio et al. 2016); these re-admissions can be due to surgical or medical complications and greatly increase costs (Clair et al. 2016). One large academic center studied re-admission rates and associated cost status post TKA and discovered an 8% re-admission rate with a total average cost of $27,979 (range $4790–$40,774) for surgical complications (infection, wound complications, post-surgical pain) and average cost of $11,682 (range $3306–$24,076) for medical complications (Clair et al. 2016). Additionally, approximately 4% of TKA patients require manipulation. The most common surgical complications include infection and periprosthetic fracture while the most common medical complications are cardiovascular or pulmonary-related (Luzzi et al. 2018).

41.3.3 Revision TKA

Revision TKA will continue to increase in frequency and complexity for the next several decades. The most common diagnosis associated with revision TKA is prosthetic joint infection (PJI), followed by mechanical loosening, implant failure or breakage, and other mechanical complications of the prosthetic joint (Postler et al. 2018). Re-admission for revision TKA is also a significant cost. A recent study demonstrated that all-cause complication rate in a large cohort for patient's undergoing revision TKA was 37.2% compared to 2.5% for patient's undergoing primary TKA; the most common complication was infection (24.1%). Additionally, it was noted that index hospital cost for re-admission was approximately $7000 higher per episode of care for revision TKA re-admission when compared to primary TKA re-admission (Nichols and Vose 2016).

41

41.4 Reimbursement

> Healthcare in the United States is expensive, comprising close to 18% of the gross domestic product (GDP) expenditures (Papanicolas et al. 2018). A large part of this increase is due to the aging population and increasingly complex healthcare options.

Due to the age of the patient population undergoing TKA, CMS remains the primary payer for these surgeries. Traditionally, in the United States, surgical procedures have fallen into the fee-for-service model, in which each provider service, as well as any follow-up, generated separate payments (with the notable exception of the global period for physician services which excludes follow-up services from additional billing for 90 days).

Traditional fee-for-service models create a situation where healthcare delivery is prioritized over provision of health – thus there is little financial incentive to improve outcomes or reduce costs as each complication or re-admission generated even more revenue for a hospital system. Care coordination was uncommon in this setting. Similarly, there was no attention paid toward the use of post-acute care facilities, which billed independently of the physician practice. These trends have shifted since the onset of alternative payment models (APMs) and bundled payments with an increased emphasis on coordination of care between each provider and facility that takes care of the patient during a TKA care episode, including the surgeon, anesthesiologist, physical and occupational therapists, and nursing staff in both home nursing and inpatient settings (Rozell et al. 2016).

41.4.1 Payment Models

The comprehensive care for joint replacement (CJR) model was initiated by CMS in April 2016 and has been used in metropolitan statistical areas (MSAs) across the United States (Center for Medicare and Medicaid Innovation 2016). In addition, the CMS bundled payments for care improvement (BPCI) initiative has defined 4 categories of bundled payments (Bundled Payments for Care Improvement (BPCI) Initiative 2013). BPCI has many models, but model 2 is the most commonly used form (as described in ◘ Fig. 41.3) which includes

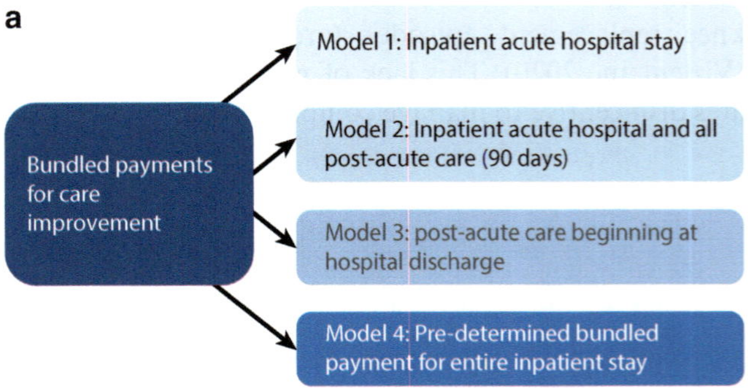

◘ **Fig. 41.3** **a, b** BPCI models. **a** The 4 versions of the BPCI model; care model 2 is the most commonly used option among total knee surgeons 35. **b** In a BPCI model 2 for TKA, billing and care are delivered as usual, with a post-hoc analysis of the spending. Participants are eligible for a repayment or a penalty based on performance throughout the program year 27

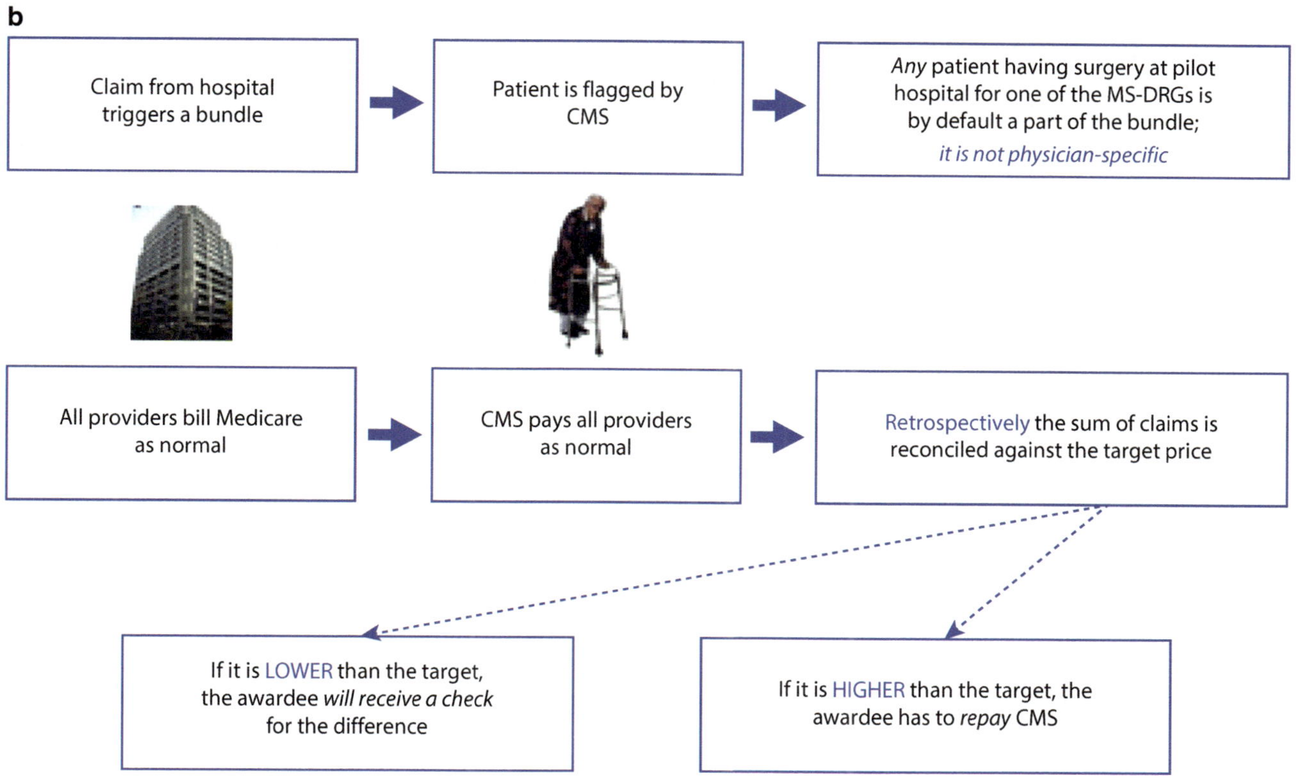

Fig. 41.3 (continued)

both upside and downside risk from the acute care episode and the post-acute phase of care.

Bundled payments have proven beneficial to all key players including the patient. They have helped to reduce costs via reduction of postoperative hospital LOS as well as the number of re-admissions. The physician's ability to effectively select patients for TKA and plan for their postoperative needs has been enhanced. As a result, overall cost has decreased and the relative value of TKA to the population has increased.

> Of note, TKA has been removed from the CMS inpatient-only (IPO) list effective January 2018, and site-neutral reimbursement is slated to begin in 2020 (Bundled Payments for Care Improvement (BPCI) Initiative 2013). These changes will have profound impact on and health systems alike as joint replacement surgery moves into the outpatient setting.

41.4.2 Limitations of New Payment Models

Bundled payments have, however, not been without their concerns. An initial concern was that bundled payments may allow for continued reimbursement reductions affecting compensation and possibly lead to decreasing quality, though multiple comparison studies of bundled payments and traditional payment models have largely mitigated this concern by demonstrating that quality does not suffer under the bundled payment model (Gray et al. 2018; Iorio et al. 2016; Dummit et al. 2016). As mentioned previously, a continued concern is that bundled payments may limit patient access due to increasingly stringent patient selection factors, a practice sometimes referred to as "cherry-picking" and "lemon-dropping" (Luzzi et al. 2018).

The two largest of these models, the BPCI and CJR, have variable financial risks to physician practices and hospitals, and it is unclear which of these mechanisms will sustain the longest-term increase in value of care.

> One may presume that a model that is voluntary and empowers physician decision-making and leadership, as in BPCI, would engender more successful long-term changes, though only time will tell.

There is no doubt that such mechanisms will drive down costs, but will they also endanger the autonomy of the orthopedic surgeon (as well as innovation and risk-taking)? Will the effect on value-based care be lasting? These are questions that will be answered in the coming years as bundled payments (will likely) become the standard across the United States. Expansion of bundled payments to smaller hospitals and less dense metropolitan statistical areas (MSAs) will likely require modifications as these "micropolitan" areas are unable to bear the financial risks of bundled payment models (Bundled Payments for Care Improvement (BPCI) Initiative 2013). Policy makers will need to take this risk into account when expanding bundle payment standards to smaller community hospitals with more diverse cases and less sub-specialization.

As previously discussed, most TKA operations are performed on patients over 60 years of age; as a result, Medicare is the primary payer for the lion's share of these procedures. It will be interesting to see the direction that private payers take over the coming years with relation to bundle payments. Although not as likely to have a large influence on total joint replacement, private payers are acutely interested in bundled payments involving younger populations such as in the maternity model (George 2018).

41.4.3 Gainsharing

Gainsharing, achieved through the identification and alignment of key stakeholders, will be essential to the success of a bundled payment model (Bosco et al. 2018). Cost savings must be shared across spheres to maintain adequate incentive for continued improvement. The financial risks must be acceptable to healthcare organizations of various sizes and revenue streams must remain steady. Hospitals cannot keep their doors open unless an adequate stream of revenue persists.

41.5 Big Data in TKA

In the world of big data, medicine must not be left behind. High-volume operations such as TKA require robust data collection that will be used in generating continued improvement for years to come. Not only will data be useful for continued improvement, it will also allow for necessary checks and balances in a system that, if too broadly applied, could lead to decreased availability of joint replacement (Navarro et al. 2018). Highly powered studies have already been used to demonstrate findings such as a decreased revision rate of TKA performed at high-volume centers compared to low-volume centers (Jeschke et al. 2017). Such studies have also shown that TKA performed at low volume centers will carry an increased risk of short-term complications. The collection of data from multiple studies is necessary for the publication of meta-analyses and level I evidence with translation for clinical practice. Easy access to this data is essential for continued production of high-quality evidence.

41.6 TKA Implants

The "Big 4" implant manufacturing companies – Stryker, Zimmer-Biomet, DePuy-Synthes, Smith & Nephew – have the majority of the market share in the world of total knee replacement implants. In an implant-driven subspecialty, it can be difficult to decipher outcomes data, oftentimes conveniently aligned with a company's marketing.

> Objective studies by third-party organizations are essential to an unbiased approach to implant characterization.

Commoditization

TKA implants comprise a significant proportion of total episode costs; in revision TKA there is yet higher implant-associated cost. It has been found that in America, implant costs vary widely; implant costs at hospitals above the 90th percentile are approximately double the implant costs of hospitals below the 10th percentile (Haas and Kaplan 2017). Generic implants have great potential for reducing costs. Much like the affordability of generic aspirin or acetaminophen, generic implants would allow for a more sustainable and affordable model for certain hospitals and populations. It has been shown that when implants are purchased from a less expensive physician-owned dealership there was no significant difference in outcomes or complications when compared to TKA with higher-cost industry-supplied implants (Baumgarten et al. 2019).

Unfortunately, there can be a drawback to commoditization. In the case of orthopedic joint replacement implants, commoditization may lead to a reduction in innovation and diminished funding for novel technologies in the treatment of end-stage osteoarthritis. Nonetheless, analysis of data surrounding the efficacy of generic TKA implants will be beneficial in the changing climate of healthcare reimbursement.

41.7 Cemented TKA

> Despite recent advances in press-fit, non-cemented TKA, a cemented knee arthroplasty remains, as of 2020, the gold standard.

Although cemented, hybrid, and non-cemented TKA all obtain similar patient-reported outcomes, non-cemented knees may have higher rates of revision than cemented based on currently available registry data

(Nugent et al. 2019). Standard cementing techniques are well established but variations exist among institutions.

41.7.1 Cementing Technique

Currently, at our institution, we primarily perform cemented TKA; press-fit implants are utilized on a case by case basis and are attending specific. Intravenous tranexamic acid is administered prior to incision. A standard medial parapatellar approach is used. Just prior to cementing, the tourniquet is inflated to achieve a pressure appropriate to patient habitus (typically 250–300 mmHg). The trial components are removed. For most TKA, two 40 g boxes of cement are adequate. A pulse lavage is used to remove debris from the bone surfaces to improve cement interdigitation. During final seating of the implants and during curing of the cement, we soak the knee with a dilute betadine solution as described by DellaValle et al., to minimize infection risk, which is both cost-efficient and powerful (Brown et al. 2012). A standard closure is used with a silver-impregnated colloidal dressing placed after closure. Early mobilization is emphasized, with the majority of patients staying in the hospital from zero to one night.

We find this approach to be the most effective in time, cost, and outcome, including patient satisfaction and infection prevention, with minimal complication profile.

41.7.2 Antibiotics in Bone Cement

Bone cement can elute antibiotics (antibiotic-laden bone cement, ALBC), and the elution properties are dependent on the amount of porosity of the cement mixture. This allows for a high local concentration of antibiotics for hours up to several days (Nugent et al. 2019). The use of ALBC in primary TKA in the United States is not standard, and from a US context it has not been proven efficacious within some clinical studies. However, the European and Australian joint registries show that commercially available antibiotic cement tends to be standard in primary TKA. For example, almost all TKAs in the United Kingdom use commercially available antibiotic cement, and up to 90% of primary TKAs in Europe use ALBC (Anagnostakos 2017).

The most common usage in the United States remains in staged revision cases. Several factors must be considered when using antibiotic cement (in particular in the context of admixing): risk for hypersensitivity exists, properties of the cement can be altered with the addition of antibiotics, and selection pressure creating drug resistance remains a possibility (albeit a limited one). In our opinion, antibiotic cement for primary joint replacement should be selectively used in patients with increased risk of infection, such as those with diabetes or other forms of immunocompromise, or prior open surgery with retained hardware.

41.8 Surgeons and the Economic Future of TKA

With changes coming secondary to advancing technology as well as increased administration and oversight, surgeons must be able to adapt and actively play a role in the economic decision-making related to providing care for patients with arthritis of the knee. Though algorithm medicine has proven beneficial in preventing errors and streamlining care, it remains the surgeon's responsibility to properly treat each unique patient. Surgeons cannot afford to take a backseat in the economic future of TKA; they must advocate with their hospitals, advocate with professional organizations, and strive to do what is right for the patient population – they must continue to innovate new care delivery models and provide increasingly high-valued care.

> As previously discussed, a "one-size-fits-all" model of bundled payments, without accounting for specific patient risk factors, would jeopardize the accessibility and quality of TKA.

Some research has focused on developing appropriate means for patient-specific, high-value payment models that will enable a continued improvement of outcomes important to patients while minimizing the use of low-efficacy treatments. One such model is the "condition-based bundle" for knee pain that has been recently implemented in both Texas and North Carolina in slightly different formats (Andrawis et al. 2019; O'Donnell et al. 2018). In these models, the goal is to utilize a team of providers to offer whatever is the most patient-centered and most favorable to long-term outcomes for a patient's knee pain in the setting of their personal health and social history.

Shared decision-making will also have substantial impact on the future of management of knee arthritis. Through shared decision-making programs, surgeons can ensure patient's needs are being met, and not the needs of the physician or the health plan. In some cases, this will involve alternative therapies, while in some it will involve bypassing much of the traditional "conservative" treatment algorithm (Sambare et al. 2017).

> The monumental increase in total joint replacement over the past few decades has led to the need for continued improvement. As the populations of developed nations continue to age, sustainable economic models are paramount.

Patients, surgeons, other providers, administrators, and policy makers should continue to strive for gainsharing that comes through improved quality, decreased cost, and an overall increase in value to our patients and to the healthcare system.

Take-Home Messages

- Management of symptomatic knee arthritis has high cost, with a substantial cost burden accrued in both the operative and non-operative phases of management; the benefit to society, however, of returning patients to work often makes TKA less costly especially for patients age 50 or younger.
- Though TKA has high economic cost, the surgery is highly effective at restoring quality-adjusted life years, a measure of cost-efficacy for medical treatments; cost-estimates vary from $18,000 to $28,000 per QALY, far below typical thresholds of $50,000 to be considered economically favorable.
- In the United States, TKA has been targeted for cost containment because of high utilization and its high proportion of health system and payer cost; this containment effort has led to the introduction of alternative payment models such as bundled payment models where providers are held to a target price for the episode costs.
- Though alternative payment models appear promising in early studies to reduce costs and maintain quality, concerns remain about the possibility that care access will be compromised and that continued cost-reduction will eventually erode the economic feasibility of caring for patients with symptomatic knee OA; future value-based programs will need to identify ways to economically reward high-value care for these patients.
- TKA implants are a significant cost associated with surgery and neutral outcomes data is necessary to show effectiveness.
- Cemented TKA remains standard in the United States despite uncemented options becoming increasingly available; the debate within the US continues whether antibiotic bone cement offers a more cost-effective alternative than plain bone cement – especially given the high costs associated with prosthetic joint infection

References

American Academy of Hip and Knee Surgeons (2019) Biologics for advanced hip and knee arthritis. American Association of Hip and Knee Surgeons. http://www.aahks.org/position-statements/biologics-for-advanced-hip-and-knee-arthritis/. Accessed 20 Dec 2019

American Academy of Orthopaedic Surgeons (2013) Clinical practice guideline on treatment of osteoarthritis of the knee. https://www.aaos.org/quality/quality-programs/lower-extremity-programs/osteoarthritis-of-the-knee/

Anagnostakos K (2017) Therapeutic use of antibiotic-loaded bone cement in the treatment of hip and knee joint infections. J Bone Jt Infect 2(1):29–37

Andrawis JP, McClellan M, Bozic KJ (2019) Bundled payments are moving upstream. In: NEJM Catalyst, Boston

Baumgarten KM, Chang PS, Looby PA, McKenzie MJ, Rothrock CP (2019) Do more expensive total knee arthroplasty prostheses provide greater improvements in outcomes over less expensive prostheses sold by a physician-owned distributorship? J Am Acad Orthop Surg 27(23):e1059–e1067

Baumgartner BT, Karas V, Kildow BJ et al (2018) Inpatient consults and complications during primary total joint arthroplasty in a bundled care model. J Arthroplast 33(4):973–975

Bedair H, Cha TD, Hansen VJ (2014) Economic benefit to society at large of total knee arthroplasty in younger patients: a Markov analysis. J Bone Joint Surg Am 96(2):119–126

Bedard NA, Dowdle SB, Anthony CA et al (2017) The AAHKS clinical research award: what are the costs of knee osteoarthritis in the year prior to total knee arthroplasty? J Arthroplast 32(9S):S8–S10. e11

Bosco JA, Harty JH, Iorio R (2018) Bundled payment arrangements: keys to success. J Am Acad Orthop Surg 26(23):817–822

Bovonratwet P, Fu MC, Tyagi V, Gu A, Sculco PK, Grauer JN (2019) Is discharge within a day of total knee arthroplasty safe in the octogenarian population? J Arthroplast 34(2):235–241

Brown NM, Cipriano CA, Moric M, Sporer SM, Della Valle CJ (2012) Dilute betadine lavage before closure for the prevention of acute postoperative deep periprosthetic joint infection. J Arthroplast 27(1):27–30

Bundled Payments for Care Improvement (BPCI) Initiative: General Information. In: (CMS) CfMaMS, ed 2013

Center for Medicare and Medicaid Innovation. Comprehensive care for joint replacement model. In: Services CfMaM, ed 2016

Clair AJ, Evangelista PJ, Lajam CM, Slover JD, Bosco JA, Iorio R (2016) Cost analysis of total joint arthroplasty readmissions in a bundled payment care improvement initiative. J Arthroplast 31(9):1862–1865

Courtney PM, Rozell JC, Melnic CM, Lee GC (2015) Who should not undergo short stay hip and knee arthroplasty? Risk factors associated with major medical complications following primary total joint arthroplasty. J Arthroplast 30(9 Suppl):1–4

Dibra FF, Silverberg AJ, Vasilopoulos T, Gray CF, Parvataneni HK, Prieto HA (2019) Arthroplasty care redesign impacts the predictive accuracy of the risk assessment and prediction tool. J Arthroplast 34(11):2549–2554

Dillon CF, Rasch EK, Gu Q, Hirsch R (2006) Prevalence of knee osteoarthritis in the United States: arthritis data from the Third National Health and Nutrition Examination Survey 1991-94. J Rheumatol 33(11):2271–2279

Dummit LA, Kahvecioglu D, Marrufo G et al (2016) Association between hospital participation in a medicare bundled payment initiative and payments and quality outcomes for lower extremity joint replacement episodes. JAMA 316(12):1267–1278

Fabre-Aubrespy M, Ollivier M, Pesenti S, Parratte S, Argenson JN (2016) Unicompartmental knee arthroplasty in patients older than 75 results in better clinical outcomes and similar survivorship compared to total knee arthroplasty. A matched controlled study. J Arthroplast 31(12):2668–2671

George J (2018) IBC, Rothman sign long-term deal. In: Philadelphia Business Journal, Philadelphia

Gogineni HC, Gray CF, Prieto HA, Deen JT, Boezaart AP, Parvataneni HK (2019) Transition to outpatient total hip and knee arthroplasty: experience at an academic tertiary care center. Arthroplast Today 5(1):100–105

Gray CF, Prieto HA, Duncan AT, Parvataneni HK (2018) Arthroplasty care redesign related to the Comprehensive Care for Joint Replacement model: results at a tertiary academic medical center. Arthroplast Today 4(2):221–226

Haas DA, Kaplan RS (2017) Variation in the cost of care for primary total knee arthroplasties. Arthroplast Today 3(1):33–37

Hutt JR, Craik J, Phadnis J, Cobb AG (2015) Arthroscopy for mechanical symptoms in osteoarthritis: a cost-effective procedure. Knee Surg Sports Traumatol Arthrosc 23(12):3545–3549

Iorio R, Clair AJ, Inneh IA, Slover JD, Bosco JA, Zuckerman JD (2016) Early results of medicare's bundled payment initiative for a 90-day total joint arthroplasty episode of care. J Arthroplast 31(2):343–350

Jeschke E, Citak M, Gunster C et al (2017) Are TKAs performed in high-volume hospitals less likely to undergo revision than TKAs performed in low-volume hospitals? Clin Orthop Relat Res 475(11):2669–2674

Keswani A, Tasi MC, Fields A, Lovy AJ, Moucha CS, Bozic KJ (2016) Discharge destination after Total joint arthroplasty: an analysis of postdischarge outcomes, placement risk factors, and recent trends. J Arthroplast 31(6):1155–1162

Kurtz S, Ong K, Lau E, Mowat F, Halpern M (2007) Projections of primary and revision hip and knee arthroplasty in the United States from 2005 to 2030. J Bone Joint Surg Am 89(4):780–785

Losina E, Walensky RP, Kessler CL et al (2009) Cost-effectiveness of total knee arthroplasty in the United States: patient risk and hospital volume. Arch Intern Med 169(12):1113–1121; discussion 1121–1112

Luzzi AJ, Fleischman AN, Matthews CN, Crizer MP, Wilsman J, Parvizi J (2018) The "bundle busters": incidence and costs of postacute complications following total joint arthroplasty. J Arthroplast 33(9):2734–2739

Navarro SM, Wang EY, Haeberle HS et al (2018) Machine learning and primary total knee arthroplasty: patient forecasting for a patient-specific payment model. J Arthroplast 33(12):3617–3623

Nichols CI, Vose JG (2016) Clinical outcomes and costs within 90 days of primary or revision total joint arthroplasty. J Arthroplast 31(7):1400–1406. e1403

Nugent M, Wyatt MC, Frampton CM, Hooper GJ (2019) Despite improved survivorship of uncemented fixation in total knee arthroplasty for osteoarthritis, cemented fixation remains the gold standard: an analysis of a National Joint Registry. J Arthroplast 34(8):1626–1633

O'Donnell J, Saunders RS, Japinga M et al (2018) Expanding payment reforms to better incentivize chronic care for degenerative joint disease. In: Health affairs blog, vol 2020. Health Affairs

Pabinger C, Lothaller H, Geissler A (2015) Utilization rates of knee-arthroplasty in OECD countries. Osteoarthr Cartil 23(10):1664–1673

Papanicolas I, Woskie LR, Jha AK (2018) Health care spending in the United States and other high-income countries. JAMA 319(10):1024–1039

Parvizi J, Huang R, Restrepo C et al (2017) Low-dose aspirin is effective chemoprophylaxis against clinically important venous thromboembolism following total joint arthroplasty: a preliminary analysis. J Bone Joint Surg Am 99(2):91–98

Pinto D, Robertson MC, Hansen P, Abbott JH (2012) Cost-effectiveness of nonpharmacologic, nonsurgical interventions for hip and/or knee osteoarthritis: systematic review. Value Health 15(1):1–12

Postler A, Lutzner C, Beyer F, Tille E, Lutzner J (2018) Analysis of total knee arthroplasty revision causes. BMC Musculoskelet Disord 19(1):55

Rozell JC, Courtney PM, Dattilo JR, Wu CH, Lee GC (2016) Should all patients be included in alternative payment models for primary total hip arthroplasty and total knee arthroplasty? J Arthroplast 31(9 Suppl):45–49

Sambare T, Uhler L, Bozic KJ (2017) Shared decision making: time to get personal. In: NEJM Catalyst. New England Journal of Medicine, Boston

Santaguida PL, Hawker GA, Hudak PL et al (2008) Patient characteristics affecting the prognosis of total hip and knee joint arthroplasty: a systematic review. Can J Surg 51(6):428–436

Smith WB 2nd, Steinberg J, Scholtes S, McNamara IR (2017) Medial compartment knee osteoarthritis: age-stratified cost-effectiveness of total knee arthroplasty, unicompartmental knee arthroplasty, and high tibial osteotomy. Knee Surg Sports Traumatol Arthrosc 25(3):924–933

Tessier JE, Rupp G, Gera JT, DeHart ML, Kowalik TD, Duwelius PJ (2016) Physicians with defined clear care pathways have better discharge disposition and lower cost. J Arthroplast 31(9 Suppl):54–58

Turkiewicz A, Petersson IF, Bjork J et al (2014) Current and future impact of osteoarthritis on health care: a population-based study with projections to year 2032. Osteoarthr Cartil 22(11):1826–1832

Vizient Inc (2020) Vizient DRG Compare- 469 470. Vizient, Inc. https://www.vizientinc.com. Accessed 6 Feb 2020

Wu CH, Gray CF, Lee GC (2014) Arthrodesis should be strongly considered after failed two-stage reimplantation TKA. Clin Orthop Relat Res 472(11):3295–3304

Conceptualizing the Problem of Cost in Cemented Total Knee Arthroplasty

Kenoma Anighoro and Kevin J. Bozic

Contents

E. Hansen, K.-D. Kühn (eds.), *Essentials of Cemented Knee Arthroplasty*,
https://doi.org/10.1007/978-3-662-63113-3_42

42.1 Introduction

Substantial research and press attention have been focused on the drivers of increasing health care costs in recent years. In the United States, it is commonly cited that economic activity in the health care sector accounts for nearly a fifth of total GDP (Papanicolas et al. 2018). It is also often pointed out that many individuals are overburdened by medical bills, some of whom have been bankrupted by health care treatment costs (Brill 2015). This is weighed against the apparent lack of superiority of US health outcomes when compared with those of other OECD countries. These realities are intertwined but not interchangeable. In some publications, "cost" refers to overall economic activity in the health care sector (i.e., societal cost); alternatively, the term may refer to revenues accrued to health systems via claim reimbursements (i.e., payer costs); or to costs borne by patients themselves (i.e., out of pocket costs). It is interesting to note, however, that other economic sectors which constitute significant swaths of economic output are not considered as "costs", per se. For example, we do not generally speak in terms of "automobile costs" or "food and beverage costs" when referencing the aggregate market capitalizations of companies in those sectors. Nor do we refer to consumer prices in these markets as costs.

> The various stakeholders in the health care system – patients, payers, purchasers, physicians, suppliers, health care systems, and society – experience costs differently. When the type of cost and relevant stakeholder are not specified, there can be a conflation of cost, revenue, and profit.

Any discussion of cost must start with identifying the stakeholder bearing that cost.

> From the business perspective, the cost of a product or service would encapsulate raw supply and personnel costs required for its production.

Because costs to other stakeholders are by nature "downstream", it is useful to have a clear understanding of the true cost to the entity delivering the service.

This chapter's discussion of cost will explore total knee arthroplasty (TKA) cost in terms of the fundamental inputs essential for the provision of the service by the health care institution. We make the assumption that the impact on other stakeholders, including the patient, would be derived from the business costs.

42.2 Methods for Assessing Cost in TKA

From an institutional perspective, cost in TKA may be assessed in several ways. Many examples in the literature provide estimates of cost extrapolated from insurance charges or payer reimbursements, because this data can be extracted fairly easily (Ong et al. 2006). By aggregating reimbursements for procedures for a given time period and multiplying an expected cost/revenue ratio, a workable cost estimate can be produced (Stargardt 2008). These rates, reimbursements, and cost/revenue ratios are components of institutional chargemasters, which are proprietary rubrics of cost, payment, and charge information for health care systems. They are highly variable between institutions as there is usually a large discrepancy between charge and reimbursement, and even a greater discrepancy between reimbursement and actual cost. The discrepancies arise as a result cost shifting, multilateral contract negotiations between suppliers, payers, and providers, and the existence of moral hazard due to the existence of third-party payers. The heterogeneity of these rubrics would make them poor sources for universally applicable financial information. To simplify the cost discussion here, we will avoid using references to charge, reimbursement, or revenue. We will instead attempt to identify true costs.

Intuitively, the cost of TKA is based on the cost of direct or indirect supply costs and personnel costs (i.e., salaries).

> The true cost of medical services is generally difficult to accurately measure due to the high level of human processing required to furnish medical services, and the inherent variability of the processing methods used.

Fortunately, in the realm of TKA, many of the inputs have become standardized and certain general expectations can be assumed. Ongoing research continues to illuminate areas of potential standardization to decrease the variability in total joint arthroplasty care. Because of this reality, we have hope of assessing the cost of TKA in a manner that may be relevant to a variety of different settings.

There are two primary methods by which costs are accounted in health care settings:

- traditional accounting, and
- time-driven activity-based accounting (Palsis et al. 2018; Akhavan et al. 2016).

> In traditional accounting, total expenses are calculated from overall business activity for a given period of time and these costs are allocated to departments – called cost centers – based on their average proportionate utilization.

This is a "top-down" accounting process which relies on assumptions about how departments generate certain expenses.

> In time-driven activity-based accounting, all business processes are broken down into their component steps by creating detailed process maps from observation. The personnel and resource time dedicated to each of the steps is determined, and the cost of the overall process is calculated.

The per-minute cost of each resource (e.g., operating room, operating table, etc.) and personnel (e.g., circulating nurse, surgical technician, etc.) is generated and a more granular service cost may be calculated in a "bottom-up" fashion.

This method offers a more granular cost estimate, but a shortcoming of this accounting is that total costs will only be as robust as the process maps they are based on, and distributive costs which are shared by all patients could be missed – for example, the cost of maintaining a sterile processing center, a responsive IT department, stocked operating room inventory, or a cleanly atmosphere – as they cannot be easily attributed to a particular patient or service experience.

To simplify discussions of cost in terms of surgical resource utilization, a report in the *Journal of the American Medical Association* in 2018 by Childers et al. sought to determine an average cost per operating room minute (Childers and Maggard-Gibbons 2018). Their estimate was calculated from total yearly expenses attributed to the surgery and recovery departments of 302 California-based hospitals divided by the respective aggregate surgery times for the same year. Using this method, they found that, on average, OR services cost \$36 to \$37 per minute across all activities. Notably, this estimate excluded surgeon, anesthesia, radiology, implant, or special equipment costs.

42.3 Comparing Costs of Cemented and Non-cemented TKA

> In the case of cemented TKA vs. non-cemented TKA, the most significant cost differences result from materials.

Assuming that team composition and other equipment are more or less unchanged, the cost differential is driven primarily by the cost of tools, disposables, and implants. *Cemented TKA* requires the use of cement, associated disposables, and the implants themselves.

Non-cemented arthroplasty obviates the need for cement but the implants are produced by alternate manufacturing methods to enhance their bony fixation such as tantalum augmentation, porositization, and/or hydroxyapatite coating (Kamath et al. 2011; Harwin et al. 2013).

> Cementless implants are sold at a premium presumably to compensate the more specialized manufacturing processes necessary for their production.

The study by Lawrie et al. provided useful cost estimates and analysis regarding cemented and cementless TKA comparisons (Lawrie et al. 2019). In their study they reported that the premium for a cementless implant can be around \$366 (differing of course by implant manufacturer and negotiated price agreements). On the other hand, PMMA cement and associated disposables could cost about \$325. If antibiotic-loaded cement were deemed necessary, this would represent yet more cost – an additional \$175 per 40 g over non-antibiotic PMMA.

Some studies have demonstrated that the cost of cement can be decreased dramatically by routinely limiting quantity per case. Yan et al. found that during routine TKA only about 30 g of cement were retained while about 90 g were wasted, representing a significant opportunity for waste and cost reduction (Yan et al. 2018). Modifying cement protocol can generally have a significant impact on reducing cost while obtaining the desired result (Kee et al. 2018).

Lawrie et al. demonstrated that even when considering the upfront cost parity of the implants and materials, there was a benefit in terms of operative time from omitting the cement curing process.

> Non-cemented TKAs were of shorter duration by about 10 min in their study (Harwin et al. 2013). When quantifying cost in terms of OR minutes, this would yield real cost differences and significant aggregate savings from personnel and equipment costs.

The time savings may also result in a reduction in rates of adverse outcomes, as some studies have reported that decreased operative time in TKA is associated with decreased rates of infection and lengths of stay (George et al. 2018; Sodhi et al. 2019). Other studies suggest that these time savings may not have a clinical impact after a threshold of 100–120 min operative time (Pugely et al. 2015; Ravi et al. 2019). From an institutional perspective, time savings of about 10 min per case could reduce the opportunity cost, increasing the likelihood that more such services could be rendered in a given time frame (Chatterjee et al. 2009). The decreased time would allow personnel to pursue other essential activities and minimize personnel exhaustion, and improve patient outcomes.

> Implant costs generally account for a substantial proportion of overall TKA costs, as high as a third of overall episode cost – even when perioperative care is included (Carducci et al. 2019).

This aspect of cost depends in large part on negotiated prices between the vendor and the institution. The study by Robinson et al. demonstrated that a substantial portion of intra- and inter-hospital TKA cost variation (97.5% of total variation) could be attributed to non-patient factors such as procedure volume, institution teaching status, or surgeon preference (Robinson et al. 2012). This is made clear by the fact that there are significant differences in price for the same implant in different geographies. Separate from the particular features of implants and their relative production costs, categorical cost savings could be achieved by improved provider-supplier deals. Some groups have had success with collective bargaining by having multiple surgeons subscribe to a particular vendor and achieving improved purchase deals (Boylan et al. 2019).

> When considering the time horizon of TKA failure, cemented knee arthroplasty has historically performed better, and there is much more available data (Fricka et al. 2019).

Yet more recent studies which explore the long-term survival of cemented and non-cemented TKA have found more similar implant survival rates (Fricka et al. 2019). This may be due to more recent innovations in orthopedic basic science and implant manufacturing.

> Later generation non-cemented constructs appear to have high 5- to 10-year survival rates >91% with good satisfaction rates (>98%), but longer follow-up data remains limited (Drexler et al. 2012; Hardeman et al. 2006).

> Cemented TKA has much longer-run data with 15- to 20-year survival rates in excess of 85% compared to lower rates for non-cemented cohorts (Ranawat et al. 2012).

As would be expected, a revision situation adds cost that is not accounted for in the initial cost analysis. Revision surgeries are more technically demanding, requiring more personnel time and material resources than primary arthroplasty. Implant costs may be nearly 200% higher, and average surgery durations may also double (Weber et al. 2018). Revision knee arthroplasty is often associated with longer lengths of stay and higher infection rates, which account for additional costs.

> Even a small improvement in survival rate for cemented arthroplasty would confer a substantial long-term cost advantage when extrapolated over the entire patient population. It remains to be seen whether long-term survival rates of cementless implants are comparable to their cemented counterparts.

It will be essential for future studies to elucidate the difference in long-term outcomes and revision rates between these two categories of implants, and to determine which patient populations would most benefit from each type of implant.

42.4 Cost Considerations in Special Populations

Antibiotic-loaded cement may benefit some populations at higher risk of infection (e.g., revisions) in terms of infection reduction, but results in routine primary TKA are mixed (Tayton et al. 2016; King et al. 2018). Moreover, unique complications such as renal failure may be introduced by the use of antibiotic-loaded cement (Chan et al. 2019). Pre-mixed antibiotic-loaded cement currently is FDA approved only for treatment of infected total joint arthroplasty, specifically in the second phase of a two-stage revision after infection has been cleared (e.g., simplex P tobramycin; PROSTALAC is approved as a temporary hip arthroplasty implant in infection revisions). These options are not approved for infection prevention in primary TJA (Nelson 2004).

Alternatively, absorbable antibiotic coatings such as hydrogel or silver may be used as tools to reduce infection rates. In the study by Romano et al., the authors found no significant difference in overall outcome, but there was a lower rate of superficial surgical site infection with hydrogel use (Romanò et al. 2016). The long-term implications of this were unclear given the limited follow-up, an average of 14.5 months. If the difference found in this study were true, it would equate to an approximate 6% absolute risk reduction, corresponding to a number-needed-to-treat of 17. Depending on the negotiated price for the material, routine use could generate significant expense. It could be argued that it would be more cost-effective to treat patients with a short course of oral antibiotics when clinical suspicion arose. Pre-emptive use may be warranted in some subpopulations, however: Trentinaglia et al. explored the economic benefit of antibiotic-loaded cement, hydrogel coating, and silver coating in primary TKA and found that these interventions could become cost neutral if pre-surgical infection risks were 1.5%, 2.6%, and 19.2%, respectively (Trentinaglia et al. 2018).

Some TKA systems offer all-polyethylene tibial components as an alternative to standard metal-backed components.

> All-polyethylene tibial components are significantly less expensive than metal-backed components, by as much as 33%. The survivorship of all-polyethylene tibial components have been shown to be equivalent to metal-backed components, especially in the elderly population (Gustke and Gelbke 2017).

In a study by Browne et al., their team used sensitivity analysis to show that all-polyethylene tibial components could be cost-effective unless there was a > 9% increased failure rate relative to metal-backed tibia options (Browne et al. 2018). In the appropriate population, all-polyethylene tibial components may be the more cost-effective option.

Detailed exploration of unsatisfactory outcomes after TKA has led some authors to explore the potential impact of metal allergy as a cause of a subset of TKA failures.

> It is hypothesized that allergy to nickel, chromium, cobalt, or polymethylmethacralate cement may contribute to earlier aseptic failure.

To address these concerns, surgeons have considered employing alternate bearing surfaces to minimize allergen exposure and improve outcomes.

Titanium-based implants and oxidized zirconium (Oxinium) implants exist which would allow avoidance of allergenic materials. Some manufacturers also produce cobalt-chrome implants with "hypersensitivity-friendly" oxidized titanium nitride or zirconium nitride coatings, conferring the benefits of strong bearing surfaces with reduced allergenic exposure (Ajwani and Charalambous 2016). These special implants are more expensive than their standard counterparts, and long-term failure rates may be higher (Vertullo et al. 2017). The added cost may be warranted in certain patient subpopulations, however.

> Currently, there is no reliable method of identifying patients who would most benefit from hypoallergenic implants. Self-reports of metal allergy have failed to correlate with demonstrable improvements in outcome in large retrospective studies (Schmidt et al. 2019).

Skin patch testing and lymphocyte testing may more accurately identify patients with reactivity, but such testing would be costly to apply on routine basis in its current form, and positive results have not been shown to correlate with worse outcomes even when allergenic implants are used (Münch et al. 2015; Yang et al. 2019). There have been case reports, however, of substantial benefit in patients with severe sensitivities (Stathopoulos et al. 2017). It remains to be seen whether future research will illuminate the clinical relevance of metal allergy in TKA.

42.5 The Importance of Incorporating Value Measurement

Value is the essential counterpart to cost assessment.

> Value should be defined from the perspective of the ultimate health care customer – the patient. When considering options to reduce cost in health care, care must be taken to ensure that value is not compromised.

Many of the studies in the current arthroplasty literature evaluate process factors such as institutional outcomes (e.g., length of stay, home discharge rate, etc.) or event rates (e.g., revision rate, transfusion rate, infection rate, etc.) as surrogates for value, but these do not necessarily correspond to patient-perceived value (Andrawis et al. 2013). Interventions with apparently similar complication rates may in fact have significantly different clinical or functional outcomes.

> Ideally, value assessment would be based on patient-reported outcome measures (PROMs), or health status instruments, that better represent clinical effectiveness from the patient's perspective (Franklin et al. 2013).

Existing examples include the Western Ontario and McMaster Universities Osteoarthritis Index (WOMAC) or Knee Injury and Osteoarthritis Outcome Score (KOOS). Assessment of the comparative effectiveness of different TKA-related treatment modalities as measured by PROMs is not routinely included in the published literature, so it is impractical to truly compare value associated with many of the alternatives considered in TKA (Makhni et al. 2015). We assume here that value to patients is more-or-less similar among the options available so that they could be interchangeable. It is important to recognize that this may not be true, despite apparently similar institutional outcomes or clinical event rates.

In this chapter's discussion of cost, we take for granted that value is preserved. If we explore in more depth, we may find that some options force value tradeoffs that are not satisfactory from a patient perspective. Future research will need to explore cost and value simultaneously.

Take-Home Messages

- Cost may be interpreted differently depending on the stakeholder, so cost analysis must first identify the perspective.
- Cost accounting in health care is inconsistent and unreliable, which may thwart attempts to define cost drivers. Time-driven activity-based costing offers a solution to increase the granularity of cost accounting, but can be highly resource intensive.
- Cemented TKA has long history of success, but cementless TKA could prove to be a viable alternative based on more recently published studies. Cementless implants tend to be marginally more expensive than cemented implants but obviate the need for cement and its associated expense.
- Special populations may benefit from more expensive alternatives such as antibiotic-impregnated cement, antibiotic coatings, or nickel-sparing biomaterials, but further research is needed to determine when these should be applied.
- Value is a necessary consideration in all cost analysis. When cost is considered in isolation, efforts to reduce cost can inadvertently compromise value from a patient's perspective.

References

Ajwani SH, Charalambous CP (2016) Availability of total knee arthroplasty implants for metal hypersensitivity patients. Knee Surg Relat Res 28(4):312

Akhavan S, Ward L, Bozic KJ (2016) Time-driven activity-based costing more accurately reflects costs in arthroplasty surgery. Clin Orthop Relat Res 474(1):8–15

Andrawis JP, Chenok KE, Bozic KJ (2013) Health policy implications of outcomes measurement in orthopaedics. Clin Orthop Relat Res 471(11):3475–3481

Boylan MR et al (2019) Preferred single-vendor program for total joint arthroplasty implants: surgeon adoption, outcomes, and cost savings. JBJS 101(15):1381–1387

Brill S (2015) America's bitter pill: money, politics, backroom deals, and the fight to fix our broken healthcare system. Random House Trade Paperbacks

Browne JA et al (2018) When would a metal-backed component become cost-effective over an all-polyethylene tibia in total knee arthroplasty? Am J Orthop (Belle Mead NJ) 47(6):1–8

Carducci MP et al (2019) Variation in the cost of care for different types of joint arthroplasty. J Bone Joint Surg Am 102(5):404–409

Chan JJ et al (2019) Antibiotic-loaded bone cement in primary total knee arthroplasty: utilization patterns and impact on complications using a national database. J Arthroplast 34(7):S188–S194

Chatterjee A et al (2009) Opportunity cost: a systematic application to surgery. Surgery 146(1):18–22

Childers CP, Maggard-Gibbons M (2018) Understanding costs of care in the operating room. JAMA Surg 153(4):e176233–e176233

Drexler M et al (2012) Cementless fixation in total knee arthroplasty: down the boulevard of broken dreams–opposes. J Bone Joint Surg 94(11_Supple_A):85–89

Franklin PD, Harrold L, Ayers DC (2013) Incorporating patient-reported outcomes in total joint arthroplasty registries: challenges and opportunities. Clin Orthop Relat Res 471(11):3482–3488

Fricka KB, McAsey CJ, Sritulanondha S (2019) To cement or not? Five-year results of a prospective, randomized study comparing cemented vs cementless total knee arthroplasty. J Arthroplast 34(7):S183–S187

George J et al (2018) How fast should a total knee arthroplasty be performed? An analysis of 140,199 surgeries. J Arthroplast 33(8):2616–2622

Gustke KA, Gelbke MK (2017) All-polyethylene tibial component use for elderly, low-demand total knee arthroplasty patients. J Arthroplast 32(8):2421–2426

Hardeman F et al (2006) Cementless total knee arthroplasty with Profix: a 8-to 10-year follow-up study. Knee 13(6):419–421

Harwin SF et al (2013) Excellent fixation achieved with cementless posteriorly stabilized total knee arthroplasty. J Arthroplast 28(1):7–13

Kamath AF et al (2011) Prospective results of uncemented tantalum monoblock tibia in total knee arthroplasty: minimum 5-year follow-up in patients younger than 55 years. J Arthroplast 26(8):1390–1395

Kee JR et al (2018) Standardization of acrylic bone cement mixing protocols for total knee arthroplasty results in cost savings. Orthopedics 41(5):e671–e675

King JD et al (2018) The hidden cost of commercial antibiotic-loaded bone cement: a systematic review of clinical results and cost implications following total knee arthroplasty. J Arthroplast 33(12):3789–3792

Lawrie CM et al (2019) The cost of implanting a cemented versus cementless total knee arthroplasty. Bone Joint J 101(7_Supple_C):61–63

Makhni EC et al (2015) What are the strength of recommendations and methodologic reporting in health economic studies in orthopaedic surgery? Clin Orthop Relat Res 473(10):3289–3296

Münch HJ et al (2015) The association between metal allergy, total knee arthroplasty, and revision: study based on the Danish Knee Arthroplasty Register. Acta Orthop 86(3):378–383

Nelson CL (2004) The current status of material used for depot delivery of drugs. Clin Orthop Relat Res 427:72–78

Ong KL et al (2006) Economic burden of revision hip and knee arthroplasty in Medicare enrollees. Clin Orthop Relat Res 446:22–28

Palsis JA et al (2018) The cost of joint replacement: comparing two approaches to evaluating costs of total hip and knee arthroplasty. JBJS 100(4):326–333

Papanicolas I, Woskie LR, Jha AK (2018) Health care spending in the United States and other high-income countries. JAMA 319(10):1024–1039

Pugely AJ et al (2015) The incidence of and risk factors for 30-day surgical site infections following primary and revision total joint arthroplasty. J Arthroplast 30(9):47–50

Ranawat CS et al (2012) Cementless fixation in total knee arthroplasty: down the boulevard of broken dreams–affirms. J Bone Joint Surg 94(11_Supple_A):82–84

Ravi B et al (2019) Surgical duration is associated with an increased risk of periprosthetic infection following total knee arthroplasty: a population-based retrospective cohort study. EClinicalMedicine 16:74–80

Robinson JC et al (2012) Variability in costs associated with total hip and knee replacement implants. JBJS 94(18):1693–1698

Romanò CL et al (2016) Does an antibiotic-loaded hydrogel coating reduce early post-surgical infection after joint arthroplasty? J Bone Joint Infect 1:34

Schmidt KJ et al (2019) Self-reported metal allergy and early outcomes after total knee arthroplasty. Orthopedics 42(6):330–334

Sodhi N et al (2019) Operative times can predict and are correlated with lengths-of-stay in primary total knee arthroplasty: a nationwide database study. J Arthroplast 34(7):1328–1332

Stargardt T (2008) Health service costs in Europe: cost and reimbursement of primary hip replacement in nine countries. Health Econ 17(S1):S9–S20

Stathopoulos IP et al (2017) Revision total knee arthroplasty due to bone cement and metal hypersensitivity. Arch Orthop Trauma Surg 137(2):267–271

Tayton ER et al (2016) The impact of patient and surgical factors on the rate of infection after primary total knee arthroplasty: an analysis of 64 566 joints from the New Zealand Joint Registry. Bone Joint J 98(3):334–340

Trentinaglia MT et al (2018) Economic evaluation of antibacterial coatings on healthcare costs in first year following total joint arthroplasty. J Arthroplast 33(6):1656–1662

Vertullo CJ et al (2017) Twelve-year outcomes of an oxinium total knee replacement compared with the same cobalt-chromium design: an analysis of 17,577 prostheses from the Australian Orthopaedic Association National Joint Replacement Registry. JBJS 99(4):275–283

Weber M et al (2018) Revision surgery in total joint replacement is cost-intensive. Biomed Res Int 2018:8987104

Yan JR et al (2018) Cement waste during primary total knee arthroplasty and its effect on cost savings: an institutional analysis. Cureus 10(11):e3637

Yang S et al (2019) Lymphocyte transformation testing (LTT) in cases of pain following total knee arthroplasty: little relationship to histopathologic findings and revision outcomes. JBJS 101(3):257–264

Cementing Technique

Contents

Polymethylmethacrylate Cements for Endoprosthetics

Klaus-Dieter Kühn

Contents

E. Hansen, K.-D. Kühn (eds.), *Essentials of Cemented Knee Arthroplasty*,
https://doi.org/10.1007/978-3-662-63113-3_43

43.1 Introduction

PMMA bone cements have been successfully used in surgery for over 60 years to anchor artificial joints, and as a local drug carrier. As a two-component system, the liquid monomer is mixed with the polymer powder before use in a suitable mixing bowl or in a mixing system to form a homogeneous dough. The cement dough can have a high, medium, or low viscosity (HV, MV, LV), depending on the composition of the bone cement used (Lewis 1997; Kühn et al. 2005a; Kühn 2014; Bistolfi et al. 2019). LV cements are preferably used in the spine to fill vertebral bodies with a thin injection needle (Lewis 2006). In a few countries, LV cements are also found in knee endoprosthetics, although registry data point out that LV cements show lower survival rates. The "trans-atlantic paradox" shows the different attitudes of surgeons in the United States and in Europe regarding the use of local antibiotics via ALBC. ALBC is routinely used in primary interventions in Europe, while plain bone cement (PBC) is used in the United States (Sanz-Ruiz et al. 2017). An actual review of the National Joint Registry of England and Wales including over 700,000 total knee arthroplasties (TKAs) demonstrated the use of ALBC was associated with a decreased risk of revision as compared to TKAs implanted with PBC. ALBC was associated with a 19% lower rate of septic and aseptic revision as compared to PBC (Jameson et al. 2019). Furthermore, the additional cost of ALBC per TKA case is \$300–\$500 as compared to PBC. The additional cost of ALBC in 115 patients would be \$34,000–\$57,000. Given the average cost of treating one periprosthetic joint infection (PJI) is approximately \$100,000 the use of ALBC potentially results in significant cost savings (Jameson et al. 2019; Sanz-Ruiz et al. 2020).

HV cements, together with the MV version, are used worldwide as anchoring material in over 90% of artificial joints. Highly viscous cements can, therefore, be described as a "gold standard", especially in combination with suitable antibiotics to prevent periprosthetic infections (Colas et al. 2015; Chan et al. 2019).

> High-viscosity PMMA cements are mainly used in large joints, whereas the use of low viscosity is relatively rare.

> ALBC is used in most primary procedures to prevent periprosthetic infections. ALBCs reduce the risk of biofilm formation on the implant surface. Antibiotics only have an adjuvant function, the therapy is the surgery!

The modern cementing technique allows for the clinician to mix the cements in partially (e.g., SMART Mix®, CEMVAC®, MixeVac®) or completely closed cementing systems (e.g., PALAMIX®, PALACOS® R+G PRO, CEMVAC®). For the surgeon, the point in time when the cement paste is ready for application is crucial. In addition, a sufficient processing width is desired by most users. The complete setting of the cement paste should not take too long, since the duration of surgery has a significant influence on the effectiveness of a treatment. However, in surgical practice, different operations are carried out in parallel, so that such key figures alone are of little significance. In addition, quality should take precedence over speed; effectiveness is ultimately measured by the overall success, which in the case of anchored artificial joints is reflected in the long-term survival of the implants.

> Modern cementing technology today offers completely closed cementing systems in which the application phase of the dough is defined.

Cemented prostheses show the best survival rates in patients who were treated with local antibiotic treatment with broad-spectrum antibiotics in addition to systemic antibiotics during surgery. This ensures that hematogenically dispersed bacteria and those found on the skin are significantly reduced by systemic administration of antibiotics while local antibiotic administration builds up a protective shield as a colonization barrier around the implant. This sensible prophylactic approach has led to infection rates remaining at a relatively low level to this day (Buchholz et al. 1981; Phillips et al. 2006; Jameson et al. 2019; Zhang et al. 2019) (▶ Sect. 43.2). Therapeutically, local administration of antibiotics is usually used in combination with systemic antibiotics. Narrow-spectrum antibiotics are combined with ALBC containing broad-spectrum antibiotics because the elution behavior is significantly improved by synergy (Kühn 2014). The elution properties of commercially available ALBCs also vary considerably and valid release data are only available for a few products. PALACOS®R+G was approved as a drug at the end of the 1960s and publications on the comparatively excellent elution behavior of gentamicin from the cement matrix were submitted to the health authorities for approval. When determining the elution behavior, a reproducible method must be used.

Unfortunately, many data presented in the literature are difficult to compare. There are microbiological limits to the number of inhibition tests, which often go unnoticed. Recent studies show marginal differences in the inhibition peak test of PMMA cements (Squire et al. 2008) and low antibiotic releases below the minimal inhibitory concentration (MIC) after 24 h (Meyer et al. 2011). Our own investigations on elution and on inhibition yard tests show large differences between the PMMA cements on the market (Kühn 2018).

> Broad-spectrum antibiotics (antibiotics with broad efficacy) should be used systemically (e.g., cephalosporins) and locally (e.g., aminoglycosides) for prophylaxis; narrow-spectrum antibiotics (antibiotics with narrow efficacy) (e.g., vancomycin against MRSA) should be used in a targeted therapy.

Today, ALBCs – especially revision cements with more than one antibiotic – are hardly ever approved as Class III medical devices, not least because the requirements for certification are disproportionately high – much to the disadvantage of patients and surgeons. In surgical practice, antibiotics are, therefore, manually added to the cement, in the best case depending on the patient's as well as the hospital's antibiogram. However, manual mixing also involves some risks and the surgeon bears responsibility in this "off label" use.

> PMMA bone cements were used to be medicinal products and were redefined as medical devices in 1998. When antimicrobial agents are added manually, the medical device is modified and the surgeon bears responsibility in this "off label" use.

43.2 History

PMMA bone cements were developed based on dental materials (Smith 2005; Smith and Bains 1956; Kühn 2014). Initially, some changes in formulation were marginal. However, with increasing interest from surgeons, the original dental products were increasingly adapted to the requirements as anchoring material for artificial joints. The formulation in the two older products PALACOS®R and Simplex®P has probably not changed significantly over the decades. In contrast, the formulation of many other products on the market has changed over the years, sometimes significantly. Under pharmaceutical legislation this would only have been possible to a very limited degree. However, this has been facilitated under the Medical Device Directive via change notifications, of which some manufacturers make use. Just replacing the polymers leads to a change of about 80–90% of the formulation, resulting in a completely new product. Chemically similar polymers are not identical in their properties, therefore, changing polymers without clinical data involves considerable risks. For that reason, only a few PMMA bone cements were commercially available before 1998, and the formulations had to be stated exactly on the packaging and in the package insert.

> Chemically similar polymers or co-polymers are not identical in their properties.

At that time, all individual components of the liquid monomer and polymer powder were regarded as medicinal products. Requirements and handling of these medicinal products were strictly regulated by Good Manufacturing Practices (GMP). Only a few manufacturers of bone cements had a license as pharmaceutical companies that could produce and distribute such products. With the changeover to the Medical Device Directive, PMMA bone cements were no longer subject to pharmaceutical legislation. Today, numerous cements are commercially available and while they all may seem to be very much alike, the only thing they have in common is the basic chemical principle of radical polymerization.

> PMMA bone cements were developed based on dental materials. Older products such as Simplex®P and Palacos®R have probably still retained their basic formulation to this day.

The first ALBC was Palacos®R with added gentamicin. Buchholz et al. (1984), together with Heraeus (Kulzer), added various amounts of gentamicin powder to the Palacos powder in the late 1960s and tested the release behavior of the incorporated active ingredient. Gentamicin was very well released from the Palacos matrix. The success story of ALBC in endoprosthetics via Palacos®R+G (former Refobacin®, Palacos®R, Palacos®R cum Gentamicin, and Palacos®R with Gentamicin) began with Heraeus (Kulzer), who started out marketing their products themselves, but later outsourced marketing to various distribution partners (Merck, Schering-Plough, Smith & Nephew, Biomet, Zimmer) (Kühn 2007, 2014). In 2017, the Australian Orthopedic Association (AOA) published a supplementary report on bone cement in hip and knee arthroplasty. The report covered 293,025 primary TKA procedures and 9753 revisions between 1999 and 2015 (AOA 2019).

> Palacos®R+G (syn. Refobacin®, Palacos®R, Palacos®R with Gentamicin) was the first ALBC on the market (1969). The use of Palacos®R+G reduced the infection rate (■ Fig. 43.1) of initially almost double-digit percentages to below 1% (Buchholz et al. 1981; Phillips et al. 2006).

In addition to gentamicin (PALACOS®, Simplex®, SmartSet® etc.), tobramycin (Simplex®), erythromycin and colistin (Simplex®), clindamycin (PALACOS®), and vancomycin (PALACOS® and others) are commercially used in ALBC. The so-called "revision cements" include Copal®G+C, Copal®G+V, Antibiotic Simplex with Erythromycin and Colistin, and VancoGenx. Copal® products, in particular, are often used today as the basis for cemented revision procedures in

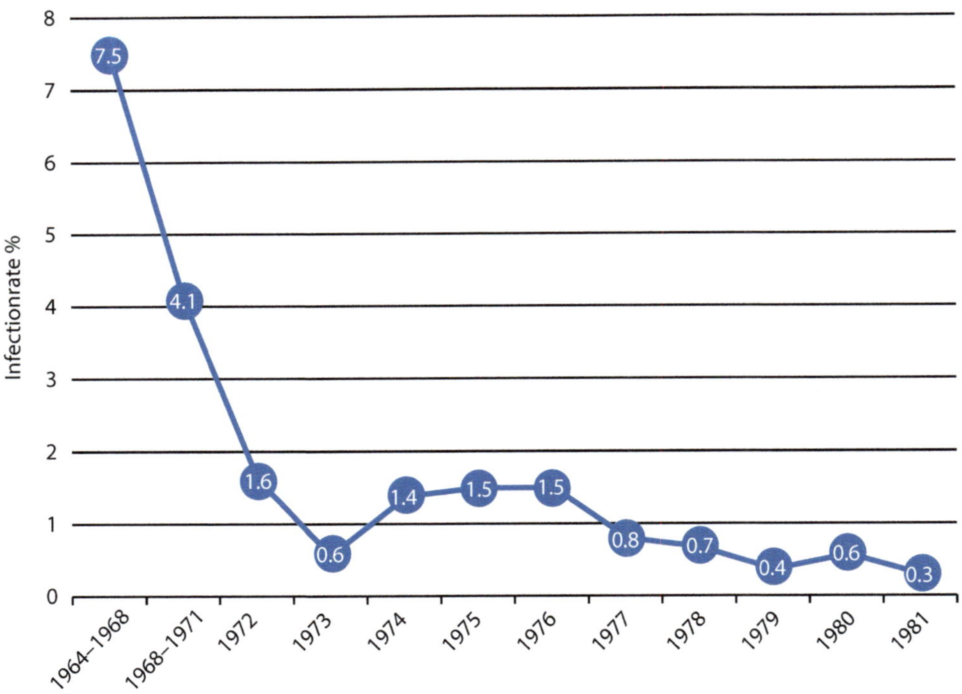

Fig. 43.1 Reduction rate of infections after introduction of PALACOS®R+G in the market below than 1%. (Data according to Buchholz et al. 1981; Phillips et al. 2006). The use of local antibiotics has also led to a drastic reduction in the risk of infection

one-stage and multiple-stage surgery (Kendoff et al. 2015; Sprowson et al. 2016; Kühn 2018). The combinations are adapted to the surgical practice. Microbiotic analyses in antibiograms show which active ingredients eliminate the detected germs. Intelligent combinations include gentamicin with vancomycin and gentamicin with clindamycin. Different synergies can be observed with gentamicin and vancomycin. While vancomycin, in particular, is more effective against certain germs in the presence of gentamicin, vancomycin elution is also increased in the presence of gentamicin. The molecule gentamicin acts as a "backpack" carrying the large molecule vancomycin out of the cement matrix.

> Revision cements contain combinations of antibiotics with intelligent synergistic effects which increase the clinical effectiveness and elution properties.

Clindamycin in combination with gentamicin has the synergistic advantage of being effective against about 90% of all relevant germs found in joint infections. This extension of the spectrum of action has, among other things, prompted clinics to use this combination in cement in high-risk patients in primary surgery (Adelaziz et al. 2019). Gentamicin and clindamycin are also released particularly well from PMMA cement as low-molecular-weight hydrophilic agents.

> Active ingredient combinations effectively prevent the development of resistance as the different antibiotics damage the bacterial cell at different targets.

Active ingredient combinations have already been successfully used for many serious diseases. Microbiologically, combinations of antibiotics of different antibiotic classes in surgery still have an important effect based on the different targets at which the respective antibiotics attack bacteria. By evolution, each administration of antibiotics can result in the accidental development of resistant bacteria. However, if antibiotics attack the bacteria in two different ways at once, the potential development of resistance is significantly reduced.

43.3 Cement Viscosity

PMMA bone cements consist of two essential components, the liquid monomer and the polymer powder. Monomers include the basic substance of all PMMA cements, methylmethacrylate (MMA), as well as the activator for radical polymerization, di-methyl-para-toluidine (DmpT), hydroquinone (HQ) as a radical scavenger and, if necessary, a dye (e.g., chlorophyll). The polymer powder contains homo- or co-polymers which have a significant influence on

- the properties of the cement later anchored in the body,
- the initiator benzoyl peroxide (BPO) which together with the DmpT of the liquid initiates polymerization,
- an X-ray contrast medium (zirconium dioxide [ZO] or barium sulfate [BS]),

- a dye, and
- in the case of ALBCs, one or two antibiotics (Bistolfi et al. 2019).

Polymer powder and monomer liquid are usually available in a ratio of 2:1, the polymer powder in a sterile bag and the liquid in a sterile amber glass ampoule. The polymer powder is sterilized by γ-radiation or ethylene oxide, the liquid is sterile-filtered. The sterilization process of the polymer powder has a significant influence on the polymer properties. The molecular weight of the polymers is significantly reduced by γ-rays, and the handling properties and viscosity are also influenced (Lewis and Mladsi 1998; Deb 2008; Kühn et al. 2005b). Ethylene oxide (Eto) sterilization, on the other hand, shows almost no interaction with the polymer. The following parameters change by γ-irradiation of the powder (sterile) compared to the non-sterile powder:

Influence of γ-Irradiation on Polymer Powder
- Powder color: slightly changed (white to slightly grey)
- Doughing time (much later)
- Working time (extended)
- Setting time (much later)
- Viscosity profile (changed)
- Molecular weight (significantly reduced, approx. 50%)
- ASTM/ISO standard mechanicals (initially high, then significantly reduced by aging)
- Aging (increased)

Mixing the components results in a homogeneous dough. However, mixing also means energy input: The stronger the mixing process, the shorter the handling properties of the cement used. Furthermore, the viscosity behavior of PMMA cements is essentially influenced by the following properties:

Factors Influencing PMMA Viscosity
- Ambient temperature
- Component temperature (e.g., cooled cement)
- Mixing procedure (e.g., speed of mixing)
- Powder–liquid ratio
- BPO(initiator)–DmpT(activator) ratio
- Physical properties of the polymer powder (surface of the beads)
- Swelling behavior of the powder with MMA
- Chemical properties (composition of the polymers/co-polymers)
- Mixing device (e.g., vacuum, speed, nozzle shape)

> The sterilization of the polymer powder has a significant influence on the cement properties. γ-Rays change polymers permanently and lead to accelerated aging; ethylene oxide does not change the polymer.

Charnley (1970) concluded, the more powerfully and the longer the cement components are mixed, the more porous the cement will be in the dough phase. This particularly applies to the mixing of low-viscosity cements. LV cements are quickly mixed homogeneously, so no additional energy input is required. When mixing LV cement under vacuum, it should be noted that too high a vacuum can cause the monomer to boil and thereby form numerous and sometimes large gas bubbles in the cement.

> With low-viscosity PMMA cements, the liquid monomer can be brought to the boiling point in vacuum and many air bubbles can be formed in the cement paste.

A study by Buller et al. (2020) showed higher odds of aseptic loosening by using HV cements compared to LV cements with a higher exothermic reaction of HV cements (Webb and Spencer 2007). The authors report results with Simplex®HV; PALACOS®R served as reference. However, in contrast to PALACOS®R, Simplex®HV has a significantly lower viscosity, so tendencies toward aseptic loosening were found with the LV material, but not with the HV cement.

The results of Buller et al. (2020) are in strong contrast to the register data of the National Joint Registry (NJR) (Jameson et al. 2019) and Northern European countries, which show best survival rates (Kaplan Mayer Curve) with HV PMMA cements (Espehaug et al. 2002) (■ Fig. 43.2).

> High-viscosity PMMA cements are used in cemented endoprosthetics in about 90% of all major joint operations and are considered the gold standard. Independent register data show superior survival rates of HV cements compared to LV cements.

T_{max} of cements especially depends on the MMA and BPO content of the PMMA cement used. While the MMA content of many cements is similar (powder–liquid ratio 2:1), the BPO content can vary considerably. Especially Simplex®P has the highest BPO content on the market and, therefore, tends to have a higher setting temperature.

> T_{max} of PMMA cements is not determined by viscosity but by the amount of MMA and BPO.

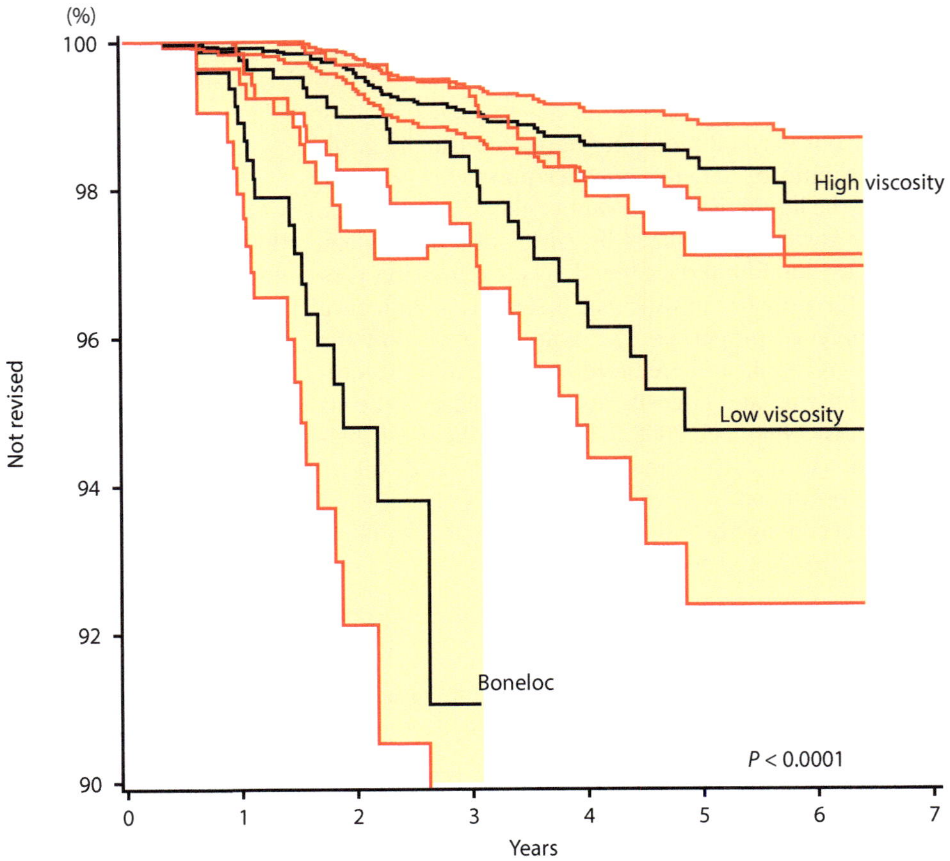

Fig. 43.2 Cemented prostheses anchored with HV cements show best survival rates

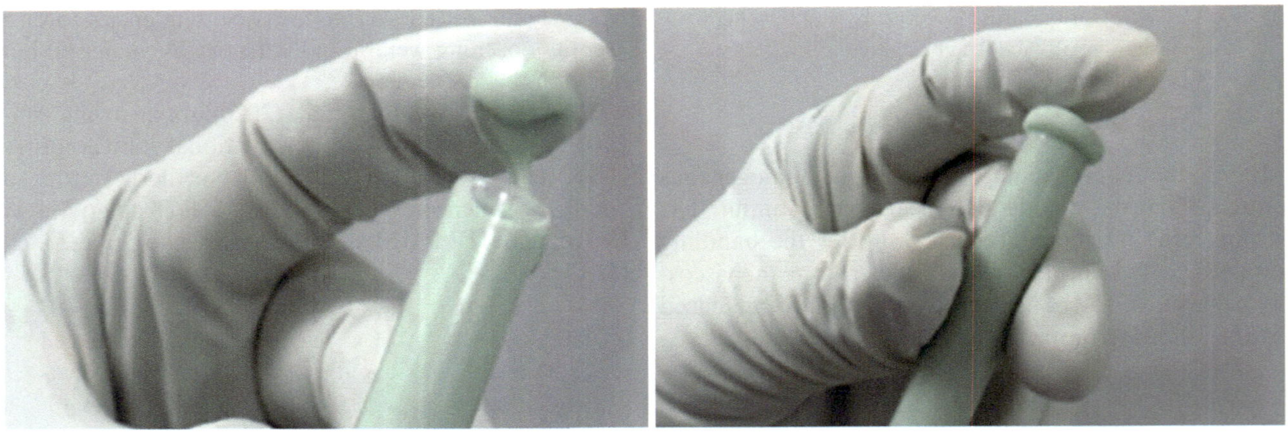

Fig. 43.3 "Doctor's finger test" according to ASTM F451/ISO 5833. Sticky cement dough (*left*) and cement reaching the doughing time of PMMA cements (*right*)

43

43.4 Flow Behavior and Intrusion

Ideally, bone cements are used when the cement is no longer sticky. The standards ASTM 451 and ISO 5833 valid for PMMA bone cements have specified a "doctor's finger test" for this purpose (ASTM F451-99a 2014; ISO 5833 2002) (Fig. 43.3). ASTM standard tests are done at 20 °C, ISO standard tests at 23 °C (Table 43.1). The mean value of a double determination of one package each (40 g/20 mL) is determined as doughing time (DT).

Table 43.1 Doughing time mean of 4 commercial PMMA cements according to ASTM 451 and ISO 5833

Cement	ASTM 451 at 20 °C	ISO 5833 at 23°
Palacos®R	75 s	55 s
SmartSet® HV	75 s	65 s
Palacos® MV	135 s	80 s
Simplex®P	300 s	220 s

> Doughing time is a measure of the ideal time for cement application in the body and is defined as the time when the cement dough is no longer sticky.

This so-called doughing time has historically been defined as a measure of the ideal time for manual cementing of the bone. When the standard was introduced, considerable fluctuations in results obtained were already noted. This was due to the fact that in Europe doughing time was measured with a glass rod and in the United States with a finger in a latex glove. In addition, measurements were also made at different ambient temperatures.

Considerable differences were found between the various cements. At that time, Simplex®P had a DT about 4 min longer than that of Palacos®R. The standards committee explained this by the different viscosity progression of the cements.

> Historically, doughing time has been tested to determine the time when the cement dough is no longer sticky after start of mixing. When using closed cementing systems without cement contact, doughing time again becomes important.

With the introduction of modern cementing technique, DT was no longer considered important at first. However, with the introduction of many new PMMA cements with unknown handling properties, it became clear that DT also represents a check on whether the cement was produced in accordance with the specifications. In addition, when using closed cementing systems, contact with the cement dough may be absent and thus a direct manual determination/estimation of when the dough is tack-free can be made.

43.5 Doughing Time and Intrusion

The doughing time of PMMA cement is carried out in a double determination with a powder-free latex glove. For this purpose, the cement is not extruded, but only stripped at the top of the nozzle, so that the monomer does not evaporate too quickly and distort the results (Fig. 43.3). Cement units are conditioned at 20 °C/23 °C ± 1 °C. Subsequently, the DT is determined according to ASTM F451/ISO 5833. Directly after the determination of DT, the intrusion is determined 1 min, 2 min, and 3 min after the tested DT.

Compared to the 3 other PMMA cements investigated, Palacos®MV has a different mixing ratio of 44 g/20 mL. This 10% difference in mass may significantly influence our test results.

Simplex®P cement dough is known to be tack-free on the surface earlier while on the inside the dough clearly is still sticky. Therefore, the DT of Simplex®P cannot be determined beyond doubt. The manufacturer also refers to this phenomenon in the package insert and recommends that surgeons process Simplex®P only after 3–4 min.

> DT values according to ASTM 451 and ISO 5833 are not comparable, since the measurement is made at different component and ambient temperatures. In addition, cements may already be tack-free on the surface, while the dough is still sticky on the inside (e.g., Simplex®P).

The determination of intrusion is mainly based and influenced on the results of the DT determination, as the measurement is performed 1 min after reaching DT. For this purpose, the cement is placed in a cylindrical form with 4 holes of 1 mm of diameter each and pressed into the 4 holes with a punch pressure of 49 N. The measurement is carried out according to ISO at 23 °C or according to ASTM at 20 °C. Shaped bodies with 4 holes and the corresponding pins are produced. The height of the pins in mm corresponds to the intrusion (Fig. 43.4).

However, as mentioned above, not every cement is ready for application after reaching the DT according to the standard determination. This is due to the behavior of some polymers or co-polymers and their interaction with the starter system (BPO-DmpT) for polymerization. For example, Simplex®P contains a styrene co-polymer and the BPO is polymerized into polymer beads. This reduces quick availability of the BPO. In many other PMMA cements, the BPO is freely present in the polymer and is immediately available. The voluminous styrene-containing co-polymer powder of Simplex®P is wetted by the monomer liquid with a time delay, which may also be a reason why the cement paste produced is initially dry. The dry top layer of the dough apparently results in Simplex®P being free of surface tackiness according to ASTM or ISO, while the dough still is quite sticky on the inside. Therefore, additional waiting time is recommended for the application, so that the cement can optimally be used.

> The optimum time for cement application in the bone is associated with a certain viscosity. The dough should be tack-free and able to withstand bleeding pressure.

However, this also means that the intrusion of Simplex®P cannot be determined at the time of DT according to ASTM or ISO, but only after an addi-

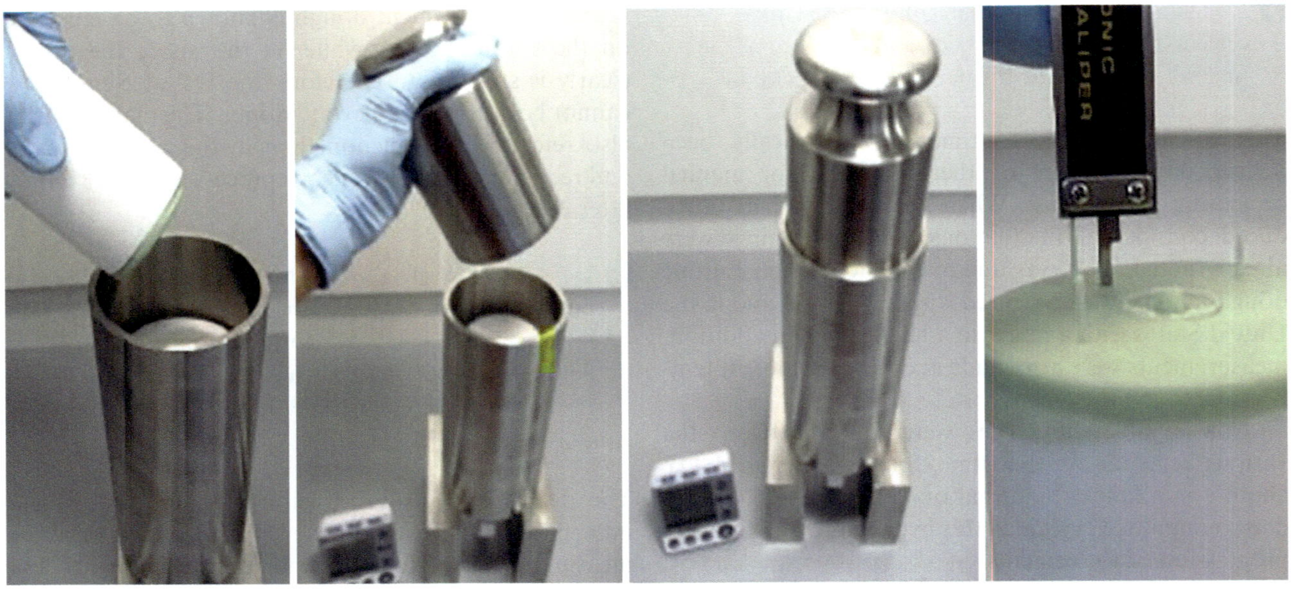

Fig. 43.4 Intrusion measurement and specimen with 4 holes to detect the intrusion (in mm) 4-times

Table 43.2 Intrusion measurement [mm] according to ASTM F451/ISO 5833 at 20 °C, intrusion at the time after doughing state is reached [min]

Product	1 min	2 min	3 min
Palacos®R	11.4 mm	10.1 mm	3.1 mm
SmartSet HV	11.7 mm	4.8 mm	2.9 mm
Palacos MV	16.8 mm	8.2 mm	2.1 mm
Simplex P	15.4 mm	7.5 mm	2.2 mm

tional waiting phase recommended by the manufacturer (+3–4 min). Since the intrusion capacity of the cements should represent cement penetration into the cancellous bone at the time of application (+1 min), intrusion results can only be compared if the operative basis – i.e., the start of the application phase – applies.

Theoretically, all PMMA-based bone cements should have a comparable viscosity at the optimal application time, which leads to comparable penetration into the cancellous bone (Table 43.2).

43

While the mixing systems used in the operating room can influence DT and intrusion, the waiting time after reaching DT is highly essential. With high-viscosity Palacos®R, the ASTM/ISO intrusions are between 4 mm and 6 mm. Without taking the waiting time into account, Simplex®P has penetration depths of 8–12 mm (Fig. 43.5a).

However, if the waiting time of 3–4 min recommended the manufacturer is considered after DT, intrusion of Simplex®P is comparable (approx. 4 mm) to that of highly viscous Palacos®R (Fig. 43.5b) because then the viscosity of both cements is comparable (Table 43.2)!

> If used correctly, Simplex®P and Palacos®R show comparable intrusion in the bone.

The use of low-viscosity PMMA cements is often linked to easy mixability and ideal interdigitation with the cancellous bone (Lewis and Carroll 2002). Theoretically, low-viscosity bone cements can only have a better penetration depth into the bone if they are introduced to the body too early, i.e., if they are not applied correctly! Regardless of the classification HV, MV, or LV cements, the use of these cements in the body is always associated with a comparable viscosity. The technical basis for this is the determination of DT. If LV cements are applied too early (before DT is reached) there is a risk of the dough pouring out. In this phase, LV cement cannot withstand the bleeding pressure yet, and mixing of cement and blood can easily occur. This leads to a lasting mechanical weakening of the cement matrix. In addition, cement constituents can more easily enter the venous system and thus increase the risk of embolism.

> Low-viscosity bone cements are often introduced to the body too early. This is associated with higher risks of embolism and necrosis. Blood can easily mix with the cement dough and significantly weaken the cement matrix after setting.

In a so-called bleeding apparatus, Lee (2005) explained that the bleeding pressure will force LV cement brands out of the bone and blood can be entrapped in the cement dough. Because of the low DT and short working time, LV cements are often applied too early to the body. In addition, vacuum mixing of LV cements may be performed only under a low vacuum of approxi-

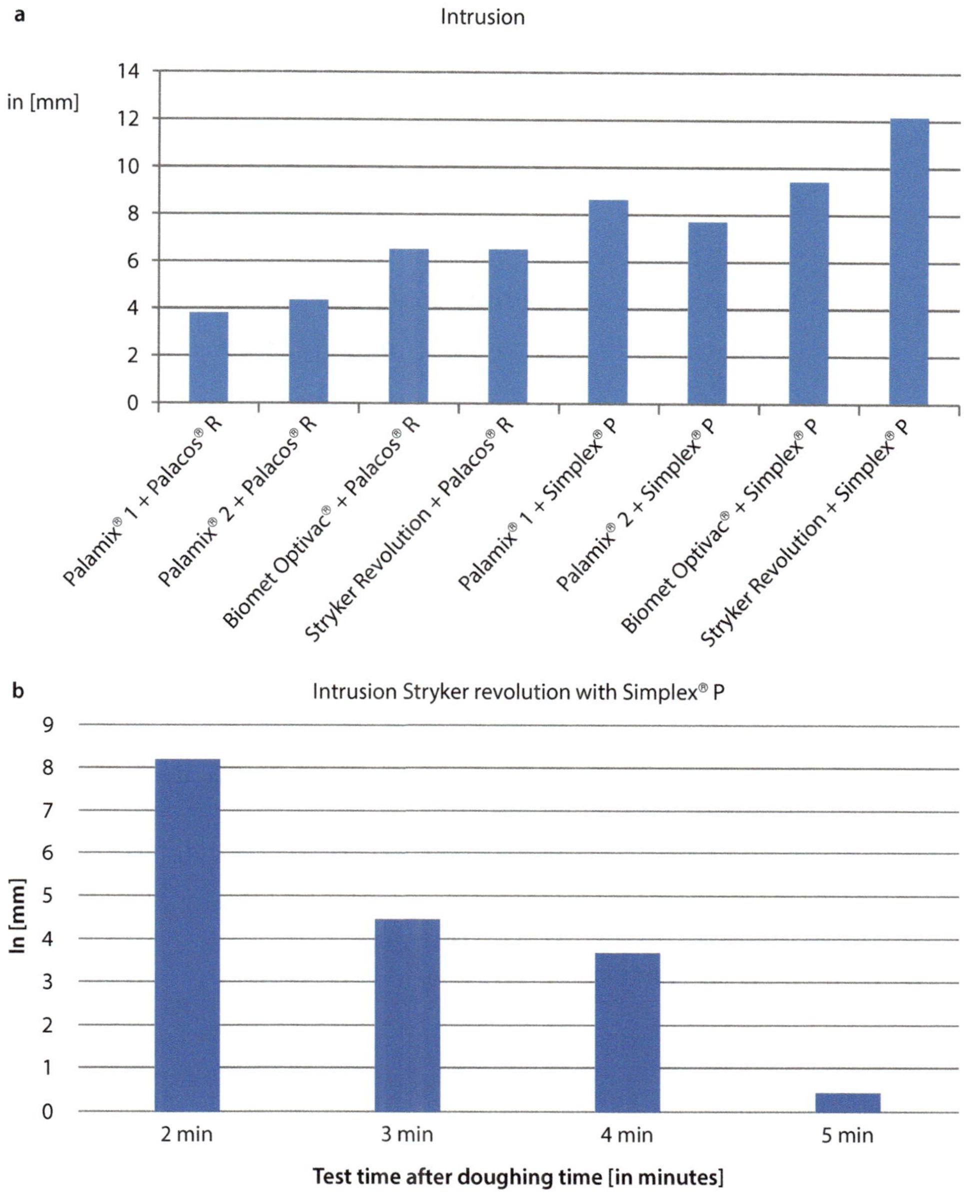

Fig. 43.5 **a** Comparison of intrusion according to ASTM F451/ISO 5833 after mixing of Palacos®R and Simplex®P in various mixing systems. **b** Intrusion of Simplex®P 2, 3, 4 and 5 min after reaching DT

mately 550 mbar. However, such a low vacuum will not be sufficient to fully eliminate the pores in the dough (Draenert et al. 1999). Therefore, vacuum mixing at room temperature at a pressure of 15 mbar will result in a boiling monomer due to its vapor pressure being a function of temperature.

Furthermore, too deep an intrusion into the bone can be associated with a high cement surface in the bone, which carries an additional necrotic risk. The drainage systems (bloodstream, metallic prosthesis, tissue) can then no longer neutralize the heat development of the deeper-lying cement.

43.6 PMMA Cement When Loaded with Antibiotics Serves as an Active Drug Carrier Reducing Infection Rates and Mortality

Periprosthetic joint infection and cancer can share similar traits (Benharroch and Osyntsov 2012). Mortality rates in oncology have been carefully documented and declined. On the other hand, mortality rates of PJI are often underreported. In 2013, the American Cancer Society published a comparison of deaths from vari-

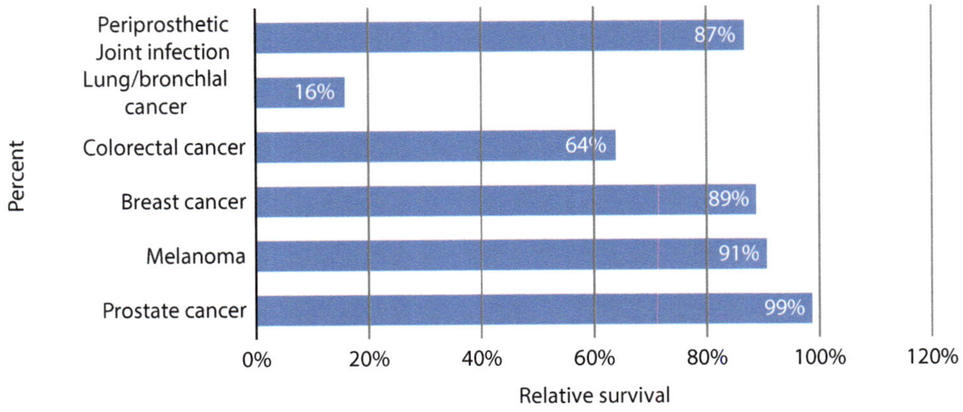

Fig. 43.6 Comparison of mortality from PJI with other serious illnesses. (Data according to Zmistowski et al. 2013)

ous cancers and after PJI. According to this source, the percentage of patients dying from PJI complications is comparable to the percentage of patients dying from breast cancer (Fig. 43.6). About a quarter of all patients treated for PJI die within 5 years (Zmistowski and Parvizi 2013; Hotchkiss and Moldawer 2014).

> Mortality from PJI is comparable to that from breast cancer.

Zmistowski et al. (2013) described the risk of 1-year mortality due to PJI in comparison with other serious illnesses. They concluded that mortality was significantly higher ($p < 0.001$) in patients with PJI compared with those undergoing aseptic revision arthroplasty at 90 days (3.7% vs. 0.8%), 1 year (10.6% vs. 2.0%), 2 years (13.6% vs. 3.9%), and 5 years (25.9% vs. 12.9%).

> Periprosthetic infections and oncological diseases have common features. In many cases, this also includes malnutrition which often massively impairs the further course of the disease and is often unnoticed.

43.7 Malnutrition as an Underestimated Risk Factor for Deep Wound Infection

Malnutrition has been shown to be an independent risk factor for multiple postsurgical complications following TJA, in addition to increasing postoperative mortality (Kamath et al. 2017). However, malnutrition is thought to impair wound healing and prolong inflammation by reducing collagen synthesis and fibroblast proliferation.

> When admitted to hospital 30–55% of hospitalized patients are malnourished (Támer et al. 2009).

Table 43.3 Malnutrition as an independent risk factor: retrospective study of 4551 revision total knee arthroplasty patients (Kamath et al. 2017)

Albumin <3.5 g/dL	OR
Any complication	2.74
Wound infection	2.57
Deep wound SSI	2.30
Pneumonia	2.84
Urinary tract infection	3.01
Acute renal failure	7.89
Sepsis	5.3

Even worse, 70% of patients are even more malnourished when discharged from hospital (Table 43.3).

> Malnutrition is a modifiable risk factor which causes 2.5 times more wound infections and 8 times more acute renal failures (ARF).

Usually, PJIs are initiated during or immediately after the surgery (Nasser 1999). The seed for PJIs is usually laid perioperatively, significantly influenced by the hygiene habits in the operating theatre and the operating algorithm of the hospital. Therefore, the strategical focus is on the prevention of infections, especially dreaded biofilm formation (Shahi and Eajazi 2015; Althans et al. 2017). In addition to a systemic administration of antibiotics, ALBCs play a special and meaningful role. In a meta-analysis of a large patient population, Parvizi et al. (2008) were able to show that the risk of infection can be reduced by >50% in primary interventions using ALBC (Fig. 43.7). Colas et al. (2015) also see the lowest risk of infection when using ALBC.

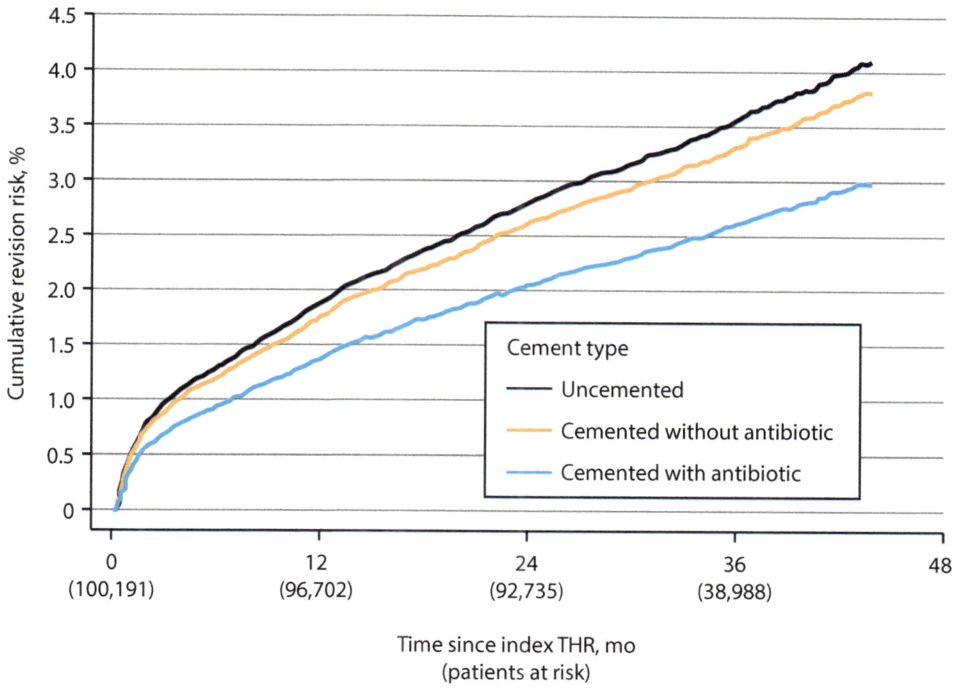

Fig. 43.7 Cumulative revision risk according to cement type. Patients at risk are given at baseline and yearly in the first 3 years. At the maximum follow-up time of 44 months there were 5378 patients at risk at 44 months of follow-up. *THR* total hip replacement

> PJIs are usually initiated perioperatively. The seed for infections is laid perioperatively. Prophylactic use of systemic antibiotics reduces hematogenically spreading germs. Locally applied antibiotics in cement reduce the risk of biofilm formation.

Systemic doses of antibiotics (1.5–2.0 g) are administered approx. 20–30 min before the incision. They serve to lower the number of possible germs in the blood and thus significantly reduce the risk of infection. Systemically administered antibiotics are readily available to the body and are rapidly distributed through the bloodstream. However, areas that are difficult to access and have poor blood circulation are less penetrated, so that smaller amounts of antibiotics get there. This is particularly noticeable in the bone near the joints, which in a healthy state may also receive nutrition from the movement of the cartilage. The cartilage in turn reacts sensitively to antibiotics and may be rapidly damaged by certain active substances.

However, a destroyed joint with considerable cartilage damage requires an antibiotic cover to prevent infection. Systemic administration of antibiotics often is not sufficient, so that an additional local administration of antibiotics (0.5–2.0 g) is necessary in order to penetrate joint areas with poor blood supply. Local antibiotics are delivered directly via the bone into the joint in a protracting manner and keep antibiotic levels stable over a reasonable period of time.

The release of antibiotics from the respective cement matrix varies greatly in PMMA cements available around the world. It is not the cements with the highest dosage of antibiotics (1 g/40 g) that release well, but rather the cements containing particularly low antibiotic quantities (0.5 g/40 g). The quality of the active ingredient used (physical properties of the surface) and the hydrophilicity (polymers or co-polymers in the cement) play a central role (Kühn 2007, 2014).

> Commercially available bone cements release anti-infective agents in very different ways. Diffusion depends on the surface and the fluid absorption capacity of the matrix.

43.8 Metabolization of Antibiotics

Reactions such as biotransformation of antibiotics to bacteria can be bacteriostatic (inhibition of bacterial reproduction) or bactericidal (killing of bacteria). Antibiotics attack bacterial structures and influence mechanisms of the bacterial cell, i.e., antibiotics can directly attack the murine structure of the bacterial cell or influence the structure of the murine layer. Mechanisms of protein synthesis can be disturbed, which is necessary for the bacterial cell to multiply. Antibiotics support the immune system by massively reducing pathogenic germs. Thus the immune system is able to sustainably fight the infection.

> Anti-infective agents reduce the number of germs and thus support the immune system. They do not heal the infection.

ALBCs only release about 10% of the added antibiotics. Diffusion does not allow the elution of antibiotic particles deeper in the cement matrix, as the distance is too long, or body fluids can hardly penetrate the hardened cement. The better the absorption of body fluids into the matrix – which is mainly dependent on the hydrophilicity of the polymers or copolymers used – the better the release of antibiotics. The concentration of antibiotics introduced into the cement (1 g/40 g polymer or 0.5 g/40 g polymer) is, therefore, very low. With an addition of 1 g of antibiotics, only 0.1 g is released over a period of several weeks, while 0.5 g releases only 0.05 g.

> PMMA bone cements release only 10% of the active ingredients used.

Antibiotic metabolism in the body can vary considerably. Aminoglycosides, for example, are not metabolized and are chemically very stable and not very sensitive to heat and oxygen. Gentamicin and tobramycin form ionic interactions with proteins, bind to the 30-S subunit of the ribosome, and become available to the body again after decay of the bacteria. In contrast to other antibiotics, aminoglycosides are excreted via the kidneys over a longer period of time due to their prolonged availability. Due to the lack of metabolism, aminoglycosides are nephrotoxic (and ototoxic) and can be detected in low concentrations in blood and urine. Glycopeptide antibiotics like vancomycin can cause similar toxic effects as aminoglycosides. Amerstorfer et al. (2017) used a novel surgical technique to increase the local antibiotic vancomycin concentration (superficial vancomycin coating, SVC) without the risk of systemic side effects.

Nephrotoxic reactions are not to be expected with locally applied aminoglycosides. While concentrations are very low, excretion is delayed and occurs over a period of time. In addition, in bone and in blood coagulates antibiotic depots are formed with various locally administered antibiotics. Chan et al. (2019) analyzed 1,180,270 US patients treated with ALBCs and assumed that there was an increased risk for kidney injury. However, while the raw data might correlate with ALBCs, after controlling for other variables known to cause renal failure ALBC association with renal failure was no longer statistically significant.

> Antibiotic combinations are microbiologically intelligent solutions for fighting infections. Synergistic effects extend the spectrum as well as the effect.

In contrast, ß-lactams are metabolized very rapidly. They bind to side chains and form irreversible bonds. The 4-carbon-ring, which is a characteristic of all ß-lactam antibiotics, is hydrolyzed and the molecule is inactivated. As a result, the molecule residues which are no longer active are excreted.

Take-Home Messages

- PMMA bone cements were developed on the basis of dental materials and were regarded as medicinal products until 1998. Older products such as Simplex®P and Palacos®R have probably still retained their basic formulation to this day. Highly viscous PMMA cements containing antibiotics are mainly used for large joints and are considered the gold standard. Independent register data show superior survival rates of HV cements compared to LV cements.
- Low-viscosity bone cements are often introduced to the body too early. This is associated with higher risks of embolism and necrosis.
- T_{max} of PMMA cements is not determined by viscosity but by the amount of MMA and BPO.
- Doughing time (DT) is a measure of the ideal time for cement placement in the body and is defined by the superficial tackiness of the cement paste. The viscosity of the DT is high enough to withstand the bleeding pressure.
- Simplex®P and Palacos®R show comparable intrusion into the bone when used correctly.
- Palacos®R+G (syn. Refobacin®Palacos®R, Palacos®R with Gentamicin) was the first ALBC on the market (1969). The evidence is the rapid reduction of an almost double-digit infection rate to below 1%.
- As a legal consequence of customized addition of antibiotics, the surgeon becomes the responsible manufacturer of the cement and thus assumes liability for product quality.
- The seed for infections is laid perioperatively. Prophylactic use of systemic AB reduces hematogenically spreading germs. Locally applied antibiotics in the cement reduce the risk of biofilm formation.
- Commercially available bone cements release anti-infective agents in very different ways. Diffusion depends on the surface and the fluid absorption capacity of the matrix
- PMMA bone cements release only 10% of the active ingredients used. The higher the active ingredient elution (spacer, manual addition), the greater the potential of side effects.

- Broad-spectrum antibiotics should be used systemically (e.g., cephalosporins) and locally (e.g., aminoglycosides) for prophylaxis; narrow-spectrum antibiotics (e.g., vancomycin) should be used in a targeted therapy.
- Revision cements contain antibiotic combinations with intelligent synergistic effects that increase effectiveness and elution.
- Combinations of active substances have a lasting effect against the development of resistance because different antibiotics destroy the bacterial cell at different targets.
- Mortality from PJI is comparable to that from breast cancer.
- The most robust modifiable risk factor for postoperative infection is malnutrition.

43.9 Manual Admixing of Anti-microbials

Industrially added active ingredients and their homogeneity in the cement and their influence on cement properties (mechanical stability, handling properties, hardening, and elution behavior) must be validly evaluated by the manufacturer as part of the certification process. In the case of ALBCs approved for marketing, the concentrations of the active ingredients are low (low-dose), whereas in the case of revision cements the amount of active ingredient in the polymer is higher.

Often no valid data can be provided for the manual addition of anti-infectives, especially since the dosed amounts vary between clinics. In the case of manual addition, not more than 4 g of active ingredient per 40 g of polymer should be dosed, because otherwise homogeneous distribution is more difficult and mechanical stability is significantly reduced (Frommelt 2007; Kühn et al. 2016). However there also are exceptions to this rule: some active ingrdient combinationss (8g piperacillin/tazobactam to 40g Palacos(R)R+G) only have minor influence on the mechanical stabiligy, whereas an addition of vancomycin has a negative effect on the mechanical characteristics even in low concentrations.

> Manual addition of anti-infectives can considerably influence cement properties. However, this relationship is variable in that some combinations improve while others worsen cement properties. Ultimately, in these cases the surgeon is the manufacturer by law.

Manual addition of active ingredients is also not synonymous with poorer drug release (Bistolfi et al. 2019). An inhomogeneous distribution of active ingredients – especially large active ingredient particles on the surface of the matrix – can even promote release. However, at such "active ingredient nests" PMMA cement can break more easily and by no means meet the standards relevant to bone cement.

References

Adelaziz H, von Förster G, Kühn KD et al (2019) Minimum 5 years follow-up after gentamicin and clindamycin loaded PMMA cement in total joint arthroplasty. J Med Microbiol 68:475–479

Althans V, Veve MP, Davis SL (2017) Trowels and tribulations: a review of antimicrobial-impregnated bone cements in prosthetic joint surgery. Pharmacotherapy 37:1565–1577

Amerstorfer F, Fischerauer S, Sadoghi P et al (2017) Superficial vancomycin coating of bone cement in orthopedic revision surgery: a safe technique to enhance local antibiotic concentrations. J Arthroplast 32(5):1618–1624. https://doi.org/10.1016/j.arth.2016.11.042

AOA (Australian Orthopaedic Association National Joint Registry) (2019) Figures KT34–35: cumulative percent revision of primary total knee replacement by fixation (primary diagnosis OA), pp 246–249

ASTM F451-99a (2014) Standard specification for acrylic bone cement. ASTM International, West Conshohocken. www.astm.org. https://doi.org/10.1520/F0451-99AR07E01

Benharroch D, Osyntsov L (2012) Infectious diseases are analogous with cancer. Hypothesis and implications. J Cancer 3:117–121. https://doi.org/10.7150/jca.3977

Bistolfi A, Ferracini R, Albanese C et al (2019) PMMA-based bone cements and the problem of joint arthroplasty infection: status and new perspectives. Materials (Basel) 12(23):4002. https://doi.org/10.3390/ma12234002

Buchholz HW, Elson RA, Engelbrecht E et al (1981) Management of deep infection of total hip replacement. J Bone Joint Surg Br 63-B(3):342–353

Buchholz HW, Elson RA, Heinert K (1984) Antibiotic-loaded acrylic cement: a current concept. Clin Orthop Relat Res 190:96–108

Buller LT, Rao V, Chiu Y et al (2020) Primary total knee arthroplasty performed using high-viscosity cement is associated with higher odds of revision for aseptic loosening. J Arthroplast 35(6S):S182–S189. https://doi.org/10.1016/j.arth.2019.08.023

Chan FY, Robinson J, Poeran J et al (2019) Antibiotic-loaded bone cement in primary total knee arthroplasty: utilization patterns and impact on complications using a national database. J Arthroplast 34:188–194

Charnley J (1970) Acrylic cement in orthopaedic surgery. Churchill Livingstone, London

Colas S, Collin C, Piriou P, Zureik M (2015) Association between total hip replacement characteristics and 3-year prosthetic survivorship. A population-based study. JAMA Surg 150(10):979–988. https://doi.org/10.1001/jamasurg.2015.1325

Deb S (2008) Orthopaedic bone cements. Kings College/Woodhead Publishing, London/Cambridge

Draenert K, Dreanert Y, Garde U, Ulrich C (1999) Manual of cementing technique. Springer, Berlin/Heidelberg/New York

Espehaug B, Furnes O, Havelin LI et al (2002) The type of cement and failure of total hip replacements. J Bone Joint Surg Br 84(6):832–838

Frommelt L (2007) Antibiotic choices in the surgery – local therapy using antibiotic-loaded bone cement. In: Walenkamp GHIM (ed) Local antibiotics in arthroplasty. State of the art from an interdisciplinary view. Thieme, Stuttgart, pp 59–64

Hotchkiss R, Moldawer L (2014) Parallels between cancer and infectious disease. N Engl J Med 371(4):380–383. https://doi.org/10.1056/NEJMcibr1404664

ISO 5833 (2002) Implants for surgery – acrylic resin cements. Orthopaedic application. Beuth. https://www.beuth.de

Jameson E, Asaad A, Diament M et al (2019) Antibiotic-loaded bone cement is associated with a lower risk of revision following primary cemented total knee arthroplasty. Bone Joint Surg Br 101(B):1331–1347

Kamath AF, Nelson CL, Elkassabany N et al (2017) Low albumin is a risk factor for complications after revision total knee arthroplasty. J Knee Surg 30(03):269–275. https://doi.org/10.1055/s--0036-1584575

Kendoff DA, Gehrke T, Stangenberg P et al (2015) Bioavailability of gentamicin and vancomycin released from an antibiotic containing bone cement in patients undergoing a septic one-stage total hip arthroplasty (THA) revision: a monocentric open clinical trial. Hip Int 26(1):90–96. https://doi.org/10.5301/hipint.5000307

Kühn KD (2007) Antibiotic loaded bone cements – antibiotic release and influence on mechanical properties. In: Walenkamp GHIM (ed) Local antibiotics in arthroplasty. State of the art from an interdisciplinary view. Thieme, Stuttgart, pp 47–58

Kühn KD (2014) PMMA cements. Springer, Berlin/Heidelberg/New York

Kühn KD (ed) (2018) Management of periprosthetic joint infection. A global perspective on diagnosis, treatment options, prevention strategies and their economic impact. Springer, Berlin/Heidelberg/New York

Kühn KD, Ege W, Gopp U (2005a) Acrylic bone cements: composition and properties. J Orthop Clin North Am 36(1):17–28

Kühn KD, Ege W, Gopp U (2005b) Acrylic bone cements: mechanical and physical properties. Composition and properties. J Orthop Clin North Am 36(1):29–39

Kühn KD, Lieb E, Berberich C (2016) PMMA bone cement: what is the role of local antibiotics. Matrise Orthopaedic, Proceeding of N°243, commission paritaire 1218T86410. ISSN:1148 2362, pp 12–18

Lee C (2005) Properties of acrylic bone cement: the mechanical properties of PMMA bone cement. In: Breusch S, Malchau H (eds) The well-cemented total hip arthroplasty. Springer, Berlin/Heidelberg/New York, pp 119–124

Lewis G (1997) Properties of acrylic bone cement: state of the art review. J Biomed Mater Res 38:155–182

Lewis G (2006) Injectable bone cements for use in vertebroplasty and kyphoplasty: state-of-the-art review. J Biomed Mater Res Part B App Biomater 76(2):456–468. https://doi.org/10.1002/jbm.b.30398

Lewis G, Carroll M (2002) Rheological properties of acrylic bone cement during curing and the role of the size of the powder particles. J Biomed Mater Res 63(2):191–199. https://doi.org/10.1002/jbm.10127

Lewis G, Mladsi S (1998) Effect of sterilization method on properties of Palacos R acrylic bone cement. Biomaterials 19:117–124

Meyer J, Piller G, Spiegel CA et al (2011) Vacuum-mixing significantly changes antibiotic elution characteristics of commercially available antibiotic impregnated bone cements. J Bone Joint S 93(22):2019–2056

Nasser S (1999) The incidence of sepsis after total hip replacement arthroplasty. Semin Arthroplast 5(4):153–159

Parvizi J, Saleh KJ, Ragland PS et al (2008) Efficacy of antibiotic-impregnated cement in total hip replacement. Acta Orthop 79(3):335–341. https://doi.org/10.1080/17453670710015229

Phillips JE, Crane TP, Noy M et al (2006) The incidence of deep prosthetic infections in a specialist orthopaedic hospital: a 15-year prospective survey. J Bone Joint Surg Br 88(7):943–948

Sanz-Ruiz S, Matas-Dies JA, Sanchez-Somolinos M et al (2017) Is the commercial antibiotic-loaded bone cement useful in prophylaxis and cost saving after knee and hip joint arthroplasty? The transatlantic paradox. J Arthroplast 32(4):1095–1099

Sanz-Ruiz P, Matas-Diez JA, Villanueva-Martínez M et al (2020) Is dual antibiotic-loaded bone cement more effective and cost-efficient than a single antibiotic-loaded bone cement to reduce the risk of prosthetic joint infection in aseptic revision knee arthroplasty? J Arthroplast 35(12):3724–3729. https://doi.org/10.1016/j.arth.2020.06.045.2020.06.045

Shahi A, Eajazi (2015) A prevention of periprosthetic joint infection. Pre- and intraoperative considerations. Orthopedics 38(4):219–221

Smith DC (2005) The genesis and evolution of acrylic bone cement. Orthop Clin North Am 36(1):1–10. https://doi.org/10.1016/j.ocl.2004.06.012. PMID: 15542117

Smith DC, Bains MED (1956) The detection and estimation of residual monomer in polymethyl methacrylate. J Dent Res 35:16–24

Sprowson AP, Jensen C, Chambers S et al (2016) The use of high-dose dual-impregnated antibiotic-laden cement with hemiarthroplasty for the treatment of a fracture of the hip. Bone Joint J 98(B):1534–1541

Squire MW, Ludwig BJ, Thompson JR et al (2008) Premixed antibiotic bone cement: an in vitro comparison of antimicrobial efficacy. J Arthroplast 23(6):1104

Támer LG, Ruiz López MD, Pérez de la Cruz AJ (2009) Desnutrición hospitalaria: relación con la estancia media y la tasa de reingresos prematuros [Hospital malnutrition: relation between the hospital length of stay and the rate of early readmissions]. Med Clin (Barc) 132(10):377–384. https://doi.org/10.1016/j.medcli.2008.06.008. Epub 2009 Mar 5. PMID: 19268323

Webb JCJ, Spencer RF (2007) The role of polymethylmethacrylate bone cement in modern orthopaedic surgery. J Bone Joint Surg Br 89(B):851–857. https://doi.org/10.1302/0301-620X.89B7.19148

Zhang J, Zhang XY, Jiang FL et al (2019) Antibiotic-impregnated cement for preventing infection in patients receiving total hip and knee replacement. Medicine (Baltimore) 98(49):e18068

Zmistowski B, Parvizi J (2013) A quarter of patients treated for PJI dead within 5 years (01/2013). Orthopedics Today. https://www.healio.com/news/orthopedics/20130104/a-quarter-of-patients-treated-for-pji-dead-within-5-years

Zmistowski B, Karam JA, Durinka JB et al (2013) Periprosthetic joint infection increases the risk of one-year mortality. J Bone Joint Surg Am 95(24):2177–2184. https://doi.org/10.2106/JBJS.L.00789

The Principles of Total Knee Arthroplasty Cementing Technique – A Japanese Perspective

Takao Kodama

Contents

E. Hansen, K.-D. Kühn (eds.), *Essentials of Cemented Knee Arthroplasty*,
https://doi.org/10.1007/978-3-662-63113-3_44

44.1 Introduction

Total knee arthroplasty (TKA) has become a common procedure with approximately 80,000 cases per year in Japan. But, unfortunately, compared to the more sophisticated cementing technique in total hip arthroplasty, it is not an exaggeration to say that there are no standardized methods of the TKA cementing technique taught in educational programs. It is assumed that many orthopedic surgeons have learned the technique from their seniors and kept using it in the same way since ever. It is indispensable to understand the difference between the types of cements and characteristics. A profound knowledge on the cementing technique improves the clinical results of the TKA cementing method, which especially has an impact on the strength of fixation. Important factors are

- the timing of cement application to the implant and bone,
- pressurized packing of the cement to the bone with adequate pretreatment of the bone marrow, and
- prevention of fatty or blood-mediated contamination at the cement application site and the cement interface.

This chapter humbly explains the important points of TKA cementing technique step by step.

44.2 Factors Involved in TKA Long-Term Results

First, let's have a look at the recent National Joint Registry (Australian Orthopaedic Association National Joint Replacement Registry 2017; National Joint Registry for England and Wales 2017). It can be seen that long-term survivorship exceeding 90% has been reported in most of the major manufacturers' implants with follow-up of more than 10 years. This is mainly due to the fact that compared to 10 years ago, polyethylene insert wear and osteolysis have decreased markedly due to improvements in materials and locking mechanisms (Sharkey et al. 2014). Furthermore, due to the improvement of surgical technique, TKA revisions caused by malalignment and instability have also decreased (Sharkey et al. 2014). On the other hand, loosening and infection as a cause for revisions have increased, relatively (Australian Orthopaedic Association National Joint Replacement Registry 2017; Sharkey et al. 2014). The major reason for revision surgery within the first year post-op is periprosthetic joint infection, but after 1 year post-op, loosening becomes the major cause (National Joint Registry for England and Wales 2017). In conclusion, the cementing technique has the most significant influence on long-term results of TKA in recent years.

> Therefore, prevention of loosening by applying a correct cementing technique leads to further improvement of TKA performance.

44.2.1 Types of Loosening

There are two types of loosening:

- loosening between bone and cement,
- loosening between implant and cement.

Loosening between bone and cement can be regarded as radiolucent lines on X-ray, and the main cause is considered to be an insufficient penetration of cement into bone.

> In other words, insufficient preparation of the bone bed and lack of thorough pressurization become the main reasons for loosening (Guha et al. 2008).

Contrary to this, loosening between implant and cement appears in the form of so-called debonding; diagnosis with X-ray is often difficult. Debonding occurs when adhesion of the cement to the implant is insufficient. Some surgeons consider debonding as a problem of implants (Foran et al. 2011; Arsoy et al. 2013; Bonutti et al. 2017) or type of cement used (Hazelwood et al. 2015) but this is absolutely not the case. It is a matter of cementing technique.

> Reasons for debonding are either a delay of cement application to the implant, an insufficient cement application range, or bone marrow fluid contamination.

44.2.2 Special Characteristics of Bone Cements

It must be understood first that cement is not just a glue, but a filler material. One has to be aware that the PMMA dough is a material having a micro-interlock mechanism: It will enter a fine gap and, once set, will not come off. For example, while hardening the cement does not bond to the smooth surface of polyethylene or the joint replacement surface. It penetrates into cancellous bone and rough surface of implants and cures there.

> It is necessary to understand that bone cement is a filler material with a "cannot-come-loose" characteristic.

44.2.3 Concept of Contamination

From the concept that cement is a filler material which penetrates into small gaps, cures there, and cannot come loose again, it is easy to comprehend that it can attach to rough but not to smooth surfaces. Even if the surface is rough, but there is a fluid membrane on it that intervenes, the strength of fixation deteriorates considerably.

Bone marrow fluid in which water, blood, and fat are mixed is an enemy of cement. If the cement anchoring surface is wetted with bone marrow fluid, this is called contamination. Fat and blood contamination will significantly decrease the fixation force (Report Tensile-adhesion properties of Biomet Bone Cement R 2017).

> Hence, it is necessary to minimize contamination while cementing.

44.2.4 Cement Types and Curing

PMMA cements differ significantly with regard to viscosity. Depending on their viscosity bone cements are classified into 3 types:

- low-viscosity (LV) cement,
- medium-viscosity (MV) cement,
- high-viscosity (HV) cement.

Ease of handling, working time, and penetrability into cancellous bone differ due to the difference in cement properties depending on viscosity. Currently, the most widely used cements in Japan are medium-viscosity Surgical Simplex P, CMW Endurance, and high-viscosity Palacos – all unloaded with antibiotics. Penetration into cancellous bone is better as viscosity decreases and penetration becomes deeper as injection pressure is increased (Rey et al. 1987) (Fig. 44.1). However, even if high-viscosity cement is pressed hard at an early stage, cement penetration becomes deeper. The curing process of cement is conveniently divided into 4 phases (Fig. 44.2).

1. Starting with the mixing phase the cement is still mostly in a liquid state.
2. The next phase is called liquid phase or waiting phase, and at this phase, the cement is still sticky to the gloves.
3. Over time, it will enter the working phase. In this phase the cement does not stick to gloves and becomes easy to handle.
4. Finally, the setting phase advances to the curing progress. MV cement has a long waiting phase and a short working phase. Conversely, HV cement has short waiting phase and immediately enters the working phase.

> Many surgeons believe that cement application to the implant must be done during the working phase, which is wrong; it should be done in the waiting phase. Meaning that it is necessary to start applying the cement in a phase when it is still sticky.

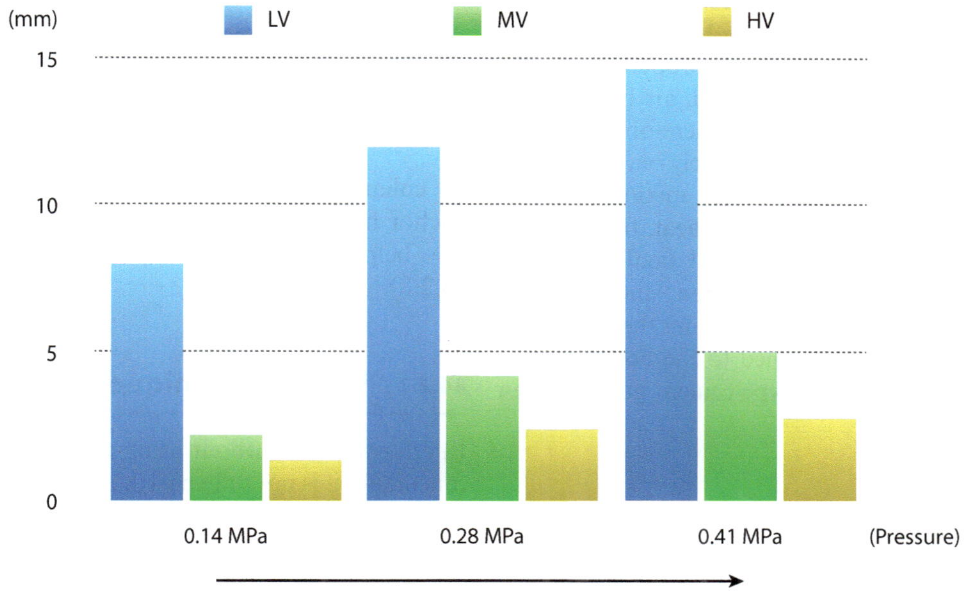

Fig. 44.1 Penetration of cement to bone marrow. Low-viscosity cement with pressurization had highest penetration. *LV* low viscosity, *MV* medium viscosity, *HV* high viscosity. (Data according to Rey et al. (1987))

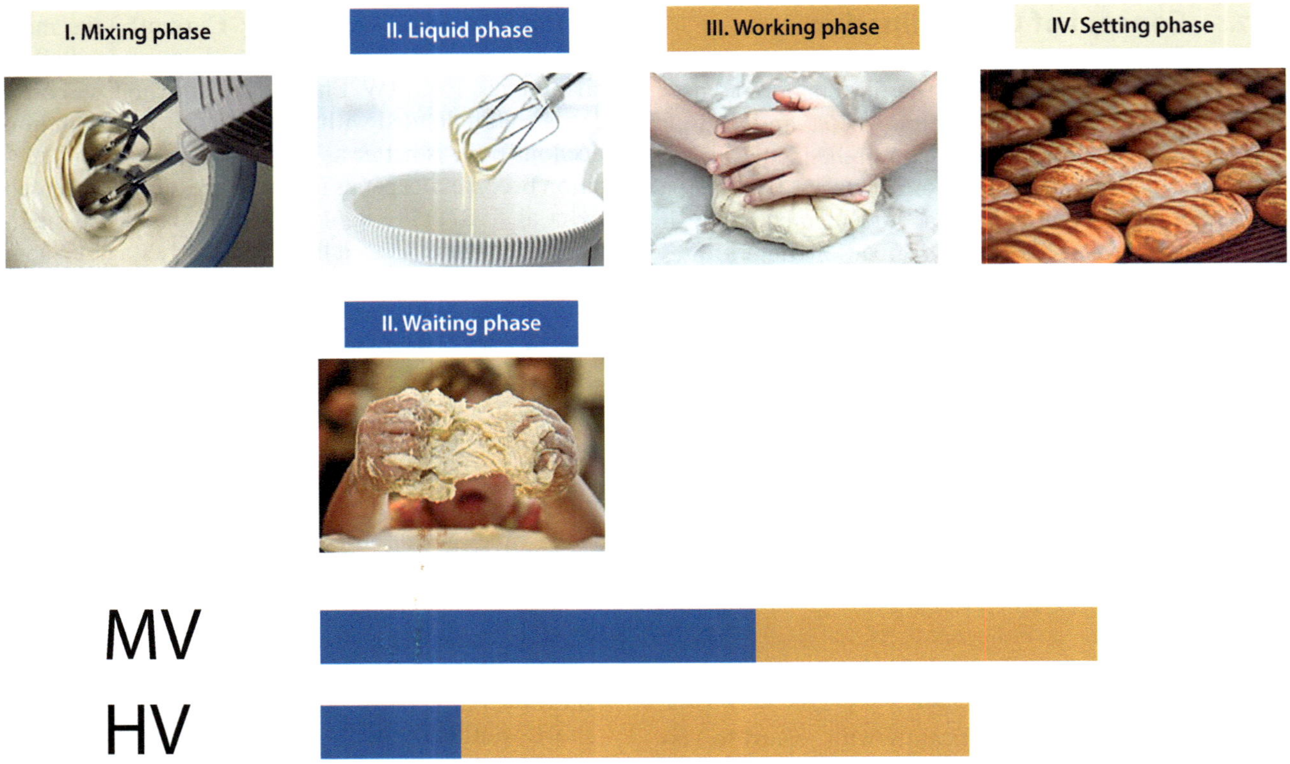

Fig. 44.2 Cement curing and different characteristics of medium- and high-viscosity cement. *MV* medium viscosity, *HV* high viscosity

44.2.5 Preparation of Cement – Mixing

Although cement mixing is often done using inexpensive open bowls, this method has the problem of the medical worker's exposure to the monomer. Therefore, vacuum mixing has been recommended recently. Furthermore, mixing under vacuum reduces air bubbles in the cement which leads to better mechanical properties of the cement. When mixing at higher speed, air bubbles and voids of cement can easily form. Therefore, it is suggested to move the handle approximately once every second and mix slowly. Furthermore, mixing too fast enhances friction which creates more heat, thus accelerates the polymerization process, and finally leads to faster setting of the cement. In addition, since contamination can be prevented by not touching the cement by hand and pressure can be applied to the bone marrow, the cartridge vacuum mixing type cement gun has been widely used.

44.2.6 Strength of Cement Fixation

To enhance the overall strength of fixation, it is important to simultaneously increase the fixation strength between cement and implant and between cement and bone. The strength of bonding between implant and cement depends on the quality of the surface of the implant and the timing of cement application.

> Applying cement to the implant in the soft waiting phase leads to enhancement of fixation strength (Report Tensile-adhesion properties of Biomet Bone Cement R 2017; Billi et al. 2014) (Fig. 44.2), and the strength of fixation increases even more when applied to stem and keel simultaneously (Billi et al. 2014).

To enhance fixation strength, it is important to drill anchor holes and thoroughly wash and dry bone marrow before pressure-packing of the cement (▶ Sect. 44.2.8).

44.2.7 Using a Tourniquet while Cementing

I perform TKA without using a tourniquet. Without a tourniquet it is not only possible to prevent deep venous thrombosis and to ensure reliable hemostasis during surgery, but there is also the advantage that the local antibiotic concentration is sufficiently increased. On the other hand, since there is the problem of contamination by bone marrow fluid, the tourniquet is inflated for 20 min only during washing, drying, and cementing.

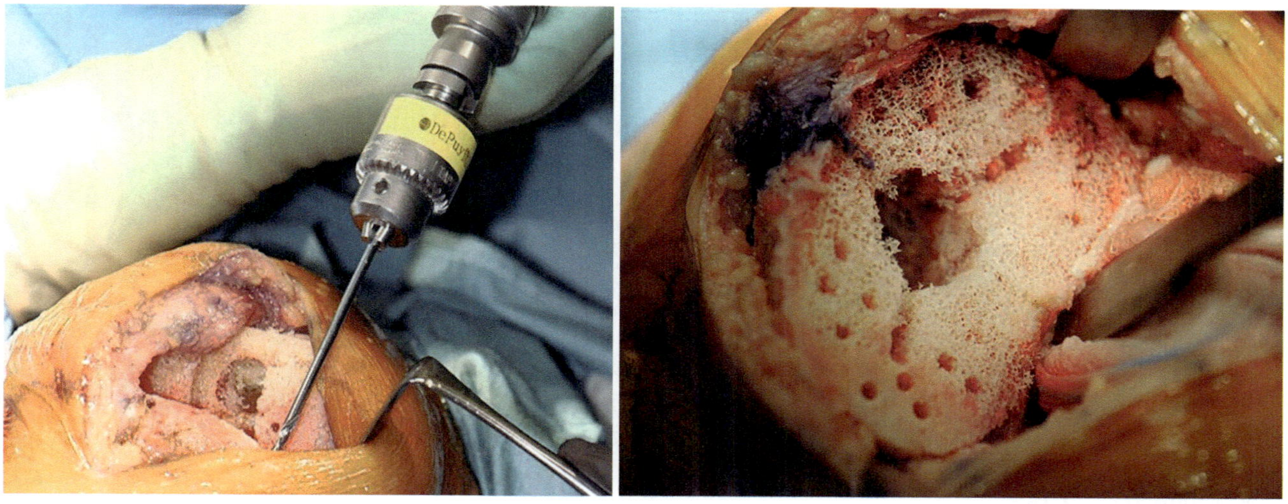

Fig. 44.3 Drilling of anchor holes

44.2.8 Preparation of the Cement Bone Bed

Preparation of the cement bone bed consists of drilling, washing, and drying in order to enhance the strength of fixation between cement and bone.

> Drilling of the osteotomy surface is effective to increase the fixation force between cement and bone.

Because cement does not infiltrate into the sclerotic bone, sufficient drilling is necessary. It is also necessary to drill the surrounding surface in order to increase the contact area between bone and cement (Fig. 44.3).

Sufficient washing is necessary to prevent contamination of bone marrow fluid, and pulsed lavage is effective for this purpose.

> It has been reported that pulsed lavage increases the thickness of the cement mantle, and as a result the pullout strength of the implant doubles (Schlegel et al. 2011).

> After washing, it is important to sufficiently dry the bone marrow including the bottom of the stem hole.

It is possible to remove bone marrow fluid from the surface of cancellous bone with sponge tapping, whereas this cannot be done at the stem hole, so that extensive suction is needed. I use Carbo Jet to blow away bone marrow fluid at the deeper bone levels and thus an even stronger bonding between bone and cement can be achieved.

> To prevent contamination, changing the glove just before cementing is recommended after the washing and drying process has been done.

44.2.9 Cement Coating

44.2.9.1 Implant

The fixation force between cement and implants becomes strongest by applying cement to the implant at an earlier time and under the condition without contamination (Report Tensile-adhesion properties of Biomet Bone Cement R 2017; Billi et al. 2014).

> Therefore, it is important to directly apply the cement to the implant from the cement gun while the cement is still soft (in the waiting phase) (Fig. 44.4).

At this point the cement application surface of the implant should never be touched with hands, i.e., prevention of contamination by gloves stained with bone marrow fluid. The application of cement to the implant in a phase where it is still soft enhances fixation strength and also cement coating on the implant surface occurs, this protects the implant from being contaminated with bone marrow fluid. There are some surgeons who do not apply the cement on the tibial stem and keel, because they fear that it will be difficult to remove the implant during revision surgery. But it is wrong not to apply the cement to the stem and keel, because it will rather increase the risk of loosening.

> Cementing the stem and keel is actually better because this will improve the fixation strength, and dramatically reduces loosening.

44.2.9.2 Bone

Try applying the cement on the cutting surface of the bone after washing and drying thoroughly. At the time of cementing on the tibial side, since cement is still in the waiting phase, inject cement with the gun nozzle directly

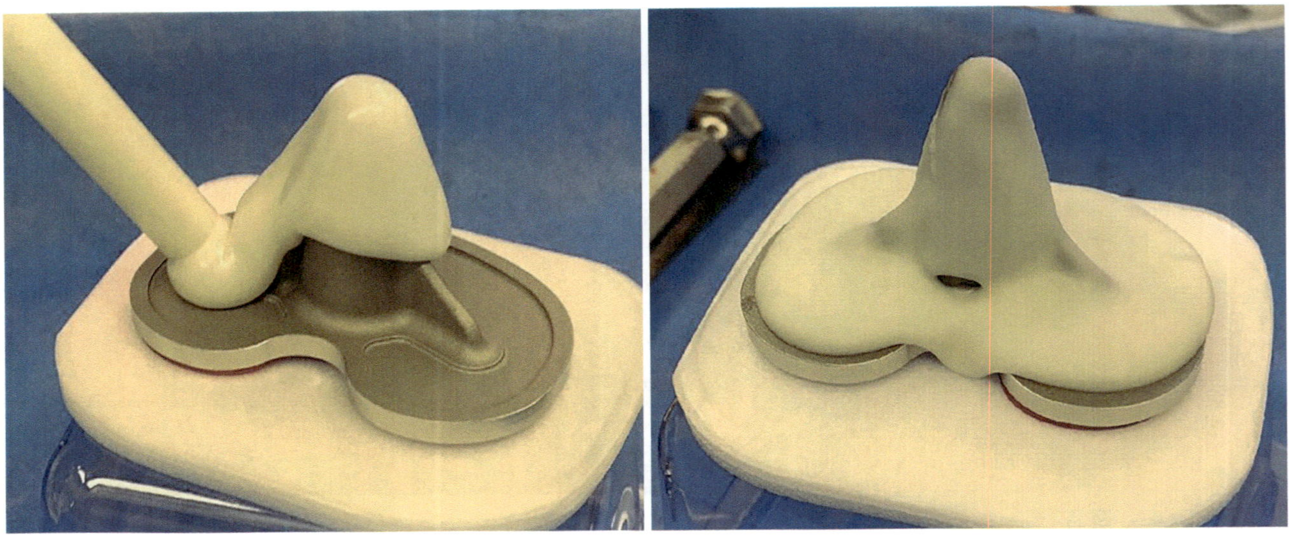

Fig. 44.4 Cement coating of the implant in the waiting phase

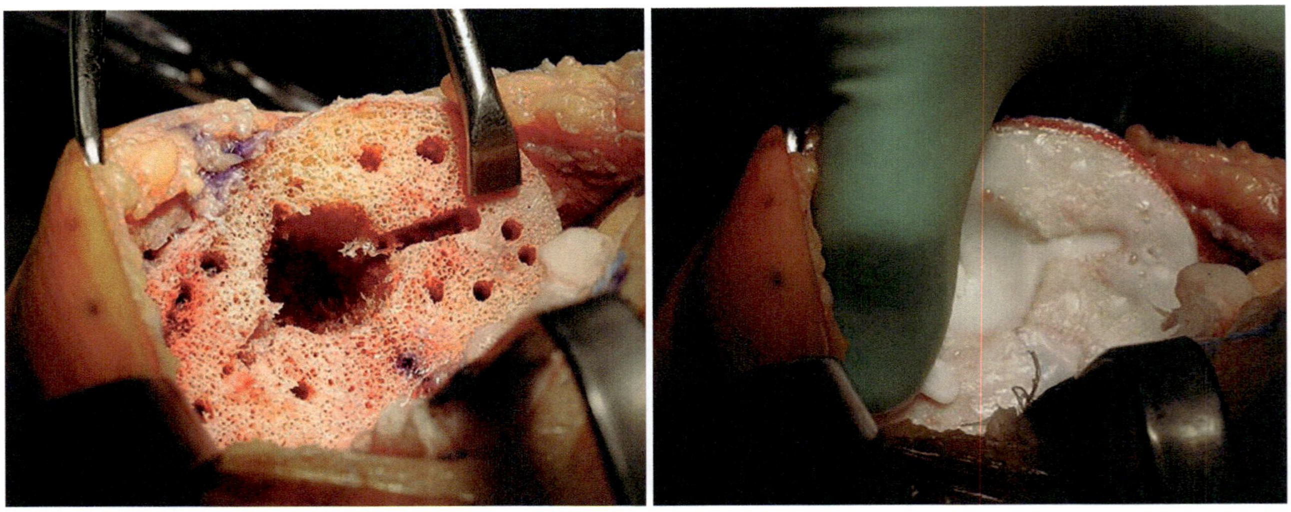

Fig. 44.5 Finger packing of the cement after meticulous washing and drying

against the cutting surface with pressure, followed by finger packing (Fig. 44.5). Finger packing might increase the risk of aseptic loosening due to contamination of the bone cement surface. It would be necessary not to touch the cement with contaminated gloves to avoid any additional risk.

> If finger packing would be needed, prior to this please change gloves.

In the waiting phase, it is better to slightly wet the belly of the thumb with a wet sponge before pressing the cement. This will prevent the cement from sticking to the glove. Even if fat is applied to gloves, cement does not adhere, but this should not be done. Water can almost be removed from the cement surface by tapping with a dry sponge after finger packing; in contrast, fat cannot be removed and will cause contamination. If bone marrow fluid has been blown off with the Carbo Jet, as described above, the bone marrow fluid will not ooze out while pressing the cement in. The same technique is used for the patella and femur.

44.2.10 Cementing Technique

44.2.10.1 Tibia

Since the tibial surface has a stem hole which is connected to the bone marrow, an increase in bone marrow pressure is observed during implant insertion. If the implant is inserted with the bone marrow fluid accumulated in the tibial stem hole or with the bone marrow

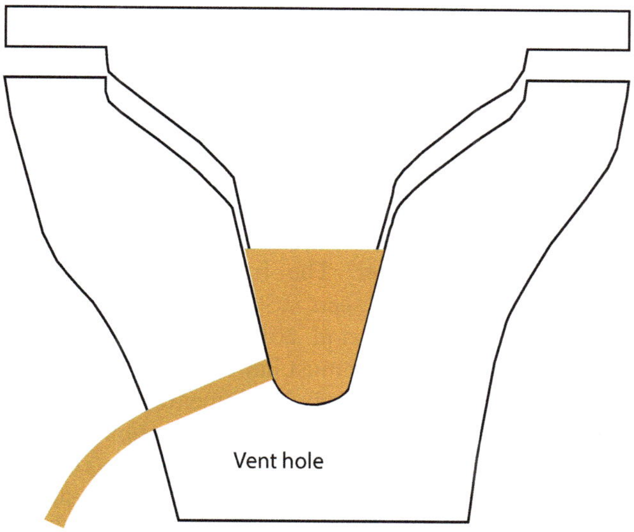

Fig. 44.6 Drilling of a vent hole to avoid contamination with bone marrow fluid

fluid remaining in the cancellous bone, the bone marrow pressure will rise and bone marrow fluid will penetrate the cement mantle layer and cause contamination.

> Therefore, it is advisable to drill a vent hole at the distal end of the stem hole in order to drain bone marrow fluid (Fig. 44.6).

At the time of cementing, bone marrow fluid remaining in the cancellous bone goes out through the vent hole which is useful for prevention of contamination. I usually drill a vent hole from the proximal-medial side of the tibial tubercle aiming at the tip of the stem hole.

44.2.10.2 Femur

The big difference between tibia and femur is that usually there is no stem hole in the femur, i.e., contamination is very low when inserting the femoral component without stem, because the rise in cancellous bone pressure is smaller as seen when inserting the tibial stem. However, after drilling, careful washing, and drying are performed, cement the implant. At this point the medium-viscosity cement is usually in the working phase and is often difficult to inject from the cement gun, so that the cement is finger-packed directly to the cancellous bone with clean gloves. After packing the cement with your fingers, tap the surface with a dry sponge to remove the bone marrow fluid that has exuded to the cement surface.

> Care should be taken when directly applying cement to the posterior condyle of the femur as it can push the cement proximally and create loose cement bodies when inserting the implant. Therefore, it seems to be safe to cement the posterior condyle of the femur only on the implant side.

In the case of the posterior stabilized (PS) model, whether or not to apply cement to the PS box is a problem, and the majority of surgeons do not seem to do this. I have not applied cement to the PS box, although it does not seem to cause any loosening.

44.2.10.3 Cement Pressurization and Cement Removal

> Hammering the femoral component to the end is difficult. Therefore, after striking to some extent, insert a trial insert, extend the knee, and apply axial pressure.

Then try to gently apply axial pressure, avoid varus/valgus pressure, and avoid flexing the knee. When applying varus/valgus pressure while the cement is still soft, a difference in bone marrow pressure between the medial and lateral side occurs, and as a result, bone marrow fluid may rise up to the implant side due to pumping action. If the cement is not applied on the implant in the liquid phase, the rising bone marrow liquid will enter the implant–cement interface. This leads to contamination and can possibly become a source of debonding, so be careful. Should bone marrow fluid not come out from cement–bone interface but only from the vent hole when applying axial pressure, it can be said that your cementing technique is excellent and contamination could be minimized.

Do not remove left over cement by pulling out but with the image of cutting. I usually cut off left over cement with the spatula that was originally used to strip the yellow ligament of the spine.

44.2.10.4 Patella

If you are an expert, it is possible to cement tibia, femur, and patella with one cement pack of 80 g. If you are unfamiliar with the operation, cement the tibia first using 40–50 g of cement and wait until it cures. Then take another pack and cement femur and patella. Use pulsatile lavage first and then thoroughly dry the bone marrow. If it is possible use Carbo Jet on the patella just before cementing. After finger packing the cement, wipe the surface to decrease contamination, push the implant with the cement already applied on it well into the surface, and let it bond. Use a patella clamp and patiently wait until cement cures.

44.3 Discussion

Unlike in the case of THA, TKA does not have systematic cement educational programs. It is assumed that many orthopedic surgeons have learned the technique from their seniors and kept using them the same way since ever. This is why there are many surgeons who just believe in wrong information such as:

- "It is correct to apply cement only on one of both, either the bone or the implant."
- "It is better to not apply cement on the stem and keel, because removal harder in case of revision."
- "It is correct to wait until the working phase, cementing should not be started when the cement is still sticky."
- "It is easier to handle cement after applying bone marrow fat to the gloves."

Of course, there might not be only one absolutely right way of cementing TKA, but in this chapter I introduced the method that at present seems to be most correct. It is well known that fixation strength is better the thicker the cement mantle is (Uhlenbrock et al. 2012). Walker et al. (1984) state that the thickness of cement necessary to capture the transverse trabeculae is at least 2–3 mm, and based on that, a cement mantle of 3–4 mm is recommended.

> The frequency of radiolucency is higher with a cement mantle thickness of 2.4 mm than with 5 mm (Lutz et al. 2009), so I aim for a cement mantle thickness of 3–5 mm.

The theory of Huiskes et al. (1981) presented at the 1981 ORS Scientific Conference that cement mantles thicker than 5 mm can cause thermal osteonecrosis has long been cited. However, Vertullo et al. (2016) reported that the average maximum temperature in the cement mantle remained at 39.13 °C, regardless of the thickness of the cement mantle, and it was reported that the temperature was lower than 47 °C, which is thought to be the temperature causing necrosis. In my own experience a cement mantle >5 mm often occurs in osteoporotic Japanese patients, but as a result not any bone necrosis was appearing around the area. So it cannot be clearly proved clinically that a mantle >5 mm poses a risk for bone necrosis.

In order to secure the cement mantle, using a cement gun is effective in addition to pulse lavage and drying with Carbo Jet. Compared to finger packing alone, it is reported that the cement mantle doubles in thickness when it is pressurized with a cement gun (Lutz et al. 2009). Therefore, the tibia which is thought to be easily contaminated is cemented first using a cement gun and finger packing. Then, the femur and patella are cemented with finger packing. It is much safer for surgeons who are not familiar with TKA to perform cementing in two stages.

44

▫ Table 44.1 summarizes the reports of previous tibial component loosening. Various types of implants were used, and high-viscosity cement was mainly used in the literature cited; references 1–5 (Foran et al. 2011; Arsoy et al. 2013; Hazelwood et al. 2015; Kopinski et al. 2016; Bonutti et al. 2017) state that all causes of loosening are either due to implants or high-viscosity cement. All of the references 1–5 (Foran et al. 2011; Arsoy et al. 2013; Hazelwood et al. 2015; Kopinski et al. 2016; Bonutti et al. 2017) reported loosening between cement–implant interfaces, the so-called debonding. Technical errors are involved in debonding as repeatedly mentioned in this chapter. The frequency of reported debonding ranges between 0.36% (Hazelwood et al. 2015) and 1.9% (Arsoy et al. 2013), which is quite high, and some technical error must have been involved. Only reference 6 (Crawford et al. 2017) mentions details of cementing technique, and from the description contents it was confirmed that cementing is properly performed in this facility. When correctly cemented, the frequency of loosening of the tibial component is as low as 0.054% (Crawford et al. 2017).

Finally, a list of causes for revision surgery at our hospital is presented in ▫ Table 44.2. Surgery was performed after April 2005, and 1943 TKA knees with a minimum follow-up period of 1 year or more were evaluated. Infection was the most frequent cause for revision surgery (frequency 0.26%). In Japan antibiotic-loaded bone cement (ALBC) is only used in revision cases, so my revision rate (0.26%) has been calculated with infection cases without ALBC use. Loosening of the femoral component was seen in one case (debonding between cement and implant, frequency 0.05%), and loosening of the tibial component was seen in one case (loosening between cement and bone, frequency 0.05%). These 2 cases occurred, before the Carbo Jet was introduced. After the introduction of Carbo Jet in March 2012, we have not experienced any more loosening.

▪ Conclusion

The correct knowledge about cementing technique is the major issue linked to prevent implant loosening. The coordination of time during cement application is a major part of the TKA cementing technique. Increased mechanical stability due to fixation between implant and cement could be achieved when cement is applied during the waiting phase. Additionally, rigorous cleaning and drying of bone marrow before cementing ameliorates the positive results. If finger packing is applied to the bone in an early phase the thickness of the cement mantle will increase by up to 3–5 mm. Fixation between bone and cement is enhanced, which has been linked to prevent loosening. The most important thing is to prevent a mixture of blood and fat from entering the surroundings of the cement at the application sites – in other words: *Prevention of contamination is the key*. If contamination occurs, stability will be significantly

Table 44.1 Tibial component loosening

Author (Year)		Number Frequency	Implant	Location of Loosening	Type of Cement Product	Cement Application
1	Foren (2011)	8/529 1.5%	Nex Gen MIS tibia	Cement-implant	HV Palacos	Bone
2	Arsoy (2013)	25/1337 1.9%	Nex Gen LPS3°	Cement-implant	MV Smplex (heated)	Unknown
3	Hazlewood (2015)	11/3048 0.36%	Genesis Legion PFC Sigma RPF	Cement-implant	HV Depuy & Palacos	Bone implant
4	Kopinski (2016)	13 Unknown	Vanguard CR8, PS5	Cement-implant	HV Cobalt 12, Depuy 1	Unknown
5	Bonutti (2017)	15 Unknown	ATTUNE	Cement-implant	Unknown	Unknown
6	Crawford (2017)	1/1851 0.054%	Vanguard	Unknown	HV Cobalt & Palacos	Bone implant

Table 44.2 Cause of revisions

Number of TKAs	1943
Insert dislocation	1
Instability	1
Periprosthetic fracture	1
Infection	5
Femoral loosening	1
Tibial loosening	1

Revision rate due to loosening 2/1943 = 0.1%; revision rate due to loosening after Carbo Jet use 0%

decreased which is associated with an earlier loosening of the implant. The so-called debonding is not a problem caused by the implant but is rather due to contamination of the space between implant and cement – in other words: The problem often arises according to the cementing technique. It has to be kept in mind that bone cement is not a mere glue, but a material with a micro-interlock mechanism. Bone cement is a space-filling material which, once infiltrated into the grainy space and hardened, will be difficult to pull out.

Take-Home Messages

- To enhance fixation strength, it is important to drill anchor holes and thoroughly wash and dry bone marrow including the bottom of the stem hole.
- Drill a vent hole at the distal end of the stem hole to drain bone marrow fluid.
- Never touch the cementing surface of the implant.
- Directly apply the cement to the implant, including stem and keel, from the cement gun while the cement is still soft.
- Change the glove just before cementing, finger pack the cement, and tap the surface with a dry sponge to remove bone marrow fluid.
- Insert a trial insert, extend the knee, and apply axial pressure without moving.

References

Arsoy D et al (2013) Aseptic tibial debonding as a cause of early failure in a modern total knee arthroplasty design. Clin Orthop Relat Res 471:94–101

Australian Orthopaedic Association National Joint Replacement Registry Annual report (2017)

Billi F et al Transactions of the ORS 2014. Annual meeting, New Orleans, LA, #1854. Factors influencing the initial strength of the tibial tray-PMMA cement bond

Bonutti PM et al (2017) Unusually high rate of early failure of tibial component in ATTUNE total knee arthroplasty system at implant-cement interface. J Knee Surg 30:435–439

Crawford DA et al (2017) Low rates of aseptic tibial loosening in obese patients with use of high-viscosity cement and standard tibial tray: 2-year minimum follow up. J Arthroplast 32: S183–S186

Foran JR et al (2011) Early aseptic loosening with a precoated low-profile tibial component. J Arthroplast 26(8):1445–1450

Guha AR et al (2008) Radiolucent lines below the tibial component of a total knee replacement (TKR) – a comparison between single and two-stage cementation techniques. Int Orthop 32(4): 453–457

Hazelwood KJ et al (2015) Case series report: early cement-implant interface fixation failure in total knee replacement. Knee 22: 424–428

Huiskes R et al (1981, February) Thermal injury of cancellous bone following pressurized penetration of acrylic cement. Proc. Orthop Res Soc Las Vegas, Nevada. p 134

Kopinski JE et al (2016) Failure at the tibial cement-implant interface with the use of high-viscosity cement in total knee arthroplasty. J Arthroplast 31:2579–2582

Lutz MJ et al (2009) The effect of cement gun and cement syringe use on the tibial cement mantle in total knee arthroplasty. J Arthroplast 24:461–467

National Joint Registry for England and Wales, 14th Annual Report (2017)

Report Tensile-adhesion properties of Biomet Bone Cement R on 30 grit blasted CoCr, test number ATS LAB#17–25539, issued Dec 2017. Data on file at Zimmer Biomet, Internal Laboratory Testing. Laboratory testing is not necessarily indicative of clinical performance

Rey RM et al (1987) A study of intrusion characteristics of low viscosity cement Simplex-P and Palacos Cements in a bovine cancellous bone model. Clin Orthop Relat Res 215:272–278

Schlegel UJ et al (2011) Pulsed lavage improves fixation strength of cemented tibial components. Int Orthop 35:1165–1169

Sharkey PF et al (2014) Why are total knee arthroplasties failing today- has anything changed after 10 years? J Arthroplast 29:1774–1778

Uhlenbrock AG et al (2012) Influence of time in-situ and implant type on fixation strength of cemented tibial trays- a post mortem retrieval analysis. Clin Biomech 27:929–935

Vertullo CJ et al (2016) Thermal analysis of tibial cement interface with modern cementing technique. Open Orthop J 10:19–25

Walker PS et al (1984) Control of cement penetration in total knee arthroplasty. Clin Orthop Relat Res 185:155–164

Influence of Cement Storage Temperature on Its Viscosity and Penetration Depth in the Tibia During Total Knee Arthroplasty

Maarten Verheyden, Dries Van Doninck, Frank Verheyden, and Klaus-Dieter Kühn

Contents

E. Hansen, K.-D. Kühn (eds.), *Essentials of Cemented Knee Arthroplasty*,
https://doi.org/10.1007/978-3-662-63113-3_45

45.1 Introduction

Cemented total knee arthroplasty (TKA) remains the gold standard treatment for end-stage osteoarthritis of the knee joint and has a survivorship over 90% at 15 years follow-up (Dixon et al. 2005; Fetzer et al. 2002; Furnes et al. 2002; Parsch et al. 2009; Berger et al. 2001). Aseptic loosening still is one of the main reasons for failure of TKA. Early aseptic loosening can be attributed to surgical error and, therefore, creates room for improvement. In early aseptic loosening the tibial component is often involved. Early aseptic loosening is assumed to be the consequence of micromotion at the bone–cement or the cement–prosthesis interface (Jacobs et al. 1994). Since an increasing number of TKA surgeries are performed in younger, more active patients it is important to reduce the number of revision TKA procedures due to aseptic loosening.

PMMA cement has been used in TKA for more than half a century (Ahmad and Kohl 2015; Haboush 1953). The chemical composition of such cements is that of PMMA or co-polymers of PMMA. PMMA cement is used as a combination of a polymer powder and a monomer liquid. When the two components are mixed, a polymerization process occurs. After mixing, viscosity changes over time from a liquid state into a workable dough-like state and, finally, the cement becomes completely solid (Jaeblon 2010; Knets et al. 2007; Kühn et al. 2005a, b; Kühn 2014).

> In TKA a perfect cementing technique is very important (Ritter et al. 1994; Miskovsky et al. 1992). One aspect of this technique is the viscosity of the bone cement during application.

Viscosity is important since it is one of the factors influencing the penetration depth into cancellous bone. Bert et al. (Bert and McShane 1998) measured micromotion at the bone–cement interface in an in vitro model. With a 1 mm cement mantle under the tibial tray, they found significant micromotion at the bone–cement interface. Increasing the cement mantle to 3 mm thickness resulted in a stable fixation of the tibial component without micromotion. Walker et al. noted that 3 mm of cement penetration is necessary to achieve microlock at the bone–cement interface with engagement of at least one level of transverse bone trabeculae and sufficient engagement in the vertical bone channels (Walker et al. 1984).

Furthermore, PMMA polymerization is an exothermic reaction which can lead to thermal osteonecrosis during cementing the TKA components. Animal models show thermonecrosis of the bone at temperatures >53 °C when applied for at least 1 min (Albrektsson and Eriksson 1985). Thermal osteonecrosis during total hip arthroplasty has been documented extensively (Whitehouse et al. 2014). In 1981, Huiskes et al. stated that there is a significant risk of thermal osteonecrosis with cement penetration of more than 5 mm (Huiskes and Sloof 1981). Vertullo et al. recently stated that with modern cementing techniques there is no correlation between cement penetration depth and maximum cement mantle temperature (Vertullo et al. 2016). These techniques were developed to increase cement penetration without creation of thermonecrosis. They include negative pressure intrusion (Banwart et al. 2000), cement pressurization (Kim et al. 1984), and pulsed lavage to decrease the temperature of the bone (Walker et al. 1984). Nevertheless, Vertullo et al. advised for further investigations because of migration of some cemented tibial trays due to thermally induced bone remodeling.

> In conclusion, currently a cement penetration depth between 3 mm and 5 mm is generally accepted to be ideal.

Since initial cement temperature influences polymerization speed, it will influence cement viscosity over time and eventually influence cement penetration depth. The aim of the study presented in the following was to evaluate the influence of bone cement storage temperature on the penetration depth in the tibia during TKA surgery.

45.2 Materials and Methods

The study was performed using a specifically developed open-pore composite sawbone model (item 1117-130, Sawbones, Malmo, Sweden), mimicking the open cell structure of the proximal tibial cancellous bone. 35 bone models were used for the tests, each identical in size and composition. The models consisted of an anatomical replica of the proximal tibia composed of a fiber-filled epoxy cortex injected around an open-pore polyurethane foam. This model has been validated previously with respect to the structural properties (Cristofolini and Viceconti 2000; Heiner and Brown 2001). The cell structure was identical in all models (cell size 1.5–2.5 mm, porosity >95%).

The sawbones (n = 35) were prepared for a size 5 tibial component of the Genesis II® PS knee prosthesis (Smith & Nephew, Memphis, TN, USA) with the standard cutting block, following standard surgical technique.

Two groups were evaluated regarding the influence of bone cement storage temperature on penetration depth into the proximal tibia:

1. *The "high viscosity" group*: The monomer and the powder (Palacos®R, Heraeus Medical, Wehrheim, Germany) were stored at 18 °C (n = 18).
2. *The "low viscosity" group*: The monomer and the powder (Palacos®R, Heraeus Medical, Wehrheim, Germany) were stored at 6 °C and only removed from the temperature-controlled environment immediately before cement mixing (n = 17).

The manufacturer instructs to store Palacos®R cement <25 °C (Heraeus Medical GmbH 2017).

The cement was prepared in a controlled environment of 18 °C and 70% relative humidity. PMMA cement polymerization from mixing to setting is divided into 4 phases:

- mixing,
- doughing phase,
- working phase,
- hardening phase.

The doughing phase is characterized by low viscosity, in which the mixture fails to separate from a gloved finger ("doctor's finger test" according to ISO 5833). In the working phase, the cement can be handled without adherence. The hardening phase is the time in which cement sets, cannot be shaped, and forms a solid structure (Haas et al. 1975). 20 g of cement powder and 10 ml of monomer were mixed manually without the use of a vacuum mixing system following the instructions of the manufacturer, and the cement was applied with a spatula in equal parts of 10 g on both the tibial component and the tibial bone. Immediately before cement application, vaseline was applied on the under-surface of the tibial baseplate to facilitate component removal for the analyses. Cement was applied as soon as the working phase was reached (positive doctor's finger test). In the low-viscosity group application of the cement and finally cementing the components started at 3 min; in the high-viscosity group cementing started at 6 min. Each component was placed onto the tibia and impacted 12 times until it was fully seated on the tibial surface. All impactions were performed by the same investigator. Van Lommel et al. showed that it is possible to carry out a series of impactions in a very reproducible manner (Vanlommel et al. 2010). During the setting phase of the cement, a constant force of 50 N along the long axis of the tibia was applied by a weight for 15 min. In all cases, excess cement was removed using a curette. After total polymerization of the cement – at 20 min – the component was removed by a gentle tap.

This action was repeated for the "room temperature" cement group at 3 – 3.5 – 3.75 – 4 – 4.5 – 5.25 – 6 – 6.5 min and for the "cold temperature" cement group at 6–7.25 – 8 – 8.25 – 8.5 – 9 min.

The specimens were then cut in the sagittal plane using a band saw. For this purpose, the model was fixed into a specifically manufactured clamp to hold the tibia in the correct orientation and position during cutting to maximize reproducibility. A slow cutting speed was used to prevent damage to the surfaces. The cut surfaces were subsequently cleaned with pressured air and grinded with sandpaper (grit 800) to remove debris.

Digital high-resolution (600 dpi) pictures were taken of all sections together with a measuring scale using a Nikon D200 camera with a 105 mm, 1:2.8 G objective. The images were imported into CorelDRAW, and the cement that was present at the outer surface of the bone was excluded from the analysis (since it should not be considered as having penetrated into the cancellous structure).

Finally, all composite pictures were imported into Corel PHOTO-PAINT 9 to quantify cement penetration. This was done for the medial and lateral sagittal cut. The cement layer in each of these zones was identified manually using the Magic Wand tool. This tool automatically defines irregularly shaped selections which include all adjacent pixels that are similar in color (defined by their hue) to the selected pixel. The hue tolerance was chosen to be 10. The predefined region was evaluated by the operator, and if necessary, extra regions were added or removed to fit the cement layer as closely as possible. The number of pixels in the final selection was used to calculate the area of the cement layer in the investigated zone, and the average penetration depth was calculated from this area by dividing it by the length of the cut for that zone. ◘ Figure 45.1 shows the cut sawbones.

Statistical analysis was performed using the unpaired 2-tailed Student's t-test in Minitab. The reproducibility studies performed by Vaninbrouckx et al. showed it to be possible to evaluate penetration depth with the described procedure with an average inter-operator precision of less than 0.5 mm (Vaninbroukx et al. 2009).

45.3 Results

◘ Figure 45.2 shows the time between cement mixing and application in relation to penetration depth into the proximal tibia for both temperature groups. There is a tendency for reduction of cement penetration with longer time, but this correlation is only statistically significant for the cement at room temperature (R^2 = 0.49, p = 0.001). The relation between cement penetration in this group is

$$d_p = 4.94 - 0.39 \cdot t$$

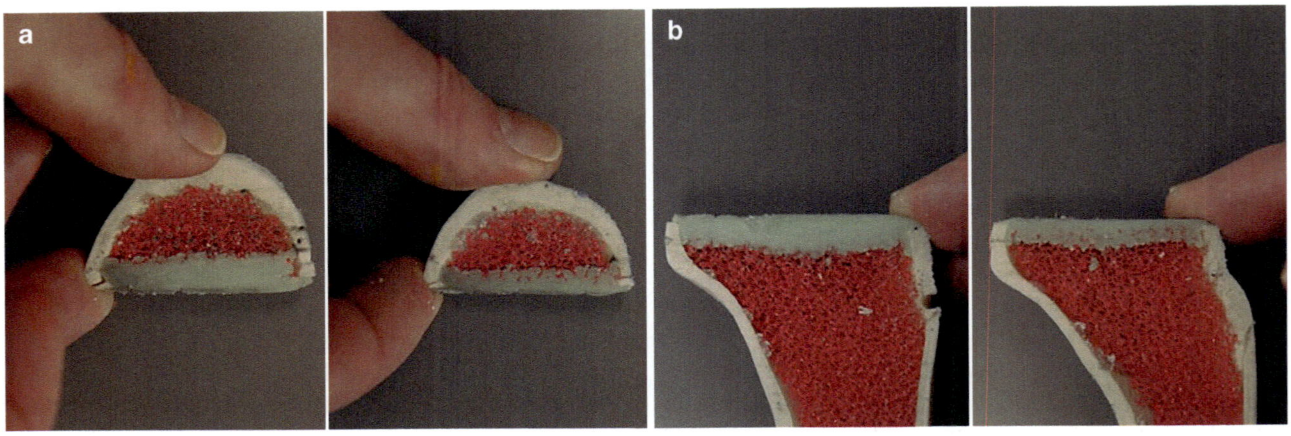

Fig. 45.1 **a** Cemented sawbone, cut on the medial side; thick cement mantle (*left*), thin cement mantle (*right*). **b** Cemented sawbone, cut on the lateral side; thick cement mantle (*left*), thin cement mantle (*right*)

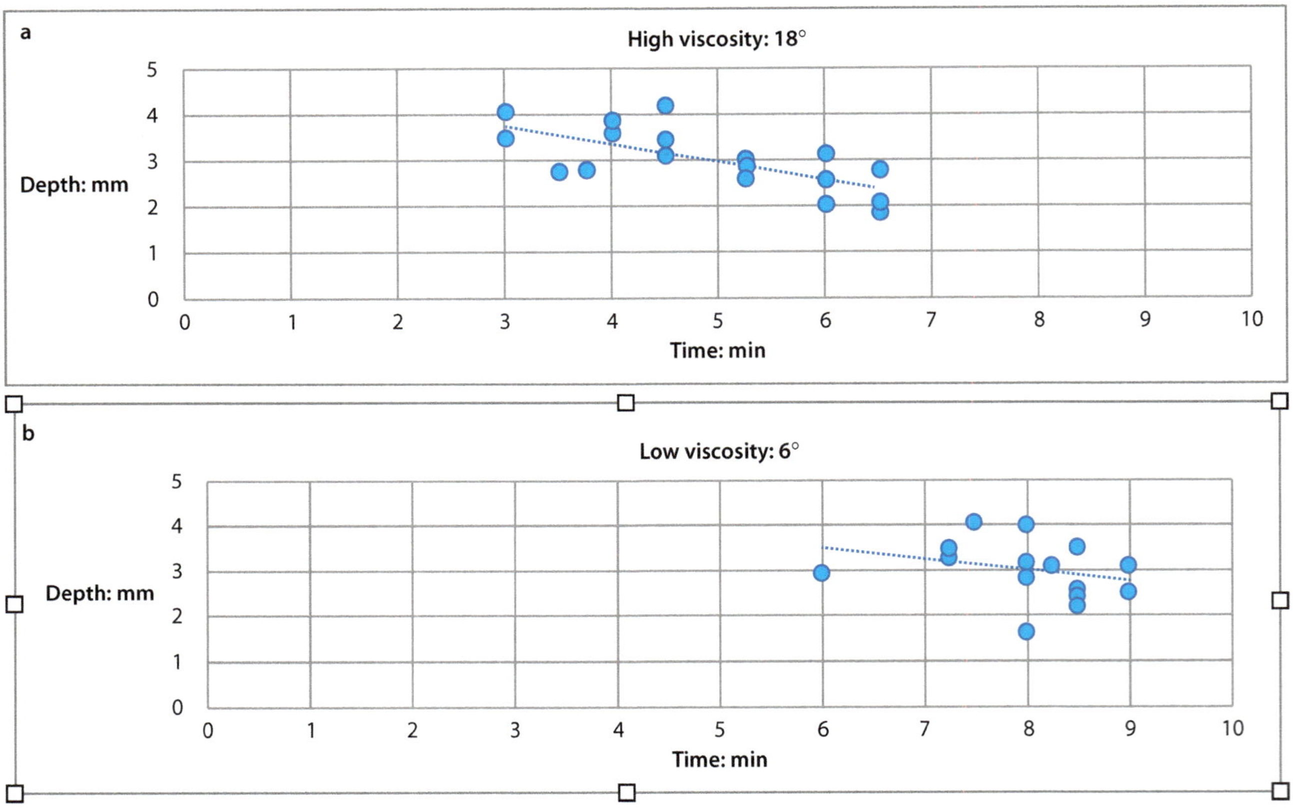

Fig. 45.2 **a** Cement intrusion of high-viscosity cement. **b** Cement intrusion of low-viscosity cement

where d_p is the penetration depth in mm and t is the amount of time after the start of mixing in minutes.

No significant difference was found between penetration depth on the medial and lateral side ($p = 0.37$) which suggests a symmetrical cementing technique. Figure 45.1 shows the average penetration depth between the medial and lateral side of each sawbone. No further distinction will be made between medial and lateral measurements.

As noted earlier, the doughing phase is defined as the time between mixing and the working phase. In this phase, bone cement is not yet ready to use. The working phase is defined as the time window in which cement can be handled without adherence. During this phase the components can be cemented onto the bony surfaces. The optimal working phase was defined as the part of the working phase that resulted in an optimal penetration depth of 3–5 mm. Based on the trendlines fitting the experimental data, in the "low-viscosity" group, a penetration depth of 3–5 mm was achieved between 6 min and 8.3 min. In the "high-viscosity" group an optimal penetration depth was from 3.1 up to 5 min. The duration of the optimal working phase was 2.3 min in the "cold cement" group compared with 1.9 min in the "room temperature cement" group. The difference between the working phases of both groups is 24 s. This difference is, however, not statistically different.

A clear difference in doughing phase was found between both groups. In the "cold cement" group, the duration of the doughing phase was 6 min, compared to 3 min in the "room temperature cement" group.

◘ Figure 45.2 shows penetration depth over time. It demonstrates the longer doughing phase in the "low-viscosity" group and the small difference in optimal working phase between both groups. There is a greater variation in penetration depth in the "high viscosity" group at the end of the working phase.

45.4 Discussion

In this in vitro study, we were able to achieve reproducible conditions during cementing the tibial components. Identical open pore sawbones were used as well as identical impaction and a standardized axial compression force of 50 N after cement was applied. The absence of blood and fat at the bone–cement interface for all measurements was important since it influences tensile and shear strengths of the bone–cement interface (Majkowski et al. 1993, 1994). In vivo, different blood pressures and cleaning of the bone surfaces result in different amounts of blood and fat at the bone–cement interface. Open pore artificial sawbone models were used since previous studies showed the accuracy of this model to imitate the normal cancellous bone structure of the proximal tibia (Cristofolini and Viceconti 2000; Heiner and Brown 2001).

> This is important because penetration depth is proportional to the pore diameter of cancellous bone (Walker et al. 1984).

Comparable intrusion behavior in both viscosity groups results in an insertion of the cements at a time of having an adequate viscosity. The doughing time of most of the cements on the market is important for surgeons to determine the timing for application. Some cements are characterized by a sticky behavior. They show only superficial doughing whereas the inner cement dough is sticky and not ready for application. Simplex®P (Stryker), a medium-viscosity cement, showed an intrusion 1 min after reaching the doughing time of approx. 7 mm tested according to ASTM or ISO 5833. Unfortunately, Simplex®P should not be used at this early phase because of its inner low-viscosity cement dough. Stryker informs surgeons not to use Simplex®P too early and recommends to wait for 3–4 min until the doughing time. Then Simplex®P has a comparable inner viscosity to other high-viscosity cements. The consequence is that the intrusion does not differ from other PMMA cements.

> High cement intrusion into the spongious bone correlates with an unfavorable relationship of cement and bone. During polymerization of the cement, the risk of necrotic properties will increase because more cement penetrates the bone and the setting heat cannot easily derive (Kühn 2014).

We found a 24 s difference in optimal working phase in favor of the "high viscosity" group (6 °C), although the difference was not statistically significant. This is in contradiction with the common assumption that working time using cooled cement is much longer. On the other hand, the sticky phase is significantly longer in the "high viscosisty" group meaning in this group one should wait longer before starting to cement the components. The scrub nurse should be aware of this fact and adapt the timing for starting to prepare the cement. Storing the cement at 6 °C has the advantages that the working phase is nearly half a minute longer and it offers a constant working condition independent of storage room temperature. Room temperature in the storing room might change over time thus changing the characteristics of the PMMA cement. Therefore, cementing conditions in this group might differ.

> Since "storing temperature" influences the length of the doughing phase; we stress the need to store bone cement in a temperature-controlled environment.

During surgery, it is important to know how much time there is between mixing and the beginning of the working phase. Since the operating room temperature influences polymerization speed of bone cement as well it is also important to maintain this temperature stable over time. Direct sunlight could heat the stored bone cement above 25 °C resulting in a shorter sticky phase and a shorter working phase. This could lead to problems during cementing. Therefore, it is important not to store bone cement in direct sunlight. In this study, we only examined penetration depth with bone cement stored at 6 °C compared with bone cement stored at 18 °C. The results might be different for other storing temperatures.

In conclusion, cooled cement ("high-viscosity" group) has a significantly longer doughing phase as compared to non-cooled cement ("low-viscosity" group) and a working time which is 24 s longer. This study comparing cementing of a tibial component using cement of either 6 °C or 18 °C shows that both groups have different working times and eventually reach identical cement penetration depths.

The advantages of using cement cooled at 6 °C in a refrigerator are that it offers uniform cement conditions independent of storage room temperature which might change during the seasons and that working time is nearly half a minute longer.

Take-Home Messages

- High-viscosity cements have a shorter doughing time compared to low-viscosity cements.
- High-viscosity cements have a longer working phase compared to low-viscosity cements.
- Cooling cement components of a high-viscosity cement results in a postponed doughing time and has only minor effects on its working behavior.
- Intrusion of high-viscosity cement and cooled cement is comparable.
- Some cements with high intrusion according to ASTM or ISO cannot be used after reaching the doughing time. The inner viscosity is too low. The manufacturer usually will inform the surgeons accordingly.
- High cement intrusion into the spongious bone might have the disadvantage of a higher risk of necrosis.

References

Ahmad SS, Kohl S (2015) 48 The optimal cementing technique in total knee replacement. In: The unhappy total knee replacement. Springer, pp 575–580

Albrektsson T, Eriksson A (1985) Thermally induced bone necrosis in rabbits: relation to implant failure in humans. Clin Orthop Relat Res 195:311–312

Banwart JC, McQueen DA, Friis EA, Graber CD (2000) Negative pressure intrusion cementing technique for total knee arthroplasty. J Arthroplast 15(3):360–367

Berger RA, Rosenberg AG, Barden RM, Sheinkop MB, Jacobs JJ, Galante JO (2001) Long-term followup of the Miller-Galante total knee replacement. Clin Orthop Relat Res 388:58–67

Bert JM, McShane M (1998) Is it necessary to cement the tibial stem in cemented total knee arthroplasty? Clin Orthop Relat Res 356:73–78

Cristofolini L, Viceconti M (2000) Mechanical validation of whole bone composite tibia models. J Biomech 33(3):279–288

Dixon MC, Brown RR, Parsch D, Scott RD (2005) Modular fixed-bearing total knee arthroplasty with retention of the posterior cruciate ligament. J Bone Joint Surg Am 87(3):598–603

Fetzer GB, Callaghan JJ, Templeton JE, Goetz DD, Sullivan PM, Kelley SS (2002) Posterior cruciate–retaining modular total knee arthroplasty: a 9-to 12-year follow-up investigation. J Arthroplast 17(8):961–966

Furnes O, Espehaug B, Lie SA, Vollset SE, Engesæter LB, Havelin LI (2002) Early failures among 7,174 primary total knee replacements: a follow-up study from the Norwegian Arthroplasty Register 1994-2000. Acta Orthop Scand 73(2):117–129

Haas SS, Brauer GM, Dickson G (1975) A characterization of polymethylmethacrylate bone cement. J Bone Joint Surg Am 57(3):380–391

Haboush EJ (1953) A new operation for arthroplasty of the hip based on biomechanics, photoelasticity, fast-setting dental acrylic, and other considerations. Bull Hosp Joint Dis 14(2):242–277

Heiner AD, Brown TD (2001) Structural properties of a new design of composite replicate femurs and tibias. J Biomech 34(6):773–781

Heraeus Medical GmbH. PALACOS® R+G pro – instruction for use. Retrieved 12 Feb 2017 from https://www.heraeus.com/media/media/hme/doc_hme/products_hme/palacos_bone_cement/pro/PALACOS_RG_pro_IFU.pdf

Huiskes R, Sloof TJ (1981) Thermal injury of cancellous bone, following pressurised penetration of acrylic bone cement. In: Proc 27th Orthop Res Soc, Las Vegas. p 134

Jacobs JJ, Shanbhag A, Glant TT et al (1994) Wear debris in total joint replacements. J Am Acad Orthop Surg 2:212

Jaeblon T (2010) Polymethylmethacrylate: properties and contemporary uses in orthopaedics. J Am Acad Orthop Surg 18(5):297–305

Kim YH, Walker PS, Deland JT (1984) A cement impactor for uniform cement penetration in the upper tibia. Clin Orthop Relat Res 182:206–210

Knets I, Krilova V, Cimdins R, Berzina L, Vitins V (2007) Stiffness and strength of composite acrylic bone cements. J Achiev Mater Manuf Eng 20(1–2):135–138

Kühn K-D (2014) PMMA cements. Springer, Heidelberg, ISBN 978-3-642-41535-7

Kühn K-D, Ege W, Gopp U (2005a) Acrylic bone cements: composition and properties. Orthop Clin North Am 36:17–28

Kühn K-D, Ege W, Gopp U (2005b) Acrylic bone cements: mechanical and physical properties. Orthop Clin North Am 36:29–39

Majkowski RS, Miles AW, Bannister GC, Perkins J, Taylor GJ (1993) Bone surface preparation in cemented joint replacement. Bone Joint J 75(3):459–463

Majkowski RS, Bannister GC, Miles AW (1994) The effect of bleeding on the cement-bone interface: an experimental study. Clin Orthop Relat Res 299:293–297

Miskovsky C, Whiteside LA, White SE (1992) The cemented unicondylar knee arthroplasty. An in vitro comparison of three cement techniques. Clin Orthop Relat Res (284):215–220

Parsch D, Krüger M, Moser MT, Geiger F (2009) Follow-up of 11–16 years after modular fixed-bearing TKA. Int Orthop 33(2):431–435

Ritter MA, Herbst SA, Keating EM, Faris PM (1994) Radiolucency at the bone-cement interface in total knee replacement. The effects of bone-surface preparation and cement technique. J Bone Joint Surg Am 76(1):60–65

Vaninbroukx M, Labey L, Innocenti B, Bellemans J (2009) Cementing the femoral component in total knee arthroplasty: which technique is the best? Knee 16(4):265–268

Vanlommel J, Porteous AJ, Hassaballa MA, Luyckx JP, Bellemans J (2010) Iatrogenic surface damage during femoral component impaction in total knee arthroplasty. Knee 17(1):43–47

Vertullo CJ, Zbrojkiewicz D, Vizesi F, Walsh WR (2016) Thermal analysis of the tibial cement interface with modern cementing technique. Open Orthop J 10:19–25

Walker PS, Soudry M, Ewald FC et al (1984) Control of cement penetration in total knee arthroplasty. Clin Orthop Relat Res 185:155–164

Whitehouse MR, Atwal NS, Pabbruwe M, Blom AW, Bannister GC (2014) Osteonecrosis with the use of polymethylmethacrylate cement for hip replacement: thermal-induced damage evidenced in vivo by decreased osteocyte viability. Eur Cell Mater 27: 50–62

Antibiotic-Loaded Bone Cement: Pro

Matthew W. Squire

Contents

E. Hansen, K.-D. Kühn (eds.), *Essentials of Cemented Knee Arthroplasty*,
https://doi.org/10.1007/978-3-662-63113-3_46

46.1 Introduction

Total knee arthroplasty (TKA) is one of the most successful orthopedic procedures to date (Price et al. 2018). The number of TKAs performed worldwide continues to exponentially increase and has been estimated to be more than two million procedures per annum (Kurtz et al. 2011). When done for appropriate patients and conditions, TKA predictably reduces pain, improves function, and increases patient quality of life (Rocha de Silva et al. 2014).

Fixation of the TKA prosthesis to bone remains an area of active investigation and improvement. Cementing using polymethylmethacrylate (PMMA) bone cement still is the most common method by which TKA prosthetic components are affixed to the bone (Abdel and Berry 2019; National Joint Registry 2019; Australian Orthopaedic Association Joint Replacement Registry 2019a). When used for TKA, PMMA has demonstrated exemplary results. Currently, cemented TKA is the "gold standard" and accounts for greater than 95% of TKAs performed worldwide (National Joint Registry 2019; Australian Orthopaedic Association Joint Replacement Registry 2019b; Nugent et al. 2019).

Unfortunately, a small percentage of TKAs will suffer from early failure due to infectious and non-infectious causes and require revision surgery. Due to the large number of TKAs performed annually, the small percentage of TKAs requiring revision results in a substantial absolute number of revision surgeries. TKA revision surgery is costly, causes significant patient morbidity, and is not uniformly successful (Bozic et al. 2010; Salah et al. 2003). Consequently, surgical techniques and materials able to reduce the incidence of revision surgery are of paramount importance. Antibiotic-loaded bone cement (ALBC) is a material that has the potential to significantly reduce the burden of TKA revision and is, therefore, the focus of current research and debate.

46.2 Historical Context

Early arthroplasty surgeons noted prosthetic joint infection (PJI) was a relatively common and disastrous cause of THA and TKA failure. In the 1970s, it was noted ALBC use during THA could reduce the incidence of PJI (Buchholz et al. 1984). ALBC was also being used to treat THA PJI with great success (Buchholz et al. 1981). Therefore, it is not surprising that ALBC was later embraced during the development of modern cemented TKA techniques to both prevent and treat PJI (Best et al. 1998).

In the late 1970s and early 1980s, the incidence of early THA and TKA failures steadily decreased due to improvements in prosthetic design, biomaterials, and surgical techniques (Moran and Horton 2000). Additionally, adoption and standardization of prophylactic parenteral antibiotic administration prior to THA and TKA markedly decreased the incidence of PJI (Lidgren 2001). During this time, significantly different ALBC usage patterns emerged.

From the 1980s onward, many surgeons strongly advocated for routine ALBC use during all THA and TKA due to the excellent past performance of ALBC with respect to preventing THA PJI and revision. In contrast, other surgeons believed the impressive PJI and revision reductions that occurred were mainly attributable to improved surgical techniques and prophylactic antibiotic administration. Many of the same surgeons argued for the use of plain bone cement (PBC) without added antibiotics during cemented THA and TKA. This difference in opinion regarding appropriateness of ALBC utilization has persisted and continues to be debated (Parvizi et al. 2013).

It should be noted that these ALBC and PBC utilization and opinion differences evolved in an easily recognized geographic distribution. In general, most surgeons in Europe adopted routine use of ALBC for all THA and TKA surgeries while most US surgeons opted to perform THA and TKA using PBC. It is unlikely coincidental that the major PMMA producers in Europe were manufacturing predominantly ALBC while those in the United States were manufacturing predominantly PBC. It is highly probable that these commercial forces helped contribute to the current bone cement "transatlantic paradox" where ALBC is routinely used in Europe and much less commonly used in the United States (Sanz-Ruiz et al. 2017, 2020).

> Such variations in ALBC opinion and utilization have set the stage for one of the premier questions and debates in THA and TKA: Should antibiotic-loaded bone cement be used routinely for all cemented THA and TKA?

The remainder of this chapter highlights evidence-based medicine (EBM) in favor of routine ALBC use for cemented TKA and briefly addresses the efficacy of other contemporary TKA local antimicrobial delivery strategies.

46.3 Current Consensus

There is wide divergence in opinion regarding the routine use of ALBC for THA and TKA PJI prophylaxis. This was documented at the 2nd International Consensus Meeting (ICM) on Periprosthetic Joint Infection where protracted debate concerning ALBC occurred amongst more than 500 PJI treatment experts. As with all topics addressed by the meeting, a team of expert topic authors (Fillingham et al. 2019) performed a systematic literature review of ALBC and formulated a response to a question posed by the Delphi Process. The evidence-based response was then presented to the attendees for a live consensus vote. The full 2018 ICM process and meeting document can be accessed at ▶ www.ICMPhilly.com.

2018 ICM ALBC question, response, and live attendee vote are detailed below:

- *Question*: Is there sufficient evidence to support the use of antibiotic-loaded cement in primary total knee arthroplasty (TKA) or total hip arthroplasty (THA) to reduce the risk of surgical site infections/periprosthetic joint infections (SSIs/PJIs)?
- *Response*: There is no conclusive evidence to demonstrate that routine use of antibiotic-loaded cement in primary TKA or THA reduces the risk of subsequent SSIs/PJIs. Recent high-level evidence and registry data have not demonstrated a reduction in SSI/PJIs. Furthermore, the added cost, the potential for the emergence of resistant organisms, and the potential adverse effect of antibiotics on the host provide adequate reasons to refrain from routine use of antibiotic-loaded cement during primary total joint arthroplasty.
- *Attendee vote*: 38% Agree, 58% Disagree, and 4% Abstain.

The initial live vote demonstrated most PJI treatment experts in attendance believed antibiotic-bone cement could reduce the incidence of PJI. It also indicated the majority of attendees believed routine use of ALBC during THA and TKA was either acceptable or preferred. Because of the failure to reach a consensus statement with the first question, the MSIS ICM organizing committee elected to modify the question in hopes of clarifying the attendee's views on ALBC use for primary THA and TKA. The modified question and response with attendee vote are detailed below:

- *Question*: Is there a role for the use of antibiotic-impregnated cement in primary total joint arthroplasty (TJA)?
- *Response*: Antibiotic-impregnated cement may be used during primary TJA to reduce the risk of surgical site infections/periprosthetic joint infections (SSIs/PJIs). The benefits of antibiotic-impregnated cement versus its cost and other potential adverse effects may be most justified in patients at high risk of infection.
- *Attendee vote*: 93% Agree, 7% Disagree.

> The supermajority and strong consensus of this vote undoubtedly shows that the 2018 ICM attendees agree that ALBC has a role in primary THA and TKA.

Furthermore, it suggests THA and TKA PJI experts agree ALBC utilization can decrease PJI incidence. Lastly, it demonstrates the potential costs and other theoretical negative aspects of ALBC usage are outweighed by ALBC benefits.

46.4 Products and Regulations

Many different commercially pre-mixed ALBC products are distributed and available for purchase in the world. The type of antibiotic contained and concentration of antibiotic vary significantly among the different products. Therefore, it is not surprising that the antibiotic elution characteristics of these pre-mixed commercially available bone cements are unique to each specific product and the intraoperative methods by which they are mixed (Kuehn 2014).

Prior investigations comparing elution of commercially pre-mixed ALBC have been performed. Squire et al. demonstrated that the in vitro antibiotic elution properties of 5 different commercially available ALBC products rapidly changed over time with high-viscosity brands producing significantly greater duration of antimicrobial activity as compared to lower-viscosity ALBC brands (Fig. 46.1) (Squire et al. 2008).

Additionally, the investigation of Meyer et al. studying the antibiotic elution properties of 6 commercially available ALBC products showed that both ALBC brand and mixing regimen (vacuum vs. atmospheric) significantly influenced antibiotic elution intensity and duration (Meyer et al. 2011). This investigation indicates antibiotic elution of many ALBC products after 24 h is below the minimal inhibitory concentration (MIC) necessary to produce antibacterial efficacy whereas other products elute antibiotic concentrations above MIC for 3 or more days (Fig. 46.2).

> Assuming the in vitro studies above are translatable to the in vivo environment, differences in ALBC product antibiotic elution intensity and duration could have a significant impact on their ability to prevent SSI and/or PJI.

Regulatory approval for commercially pre-mixed ALBC products varies by country. While use of pre-mixed ALBC is the standard of care for primary THA and TKA in Europe and many other regions, in the United

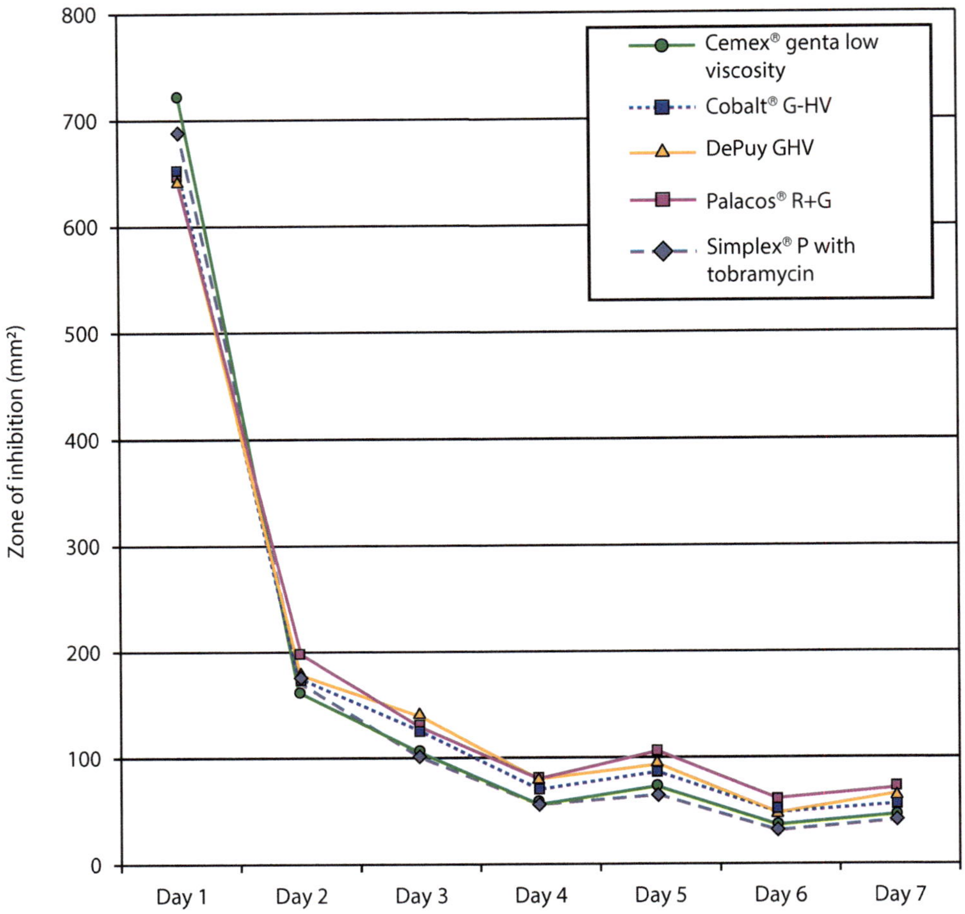

Fig. 46.1 Antimicrobial efficacy. (Squire et al. 2008, with permission from Elsevier)

States, usage of pre-mixed ALBC is Food and Drug Administration approved only for use in the second stage of a two-stage revision for known septic THA and TKA. Therefore, in the United States, routine usage for primary THA and TKA is "off-label".

ALBC can be constructed by "hand blending" of powdered antibiotics into PMMA not containing antibiotics.

> Hand-blended ALBC suffers from inconsistencies introduced by human error and results in PMMA that has variable elution and mechanical characteristics (Ferraris et al. 2010; Dunne et al. 2007; Neut et al. 2003).

Importantly, a review of physician modification of FDA-approved devices concluded that "since the device had been modified after the manufacturing process and used outside the instructions for use, the manufacturer essentially became exempt from any product liability claim" (Starnes 2013), potentially enhancing the liability of the physician in cases where patient harm is realized. Because of the excellent pre-mixed commercial products currently available, the utility of hand blending ALBC for routine primary THA and TKA PJI prophylaxis is questionable.

> It is the author's opinion that hand blending of ALBC should be reserved for infrequent clinical situations requiring local delivery of more or different antibiotics than commercially pre-mixed ALBC products can provide.

46.5 Evidence

46.5.1 Retrospective

In 2003, investigators at a French hospital compared their experience with ALBC to PBC when used during primary TKA (Eveillard et al. 2003). In this review of TKAs, ALBC containing unknown concentration of gentamicin was utilized. Clean-air rooms, pre-incision parenteral antibiotics, and iodized alcohol skin preparation were also utilized for all patients. Incidence of comorbid conditions increasing PJI incidence was not

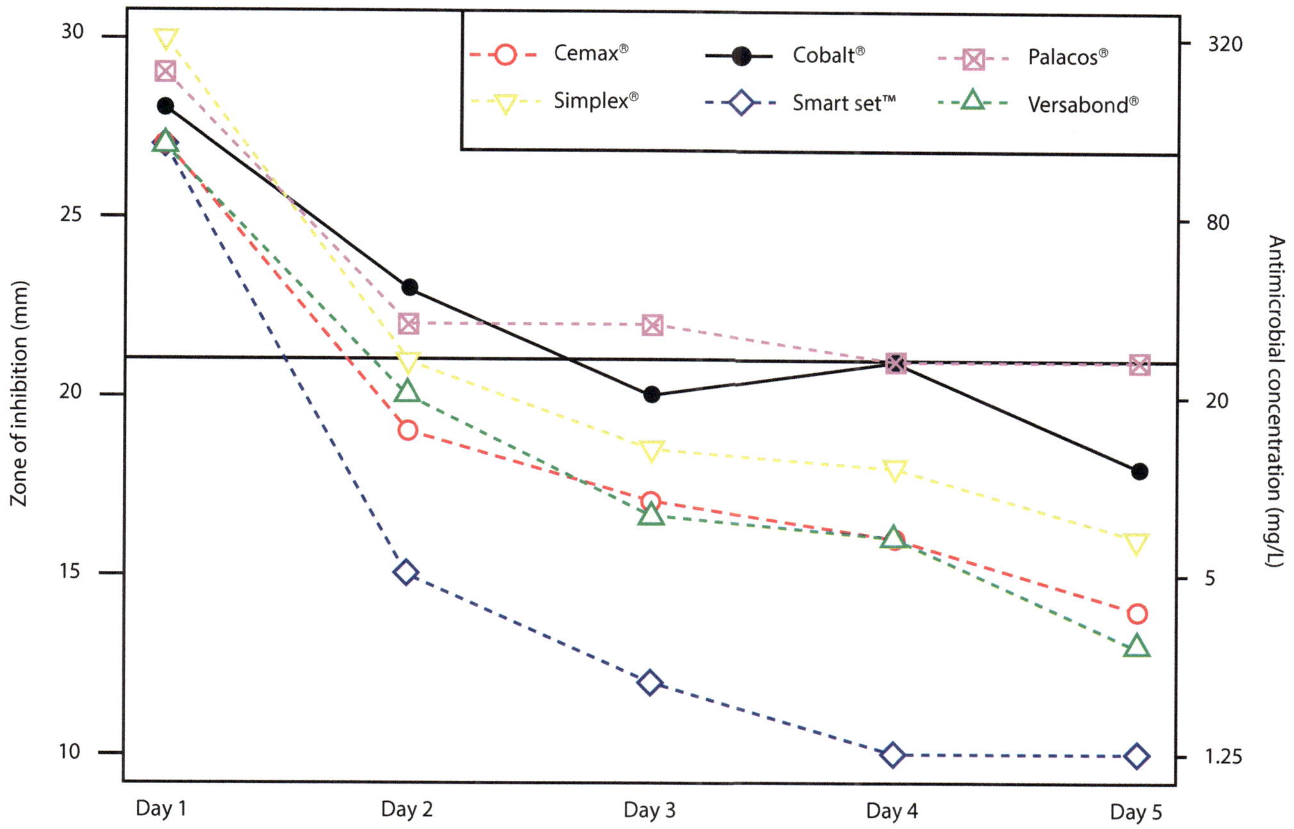

Fig. 46.2 Comparison of average zone of bacterial growth inhibition (*left*) and antibiotic concentration (*right*) for vacuum-mixed bone cements during 5-day elution study. The *horizontal line* represents the 32 mg/L susceptibility threshold. (From Meyer et al. 2011, by courtesy of Wolters Kluwer Health, Inc.)

detailed for the different groups. Minimum follow-up was 12 months and the outcome of interest was PJI. ALBC was utilized in 83 patients and PBC was utilized in 84 patients per the discretion of the faculty surgeon. PJI incidence in the ALBC group was 1.21% while the PJI incidence in the PBC group was 9.52%.

> In this investigation, ALBC demonstrated protective efficacy against PJI ($p = 0.03$); however, it should be noted the incidence of PJI for the PBC cohort was much higher than expected for primary TKA.

In a 2009 non-randomized investigation, ALBC ability to reduce PJI in 1625 consecutive TKAs performed in a Canadian institution was assessed (Gandhi et al. 2009). Analysis of the ALBC and PBC groups showed them to be demographically and clinically similar. ALBC group (814 TKA) PJI incidence was 2.2% and PBC group (811 TKA) PJI incidence was 3.1%. There were 7 fewer PJIs at 1 year in the ALBC group which is a 30% reduction in PJI. Despite this, PJI difference between ALBC and PBC groups was deemed to not be statistically significant. Examination of the statistical methodology used demonstrates the investigation was constructed to detect a 50% PJI incidence change.

> Therefore, failure to ascribe statistical significance to the observed 30% PJI reduction could very well represent a type II error and failure to recognize the efficacy of ALBC in preventing PJI.

The Kaiser Permanente Registry reported on the efficacy of ALBC from 2003 to 2007 using their large US community database of 22,889 TKAs (Namba et al. 2009). In this investigation, ALBC was used per the surgeon's discretion in 8.9% of all TKAs (2030). In this investigation, TKA PJI incidence was noted to be 1.4% in the ALBC group vs. 0.7% in the PBC cohort, and use of ALBC was found to be an independent risk factor for development of TKA PJI.

Careful examination of the study reveals significant differences in the ALBC and PBC cohorts. The ALBC cohort had statistically greater percentages of diabetics (14.5% vs. 10.3%), individuals <55 years of age (10.3% vs 7.0%), diagnoses other than osteoarthritis (10.8% vs. 7.3%), and ASA III classification patients (41.9% vs. 35.3%). Multivariate analyses performed in this investigation demonstrated all of these patient characteristics were independent risk factors for development of TKA PJI. Increased selective ALBC utilization in patients demonstrated to be at high risk for PJI is a substantial methodological and statistical bias which most likely increased the PJI incidence among the ALBC cohort.

> Despite being a large registry-driven investigation, the statistical consequences of not controlling for the above cohort disparities seriously call into question the conclusions drawn from comparing the ALBC and PBC groups.

A recent investigation published in the *Journal of Arthroplasty* details a European hospital's PJI experience when changing from PBC to commercially pre-mixed ALBC (Sanz-Ruiz et al. 2017). As reported, PMMA type was the only surgical or infection control variable changed within the institution over the study period with PBC uniformly used from 2009 to 2010 and uniform ALBC utilization from 2011 to 2012. All patients receiving either a primary TKA, THA, or hemiarthroplasty, were enrolled consecutively, and assessed for PJI at 2-year minimum follow-up. Despite the retrospective design, this study included the institutional PJI incidence for cementless hemiarthroplasty and THA during the same time period which effectively serve as control groups. ALBC utilization significantly decreased PJI incidence for all cemented groups (TKA, THA, and hemiarthroplasty).

> TKA PJI risk dropped from 3.3% to 1.3% which was a statistically significant overall risk reduction of 60%.

Similar statistically significant decreases in cemented THA and hemiarthroplasty PJI incidence were also noted. PJI incidence of the control groups (cementless THA and cementless hemiarthroplasty) demonstrated no statistical change throughout the study duration. This contemporary investigation indicates ALBC use can significantly decrease PJI incidence.

Risk stratified usage of ALBC was examined in the similarly named article published in the *Journal of Orthopedics* 2020 (Qadir et al. 2014). In this retrospective review of TKAs performed in a single center, the authors divided patients into 3 groups: PBC TKAs, ALBC TKAs, and selective ALBC TKAs (used per surgeon discretion in patient when deemed high risk). The 3 groups had statistically similar numbers of diabetics and patients with inflammatory arthritis; however, there was a trend for the selective ALBC group to have more patients with significant obesity within it.

> There were no details given regarding group-to-group distribution of other patient characteristics (e.g., malnutrition) thought to increase PJI incidence.

This investigation noted the 30-day, 6 month, and 1 year incidence of PJI among the different groups was identical. Obese patients in group 3 demonstrated a trend for increased PJI although this was not statistically significant. The conclusion of this investigation was that ALBC did not decrease PJI incidence and even selective use may not be justified. Another interpretation of this data could be that the selective ALBC group which was at the highest theoretical risk for PJI did not demonstrate an increased risk of PJI; therefore, the selective ALBC use mitigated excess PJI risk and its use was indeed justified.

A very recent analysis of 1,180,270 US patients undergoing TKA strongly supports the selective use of antibiotic-loaded bone cement (Chan et al. 2019). This study leveraged the Premier Healthcare Database, which contains administrative claims data for 20–25% of all US hospitalizations. ALBC was used in 27% of patients and was associated with both PJI prevention and lower odds of early postoperative infection (OR = 0.89; 95% CI 0.83–0.96). The investigation is unique for its extremely large patient cohort and robust multi-variate analysis including a significant number of variables known to increase PJI risks such as age, anesthesia modality, concomitant medications, smoking, obesity, and the Quan adaptation of the Charlson-Deyo index. Raw data analysis in this investigation indicated ALBC use might be correlated with acute renal failure not requiring dialysis (OR = 1.06; 95% CI: 1.02–1.11).

> However, after controlling for other variables known to cause renal failure, ALBC association with renal failure was no longer statistically significant. Likewise, ALBC use did not lead to statistically greater allergic complications or microbiome disruptions.

46.5.2 Randomized Controlled

Limited prospective randomized studies exist detailing ALBC efficacy for primary TKA PJI prevention. Existing studies have shown mixed results and are prone to type II statistical error as PJI occurs infrequently and extremely large patient cohorts are required to demonstrate a positive effect on PJI prevention.

> Unfortunately, different ALBC products were used in different studies which could be the reason different results and conclusions were reached by the authors.

One of the first randomized prospective studies demonstrating efficacy of ALBC was performed by Chiu et al. in a patient cohort of diabetic patients undergoing

TKA. He demonstrated that ALBC decreased PJI risk in this cohort by 13% (Chiu et al. 2001). Using another randomized prospective study, the same authors demonstrated that ALBC significantly decreased the incidence of PJI in a non-diabetic patient cohort (Chiu et al. 2002). Both studies indicated ALBC use decreased PJI incidence but critiques of both studies noted a relatively high baseline risk of infection.

In contrast, a Spanish group of investigators failed to find efficacy of hand-blended ALBC containing colistin and erythromycin for reducing TKA PJI in a randomized-controlled study design (Hinarejos et al. 2013). In this reasonably powered and well-designed study, PJI incidence for the ALBC and PBC groups were very similar (1.37% and 1.35%, respectively). However, the authors noted several times that even though this was a level I investigation, the results of the study are only specific to ALBC containing colistin and erythromycin and repeating the study with a different ALBC formulation might demonstrate ALBC ability to reduce the incidence of PJI.

Currently, a large prospective study entitled "Antibiotic Loaded Bone Cement in Prevention of Periprosthetic Joint Infections in Primary Total Knee Arthroplasty" is enrolling patients. In this randomized study where patients will either receive ALBC or PBC for primary TKA, the primary aim is to determine the rate of revision due to PJI for the two groups and the cost-effectiveness of ALBC. The study seeks to enroll over 11,000 patients based on power analyses demonstrating registry PJI incidence of 1.0% (ALBC) and 1.5% (PBC), respectively.

> The results of this study will be invaluable to improving our understanding the role of ALBC in primary TKA.

46.5.3 Systematic Reviews and Meta-analyses

Use of ALBC has been examined in systematic reviews and meta-analyses and has yielded conflicting results (Wang et al. 2013; Zhou et al. 2015; Schiavone Panni et al. 2016; King et al. 2018; Zhang et al. 2019). Due to lack of control groups and other deficiencies in scientific rigor, there are very few investigations examining the effect of ALBC on PJI incidence that qualify for inclusion in systematic reviews or meta-analyses. Careful examination of this literature shows it spans a broad time range (1987–2015) over which surgical environmental conditions and techniques have remarkably changed potentially skewing results. Furthermore, the types of ALBC used in the studies are quite heterogeneous (different products, antibiotics, antibiotic concentrations, as well as ALBC preparation methods) potentially introducing a confounding influence on results. Lastly, because of the low number of quality studies available, subtle differences in investigation exclusion and inclusion criteria can produce profound differences in results and conclusions.

An Italian group of authors performed a systemic review of ALBC efficacy for reducing TKA PJI incidence in 2016 (Schiavone Panni et al. 2016). Literature search returned 260 articles which were then narrowed to 6 publications. The pooled patient number included in the review was 6300. Significant methodological deficiencies in the included studies were identified which included but were not limited to heterogeneity in ALBC product type, differences in patient comorbidities, as well as poor patient randomization and blinding practices. This systematic review concluded ALBC was not protective for preventing TKA PJI. Two included investigations demonstrated ALBC to be protective against TKA PJI (Chiu, Eveillard) while four studies did not (Gandhi, Namba, Hinarejos, Wang). Only two randomized controlled studies could be identified and were included in this systematic review, one of which demonstrated efficacy of ALBC for the prevention of TKA PJI (Chiu) and the other one did not (Hinarejos). It should be noted that more than two-thirds of the pooled patients included in this review were derived from two retrospective studies with the lowest methodological quality scores both of which did not demonstrate efficacy of ALBC for preventing TKA PJI (Namba, Wang).

The most recent meta-analysis on ALBC efficacy in PJI prevention was published in 2019 (Zhang et al. 2019). This investigation narrowed initial search from 1049 potential studies to 10 randomized controlled trials (RCT) or cohort studies providing 13,909 THA and TKA patients for analysis. The date range for the included studies was 1981–2017. Within this meta-analysis, there were 3 randomized controlled trials (RCT) with 2287 patients which compared SSI/PJI incidence between patient groups receiving prophylactic antibiotics at the time of surgery to those receiving ALBC but no systemic antibiotics at the time of surgery. While the PJI incidence was lower within this ALBC subgroup (OR 0.34, CI: 0.14–0.89) the SSI incidence was higher within the ALBC group (OR 1.53, CI: 1.11–2.11) as compared to the prophylactic antibiotic group.

- When the studies not providing systemic prophylactic antibiotics were removed and compared ALBC+prophylactic antibiotics to prophylactic antibiotics alone, SSI odds ratio for the ALBC+prophylactic antibiotic group was 0.68 (CI: 0.52–0.88).

- When all 10 studies were included comparing THA and TKA PJI incidence in patients receiving ALBC with those that did not receive ALBC the OR markedly favored the ALBC group (OR 0.52, CI: 0.39–0.71).
- When only TKA PJI was considered, again the odds ratio favored ALBC (OR 0.62, CI: 0.45–0.87).

46.5.4 Registry

Registry Data

In 2017, the Australian Orthopaedic Association published a supplementary report on bone cement in hip & knee arthroplasty using their national registry (Australian Orthopaedic Association 2017). This report covered 293,025 primary TKA procedures and 9753 revisions between 1999 and 2015.

> In this analysis of total knee replacements, use of plain cement was associated with a statistically higher rate of revision (HR = 1.06; $p = 0.038$) as compared to ALBC.

Recently, a review of the National Joint Registry of England and Wales including over 700,000 TKAs demonstrated use of ALBC was associated with a decreased risk of revision as compared to TKAs implanted with PBC (Jameson et al. 2019). In this study many variables thought to be potential biases were controlled and separately examined.

> The conclusion of the article was that ALBC was associated with a 19% lower rate of septic and aseptic revisions as compared to PBC.

Importantly, this analysis allowed determination of the number of patients who would have to receive ALBC before one PJI was prevented. The so-called number-needed-to-treat (NNT) was 115, i.e., one PJI would be prevented for every 115 patients receiving ALBC. From this NNT, cost-effectiveness can be estimated for a large population.

> Assuming the additional cost of ALBC per TKA case is $300–500 USD as compared to PBC, the additional cost of ALBC in 115 patients would be $34,000–57,000 USD. Because the average cost of treating one PJI is approx. $100,000 USD, use of ALBC in this study would result in significant cost savings.

A report on 43,149 knee replacement cases from the Finnish Registry examined the impact of antibiotic delivery on re-operations for infections in primary and revision knees (Jamsen et al. 2009). The investigators looked at the impact of different antibiotic delivery strategies. In this analysis, systemic administration with ALBC demonstrated the lowest risk of revision for PJI in both primary and revision TKA. When compared to the systemic antibiotic with ALBC group, primary TKAs performed with systemic antibiotics only demonstrated a hazard ratio of 1.42 (95% CI: 1.08–1.88) for re-operation due to PJI. For revision TKA, only using systemic antibiotics increased the odds of re-operation for PJI by 2.12 (95% CI: 1.14–3.92).

For completeness, it is important to acknowledge both the Canadian and New Zealand Registry data with respect to ALBC and primary TKA. Data from these registries have been cited as evidence that ALBC usage does not prevent PJI or improve TKA outcomes. Understanding ALBC utilization, statistical nuances, and idiosyncratic findings of these registries are important to better understand the role of ALBC for primary TKA.

The Canadian Registry examined 36,681 primary TKA cases from 2003 to 2008 of which 45% were implanted with ALBC (Bohm et al. 2013). The multivariate analysis of this registry, which controlled for age, sex, diabetes, and Charlson Comorbidity Index score indicated ALBC did not statistically alter the odds of needing TKA revision at 2 years (HR = 1.066; 95% CI: 0.90–1.27). However, and importantly, this registry analysis noted the hazard ratio for primary TKA revision was lower for surgeons who uniformly utilized ALBC (HR 1.04, 95% CI: 0.86–1.44) as compared to surgeons selectively utilizing ALBC (HR 1.19, CI: 0.75–1.90).

> This curious paradox indicates all confounding variables may not have been adequately identified or controlled during registry data analysis and could be used to promote increased ALBC usage in the Canadian TKA population.

The New Zealand registry examined 64,566 primary TKAs performed between 1999 and 2012. Approximately, two-thirds of the patients in the New Zealand registry received a low-viscosity ALBC product with less than optimal antibiotic elution characteristics. Multivariate analysis of this registry data indicated ALBC was a significant predictor of PJI at 6 months (OR = 1.93; $p = 0.008$) but not at 12 months. Unfortunately, this investigation included few patient risk factors correlated with PJI (BMI and prior surgery) and the authors acknowledge the increased PJI hazard rate with ALBC use is likely a direct result of selective ALBC use in patients at increased risk for PJI.

> Because of the ALBC product utilized and suboptimal statistical control of confounding variables known to be correlated with PJI, caution should be exercised when drawing ALBC efficacy conclusions from this investigation.

46.6 Cost-Effectiveness

The economic ramifications for ALBC utilization differ among geographic markets. The main variables required to compute ALBC cost-effectiveness are:

- PJI incidence (hospital and/or health system),
- PJI treatment cost ($100,000 USD),
- ALBC product cost in comparison to PBC product.

In general, as the absolute price difference between ALBC and PBC decreases so does the institutional PJI incidence required to make the use of ALBC cost neutral or cost beneficial. Geographically, the cost of ALBC is the greatest in the US healthcare marketplace, which more likely than not accounts for US vs. non-US reported differences in ALBC cost-effectiveness.

ALBC pricing within the US healthcare marketplace has consistently trended downward so that the average cost difference of two ALBC packs compared to two PBC packs is now less than $300 (Mendenhall & Associates). Theoretically, at this cost, ALBC would have to decrease PJI incidence by one TKA per 333 TKAs (0.3%) to make its use cost neutral or to demonstrate cost savings.

46.7 Safety

The main safety concerns with use of antibiotic-loaded bone cement pertains to kidney damage and antibiotic resistance. As previously discussed, a study of 1,184,270 US TKA insurance claims found that ALBC use was associated with a slight increase in acute renal failure in one analysis (OR = 1.06; 95% CI: 1.02–1.11) but this finding could not be replicated in subsequent sensitivity analyses and ALBC was not associated with a significant increase in the need for acute dialysis (Chan et al. 2019).

In a separate study of 2775 arthroplasty procedures performed in Belfast, Northern Ireland, from 2015 to 2016, patients undergoing cementless arthroplasty received intravenous cefuroxime and gentamicin while patients with cemented arthroplasty received intravenous cefuroxime and localized administration of gentamicin via ALBC (Tucker et al. 2018).

> Patients receiving systemic gentamicin were observed to have twice the rate of acute kidney injury as compared to patients receiving gentamicin-impregnated ALBC (OR = 2.118; $p = 0.004$).

In 2014, the Rothman Institute reported on how ALBC impacted antimicrobial resistance patterns among patients who developed PJI (Hansen et al. 2014). The Rothman Institute switched from PBC to ALBC in 2003 allowing comparison of a cementless THA cohort over the entire study duration, PBC cohort prior to 2003, and ALBC cohort after 2003. With the switch to ALBC, they observed a 65% institutional reduction in the incidence of PJI for cemented arthroplasties (2.0% to 0.7%). Over the same time period, the PJI incidence in cementless hips only decreased by 33% (0.6% to 0.4%).

Investigators also examined the change in infective organism and antimicrobial resistance profiles for patients who developed culture-positive PJI ($n_{TKA} = 120$; $n_{THA} = 54$). After the initiation of routine ALBC use, the causative organism did not change significantly ($p > 0.1$). Additionally, while methicillin-resistance increased in cementless hips after 2003, the incidence of methicillin-resistant *Staphylococcus aureus* significantly decreased in patients receiving ALBC (40% vs. 18%, $p = 0.048$). The incidence of methicillin-resistant *S. epidermidis* was unchanged over this time period ($p = 0.6$). Non-significant decreases in tetracycline and erythromycin resistance rates were also observed.

A presentation at the 2019 AAOS Annual Meeting supports the findings of the Rothman Institute (Schmitt et al. 2019). This study from Loyola University also investigated causative organisms and antimicrobial resistance patterns amongst patients treated at their academic medical center over 20 years who developed PJI.

> In 32 patients with 36 cases of PJI, ALBC was not observed to significantly alter the organism causative of PJI, increase the risk of antibiotic resistance, or alter the pattern of antimicrobial resistance.

46.8 Alternative Local Therapy

Wound cavity administration of antimicrobial and antibiotic compounds following TKA implantation but before arthrotomy closure is an area of active research. In essence, the goal of these treatments is similar to that of ALBC which is to sterilize the wound cavity and eradicate any bacteria introduced into the wound at the time of surgery. To date, limited evidence is available regarding the efficacy of such treatments (Edmiston et al. 2018; Heckmann et al. 2019).

> Most investigations promoting such treatments suffer from very small patient numbers, inadequate follow-up intervals, retrospective study design, etc., which has significantly limited the ability to draw solid statistical conclusions from these studies.

The most popular topics discussed are the use of
- povidone-iodine soaks,
- intra-articular application of vancomycin powder,
- dilute chlorhexidine irrigation.

All treatments have surgical literature that both supports and refutes their ability to modify SSI incidence and there is some literature to assess their effectiveness in altering the incidence of PJI (Brown et al. 2012; Cichos et al. 2019; Hart et al. 2019; Heckmann et al. 2019; Iorio et al. 2020). All treatments have advocates and opponents whose views are largely based upon expert opinion and anecdotal experience.

Intra-articular vancomycin application following TKA was recently noted to increase the wound complication rate with no ability to decrease PJI incidence, which is contrary to literature supporting its use in hip arthroplasty and spine surgery (Dial et al. 2018; Ghobrial et al. 2015). Povidone-Iodine irrigation for THA and TKA has been widely embraced but concerns regarding its preparation and efficacy remain (Hart et al. 2019). The combination of intra-articular povidone-iodine washes followed by vancomycin powder application prior to arthrotomy closure in high-risk THA patients has recently been investigated and the authors conclude this approach has the ability to decrease PJI incidence (Iorio et al. 2020). Dilute chlorhexidine irrigation has the potential to decrease bacterial contamination of the wound but its ability to decrease PJI incidence is to date unproven (Smith et al. 2015; Frisch et al. 2017; Driesman et al. 2020).

Because the soft tissue envelope around the knee is much more tenuous than the hip, adverse tissue responses to intra-articular treatments as described above can be disastrous (Osei et al. 2016). Allergies, sensitivities, and soft tissue compromise as a result of local administration of powdered vancomycin, povidone-iodine, and chlorhexidine have all been noted albeit rare (Krautheim et al. 2004; Ghobrial et al. 2015; Su et al. 2016).

> Adoption of these strategies for PJI reduction should balance their potential ability to reduce PJI against potential for sterile field compromise during preparation and complications that can be precipitated by the treatment.

Take-Home Messages

- Hand-blended ALBC suffers from inconsistencies introduced by human error and results in PMMA that has variable elution and mechanical characteristics.
- Commercially premixed ALBCs have a predictable, uniform release.
- According to registry data of Australian Orthopaedic Association (2017), the use of plain cement was associated with a statistically higher rate of revision (HR = 1.06; 0 = 0.038) as compared to ALBC.
- Because the average cost of treating one PJI is approximately \$100,000 USD, the use of ALBC in this study would result in significant cost savings.
- The frequently discussed acute renal insufficiency finding could not be replicated in subsequent sensitivity analyses and ALBC was not associated with a significant increase in the need for acute dialysis.
- ALBC was not observed to significantly alter the organism causative of PJI, increase the risk of antibiotic resistance, or alter the pattern of antimicrobial resistance.

References

Abdel MP, Berry DJ (2019) Current practice trends in primary hip and knee arthroplasties among members of the American Association of Hip and Knee Surgeons: a long-term update. J Arthroplast 34(7S):S24–S27

Australian Orthopaedic Association (2017) Supplementary report: cement in hip & knee arthroplasty. Figure C7: Cumulative percent revision of cemented primary total knee replacement by cement type (Primary Diagnosis OA). p 13

Australian Orthopaedic Association National Joint Registry (2019a) Annual report 2019. Figure KT4: Primary total knee replacement by fixation, p 210. https://aoanjrr.sahmri.com

Australian Orthopaedic Association National Joint Registry (2019b) Annual report 2019. Figures KT34–35: Cumulative percent revision of primary total knee replacement by fixation (Primary Diagnosis OA), pp 246–249. https://aoanjrr.sahmri.com

Best AJ, Fender D, Harper WM et al (1998) Current practice in primary total hip replacement: results from the National Hip Replacement Outcome Project. Ann R Coll Surg Engl 80(5): 350–355

Bohm E, Zhu N, de Guia N et al (2013) Does adding antibiotics to cement reduce the need for early revision in total knee arthroplasty. Clin Orthop Relat Res 472(1):162–168

Bozic KJ, Kurtz SM, Lau E et al (2010) The epidemiology of revision total knee arthroplasty in the United States. Clin Orthop Relat Res 468:45–51
Brown NM, Cipriano CA, Moric M et al (2012) Dilute betadine lavage before closure for the prevention of acute postoperative deep periprosthetic joint infection. J Arthroplast 27(1):27–30
Buchholz HW, Elson RA, Engelbrecht E et al (1981) Management of deep infection of total hip replacement. J Bone Joint Surg Br 63-B(3):342–353
Buchholz HW, Elson RA, Heinert K (1984) Antibiotic-loaded acrylic cement: current concepts. Clin Orthop Relat Res 190:96–108
Chan JJ, Robinson J, Poeran J et al (2019) Antibiotic-loaded bone cement in primary total knee arthroplasty: utilization patterns and impact on complications using a national database. J Arthroplast 34(7S):S188–S194
Chiu FY, Lin CF, Chen CM et al (2001) Cefurozime-impregnated cement at primary total knee arthroplasty in diabetes mellitus: a randomized, prospective study. J Bone Joint Surg Br 839b:691–695
Chiu FY, Chen CM, Lin CFJ, Lo WH (2002) Cefuroxime-impregnated cement in primary total knee arthroplasty; a prospective, randomized study of three hundred and forty knees. J Bone Joint Surg Am 84(5):759–762
Cichos KH, Andrews RM, Wolschendorf F et al (2019) Efficacy of intraoperative antiseptic techniques in the prevention of periprosthetic joint infection: superiority of betadine. J Arthroplast 34(7S):S312–S318
Dial BL, Lampley AJ, Green CL, Hallows R (2018) Intrawound vancomycin powder in primary total hip arthroplasty increases rate of sterile wound complications. Hip Pelvis 30(1):37–44
Driesman A, Shen M, Feng JE et al (2020) Perioperative chlorhexidine gluconate wash during joint arthroplasty has equivalent periprosthetic joint infection rates in comparison to betadine wash. J Arthroplast 35(3):845–848
Dunne N, Hill J, Mcafee P et al (2007) In vitro study of the efficacy of acrylic bone cement loaded with supplementary amounts of gentamicin: effect on mechanical properties, antibiotic release, and biofilm formation. Acta Orthop 78(6):774–785
Edmiston CE, Spencer M, Leaper D (2018) Antiseptic irrigation as an effective interventional strategy for reducing the risk of surgical site infections. Surg Infect 19(8):774–780
Eveillard M, Mertl P, Tramier B, Francois EB (2003) Effectiveness of gentamicin-impregnated cement in the prevention of deep wound infection after primary total knee arthroplasty. Infect Control Hosp Epidemiol 24(10):778–780
Ferraris S, Miola M, Bistolfi A et al (2010) In vitro comparison between commercially and manually mixed antibiotic-loaded bone cements. J Appl Biomater Biomech 8(3):166–174
Fillingham Y, Greenwald AS, Grenier J et al (2019) Hip and knee section, local antimicrobials: proceedings of international consensus on orthopedic infections. J Arthroplast 34(2S):S289–S292
Frisch NB, Kadri OM, Tenbrunsel T et al (2017) Intraoperative chlorhexidine irrigation to prevent infection in total hip and knee arthroplasty. Arthroplast Today 3(4):294–297
Gandhi R, Razak F, Pathy R et al (2009) Antibiotic bone cement and the incidence of deep infection after total knee arthroplasty. J Arthroplast 24(7):1015–1018
Ghobrial GM, Cadotte DW, Williams K et al (2015) Complications from the use of intrawound vancomycin in lumbar spine surgery: a systematic review. Neurosurg Focus 39(4):E11
Hansen EN, Adeli B, Kenyon R, Parvizi J (2014) Routine use of antibiotic laden bone cement for primary total knee arthroplasty: impact on infecting microbial patterns and resistance profiles. J Arthroplast 29(6):1123–1127
Hart A, Hernandez NM, Abdel MP et al (2019) Povidone-iodine wound lavage to prevent infection after revision total hip and knee arthroplasty: an analysis of 2,884 cases. J Bone Joint Surg Am 101(13):1151–1159
Heckmann ND, Mayfield CK, Culvern CN et al (2019) Systematic review and meta-analysis of intrawound vancomycin in total hip and total knee arthroplasty: a call for a prospective randomized trial. J Arthroplast 34(8):1815–1822
Hinarejos P, Guirro P, Leal J et al (2013) The use of erythromycin and colistin-loaded cement in total knee arthroplasty does not reduce the incidence of infection: a prospective randomized study in 3000 knees. J Bone Joint Surg Am 95(9):769–764
Iorio R, Yu S, Anoushiravani AA et al (2020) Vancomycin powder and dilute povidone-iodine lavage for infection prophylaxis in high-risk total joint arthroplasty. J Arthroplast 35(7):1933–1936
Jameson SS, Asaad A, Diament M et al (2019) Antibiotic-loaded bone cement is associated with a lower risk of revision following primary cemented total knee arthroplasty. Bone Joint Surg Br 101-B:1331–1347
Jamsen E, Huhtala H, Puolakka T, Moilanen T (2009) Risk factors for infection after knee arthroplasty. J Bone Joint Surg Am 91(1):38–47
King JD, Hamilton DH, Jacobs CA, Duncan ST (2018) Antibiotic-loaded bone cement: a systematic review of clinical results and cost implications following total knee arthroplasty. J Arthroplast 33(12):3789–3792
Krautheim AB, Jermann THM, Bircher AJ (2004) Chlorhexidine anaphylaxis: case report and review of the literature. Contact Dermatitis 50(3):113–116
Kuehn KD (2014) PMMA cement as a drug carrier in PMMA cements. Springer, Berlin/Heidelberg/New York
Kurtz SM, Ong KL, Lau E et al (2011) International survey of primary and revision total knee replacement. Int Orthop 35(12):1783–1789
Lidgren L (2001) Joint prosthetic infections: a success story. Acta Orthop Scand 72:553
Meyer J, Piller G, Spiegel CA et al (2011) Vacuum-mixing significantly changes antibiotic elution characteristics of commercially available antibiotic-impregnated bone cements. J Bone Joint Surg 93(22):2049–2056
Moran CG, Horton TC (2000) Total knee replacement: the joint of the decade. BMJ 320(7328):820
Namba RS, Chen Y, Paxton EW et al (2009) Outcomes of routine use of antibiotic-loaded bone cement in primary total knee arthroplasty. J Arthroplast 24(6S):44–47
National Joint Registry for England, Wales, Northern Ireland and the Isle of Man (2019) Table 3.26: Kaplan-Meier estimates of cumulative revision (95% CI) by gender, age, fixation, constraint and bearing. 16th Annual Report 2019. p 128
Neut D, van de Belt H, van Horn JR et al (2003) The effect of mixing on gentamicin release from polymethylmethacrylate bone cements. Acta Orthop 74(6):670–676
Nugent M, Wyatt MC, Frampton CM, Hooper GJ (2019) Despite improved survivorship of uncemented fixation in total knee arthroplasty for osteoarthritis, cemented fixation remains the gold standard: an analysis of a National Joint Registry. J Arthroplast 34(8):1626–1633
Osei DA, Rebehn KA, Boyer MI (2016) Soft-tissue defects after total knee arthroplasty: management and reconstruction. J Am Acad Orthop Surg 24(11):769–779
Parvizi J, Gehrke T, Chen AF (2013) Proceedings of the international consensus on periprosthetic joint infection. Bone Joint J 95-B(11):1450–1452
Price AJ, Alvand A, Troelsen A et al (2018) Knee replacement. Lancet 392(10158):1672–1682

Qadir R, Sanbir S, Ochsner JL et al (2014) Risk stratified usage of antibiotic-loaded bone cement for primary total knee arthroplasty: short term infection outcomes with a standardized cement protocol. J Arthroplast 29(8):1622–1624
Rocha de Silva R, Santos AAM, Carvalho JS Jr, Matos MA (2014) Quality of life after total knee arthroplasty: systemic review. Rev Bras Ortop 49(5):520–527
Salah KJ, Hoeffel DP, Kassim RA, Burstein G (2003) Complications after revision total knee arthroplasty. JBJS 85-A(Suppl 1):71–74
Sanz-Ruiz S, Matas-Dies JA, Sanchez-Somolinos M et al (2017) Is the commercial antibiotic-loaded bone cement useful in prophylaxis and cost saving after knee and hip joint arthroplasty? The transatlantic paradox. J Arthroplast 32(4):1095–1099
Sanz-Ruiz P, Matas-Diez JA, Villanueva-Martínez M et al (2020) Is dual antibiotic-loaded bone cement more effective and cost-efficient than a single antibiotic-loaded bone cement to reduce the risk of prosthetic joint infection in aseptic revision knee arthroplasty? J Arthroplast 35(12):3724–3729. https://doi.org/10.1016/j.arth.2020.06.045
Schiavone Panni A, Corona K et al (2016) Antibiotic-loaded bone cement reduces risk of infections in primary total knee arthroplasty? A systematic review. Knee Surg Sports Traumatol Arthrosc 24(10):3168–3174
Schmitt D, Killen C, Murphy M et al (2019) The impact of antibiotic-loaded bone cement on antibiotic resistance in periprosthetic knee infections. AAOS Annual Meeting. Las Vegas, 12–16 March 2019; Abstract 3595
Smith DC, Maiman R, Schwechter EM et al (2015) Optimal irrigation and debridement of infected total joint implants with chlorhexidine gluconate. J Arthroplast 30(10):1820–1822
Squire MW, Ludwig BJ, Thompson JR et al (2008) Premixed antibiotic bone cement: an in vitro comparison of antimicrobial efficacy. J Arthroplast 23(6):1104
Starnes BW (2013) A surgeon's perspective regarding the regulatory, compliance, and legal issues involved with physician-modified devices. J Vasc Surg 57(3):829–831
Su D, Zhao H, Hu J et al (2016) TRPA1 and TRPV1 contribute to iodine antiseptics-associated pain and allergy. EMBO Rep 17(10):1422–1430
Tucker A, Hegarty P, Magill PJ et al (2018) Acute kidney injury after prophylactic cefuroxime and gentamicin in patients undergoing primary hip and knee arthroplasty – a propensity score-matched study. J Arthroplast 33:3009–3015
Wang J, Zhu C, Cheng T et al (2013) A systematic review and meta-analysis of antibiotic-impregnated bone cement use in primary total hip or knee arthroplasty. PLoS One 8(12):e82745
Zhang J, Zhang XY, Jiang FL et al (2019) Antibiotic-impregnated cement for preventing infection in patients receiving primary total hip and knee replacement. Medicine (Baltimore) 98(49):e18068
Zhou Y, Li L, Zhou Q, Yuan S et al (2015) Lack of efficacy of prophylactic application of antibiotic-loaded bone cement for prevention of infection in primary total knee arthroplasty: results of a meta-analysis. Surg Infect 16(2):183–187

Antibiotic-Loaded Bone Cement: Con

Shayan Hosseinzadeh, Hugh Gorman, and Antonia F. Chen

Contents

In the following chapter, the authors unveil the Cons of ALBC in knee arthroplasty. The task for the authors was to consistently and scientifically argue according to the clinical use of ALBC. The compiled arguments do not always represent the opinion of the author.

E. Hansen, K.-D. Kühn (eds.), *Essentials of Cemented Knee Arthroplasty*,
https://doi.org/10.1007/978-3-662-63113-3_47

47.1 Introduction

The overall rate of infection after TKA is approximately 1–2% (Garvin and Konigsberg 2011; Kurtz et al. 2010; Zimmerli et al. 2004), but the rates have decreased in the last decade due to patient optimization, the appropriate use of systemic and local antibiotics, and implementing decolonization protocols (Hansen et al. 2014). Deep infection rates are controversial, as they might be as low as 1–2% even without the use of ALBC (ALBC) (Hinarejos et al. 2015; Qadir et al. 2014). ALBC has the potential of localized antibiotic delivery directly at the surgical site and is widely used for the prophylaxis and treatment of orthopedic infections after TKA. From the first introduction of the concept by Bucholz and Engelbrecht in 1970 (Kleppel et al. 2017), ALBC has become a popular method of managing periprosthetic joint infections (PJIs) after TKA with the result of significant reduction of PJI infection rate (Abdelaziz et al. 2019; Espehaug et al. 1997). Classically ALBC is used in one- or two-stage exchange revision arthroplasty with static or articulating spacers, rods, beads, or any custom-made spacers (Chan et al. 2019).

Desirable characteristics of an appropriate antibiotic admixed into bone cement, which is an "off label" use, are

- availability in powder form,
- bactericidal effects at low concentrations,
- wide-spectrum bacterial coverage,
- a prolonged period of elution in high concentration,
- thermal stability,
- low serum protein binding,
- a low risk of delayed allergy and delayed hypersensitivity,
- low impact on cement mechanical properties (Anagnostakos and Kelm 2009).

Glycopeptides and aminoglycosides that are often manually admixed to PMMA are the antibiotic groups that meet most of these criteria. Interestingly, their combination provides wide bacterial spectrum coverage, while maintaining appropriate elution kinetics (Anagnostakos 2017).

However, the lack of clinical evidence reporting that routine use of ALBC in primary TKA actually reduces infection rates has led to an overall decrease in the use of ALBC in recent years, especially among medium- to large-sized hospitals (Chan et al. 2019). While ALBC is able to provide antibiotic prophylaxis in primary TKA, it is not without flaws. Re-infection or development of infection resistance, an allergic reaction, and renal or hepatic failure are all possible complications to be discussed (Anagnostakos 2017). Increased cost, mechanical loosening, and subsequent TKA failures are among other concerns (Chan et al. 2019). In this chapter, the potential cons of using ALBC after admixing antibiotics in primary TKA in the USA will be described.

47.2 Decreased Mechanical Strength

A rise in temperature during the bone cement polymerization reaction starts as an air bubble formation in the cement that results in some porosity in the cement structure (Hinarejos et al. 2015). The final cement porosity depends on the cement composition, manipulation method, and cement viscosity (Van De Belt et al. 2001). Although cement porosity increases the antibiotic release capacity, if any antibiotics are added to its structure, it causes a decrease in mechanical properties (Alentorn-Geli et al. 2015). ALBC can be hand-mixed, which increases the porosity and elution kinetics of the antibiotics, or can be mixed in a standardized manner by vacuum mixing that improves the tensile fatigue strength (Chen and Parvizi 2014).

> As a legal consequence of the customized addition of antibiotics, the surgeon becomes the responsible manufacturer and thus assumes liability for the product quality (Kühn et al. 2018).

Different mechanical effects of each antibiotic dose level in ALBCs are summarized in Fig. 47.1 (Gogus et al. 2002; Lautenschlager et al. 1976; Moran et al. 1979).

In vitro studies have suggested that even adding small quantities of antibiotic powder to polymethylmethacrylate (PMMA) decreases the tensile and compressive strengths of the bone cement, which continues to decline by increasing the dose of antibiotics (Lautenschlager et al. 1976).

> Unfortunately, the ideal amount of antibiotic to be used in ALBC has not yet been determined (Kleppel et al. 2017).

It has been shown, however, that higher dosages of antibiotic impregnation in cement spacers (>4 g of antibiotic powder per 40 g cement) can result in greater mechanical issues such as prosthetic loosening and fracture or dislocation of spacers (Anagnostakos 2017). Lower doses (<1 g of antibiotic powder per 40 g cement) of antibiotic impregnation leads to less mechanical loosening, but may contribute to poor elution and weaker antimicrobial properties, eventually leading to antibiotic

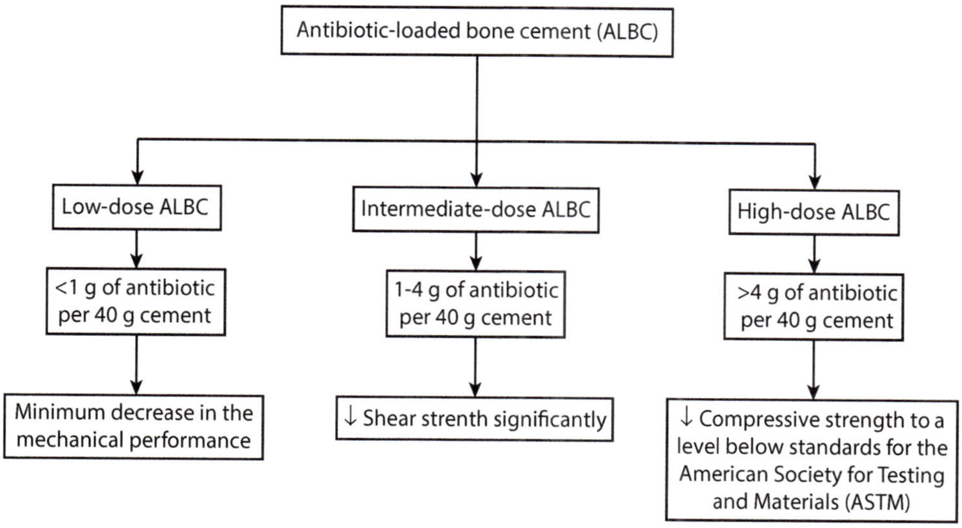

Fig. 47.1 Variations in mechanical performance among different antibiotic dose levels

resistance and infection (Anagnostakos 2017) and increased probability of obtaining a negative culture whenever subsequent aspirations are performed (Chen and Parvizi 2014). Given this detrimental effect on the mechanical properties of the cement, it is widely accepted that high-dose ALBC (>4 g per 40 g of cement) should only be used in temporary cement spacers or beads used in the treatment of prosthetic infections, while low doses (<1 g per 40 g of cement) can be used for prophylactic ALBC since the principal aim of the implants is fixation and maintenance of mechanical properties (Bistolfi et al. 2011; Dunne et al. 2008; Klekamp et al. 1999). The above-mentioned negative effects of antibiotics on cement mechanical properties could even arise with lower doses of imipenem. It is also important to take into consideration that different orthopedic cement brands elute differently (Slane et al. 2018).

47.3 Antibiotic Resistance

The risk of developing any antibiotic resistance may be less for locally delivered antibiotics, because the pharmacokinetics of local antibiotics are associated with generally lower systemic levels compared to systemic antibiotics.

However, even though most locally delivered antibiotics drop below the detectable threshold after 2 days depending on the cement brand (Kendoff et al. 2016; Wahlig and Dingeldein 1980), if any resistant bacterial strain survives the initial elution peak, a selection process occurs.

Hendriks et al. studied this concept by mimicking the space between ALBC and bone tissue in a gap model investigation, in which all susceptible *Staphylococcus epidermidis* bacteria were killed by the antibiotic released from the cement, but bacteria were able to survive if challenged with resistant *S. epidermidis* mutant strains (Hendriks et al. 2005).

In another study, Thornes et al. demonstrated in an animal model that infection reduction in ALBC led to an increase in antibiotic resistance when the infection was not properly eradicated (Thornes et al. 2002). It has been shown that approximately 8% of the antibiotic content in ALBC is quickly released immediately after surgery, followed by an ineffective low-dose release below the minimum inhibitory concentration that can allow for the development of mutational resistance in bacteria (Hendriks et al. 2005; Hinarejos et al. 2015; Van De Belt et al. 2001). The use of gentamicin-impregnated cement for primary TKA led to the development of resistant coagulase-negative Staphylococci in one study (Neut et al. 2001). Aminoglycosides have higher rates of resistance if the spacer is used in two-stage revision arthroplasties, confirming the risk of resistant mutant strains selection when using ALBC (Corona et al. 2014). Nevertheless, Sprowson et al. (2016) described a significantly lower resistance tendency while using different antibiotics that had different modes of action.

Contributing factors for re-infection or infection persistence are

- the general condition of the patient,
- the virulence of the causative bacteria,
- inadequate systemic antibiotic therapy,
- insufficient debridement of infected and necrotic tissue,

- wrong antibiotic choice for impregnation,
- implant surface biofilm formation,
- the lack of definitive infection eradication before prosthesis re-implantation (Anagnostakos 2017).

Furthermore, residual ALBC might also be significantly associated with the persistence of infection, which was eventually treated with resection arthroplasty (Buttaro et al. 2004; Mcdonald et al. 1989). The majority (90%) of these patients can clear the infection after the residual ALBC has been removed (Anagnostakos 2017). Tyas et al. (2018) observed a significantly lower infection rate with the use of high-dose dual-antibiotic cement (HDDAC) compared to low-dose single-antibiotic cement (LDSAC), with a trend to a lower rate of resistance with the use of high-dose dual-antibiotic cement. However, there were increases in the proportion of resistant cases, most notably to clindamycin and ciprofloxacin in Gram-positive organisms (Table 47.1), possibly reflecting the higher number of *S. epidermidis* in the high-dose dual-antibiotic cement group. While the differences in the study were not found to be statistically significant, the findings were reassuring for those using high-dose dual-antibiotic cement to prevent SSI in hip hemiarthroplasty (Tyas et al. 2018).

Since 1980 (Josefsson et al. 1981) until 2016 (Amerstorfer et al. 2017) even locally applied high-dose vancomycin did not result in nephrotoxicity. Amerstorfer et al. showed that high superficial vancomycin coating of bone cement is an effective technique to enhance local concentrations of vancomycin without contributing to systemic side effects (Amerstorfer et al. 2017).

Table 47.1 Percentages of microorganism resistance to low-dose single antibiotic- (LDSAC) and high-dose dual antibiotic-impregnated cements (HDDAC) in Gram-positive and Gram-negative bacteria

Antibiotic	LDSAC organism resistance (%)	HDDAC organism resistance (%)
Gram-Positive microorganisms		
Amoxicillin	60.00	40.00
Ciprofloxacin	64.00	100.00
Clindamycin	36.36	96.30
Daptomycin	0.00	0.00
Erythromycin	69.70	100.00
Flucloxacillin	81.48	95.24
Fusidic acid	33.33	50.00
Gentamicin	65.63	92.59
High-level gentamicin	100.00	50.00
Linezolid	0.00	0.00
Rifampicin	11.11	13.64
Teicoplanin	22.58	26.92
Tetracycline	46.43	60.00
Tigecycline	0.00	0.00
Trimethoprim	78.57	81.48
Vancomycin	0.00	3.70
Gram-Negative microorganisms		
Amoxicillin	66.64	83.33
Aztreonam	14.29	0.00
Ceftazidime	30.00	16.67
Cefuroxime	33.33	60.00
Ciprofloxacin	15.38	12.50
Co-amoxiclav	30.00	50.00
Ertapenem	0.00	20.00
Gentamicin	35.71	12.50
Meropenem	0.00	0.00
Piperacillin-Tazobactam	0.00	14.29
Tigecycline	37.50	50.00
Trimethoprim	50.00	33.33

47.4 Acute Renal Failure

Several cases have resulted in acute renal failure (ARF) as a complication when using a high dosage of antibiotics. With utilization rates of around 30%, Chan et al. found that ALBC reduced odds for early postoperative infection and increased odds for kidney injury (Chan et al. 2019).

Staphylococci are the most common bacteria causing orthopedic-related infections.

The 3 most commonly used antibiotics in ALBC are vancomycin, gentamicin, and tobramycin, all of which have the potential for inducing a renal toxicity crisis (Eveillard et al. 2003; Randelli et al. 2010).

Experimental investigations have also found that gentamicin decreases the alkaline phosphates levels in osteoblasts derived from trabecular bone, suggesting a cellular toxicity effect (Edin et al. 1996; Ince et al. 2007).

Approximately half of the patients in a study had detectable aminoglycosides in their serum after using ALBC, including some primary TKA cases with low-dose ALBC (Kalil et al. 2012). Since many of them have a serum creatinine level elevation, measuring aminoglycoside serum concentration is recommended during the early postoperative management of these patients, although this is still controversial in the literature. Other authors like Buchholz and Engelbrecht (1970), Reed (Reed et al. 2014), Wahlig (Wahlig and Dingeldein 1980), Jämeson (Jameson et al. 2019), and Joseffson (Josefsson et al. 1981) did not find kidney injuries as a consequence of using ALBC. Parenteral application of antibiotics should be taken into account, as local antibiotics may lead to reduced serum antibiotic use.

Increased rates of ARF in primary hip and knee joint arthroplasties have been already demonstrated in the routine use of perioperative systemic renal toxic antibiotics (Bailey et al. 2014; Courtney et al. 2015). Since the antibiotic release is significantly higher in ALBC, with up to 30 days of elution postoperatively, it places patients at a higher risk of developing ARF (Chan et al. 2019). The role of ALBC in the development of postoperative ARF in revision TKA has been well established in the literature (Edelstein et al. 2018; Patel et al. 2018). ARF patients showed a return to normal serum antibiotic and creatinine levels and normal renal function after removal of the ALBC.

> However, most of the previous studies only focused on the events during hospitalization and given the long elution time of ALBC, further investigations are still required to evaluate chronic renal failure that could take longer to develop.

47.5 Infection Risk

In contrast to the established pros of ALBC use in revision TKA for PJIs, a systemic review and meta-analysis by Kleppel et al. found that the use of ALBC did not reduce infection rates after primary TKA (Kleppel et al. 2017). Furthermore, literature reviews have found that ALBC does not significantly reduce superficial infection rates (Panni et al. 2016; Voigt et al. 2016; Wang et al. 2013). Infection rates were higher in patients who received systemic prophylactic antibiotics (1.6%) compared to local ALBC (0.4%) using Palacos with gentamicin, with no evidence of nephrotoxicity or allergic reactions. Interestingly, Tayton et al. actually found an increased revision rate for PJI when using ALBC in a large Australian registry database (Tayton et al. 2016). Some have suggested that the amount of cement used in TKA settings is generally lower than the antibiotic spacers in revisions, which predispose to lower durability and lower effective antibiotic levels throughout the joint, potentially predisposing to increased PJI (Bohm et al. 2014).

47.6 Allergic Reactions

> In general, antibiotics can potentially trigger allergic reactions. Hence, the allergy history of each patient should be obtained prior to any ALBC implantation.

The possibility of an allergic reaction is higher if using cephalosporin-impregnated cement given the cross-reactivity to penicillin, which is rarely used in combination with PMMA cement because of their low thermostable properties. It is well known that a systemic hypersensitivity reaction can occur in response to extremely high vancomycin-loaded bone cement leading to a diffuse desquamating rash (Cummins et al. 2009).

47.7 Indications

Given the higher cost, controversial effectiveness, and potential complications, we only potentially recommend using ALBC in high-risk groups of patients such as immunocompromised patients and patients with diabetes (Dowsey and Choong 2009; Jämsen et al. 2010; Mraovic et al. 2011), morbid obesity (Dowsey and Choong 2009; Malinzak et al. 2009; Pulido et al. 2008), rheumatoid arthritis (Liu et al. 2003), previous history of knee infection or fracture, and those undergoing prolonged surgeries (Jämsen et al. 2009; Kurtz et al. 2010; Namba et al. 2013; Willis-Owen et al. 2010). However, a recent study indicated that the use of ALBC in primary TKA is not justified, even in the aforementioned high-risk groups of patients (Qadir et al. 2014).

Note

Infection rates have not decreased despite modern advanced education for orthopedic surgeons, their specialization, ameliorated standards of hygiene in the operation field, and an additional shorter operation time which is a possible reason for not routinely using ALBC.

Take-Home Messages

- Manual admixing of antibiotics to PMMA has potential adverse effects and should not be used routinely in primary TKA in the USA. However, if it is used, there should be less than 1 g of antibiotics per 40 g bag (low-dose) of cement.
- The risk of developing any antibiotic resistance depends on subtherapeutic concentrations of antibiotics in the environment of microorganisms. Based on the choice of antibiotic, choice of cement, and choice of antibiotic concentration, ALBC can lead to an increase in antibiotic resistance when the infection was not properly eradicated.
- Manual admixing of antibiotics to PMMA decreases mechanical strength and may result in antibiotic resistance, acute renal failure, infection risk, and allergic reactions.
- Given these complications and higher cost along with the low baseline infection rates in primary TKA at approximately 1%, we do not generally recommend using ALBC in low-risk groups of TKA patients.
- The use of appropriate manually admixed ALBC in primary TKA may be considered in high-risk patients, including immunocompromised patients, patients with diabetes, morbidly obese patients, rheumatoid arthritis patients, and patients with a previous history of knee infection or fracture.
- Acute renal failure mostly occurs when higher concentrations of antibiotics are detected in serum and urine. Systemically applied antibiotics in TKA are usually found in serum and urine, whereas antibiotics applied via ALBC are found in high local concentrations.
- As a legal consequence of customized addition of antibiotics, the surgeon becomes the responsible manufacturer of the cement and thus assumes liability for the product quality.

References

Abdelaziz H, Von Förster G, Kühn KD et al (2019) Minimum 5 years' follow-up after gentamicin- and clindamycin-loaded PMMA cement in total joint arthroplasty. J Med Microbiol 68:475–479

Alentorn-Geli E, Pelfort X, Mingo F et al (2015) An evaluation of the association between radiographic intercondylar notch narrowing and anterior cruciate ligament injury in men: the notch angle is a better parameter than notch width. Arthroscopy 31:2004–2013

Amerstorfer F, Fischerauer S, Sadoghi P et al (2017) Superficial vancomycin coating of bone cement in orthopedic revision surgery: a safe technique to enhance local antibiotic concentrations. J Arthroplast 32:1618–1624

Anagnostakos K (2017) Therapeutic use of antibiotic-loaded bone cement in the treatment of hip and knee joint infections. J Bone Jt Infect 2:29–37

Anagnostakos K, Kelm J (2009) Enhancement of antibiotic elution from acrylic bone cement. J Biomed Mater Res B Appl Biomater 90:467–475

Bailey O, Torkington MS, Anthony I et al (2014) Antibiotic-related acute kidney injury in patients undergoing elective joint replacement. Bone Joint J 96-b:395–398

Bistolfi A, Massazza G, Verné E et al (2011) Antibiotic-loaded cement in orthopedic surgery: a review. ISRN Orthop 2011:290851

Bohm E, Zhu N, Gu J et al (2014) Does adding antibiotics to cement reduce the need for early revision in total knee arthroplasty? Clin Orthop Relat Res 472:162–168

Buchholz HW, Engelbrecht H (1970) Depot effects of various antibiotics mixed with Palacos resins. Der Chirurg; Zeitschrift fur alle Gebiete der operativen Medizen 41:511–515

Buttaro M, Valentini R, Piccaluga F (2004) Persistent infection associated with residual cement after resection arthroplasty of the hip. Acta Orthop Scand 75:427–429

Chan JJ, Robinson J, Poeran J et al (2019) Antibiotic-loaded bone cement in primary total knee arthroplasty: utilization patterns and impact on complications using a National Database. J Arthroplast 34:S188–S194.e181

Chen AF, Parvizi J (2014) Antibiotic-loaded bone cement and periprosthetic joint infection. J Long-Term Eff Med Implants 24:89–97

Corona PS, Espinal L, Rodríguez-Pardo D et al (2014) Antibiotic susceptibility in gram-positive chronic joint arthroplasty infections: increased aminoglycoside resistance rate in patients with prior aminoglycoside-impregnated cement spacer use. J Arthroplast 29:1617–1621

Courtney PM, Rozell JC, Melnic CM et al (2015) Who should not undergo short stay hip and knee arthroplasty? Risk factors associated with major medical complications following primary total joint arthroplasty. J Arthroplast 30:1–4

Cummins JS, Tomek IM, Kantor SR et al (2009) Cost-effectiveness of antibiotic-impregnated bone cement used in primary total hip arthroplasty. JBJS 91:634–641

Dowsey MM, Choong PF (2009) Obese diabetic patients are at substantial risk for deep infection after primary TKA. Clin Orthop Relat Res 467:1577–1581

Dunne N, Hill J, Mcafee P et al (2008) Incorporation of large amounts of gentamicin sulphate into acrylic bone cement: effect on handling and mechanical properties, antibiotic release, and biofilm formation. Proc Inst Mech Eng H J Eng Med 222:355–365

Edelstein AI, Okroj KT, Rogers T et al (2018) Nephrotoxicity after the treatment of periprosthetic joint infection with antibiotic-loaded cement spacers. J Arthroplast 33:2225–2229

Edin ML, Miclau T, Lester GE et al (1996) Effect of cefazolin and vancomycin on osteoblasts in vitro. Clin Orthop Relat Res (333):245–251

Espehaug B, Engesaeter LB, Vollset SE et al (1997) Antibiotic prophylaxis in total hip arthroplasty. Review of 10,905 primary cemented total hip replacements reported to the Norwegian arthroplasty register, 1987 to 1995. J Bone Joint Surg 79:590–595

Eveillard M, Mertl P, Tramier B et al (2003) Effectiveness of gentamicin-impregnated cement in the prevention of deep wound infection after primary total knee arthroplasty. Infect Control Hosp Epidemiol 24:778–780

Garvin KL, Konigsberg BS (2011) Infection following total knee arthroplasty: prevention and management. J Bone Joint Surg Am 93:1167–1175

Gogus A, Akman S, Goksan SB et al (2002) Mechanical strength of antibiotic-impregnated bone cement on Day 0 and Day 15: a biomechanical study with Surgical Simplex P and teicoplanin. Acta Orthop Traumatol Turc 36:63–71

Hansen EN, Adeli B, Kenyon R et al (2014) Routine use of antibiotic laden bone cement for primary total knee arthroplasty: impact on infecting microbial patterns and resistance profiles. J Arthroplast 29:1123–1127

Hendriks J, Neut D, Van Horn J et al (2005) Bacterial survival in the interfacial gap in gentamicin-loaded acrylic bone cements. J Bone Joint Surg 87:272–276

Hinarejos P, Guirro P, Puig-Verdie L et al (2015) Use of antibiotic-loaded cement in total knee arthroplasty. World J Orthop 6:877–885

Ince A, Schütze N, Karl N et al (2007) Gentamicin negatively influenced osteogenic function in vitro. Int Orthop 31:223–228

Jameson SS, Asaad A, Diament M et al (2019) Antibiotic-loaded bone cement is associated with a lower risk of revision following primary cemented total knee arthroplasty: an analysis of 731,214 cases using National Joint Registry data. Bone Joint J 101-b:1331–1347

Jämsen E, Huhtala H, Puolakka T et al (2009) Risk factors for infection after knee arthroplasty: a register-based analysis of 43,149 cases. JBJS 91:38–47

Jämsen E, Nevalainen P, Kalliovalkama J et al (2010) Preoperative hyperglycemia predicts infected total knee replacement. Eur J Intern Med 21:196–201

Josefsson G, Lindberg L, Wiklander B (1981) Systemic antibiotics and gentamicin-containing bone cement in the prophylaxis of postoperative infections in total hip arthroplasty. Clin Orthop Relat Res 159:194–200

Kalil GZ, Ernst EJ, Johnson SJ et al (2012) Systemic exposure to aminoglycosides following knee and hip arthroplasty with aminoglycoside-loaded bone cement implants. Ann Pharmacother 46:929–934

Kendoff DO, Gehrke T, Stangenberg P et al (2016) Bioavailability of gentamicin and vancomycin released from an antibiotic containing bone cement in patients undergoing a septic one-stage total hip arthroplasty (THA) revision: a monocentric open clinical trial. Hip Int 26:90–96

Klekamp J, Dawson JM, Haas DW et al (1999) The use of vancomycin and tobramycin in acrylic bone cement: biomechanical effects and elution kinetics for use in joint arthroplasty. J Arthroplast 14:339–346

Kleppel D, Stirton J, Liu J et al (2017) Antibiotic bone cement's effect on infection rates in primary and revision total knee arthroplasties. World J Orthop 8:946–955

Kühn KD, Berberich C, Bösebeck H (2018) Bone substitute materials as local drug carriers: current status of substitutes of various origins. Der Orthopade 47:10–23

Kurtz SM, Ong KL, Lau E et al (2010) Prosthetic joint infection risk after TKA in the Medicare population. Clin Orthop Relat Res 468:52–56

Lautenschlager E, Jacobs J, Marshall G et al (1976) Mechanical properties of bone cements containing large doses of antibiotic powders. J Biomed Mater Res 10:929–938

Liu H-T, Chiu F-Y, Chen C-M et al (2003) The combination of systemic antibiotics and antibiotics impregnated cement in primary total knee arthroplasty in patients of rheumatoid arthritis--evaluation of 60 knees. J Chin Med Assoc: JCMA 66:533–536

Malinzak RA, Ritter MA, Berend ME et al (2009) Morbidly obese, diabetic, younger, and unilateral joint arthroplasty patients have elevated total joint arthroplasty infection rates. J Arthroplast 24:84–88

Mcdonald DJ, Fitzgerald JR, Ilstrup D (1989) Two-stage reconstruction of a total hip arthroplasty because of infection. J Bone Joint Surg Am 71:828–834

Moran JM, Greenwald AS, Matejczyk MB (1979) Effect of gentamicin on shear and interface strengths of bone cement. Clin Orthop Relat Res (141):96–101

Mraovic B, Suh D, Jacovides C et al (2011) Perioperative hyperglycemia and postoperative infection after lower limb arthroplasty. J Diabetes Sci Technol 5:412–418

Namba RS, Inacio MC, Paxton EW (2013) Risk factors associated with deep surgical site infections after primary total knee arthroplasty: an analysis of 56,216 knees. JBJS 95:775–782

Neut D, Van De Belt H, Stokroos I et al (2001) Biomaterial-associated infection of gentamicin-loaded PMMA beads in orthopaedic revision surgery. J Antimicrob Chemother 47:885–891

Panni AS, Corona K, Giulianelli M et al (2016) Antibiotic-loaded bone cement reduces risk of infections in primary total knee arthroplasty? A systematic review. Knee Surg Sports Traumatol Arthrosc 24:3168–3174

Patel RA, Baker HP, Smith SB (2018) Acute renal failure due to a tobramycin and vancomycin spacer in revision two-staged knee arthroplasty. Case Rep Nephrol 2018:6579894–6579894

Pulido L, Ghanem E, Joshi A et al (2008) Periprosthetic joint infection: the incidence, timing, and predisposing factors. Clin Orthop Relat Res 466:1710–1715

Qadir R, Sidhu S, Ochsner JL et al (2014) Risk stratified usage of antibiotic-loaded bone cement for primary total knee arthroplasty: short term infection outcomes with a standardized cement protocol. J Arthroplast 29:1622–1624

Randelli P, Evola FR, Cabitza P et al (2010) Prophylactic use of antibiotic-loaded bone cement in primary total knee replacement. Knee Surg Sports Traumatol Arthros 18:181–186

Reed EE, Johnston J, Severing J et al (2014) Nephrotoxicity risk factors and intravenous vancomycin dosing in the immediate postoperative period following antibiotic-impregnated cement spacer placement. Ann Pharmacother 48:962–969

Slane J, Gietman B, Squire M (2018) Antibiotic elution from acrylic bone cement loaded with high doses of tobramycin and vancomycin. J Orthop Res 36:1078–1085

Sprowson AP, Jensen C, Chambers S et al (2016) The use of high-dose dual-impregnated antibiotic-laden cement with hemiarthroplasty for the treatment of a fracture of the hip: the fractured hip infection trial. Bone Joint J 98-B:1534–1541

Tayton ER, Frampton C, Hooper GJ et al (2016) The impact of patient and surgical factors on the rate of infection after primary total knee arthroplasty: an analysis of 64,566 joints from the New Zealand Joint Registry. Bone Joint J 98-b:334–340

Thornes B, Murray P, Bouchier-Hayes D (2002) Development of resistant strains of Staphylococcus epidermidis on gentamicin-loaded bone cement in vivo. J Bone Joint Surg 84:758–760

Tyas B, Marsh M, Oswald T et al (2018) Antibiotic resistance profiles of deep surgical site infections in hip hemiarthroplasty; comparing low dose single antibiotic versus high dose dual antibiotic impregnated cement. J Bone Jt Infect 3:123–129

Van De Belt H, Neut D, Schenk W et al (2001) Staphylococcus aureus biofilm formation on different gentamicin-loaded polymethylmethacrylate bone cements. Biomaterials 22: 1607–1611

Voigt J, Mosier M, Darouiche R (2016) Antibiotics and antiseptics for preventing infection in people receiving revision total hip and

knee prostheses: a systematic review of randomized controlled trials. BMC Infect Dis 16:749
Wahlig H, Dingeldein E (1980) Antibiotics and bone cements: experimental and clinical long-term observations. Acta Orthop Scand 51:49–56
Wang J, Zhu C, Cheng T et al (2013) A systematic review and meta-analysis of antibiotic-impregnated bone cement use in primary total hip or knee arthroplasty. PLoS One 8:e82745
Willis-Owen C, Konyves A, Martin D (2010) Factors affecting the incidence of infection in hip and knee replacement: an analysis of 5277 cases. J Bone Joint Surg 92:1128–1133
Zimmerli W, Trampuz A, Ochsner PE (2004) Prosthetic-joint infections. N Engl J Med 351:1645–1654

Enhancement of Release Profile of Antibiotic from Antibiotic-Loaded Poly(methyl methacrylate) Bone Cement for Anchoring of Total Joint Arthroplasties: A State-of-the-Art Review

Gladius Lewis

Contents

E. Hansen, K.-D. Kühn (eds.), *Essentials of Cemented Knee Arthroplasty*,
https://doi.org/10.1007/978-3-662-63113-3_48

48.1 Introduction

In current clinical practice involving the use of antibiotic-loaded bone cements (ALBCs) for preventing or managing/treating prosthetic joint infection (PJI) in total joint arthroplasty (TJA), one of two approaches is taken. In one, a commercially formulated ALBC brand approved by a relevant regulatory agency (such as the US Food and Drug Administration) (hereafter referred to as "approved cement brand") is used (Jiranek et al. 2006) and, in the other approach, a surgeon-directed (custom) formulation is prepared (Lewis et al. 2010).

> Regardless of the approach used, one shortcoming of ALBC is widely acknowledged. This is that the antibiotic release profile (amount released and duration of release) is sub-optimal.

Antibiotic Release Profile

Specifically, it is characterized by:

- An initial burst phase (a high-release-rate phase), in which surface-held antibiotic particles are released
- Followed by a phase in which the release rate decreases markedly
- An exhaustion phase (one in which release reduces to a very low, non-therapeutically effective level and, eventually, stops)

Typically, the burst phase occurs during the first ~0.33 to ~8 days and the exhaustion phase starts after ~4 to ~67 days (Kuechle et al. 1991; Penner et al. 1999; van de Belt et al. 2000; Neut et al. 2003; Kaplan et al. 2012; Samuel et al. 2012; Lee et al. 2016; Paz et al. 2015; Al Thaher et al. 2018; Meeker et al. 2019; Miller et al. 2011) (◘ Fig. 48.1). Additionally, the cumulative released amount is very low ($\leq$ ~5% of the initial mass of the antibiotic in the cement powder after ~168 h release in 1X phosphate buffered saline (PBS) solution, at 37 °C (Kuechle et al. 1991; Penner et al. 1999; van de Belt et al. 2000; Neut et al. 2003; Kaplan et al. 2012; Samuel et al. 2012; Lee et al. 2016; Paz et al. 2015; Al Thaher et al. 2018; Meeker et al. 2019; Miller et al. 2011)).

In other words, most of the antibiotic remains trapped in the cement (presumably in the matrix).

> Thus, there is scope for enhancing antibiotic release profile (◘ Fig. 48.1).

This review is a critical examination of the state-of-the-art in the full scope of methods that have been presented in the literature for enhancing antibiotic release profile. There are two caveats attached to the review. First, while its predominant focus is the literature on ALBCs intended for use in a structural application (i.e., the bed for anchoring of primary or revision TJAs), it includes brief consideration of the literature on uses of ALBC in spacers and beads because these devices are used in treatment of PJI via revision arthroplasty (Guild et al. 2014; Likine and Seligson 2019). Second, the review does not include the literature on ALBCs that contain more than one antibiotic (Parra-Ruiz et al. 2017; Boelch et al. 2018).

The review opens with a summary of the values of 3 indices of antibiotic release from specimens of commercially formulated ALBC ("baseline indices"). This summary is needed to establish a baseline against which enhancement methods can be assessed. In the next section, salient features of 10 different elution enhancement methods/approaches are presented, with the section ending with a compact presentation of the rationale used to select the most promising of these methods. The review ends with a summary of the most key points made ("take-home messages").

48.2 Baseline Release Profile Characteristics

Three indices of the release of an antibiotic are presented:

1. The duration of the burst phase (DBPH)
2. The time at the start of the exhaustion phase (TSEP)
3. The normalized cumulative amount of antibiotic released at the end of the test (NCAR).

> The baseline values of these indices show a wide spread (◘ Table 48.1).

This is to be expected given that antibiotic release is a function of a large number of intrinsic variables (such as antibiotic used, composition of the powder of the basis cement, and method used to mix antibiotic and cement powder) and extrinsic variables (such as cement storage conditions [temperature and time] and method used to mix the solid constituents [antibiotic + cement powder mixture] and the cement liquid).

Additionally, there is a wide variation in release determination protocol used, especially in terms of

- Composition of the test solution (e.g., phosphate-buffered saline (PBS) solution, solution of NaCl with Tween20®, and Ringer's solution

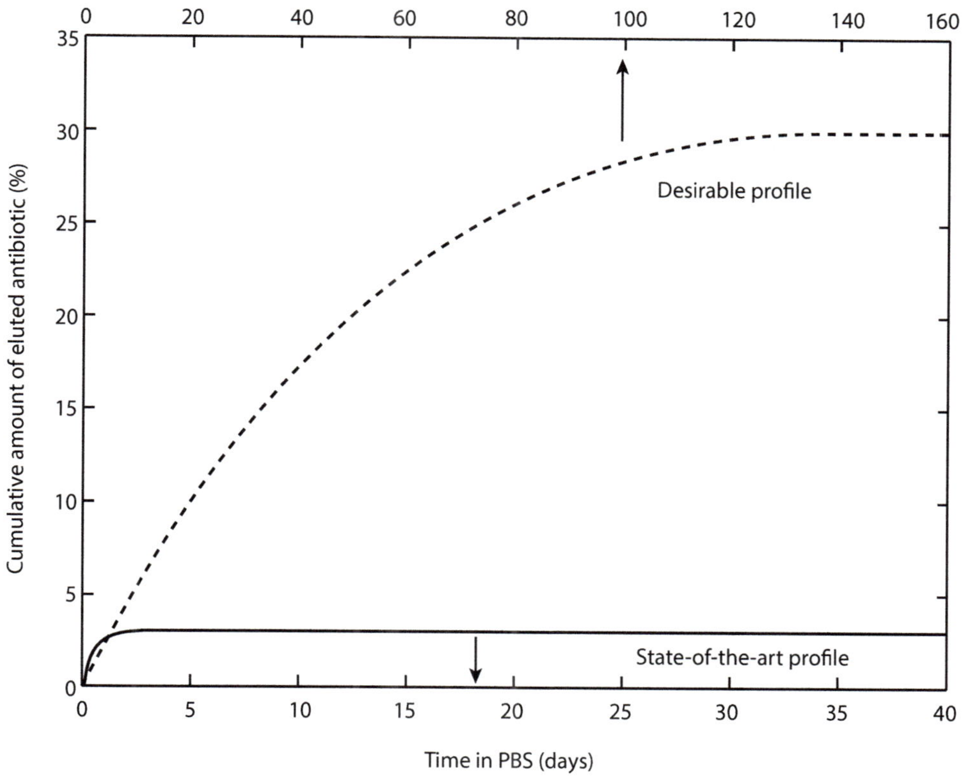

Fig. 48.1 State-of-the-art and desirable profiles of antibiotic release from ALBC specimen

Table 48.1 Summary of values of 3 indices of release of antibiotic from specimens of commercially formulated ALBC

Index	Value	Reference
Duration of burst phase[a] [days]	0.33–8.00	Kuechle et al. (1991)
		Penner et al. (1999)
		van de Belt et al. (2000)
		Neut et al. (2003)
		Kaplan et al. (2012)
		Samuel et al. (2012)
		Lee et al. (2016)
		Paz et al. (2015)
		Al Thaher et al. (2018)
		Meeker et al. (2019)
Start of exhaustion phase[b] [days]	3–67	Kuechle et al. (1991)
		Penner et al. (1999)
		van de Belt et al. (2000)
		Neut et al. (2003)
		Kaplan et al. (2012)
		Samuel et al. (2012)
		Lee et al. (2016)
		Paz et al. (2015)
		Al Thaher et al. (2018)

(continued)

Table 48.1 (continued)

Index	Value	Reference
Mean cumulative mass of antibiotic released at end of test period per PBS volume used in test per wt./wt.% of antibiotic in blended powder mixture (cement powder + antibiotic powder)[c] [mg $mL^{-1}\%^{-1}$]	0.004	Samuel et al. (2012)
	0.02	Paz et al. (2015)
	0.12	Lee et al. (2016)
	0.70	Kaplan et al. (2012)
	1.31	Penner et al. (1999)
Mean cumulative mass of antibiotic released at end of test period as % of mass of antibiotic in blended powder mixture (cement powder + antibiotic)[c] [wt./wt.%]	0.001	Samuel et al. (2012)
	0.025	Paz et al. (2015)
	0.50	Kaplan et al. (2012)
	0.75	Lee et al. (2016)
	0.80	Miller et al. (2011)
	1.55	Penner et al. (1999)

[a]Duration of burst phase (DBPH)
[b]Time at start of exhaustion phase (TSEP)
[c]Normalized cumulative amount of antibiotic released at end of test (NCAR)

- Volume of test solution used (e.g., 1 mL, 3 mL, and 5 mL)
- Method used to determine the amount of antibiotic released (e.g., high-performance liquid chromatography, ultraviolet-visible spectroscopy, and clinical analyzer with a homogene enzyme immunoassay)
- The parameters used to express the determined amount of antibiotic released (unnormalized [e.g., mg] or normalized [e.g., μg mL^{-1}, μg cm^{-2} h^{-1}, and ratio of amount of released antibiotic to amount of antibiotic in starting powder, expressed as wt./wt.%]).

48.3 Enhancement Methods

48.3.1 Additive(s) to Cement Powder

An assortment of additives have been used, namely:

Additives to Cement Powder

- A soluble poragen (such as dextran, xylitol, glycine, sucrose, erthyritol, lactose, $CaCO_3$, gelatin sponge, ceramic capsules, bioactive borate glass particles, an antimicrobial peptide [Dhvar-5])
- A surfactant-stabilized emulsifier
- Dried mesoporous silica nanoparticles(MSNP)-containing slurry
- Poly(D,l-lactic-co-glycolic) acid (PDLA) nanoparticles
- Silica nanoparticles loaded with an antibiotic (gentamicin sulfate) (McLaren et al. 2006, 2007; Virto et al. 2003; Frutos et al. 2010; Matos et al. 2015; Nugent et al. 2010; Salehi et al. 2013; Slane et al. 2014; Chang et al. 2014; Bitsch et al. 2015; Wu et al. 2016; Funk et al. 2018; Faber et al. 2005; Shen et al. 2011; Letchmanan et al. 2017; Perni et al. 2019)

Among the mechanisms put forward for the enhancement effect of these agents are:

- Increase of the porosity of the cement, thereby creating a porous network through which the test solution permeates the cement matrix and dissolves the antibiotic located deep within the matrix (Kuechle et al. 1991; McLaren et al. 2007; Nugent et al. 2010; Salehi et al. 2013; Slane et al. 2014).
- Modulation of the release of the antibiotic (addition of an additive creates an irregular surface of the cement, characterized by a series of "ink well" pores and voids) (Virto et al. 2003; Frutos et al. 2010).
- Dissolution of the antibiotic particles present on the surface of the specimen (Matos et al. 2015).
- Dissolution of the cement matrix, which creates a porous network within the matrix, which, in turn, allows release of the antibiotic from zones deep

within the matrix (Virto et al. 2003; Faber et al. 2005).

- A surfactant-stabilized formulation allowing the antimicrobial to be loaded without separation during polymerization, leading to a homogeneous matrix which, in turn, facilitates the release of the antibiotic (Miller et al. 2011).
- Nanoparticles facilitating formation of a nano-network path for diffusion of the antibiotic from the cement matrix, from which it is released (Shen et al. 2011; Letchmanan et al. 2017).
- Decreased porosity of the matrix caused by degradation of microparticles of a polymer (Parra-Ruiz et al. 2017).
- Release of the antibiotic from the coating on silica nanoparticles, followed by migration of these particles through the bone cement matrix (Al Thaher et al. 2018).

48.3.2 Additive to Cement Liquid

An experimental ALBC formulation was prepared in which the liquid of an approved gentamicin-loaded ALBC brand was modified by including gentamicin that has been incorporated into extruded liposomes coated with a non-toxic, neutral surfactant, but the powder was the same as that for an approved ALBC brand (LIPO cement) (Ayre et al. 2016). Cumulative gentamicin released from LIPO cement specimens was more than from specimens of control cement (no liposomal gentamicin added). These results were explained by the fact that LIPO cement had a series of small, well-dispersed pores, which, ultimately, facilitated gradual and controlled release of the gentamicin; in contrast, the control cement had large, random pores (caused by the release of surface agglomerates of the antibiotic) that allowed a less controlled release of the gentamicin. DBPH was about the same in both sets of specimens (~6 h) as was TSEP (~30 days) (Ayre et al. 2016).

48.3.3 Direct Impregnation of Antibiotic

An experimental ALBC was obtained by loading gentamicin into halloysite nanotubes ("gentamicin-loaded halloysite nanotubes" [GHNs]) (GHN cement) (Wei et al. 2012). Release of gentamicin from GHN cement specimens was markedly slower than from specimens of the control cement (no GHNs added) (Wei et al. 2012). It was postulated that the halloysite nanotubes isolate the gentamicin from the cement liquid and act as nanocontainers for slow release of the gentamicin (Wei et al. 2012).

A series of experimental gentamicin-loaded bone cement formulations were obtained by loading gentamicin into 4 nanostructured materials (MSNPs, hydroxyapatite nanorods [HANRs], carbon nanotubes [CNTs], and TiO_2 nanotubes [TNTs]) (Shen et al. 2016, 2019). The loaded nanoparticles were then dried, ground, and added to the powder of a commercially formulated plain cement brand (NANO cement). The control cement was a commercially formulated ALBC brand.

> At each time point during the course of the study, gentamicin released from NANO cement specimens was significantly more than from control cement specimens.

In the case of results from cement that contained MSNPs or TNTs, the explanation was the same as that given in an earlier report for MSNP-containing cement (Shen et al. 2011) but no explicit explanations were put forward for the results for the cements that contained either HANRs or CNTs. Furthermore, DBPH for NANO cement specimens was ~7 times longer and TSEP ~3 times longer compared to the corresponding values for control cement specimens (Shen et al. 2016, 2019).

48.3.4 Method of Mixing Antibiotic Powder and Cement Powder

When a cement powder and gentamicin were blended using a proprietary method ("industrial addition"), gentamicin released was significantly more than when they were blended using a manual method (Neut et al. 2003). The trend, which was the same regardless of the antibiotic loading (2.1 or 4.2 wt./wt.%), was attributed to the manual mixing producing a mixture that is less homogenous than was obtained when industrial addition was used .(Neut et al. 2003).

Two variants of a high-antibiotic-loading experimental formulation were prepared. For the first, vancomycin powder was manually mixed with the powder of an approved plain cement brand (MAN method). For the second variant, the cement powder and liquid were mixed by a manual method to produce a dough to which the antibiotic was added without breaking up the chunks ("dough-phase-mixing" [DPM] method) (Miller et al. 2012).

> Cumulative amount of antibiotic released was significantly more when DPM specimens were used than when MAN specimens were used (Miller et al. 2012), which was attributed to the fact that in the DPM method, antibiotic chunks that survived functioned as a poragen (Miller et al. 2012).

48.3.5 Method of Mixing Blended Cement Powder and Cement Liquid

When a mechanical foaming device was used to mix the powder and liquid of an experimental cefazolin-loaded bone cement, the cumulative amount of cefazolin released over the course of 1 week was significantly more than when the constituents were manually mixed in an open bowl (Shiramizu et al. 2008). Total specimen porosity and cumulative amount of cefazolin released were moderately but significantly correlated (Shiramizu et al. 2008).

For 6 commercially formulated gentamicin-loaded brands (each with antibiotic loading of 2.1 wt./wt.% or 4.2 wt./wt.%), the influence of the method used to mix the cement powder and liquid (in a bowl open to the ambient atmosphere [HM mixing] vs. in the mixing cartridge of a vacuum-mixing system [VM mixing]) on cumulative amount of gentamicin released depends on the brand (Neut et al. 2003). Thus, for 3 of the brands, significantly more gentamicin was released from HM specimens than from their VM counterparts; for 2 of the brands, gentamicin release from HM specimens was more than from VM specimens but not significantly so; and for 1 brand, more gentamicin was released from VM specimens than from HM specimens (Neut et al. 2003). The lattermost results were attributed to an increase in the number and distribution of micropores in the specimens (diameter <1 mm), which were formed during polymerization (Neut et al. 2003). It was argued that the results were consistent with

- The observation that VM led to significant reduction in both the number and size of large voids in the specimens
- The postulate that long-term release of antibiotics was determined by large pores (Neut et al. 2003).

Results of an investigation of influence of mixing method on antibiotic release from 6 commercially formulated brands (5 loaded with gentamicin and 1 with tobramycin) (loading: 2.5 wt./wt.%) indicated that, for low antibiotic-loading brands, vacuum mixing is beneficial to 1 of the 2 high-viscosity brands but not beneficial to the low-viscosity brand and its influence on 2 of the 3 medium-viscosity brands is unclear (Meyer et al. 2011).

48.3.6 Application of Ultrasound

A number of variants of ultrasound (US) have been used, these being

- Low-intensity-low frequency
- Pulsed
- Continuous-wave
- Delayed pulse-wave
- Continuous watt-level
- Intermittent watt-level
- Microbubbles-mediated (addition of a microbubbles contrast agent to the antibiotic release test solution and regular refreshment during the release test) (MBMUS) (Hendriks et al. 2003; Ensing et al. 2005; Yan et al. 2005; Cai et al. 2007, 2008, 2017; Lin et al. 2015; Wendling et al. 2019)

In addition, the influence of frequency and duration of US has been the subject of one study (Wendling et al. 2019). In general, marked enhancement of amount of antibiotic released from US-treated specimens was reported, varying from ~25% to ~400% (Hendriks et al. 2003; Ensing et al. 2005; Yan et al. 2005; Cai et al. 2007, 2008, 2017; Lin et al. 2015; Wendling et al. 2019).

> The postulated mechanism of enhancement of antibiotic release by exposure to US may be summarized as follows: Cavitation, caused by the low- and high-pressure areas in the fluid, leads to formation of microstreams (Yan et al. 2005).

Microstreams (1) facilitate transport of the test solution via pores in the cement matrix and (2) produce a high shear stress at the antibiotic–cement matrix interface, causing detachment of antibiotic particles (Hendriks et al. 2003; Cai et al. 2008, 2017; Lin et al. 2015). Vancomycin release enhancement by intermittent watt-level ultrasonication is postulated to be associated with stable cavitation and radiation pressure, which generated multidirectional acoustic microstreams (Cai et al. 2008). These microstreams produced a high shear stress at the vancomycin powder–cement matrix interface, which facilitated detachment of vancomycin grains from the surface and, then, during the rest period, these grains diffuse out of the craters and pores that are created in the specimen during the application of the ultrasonication (Cai et al. 2008). Enhanced vancomycin release profile when MBMUS specimens were used was attributed to stable cavitation and associated ultrasonic pressure produced by exposure to US (Cai et al. 2017), increased rate of mass transfer from the cement matrix (Cai et al. 2017), and rupture of microbubbles by exposure to US, which increased microstream stress and shear stress (Lin et al. 2015).

48.3.7 Alteration of Surface Pattern

An increase in the surface area-to-volume ratio of a specimen (achieved through the application of hemispherical ridges to each side of a rectangular test specimen) resulted in increase in vancomycin release although this increase was only significant over the first week of an 8-week test period, which approximates to the duration of the burst phase (Masri et al. 1995).

48.3.8 Timing of Addition of Antibiotic Powder to Cement Powder

Two sets of specimens were fabricated, with those in the first set fabricated from cement prepared in the standard method (i.e., manually mix the powder of an approved plain cement brand and vancomycin, then add the liquid of the approved plain cement brand, and, then, mix the resulting dough under vacuum ["standard method"]) (Amin et al. 2012). For the second set, the powder and liquid of the plain cement brand were mixed under vacuum after which the vacuum was removed, and the antibiotic was added to the dough, which was then mixed for an additional time under vacuum ("delayed antibiotic addition method") (Amin et al. 2012).

> Cumulative vancomycin released from delayed antibiotic addition method specimens was significantly more than that from standard method specimens.

This result was attributed to the possibility that delayed addition of the antibiotic leads to decreased interference of the vancomycin with the initial polymerization process and, hence, increased porosity of the specimens (Amin et al. 2012).

In the study by Wendling et al. (2016) the two study groups comprised specimens fabricated from cement prepared as follows:

- Vancomycin powder was mixed with the powder of an approved plain cement brand and, then, the liquid of the brand was added (STANDARD group).
- The powder and liquid of the approved plain cement brand were mixed for 60 s and, then, vancomycin was added, followed by 30 s of mixing (DELAYED group).

Initial vancomycin release (determined after 1 day of the test) from the DELAYED group specimens was significantly more than from the STANDARD group specimens. However, starting at day 2 until the end of the release test period (10 days), the vancomycin amount released from both groups of specimens was practically the same (Wendling et al. 2016).

48.3.9 State of Antibiotic upon Addition to Cement Liquid

Two sets of specimens were fabricated using cement prepared as follows:

- Vancomycin powder was mixed with the powder of an approved plain cement brand and, then, the liquid of the plain brand was added (SOLID group).
- Vancomycin powder was added to distilled water, the solution vortexed for 30 s and then added to the liquid of the plain cement, the whole blend mixed manually, and the powder of the plain cement brand was added and the final blend was mixed manually for 2 min (SOLUTION group) (Chang et al. 2014).

While NCAR was significantly higher from SOLUTION group specimens than from SOLID group specimens, the difference in DBPH was not significant (Chang et al. 2014).

48.3.10 Combination Technique

With respect to the aforementioned study by Wendling et al. (2016) after fabrication, the specimens in both study groups were exposed to low-frequency US for various times (t). At $t = 5$ min or 45 min, significantly more vancomycin was released from DELAYED group specimens compared to that from STANDARD group specimens (Wendling et al. 2016).

Two experimental cement formulations were the subject of a study by Frutos et al. (2002)

- For the first, gentamicin powder was added to the powder of an approved plain cement brand ("GS-powder blend"; control cement) and the liquid was that for the plain cement brand.
- For the second, the powder consisted of the GS powder blend and a polymer (poly(N-vinyl-2-pyrrolidone) [PVP]) and the liquid consisted of the liquid of the plain cement brand and another monomer, (2-hydroxethyl methacrylate) ([HEMA] PVP + HEMA cement).

At each time point during the course of the release study, gentamicin released from PVP + HEMA cement specimens was markedly more than from control cement specimens.

> This was attributed to dissolution of PVP within the HEMA matrix, creating a series of interconnected pores through which the gentamicin was released (Frutos et al. 2002).

48.4 Overview

Where the relevant data were given in the literature reports reviewed in the preceding sub-section, values of TSEP and NCAR when an enhancement method was used and when one was not used were calculated. On the basis of these calculated values and, taking into account the number of reported studies reviewed for each of the enhancement methods, it appears that the two most effective enhancement methods are additive(s) to the cement powder (mean increase in TSEP = 200%; mean increase in NCAR = 420%) and direct impregnation of the antibiotic into the cement powder (mean increase in TSEP = 120%; mean increase in NCAR = 1100%).

Take-Home Messages

- A shortcoming of the current generation of ALBCs – perhaps, the principal one – is the sub-optimal profile of release of the antibiotic from specimens of the cement in in vitro antibiotic release tests. Two elements of this profile are
  - An initial burst phase (occurs between hours and a few days) followed by a marked decrease in the release rate and, then, exhaustion of release (after, typically, ~25 days).
  - Cumulative amount of antibiotic released at the end of test (typically, ~40 days) is no more than ~5% of the starting mass of the antibiotic in the cement.
- From among the large assortment of methods or approaches used to enhance antibiotic release profile, as presented in the literature, it appears that the most effective ones are incorporation of additive(s) into the cement powder and direct impregnation of the antibiotic into the cement powder.

References

Al Thaher Y, Yang L, Jones SA, Perni S, Prokopovich P (2018) LbL-assembled gentamicin delivery system for PMMA bone cements to prolong antimicrobial activity. PLoS One 13(12):e0207753. https://doi.org/10.1371/journal.pone.0207753

Amin TJ, Lamping JW, Hendricks KJ, McIff TE (2012) Increasing the elution of vancomycin from high-dose antibiotic-loaded bone cement: a novel preparation technique. J Bone Joint Surg Am 94:1946–1951

Ayre WN, Birchall JC, Evans SL, Denyer SP (2016) A novel liposomal drug delivery system for PMMA bone cements. J Biomed Mater Res Part B 104B:1510–1524

Bitsch RG, Kretzer JP, Vogt S, Buchner H, Thomsen MN, Lehner B (2015) Increased antibiotic release and equivalent biomechanics of a spacer cement without hard radio contrast agents. Diagnos Microbiol Infect Dis 83:203–209

Boelch SP, Rueckl K, Fuchs C, Jordan M, Knauer M, Steinert A, Rudert M, Luedemann M (2018) Comparison of elution characteristics and compressive strength of biantibiotic-loaded PMMA bone cement for spacers: Copal® Spacem with gentamicin and vancomycin versus Palacos® R+G with vancomycin. Biomed Res Int 2018:1–5. Article ID: 4323518

Cai X-Z, Yan S-G, Wu H-B, Dai X-S, Chen H-X, Yan R-J, Zhao X-H (2007) Effect of delayed pulse-wave ultrasound on local pharmokinetics and pharmodynamics of vancomycin-loaded acrylic bone cement in vivo. Antimicrob Agents Chemotherap 51:3199–3204

Cai X-Z, Chen X-C, Yan S-G, Ruan Z-R, Yan R-J, Ji K, Xu J (2008) Intermittent watt-level ultrasonication facilitates vancomycin release from therapeutic acrylic bone cement. J Biomed Mater Res Part B Appl Biomater 90B:11–17

Cai Y, Wang J, Liu X, Wang R, Xia L (2017) A review of the combination therapy of low frequency ultrasound with antibiotics. BioMed Res Int 2017:1–14. Article ID: 2317846

Chang YH, Tai CL, Hsu HY, Hsieh PH, Lee MS, Ueng SWN (2014) Liquid antibiotics in bone cement: an effective way to improve the efficiency of antibiotic release in antibiotic loaded bone cement. Bone Joint Res 3:246–251

Ensing GT, Hendriks JGE, Jongsma JE, van Horn JR, van der Mei HC, Busscher HJ (2005) The influence of ultrasound on the release of gentamicin from antibiotic-loaded acrylic beads and bone cements. J Biomed Mater Res Part B Appl Biomater 75B:1–5

Faber C, Hoogendoorn RJW, Lyaruu DM, Stallman HP, van Marle J, van Nieuw AA, Smit TH, Wuisman PIJM (2005) The effect of the antimicrobial peptide, Dhvar-5, on gentamicin release from a polymethyl methacrylate bone cement. Biomaterials 26:5717–5726

Frutos P, Diez-Pena E, Frutos G, Barrales-Rienda JM (2002) Release of gentamicin sulphate from a modified commercial bone cement. Effect of (2-hydroxyethyl methacrylate) comonomer and poly(N-vinyl-2-pyrrolidone) additive on release mechanism and kinetics. Biomaterials 23:3787–3792

Frutos G, Pastor JY, Martinez N, Virto MR, Torrado S (2010) Influence of lactose addition to gentamicin-loaded acrylic bone cement on the kinetics of release of the antibiotic and the cement properties. Acta Biomater 6:804–811

Funk GA, Burkes JC, Cole KA, Rahaman MN, McIff TE (2018) Antibiotic elution and mechanical strength of PMMA bone cement loaded with borate bioactive glass. J Bone Joint Infect 3:187–196

Guild GN, Baohua W, Scuderi GR (2014) Articulating vs. static antibiotic impregnated spacers in revision total knee arthroplasty for sepsis; a systematic review. J Arthroplast 29:558–563

Hendriks JGE, Ensing GT, van Horn JR, Lubbers J, van der Mei HC, Busscher HJ (2003) Increased release of gentamicin from acrylic bone cements under influence of low-frequency ultrasound. J Control Release 92:369–374

Jiranek WA, Hanssen AD, Greenwald AS (2006) Antibiotic-loaded bone cement for infection prophylaxis in total joint replacement. J Bone Joint Surg Am 88:2487–2500

Kaplan L, Kurdziel M, Baker KC, Verner J (2012) Characterization of daptomycin-loaded antibiotic cement. Orthopedics 35:e503–e509

Kuechle DK, Landon GC, Musher DM, Noble PC (1991) Elution of vancomycin, daptomycin, and amikacin from acrylic bone cement. Clin Orthop Relat Res 264:302–308

Lee S-H, Tai C-L, Chen S-Y, Chang C-H, Chang Y-H, Hsieh P-H (2016) Elution and mechanical strength of vancomycin-loaded bone cement: in vitro study of the influence of brand combination. PLoS One 11(11):e0166545. Published 2016 Nov 17. https://doi.org/10.1371/journal.pone.0166545

Letchmanan K, Shen S-C, Ng WK, Kingshuk P, Shi Z, Wang W, Tan RBH (2017) Mechanical properties and antibiotic release characteristics of poly(methyl methacrylate)-based bone cement formulated with mesoporous silica nanoparticles. J Mech Beh Biomed Mater 72:163–170

Lewis G, Brooks JL, Courtney HS, Li Y, Haggard WO (2010) An approach for determining antibiotic loading for a physician-directed antibiotic-loaded PMMA bone cement formulation. Clin Orthop Relat Res 468:2092–2100

Likine EF, Seligson D (2019) Rifampin and tobramycin combination with PMMA antibiotic cement. Eu J Orthop Surg Traumatol 29:499–500

Lin T, Cai X-Z, Shi M-M, Ying Z-M, Hu B, Zhou C-H, Wang W, Shi Z-L, Yan S-G (2015) In vitro and in vivo evaluation of vancomycin-loaded PMMA bone cement in combination with ultrasound and microbubbles-mediated ultrasound. BioMed Res Int 2015:1–7. Article ID: 309739

Masri BA, Duncan CP, Beauchamp CP, Paris NJ, Arntorp J (1995) Effect of varying surface patterns on antibiotic elution from antibiotic-loaded bone cement. J Arthroplast 10:453–459

Matos AC, Ribeiro IAC, Guedes RC, Pinto R, Vaz MA, Goncalves LM, Almeida AJ, Bettencourt AF (2015) Key-properties outlook of a levofloxacin-loaded acrylic bone cement with improved antibiotic delivery. Int J Pharm 485:317–328

McLaren AC, McLaren SG, Smeltzer M (2006) Xylitol and glycine fillers increase permeability of PMMA to enhance elution of daptomycin. Clin Orthop Relat Res 451:25–28

McLaren AC, McLaren SG, Hickmon MK (2007) Sucrose, xylitol, and erythritol increase PMMA permeability for depot antibiotics. Clin Orthop Relat Res 461:60–63

Meeker DG, Cooper KB, Renard RL, Mears SC, Smeltzer MS, Barnes CL (2019) Comparative study of antibiotic elution profiles from alternative formulations of polymethylmethacrylate bone cement. J Arthroplast 34:1458–1461

Meyer J, Piller G, Spiegel CA, Hetzel S, Squire M (2011) Vacuum-mixing significantly changes antibiotic elution characteristics of commercially-available antibiotic-impregnated bone cements. J Bone Joint Surg 93:2049–2056

Miller RB, McLaren A, Leon CM, Vernon BL, McLemore R (2011) Surfactant-stabilized emulsion increases gentamicin elution from bone cement. Clin Orthop Relat Res 469:2995–3001

Miller R, McLaren A, Leon C, McLemore R (2012) Mixing method affects elution and strength of high-dose ALBC: a pilot study. Clin Orthop Relat Res 470:2677–2683

Neut D, van de Belt H, van Horn JR, van der Mei HC, Busscher HJ (2003) The effect of mixing on gentamicin release from polymethylmethacrylate bone cements. Acta Orthop Scand 74:670–676

Nugent M, McLaren A, Vernon B, McLemore R (2010) Strength of antimicrobial bone cement decreases with increased poragen fraction. Clin Orthop Relat Res 468:2101–2106

Parra-Ruiz FJ, Gonzalez-Gomez A, Fernandez-Gutierrez M, Parra J, Garcia-Garcia J, Azuara G et al (2017) Development of advanced biantibiotic loaded bone cement spacers for arthroplasty associated infections. Int J Pharm 522:11–20

Paz E, San-Ruiz P, Abenojar J, Vaquero-Martin J, Forriol F, Del Real JC (2015) Evaluation of elution and mechanical properties of high-dose antibiotic-loaded bone cement: comparative "in vitro" study of the influence of vancomycin and cefazolin. J Arthroplast 30:1423–1429

Penner MJ, Duncan CP, Masri BA (1999) The in vitro elution characteristics of antibiotic-loaded CMW and Palacos-R bone cements. J Arthroplast 14:209–213

Perni S, Caserta S, Pasquino R, Jones SA, Prokopovich P (2019) Prolonged antimicrobial activity of PMMA bone cement with embedded gentamicin-releasing silica nanocarriers. ACS Appl Bio Mater 2:1850–1861

Salehi A, Cox Parker A, Lewis G, Courtney HS, Haggard WO (2013) A daptomycin-xylitol-loaded polymethylmethacrylate bone cement: how much xylitol should be used? Clin Orthop Relat Res 471:3149–3157

Samuel S, Mathew BS, Veeraraghavan B, Fleming DH, Chittaranjan SB, Prakask JAJ (2012) In vitro study of elution kinetics and bio-activity of meropenem-loaded acrylic bone cement. J Orthopaed Traumatol 13:131–136

Shen S-C, Ng WK, Shi Z, Chia L, Neoh KG, Tan RBH (2011) Mesoporous silica nanoparticle-functionalized poly(methyl methacrylate)-based bone cement for effective antibiotics delivery. J Mater Sci Mater Med 22:2283–2292

Shen S-C, Ng WK, Dong Y-C, Ng J, Tan RBH (2016) Nanostructured material formulated acrylic bone cements with enhanced drug release. Mater Sci Eng C 58:233–241

Shen S-C, Letchmanan K, Chow PS, Tan RBH (2019) Antibiotic elution and mechanical property of TiO_2 nanotubes functionalized PMMA-based bone cements. J Mech Beh Biomed Mater 91:91–98

Shiramizu K, Lovric V, Leung A, Walsh WR (2008) How do porosity-inducing techniques affect antibiotic elution from bone cement? An in vitro comparison between hydrogen peroxide and a mechanical mixer. J Orthopaed Traumatol 9:17–22

Slane JA, Vivano JF, Rose WE, Squire MW, Ploeg H-L (2014) The influence of low concentrations of a water soluble poragen on the material properties, antibiotic release, and biofilm inhibition of an acrylic bone cement. Mater Sci Eng C 42:168–176

van de Belt H, Neut D, Uges DRA, Schenk W, van Horn JR, van der Mei HC, Busscher HJ (2000) Surface roughness, porosity and wettability of gentamicin-loaded bone cements and their antibiotic release. Biomaterials 21:1981–1987

Virto MR, Frutos P, Torrado S, Frutos G (2003) Gentamicin release from modified acrylic bone cements with lactose and hydroxypropylmethylcellulose. Biomaterials 24:79–87

Wei W, Abdullayev E, Hollister A, Mills D, Lvov YM (2012) Clay nanotube/poly(methyl methacrylate) bone cement composites with sustained antibiotic release. Macromol Mater Eng 297:645–653

Wendling A, Mar D, Wischmeier N, Anderson D, McIff T (2016) Combination of modified mixing technique and low frequency ultrasound to control the elution profile of vancomycin-loaded acrylic bone cement. Bone Joint Res 5:26–32

Wendling AC, Mar DE, Burkes JC, McIff TE (2019) Effect of ultrasound frequency and treatment duration on antibiotic elution from polymethylmethacrylate bone cement. Kans J Med 12:45–49

Wu K, Chen Y-C, Hsu Y-M, Chang C-H (2016) Enhancing drug release from antibiotic-loaded bone cement using porogens. J Am Acad Orthop Surg 24:188–195

Yan SY, Cai X, Yan W, Dai X, Wu H (2005) Continuous wave ultrasound enhances vancomycin release and antimicrobial efficacy of antibiotic-loaded acrylic bone cement *in vitro* and *in vivo*. J Biomed Mater Res Part B Appl Biomater 82B:57–64

Tourniquet Use in Cemented Total Knee Arthroplasty

Carl L. Herndon and H. John Cooper

Contents

E. Hansen, K.-D. Kühn (eds.), *Essentials of Cemented Knee Arthroplasty*,
https://doi.org/10.1007/978-3-662-63113-3_49

49.1 Introduction

The word tourniquet, which is derived from the French word *tourner*, meaning *turn*, has been used to describe any device that restricts blood flow to a limb. Historically, tourniquets were first employed in the ancient Roman Empire during battle to control hemorrhage (Noordin et al. 2009; Welling et al. 2012). Cushing was the first to describe the use of a pneumatic tourniquet in 1904, in order to maintain hemostasis but not over-compress the limb to limit peripheral nerve compression injuries related to the elastic tourniquets of the day (Cushing 1904). Since that time, tourniquet use has flourished in various surgical fields, and they are used very commonly in orthopedics. This chapter will specifically focus on its use in cemented total knee arthroplasty (TKA).

The use of tourniquet in TKA has become a topic of considerable controversy in recent years, with many articles espousing the benefits, risks, and alternatives to tourniquet use (Arthur and Spangehl 2019).

Proposed benefits of tourniquet use include

- Better operative visualization
- Less blood loss
- Shorter operative times
- Possibly deeper cement mantle penetration (Goel et al. 2019; Alcelik et al. 2012; Zhou et al. 2017; Pfitzner et al. 2016)

Described disadvantages include

- Delayed bleeding and wound complications
- Increased postoperative pain and reduced function
- Increased muscle inflammation
- Decreased muscle strength
- Thromboembolism
- Peripheral nerve injury
- Patellar maltracking
- Skin burns
- Thigh adipose tissue necrosis (Zhang et al. 2017; Alcelik et al. 2012; Ozkunt et al. 2018; Huang et al. 2015; Dennis et al. 2016; Tai et al. 2011; Berman et al. 1998; Husted et al. 2010; Husted and Jensen 2005)

A wide breadth of studies has been performed evaluating these issues, but much controversy still exists in terms of whether or not to use tourniquets, if so, for how long, at what inflation pressure, and what are the clinical outcomes of these various permutations. We will attempt to address these questions below.

49.2 Blood Loss

Intuitively, it makes sense that a tourniquet would reduce blood loss during TKA. However, this fact has been well-studied, and the results are not definitive. When reviewing the literature regarding blood loss in TKA, it is important to highlight the various ways in which blood loss is defined in various reports. Estimated blood loss is usually just that, an estimation made by the surgeon of how much blood was absorbed by sponges and suctioned from the wound throughout the case. Postoperative blood loss is typically measured with the use of an intra-articular drain left in the wound upon closure. Finally, hidden blood loss is often referred to as the blood that is lost on the drapes, or remains in the knee. The sum of these three losses is often referred to as total blood loss. In addition to these empiric measures, there are also several formulas for calculating blood loss based on hemoglobin, such as Gross's formula (Gross 1983).

> When discussing blood loss in TKA, it is very important to distinguish between the various methods of reporting blood loss.

Several systematic reviews and meta-analyses have evaluated studies that focus on blood loss in TKA with and without tourniquet. In one, Alcelik et al. found both intraoperative and total blood loss to be less in the tourniquet group compared to no tourniquet (Alcelik et al. 2012). Similarly, Smith et al. performed a pooled analysis of over 1000 TKAs and found an average of 269 mL more intraoperative blood loss in the non-tourniquet group (Smith and Hing 2010). Although these results point to less intraoperative blood loss with a tourniquet, postoperative and total blood loss is less clear. In another systematic review and meta-analysis, Jiang et al. pooled data for 1450 TKAs and noted no difference in postoperative, total, or calculated blood loss (Jiang et al. 2015). Similarly, Li et al. found in their review of 15 randomized-controlled trials (RCTs) that although there was less intraoperative blood loss using a tourniquet, postoperative blood loss was higher, and, therefore, there was no difference in total blood loss (Li et al. 2014). Zhang et al., in another meta-analysis, noted that there was no difference in postoperative or total blood loss and that transfusion rates were equivalent between groups (Zhang et al. 2014a). Schnettler et al. actually showed a paradoxical increase in total blood loss with a tourniquet compared to without (Schnettler et al. 2017). In a more recent study, however, Goel et al. showed less calculated total blood loss in the tourniquet group compared to the non-tourniquet group (Goel et al. 2019).

These studies all specifically evaluated blood loss whether or not a tourniquet was used, but there are also several strategies for timing of tourniquet use to use it selectively during the case, rather than throughout. Again, one would intuit that having the tourniquet released at any point during the case would increase blood loss. One meta-analysis by Huang et al. corroborated that thinking, showing that releasing the tourniquet prior to wound closure increased blood loss significantly (Huang et al. 2015). Additionally, Mittal et al. performed an RCT using a tourniquet just during cementation vs. prior to incision through the end of cementation. They stopped their study early due to a higher rate of transfusion in the selective tourniquet group, and found no significant difference in Oxford Knee Score at 10 weeks, nor improved function.

> Based on their findings, they concluded that tourniquets should be utilized at least through the cementation step of the case (Mittal et al. 2012).

However, the point in the operation where the tourniquet is deflated may also influence outcomes. One concern with leaving the tourniquet inflated through final closure is that of delayed bleeding, in which unrecognized small vessels that are not coagulated during the case can continue to bleed intra-articularly immediately postoperatively. This hemarthrosis can cause complications such as wound breakdown and dehiscence and poorer patient outcomes due to pain and swelling and consequent difficulty with rehabilitation exercises. A meta-analysis by Rama et al. found just that: Releasing the tourniquet to achieve meticulous hemostasis prior to closure resulted in increased intraoperative blood loss, but reduced postoperative complications by 3% (Rama et al. 2007). A similar meta-analysis by Zhang et al. found that early release of the tourniquet was associated with greater blood loss but fewer complications (Zhang et al. 2014b). Fan et al. showed in an RCT that there was no difference in total measured blood loss or hemoglobin in patients undergoing TKA with a tourniquet throughout the procedure vs. those with a tourniquet inflated from cementation through closure (Fan et al. 2014).

Additionally, Wang et al. performed staged bilateral TKAs in 50 patients, and they had each knee randomized to either long duration tourniquet (start of the case through cementation) vs. short duration (only during cementing). They found that there was less total and intraoperative blood loss in the long duration group, but higher hidden and postoperative blood loss in the short duration group (Wang et al. 2017). In a meta-analysis pooling 440 TKAs, another group also found that long duration tourniquet use decreased intraoperative and total blood loss, but that short duration use does not increase the need for transfusion or operative time (Wang et al. 2018). An RCT by Tarwala et al. showed no difference in operative time, postoperative pain scores, amount of pain medication required, hemoglobin change, range of motion, or total blood loss between groups of patients with a tourniquet used throughout the case compared to only during cementation. They did note one case of compartment syndrome related to the tourniquet, while no complications were reported in the no tourniquet group (Tarwala et al. 2014).

> Further confusing the matter, not only are there different strategies for the amount of time during the case that the tourniquet is inflated, but also differences in inflation pressure.

The tradeoff with pressure is that it must be high enough to restrict blood flow, but pressures too high may cause other adverse effects such as myonecrosis or increased postoperative pain (Dennis et al. 2016). Ishii and Matsuda performed an RCT evaluating this issue in cementless TKAs. They randomized patients to either 300 mmHg or systolic blood pressure + 100 mmHg, and found no differences in intraoperative or postoperative blood loss, suggesting that as long as the tourniquet is inflated to sufficiently restrict blood flow, that the effect of pressure on blood loss is not significant (Ishii and Matsuda 2005).

> There is a great deal of heterogeneity in the literature studying tourniquet use in TKA. From different timings to different pressures, and different combinations of those factors, it is difficult to make any strong conclusions.

With that said, the current literature does suggest that the use of tourniquet likely does reduce intraoperative blood loss, but its effect on postoperative and total blood loss are less clear. Further, and more standardized, study is needed to assess these issues.

49.3 Visualization

It is impossible for any surgeon to perform a good TKA without adequate visualization. It is sensible to think that utilizing a tourniquet would aid in visualization by reducing the blood in the operative field, thereby aiding the surgeon in correctly identifying anatomical landmarks and correctly positioning components. This has been recently studied by Goel et al. in an RCT of patients undergoing TKA with and without a tourniquet. They noted that a statistically higher percentage of surgeons performing TKA with the use of a tourniquet had "no difficulty" with visualization throughout the case compared to those performing the case without a tourniquet (Goel et al. 2019). However, it is worth noting that over half of the cases performed without a tourniquet either had "no difficulty" or "some difficulty, but did not affect the case", which raises the question of how important this finding may be. This has been further corroborated in the arthroscopy literature, as Kirkley et al. also

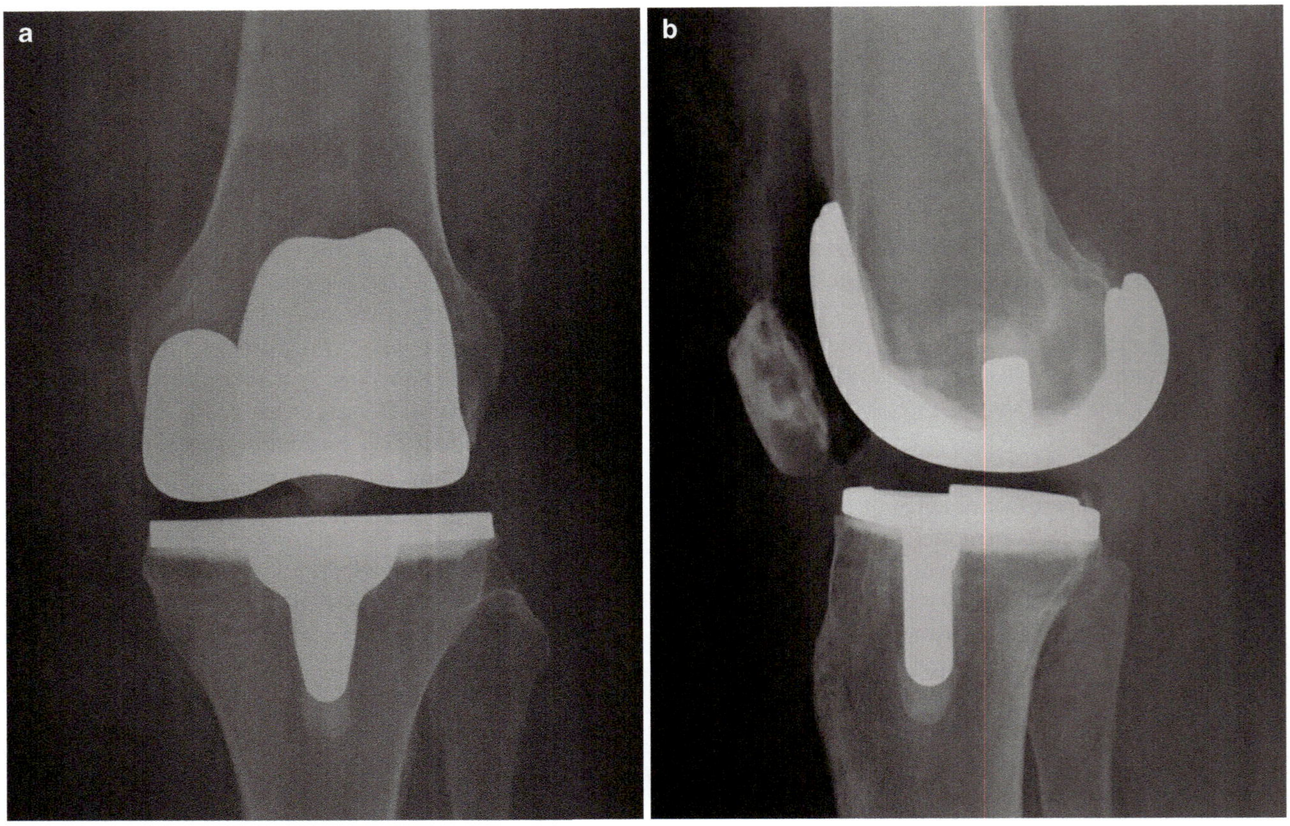

Fig. 49.1 **a** Anteroposterior and **b** lateral radiograph of a left primary TKA showing excellent cement mantle penetration

reported that surgeons performing knee arthroscopy reported that visualization was improved with the use of a tourniquet (Kirkley et al. 2000).

In our experience, it is infrequent to have a case where the lack of a tourniquet produces enough of an issue with visualization as to hamper the progress or outcome of the case.

> In fact, the tourniquet can at times further hinder visualization by being a venous tourniquet and allowing more blood to pool in the operative extremity.

49.4 Cementation

Cement mantle penetration is essential for the long-term success of a primary TKA (Fig. 49.1). Greater cement mantle penetration has been shown to provide increased implant survival and stability (Bert and McShane 1998; Peters et al. 2003; Walker et al. 1984). Aseptic loosening, a leading cause for revision TKA (Dalury et al. 2013), is a devastating complication that usually occurs at the bone–cement interface (Maistrelli et al. 1995).

> In order to avoid this, surgeons must be meticulous and systematic in their preparation of the bone in order to minimize blood at the bony surface and allow for a strong cement bond (Ritter et al. 1994; Bannister and Miles 1988; Clarius et al. 2009; Gruen et al. 1976; Krause et al. 1982; Majkowski et al. 1994).

Historically, one reason for tourniquet use was to facilitate this vital step. However, with modern protocols and the advent and wide adoption of tranexamic acid (TXA) in TKA (Franchini et al. 2018), blood loss has been reduced, transfusion rates have plummeted, and requiring a tourniquet to maintain a bloodless bone–cement interface may no longer be required (Zhang et al. 2012; Gomez-Barrena et al. 2014; Shemshaki et al. 2015; Huang et al. 2015; Herndon et al. 2019; Ozkunt et al. 2018; Jawhar et al. 2018). Additionally, novel interventions such as the addition of sterile carbon dioxide gas to further aid in drying the bony surfaces have been promising (Gapinski et al. 2019). Yet the need for a deep cement mantle, and, therefore, a clean surgical field, has inspired many surgeons to continue to utilize the tourniquet for at least cementation during the case.

Specifically evaluating the role and timing of tourniquet use on cement mantle penetration, Pfitzner et al. performed an RCT evaluating the cement mantle penetration of patients undergoing TKA with and without tourniquet. They found that tourniquet use did increase the average cumulative cement mantle penetration by 1.2 mm, but found that postoperative pain scores were higher (Pfitzner et al. 2016). Contrary to their findings, in a more recent cohort, Herndon et al. showed that in patients receiving TXA, there was no difference in cement mantle penetration whether or not a tourniquet was used (Herndon et al. 2019). Similarly, an RCT by Ozkunt et al. randomized patients to one of three arms: tourniquet throughout the case, only during cement, or none at all. They found no difference in cement mantle penetration, postoperative drainage, or transfusions. However, they did note higher pain scores and lower Knee Society Scores in the group that had a tourniquet throughout the case compared to both other groups (Ozkunt et al. 2018). Finally, Vertullo and Nagarajan also noted no difference in cement penetration in patients who had tourniquets inflated during cementation vs. not at all (Vertullo and Nagarajan 2017).

To further quantify the effect of cementation on implant migration, roentgen stereophotogrammetric analysis (RSA) has been utilized. This method uses 1 mm radio-opaque tantalum beads implanted in the bone surrounding an implant to detect small changes in implant position and micromotion over time in a three-dimensional way. Ledin et al. and Ejaz et al. both performed studies using RSA to evaluate the tibial component 2 years postoperatively and found no difference in tibial component micromotion or migration whether or not a tourniquet was used (Ejaz et al. 2015; Ledin et al. 2012). Similarly, Molt et al. found no difference in tibial component translation or rotation in TKAs done with a tourniquet compared to those done without one (Molt et al. 2014). These results suggest that the equivalent cement mantle at the time of surgery afforded to both tourniquet and tourniquetless TKAs does extrapolate to equivalent implant stability in at least the short term.

> This current body of literature suggests that inflation of the tourniquet at any point during the procedure, including during the vital cementation step, has little effect on cement penetration or implant stability, and may be unnecessary.

49.5 Pain and Clinical Outcomes

The pervading hypothesis is that use of a tourniquet, with its constant and strong pressure to the thigh during surgery, may have deleterious effects on postoperative pain, muscle strength and function, and, therefore, negatively affect patient outcomes following TKA. These issues have also been well studied. Dennis et al. showed that quadriceps strength was 14% greater at 3 weeks postoperatively and 7% greater at 3 months when no tourniquet was used (Dennis et al. 2016). Guler et al. found that patients who underwent TKA with a tourniquet had a 20% loss of quadriceps muscle volume at 1 month postoperatively compared to the contralateral limb, and found no difference in patients who underwent TKA without a tourniquet (Guler et al. 2016). Relating to these results, Chen et al. found that patients who had a tourniquet used throughout their case had significantly greater thigh pain on postoperative day (POD) 3 compared to patients in which the tourniquet was only used after bony cuts were made. Further, Huang et al. found that tourniquet patients had more knee pain until POD 5, and this was associated with decreased range of motion (Huang et al. 2017). Li et al. also showed that the use of tourniquet reduced knee flexion at POD 1 and POD 3, but found no difference by POD 7 (Li et al. 2009). Those patients were also better able to perform a straight leg raise at those time points.

Contrary to these results, Singh et al. found no difference in postoperative range of motion between patients with selective tourniquet use and those in which a tourniquet was not used (Singh et al. 2015). Additionally, Goel et al. found no difference in postoperative pain, range of motion, patient-reported outcome scores, or functional tests including the timed up and go test and the stair climb test at any time point immediately postoperatively, at 4–6 weeks, or 6–8 months postoperatively in patients having undergone TKA with a tourniquet compared to those who underwent TKA without one (Goel et al. 2019). Finally, Jawhar et al. showed no difference between tourniquet and no tourniquet groups in any patient-reported outcome measure, strength measurement, or patient satisfaction following TKA (Jawhar et al. 2019).

> These conflicting data are difficult to reconcile. In the authors' anecdotal experience it does seem that patients having undergone TKA without the use of a tourniquet do recover more quickly and with less thigh pain compared to those who have a tourniquet, but more study is warranted on this issue.

49.6 Complications Related to Tourniquet Use

As with anything, tourniquet use is not without potential complications. Deep venous thromboembolism (DVT) and associated pulmonary embolism (PE), peripheral nerve compression injury, and metabolic disturbance and subsequent wound healing issues have all been investigated.

In terms of thromboembolism, research has demonstrated increased rates of thrombosis and fibrinolysis after tourniquet release during TKA (Reikerås and Clementsen 2009), but other studies have shown a protective effect of tourniquet use. Aglietti et al. showed that there were greater concentrations of thrombin in the group not using a tourniquet and higher levels of fibrinolysis (less clot formation) in the group using a tourniquet in a study of 20 patients undergoing TKA (Aglietti et al. 2000). Clinically, Fahmy and Patel showed a decreased rate of DVT after TKA with a tourniquet, which was attributed to this increased fibrinolytic activity (Fahmy and Patel 1981).

Many studies have also evaluated the rate of DVT in patients undergoing TKA with and without tourniquet, and the results are mixed. Some show no difference in DVT rate between groups (Alcelik et al. 2012; Li et al. 2014; Tie et al. 2016; Zan et al. 2015), while others show a small increase in DVT rate with the use of tourniquet (Jiang et al. 2015; Huang et al. 2015; Goel et al. 2019). As mentioned before, these groups are heterogeneous and contain multiple permutations of tourniquet use, which makes extrapolating these results challenging.

In addition to thromboembolic events, local complications are also possible as a result of tourniquet use. Several animal studies have shown that peripheral nerve injury, including myelin sheath compromise and Schwann cell hypertrophy, and muscular damage leading to weakness occur with prolonged tourniquet use (Nitz and Matulionis 1982; Ochoa et al. 1972; Mohler et al. 1999). In clinical studies, Olivecrona et al. noted 1 out of 20 patients had electromyography (EMG) changes postoperatively after TKA with a tourniquet that was inflated to 294 mmHg (Olivecrona et al. 2013). Additionally, in a retrospective review of over 1000 patients, Horlocker et al. showed that the chance for peroneal and tibial nerve palsies was significantly more common in patients with cumulative tourniquet time over 150 min, even if that time was interrupted by 20–30 min breaks to allow for reperfusion of the limb (Horlocker et al. 2006).

> With that said, there is no research to our knowledge that definitively shows optimal tourniquet time in terms of peripheral nerve injury.

In addition to nervous structures, the TKA wound bed is also affected by the use of a tourniquet, and it has been theorized that a reduction in perfusion may adversely affect the local healing process. Clarke et al. investigated whether tourniquet pressure had any effect on local tissue oxygenation. They used three arms: no tourniquet, a low-pressure tourniquet (225 mmHg), and high-pressure tourniquet (350 mmHg). They found that all patients had a reduction in oxygen tension at the wound site in the first postoperative week, but it was significantly lower with the high-pressure tourniquet compared to both other groups (Clarke et al. 2001). This decrease in oxygen tension at the wound surface may or may not have a clinical correlation though. Multiple other studies have evaluated perioperative complications, including wound healing issues and the need to return to the operating room for further surgery and seen no difference between tourniquet and no tourniquet groups (Goel et al. 2019; Jawhar et al. 2019), but these studies are not powered to sufficiently answer this clinical question, as complications like this are fortunately rare.

49.7 Authors' Current Protocol

The current practice of the senior author is to not place or inflate a tourniquet at all during either primary or revision TKA. Prior to incision, 1 g of TXA is administered, and a second dose is administered at the time of closure. We prefer to perform cemented TKA and utilize a combination of suction and dry sponges to prepare the bone surfaces immediately prior to cementation, and then manually pressurize the cement into the cancellous bone. Intra-articular drains are not routinely placed, and aspirin is our drug of choice for DVT prophylaxis, unless the patient has a contraindication or is on another agent at baseline for another medical issue, such as atrial fibrillation.

Conclusion

Tourniquet use in TKA remains controversial. Many studies have attempted to address various questions regarding its use, the timing of its use, and the benefits and pitfalls. The body of literature is limited by multiple permutations of groups which makes definitive conclusions difficult to draw. Regardless of whether or not a tourniquet is used, proper placement of components and good cementation technique are paramount to both short-term and long-term outcomes following TKA.

Take-Home Messages

- Tourniquet use likely reduces intraoperative blood loss during TKA. The effects on postoperative and total blood loss are less clear.
- Tourniquet use likely improves intraoperative visualization, but not using one does not necessarily make visualization difficult enough to affect the outcome of the case.
- With the adoption of TXA and novel methods of preparing the cut bone surface for cement pressurization, a tourniquet is not necessary for obtaining a high-quality cement mantle, and RSA studies in the short term show no increased implant micromotion or migration.
- Although basic science data shows and it intuitively makes sense that tourniquet use would be associated with increased thigh pain and decreased patient outcomes, this has not been consistently demonstrated in recent literature.
- The data regarding complications of tourniquet use, namely DVT, nerve injury, and wound-healing issues is underpowered and inconclusive.
- Whatever the choice of the operating surgeon regarding using a tourniquet, ensuring proper implant placement and a quality cement mantle is of upmost importance. With a lack of definitive evidence one way or the other, surgeons should proceed with whatever they are comfortable with and what allows them to perform the best technical surgery.

References

Aglietti P, Baldini A, Vena LM, Abbate R, Fedi S, Falciani M (2000) Effect of tourniquet use on activation of coagulation in total knee replacement. Clin Orthop Relat Res 371:169–177

Alcelik I, Pollock RD, Sukeik M, Bettany-Saltikov J, Armstrong PM, Fismer P (2012) A comparison of outcomes with and without a tourniquet in total knee arthroplasty: a systematic review and meta-analysis of randomized controlled trials. J Arthroplast 27(3):331–340

Arthur JR, Spangehl MJ (2019) Tourniquet use in total knee arthroplasty. J Knee Surg 32(8):719–729. https://doi.org/10.1055/s-0039-1681035

Bannister GC, Miles AW (1988) The influence of cementing technique and blood on the strength of the bone-cement interface. Eng Med 17(3):131–133

Berman AT, Parmet JL, Harding SP, Israelite CL, Chandrasekaran K, Horrow JC, Singer R, Rosenberg H (1998) Emboli observed with use of transesophageal echocardiography immediately after tourniquet release during total knee arthroplasty with cement. JBJS 80(3):389–396

Bert JM, McShane M (1998) Is it necessary to cement the tibial stem in cemented total knee arthroplasty? Clin Orthop Relat Res 356:73–78

Clarius M, Hauck C, Seeger JB, James A, Murray DW, Aldinger PR (2009) Pulsed lavage reduces the incidence of radiolucent lines under the tibial tray of Oxford unicompartmental knee arthroplasty: pulsed lavage versus syringe lavage. Int Orthop 33(6):1585–1590. https://doi.org/10.1007/s00264-009-0736-y

Clarke MT, Longstaff L, Edwards D, Rushton N (2001) Tourniquet-induced wound hypoxia after total knee replacement. J Bone Joint Surg 83(1):40–44

Cushing H (1904) Pneumatic tourniquets with special reference to their use in craniotomies. Med News 84:557–557

Dalury DF, Pomeroy DL, Gorab RS, Adams MJ (2013) Why are total knee arthroplasties being revised? J Arthroplast 28(8):120–121

Dennis DA, Kittelson AJ, Yang CC, Miner TM, Kim RH, Stevens-Lapsley JE (2016) Does tourniquet use in TKA affect recovery of lower extremity strength and function? A randomized trial. Clin Orthop Relat Res 474(1):69–77

Ejaz A, Laursen AC, Jakobsen T, Rasmussen S, Nielsen PT, Laursen MB (2015) Absence of a tourniquet does not affect fixation of cemented TKA: a randomized RSA study of 70 patients. J Arthroplast 30(12):2128–2132

Fahmy NR, Patel DG (1981) Hemostatic changes and postoperative deep-vein thrombosis associated with use of a pneumatic tourniquet. J Bone Joint Surg Am 63(3):461–465

Fan Y, Jin J, Sun Z, Li W, Lin J, Weng X, Qiu G (2014) The limited use of a tourniquet during total knee arthroplasty: a randomized controlled trial. Knee 21(6):1263–1268

Franchini M, Mengoli C, Marietta M, Marano G, Vaglio S, Pupella S, Mannucci PM, Liumbruno GM (2018) Safety of intravenous tranexamic acid in patients undergoing majororthopaedic surgery: a meta-analysis of randomised controlled trials. Blood Transfus 16(1):36–43. https://doi.org/10.2450/2017.0219-17

Gapinski ZA, Yee EJ, Kraus KR, Deckard ER, Meneghini RM (2019) The effect of tourniquet use and sterile carbon dioxide gas bone preparation on cement penetration in primary total knee arthroplasty. J Arthroplast 34(8):1634–1639. https://doi.org/10.1016/j.arth.2019.03.050

Goel R, Rondon AJ, Sydnor K, Blevins K, O'Malley M, Purtill JJ, Austin MS (2019) Tourniquet use does not affect functional outcomes or pain after total knee arthroplasty: a prospective, double-blinded, randomized controlled trial. J Bone Joint Surg Am 101(20):1821–1828. https://doi.org/10.2106/jbjs.19.00146

Gomez-Barrena E, Ortega-Andreu M, Padilla-Eguiluz NG, Pérez-Chrzanowska H, Figueredo-Zalve R (2014) Topical intra-articular compared with intravenous tranexamic acid to reduce blood loss in primary total knee replacement: a double-blind, randomized, controlled, noninferiority clinical trial. J Bone Joint Surg Am 96(23):1937–1944. https://doi.org/10.2106/JBJS.N.00060

Gross JB (1983) Estimating allowable blood loss: corrected for dilution. Anesthesiology 58:277–280

Gruen TA, Markolf KL, Amstutz HC (1976) Effects of laminations and blood entrapment on the strength of acrylic bone cement. Clin Orthop Relat Res 119:250–255

Guler O, Mahirogullari M, Isyar M, Piskin A, Yalcin S, Mutlu S, Sahin B (2016) Comparison of quadriceps muscle volume after unilateral total knee arthroplasty with and without tourniquet use. Knee Surg Sports Traumatol Arthrosc 24(8):2595–2605

Herndon CL, Grosso MJ, Sarpong NO, Shah RP, Geller JA, Cooper HJ (2019) Tibial cement mantle thickness is not affected by tourniquetless total knee arthroplasty when performed with tranexamic acid. Knee Surg Sports Traumatol Arthrosc. https://doi.org/10.1007/s00167-019-05559-3

Horlocker TT, Hebl JR, Gali B, Jankowski CJ, Burkle CM, Berry DJ, Zepeda FA, Stevens SR, Schroeder DR (2006) Anesthetic, patient, and surgical risk factors for neurologic complications after prolonged total tourniquet time during total knee arthroplasty. Anesth Analg 102(3):950–955

Huang Z, Ma J, Zhu Y, Pei F, Yang J, Zhou Z, Kang P, Shen B (2015) Timing of tourniquet release in total knee arthroplasty. Orthopedics 38(7):445–451. https://doi.org/10.3928/01477447-20150701-06

Huang Z, Xie X, Li L, Huang Q, Ma J, Shen B, Kraus VB, Pei F (2017) Intravenous and topical tranexamic acid alone are superior to tourniquet use for primary total knee arthroplasty: a prospective, randomized controlled trial. JBJS 99(24):2053–2061

Husted H, Jensen TT (2005) Influence of the pneumatic tourniquet on patella tracking in total knee arthroplasty: a prospective randomized study in 100 patients. J Arthroplast 20(6):694–697

Husted H, Hansen HC, Holm G, Bach-Dal C, Rud K, Andersen KL, Kehlet H (2010) What determines length of stay after total hip and knee arthroplasty? A nationwide study in Denmark. Arch Orthop Trauma Surg 130(2):263–268. https://doi.org/10.1007/s00402-009-0940-7

Ishii Y, Matsuda Y (2005) Effect of tourniquet pressure on perioperative blood loss associated with cementless total knee arthroplasty: a prospective, randomized study. J Arthroplast 20(3):325–330

Jawhar A, Stetzelberger V, Kollowa K, Obertacke U (2018) Tourniquet application does not affect the periprosthetic bone cement penetration in total knee arthroplasty. Knee Surg Sports Traumatol Arthrosc 27(7):2071–2081

Jawhar A, Skeirek D, Stetzelberger V, Kollowa K, Obertacke U (2019) No effect of tourniquet in primary total knee arthroplasty on muscle strength, functional outcome, patient satisfaction and health status: a randomized clinical trial. Knee Surg Sports Traumatol Arthrosc 28(4):1045–1054

Jiang F-z, Zhong H-m, Hong Y-c, Zhao G-f (2015) Use of a tourniquet in total knee arthroplasty: a systematic review and meta-analysis of randomized controlled trials. J Orthop Sci 20(1):110–123

Kirkley A, Rampersaud R, Griffin S, Amendola A, Litchfield R, Fowler P (2000) Tourniquet versus no tourniquet use in routine knee arthroscopy: a prospective, double-blind, randomized clinical trial. Arthroscopy: J Arthrosc Relat Surg 16(2):121–126

Krause WR, Krug W, Miller J (1982) Strength of the cement-bone interface. Clin Orthop Relat Res 163:290–299

Ledin H, Aspenberg P, Good L (2012) Tourniquet use in total knee replacement does not improve fixation, but appears to reduce final range of motion: a randomized RSA study involving 50 patients. Acta Orthop 83(5):499–503

Li B, Wen Y, Wu H, Qian Q, Lin X, Zhao H (2009) The effect of tourniquet use on hidden blood loss in total knee arthroplasty. Int Orthop 33(5):1263–1268

Li X, Yin L, Chen Z-Y, Zhu L, Wang H-L, Chen W, Yang G, Zhang Y-Z (2014) The effect of tourniquet use in total knee arthroplasty: grading the evidence through an updated meta-analysis of randomized, controlled trials. Eur J Orthop Surg Traumatol 24(6):973–986

Maistrelli GL, Antonelli L, Fornasier V, Mahomed N (1995) Cement penetration with pulsed lavage versus syringe irrigation in total knee arthroplasty. Clin Orthop Relat Res 312:261–265

Majkowski RS, Bannister GC, Miles AW (1994) The effect of bleeding on the cement-bone interface. An experimental study. Clin Orthop Relat Res 299:293–297

Mittal R, Ko V, Adie S, Naylor J, Dave J, Dave C, Harris IA, Hackett D, Ngo D, Dietsch S (2012) Tourniquet application only during cement fixation in total knee arthroplasty: a double-blind, randomized controlled trial. ANZ J Surg 82(6):428–433

Mohler LR, Pedowitz RA, Lopez MA, Gershuni DH (1999) Effects of tourniquet compression on neuromuscular function. Clin Orthop Relat Res 359:213–220

Molt M, Harsten A, Toksvig-Larsen S (2014) The effect of tourniquet use on fixation quality in cemented total knee arthroplasty a prospective randomized clinical controlled RSA trial. Knee 21(2):396–401

Nitz AJ, Matulionis DH (1982) Ultrastructural changes in rat peripheral nerve following pneumatic tourniquet compression. J Neurosurg 57(5):660–666

Noordin S, McEwen JA, Kragh CJF Jr, Eisen A, Masri BA (2009) Surgical tourniquets in orthopaedics. JBJS 91(12):2958–2967

Ochoa J, Fowler TJ, Gilliatt RW (1972) Anatomical changes in peripheral nerves compressed by a pneumatic tourniquet. J Anat 113(Pt 3):433

Olivecrona C, Blomfeldt R, Ponzer S, Stanford BR, Nilsson BY (2013) Tourniquet cuff pressure and nerve injury in knee arthroplasty in a bloodless field: a neurophysiological study. Acta Orthop 84(2):159–164

Ozkunt O, Sariyilmaz K, Gemalmaz HC, Dikici F (2018) The effect of tourniquet usage on cement penetration in total knee arthroplasty: a prospective randomized study of 3 methods. Medicine 97(4):e9668

Peters CL, Craig MA, Mohr RA, Bachus KN (2003) Tibial component fixation with cement: full- versus surface-cementation techniques. Clin Orthop Relat Res 409:158–168. https://doi.org/10.1097/01.blo.0000058638.94987.20

Pfitzner T, von Roth P, Voerkelius N, Mayr H, Perka C, Hube R (2016) Influence of the tourniquet on tibial cement mantle thickness in primary total knee arthroplasty. Knee Surg Sports Traumatol Arthrosc 24(1):96–101. https://doi.org/10.1007/s00167-014-3341-6

Rama KRBS, Apsingi S, Poovali S, Jetti A (2007) Timing of tourniquet release in knee arthroplasty: meta-analysis of randomized, controlled trials. J Bone Joint Surg Am 89(4):699–705

Reikerås O, Clementsen T (2009) Time course of thrombosis and fibrinolysis in total knee arthroplasty with tourniquet application. Local versus systemic activations. J Thromb Thrombolysis 28(4):425

Ritter MA, Herbst SA, Keating EM, Faris PM (1994) Radiolucency at the bone-cement interface in total knee replacement. The effects of bone-surface preparation and cement technique. J Bone Joint Surg Am 76(1):60–65

Schnettler T, Papillon N, Rees H (2017) Use of a tourniquet in total knee arthroplasty causes a paradoxical increase in total blood loss. JBJS 99(16):1331–1336

Shemshaki H, Nourian SM, Nourian N, Dehghani M, Mokhtari M, Mazoochian F (2015) One step closer to sparing total blood loss and transfusion rate in total knee arthroplasty: a meta-analysis of different methods of tranexamic acid administration. Arch Orthop Trauma Surg 135(4):573–588. https://doi.org/10.1007/s00402-015-2189-7

Singh G, Han F, Kaki RR, Shen L, Nathan SS (2015) Does limited tourniquet usage in primary total knee arthroplasty result in better functional outcomes? Ann Acad Med Singap 44(8):302–306

Smith TO, Hing CB (2010) Is a tourniquet beneficial in total knee replacement surgery?: a meta-analysis and systematic review. Knee 17(2):141–147

Tai T-W, Lin C-J, Jou I-M, Chang C-W, Lai K-A, Yang C-Y (2011) Tourniquet use in total knee arthroplasty: a meta-analysis. Knee Surg Sports Traumatol Arthrosc 19(7):1121–1130

Tarwala R, Dorr LD, Gilbert PK, Wan Z, Long WT (2014) Tourniquet use during cementation only during total knee arthroplasty: a randomized trial. Clin Orthop Relat Res 472(1):169–174

Tie K, Qi Y, Hu D, Wang H, Chen L (2016) Effects of tourniquet release on total knee arthroplasty. Orthopedics 39(4):e642–e650

Vertullo CJ, Nagarajan M (2017) Is cement penetration in TKR reduced by not using a tourniquet during cementation? A single blinded, randomized trial. J Orthop Surg 25(1): 2309499016684323

Walker PS, Soudry M, Ewald FC, McVickar H (1984) Control of cement penetration in total knee arthroplasty. Clin Orthop Relat Res 185:155–164

Wang K, Ni S, Li Z, Zhong Q, Li R, Li H, Ke Y, Lin J (2017) The effects of tourniquet use in total knee arthroplasty: a randomized, controlled trial. Knee Surg Sports Traumatol Arthrosc 25(9):2849–2857. https://doi.org/10.1007/s00167-015-3964-2

Wang C, Zhou C, Qu H, Yan S, Pan Z (2018) Comparison of tourniquet application only during cementation and long-duration tourniquet application in total knee arthroplasty: a meta-analysis. J Orthop Surg Res 13(1):216. https://doi.org/10.1186/s13018-018-0927-6

Welling DR, McKay PL, Rasmussen TE, Rich NM (2012) A brief history of the tourniquet. J Vasc Surg 55(1):286–290

Zan PF, Yang Y, Fu D, Yu X, Li GD (2015) Releasing of tourniquet before wound closure or not in total knee arthroplasty: a meta-analysis of randomized controlled trials. J Arthroplast 30(1):31–37

Zhang H, Chen J, Chen F, Que W (2012) The effect of tranexamic acid on blood loss and use of blood products in total knee arthroplasty: a meta-analysis. Knee Surg Sports Traumatol Arthrosc 20(9):1742–1752. https://doi.org/10.1007/s00167-011-1754-z

Zhang W, Li N, Chen S, Tan Y, Al-Aidaros M, Chen L (2014a) The effects of a tourniquet used in total knee arthroplasty: a meta-analysis. J Orthop Surg Res 9(1):13

Zhang W, Liu A, Hu D, Tan Y, Al-Aidaros M, Pan Z (2014b) Effects of the timing of tourniquet release in cemented total knee arthroplasty: a systematic review and meta-analysis of randomized controlled trials. J Orthop Surg Res 9:125. https://doi.org/10.1186/s13018-014-0125-0

Zhang P, Liang Y, He J, Fang Y, Chen P, Wang J (2017) Timing of tourniquet release in total knee arthroplasty: a meta-analysis. Medicine (Baltimore) 96(17):e6786. https://doi.org/10.1097/MD.0000000000006786

Zhou K, Ling T, Wang H, Zhou Z, Shen B, Yang J, Kang P, Pei F (2017) Influence of tourniquet use in primary total knee arthroplasty with drainage: a prospective randomised controlled trial. J Orthop Surg Res 12(1):172

Complications

Contents

Perioperative Thromboembolic Events

Steven D. Donohoe and Jeremy Gililland

Contents

E. Hansen, K.-D. Kühn (eds.), *Essentials of Cemented Knee Arthroplasty*,
https://doi.org/10.1007/978-3-662-63113-3_50

50.1 Introduction

Fat embolism syndrome (FES) and bone cement implantation syndrome (BCIS) are two clinical entities in the spectrum of embolic syndromes characterized by hypoxia, hypotension, cardiac arrhythmias, increased pulmonary vascular resistance, and occasionally cardiac arrest that occur when the marrow contents are exposed during trauma or manipulated during surgery (Eriksson et al. 2011). While often thought of as separate entities, there is no definitive evidence that these are distinct.

Parvizi et al. reviewed 23 patients who died suddenly while undergoing hip arthroplasty at their institution. They observed that all of these deaths occurred during cemented total hip arthroplasty or cemented hemiarthroplasty. Autopsy performed on 13 of these patients found bone marrow microemboli in the lungs of 11 of the 13 patients, and methylmethacrylate in the lungs of 3 of 13 patients (Parvizi et al. 1999). Markel et al. performed TKAs on canines and collected embolic debris from the lungs of the dogs after sacrifice. They hypothesized that they would find mixed embolic debris within the canine lungs; instead, they found that the primary constituent of embolic debris was marrow elements with little to no cement debris (Markel et al. 1999). Further, it has been shown that there is a paucity of literature looking at BCIS as a distinct clinical entity (Donaldson et al. 2009). For this reason, this chapter will refer to this condition as a single disease state called fat embolism syndrome (FES).

In an effort to present a comprehensive review, we believe that a description of the history of this syndrome is warranted. Scientific interest in FES started hundreds of years ago. Lower developed an animal model 300 years ago by injecting milk intravenously into dogs and then studying the effects. In the early nineteenth century, Magendie injected oil into an animal model and then described the properties of embolized fat globules in the pulmonary capillaries. Shortly after Magendie's publication, Virchow demonstrated that a similar injection could lead to pulmonary edema (Tzioupis and Giannoudis 2011). Zenker first described this phenomenon in humans when he reported on the presence of fat globules in the lung capillaries of a railroad worker who had died of a crush injury (Bulger et al. 1997). Up to this time, all published studies report on the presence of pulmonary fat droplets post-mortem.

> This is important because there is a distinction between fat embolism (FE) and fat embolism syndrome (FES).

FE refers to any time that fat globules are found in the circulation or in lung tissue. FES refers to a clinical syndrome characterized by a consistent pattern of signs and symptoms including respiratory distress, neurological compromise, and petechial rash. Von Bergmann first described the symptoms of FES in 1873 when he reported on a patient who fell from a roof and suffered a comminuted femur fracture. Two days following the injury, the patient developed confusion, dyspnea, petechiae, and ultimately expired less than 1 day after symptom onset. A large pulmonary fat embolus was found at the time of autopsy (Tzioupis and Giannoudis 2011).

> In spite of the long history of interest and study into FES, it is still fairly poorly understood.

50.2 Clinical Manifestations and Pathophysiology

The Main Manifestations of FES

- Respiratory distress
- Neurologic changes
- Petechial rash

There is a spectrum of *pulmonary manifestations* of FES. Acute cardiopulmonary collapse can occur, and this results from a rush of large fat emboli causing altered pulmonary vascular resistance, decreased systemic blood pressure and cardiac output, and a drop in intraoperative arterial oxygen saturation (Christie et al. 1995; Winn et al. 1987). The other pulmonary manifestations of FES are typically more insidious. There is a delay of 12–72 h and then patients will develop respiratory dysfunction and hypoxemia. This occurs because the lungs are the first organs to filter the embolic load, and there are local mechanical and biochemical mechanisms that result in impaired oxygen transfer to hemoglobin. An increase in alveolar dead space (alveoli that are ventilated but not perfused) occurs because the alveolar capillaries are mechanically occluded by fat particles, but this does not account completely for the hypoxemia. There is also abnormal mixing of arterial and venous blood in the lung. This mechanism is unclear but it could be due to extensive hemorrhage or edema from cytokine cascades leading to alveolar consolidation, and perfused but non-ventilated alveoli (Moore and Moore 1995).

The *neurological manifestations* of FES also cover a broad spectrum. These can range anywhere from the inability to awaken a patient at the conclusion of an operation, to generalized postoperative encephalopathy, to focal neurological signs mimicking acute hypoxia. These symptoms will typically resolve with time and supportive care but there can be persistent cognitive,

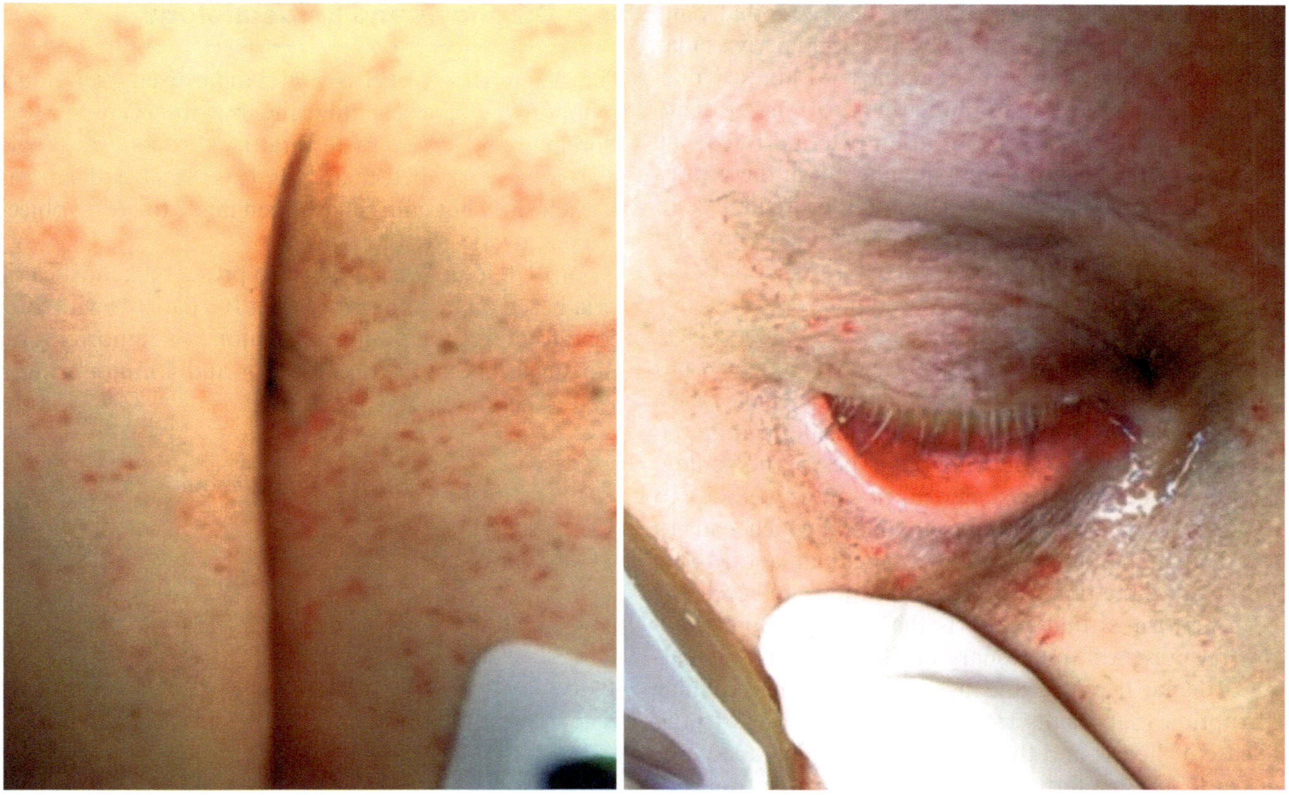

Fig. 50.1 Axillary and conjunctival petechiae. (Fenire (2014), with permission)

personality, and conversational changes (Byrick et al. 2001; Dive et al. 2002; Sulek et al. 1999; Yeon et al. 2003). Postoperative confusion and delirium in the absence of pulmonary and dermatologic manifestations may result from fat embolism (Cox et al. 2011). Studies have demonstrated that the incidence of cerebral fat embolism can range anywhere from 60% to 100% of patients after arthroplasty, and 40–75% of those patients had a measurable decrease in cognitive function in the early postoperative period (Sulek et al. 1999; Rodriguez et al. 2005).

The presence of *skin manifestations* of FES may correlate with the severity of the syndrome. The petechial rash is considered to be pathognomonic for FES and is frequently the last of the triad to appear. The rash does not appear on the posterior side of the body, and it has been postulated that this is the result of the low density of lipid droplets causing them to "rise up" in a supine patient. The rash is also most frequently seen in conjunctiva, oral mucous membranes, and the skin folds of the anterior neck and axillae. This is likely because the droplets accumulate in the aortic arch and are transported to the anterior and cranial structures via the subclavian and carotid vessels (Fig. 50.1) (Tachakra 1976).

> The pathophysiology of FES is not well-defined. There have been attempts to define the mechanism by which the syndrome initiates and propagates to systemic manifestations, but there is still uncertainty.

At the time of autopsy, patients will frequently have marrow contents found in their lungs but will not have shown any signs of FES prior to death. This makes it difficult to determine which patients with FE will develop FES. Attempts have been made to describe the pathophysiology. In 1924, Gauss proposed his mechanical theory. He believed that visceral trauma, and long bone trauma or manipulation led to 3 distinct stages of pathogenesis:

- First, that the injury produced sufficient disorganization of the supporting tissue stroma to release free fat into an uncontained area.
- Second, that the injury caused rupture of veins in the area.
- Third, that some mechanism occurs by this liberated fat is passed into the open ends of blood vessels.

He acknowledged that this theory does not seem to make sense given the fact that veins have weak flexible walls and would be difficult to pressurize fat globules into the flimsy open ends. However, he argues that veins in longs bones are different. They have rigid perivascular sheaths because they are contained within calcified tubules. This allows the injured ends to remain open, and both positive pressure from an external force (the injury) and the negative pressure inherent in the venous system can introduce fat droplets into the circulation. In arthroplasty, a rapid increase in intramedullary pressure after manipulating the endosteum can force fat into the veins and into systemic circulation (Gauss 1924).

Lehman and Moore challenged Gauss's theory. They report cases of fat embolism present in patients with non-traumatic causes of death. These include death from cardiorenal disease, post-influenzal pneumonia, eclampsia, diabetes, and different types of poisoning. They proposed that a systemic insult causes the body to mobilize its fat stores into the circulation which leads to a systemic inflammatory response (Lehman and Moore 1927). Since the time of these publications, research has been performed that supports their theory. Bone marrow fat present in pulmonary capillaries leads to localized edema, hypoxia, and hypoperfusion. The cellular disruption that results from this sequence leads to the release of lipase, and the fat globules are degraded into glycerol and free fatty acids. A cytokine cascade ensues and there are increased levels of TNF-alpha, IL-1, IL-6, and IL-8 which can lead to acute respiratory distress syndrome (ARDS). These proinflammatory cytokines can also act on vasoactive mediators, the complement cascade, and the coagulation cascade. In extreme cases, this can progress to disseminated intravascular coagulation (DIC) (Peltier 1988; Botha et al. 1995; Colotta et al. 1992; Rose and Marzi 1998).

> It is important to note that these extreme cases usually involve multiply injured patients, and to our knowledge, there are no published reports of FES-induced ARDS or DIC following hip or knee arthroplasty.

It has long been thought that the systemic effects of FES could only occur in the presence of a patent foramen ovale (PFO). It has been estimated that a PFO is present in 20–25% of the general population but is only clinically significant in approximately 6% of people. It has also been postulated that the extrapulmonary manifestations do not occur solely because of a right-to-left cardiac shunt but can also result from fat being forced through the pulmonary capillary barrier (Palmovic and McCarroll 1965). This is why FES can be observed in patients without a PFO (Gurd 1970).

50.3 Diagnosis and Epidemiology

The diagnosis of FES is not standardized. It is most commonly diagnosed clinically by observing for the aforementioned triad of respiratory distress, neurologic symptoms, and a petechial rash. It is usually a diagnosis of exclusion, but efforts have been made to create objective diagnostic criteria.

In 1970, Gurd was the first to present diagnostic criteria based on his experience with 100 patients with long bone fractures (he designates major and minor criteria and suggests that at least 1 major and 4 minor criteria need to be present) (Gurd 1970):

Gurd Criteria (Tzioupis and Giannoudis 2011)

- *Major criteria:*
  - Petechial rash: axillary or subconjunctival petechia
  - Respiratory symptoms: positive radiographic changes; hypoxemia ($PaO_2 < 60$ mmHg, $FiO_2 < 0.4$)
  - Cerebral depression disproportionate to hypoxemia
  - Pulmonary edema
- *Minor criteria:*
  - Tachycardia (>110 beats/min)
  - Pyrexia (<38.5 °C)
  - Retinal fat or petechiae
  - Presence of urinary fat globules
  - Sudden drop in Hg level or platelet values
  - High erythrocyte sedimentation rate
  - Fat globules in the sputum
  - Urinary incontinence

FES = 1 major +4 minor + fat macroglobulinemia.

Lindeque studied a group of 55 patients with long bone fractures, and developed diagnostic criteria based on respiratory symptoms (Tzioupis and Giannoudis 2011):

Lindeque Criteria (Tzioupis and Giannoudis 2011)

- Sustained $PaO_2 < 8$ kPa
- Sustained $PCO_2 < 7.3$ kPa or pH < 7.3
- Sustained respiratory rate >35 breaths/min, despite sedation
- Increased work of breathing: dyspnea, accessory muscle use, tachycardia, and anxiety

Schonfeld developed criteria based on his opinion of the most important features. He variably weighted these findings according to observed specificity and set a cut-off value above which a patient was diagnosed with FES (Tzioupis and Giannoudis 2011):

Schonfeld's Criteria (Tzioupis and Giannoudis 2011) – A Score > 5 Is Diagnostic of FES

- Diffuse petechiae
- Chest X-ray changes (alveolar infiltrates)
- Hypoxemia (PaO2 < 9.3 kPa)
- Confusion
- Fever (>38 °C)
- Heart rate (120 beats/min)
- Tachypnea (>30 bpm)

FE index = 5 or more points.

> It is important to note that none of these systems have been prospectively validated.

Laboratory tests are not helpful in the diagnosis of FES. Patients will commonly demonstrate anemia, thrombocytopenia, and elevated inflammatory markers but no set criteria have been established to guide use of these tests for diagnosis. Patients can be hypocalcemic because serum lipase can bind calcium. Albumin also binds free fatty acids (FFAs) so it is possible to see a decrease in serum albumin (Markel et al. 1999). Prakash et al. measured IL-6 levels in patients diagnosed with FES by Gurd criteria and found elevated serum levels. They concluded that this could be a useful adjunct (Prakash et al. 2013).

Bronchoalveolar lavage can be used to assess for fat in the lungs; although the presence of fat in the lungs is non-specific. Karagiorga et al. compared BAL results in patients with FES and ARDS and found that patients with FES had >30% alveolar macrophages with lipid inclusions while patients with ARDS only had about half that number. They also reported that there are significantly elevated total cholesterol and lipid ester levels in patients with FES as compared to patients with ARDS (Prakash et al. 2013).

Imaging studies can also aid in diagnosis of FES. Chest radiographs (Fig. 50.2) will show bilateral diffuse or patchy opacities, but the findings are non-specific and can be seen in numerous other clinical entities (Newbigin et al. 2016a). Computed tomography has far more specific findings. Newbigin et al. describe a "crazy paving" pattern characterized by patchy ground-glass opacities and consolidation with interlobular thickening (Newbigin et al. 2016a) (Fig. 50.3). This same group demonstrated that the severity of these findings correlates with disease severity (Newbigin et al. 2016b). Because of the frequency of neurological symptoms, head imaging has also been used diagnostically. Computed tomography of the head is frequently normal, but magnetic resonance imaging has some sensitive findings. T2-weighted images will often show a "starfield pattern" with multiple small, hyperintense lesions in the periventricular, subcortical, and deep white matter. This appearance is described as looking similar to diffuse axonal injury (DAI), except that lesions in DAI are found at the gray–white matter junction (Kuo et al. 2014).

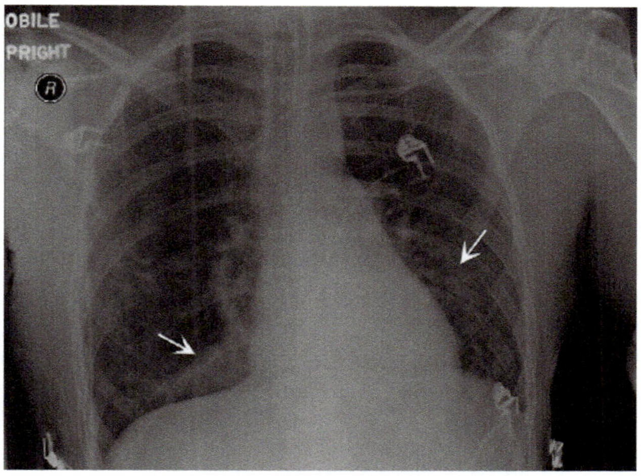

Fig. 50.2 Chest radiograph demonstrating patchy, ill-defined opacities in the perihilar and lower lobe regions. (Reprinted from Newbigin et al. © 2016, with permission from Elsevier) (Newbigin et al. 2016b)

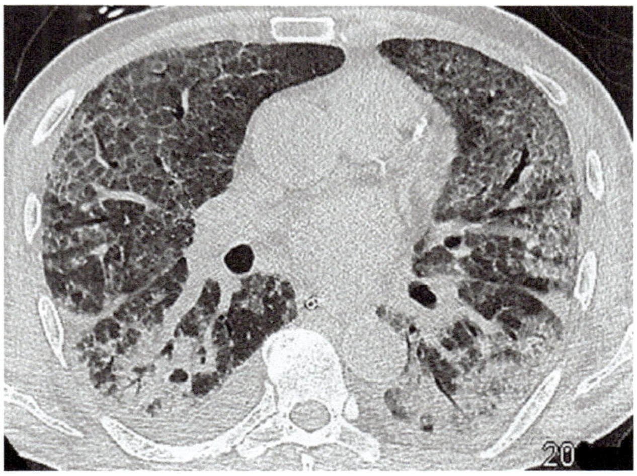

Fig. 50.3 CT chest demonstrating ground-glass opacities and interlobular septal thickening characterizing the crazy-paving pattern in the anterior lungs. (Reprinted from Newbigin et al. © 2016, with permission from Elsevier) (Newbigin et al. 2016b)

The epidemiology of FES is based on multiple studies of small groups of patients. Fat and other embolic material in the peripheral circulation during orthope-

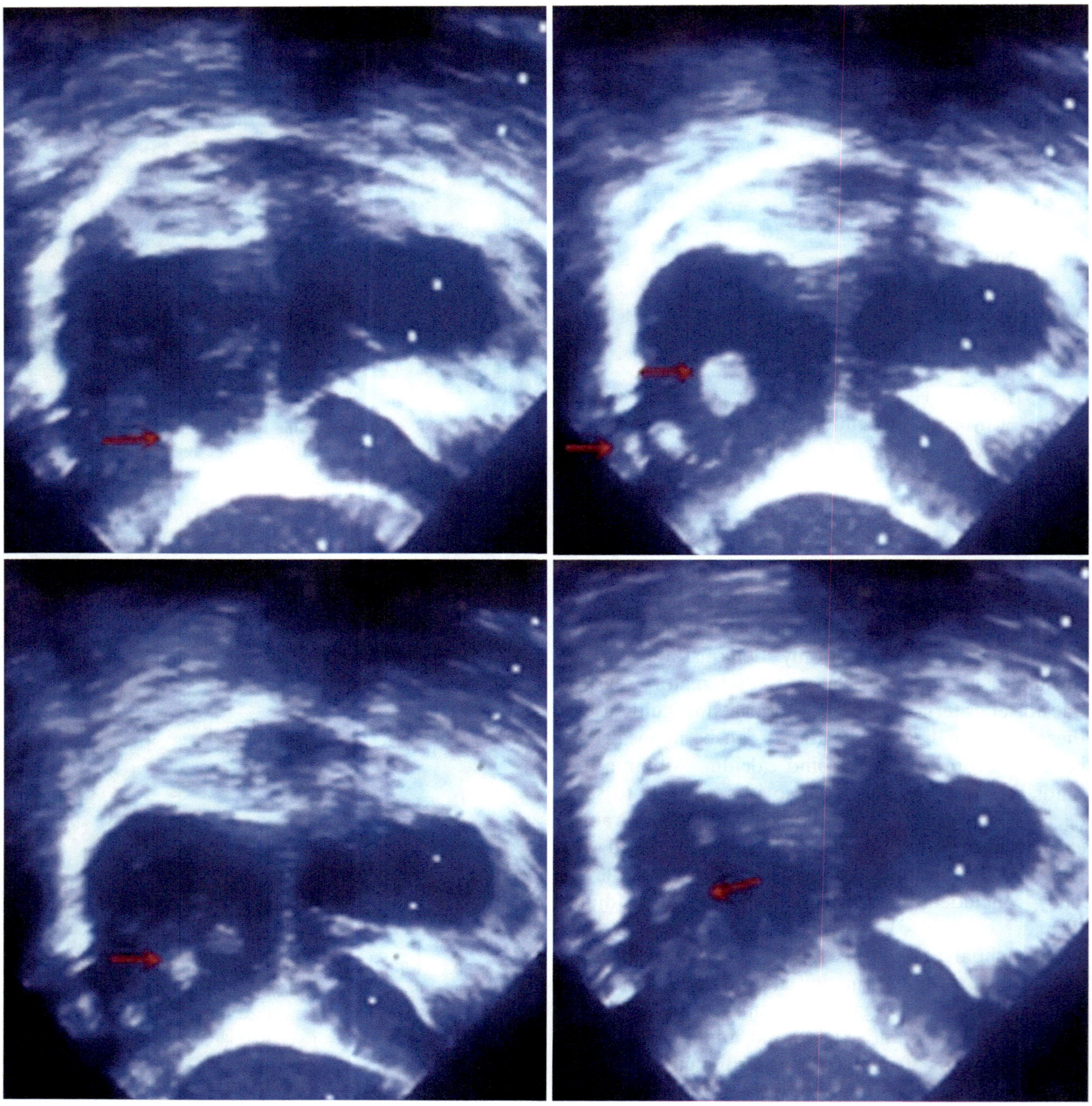

Fig. 50.4 TEE demonstrating multiple large embolic particles following release of pneumatic thigh tourniquet during TKA. (From Lu et al. 2017, by courtesy of Wolters Kluwer Health, Inc.) (Lu et al. 2017)

dic surgery is a common occurrence. Transesophageal echocardiograms (TEE) have been used during orthopedic procedures to observe the passage of embolic loads through the heart. Christie et al. reported on their findings utilizing TEE during 111 orthopedic procedures, including cemented and uncemented hip arthroplasty. They found echogenic material traveling through the heart in 87% of procedures. They confirmed it was fat embolism by sampling blood from the right atrium in a subset of patients. They found that 43% of the patients had emboli larger than 1 cm (Rodriguez et al. 2005). Another group performed TEE during 59 cemented total knee arthroplasties (TKA) (Berman et al. 1998). They observed showers of echogenic material in the right atrium and right ventricle of all patients after tourniquet release. They noted an average decrease in mixed venous oxygen saturation, increase in pulmonary arterial pressure, and increase in pulmonary vascular resistance index (Fig. 50.4) (Berman et al. 1998). Neither of these studies commented on whether any of the study patients went on to develop FES.

Kim et al. studied the prevalence of fat embolism, hemodynamic compromise, hypoxemia, and mental status changes in patients undergoing unilateral and simultaneous bilateral THA. This included both cemented and uncemented stems, and the simultaneous bilateral group was compared to a cohort undergoing unilateral THA. They analyzed right atrial blood samples in these patients and reported the presence of fat globules in 54% of the patients in the bilateral group compared with 49% of patients in the unilateral group. They also reported the presence of fat globules in 34% of patients in the cemented stem group, and 44% of patients in the uncemented stem group. Four patients with marrow cells in their blood samples developed diffuse encephalopathy, agitation, and confusion that lasted for approximately 24 h (Kim et al. 2002).

> While fat emboli are frequently seen, the incidence of FES is much lower.

Kim published results on 100 patients undergoing simultaneous bilateral cemented or cementless TKA, or unilateral cemented or cementless TKA. He obtained blood samples from the right atrium and radial artery at various points in the operation where an embolic load would be produced. He observed neurological changes and marrow cells in blood samples of 2 patients in the unilateral TKA group and 4 patients in the bilateral TKA group (Kim 2001). Apart from this study, there is a paucity of good data in the arthroplasty literature on the incidence of FES. Bulger et al. retrospectively reviewed patients with long bone fractures from their institutional database over a 10-year period and reported an incidence of 0.9% using the Gurd criteria (Bulger et al. 1997). Stein et al. reviewed the National Hospital Discharge Survey over a 26-year period. This included over one billion patients, and among all fracture patients the incidence of FES was only 0.17% (Stein et al. 2008).

50.4 Prevention

> There are means of preventing FE and FES during arthroplasty.

Because marrow contents are more aggressively manipulated during THA, the majority of the published literature focuses on risk reduction in THA. However, there are a number of studies looking at ways to prevent FES in TKA.

> It has been shown that the peak of embolic activity occurs in the first minute after tourniquet release (Kato et al. 2002; Parmet et al. 1994). This is when patients are at highest risk for encountering a large embolic load in the pulmonary system.

Several studies have been performed to determine ways to mitigate the risk during this critical period. One method that has been studied involves attempting to reduce intramedullary pressures and the resultant embolic load has been published. Amro et al. performed TKA on cadavers. Half of the specimens had the intramedullary femoral guide rod placed with no suction, and half with suction of the canal prior to placement of the guide rod. They recorded a significant decrease in intramedullary pressure with the use of canal suction. They then randomized 24 patients undergoing TKA into a suction or non-suction group. They identified the presence of embolic showers using TEE. They reported a decrease in embolic load in the suction group, and further, 2 of the patients in the non-suction group exhibited transient postoperative confusion (Amro et al. 2001). Zhao et al. built on this and randomized 30 patients to undergo cemented TKA in a conventional manner or with the use of canal irrigation prior to instrumentation. They recorded embolic activity in the heart with TEE and saw a significant decrease in embolic load in the irrigation group (Zhao et al. 2015). Van Gorp et al. looked at the use of a Reamer-Irrigator-Aspirator prior to insertion of the femoral intramedullary alignment rod during TKA. They simulated TKAs on 14 cadaveric femurs and measured intramedullary canal pressures. They reported a decrease in intramedullary pressure of 86% proximally and 87% distally after using the RIA system (Van Gorp et al. 2009).

Multiple studies have been performed looking at the impact of computer-assisted navigation on embolic load.

> The theory is that navigated knees do not require penetration of the femoral canal and this should lessen the embolic load.

The literature on this is somewhat mixed. Kim et al. analyzed blood samples from the right atrium and radial artery in 26 navigated TKAs and 210 standard TKAs and found no difference in the presence of fat globules and marrow contents between the two groups (Kim et al. 2008). O'Connor et al. used TEE to monitor the right atrium of patients in navigated and standard TKA after tourniquet release. They used a standardized grading system to grade the embolic load and found no difference between the two groups (O'Connor et al. 2010).

Church et al. performed a very similar study with longer TEE recording times and a slightly different grading system from O'Connor, and they found a significant decrease in embolic load in the navigated TKA group (Church et al. 2007). Kalairajah et al. demonstrated a significant difference in the presence and number of cerebral microemboli between standard and navigated TKA patients (Kalairajah et al. 2006). Interestingly, they did report small, cerebral microemboli in half of the navigated group. They state that this occurred at the time of insertion of the trial prosthesis, which suggests that even with the use of navigation the production of embolic material is not reduced to zero. Malhotra et al. randomized patients into two groups, a conventionally instrumented group and a computer-assisted group. They invasively monitored with the use of TEE and pulmonary artery catheter. There was a statistically significant decrease in the embolic load in the computer-assisted group. In addition, they identified fat emboli in the blood of 5/28 patients in the conventional group, and 1/29 in the computer-assisted group. They concluded that while there was statistically significant difference in embolic load, there was no clinical difference between the two groups (Malhotra et al. 2015).

50.5 Treatment

> Treatment of FES is primarily supportive.

Current recommendations are based on case reports and physiological principles. Patients with suspected FES should be put on 100% supplemental oxygen. If there is cardiovascular collapse, it should be considered right-sided heart failure and treated as such (Byrick 1997; Pietak et al. 1997). It is also recommended to aggressively resuscitate with intravenous fluids (Pietak et al. 1997; Patterson et al. 1991). There have been more recent studies attempting to elucidate the role of the renin-angiotensin pathway, and if alterations to this pathway can prevent or treat FES. Macrophages in the lung take up fat molecules, release renin, and this leads to increased levels of the pro-fibrotic, pro-inflammatory angiotensin. Fletcher et al. treated rats with the renin inhibitor aliskiren and then induced FES. They found that rats treated with aliskiren showed decreased fat content in vessels compared with control rats (Fletcher et al. 2017). Other groups have studied the role of prophylactic corticosteroids to reduce the incidence and severity of FES. A meta-analysis performed in 2009 suggested that prophylactic steroids could reduce the risk of FES by 78% (Bederman et al. 2009). A systematic review from 2012 showed a similar benefit with the use of steroids. They reported that 9/223 patients receiving a steroid developed FES compared with 60/260 in the control group. This difference was shown to be statistically significant. Unfortunately, there was marked heterogeneity in prophylaxis protocols among the different studies and no firm recommendations could be made (Sen et al. 2012). However, recent data has demonstrated a beneficial role of perioperative corticosteroid administration on postoperative pain and nausea (Xing et al. 2017; Kardash et al. 2008; Samona et al. 2017), and on reduction of postoperative circulation of acute phase reactants (Samona et al. 2017; Brekke et al. 2019; Smith et al. 2006).

> While the meta-analysis and systematic reviews could not give strong recommendations on routine use of steroid prophylaxis for FES, perioperative steroid use is becoming more common in primary knee arthroplasty and could have an added, protective effect against FES.

Conclusion

FES is rare in TKA. The clinical manifestations usually involve some combination of respiratory compromise, neurological manifestations, and a petechial rash. FES can occur as the result of instrumenting the femur, but it can also occur as the result of impacting cemented components. The first minute after tourniquet release is when the highest embolic load has been observed. Treatment is supportive and symptoms will usually resolve with time. Preventative measures include irrigating or suctioning the femoral canal prior to instrumentation, use of computer navigation to avoid entering the canal, and there may be a protective effect with the use of corticosteroids. While FES can occur in patients with normal hearts, extra care should be taken in patients with patent foramen ovale or other right-to-left shunts.

Take-Home Messages

- Fat embolism syndrome in TKA is a rare occurrence.
- The pathophysiology is still not fully understood, but systemic manifestations can occur in the absence of a patent foramen ovale.
- This is a diagnosis of exclusion, but there is a classic triad of respiratory compromise, neurological changes, and a petechial rash.
- Treatment is supportive and should be approached as if the patient is suffering from right-sided heart failure.
- Preventive measures include suctioning the femoral canal prior to instrumentation, use of navigation or robotics in high-risk patients, and there may be a role for corticosteroid prophylaxis.

References

Amro RR, Nazarian DG, Norris RB et al (2001) Suction instrumentation decreases intramedullary pressure, pulmonary embolism during total knee arthroplasty. Univ Penn Orthop J 14:55–59

Bederman SS, Bhandari M, McKee MD, Schemitsch EH (2009) Do corticosteroids reduce the risk of fat embolism syndrome in patients with long-bone fractures? A meta-analysis. Can J Surg 52:386–393

Berman AT, Parmet JL, Harding SP et al (1998) Emboli observed with use of transesophageal echocardiography immediately after tourniquet release during total knee arthroplasty with cement. J Bone Joint Surg Am 80:389–396

Botha AJ, Moore FA, Moore EE et al (1995) Post-injury neutrophil priming and activation: an early vulnerable window. Surgery 118:358–365

Brekke AC, Amaro EJ, Posey SL et al (2019) Do corticosteroids attenuate the peri-operative acute phase response after total knee arthroplasty? J Arthroplast 34:27–35

Bulger EM, Smith DG, Maier RV, Jurkovich GJ (1997) Fat embolism syndrome: a 10-year review. Arch Surg 132:435–439

Byrick RJ (1997) Cement implantation syndrome: a time limited embolic phenomenon. Can J Anaesth 44:107–111

Byrick RJ, Korley RE, McKee MD et al (2001) Prolonged coma after unreamed, locked nailing of femoral shaft fracture. Anesthesiology 94:163–165

Christie J, Robinson CM, Pell AC, McBirnie J, Burnett R (1995) Transcardiac echocardiography during invasive intramedullary procedures. J Bone Joint Surg Br 77:450–455

Church JS, Scadden JE, Gupta RR et al (2007) Emboli phenomena during computer-assisted and conventional total knee replacement. J Bone Joint Surg Br 89:481–485

Colotta F, Re F, Polentarutti N et al (1992) Modulation of granulocyte survival and programmed cell death by cytokines and bacterial products. Blood 80:2012–2020

Cox G, Tzioupis C, Calori GM, Green J et al (2011) Cerebral fat emboli: a trigger of post-operative delirium. Injury S4:S6–S10

Dive AM, Dubois PE, Ide C et al (2002) Paradoxical cerebral fat embolism: an unusual cause of persistent unconsciousness after orthopedic surgery. Anesthesiology 96:1029–1031

Donaldson AJ, Thomson HE, Harper NJ, Kenny NW (2009) Bone cement implantation syndrome. Br J Anaest 102:12–22

Eriksson EA, Pellegrini DC, Vanderkolk WE, Minshall CT et al (2011) Incidence of pulmonary fat embolism at autopsy: an undiagnosed epidemic. J Trauma 71:312–315

Fenire M (2014) Fat embolism syndrome. SWRCCC 2(5):21–23

Fletcher AN, Molteni A, Ponnapureddy R et al (2017) The renin inhibitor aliskiren protects rat lungs from the histopathologic effects of fat embolism. J Trauma Acute Care Surg 82:338–344

Gauss H (1924) The pathology of fat embolism. Arch Surg 9:593–605

Gurd AR (1970) Fat embolism: an aid to diagnosis. J Bone Joint Surg Br 52:732–737

Kalairajah Y, Cossey AJ, Verrall GM et al (2006) Are systemic emboli reduced in computer-assisted knee surgery? A prospective, randomized clinical trial. J Bone Joint Surg Br 88:198–202

Kardash KJ, Sarrazin F, Tessler MJ, Velly AM (2008) Single-dose dexamethasone reduces dynamic pain after total hip arthroplasty. Anesth Analg 106:1253–1257

Kato N, Nakanishi K, Yoshino S, Ogawa R (2002) Abnormal echogenic findings detected by transesophageal echocardiography and cardiorespiratory impairment during total knee arthroplasty with tourniquet. Anesthesiology 97:1123–1128

Kim YH (2001) Incidence of fat embolism syndrome after cemented or cementless bilateral simultaneous and unilateral total knee arthroplasty. J Arthroplast 16:730–739

Kim YH, Oh SW, Kim JS (2002) Prevalence of fat embolism following bilateral simultaneous and unilateral hip arthroplasty performed with or without cement: a prospective, randomized clinical study. J Bone Joint Surg Am 84:1372–1379

Kim YH, Kim JS, Hong KS et al (2008) Prevalence of fat embolism after total knee arthroplasty performed with or without computer navigation. J Bone Joint Surg Am 90:123–128

Kuo KH, Pan YJ, Lai YJ, Cheung WK, Chang FC, Jarosz J (2014) Dynamic MR imaging patterns of cerebral fat embolism: a systematic review with illustrative cases. AJNR Am J Neuroradiol 35:1052–1057

Lehman EP, Moore RM (1927) Fat embolism: including experimental production without trauma. Arch Surg 14:621–662

Lu K, Xu M, Li W et al (2017) A study on dynamic monitoring, components, and risk factors of embolism during total knee arthroplasty. Medicine 96(51):e9303. https://journals.lww.com/md-journal/pages/default.aspx

Malhotra R, Singla A, Lekha C, Kumar V et al (2015) A prospective randomized study to compare systemic emboli using computer-assisted and conventional techniques of total knee arthoplasty. J Bone Joint Surg Am 97:889–894

Markel DC, Femino JE, Farkas P, Markel SF (1999) Analysis of lower extremity embolic material after total knee arthroplasty in a canine model. J Arthroplast 14:227–232

Moore FA, Moore EE (1995) Evolving concepts in the pathogenesis of postinjury multiple organ failure. Surg Clin North Am 75:257–277

Newbigin K, Souza CA, Torres C et al (2016a) Fat embolism syndrome: state-of-the-art review focused on pulmonary imaging findings. Respir Med 113:93–100

Newbigin K, Souza CA, Armstrong M et al (2016b) Fat embolism syndrome: do the CT findings correlate with clinical course and severity of symptoms? A clinical radiological study. Eur J Radiol 85:422–427

O'Connor MI, Broderson MP, Feinglass NG et al (2010) Fat emboli in total knee arthroplasty: a prospective randomized study of computer-assisted navigation versus standard surgical technique. J Arthroplast 25:1034–1040

Palmovic V, McCarroll JR (1965) Fat embolism in trauma. Arch Pathol 80:630–635

Parmet JL, Horrow JC, Singer R, Berman AT, Rosenberg H (1994) Echogenic emboli upon tourniquet release during total knee arthroplasty: pulmonary hemodynamic changes and embolic composition. Anesth Analg 79:940–945

Parvizi J, Holiday AD, Ereth MH, Lewallen DG (1999) Sudden death during primary hip arthroplasty. Clin Orthop Relat Res 369:39–48

Patterson B, Healey J, Cornell C, Sharrock N (1991) Cardiac arrest during hip arthroplasty with a cemented long-stem component. A report of seven cases. J Bone Joint Surg 73:271–277

Peltier LF (1988) Fat embolism. A perspective. Clin Orthop Relat Res 232:263–270

Pietak S, Holmes J, Matthews R, Petrasek A, Porter B (1997) Cardiovascular collapse after femoral prosthesis surgery for acute hip fracture. Can J Anesth 44:198–201

Prakash S, Sen RK, Tripathy SK, Sen IM, Sharma RR, Sharma S (2013) Role of interleukin- 6 as an early marker of fat embolism syndrome: a clinical study. Clin Orthop Relat Res 471:2340–2346

Rodriguez RA, Tellier A, Grabowski J et al (2005) Cognitive dysfunction after total knee arthroplasty: effects of intraoperative

cerebral embolization and postoperative complications. J Arthroplast 20:763–771
Rose S, Marzi I (1998) Mediators in polytrauma-pathophysiological significance and clinical relevance. Langenbeck's Arch Surg 383:199–208
Samona J, Cook C, Krupa K, Swatsell K, Jackson A, Dukes C et al (2017) Effect of intraoperative dexamethasone on pain scores and narcotic consumption in patients undergoing total knee arthroplasty. Orthop Surg 9:110–114
Sen RK, Tripathy SK, Krishnan V (2012) Role of corticosteroid as a prophylactic measure in fat embolism syndrome: a literature review. Musculoskelet Surg 96:1–8
Smith C, Erasmus P, Myburgh K (2006) Endocrine and immune effects of dexamethasone in unilateral total knee replacement. J Int Med Res 34:603–611
Stein PD, Yaekoub AY, Matta F, Kleerekoper M (2008) Fat embolism syndrome. Am J Med Sci 336:472–477
Sulek CA, Davies LK, Enneking K, Gearen PA, Lobato EB (1999) Cerebral microembolism diagnosed by transcranial Doppler during total knee arthroplasty: correlation with transesophageal echocardiography. Anesthesiology 91:672–676
Tachakra SS (1976) Distribution of skin petechiae in fat embolism rash. Lancet 7954:284–285
Tzioupis CC, Giannoudis PV (2011) Fat embolism syndrome: what have we learned over the years? Trauma 13:259–281
Van Gorp CC, Falk JV, Kmiec SJ, Siston RA (2009) The reamer/irrigator/aspirator reduces femoral canal pressure in simulated TKA. Clin Orthop Relat Res 467:805–809
Winn R, Maunder R, Harlan J (1987) Lung lymph flow after bone marrow injection into goats was reduced by indomethacin. J Appl Physiol 62:762–767
Xing LZ, Li L, Zhang LJ (2017) Can intravenous steroid administration reduce postoperative pain scores following total knee arthroplasty? Medicine 96:e7134
Yeon HB, Ramappa A, Landzberg MJ, Thornhill TS (2003) Paradoxic cerebral embolism after cemented knee arthroplasty: a report of 2 cases and prophylactic option for subsequent arthroplasty. J Arthroplast 18:113–120
Zhao J, Zhang J, Ji Z et al (2015) Does intramedullary canal irrigation reduce fat emboli? A randomized clinical trial with transesophageal echocardiography. J Arthroplast 30:450–455

Current State of the Art for Prophylactic Treatment of Thromboembolic Events After TKA

Jean-Yves Jenny

Contents

E. Hansen, K.-D. Kühn (eds.), *Essentials of Cemented Knee Arthroplasty*,
https://doi.org/10.1007/978-3-662-63113-3_51

51

51.1 Introduction

Potent anticoagulants are generally considered mandatory for venous thromboembolism (VTE) prevention after most surgical procedures, and especially after total knee arthroplasty (TKA). In most countries, potent anticoagulant agents such as low-molecular-weight heparin (LMWH) and direct oral anticoagulant agents (DOA) are recommended. However, iatrogenic complications may occur and overcome the benefit of prevention. Furthermore, the acceleration of postoperative rehabilitation ("fast-track surgery") might decrease the risk of VTE. Some surgeons currently suggest to use alternate treatments instead of potent anticoagulants for VTE prevention after TKA. The goal of this chapter is to analyze the existing literature about the prevention of VTE events after TKA and to provide a rationale for clinical practice.

51.2 Current Recommendation

According to the recommendations of the Société Française d'Anesthésie-Réanimation (SFAR) and their 2011 update, anti-thrombotic prophylaxis after TKA should be based on the administration of LMWH or DAO (Samama et al. 2006, 2011). The American College of Chest Physicians (ACCP) suggested the same agents in their previous recommendation [X]. However, this society recently updated these recommendations (Falck-Ytter et al. 2012), and currently recommends that either LMWHs, unfractionated heparin, DAOs, aspirin, or conventional oral anticoagulants be used with the same strength of recommendation; the use of intermittent pneumatic compression is routinely recommended as well. The American College of Orthopaedic Surgeons (AAOS) does not comment on the choice between these options (Mont et al. 2011; Jacobs et al. 2012). Recent recommendations published by the European Society for Anaesthesiology (ESA) state that aspirin is probably slightly less effective than standard LMWH or DOA therapy, but is associated with fewer minor or even major bleeding complications (Jenny et al. 2018; Venclauskas et al. 2018). These ESA recommendations recommend the use of intermittent pneumatic compression when aspirin is used as a thromboprophylaxis agent (Venclauskas et al. 2018).

51.3 Why Aspirin?

Nowadays, aspirin is widely used to prevent arterial thrombotic events, mainly stroke or myocardial infarction (Vandvik et al. 2012). It is inexpensive, does not require monitoring, and does not accumulate in patients with renal insufficiency (Eikelboom et al. 2012). Until the publication of the 9th American College of Chest Physicians Guidelines (ACCP 2012; Falck-Ytter et al. 2012), most international guidelines recommended against its use for VTE prophylaxis after TKA (Samama et al. 2006; Geerts et al. 2008).

> However, aspirin may be efficient against VTE as well. Two recent comprehensive reviews have recently summarized the different mechanisms of action of aspirin in order to try to explain why it may be useful for VTE prophylaxis (Becattini and Agnelli 2014; Undas et al. 2014).

The classical principal activity of aspirin is represented by the permanent inactivation of the cyclo-oxygenase activity of prostaglandin H synthase 1 (COX-1). Furthermore, aspirin may interfere with thrombin formation, may act on the expression of tissue factor on monocytes/macrophages, may also reduce thrombin generation by acetylating prothrombin and/or platelet membrane components.

Low-dose aspirin may also modify the size of fibrin fibers while leading to the formation of thicker fibers and larger network pores, increasing clot permeability, as also observed with direct oral anticoagulants. Aspirin might impair the acetylation of fibrinogen and induce enhanced clot lysis, although this has not been confirmed in all clinical settings, for example, diabetes. Aspirin also inhibits factor XIII activation, which may lead to a decrease in the stability of fibrin clots.

51.4 Effectiveness of Aspirin After TKA

The 9th American College of Chest Physicians' (ACCP) guidelines of 2012 recommend the use of aspirin in patients undergoing TKA for a minimum of 10–14 days (Grade 1B) (Falck-Ytter et al. 2012). These recommendations are mainly based on the Pulmonary Embolism Prevention (PEP) trial (Pulmonary Embolism Prevention, PEP. Trial Collaborative Group 2000). There was a 28% relative risk decrease in symptomatic DVT. There was no decrease in fatal pulmonary embolism. There was no difference in bleeding. But patients in this trial were operated for total hip arthroplasty (THA) and hip fracture surgery (HFS).

Since 2012, one systematic review was published in 2015, including 3 meta-analyses and 3 prospective randomized controlled trials (RCT) with 46,254 patients operated mainly for THA, TKA, and HFS (Sahebally et al. 2015). All studies included were published prior to 2012, and the PEP trial was also included. Although some results were conflicting, aspirin was considered to be more effective than placebo in primary VTE prevention. No recent data are available for TKA.

Very recently, Wilson et al. (2016) performed another systematic review of 13 studies, some of them published from 2012 to 2015. They reported that there was insufficient evidence from trials with moderate to severe risk of bias being present to suggest that aspirin was more or less effective than LMWH, warfarin, or dabigatran for the prevention of VTE in TKA or THA. Compared with aspirin, rates of asymptomatic DVT in TKA may be reduced with rivaroxaban, but insufficient evidence existed to demonstrate an effect on the incidence of symptomatic DVT. Compared with aspirin, there was evidence of more wound complications following THA and TKA with dabigatran and in TKA with rivaroxaban. Some studies highlighted concerns over bleeding complications and efficacy of aspirin (Ogonda et al. 2016).

As a conclusion, they suggested that aspirin may be considered a suitable alternative to other thromboprophylactic agents following THA and TKA.

51.5 Cost-Effectiveness Ratio of Aspirin After TKA

In the ACCP 2012 guidelines, LMWH was recommended over aspirin in patients undergoing TKA (Grade 2C) (Falck-Ytter et al. 2012). These recommendations are based on two trials of low quality (one published article and one abstract only) including 469 patients (Westrich et al. 2006). The pooled results showed an increased risk of symptomatic DVT (RR 1.87; 95% CI 1.3–2.7) in the aspirin group. Pulmonary embolism could not be evaluated. There was no reported death or major bleeding.

Since 2012, 3 systematic reviews were published. Drescher et al. (2014) included 8 prospective RCTs and 1408 patients. All studies included were published prior to 2012. There was no difference in the occurrence of DVT between aspirin and anticoagulants. There was a non-significant trend favoring anticoagulation following hip fracture repair. The risk of bleeding was lower with aspirin than anticoagulants following hip fracture repair, with a non-significant trend favoring aspirin after arthroplasty. Rates of pulmonary embolism were too low to provide reliable estimates. Compared with anticoagulation, aspirin may be associated with a higher risk of DVT following hip fracture repair, although bleeding rates were substantially lower. Aspirin was similarly effective after lower extremity arthroplasty and may be associated with a lower bleeding risk.

Sahebally et al. (2015) included one meta-analysis, 5 prospective RCTs, and one prospective study with 9599 patients (2 recent studies). Although results were conflicting, aspirin was considered to be as effective as LMWH in primary VTE prevention and may reduce bleeding.

Lieberman et al. (2017) collected 21 studies including 34,764 patients. Prophylactic treatments used were LMWH (13,590 patients), oral factor Xa inhibitors (6609 patients), oral direct thrombin inhibitors (5965 patients), indirect factors Xa/IIa inhibitors (3444 patients), aspirin (2427 patients), warfarin (489 patients), mobile compression device (199 patients), and placebo (2041 patients). Across all included studies, the estimated rate of pulmonary embolism was 0.21%, and was consistent throughout the 17 years spanning these RCTs. The authors suggested that no prophylactic treatment was able to decrease the risk of pulmonary embolism significantly.

The Intermountain Joint Replacement Center Writing Committee (2012) included 696 cases of elective THA or TKA and compared aspirin with warfarin or LMWH. DVT was diagnosed by a questionnaire and confirmed by imaging if necessary. There was an increased rate of DVT in the aspirin group (8 vs. 1%, $P = 0.001$). There were no differences in major or minor bleeding, or deaths.

Anderson et al. (2013) included 778 cases of elective THA and compared aspirin with LMWH. The method of diagnosis of DVT was not clearly described. Aspirin was neither inferior nor superior. There were less clinically relevant bleeding events in the aspirin group. Jiang et al. (Parvizi et al. 2017) included 120 cases of elective TKA and compared aspirin combined with mechanical measures postoperatively (60 cases) with LMWH and rivaroxaban sequentially in combination with mechanical measures postoperatively (60 cases). DVT was detected in 10 (17%) and 11 (18%) cases, respectively ($P = 0.500$). There were no symptomatic VTEs or deaths during the follow-up period.

51.6 Side-Effects of Aspirin After TKA

The PEP trial (Pulmonary Embolism Prevention, PEP. Trial Collaborative Group 2000) showed no difference in bleeding between aspirin and placebo. Since 2012, 2 systematic studies were published. Drescher et al. (2014) included 8 prospective RCTs and 1408 patients. All studies included were published prior to 2012. The risk of bleeding was lower with aspirin than anticoagulants following hip fracture repair, with a non-significant trend favoring aspirin after arthroplasty. Compared with anticoagulation, aspirin may be associated with a substantially lower bleeding risk following hip fracture repair. Similarly, aspirin may be associated with a lower bleeding risk after lower extremity arthroplasty. Sahebally et al. (2015) included one meta-analysis, 5 prospective RCTs, and one prospective study with 9599 patients (2 recent studies). Although some results were conflicting, aspirin may reduce bleeding.

The Intermountain Joint Replacement Center Writing Committee (2012) included 696 cases of elective THA or TKA and compared aspirin with warfarin or LMWH. There were no differences in major or minor bleeding, or deaths. Anderson et al. (2013) included 778 cases of elective THA and compared aspirin with LMWH. There were less clinically relevant bleeding events in the aspirin group. Jiang et al. (2014) included 120 cases of elective TKA and compared aspirin combined with mechanical measures postoperatively (60 cases) with LMWH and rivaroxaban sequentially in combination with mechanical measures postoperatively (60 cases). Patients treated with aspirin had a significant lower blood loss index. No transfusion cases were observed in either group.

51.7 Indication of Aspirin After TKA

Since 2012 and the ACCP guidelines (Falck-Ytter et al. 2012), aspirin is recommended for prevention of DVT and pulmonary embolism after TKA without patient selection (Grade 1B). However, there may be a concern about an increased risk of DVT reported in some studies.

> Although currently there are no data available about this point, it may be advantageous to exclude patients with an elevated risk of DVT from aspirin prophylaxis.

In patients with an increased risk of bleeding, no prophylaxis or the use of intermittent pneumatic compression (IPC) devices is recommended by ACCP rather than pharmacological prophylaxis (Grade 2C). No more recent data are currently available.

Although no prospective comparative RCT is currently available, prospective cohort studies suggest that the use of a rapid recovery program after THA and TKA may be associated with a low risk of DVT, irrespective of the type of DVT prophylaxis used.

Husted et al. (2010) analyzed 1977 consecutive, unselected patients who were operated for primary THA, TKA, or bilateral simultaneous TKA in a standardized fast-track set-up from 2004 to 2008. Patients received DVT prophylaxis with LMWH starting 6–8 h after surgery until discharge. All re-admissions and deaths within 30 and 90 days were analyzed using the national health register, especially concentrating on clinical DVT (confirmed by ultrasound and elevated D-dimer), pulmonary embolism, or sudden death. 3 deaths (0.15%) were associated with clotting episodes and, overall, 11 clinical DVTs (0.56%) and 6 pulmonary embolisms (0.30%) were found. During the final 2 years of the study (854 patients), when patients were mobilized within 4 h postoperatively and the duration of DVT prophylaxis was shorter (1–4 days), the mortality was 0% and the incidences of DVT were 0.60% after TKA, 0.51% after THA, and 0% after bilateral simultaneous TKA. Pulmonary embolism occurred in 0.30% of patients after TKA, 0% after THA, and 0% after bilateral simultaneous TKA.

> These data suggest that the risks of clinical DVT and of fatal and non-fatal pulmonary embolism after THA and TKA following a fast-track set-up with early mobilization, short hospitalization, and short duration of DVT prophylaxis are low.

Jørgensen et al. (2013) followed prospectively 4924 consecutive unselected unilateral primary THAs and TKAs. DVT prophylaxis included LMWH or factor Xa inhibitors only during hospitalization when length of stay was 5 days or less. Symptomatic thromboembolic events were observed in 0.84% of the patients and VTEs were observed in 0.41% during a 90-day follow-up: 5 pulmonary embolisms (0.11%) and 14 DVTs (0.30%). There were 4 (0.09%) surgery-related deaths, one of which (0.02%) was due to pulmonary embolism, and 6 (0.13%) deaths of unknown cause after discharge.

> Data suggest that the incidence of thromboembolic events is low in fast-track THA and TKA patients with length of stay 5 days or less.

Many physicians consider that the low risk of symptomatic DVT after THA and TKA followed by a fast-track program and the lower risk of bleeding might compensate for the possible higher rate of DVT after aspirin prophylaxis than with other pharmacological agents. The panel suggests that aspirin prophylaxis could be routinely associated with a rapid recovery program after THA and TKA.

The use of IPC devices is recommended by the ACCP in patients undergoing major orthopedic surgery in association with an antithrombotic agent (Grade 2C) (Falck-Ytter et al. 2012). This recommendation was based on the analysis of 5 trials including more than 2400 patients, which reported a 70% reduction in the DVT rate when IPC devices were used.

Westrich et al. (2006) performed a prospective randomized study of 275 patients undergoing unilateral TKA under spinal-epidural anesthesia (SEA), comparing IPC associated with either enoxaparin or aspirin. All patients had an in-hospital ultrasound screening test on postoperative days 3–5 and a second follow-up ultrasound 4–6 weeks after surgery. The overall DVT rates in the enoxaparin group and the aspirin group were 14.1 and 17.8% (P = not significant), respectively. When used in combination with pneumatic compression devices and SEA, enoxaparin was not superior to aspirin in preventing DVT after TKA.

51.8 Dose and Duration of Aspirin After TKA

Many different regimens have been described in the literature (Wilson et al. 2016). There is a considerable range for dose (from 75 to 1000 mg/day) and duration of treatment (from 2 days to 6 weeks). Selection criteria are not routinely provided. There is a definite trend to decrease dose (Jørgensen et al. 2013) and duration of treatment (Parvizi et al. 2017). However, the current literature does not allow a definitive recommendation concerning dose and duration of treatment and patient selection.

Eventually, is aspirin appropriate for venous thromboembolism prophylaxis after TKA?

Several authors are still reluctant to recommend the use of aspirin for VTE prophylaxis (Cohen et al. 2015). Aspirin is less potent than LMWH and the new direct anticoagulants, but the induced bleeding risk is also lower. In addition, pending the steadily decreasing VTE risk in surgical patients, the benefit:risk ratio and the duration of treatments are changing. More attention has to be given to the bleeding risk (Sharrock et al. 2008). Aspirin may be proposed in moderate-risk orthopedic patients or in highly selected high-risk patients scheduled for THA or TKA combined with an enhanced recovery procedure, or in hip fracture patients with a high bleeding risk. IPC should always be used when aspirin is prescribed as the only pharmacological agent. However, current literature does not provide a rationale for precise recommendation about management (dose, duration, follow-up parameters), interactions with other diseases and medicines, or patient and surgery selection. Data are lacking for non-orthopedic surgery patients and for intensive care patients.

51.9 Conclusion

Fast-track rehabilitation after TKA reduces the length of hospital stay (Guerra et al. 2015) and is also likely to be associated with a reduced risk of thromboembolic events. Therefore, aspirin can be used alone as an alternative to reference agents.

Take-Home Messages

- The final choice of thromboprophylactic treatment must be tailored for each patient, which also depends on several risk factors.
- Risk factors for thromboembolic events related to the patient and his surgery include (non-exhaustive list):
  - The patient's age and sex, the patient's age at surgery, morbid obesity, a personal or family history of thromboembolic events, the presence of cancer, surgery lasting more than 120 min, delayed getting up and walking, etc.
  - The presence of one or more of these risk factors would lead to a preference for treatment with LMWH or DOA.
- Possible bleeding risk factors related to the patient.
  - The presence of one or more risk factor(s) for bleeding would suggest a preference for aspirin therapy.
- A precise therapeutic regimen (dose, duration, etc.) cannot be proposed because of the wide variety of practices found in the literature.

References

Anderson DR, Dunbar MJ, Bohm ER et al (2013) Aspirin versus low-molecular-weight heparin for extended venous thromboembolism prophylaxis after total hip arthroplasty: a randomized trial. Ann Int Med 158:800–806

Becattini C, Agnelli G (2014) Aspirin for prevention and treatment of venous thromboembolism. Blood Rev 28:103–108

Cohen AT, Imfeld S, Markham J, Granziera S (2015) The use of aspirin for primary and secondary prevention in venous thromboembolism and other cardiovascular disorders. Thromb Res 135:217–225

Drescher FS, Sirovich BE, Lee A et al (2014) Aspirin versus anticoagulation for prevention of venous thromboembolism major lower extremity orthopedic surgery: a systematic review and meta-analysis. J Hosp Med 9:579–585

Eikelboom JW, Hirsh J, Spencer FA et al (2012) Antiplatelet drugs: antithrombotic therapy and prevention of thrombosis, 9th edn: American College of Chest Physicians evidence-based clinical practice guidelines. Chest 141(suppl 2):e89S–e119S

Falck-Ytter Y, Francis CW, Johanson NA, Curley C, Dahl OE, Schulman S, Ortel TL, Pauker SG, Colwell CW Jr (2012) Prevention of VTE in orthopedic surgery patients: antithrombotic therapy and prevention of thrombosis, 9th ed: American College of Chest Physicians evidence-based clinical practice guidelines. Chest 141(2 Suppl):e278S–e325S. https://doi.org/10.1378/chest.11-2404

Geerts WH, Bergqvist D, Pineo GF et al (2008) Prevention of venous thromboembolism: American College of Chest Physicians evidence-based clinical practice guidelines (8th edition). Chest 133(suppl 6):381S–453S

51

Guerra ML, Singh PJ, Taylor NF (2015) Early mobilization of patients who have had a hip or knee joint replacement reduces length of stay in hospital: a systematic review. Clin Rehabil 29:844–854

Guyatt GH, Akl EA, Crowther M, Gutterman DD, Schünemann HJ; for the American College of Chest Physicians Antithrombotic Therapy and Prevention of Thrombosis Panel (2012) Antithrombotic therapy and prevention of thrombosis, 9th ed: American College of Chest Physicians. Evidence-based clinical practice guidelines. Chest 141(Suppl):7S–47S

Husted H, Otte KS, Kristensen BB et al (2010) Low risk of thromboembolic complications after fast-track hip and knee arthroplasty. Acta Orthop 81:599–605

Intermountain Joint Replacement Center Writing Committee (2012) A prospective comparison of warfarin to aspirin for thromboprophylaxis in total hip and total knee arthroplasty. J Arthroplast 27:1–9

Jacobs JJ, Mont MA, Bozic KJ, Della Valle CJ, Goodman SB, Lewis CG, Yates AC Jr, Boggio LN, Watters WC 3rd, Turkelson CM, Wies JL, Sluka P, Hitchcock K (2012) American Academy of Orthopaedic Surgeons clinical practice guideline on: preventing venous thromboembolic disease in patients undergoing elective hip and knee arthroplasty. J Bone Joint Surg Am 94(8):746–747. https://doi.org/10.2106/JBJS.9408.ebo746

Jenny JY, Pabinger I, Samama CM, ESA VTE Guidelines Task Force (2018) European guidelines on perioperative venous thromboembolism prophylaxis: aspirin. Eur J Anaesthesiol 35(2):123–129. https://doi.org/10.1097/EJA.0000000000000728

Jiang Y, Du H, Liu J, Zhou Y (2014) Aspirin combined with mechanical measures to prevent venous thromboembolism after total knee arthroplasty: a randomized controlled trial. Chin Med J 127:2201–2215

Jørgensen CC, Jacobsen MK, Soeballe K et al (2013) Thromboprophylaxis only during hospitalisation in fast-track hip and knee arthroplasty, a prospective cohort study. BMJ Open 3:e003965

Lieberman JR, Cheng V, Cote MP (2017) Pulmonary embolism rates following total hip arthroplasty with prophylactic anticoagulation: some pulmonary emboli cannot be avoided. J Arthroplast 32:980–986

Mont MA, Jacobs JJ, Boggio LN (2011) Preventing venous thromboembolic disease in patients undergoing elective hip and knee arthroplasty. J Am Acad Orthop Surg 19:768–776

Ogonda L, Hill J, Doran E et al (2016) Aspirin for thromboprophylaxis after primary lower limb arthroplasty: early thromboembolic events and 90 day mortality in 11,459 patients. Bone Joint J 98-B:341–348

Parvizi J, Huang R, Restrepo C et al (2017) Low-dose aspirin is effective chemoprophylaxis against clinically important venous thromboembolism following total joint arthroplasty. J Bone Joint Surg 99:91–98

Pulmonary Embolism Prevention, PEP. Trial Collaborative Group (2000) Prevention of pulmonary embolism and deep vein thrombosis with low dose aspirin: pulmonary embolism prevention (PEP) trial. Lancet 355:1295–1302

Sahebally SM, Healy D, Walsh SR (2015) Aspirin in the primary prophylaxis of venous thromboembolism in surgical patients. Surgeon 13:348–358

Samama CM, Albaladejo P, Benhamou D, Bertin-Maghit M, Bruder N, Doublet JD, Laversin S, Leclerc S, Marret E, Mismetti P, Samain E, Steib A, Committee for Good Practice Standards of the French Society for Anaesthesiology and Intensive Care (SFAR) (2006) Venous thromboembolism prevention in surgery and obstetrics: clinical practice guidelines. Eur J Anaesthesiol 23(2):95–116

Samama CM, Gafsou B, Jeandel T, Laporte S, Steib A, Marret E, Albaladejo P, Mismetti P, Rosencher N (2011) Recommandations formalisées d'experts. Prévention de la maladie thromboembolique veineuse postopératoire. Actualisation 2011. Annales Françaises d'Anesthésie et de Réanimation 30:947–951

Sharrock NE, González Della Valle A, Go G et al (2008) Potent anticoagulants are associated with a higher all-cause mortality rate after hip and knee arthroplasty. Clin Orthop Relat Res 466:714–721

Undas A, Brummel-Ziedins K, Mann KG (2014) Why does aspirin decrease the risk of venous thromboembolism? On old and novel antithrombotic effects of acetyl salicylic acid. J Thromb Haemost 12:1776–1787

Vandvik PO, Lincoff AM, Gore JM et al (2012) Primary and secondary prevention of cardiovascular disease: antithrombotic therapy and prevention of thrombosis, 9th edn: American College of Chest Physicians evidence-based clinical practice guidelines. Chest 141(suppl 2):e637S–e668S

Venclauskas L, Llau JV, Jenny JY, Kjaersgaard-Andersen P, Jans Ø, ESA VTE Guidelines Task Force (2018) European guidelines on perioperative venous thromboembolism prophylaxis: day surgery and fast-track surgery. Eur J Anaesthesiol 35(2):134–138. https://doi.org/10.1097/EJA.0000000000000706

Westrich GH, Bottner F, Windsor RE et al (2006) VenaFlow plus Lovenox vs VenaFlow plus aspirin for thromboembolic disease prophylaxis in total knee arthroplasty. J Arthroplast 21(6 Suppl 2):139–143

Wilson DGG, Poole WEC, Chauhan SK, Rogers BA (2016) Systematic review of aspirin for thromboprophylaxis in modern elective total hip and knee arthroplasty. Bone Joint J 98-B:1056–1061

Aseptic Loosening – A US Perspective

Ahmed Siddiqi and Atul F. Kamath

Contents

E. Hansen, K.-D. Kühn (eds.), *Essentials of Cemented Knee Arthroplasty*,
https://doi.org/10.1007/978-3-662-63113-3_52

52.1 Introduction

Over the past decade, the number of total knee arthroplasty (TKA) procedures has doubled in the United States (US), with the greatest increases seen among younger populations (Weinstein et al. 2013). Individuals who undergo TKA at a younger age are at increased lifetime risk for complications and revision surgery. These younger patients, coupled with heavier and more active patients undergoing primary TKA, fuel the projected demand for revision TKA, which is projected to rise by 601% between 2005 and 2030 (Schroer et al. 2013; Kurtz et al. 2007). Aseptic loosening continues to be one of the leading causes of aseptic failure after primary TKA (Schroer et al. 2013; Kulshrestha et al. 2019; Calliess et al. 2015; Dalury et al. 2013; Sharkey et al. 2002, 2013). This is relevant as revision TKA places a significant economic burden on healthcare systems (Losina et al. 2012; Bhandari et al. 2012). Therefore, judicious identification and diagnosis of aseptic loosening and its management remains of paramount importance. Although aseptic loosening after TKA is a common complication, its diagnosis may be challenging due to subtleties and requires a systematic approach (◘ Fig. 52.1). This chapter focuses on the history and physical findings to diagnose aseptic loosening, patient and surgical risk factors for perioperative management, and clinical outcomes after revision TKA for aseptic loosening.

52.2 Case Example

A 75-year-old female with a past medical history of rheumatoid arthritis, diabetes mellitus, obesity, and status post right TKA performed 6 years prior presented with gradual onset of worsening knee pain and recurrent effusions. She underwent a course of physical therapy with minimal improvement. Plain radiographs from outside facility were obtained (◘ Fig. 52.2). Serum erythrocyte sedimentation rate (ESR) and C-reactive protein (CRP) were 29 mm/h and 1.2 mg/dL, respectively. A right knee arthrocentesis was performed to rule out periprosthetic joint infection. Synovial cell count was 788 WBC/mL, 68% polymorphonuclear leukocytes with negative cultures. The etiology of the progressive

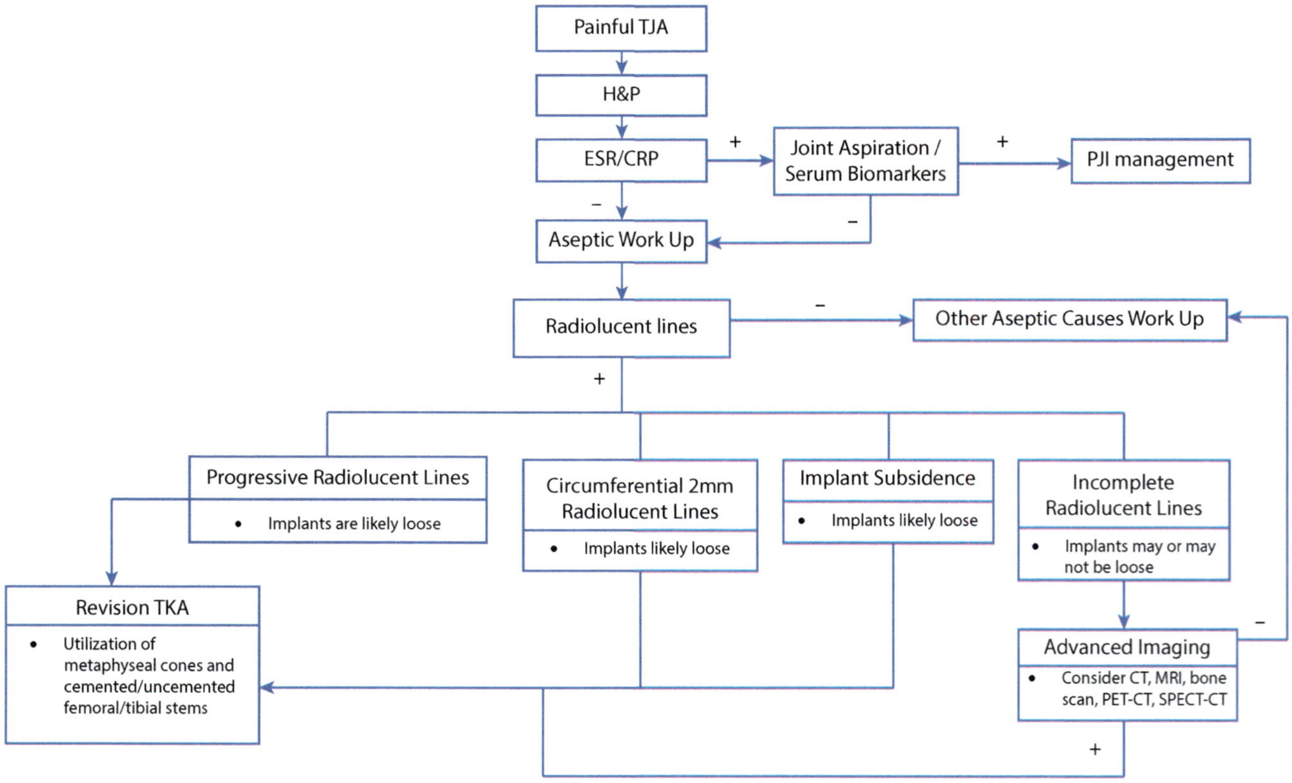

◘ **Fig. 52.1** The authors' flowchart algorithm of diagnosis and management of TKA aseptic loosening. *PJI* periprosthetic joint infection, *H&P* history and physical exam, *ESR* erythrocyte sedimentation rate, *CRP* c-reactive protein, *CT* computed tomography, *MRI* magnetic resonance imaging, *PET-CT positron emission tomography-computed tomography, SPECT-CT* single-photon emission-computerized tomography

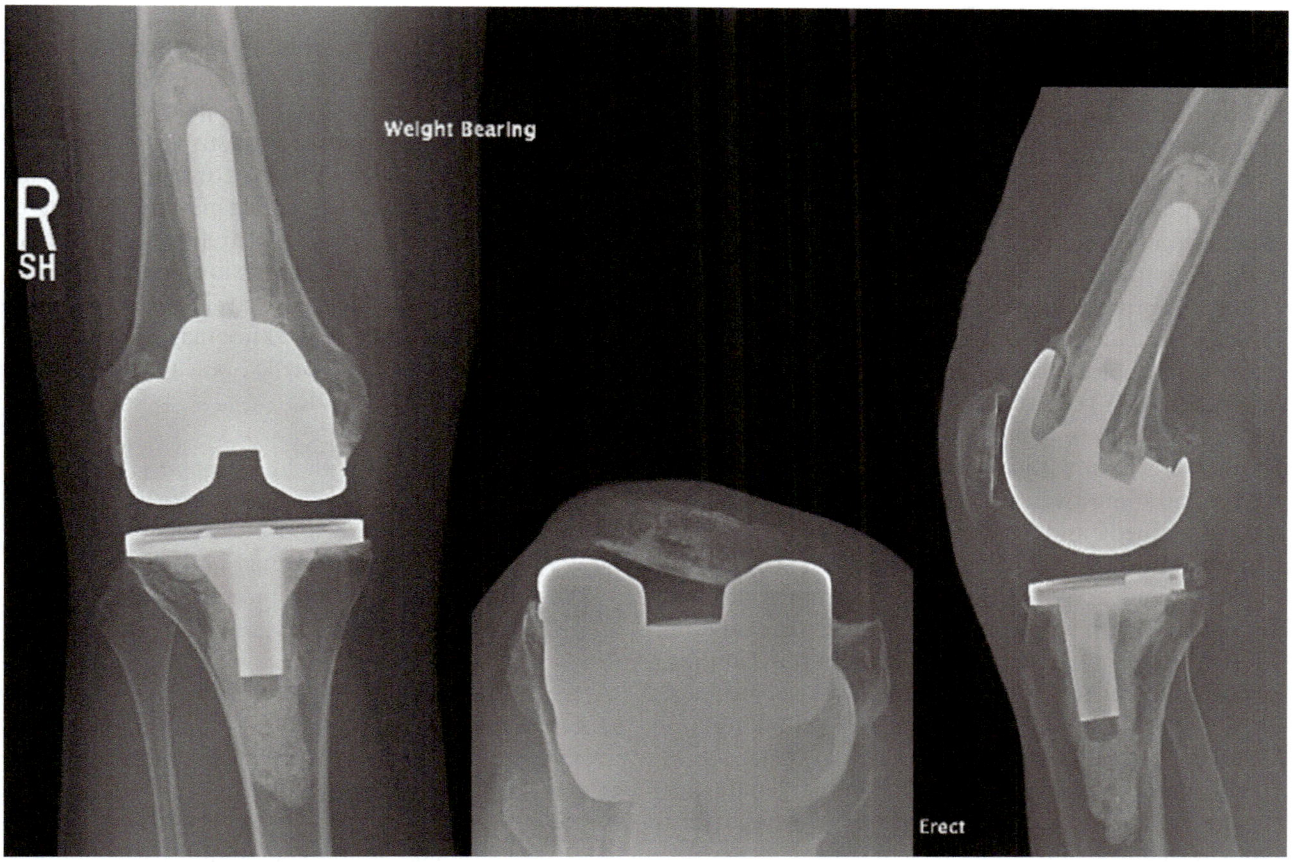

Fig. 52.2 Anteroposterior, sunrise, and lateral plain radiographs demonstrating radiolucent lines surrounding the femoral and tibial components

radiolucent lines and implant subsidence was determined to be from aseptic loosening.

52.3 Pathophysiology

Aseptic loosening is theorized to originate from excess wear particles generated in a proinflammatory state (Jiang et al. 2013; Cherian et al. 2015). The inflammatory environment stimulates a cellular response, with increased secretion of host cytokines such as tumor necrosis factor (TNF), receptor activator of nuclear factor-κB ligand (RANKL), interleukin-6 (IL-6), IL-1, and IL-11. Most of these cytokines affect osteoblast and osteoclast differentiation (Abu-Amer et al. 2007). The increased macrophage production causes local osteolysis and progressive implant loosening (Cherian et al. 2015; McLaughlin and Lee 2006). Other cofactors of aseptic loosening can be attributed to inadequate initial fixation with host bone or mechanical loss of fixation over time (Abu-Amer et al. 2007), either primary in etiology or secondary to co-existing pathology such as component malrotation and/or ligamentous instability. Other theoretical causes contributing to the acceleration of aseptic include metal hypersensitivity (Granchi et al. 2008; Teo and Schalock 2017; Eftekhary et al. 2018).

52.4 History and Physical Exam

> A thorough preoperative evaluation is essential to diagnose and determine the primary cause of TKA failure.

Patients with symptomatic TKA often present with pain, swelling, instability, and/or stiffness (Flierl et al. 2019; Higuera-Rueda and Parvizi 2015). Periprosthetic joint infection (PJI) should be ruled out in every painful TKA consultation. Early signs of loosening after TKA, rapid decline, and constant pain regardless of activity level may indicate infection. With elevation of either erythrocyte sedimentation rate (ESR) or C-reactive protein (CRP) serum marker, an arthrocentesis is warranted to rule out PJI (DIAGNOSIS AND PREVENTION OF PERIPROSTHETIC JOINT INFECTIONS CLINICAL PRACTICE GUIDELINE 2019).

The initial patient evaluation should focus on the type and duration of symptoms and associated exacerbating and/or alleviating factors. Symptoms that do not improve after surgery may be related to extrinsic sources of pain, such as degenerative disk disease and radiculopathy from the lumbar spine, hip pathology, or peripheral vascular disease (Flierl et al. 2019). Symptoms that present early after TKA (e.g., within 2 years postoperatively when PJI ruled out) are more indicative of instability and component malposition, while symptomology from osteolysis and aseptic loosening will often present years after the index surgery (Higuera-Rueda and Parvizi 2015). Patients with aseptic loosening often express time periods without pain prior to the insidious onset of their symptoms. Aseptic loosening presents with pain and progressive instability that is worse with increased activity and weight-bearing and improved with activity cessation and rest (Higuera-Rueda and Parvizi 2015; Lonner et al. 2009). Chronic effusions, difficulty with uneven surfaces and/or stairs, and activity-dependent symptoms are also consistent with mechanical issues surrounding TKA. Furthermore, start-up pain (sitting to standing) is closely correlated with loosening, whereas mechanical symptoms such as progressive "clunking" or "catching" may be from instability (Lonner et al. 2009). Improvement with pain with bracing and activity modification may also correlate with instability etiology for pain.

Additional questions should focus on the patient's perioperative experience after the index surgery including complications, prolonged antibiotic use, or wound healing difficulties.

> It is imperative to try to obtain medical records, including operative reports, implant information, hospital discharge summary, and clinical notes, to identify preoperative range of motion and deformity as well as other possible sources of pain.

Severe fixed varus deformity and flexion contracture have reported to be risk factors for early tibial loosening (Higuera-Rueda and Parvizi 2015; Windsor et al. 1989; Gonzalez and Mekhail 2004). Implant information is also vital, as certain types of implants (metal-backed patella components (Bayley et al. 1988), older cementless TKA systems (Berger et al. 2001), certain high-flexion TKA designs (Choi et al. 2018; Kim et al. 2017), and certain mobile-bearing TKA (Namba et al. 2012; Namba et al. 2014; Gøthesen et al. 2013)) have seen reports of early loosening and failure. It is also critical to identify implants for preoperative planning to ensure appropriate revision implants be present during revision surgery to prevent unnecessary removal of well-fixed components causing increased surgical complexity and bone loss.

- **Physical Exam**

Prior incisions should be carefully assessed for wound erythema, along with an assessment of the joint for fluid collections/effusion, swelling, and pain with passive range of motion. The presence of an active or healed sinus tract is indicative of PJI. Progressive stiffness and motion limited by pain and swelling may also be signs of infection. The joint should be carefully palpated for areas of point tenderness. As flexion and mid-flexion instability progresses, increased strain on surrounding soft tissues to help stabilize the knee may be determined by tenderness along the patella, pes anserine, biceps femoris, and Gerdy's tubercle.

> Key components of the physical examination should include coronal and sagittal plane stability assessment throughout range of motion (full extension; along with 30°, 60°, and 90° of flexion), gait analysis, and examination of ipsilateral hip and lumbar spine (Flierl et al. 2019; Park et al. 2016).

52.5 Imaging

52.5.1 Plain Radiographs

Initial radiographic evaluation should include weight-bearing anteroposterior (AP), lateral, and Merchant views. The images should be carefully inspected to assess fixation (cemented vs. cementless), polyethylene wear, osteolysis, radiolucent lines, patellar tracking, and overall component size and position. Initial postoperative and sequential follow-up radiographs are critical to identify any progressive radiolucent lines or implant migration. Identification of radiolucent lines can be very sensitive to radiograph obliquity as little as 4° of angulation can cause obscurity (Ecker et al. 1987). Fluoroscopically aligned radiographs may improve the beam projection for identification of subtle radiolucencies (Yamazaki et al. 2005; Vyskocil et al. 1999). Radiolucencies typically begin on the femoral/tibial component periphery at the implant–cement interface and subsequently progresses (Guha et al. 2008; Smith et al. 1999). Since cementless implants may have immediate postoperative radiolucencies at the implant–bone junction, it is critical to compare these findings from subsequent films to determine progression and/or clinical significance.

> It is important to correlate radiographic findings with the patient's history and symptoms.

Not all radiolucent lines necessarily imply component loosening (Higuera-Rueda and Parvizi 2015; Smith

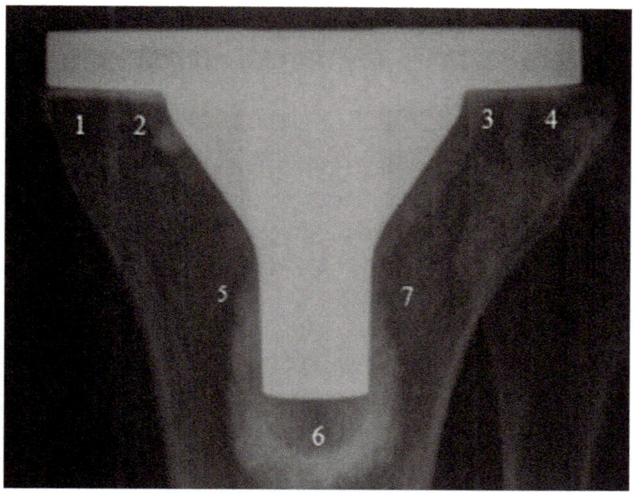

Fig. 52.3 The Knee Society Total Knee Arthroplasty Roentgenographic Evaluation and Scoring System (KSRES) divides the tibial component into 7 zones for classification of prosthesis interface issues. (Adapted from Chalmers et al. (2017), with permission from Elsevier)

et al. 1999), especially if non-progressive in nature. Non-progressive radiolucent lines less than 2 mm under the femoral or tibial component after cemented arthroplasty are likely attributed from poor cement interdigitation into the cancellous bone (Guha et al. 2008) whereas radiolucencies more than 2 mm are associated with greater rates of loosening and poor results (Ecker et al. 1987).

The Knee Society Total Knee Arthroplasty Roentgenographic Evaluation and Scoring System (KSRES), based on consensus agreement, provides guidelines for assessing both TKA component position and radiolucent lines. In evaluating radiolucent lines, the KSRES divides TKA components into 7 zones on the AP radiograph for the tibia and the lateral radiograph for the femoral component (Fig. 52.3) (Ewald 1989). The width of radiolucent lines (millimeters) from each of the 7 zones is added into a final score. The final score for each component then indicates

- No concern (score ≤4)
- Closer clinical follow-up for progression (score 5–9)
- Loose implants (score ≥10) (Ewald 1989)

> Although studies have shown good reliability and reproducibility for component evaluation using the KSRES, there is poor reliability of radiolucent lines assessment (Bach et al. 2001, 2005).

Chalmers et al. (2017) developed a novel percentage-based system, a modification of KSRES, in an attempt to detect more modern causes of TKA aseptic loosening by implant debonding. The authors determined the percent involvement of any radiolucency at the tibial bone–cement or cement–bone interface and then determined the proportion of this radiolucency to the entire implant interface. The authors then assigned a percentage score for the AP and lateral radiographs independently. Similar to KSRES, each tibial component was categorized as

- Non-concerning (10% or less of the implant interface)
- Closer clinical follow-up for progression (11–24% of the implant interface)
- Loose (25% or greater of the implant interface) (Chalmers et al. 2017)

As the complexity and variety of implants have increased over the past decade, Meneghini et al. (2015) developed a Modernized Knee Society Scoring System to be more descriptive and detailed, allowing for evaluation of multiple implant designs (Fig. 52.4). However, this evaluation system remains largely descriptive rather than predictive or prognostic in its current form.

52.5.2 Bone Scintigraphy

Three-phase bone scintigraphy, or nuclear bone scans, may be helpful in diagnosing loosening when used appropriately and after sufficient time from the index surgery. The scans have higher utility when obtained years after surgery (Claassen et al. 2014; Hochman et al. 2017; French et al. 2013; Holst et al. 2019), since positive bone scans can occur in 20% of asymptomatic knees at 1 year post-op and in 12.5% of individuals 2 years after surgery (Duus et al. 1990; Kantor et al. 1990). Increased radioisotope uptake on the delayed images but not on the blood-pool phase can be indicative of loosening rather than infection (Smith et al. 2001).

> However, these findings are often subtle and studies report that bone scintigraphy is often unable to differentiate septic from aseptic loosening (Palestro 2014; Aliabadi et al. 1989).

The use of white blood cell tagging and other nuclear medicine protocols of course improve this distinction between aseptic and septic causes for failure. Normal bone scans are the most insightful, with a high negative predictive value (Smith et al. 2001; Hofmann et al. 1990).

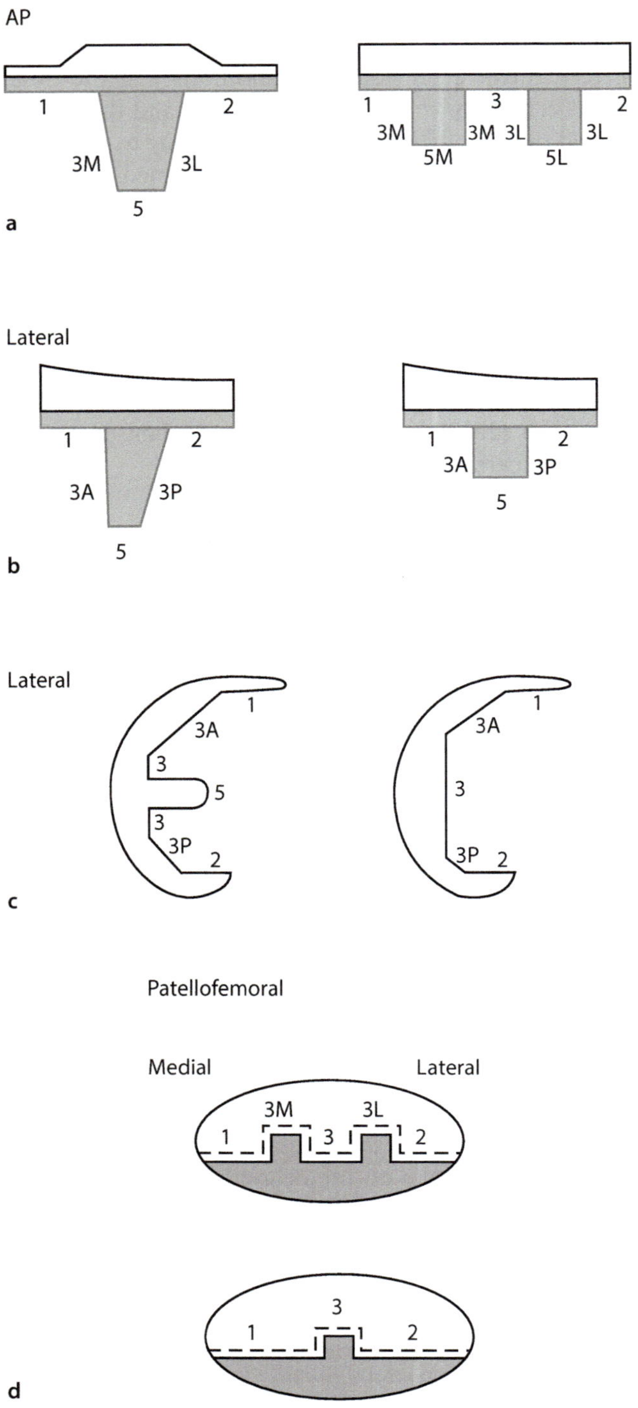

Fig. 52.4 Coronal **a** and sagittal **b** radiographic schema for keeled and two-peg implants, with zones for documentation of radiolucent lines and osteolysis. Sagittal **c** radiographic schematic of femoral implant with zones denoted for documentation of radiolucent lines and osteolysis. Patellofemoral **d** radiographic schematic of multi- or single-peg patella implant with zones denoted for documentation of radiolucent lines and osteolysis. Radiolucent lines should be denoted and documented as "partial" or "complete" and osteolysis documented in millimeters. (Adapted from Meneghini et al. (2015), with permission from Elsevier)

52.5.3 Computed Tomography (CT) and Magnetic Resonance Imaging (MRI)

Computed tomography (CT) scans can aid in defining the extent and width of osteolytic lesions that may be less apparent on plain radiographs (Higuera-Rueda and Parvizi 2015; Hochman et al. 2017).

> Conventional CT scans have a limited use to identifying loosening in the absence of lucent zones (Hochman et al. 2017). The CT scans are more insightful in assessing femoral and tibial component rotation relative to the transepicondylar/posterior condylar axis and medial third of tubercle, respectively.

Similarly, magnetic resonance imaging (MRI) in traditional methods is not validated and has low utility in the evaluation of loosening and osteolysis due to significant metal artifact. Interestingly, Fritz et al. (2015) suggested that metal artifact reduction MRI can demonstrate distinct bone–cement and cement–implant interfaces as well as fibrous membrane between implant–cement junction.

> However, it is important to note that MRIs are very sensitive to motion artifact and routine reliable reproduction of bone–cement and implant–cement interface may be unlikely.

52.5.4 Positron Emission Tomography-Computed Tomography (PET-CT)

Before gross implant motion occurs and radiographic changes are recognized, micromotion at the bone–cement or cement–implant junction causes pain and remains difficult to diagnosis (Koob et al. 2019). Plain radiographs and traditional bone scan imaging are unable to detect early micromotion sequala given their low-spatial resolution (Koob et al. 2019). Fluorodeoxyglucose (FDG) positron emission tomography-computed tomography (PET-CT) is an emerging alternative. The radiopharmaceutical FDG shows high affinity for bone and a rapid blood clearance, producing a high bone-to-background ratio in a shorter time vs. standard radioisotope tracers (Koob et al. 2019; Even-Sapir et al. 2007). Sterner et al. (2007) examined 14 patients with painful TKA and found a sensitivity of 100% for diagnosing aseptic loosening with FDG PET-CT, whereas specificity was very low at

56%. This study was the first to present the utility of FDG PET-CT imaging in the diagnosis of aseptic loosening. Few studies since have demonstrated similar high sensitivities with lower specificities, suggesting PET-CT may be an appropriate "rule out" test but not a reliable "rule in" modality (Koob et al. 2019; Delank et al. 2006; Barnsley and Barnsley 2019).

However, a meta-analysis and systematic review of 12 studies (401 patients) comparing bone scintigraphy, FDG PET-CT, single-photon emission-computerized tomography (SPECT-CT), and radionuclide arthrogram found that the most accurate modality for detection of aseptic loosening in TKA was SPECT-CT arthrography (Barnsley and Barnsley 2019). The authors found, however, that the available evidence has a high risk of bias, with the total number of patients in each modality cohort to be small.

> Further research is needed to evaluate the efficacy of FDG PET-CT and SPECT-CT in the diagnosis of TKA aseptic loosening.

52.6 Risk Factors

52.6.1 Body Mass Index

A high body mass index (BMI) has been correlated with increased rates of aseptic loosening after primary TKA (Schroer et al. 2013; Dewan et al. 2009; Issa et al. 2016; Ranawat et al. 1993; Vazquez-Vela Johnson et al. 2003; Wagner et al. 2016). Foran et al. (2004) reported on 30 TKAs in obese patients (mean BMI 34 kg/m^2) who were matched to 30 TKAs in non-obese patients at a mean 15-year long-term follow-up. There were more polyethylene insert revisions in the non-obese group vs. obese group likely attributed to higher activity levels in the non-obese cohort as demonstrated by higher Knee Society Function Scores (89 vs. 81, $p = 0.019$). The authors also found that, although not statistically significant, there was a trend for obesity to influence aseptic loosening rates. The authors suggested that increased BMI places higher stress at the bone–prosthesis interface causing earlier loosening. Furthermore, continued weight gain after primary TKA has deleterious effects (Lim et al. 2017). Lim et al. (2017) retrospectively reviewed 160 primary TKA patients who were stratified according to BMI change from primary TKA to revision arthroplasty. Sustaining a stable weight after primary TKA was protective against all-cause late revision ($p = 0.004$). Patients who gained weight were revised for aseptic loosening earlier (less than 5 years; $p = 0.020$), whereas those who reduced their BMI were revised later (greater than 10 years; $p = 0.004$).

Conversely, multiple other studies have not shown any association between obesity (BMI >30 kg/m^2) and aseptic loosening rates (Griffin et al. 1998; Krushell and Fingeroth 2007; Mont et al. 1996; Naziri et al. 2013; Whiteside and Viganò 2007). Naziri et al. (2013) evaluated 101 TKA patients with a minimum BMI of 50 kg/m^2 vs. 101 matched TKA patients with BMI less than 30 kg/m^2. There were no differences in aseptic implant survivorship (94% vs. 98%, $p = 0.28$); however, medical and surgical complication rates (14% vs. 5%, $p = 0.037$) were significantly higher in the super-obese patients compared with the non-obese matching group, respectively. Similarly, systematic review and meta-analysis by Cherian et al. (2015) of 20 studies (16 total hip arthroplasty and 5 TKA studies; 288 TKA patients) found no difference in aseptic loosening risk in patients with BMI >30 kg/m^2 compared to patients with BMI <30 kg/m^2 (odds ratio 2.28; 95% CI 0.60–8.62; $p = 0.22$). Although there was no association between obesity and aseptic loosening in this meta-analysis, the authors attributed this finding to the small cohorts in each of the included studies.

> Further research is needed to examine the role of obesity, morbid obesity, and super obesity and to determine if different subclassifications negatively influence implant survivorship and rates of aseptic loosening.

52.6.2 Diabetes Mellitus

Patients with diabetes mellitus are significantly more likely to experience adverse events perioperatively after TKA, with higher rates of re-admission, revision arthroplasty, and periprosthetic joint infection (Marchant et al. 2009; Martínez-Huedo et al. 2017; Gu et al. 2019; Lenguerrand et al. 2018; Meding et al. 2003). There is some data, albeit limited, that suggest the long-term effects of diabetes mellitus on the risk of aseptic revision and loosening after primary TKA (Meding et al. 2003; Papagelopoulos et al. 1996; Maradit Kremers et al. 2017; Watts et al. 2016). In a Kaiser Permanente Registry study of 64,017 primary TKA patients followed for a median 2.9 years, the presence of diabetes mellitus was reported as a risk factor for aseptic loosening in TKA ($p = 0.003$) (Namba et al. 2013). Similarly, at a mean 52-month follow-up, Meding et al. (2003) reported the rate of aseptic loosening of both femoral and tibial components to be higher in patients with diabetes compared to individuals without diabetes (3.6% vs. 0.4%, respectively; $p < 0.05$). Hyperglycemia during the immediate preoperative timeframe also increases the risk of aseptic revision and loosening after primary TKA

(Maradit Kremers et al. 2017). These findings may be attributed to negative systemic as well as local effects of hyperglycemia on the bone–cement/cement–implant interface (Maradit Kremers et al. 2017; Berenbaum 2011).

52.6.3 Mobile-Bearing TKA

The influence of implant design may also factor into aseptic loosening. For example, certain mobile-bearing TKA designs have been reported to have higher risk for aseptic loosening compared to fixed-bearing implants in several registry studies (Namba et al. 2012, 2014; Gøthesen et al. 2013; Graves et al. 2011). The cemented low-contact stress (LCS) mobile-bearing implant (DePuy Synthes, Warsaw, IN, USA), in particular, has a seven-fold greater risk of aseptic loosening reported in a Norwegian study (Gøthesen et al. 2013). A US registry study found similar higher aseptic loosening revision rates for the LCS tibial baseplate compared to fixed-bearing TKA designs (Namba et al. 2012). Another study comparing the Norwegian Arthroplasty Registry with the Kaiser Permanente Total Joint Replacement Registry reported similar findings (Paxton et al. 2011). Although an LCS design was used in over 33% of arthroplasty procedures in the Norwegian cohort and only 10% in the Kaiser Permanente group, both registries demonstrated higher aseptic loosening rates for the LCS TKA design. Differences in tibial under-surface manufacturing and poor cement–implant bonding have been reported as possible explanations for these outcomes (Namba et al. 2012, 2014; Gøthesen et al. 2013; Kutzner et al. 2018).

52.6.4 High-Viscosity Cement

Polymethylmethacrylate (PMMA) cement has played an integral role in TKA and implant fixation (Cawley et al. 2013). Bone cement forms a strong bond between the implant and native bone through interdigitation, while evenly distributing load (Cawley et al. 2013).

- Cement penetration of 3–4 mm in cancellous bone has been reported to be the minimum depth needed for optimal fixation (Cawley et al. 2013; Incavo et al. 1994; Johnson et al. 1983; Janssen et al. 2008). High-viscosity cement has advantages of longer working phase (Crawford et al. 2017) and increased tensile strength (Eriksson et al. 1984), but has reports of decreased intrusion depth and fixation strength (Rey et al. 1987).

The American Joint Replacement Registry (AJRR) has shown a steady increase of HVC utilization from 46% of TKAs in 2012 to 61.3% of TKAs in 2017 (Kelly et al. 2018).

There is inconclusive evidence of superiority of high-viscosity cement (HVC) over low-viscosity cement (LVC). There has been increasing concern, however, for HVC having increased risk of aseptic loosening after primary TKA (Kopinski et al. 2016; Hazelwood et al. 2015; Buller et al. 2019).

In a retrospective review of 10,014 TKA patients, Buller et al. (2019) found that aseptic loosening was significantly higher in the HVC cohort (91 of 4790; 1.9%) compared to the LVC cohort (48 of 5224; 0.92%) ($p < 0.001$) across multiple different implant types.

- The authors concluded that their study only confirmed the association between HVC and risk for aseptic loosening and did not provide a mechanism for the increased odds of failure.

- Further prospective studies in large cohorts are required to confirm the higher risk of aseptic loosening for HVC compared to LVC during primary TKA.

52.7 Revision TKA Clinical Outcomes

Historically, the overall results of revision TKA after aseptic causes, similar to septic revisions, demonstrated lower success rates compared to primary arthroplasty (Ahlberg and Lunden 1981; Bargar et al. 1980; Cameron and Hunter 1982; Kim and Finerman 1983; Bryan and Rand 1985; Thornhill et al. 1982). Additionally, patient satisfaction has been reported to be significantly lower after revision TKA vs. primary arthroplasty (Greidanus et al. 2011). Postoperative general health measures (e.g., Shortform-12), and knee-specific scores (e.g., Oxford Knee Score [OKS], Western Ontario and McMaster Universities Osteoarthritis Index [WOMAC]) have also been reported to be lower after aseptic revision TKA (Greidanus et al. 2011; Saleh et al. 2002; Hanssen and Rand 1988; Hartley et al. 2002).

With newer implant technology and improved surgical technique, the results of revision TKA after aseptic loosening have improved (Friedman et al. 1990; Baker et al. 2012; Cherian et al. 2016; Pun and Ries 2008; Sachdeva et al. 2019; Bertin et al. 1985; Schwab et al. 2005; Haas et al. 1995). Haas et al. reported that 84% (56 of 67 patients) had an excellent or good result after revision using modern modular cemented components at mean 3.5-year follow-up. Mabry et al. reported on 72 patients and found implant survivorship at 10-year long-term follow-up to be 92%.

Aside from implant longevity, patient-reported outcome measures (PROMs) after revisions performed for aseptic loosening have recently been associated with high OKS, the European Quality of Life Group (EuroQol-5D), and patient satisfaction scores compared to revisions for other aseptic causes (Baker et al. 2012). Sachdeva et al. (2019) retrospectively compared 100 aseptic revision TKA patients matched to 100 patients who underwent primary TKA with the same prosthesis. At mean 57-month follow-up in the revision group and 67-month follow-up in the primary TKA cohort, the average improvement in Knee Society Score (KSS) function scores were similar in both groups (28-point improvement, $p < 0.05$) (Sachdeva et al. 2019). The authors concluded that patients undergoing revision TKA for aseptic loosening can expect similar improvements in clinical function and outcome scores compared to primary TKA when controlling for implant type (Sachdeva et al. 2019). Similarly, Hamilton et al. (2017) reported on 53 consecutive aseptic TKA revisions (39 of 53 were revised for loosening; 74%) to total stabilized implants. Patients were evaluated preoperatively and at 6, 26, 52, and 104 weeks postoperatively using the OKS, range of motion, pain rating scale, and timed functional performance assessments (Hamilton et al. 2017). Data was compared to a matched cohort of primary TKA patients with the same outcome assessments at equivalent time points (Hamilton et al. 2017). Postoperative outcomes for revision TKA were analogous to primary TKA, with final range of motion at 2 years, pain scores, PROMs, and timed functional assessments ($p > 0.05$ for all). Post-hoc analysis demonstrated statistically significant differences between the 2 cohorts at early time points (6 weeks and 26 weeks) across all 4 outcome measures; however, there were no differences after the 6-month time point.

> In summary, revision TKA is a costly and complex surgical intervention that requires more resources than primary arthroplasty (Kurtz et al. 2005).

Although survivorship, patient health, and functional scores after revision TKA for aseptic etiology have improved over the past decade, the outcomes of revision TKA are particularly challenging to quantify, as the complexity of revision failure mode and reconstructive efforts are not well-defined. Revision arthroplasty ranges from less complex procedures such as polyethylene exchange, up to constrained/linked and megaprostheses for massive bone loss and soft tissue compromise. Patient outcomes are likely to reflect variability in host and local surgical factors, as well as various indications for surgery. Further research is needed to evaluate patient functional outcomes following revision TKA beyond only implant survivorship, as well as the rates of surgical complications for varying revision TKA complexities.

52.8 Case Example Continued

The patient presented at the beginning of the chapter (▶ Sect. 52.2) underwent a successful revision TKA with metaphyseal femoral and tibial cones and cemented femoral and tibial stems. Femoral and tibial cones were used to fill contained metaphyseal defects (◘ Figs. 52.5 and ◘ 52.6). The authors' preferred technique for reconstruction involves routine utilization of cones which allows for long-term biologic fixation as well as the utility of short cemented femoral and tibial stems which provides immediate initial implant stability (◘ Fig. 52.7) (Lachiewicz and Watters 2014). The cone–stem synergy technique is complementary with cementless stems as well. After revision arthroplasty, the patient has remained asymptomatic at 3 years postoperatively (◘ Fig. 52.8).

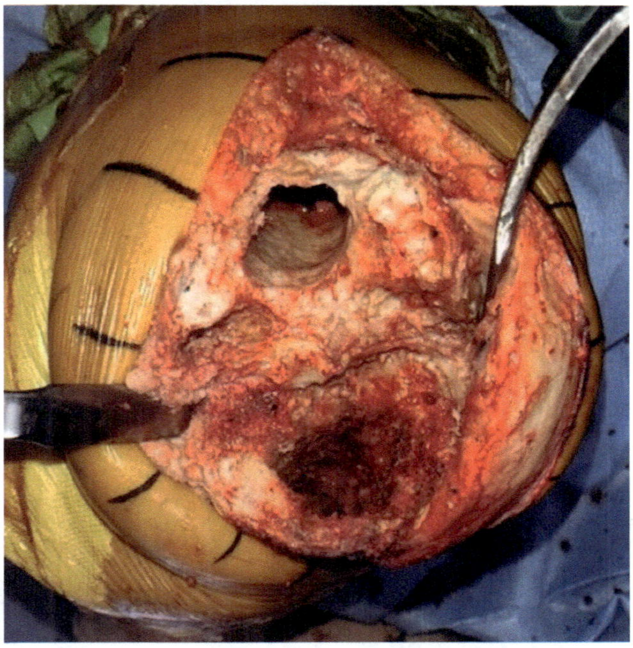

◘ **Fig. 52.5** Intraoperative clinical picture demonstrating large contained metaphyseal femoral and tibial bone defects after implant removal

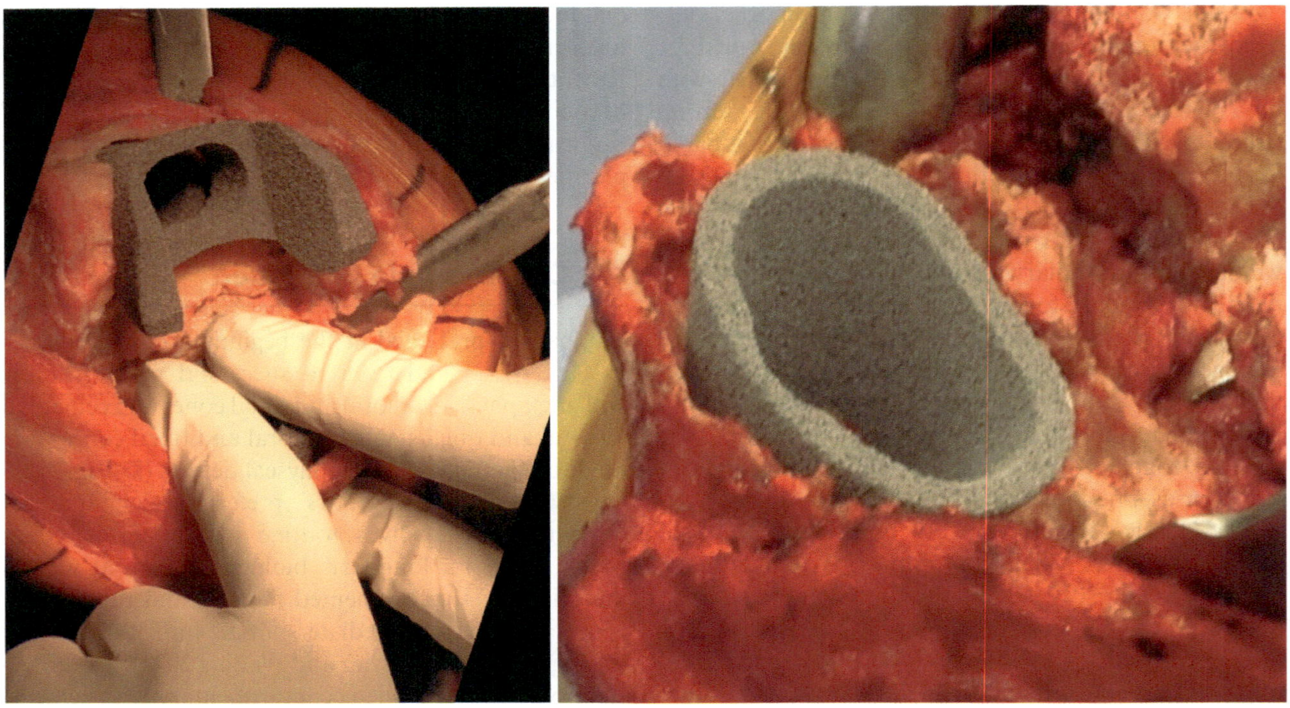

Fig. 52.6 Intraoperative clinical pictures showing placement of femoral and tibial metaphyseal cones

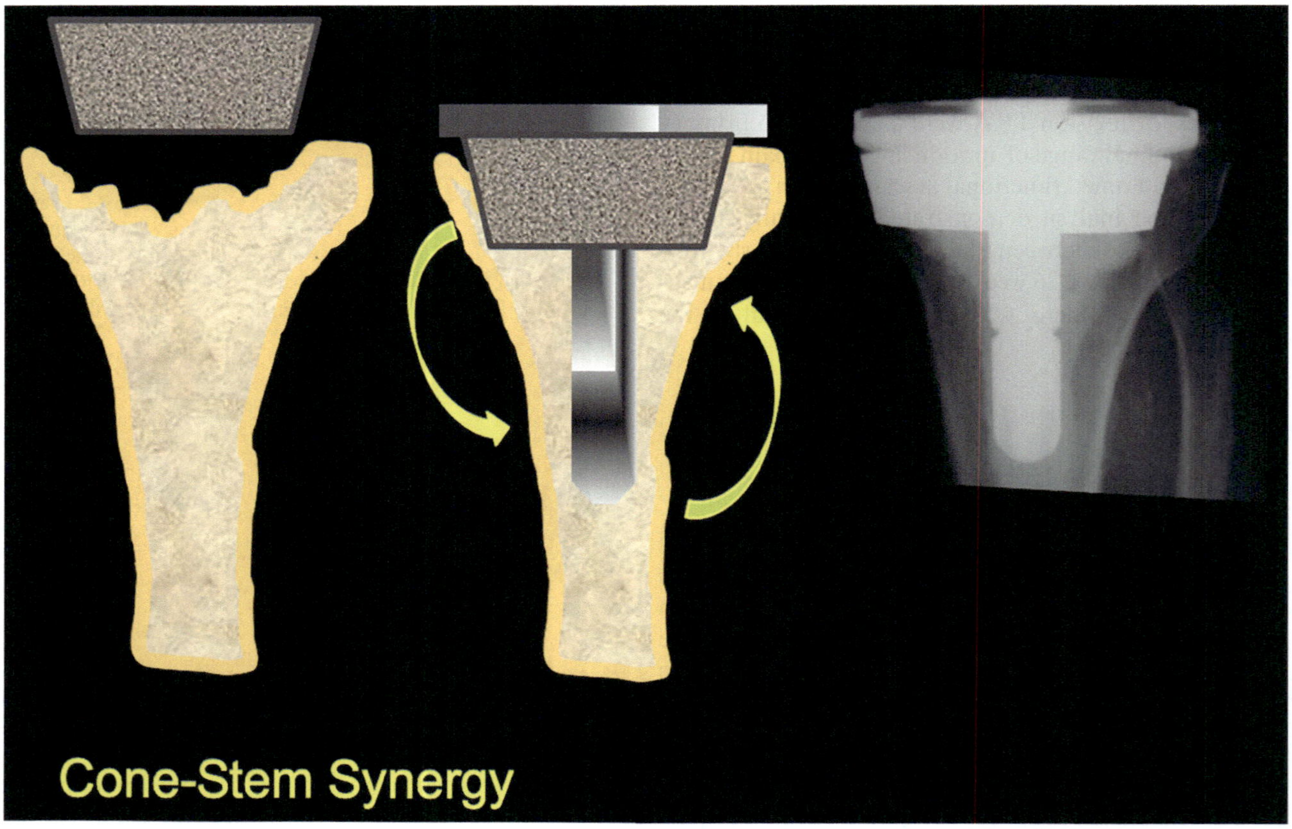

Fig. 52.7 Illustration demonstrating cone–stem synergy. The initial stability afforded by cemented stems may allow for long-term biologic fixation through the porous metal cones. The fixation at the joint level may in turn offload stresses seen by the cemented stems in the meta-diaphysis

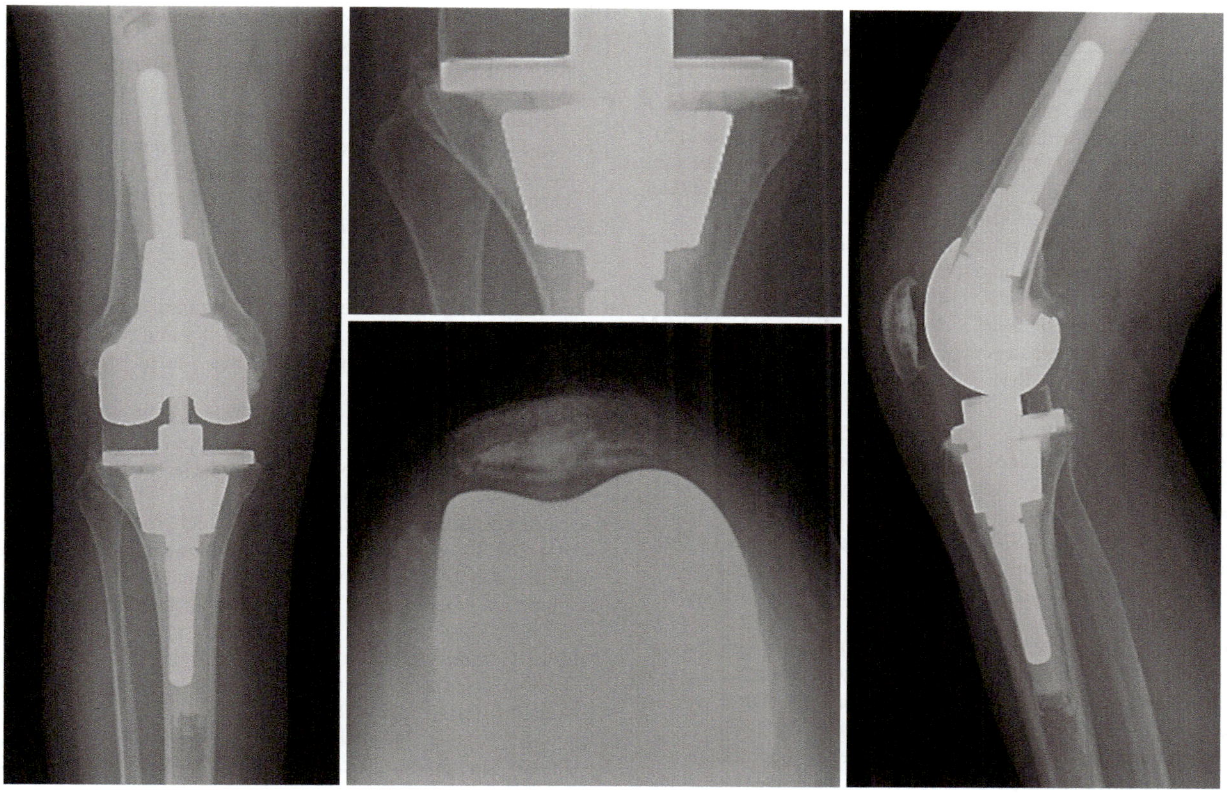

Fig. 52.8 Anteroposterior, sunrise, and lateral plain radiographs demonstrating revision TKA with femoral and tibial metaphyseal cones and short cemented femoral and tibial stems

Take-Home Messages

- Aseptic loosening continues to be one of the leading causes of failure after primary TKA.
- Patients with aseptic loosening often express time-dependent symptoms. Aseptic loosening may present with pain and progressive instability that is worse with activity and weight-bearing, while improved with rest.
- Radiolucencies on radiographic examination typically begin on the femoral/tibial component periphery at the implant–cement interface and subsequently progress. It is important to correlate radiographic findings with the patient's history and symptoms. Not all radiolucent lines necessarily imply component loosening, especially if non-progressive.
- Obesity and diabetes mellitus have been reported to be patient risk factors for aseptic loosening. With respect to diabetes, some studies highlight perioperative hyperglycemia as a bigger risk factor than elevated HbA1c for both aseptic loosening and periprosthetic joint infection.
- Certain mobile-bearing TKA designs and high-viscosity bone cement may be surgical risk factors for the increased likelihood of aseptic loosening.
- Cement penetration of 3–4 mm in cancellous bone has been reported to be the minimum depth needed for optimal fixation. High-viscosity cement has advantages of longer working phase and increased tensile strength, but has reports of decreased intrusion depth and fixation strength.
- There is inconclusive evidence of superiority of high-viscosity cement over low-viscosity cement. Further prospective studies in large cohorts are required to confirm the higher risk of aseptic loosening of high-viscosity compared to low-viscosity cement during primary TKA.
- Revision TKA is a costly and complex surgical intervention that requires more resources than primary arthroplasty. Overall results of revision TKA for aseptic causes have historically been less predictable and with lower success rates and patient satisfaction scores when compared to primary arthroplasty outcomes.
- With newer implant technology and improved surgical technique, the results of revision TKA after aseptic loosening have improved despite ongoing areas for refinement.
- Further research is needed to evaluate patient functional outcomes following revision TKA, beyond implant survivorship, as well as the rates of surgical complications for varying revision TKA complexities.

References

Abu-Amer Y, Darwech I, Clohisy JC (2007) Aseptic loosening of total joint replacements: mechanisms underlying osteolysis and potential therapies. Arthritis Res Ther. https://doi.org/10.1186/ar2170

Ahlberg A, Lunden A (1981) Secondary operations after knee joint replacement. Clin Orthop Relat Res. https://doi.org/10.1097/00003086-198105000-00022

Aliabadi P, Tumeh SS, Weissman BN, McNeil BJ (1989) Cemented total hip prosthesis: radiographic and scintigraphic evaluation. Radiology. https://doi.org/10.1148/radiology.173.1.2675184

Bach CM, Steingruber IE, Peer S, Nogler M, Wimmer C, Ogon M (2001) Radiographic assessment in total knee arthroplasty. Clin Orthop Relat Res. https://doi.org/10.1097/00003086-200104000-00022

Bach CM, Biedermann R, Goebel G, Mayer E, Rachbauer F (2005) Reproducible assessment of radiolucent lines in total knee arthroplasty. Clin Orthop Relat Res. https://doi.org/10.1097/01.blo.0000153077.79573.a4

Baker P, Cowling P, Kurtz S, Jameson S, Gregg P, Deehan D (2012) Reason for revision influences early patient outcomes after aseptic knee revision knee. Clin Orthop Relat Res. https://doi.org/10.1007/s11999-012-2278-7

Bargar WL, Cracchiolo A, Amstutz HC (1980) Results with the constrained total knee prosthesis in treating severely disabled patients and patients with failed total knee replacements. J Bone Jt Surg Ser A. https://doi.org/10.2106/00004623-198062040-00003

Barnsley L, Barnsley L (2019) Detection of aseptic loosening in total knee replacements: a systematic review and meta-analysis. Skelet Radiol. https://doi.org/10.1007/s00256-019-03215-y

Bayley JC, Scott RD, Ewald FC, Holmes GB (1988) Failure of the metal-backed patellar component after total knee replacement. J Bone Jt Surg Ser A. https://doi.org/10.2106/00004623--198870050-00005

Berenbaum F (2011) Diabetes-induced osteoarthritis: from a new paradigm to a new phenotype. Ann Rheum Dis. https://doi.org/10.1136/ard.2010.146399

Berger RA, Lyon JH, Jacobs JJ et al (2001) Problems with cementless total knee arthroplasty at 11 years followup. Clin Orthop Relat Res. https://doi.org/10.1097/00003086-200111000-00024

Bertin KC, Freeman MAR, Samuelson KM, Ratcliffe SS, Todd RC (1985) Stemmed revision arthroplasty for aseptic loosening of total knee replacement. J Bone Jt Surg Ser B. https://doi.org/10.1302/0301-620x.67b2.3980534

Bhandari M, Smith J, Miller LE, Block JE (2012) Clinical and economic burden of revision knee arthroplasty. Clin Med Insights Arthritis Musculoskelet Disord. https://doi.org/10.4137/CMAMD.S10859

Bryan RS, Rand J (1985) Indications, results, and complications of revision of total knee arthroplasty for mechanical failure. In: Total-condylar knee arthroplasty: technique, results, and complications. Springer, New York, pp 249–267

Buller LT, Rao V, Chiu YF, Nam D, McLawhorn AS (2019) Primary total knee arthroplasty performed using high-viscosity cement is associated with higher odds of revision for aseptic loosening. J Arthroplast. https://doi.org/10.1016/j.arth.2019.08.023

Calliess T, Ettinger M, Hülsmann N, Ostermeier S, Windhagen H (2015) Update on the etiology of revision TKA – evident trends in a retrospective survey of 1449 cases. Knee. https://doi.org/10.1016/j.knee.2015.02.007

Cameron HU, Hunter GA (1982) Failure in total knee arthroplasty. Mechanisms, revisions, and results. Clin Orthop Relat Res. https://doi.org/10.1097/00003086-198210000-00018

Cawley DT, Kelly N, McGarry JP, Shannon FJ (2013) Cementing techniques for the tibial component in primary total knee replacement. Bone Joint J. https://doi.org/10.1302/0301-620x.95b3.29586

Chalmers BP, Sculco PK, Fehring KA, Trousdale RT, Taunton MJ (2017) A novel percentage-based system for determining aseptic loosening of total knee arthroplasty tibial components. J Arthroplast 32(7):2274–2278. https://doi.org/10.1016/j.arth.2017.02.020

Cherian JJ, Jauregui JJ, Banerjee S, Pierce T, Mont MA (2015) What host factors affect aseptic loosening after THA and TKA? Clin Orthop Relat Res. https://doi.org/10.1007/s11999-015-4220-2

Cherian JJ, Bhave A, Harwin SF, Mont MA (2016) Outcomes and aseptic survivorship of revision total knee arthroplasty. Am J Orthop (Belle Mead NJ) 45:79–85

Choi Y-J, Lee KW, Ha J-K et al (2018) Comparison of revision rates due to aseptic loosening between high-flex and conventional knee prostheses. Knee Surg Relat Res. https://doi.org/10.5792/ksrr.17.071

Claassen L, Ettinger M, Plaass C, Daniilidis K, Calliess T, Ezechieli M (2014) Diagnostic value of bone scintigraphy for aseptic loosening after total knee arthroplasty. Technol Health Care. https://doi.org/10.3233/THC-140850

Crawford DA, Berend KR, Nam D, Barrack RL, Adams JB, Lombardi AV (2017) Low rates of aseptic tibial loosening in obese patients with use of high-viscosity cement and standard tibial tray: 2-year minimum follow-up. J Arthroplast. https://doi.org/10.1016/j.arth.2017.04.018

Dalury DF, Pomeroy DL, Gorab RS, Adams MJ (2013) Why are total knee arthroplasties being revised? J Arthroplast. https://doi.org/10.1016/j.arth.2013.04.051

Delank KS, Schmidt M, Michael JWP, Dietlein M, Schicha H, Eysel P (2006) The implications of 18F-FDG PET for the diagnosis of endoprosthetic loosening and infection in hip and knee arthroplasty: results from a prospective, blinded study. BMC Musculoskelet Disord. https://doi.org/10.1186/1471-2474-7-20

Dewan A, Bertolusso R, Karastinos A, Conditt M, Noble PC, Parsley BS (2009) Implant durability and knee function after total knee arthroplasty in the morbidly obese patient. J Arthroplast. https://doi.org/10.1016/j.arth.2009.04.024

DIAGNOSIS AND PREVENTION OF PERIPROSTHETIC JOINT INFECTIONS CLINICAL PRACTICE GUIDELINE – American Academy of Orthopaedic Surgeons; 2019

Duus BR, Boeckstyns M, Stadeager C (1990) The natural course of radionuclide bone scanning in the evaluation of total knee replacement – a 2 year prospective study. Clin Radiol. https://doi.org/10.1016/S0009-9260(05)81699-X

Ecker ML, Lotke PA, Windsor RE, Cella JP (1987) Long-term results after total condylar knee arthroplasty. Significance of radiolucent lines. Clin Orthop Relat Res. https://doi.org/10.1097/00003086-198703000-00023

Eftekhary N, Shepard N, Wiznia D, Iorio R, Long WJ, Vigdorchik J (2018) Metal hypersensitivity in total joint arthroplasty. JBJS Rev. https://doi.org/10.2106/JBJS.RVW.17.00169

Eriksson RA, Albrektsson T, Magnusson B (1984) Assessment of bone viability after heat trauma: a histological, histochemical and vital microscopic study in the rabbit. Scand J Plast Reconstr Surg Hand Surg. https://doi.org/10.3109/02844318409052849

Even-Sapir E, Mishani E, Flusser G, Metser U (2007) 18F-Fluoride positron emission tomography and positron emission tomography/computed tomography. Semin Nucl Med. https://doi.org/10.1053/j.semnuclmed.2007.07.002

Ewald FC (1989) The Knee Society total knee arthroplasty roentgenographic evaluation and scoring system. Clin Orthop Relat Res. https://doi.org/10.1097/00003086-198911000-00003

Flierl MA, Sobh AH, Culp BM, Baker EA, Sporer SM (2019) Evaluation of the painful total knee arthroplasty. J Am Acad Orthop Surg. https://doi.org/10.5435/JAAOS-D-18-00083

Foran JRH, Mont MA, Rajadhyaksha AD, Jones LC, Etienne G, Hungerford DS (2004) Total knee arthroplasty in obese patients: a

comparison with a matched control group. J Arthroplast. https://doi.org/10.1016/j.arth.2004.03.017
French TH, Russell N, Pillai A (2013) The diagnostic accuracy of radionuclide arthrography for prosthetic loosening in hip and knee arthroplasty. Biomed Res Int. https://doi.org/10.1155/2013/693436
Friedman RJ, Hirst P, Poss R, Kelley K, Sledge CB (1990) Results of revision total knee arthroplasty performed for aseptic loosening. Clin Orthop Relat Res. https://doi.org/10.1097/00003086--199006000-00031
Fritz J, Lurie B, Potter HG (2015) MR imaging of knee arthroplasty implants. Radiographics. https://doi.org/10.1148/rg.2015140216
Gonzalez MH, Mekhail AO (2004) The failed total knee arthroplasty: evaluation and etiology. J Am Acad Orthop Surg. https://doi.org/10.5435/00124635-200411000-00008
Gøthesen EB, Havelin L et al (2013) Survival rates and causes of revision in cemented primary total knee replacement: a report from the Norwegian arthroplasty register 1994–2009. Bone Jt J. https://doi.org/10.1302/0301-620X.95B5.30271
Granchi D, Cenni E, Tigani D, Trisolino G, Baldini N, Giunti A (2008) Sensitivity to implant materials in patients with total knee arthroplasties. Biomaterials. https://doi.org/10.1016/j.biomaterials.2007.11.038
Graves SE, Davidson D, Tomkins A (2011) Australian Orthopaedic Association National Joint Replacement Registry: annual report 2011
Greidanus NV, Peterson RC, Masri BA, Garbuz DS (2011) Quality of life outcomes in revision versus primary total knee arthroplasty. J Arthroplast. https://doi.org/10.1016/j.arth.2010.04.026
Griffin FM, Scuderi GR, Insall JN, Colizza W (1998) Total knee arthroplasty in patients who were obese with 10 years followup. Clin Orthop Relat Res. https://doi.org/10.1097/00003086--199811000-00006
Gu A, Wei C, Robinson H et al (2019) Postoperative complications and impact of diabetes mellitus severity on revision total knee arthroplasty. J Knee Surg. https://doi.org/10.1055/s-0038-1677542
Guha AR, Debnath UK, Graham NMK (2008) Radiolucent lines below the tibial component of a total knee replacement (TKR) – a comparison between single-and two-stage cementation techniques. Int Orthop. https://doi.org/10.1007/s00264-007-0345-6
Haas SB, Insall JN, Montgomery W, Windsor RE (1995) Revision total knee arthroplasty with use of modular components with stems inserted without cement. J Bone Jt Surg Ser A. https://doi.org/10.2106/00004623-199511000-00009
Hamilton DF, Simpson PM, Patton JT, Howie CR, Burnett R (2017) Aseptic revision knee arthroplasty with total stabilizer prostheses achieves similar functional outcomes to primary total knee arthroplasty at 2 years: a longitudinal cohort study. J Arthroplast. https://doi.org/10.1016/j.arth.2016.10.028
Hanssen AD, Rand JA (1988) A comparison of primary and revision total knee arthroplasty using the kinematic stabilizer prosthesis. J Bone Jt Surg Ser A. https://doi.org/10.2106/00004623--198870040-00003
Hartley RC, Barton-Hanson NG, Finley R, Parkinson RW (2002) Early patient outcomes after primary and revision total knee arthroplasty. A prospective study. J Bone Jt Surg Ser B. https://doi.org/10.1302/0301-620X.84B7.12607
Hazelwood KJ, O'Rourke M, Stamos VP, McMillan RD, Beigler D, Robb WJ (2015) Case series report: early cement-implant interface fixation failure in total knee replacement. Knee. https://doi.org/10.1016/j.knee.2015.02.016
Higuera-Rueda C, Parvizi J (2015) Causes and diagnosis of aseptic loosening after total knee replacement. In: Hirschman M, Becker R (eds) The unhappy total knee replacement: a comprehensive review and management guide. Springer, Cham
Hochman MG, Melenevsky YV, Metter DF et al (2017) ACR appropriateness criteria® imaging after total knee arthroplasty. J Am Coll Radiol. https://doi.org/10.1016/j.jacr.2017.08.036
Hofmann AA, Wyatt RW, Daniels AU, Armstrong L, Alazraki N, Taylor A Jr (1990) Bone scans after total knee arthroplasty in asymptomatic patients. Cemented versus cementless. Clin Orthop Relat Res (251):183–188
Holst DC, Angerame MR, Dennis DA, Jennings JM (2019) What is the value of component loosening assessment of a preoperatively obtained bone scan prior to revision total knee arthroplasty? J Arthroplast. https://doi.org/10.1016/j.arth.2019.02.065
Incavo SJ, Ronchetti PJ, Howe JG, Tranowski JP (1994) Tibial plateau coverage in total knee arthroplasty. Clin Orthop Relat Res. https://doi.org/10.1097/00003086-199402000-00011
Issa K, Harwin SF, Malkani AL, Bonutti PM, Scillia A, Mont MA (2016) Bariatric orthopaedics: Total hip arthroplasty in super-obese patients (those with a BMI of ≥50 kg/m2). J Bone Jt Surg Am Vol. https://doi.org/10.2106/JBJS.O.00474
Janssen D, Mann KA, Verdonschot N (2008) Micro-mechanical modeling of the cement-bone interface: the effect of friction, morphology and material properties on the micromechanical response. J Biomech. https://doi.org/10.1016/j.jbiomech.2008.08.020
Jiang Y, Jia T, Wooley PH, Yang SY (2013) Current research in the pathogenesis of aseptic implant loosening associated with particulate wear debris. Acta Orthop Belg 79(1):1–9
Johnson JA, Krug WH, Nahon D, Miller JE, Ahmed AM (1983) Evaluation of the load bearing capability of the cancellous proximal tibia with special interest in the design of knee implants. In: Transactions of the Annual Meeting of the Society for Biomaterials in Conjunction with the Interna
Kantor SG, Schneider R, Insall JN, Becker MW (1990) Radionuclide imaging of asymptomatic versus symptomatic total knee arthroplasties. Clin Orthop Relat Res. https://doi.org/10.1097/00003086-199011000-00021
Kelly MP, Illgen RL, Chen AF, Nam D (2018) Trends in the use of high-viscosity cement in patients undergoing primary total knee arthroplasty in the United States. J Arthroplast. https://doi.org/10.1016/j.arth.2018.07.007
Kim L, Finerman G (1983) Results of revision for aseptic failed knee arthroplasties. Orthop Trans 7:535
Kim YH, Park JW, Kim JS (2017) Do high-flexion total knee designs increase the risk of femoral component loosening? J Arthroplast. https://doi.org/10.1016/j.arth.2017.01.026
Koob S, Gaertner FC, Jansen TR et al (2019) Diagnosis of periprosthetic loosening of total hip and knee arthroplasty using 18F-Fluoride PET/CT. Oncotarget. https://doi.org/10.18632/oncotarget.26762
Kopinski JE, Aggarwal A, Nunley RM, Barrack RL, Nam D (2016) Failure at the tibial cement–implant interface with the use of high-viscosity cement in total knee arthroplasty. J Arthroplast. https://doi.org/10.1016/j.arth.2016.03.063
Krushell RJ, Fingeroth RJ (2007) Primary total knee arthroplasty in morbidly obese patients. A 5- to 14-year follow-up study. J Arthroplast. https://doi.org/10.1016/j.arth.2007.03.024
Kulshrestha V, Datta B, Mittal G, Kumar S (2019) Epidemiology of revision total knee arthroplasty: a single center's experience. Indian J Orthop. https://doi.org/10.4103/ortho.IJOrtho_127_17
Kurtz S, Mowat F, Ong K, Chan N, Lau E, Halpern M (2005) Prevalence of primary and revision total hip and knee arthroplasty in the United States from 1990 through 2002. J Bone Jt Surg Ser A. https://doi.org/10.2106/JBJS.D.02441

Kurtz S, Ong K, Lau E, Mowat F, Halpern M (2007) Projections of primary and revision hip and knee arthroplasty in the United States from 2005 to 2030. J Bone Jt Surg Ser A. https://doi.org/10.2106/JBJS.F.00222

Kutzner I, Hallan G, Høl PJ et al (2018) Early aseptic loosening of a mobile-bearing total knee replacement: a case-control study with retrieval analyses. Acta Orthop. https://doi.org/10.1080/17453674.2017.1398012

Lachiewicz PF, Watters TS (2014) Porous metal metaphyseal cones for severe bone loss: when only metal will do. Bone Jt J. https://doi.org/10.1302/0301-620X.96B11.34197

Lenguerrand E, Beswick AD, Whitehouse MR, Wylde V, Blom AW (2018) Outcomes following hip and knee replacement in diabetic versus nondiabetic patients and well versus poorly controlled diabetic patients: a prospective cohort study. Acta Orthop. https://doi.org/10.1080/17453674.2018.1473327

Lim CT, Goodman SB, Huddleston JI et al (2017) Weight gain after primary total knee arthroplasty is associated with accelerated time to revision for aseptic loosening. J Arthroplast. https://doi.org/10.1016/j.arth.2017.02.026

Lonner JH, Fehring TK, Hanssen AD et al (2009) Revision total knee arthroplasty: the preoperative evaluation. J Bone Jt Surg [Am]. https://doi.org/10.1016/S0021-9355(09)73915-3

Losina E, Thornhill TS, Rome BN, Wright J, Katz JN (2012) The dramatic increase in total knee replacement utilization rates in the United States cannot be fully explained by growth in population size and the obesity epidemic. J Bone Jt Surg Ser A. https://doi.org/10.2106/JBJS.J.01958

Maradit Kremers H, Schleck CD, Lewallen EA, Larson DR, Van Wijnen AJ, Lewallen DG (2017) Diabetes mellitus and hyperglycemia and the risk of aseptic loosening in total joint arthroplasty. J Arthroplast. https://doi.org/10.1016/j.arth.2017.02.056

Marchant MH, Viens NA, Cook C, Vail TP, Bolognesi MP (2009) The impact of glycemic control and diabetes mellitus on perioperative outcomes after total joint arthroplasty. J Bone Jt Surg Ser A. https://doi.org/10.2106/JBJS.H.00116

Martínez-Huedo MA, Jiménez-García R, Jiménez-Trujillo I, Hernández-Barrera V, del Rio LB, López-de-Andrés A (2017) Effect of type 2 diabetes on in-hospital postoperative complications and mortality after primary total hip and knee arthroplasty. J Arthroplast. https://doi.org/10.1016/j.arth.2017.06.038

McLaughlin JR, Lee KR (2006) The outcome of total hip replacement in obese and non-obese patients at 10- to 18-years. J Bone Jt Surg Ser B. https://doi.org/10.1302/0301-620X.88B10.17660

Meding JB, Reddleman K, Keating ME et al (2003) Total knee replacement in patients with diabetes mellitus. Clin Orthop Relat Res. https://doi.org/10.1097/01.blo.0000093002.90435.56

Meneghini RM, Mont MA, Backstein DB, Bourne RB, Dennis DA, Scuderi GR (2015) Development of a modern knee society radiographic evaluation system and methodology for total knee arthroplasty. J Arthroplast 30(12):2311–2314. https://doi.org/10.1016/j.arth.2015.05.049

Mont MA, Mathur SK, Krackow KA, Loewy JW, Hungerford DS (1996) Cementless total knee arthroplasty in obese patients: a comparison with a matched control group. J Arthroplast. https://doi.org/10.1016/S0883-5403(05)80009-9

Namba RS, Inacio MCS, Paxton EW et al (2012) Risk of revision for fixed versus mobile-bearing primary total knee replacements. J Bone Jt Surg Ser A. https://doi.org/10.2106/JBJS.K.01363

Namba RS, Cafri G, Khatod M, Inacio MCS, Brox TW, Paxton EW (2013) Risk factors for total knee arthroplasty aseptic revision. J Arthroplast. https://doi.org/10.1016/j.arth.2013.04.050

Namba R, Graves S, Robertsson O et al (2014) International comparative evaluation of knee replacement with fixed or mobile non-posterior-stabilized implants. J Bone Jt Surg Am Vol. https://doi.org/10.2106/JBJS.N.00466

Naziri Q, Issa K, Malkani AL, Bonutti PM, Harwin SF, Mont MA (2013) Bariatric orthopaedics: Total knee arthroplasty in super-obese patients (BMI > 50 kg/m 2). Survivorship and complications. Clin Orthop Relat Res. https://doi.org/10.1007/s11999-013-3154-9

Palestro CJ (2014) Nuclear medicine and the failed joint replacement: past, present, and future. World J Radiol. https://doi.org/10.4329/wjr.v6.i7.446

Papagelopoulos PJ, Idusuyi OB, Wallrichs SL, Morrey BF (1996) Long term outcome and survivorship analysis of primary total knee arthroplasty in patients with diabetes mellitus. Clin Orthop Relat Res. https://doi.org/10.1097/00003086-199609000-00015

Park CN, White PB, Meftah M, Ranawat AS, Ranawat CS (2016) Diagnostic algorithm for residual pain after total knee arthroplasty. Orthopedics. https://doi.org/10.3928/01477447-20160119-06

Paxton EW, Furnes O, Namba RS, Inacio MCS, Fenstad AM, Havelin LI (2011) Comparison of the Norwegian knee arthroplasty register and a United States arthroplasty registry. J Bone Joint Surg Am. https://doi.org/10.2106/jbjs.k.01045

Pun SY, Ries MD (2008) Effect of gender and preoperative diagnosis on results of revision total knee arthroplasty. Clin Orthop Relat Res. https://doi.org/10.1007/s11999-008-0451-9

Ranawat CS, Flynn WF, Saddler S, Hansraj KK, Maynard MJ (1993) Long-term results of the total condylar knee arthroplasty: a 15-year survivorship study. Clin Orthop Relat Res. https://doi.org/10.1097/00003086-199301000-00015

Rey RM, Paiement GD, McGann WM et al (1987) A study of intrusion characteristics of low viscosity cement Simplex-P and Palacos cements in a bovine cancellous bone model. Clin Orthop Relat Res. https://doi.org/10.1097/00003086-199702000-00039

Sachdeva S, Baker JF, Bauwens JE et al (2019) Can revision TKA patients achieve similar clinical functional improvement compared to primaries. J Knee Surg. https://doi.org/10.1055/s-0039-1693415

Saleh KJ, Dykes DC, Tweedie RL et al (2002) Functional outcome after total knee arthroplasty revision: a meta-analysis. J Arthroplast. https://doi.org/10.1054/arth.2002.35823

Schroer WC, Berend KR, Lombardi AV et al (2013) Why are total knees failing today? Etiology of total knee revision in 2010 and 2011. J Arthroplast. https://doi.org/10.1016/j.arth.2013.04.056

Schwab JH, Haidukewych GJ, Hanssen AD, Jacofsky DJ, Pagnano MW (2005) Flexion instability without dislocation after posterior stabilized total knees. Clin Orthop Relat Res. https://doi.org/10.1097/01.blo.0000185449.51246.d6

Sharkey PF, Hozack WJ, Rothman RH, Shastri S, Jacoby SM (2002) Why are total knee arthroplasties failing today? Clin Orthop Relat Res. https://doi.org/10.1097/00003086-200211000-00003

Sharkey PF, Lichstein PM, Shen C, Tokarski AT, Parvizi J (2013) Why are total knee arthroplasties failing today-has anything changed after 10 years? J Arthroplast. https://doi.org/10.1016/j.arth.2013.07.024

Smith S, Naima VSN, Freeman MAR (1999) The natural history of tibial radiolucent lines in a proximally cemented stemmed total knee arthroplasty. J Arthroplast. https://doi.org/10.1016/S0883--5403(99)99999-0

Smith SL, Wastie ML, Forster I (2001) Radionuclide bone scintigraphy in the detection of significant complications after total knee joint replacement. Clin Radiol. https://doi.org/10.1053/crad.2000.0620

Sterner T, Pink R, Freudenberg L et al (2007) The role of [18F]fluoride positron emission tomography in the early detection of

aseptic loosening of total knee arthroplasty. Int J Surg. https://doi.org/10.1016/j.ijsu.2006.05.002
Teo WZW, Schalock PC (2017) Metal hypersensitivity reactions to orthopedic implants. Dermatol Ther (Heidelb). https://doi.org/10.1007/s13555-016-0162-1
Thornhill TS, Dalziel RW, Sledge CB (1982) Alternatives to arthrodesis for the failed total knee arthroplasty. Clin Orthop Relat Res. https://doi.org/10.1097/00003086-198210000-00017
Vazquez-Vela Johnson G, Worland RL, Keenan J, Norambuena N (2003) Patient demographics as a predictor of the ten-year survival rate in primary total knee replacement. J Bone Jt Surg Ser B. https://doi.org/10.1302/0301-620X.85B1.12992
Vyskocil P, Gerber C, Bamert P (1999) Radiolucent lines and component stability in knee arthroplasty. Standard versus fluoroscopically-assisted radiographs. J Bone Jt Surg Ser B. https://doi.org/10.1302/0301-620X.81B1.9213
Wagner ER, Kamath AF, Fruth K, Harmsen WS, Berry DJ (2016) Effect of body mass index on reoperation and complications after total knee arthroplasty. J Bone Jt Surg Am Vol. https://doi.org/10.2106/JBJS.16.00093
Watts CD, Houdek MT, Wagner ER, Abdel MP, Taunton MJ (2016) Insulin dependence increases the risk of failure after Total knee arthroplasty in morbidly obese patients. J Arthroplast. https://doi.org/10.1016/j.arth.2015.08.026
Weinstein AM, Rome BN, Reichmann WM et al (2013) Estimating the burden of total knee replacement in the United States. J Bone Jt Surg Ser A. https://doi.org/10.2106/JBJS.L.00206
Whiteside LA, Viganò R (2007) Young and heavy patients with a cementless TKA do as well as older and lightweight patients. Clin Orthop Relat Res. https://doi.org/10.1097/BLO.0b013e31815a052c
Windsor RE, Scuderi GR, Moran MC, Insall JN (1989) Mechanisms of failure of the femoral and tibial components in total knee arthroplasty. Clin Orthop Relat Res. https://doi.org/10.1097/00003086-198911000-00005
Yamazaki T, Watanabe T, Nakajima Y et al (2005) Visualization of femorotibial contact in total knee arthroplasty using X-ray fluoroscopy. Eur J Radiol. https://doi.org/10.1016/j.ejrad.2003.09.018

Management of Extensor Mechanism Disruption After Total Knee Arthroplasty

Krit Boontanapibul, Stuart B. Goodman, and Derek F. Amanatullah

Contents

E. Hansen, K.-D. Kühn (eds.), *Essentials of Cemented Knee Arthroplasty*,
https://doi.org/10.1007/978-3-662-63113-3_53

53.1 Introduction

Extensor mechanism disruption is a dreaded and devastating complications after total knee arthroplasty (TKA). Loss of knee extension severely impairs ambulatory function and quality of life. Reconstruction of the extensor mechanism is technically demanding. Improper treatment selection for a disrupted extensor mechanism may result in continued extension lag, progressive quadriceps muscle weakness, reduced ambulatory capacity, and significant functional disability.

53.2 Case Example

A 60-year-old female presents post-primary right TKA and two-stage revision for periprosthetic joint infection 6 months ago complaining of anterior knee pain and being unable to ambulate after a fall on a flexed knee 4 months ago. She is unable to actively extend her knee. She is extremely unstable while walking. She can perform tenuous bed–chair and chair–bathroom straight-legged transfers in a knee immobilizer. Her limited activity has confined her to a wheelchair. She denies fevers or wound-related complications, including drainage or erythema. Her comorbid medical issues include prior ischemic stroke, type 2 diabetes mellitus, obesity, hypertension, and hyperlipidemia.

Physical examination of her right knee shows a warm and well-perfused limb with a well-healed anterior incision over the knee. There is no evidence of erythema or a sinus tract. There is minimal pain with a passive range of motion from 0° to 95°. The patient cannot perform active knee extension and a straight leg raise and has a 65° extension lag with a palpable defect in the quadriceps tendon.

Weight-bearing 36-inch long leg and anterior-to-posterior radiographs of the right knee show a well-fixed TKA with stemmed revision tibial component as well as deficiency of lateral collateral ligament and varus alignment as a result of extension instability with otherwise well-positioned components. Lateral radiograph of the knee shows severe patella baja, suggesting chronic soft tissue deficiency of the quadriceps tendon in the setting of a well-fixed posterior stabilized femoral component and resurfaced patella (Fig. 53.1). A knee aspiration under ultrasound guidance for routine polymorphonuclear cell count and percentage, aerobic and anaerobic culture, and a serum erythrocyte sedimentation rate and C-reactive protein are all negative and show no signs of recurrent periprosthetic joint infection.

The patient is diagnosed with a chronic postoperative extensor mechanism disruption involving the quadriceps tendon with a lateral collateral ligament insufficiency after traumatic fall on a revision right TKA in the set-

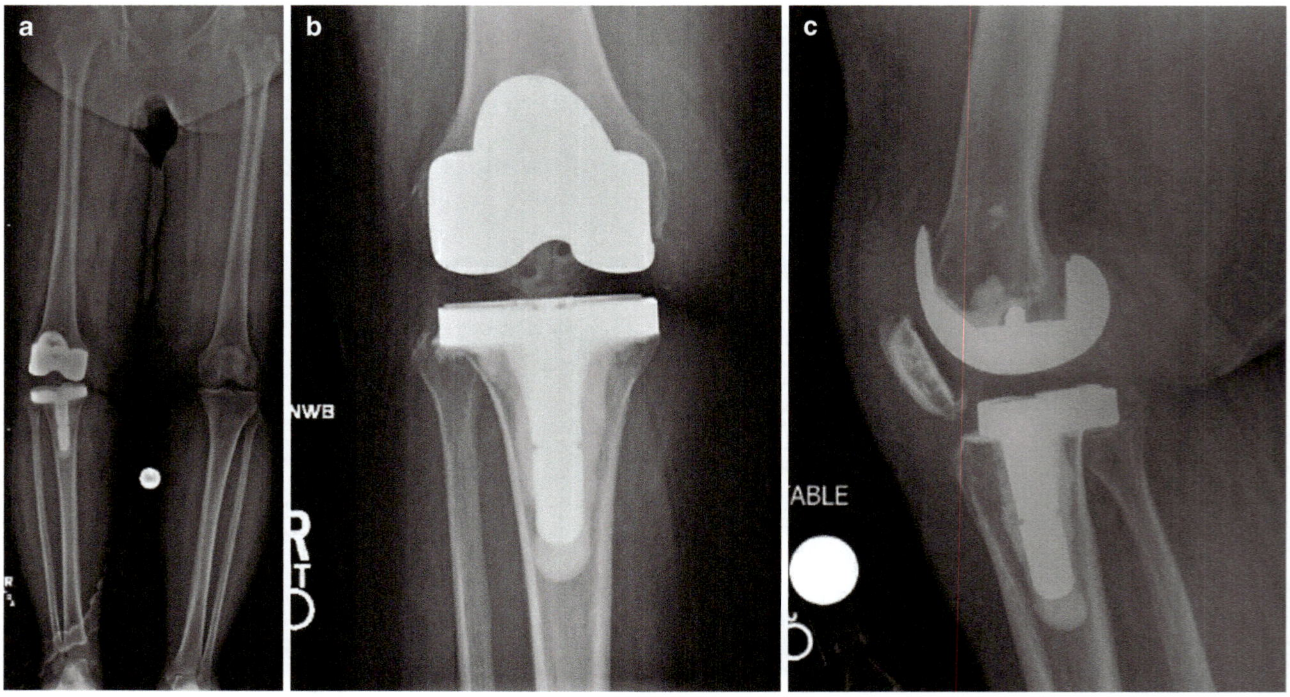

Fig. 53.1 **a** 36-inch standing long radiograph demonstrating lateral instability of right total knee. **b** Weight-bearing anterior-to-posterior radiograph of the right knee demonstrating a well-fixed revision tibial component. **c** Lateral radiograph of the right knee demonstrating severe patella baja and a well-fixed posterior stabilized femoral component and patellar resurfacing

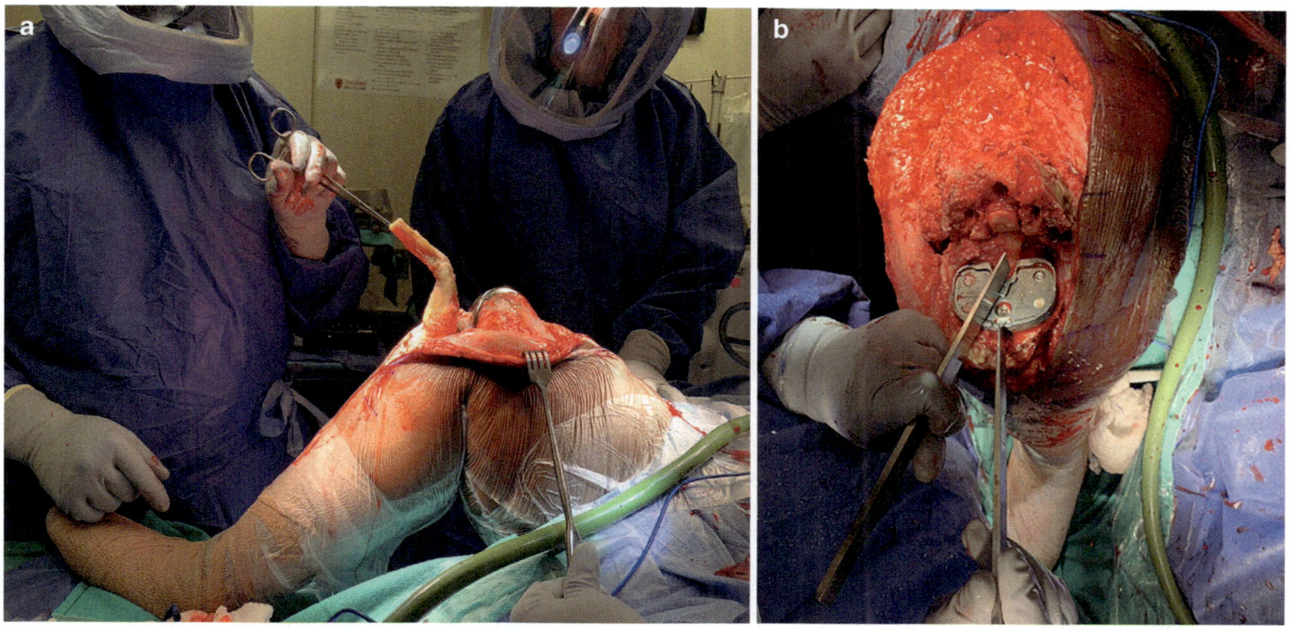

Fig. 53.2 **a** Chronic disruption of the extensor mechanism with necrotic distal quadriceps tendon, patella, and patellar tendon. **b** Severe internal rotation of tibial component

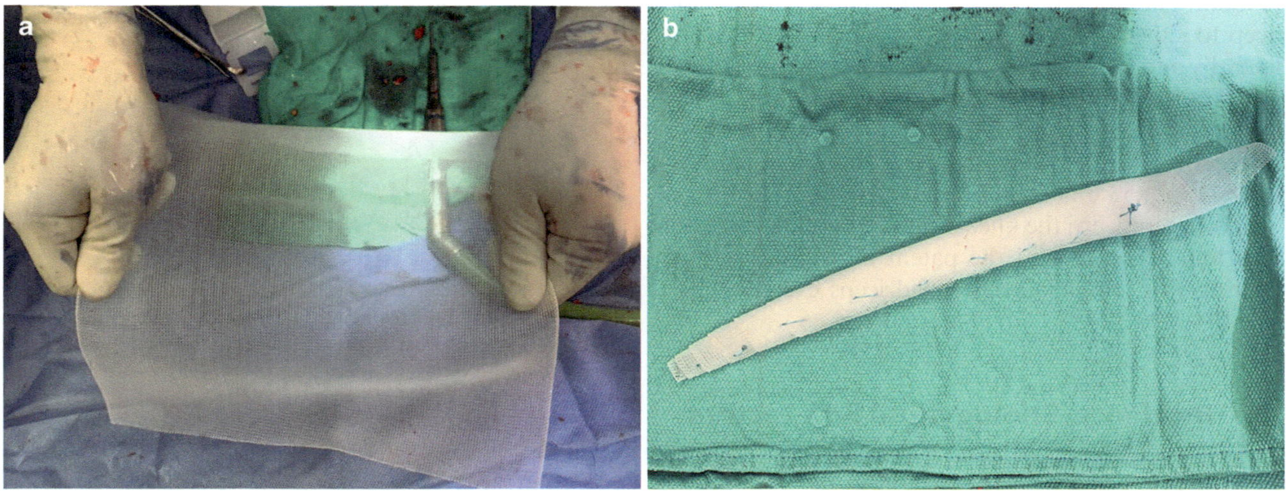

Fig. 53.3 **a** Find the less stretchable side of synthetic mesh. **b** Roll the synthetic mesh along the axis of the less stretchable side to form a 10-layer tube with 1.5–2 cm in width and secure that tube with a running #5 Ethibond suture

ting of prior periprosthetic joint infection. She undergoes revision to hinged TKA with simultaneous extensor mechanism reconstruction with synthetic mesh reconstruction of her extensor mechanism. A medial parapatellar approach and full thickness of medial and lateral subcutaneous flaps are performed. Intraoperatively, the distal quadriceps tendon, patella, and patellar tendon are necrotic and avascular for a length of 15 cm; there is complete disruption of the lateral collateral ligament at the femoral insertion and extreme internal rotation of tibial component by over 30° (Fig. 53.2). All necrotic tissue is resected, and patellectomy is performed. The revision prosthesis is removed, and the remaining bone is prepared for a cemented rotating hinge over porous cones. Synthetic mesh reconstruction is performed as described by Browne and Hanssen (2011) with the modifications described in the synthetic mesh portion of this chapter (▶ Sect. 53.5.6) for a quadriceps tendon rupture (Figs. 53.3 and 53.4).

Traditionally, after cementation, the synthetic mesh is transfixed with a 6.5 mm cortical screw if there is an implant in place and the synthetic mesh is cemented through the groove in the tibia. However, when the synthetic mesh is placed at the same time as the tibial com-

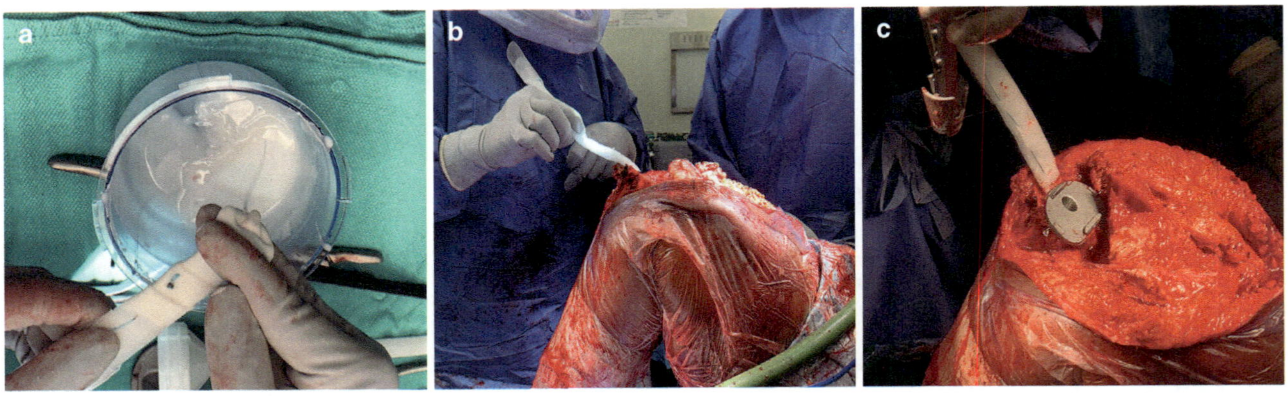

▣ **Fig. 53.4** **a** Lamination of the distal part of synthetic mesh with wet polymethylmethacrylate cement. **b** Insertion of cement-laminated synthetic mesh into the trough in the proximal tibia. **c** Cementation of the tibial component to trap the synthetic mesh within the tibial trough

ponent through a trough, and no screw is utilized. The remnants of lateral retinaculum are identified and interposed between the synthetic mesh and the tibial component to prevent abrasion between the polyethylene insert and the synthetic mesh (▣ Fig. 53.5). The proximal part of the synthetic mesh is then passed under the remnant lateral retinaculum through a tunnel from deep to superficial before being repaired to the vastus lateralis and vastus medialis in a pants-over-vest fashion. The tension of extensor mechanism is set by traction of synthetic mesh proximally and sutured with nonabsorbable #5 Ethibond in the fully extended position (▣ Fig. 53.6).

Postoperatively, the knee is immobilized in extension in a long leg cast, and the patent is made nonweight bearing with only isometric quadriceps exercises for 3 months.

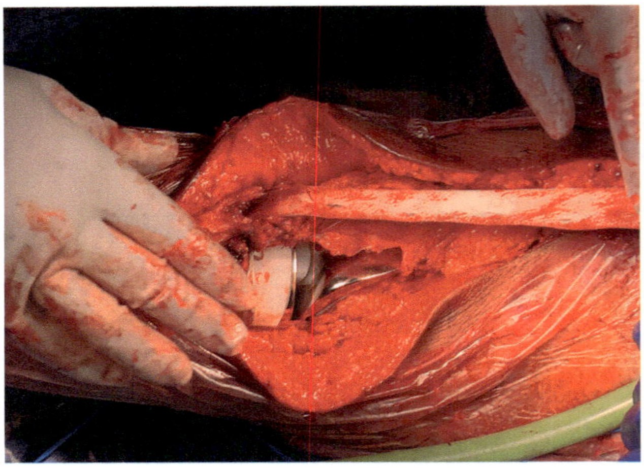

▣ **Fig. 53.5** The proximal part of the synthetic graft is passed through a tunnel in the remnant of lateral retinaculum from deep to superficial layer in order to prevent abrasion between the synthetic mesh and the polyethylene insert when motion ensues after 3 months of immobilization

53.3 Incidence, Etiology, and Risk Factors

The incidence of extensor mechanism disruption after primary TKA is between 0.2% and 2.5% (Schoderbek et al. 2006). Quadriceps tendon ruptures account for 0.1–1.1% of cases (Dobbs et al. 2005; Lynch et al. 1987), patellar tendon ruptures account for 0.2–1.0% of cases (Schoderbek et al. 2006; Lynch et al. 1987; Nam et al. 2014; Papalia et al. 2015; Rand et al. 1989), and patella fractures account for 0.7% of cases. The incidence of an extensor mechanism disruption after revision TKA is 1.8% (Berry 1999).

There are three classes of risk factors associated with an extensor mechanism disruption after TKA:

- Patient factors
- Operative factors
- Postoperative factors

▪ Patient Factors

Patients with multiple knee surgeries prior to TKA have the highest risk of an extensor mechanism disruption when compared to patients with no knee surgery prior to TKA (Crossett et al. 2002; Jaureguito et al. 1997; Nazarian and Booth 1999).

Patella baja is shortening of the patellar tendon. Prolonged casting with knee extension or surgery such as after proximal tibial osteotomy can result in patella baja. Patella baja increases the risk of patella tendon rupture after primary TKA (Nam et al. 2014; Dalury and Dennis 2003).

Long-term systemic glucocorticoid therapy and multiple intra-articular corticosteroid injections are indirectly related to the weakening of tendons and ligaments but have not been directly linked to an

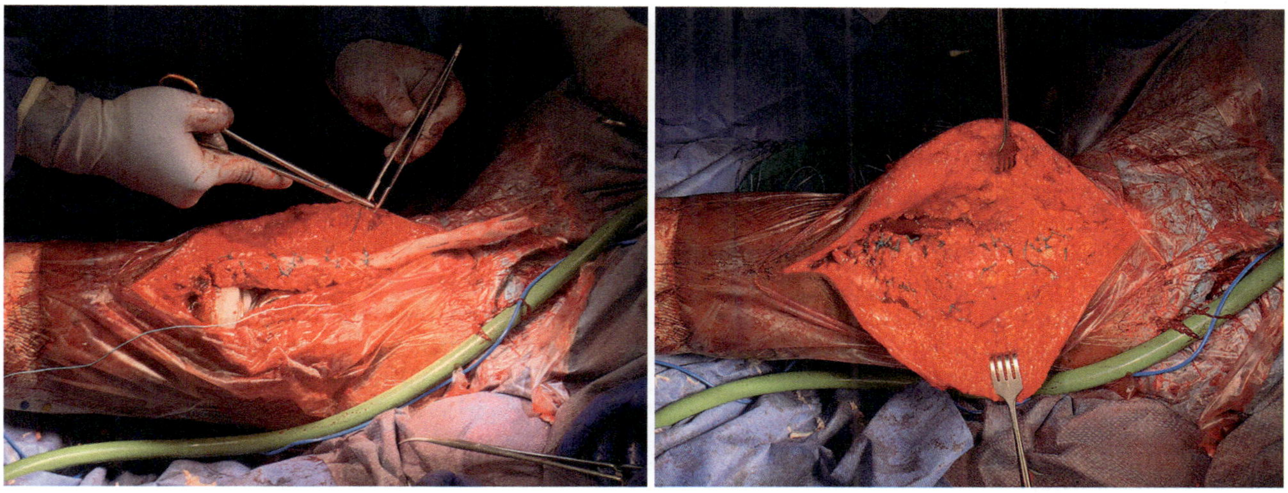

Fig. 53.6 The tension of the extensor mechanism is set in the fully extended knee position, and the proximal part of the synthetic mesh is sutured to the residual quadriceps tendon as well as vastus lateralis and rectus femoris muscles with nonabsorbable #5 Ethibond suture (*left*). The vastus medialis muscle is advanced over the synthetic mesh to cover it in a pants-over-vest fashion (*right*)

increased incidence of extensor mechanism rupture (Dobbs et al. 2005; Lynch et al. 1987; Springer and Della Valle 2008).

> Comorbid diseases, including rheumatoid arthritis, systemic lupus erythematosus, diabetes mellitus, chronic kidney disease, hyperthyroidism, obesity, and osteoporosis, increase the risk of an extensor mechanism rupture or patella fracture after primary TKA (Lynch et al. 1987; Rorabeck et al. 1998; Meding et al. 2008; Sheth et al. 2007).

Intraoperative Factors

Extensive soft tissue dissection during TKA may compromise the blood supply to the extensor mechanism. A V–Y quadriceps turndown or lateral retinacular release of the patella disrupts the superior lateral genicular artery, which may be the only remaining blood supply to the patella after medial parapatellar arthrotomy (Lynch et al. 1987; Pawar et al. 2009; Barrack 1999). Using electrocautery to strip the soft tissue surrounding the patella results in the potential compromise of the patellar vascularity and increases the risk of osteonecrosis and patella fracture (Ortiguera and Berry 2002). Intraoperative patellar tendon ruptures are often found at the tibial tubercle insertion (Nam et al. 2014; Papalia et al. 2015; Pagnano 2003) when excessive traction is performed exposing a stiff knee (Schoderbek et al. 2006; Rand et al. 1989; Dalury and Dennis 2003; Parker et al. 2003) and inadequate lysis of adhesions during exposure, especially during revision TKA (Schoderbek et al. 2006), after proximal tibial osteotomy (Nam et al. 2014; Dalury and Dennis 2003), or prior extensor realignment procedure (Schoderbek et al. 2006; Lynch et al. 1987; Nam et al. 2014; Pagnano 2003; Bates and Springer 2015). Patellar eversion during the exposure of a stiff knee may increase the traction force on the patellar tendon with the knee flexed and initiate a patellar tendon avulsion (Crossett et al. 2002; Nazarian and Booth 1999).

Excessive patellar resection for the purpose of patellar resurfacing increases the risk of a patella fracture (Schoderbek et al. 2006; Nam et al. 2014; Papalia et al. 2015; Parker et al. 2003; Emerson et al. 1994; Lie et al. 2005). Patients whose remaining patellar thickness was 11 mm had higher strain and a greater risk of patella fracture when compared to patients with 13 mm or 16 mm of remaining patellar thickness (Lie et al. 2005). Patients with a patellar thickness of less than 12 mm after TKA increased the risk of a patella fracture by 60% compared to a patellar thickness of 12 mm or greater.

Patellar tilt after TKA may increase the risk of a patella fracture as a result of abnormal eccentric loading within the patellofemoral compartment (Berger et al. 1998; Figgie et al. 1989; Seo et al. 2012). Several case series demonstrate that internal rotation of the femoral or tibial components as well as lateralization of the patellar component increases the load within the patellofemoral joint, increasing the probability of lateral patellar subluxation resulting in disruption of the extensor mechanism or a patella fracture (Crossett et al. 2002; Nazarian and Booth 1999; Seo et al. 2012; Jaureguito et al. 1997).

Postoperative Factors

Extensor mechanism disruption after TKA can develop traumatically after a fall with the knee in a flexed position or without trauma as a result of pathologic muscle or tendon deterioration.

53.4 Diagnosis and Treatment Options

A complete disruption of the extensor mechanism is relatively easy to diagnose because of the presence of a large extensor lag. A patient with a traumatic extensor mechanism disruption often presents with sudden anterior knee pain and swelling after falling with the knee in the flexed position. An extensor lag is present if the patient cannot perform a straight leg raise, but the knee can be extended passively. A palpable gap in the extensor mechanism can usually be felt at the location of pain and swelling.

Incomplete disruption of the extensor mechanism is often more difficult to diagnose because the deficit may only be present when patients perform activities such as climbing stairs or walking. The physical examination may reveal anterior knee pain, swelling, poor quadriceps strength, or a mild extensor lag.

Anterior-to-posterior, lateral with 30° of flexion, and patellar skyline radiographic views can be diagnostic for a patella fracture or tendon rupture when compared to the normal side. The Insall–Salvati ratio measures the ratio between the length of patellar tendon (LT) and the diagonal length of patella (LP). If the value of LT/LP is >1.2, this indicates patella alta, which occurs after a patellar tendon tear. If the LT/LP value is <0.8, this indicates patella baja, but may not be evident with a quadriceps tendon tear. The skyline view indicates the thickness of patellar bone stock, the alignment of patellar component within the trochlear groove, and patella tilt from an incomplete rupture at the insertion of the vastus medialis obliquus muscle.

Ultrasound or magnetic resonance imaging (MRI) can help in diagnosing an incomplete patellar or quadriceps tendon rupture. However, it should be noted that ultrasound is operator-dependent, and MRI without metal suppression techniques can be difficult to interpret due to metal artifacts.

> The treatment of an extensor mechanism disruption depends on the anatomical position of the disruption (patellar tendon, patella fracture, and quadriceps tendon), the time of the disruption (intraoperative or postoperative), and the extent of the extensor lag (complete or incomplete).

53.5 Patellar Tendon Rupture

An intraoperative patellar tendon rupture occurs during the exposure of a stiff knee. Direct repair of the patellar tendon through drill holes, staple fixation, or suturing anchors will not provide enough strength. Direct repair without augmentation will result in extension lag and a high re-rupture rate (Schoderbek et al. 2006; Rand et al. 1989; Browne and Hanssen 2011). There are many augmentation techniques, including auto- and allograft tendon, local muscle transfer, and synthetic mesh.

> Reconstruction is the gold standard for treating acute or chronic complete postoperative patella tendon rupture.

There is also no role for direct repair of acute or chronic complete postoperative disruptions alone because of the significant proximal retraction of the patella from the force of quadriceps combined with devascularization of the soft tissues.

Patellar Tendon Rupture—Reconstructive Treatment Options

- Semitendinosus with or without gracilis tendon autograft (Rand et al. 1989; Cadambi and Engh 1992; Järvelä et al. 2005)
- Medial gastrocnemius flap (Jaureguito et al. 1997; Busfield et al. 2004)
- Achilles tendon allograft (Crossett et al. 2002; Nazarian and Booth 1999; Parker et al. 2003; Emerson et al. 1994; Lim et al. 2017; Ares et al. 2014; Diaz-Ledezma et al. 2014; Barrack et al. 2003; Burnett et al. 2006; Emerson et al. 1990; Rosenberg 2012; Leopold et al. 1999)
- Extensor mechanism allograft (Crossett et al. 2002; Nazarian and Booth 1999; Parker et al. 2003; Emerson et al. 1990, 1994; Lim et al. 2017; Ares et al. 2014; Diaz-Ledezma et al. 2014; Barrack et al. 2003; Burnett et al. 2006; Rosenberg 2012; Leopold et al. 1999)
- Synthetic mesh (Jaureguito et al. 1997; Busfield et al. 2004; Browne and Hanssen 2011; Aracil et al. 1999; Fernandez-Baillo et al. 1993; Fujikawa et al. 1994; Fukuta et al. 2003)

53.5.1 Nonoperative Management

Nonoperative management of complete extensor mechanism disruptions commonly results in unsatisfactory outcomes (Rand et al. 1989). However, nonoperative treatment by immobilization with a knee brace that locks in extension may be considered in elderly, sedentary patients who have low functional demands, patients that are dependent on gait aids, or poor candidates for the surgical treatment.

Incomplete postoperative patellar tendon ruptures that do not have an extensor lag indicate that the surrounding retinaculum is intact and can be treated nonoperatively by immobilization with a long leg cast or locked hinged brace for 8–12 weeks and a nonweight-bearing interval for at least 8 weeks with isometric quadriceps exercise. After 8 weeks, the cast can be removed, and the patient can begin with an active motion from 0° to 30° in the hinged knee brace. The range of motion can be increased within the knee brace in 30° increments every 2 weeks until motion exceeds 90°.

53.5.2 Semitendinosus Tendon Autograft

The semitendinosus muscle originates from the ischial tuberosity, and its distal tendon inserts at the pes anserinus. Cadambi et al. (Cadambi and Engh 1992) reported augmenting a direct repair of the patellar tendon by using autograft semitendinosus tendon. A tendon stripper is used to harvest the distal tendinous portion of the semitendinosus through a posteromedial incision after exposure of the semitendinosus insertion by elevating the sartorius fascia. After autograft harvest, a 0.625 cm (1/4 inch) hole is drilled horizontally across the lower pole of the patella.

> Care is taken to not disturb the patellar component, if present.

The proximal autograft is inserted through the transverse patellar bone drill hole from the medial to lateral side. After autograft passage, the residual autograft is sutured back to the semitendinosus insertion to form a reinforced triangle (Fig. 53.7a).

When the length of the semitendinosus tendon is insufficient for reconstruction, the proximal end of the gracilis tendon from midthigh can be detached to lengthen and support the semitendinosus tendon graft by suturing it to the residual semitendinosus insertion on the lateral aspect of the patella to complete the triangle.

If there is no bone space for a drill hole through the patella, the autograft can be passed through the quadriceps tendon. However, this may induce patellar tilt by retracting the proximal pole of the patella. To compensate, the surgeon may advance the vastus medialis muscle and medial quadriceps tendon to reinforce the reconstruction and correct any patellar tilt.

The tension of the autograft should be reconstructed when the patella is aligned at the top of the femoral flange and centered in the trochlear groove with the knee in full extension. Autograft augmentation of the patellar tendon has satisfactory outcomes with a mean residual extension lag of 4° and a mean knee flexion of 80° (Cadambi and Engh 1992).

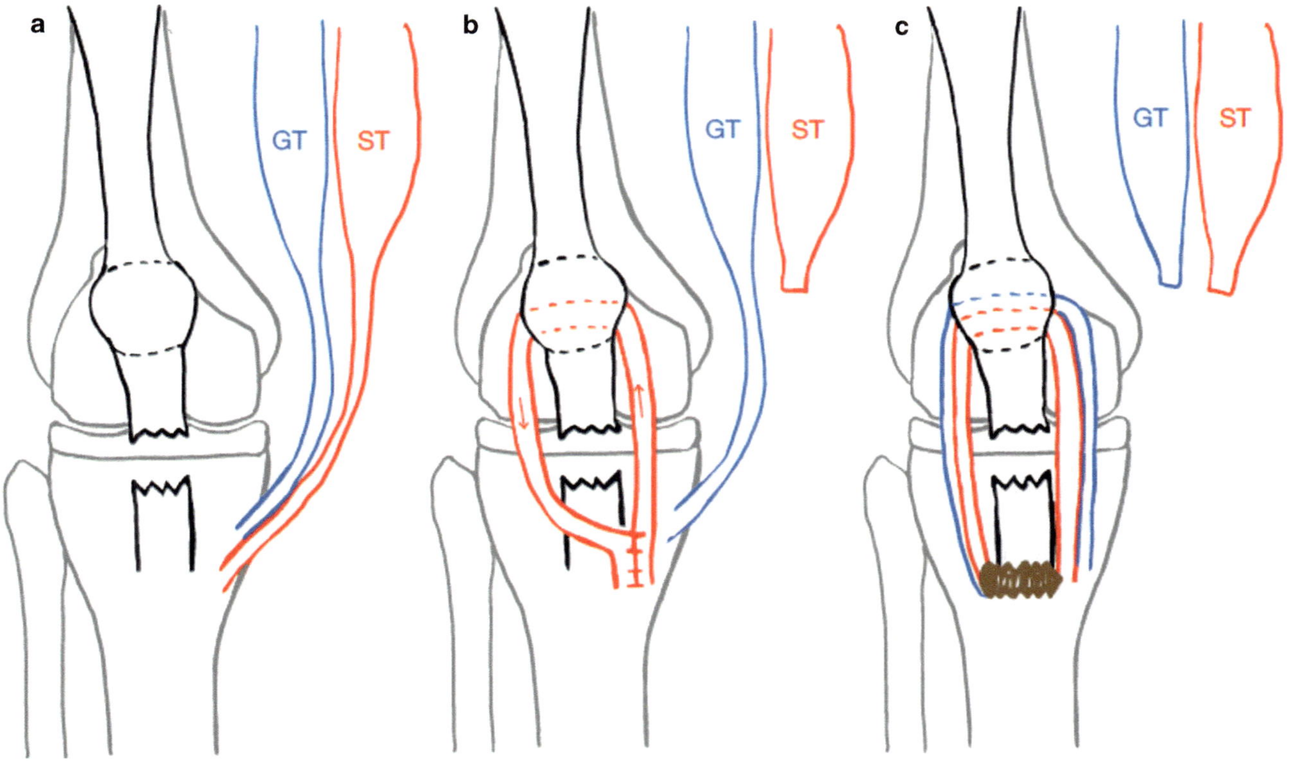

Fig. 53.7 **a** Illustration of the anterior aspect of the knee with patellar tendon rupture after TKA. **b** The semitendinosus tendon (*ST*) is harvested to augment the patellar tendon as described by Cadambi and Engh (1992). **c** The semitendinosus (*ST*) and gracilis tendons (*GT*) are harvested and fixed with an interference screw and tibial tunnel as described by Jarvela (Jarvela et al. 2005)

However, since Cadambi et al. (Cadambi and Engh 1992) described this method, there is only a case report from Jarvela et al. (2005), who augmented the patellar tendon with dual semitendinosus and gracilis tendons. After the dual grafts were passed through the patellar tunnel, they were secured to the tibia through a lateral-to-medial tunnel with an interference screw and staple. This modified technique, at 1 year, had no extension lag and a mean postoperative knee flexion of 80° (◘ Fig. 53.7b).

53.5.3 Medial Myofascial Gastrocnemius Rotational Flap

A medial gastrocnemius flap may be used to provide soft tissue coverage to the anterior medial knee and reinforce a disrupted patellar tendon. Jaureguito et al. (1997) first described using a medial gastrocnemius flap technique for extensor mechanism reconstruction. The distal end of the medial gastrocnemius muscle is detached from the intermuscular septum and Achilles tendon at the musculotendinous junction. The medial branch of the sural artery, which is the main blood supply of the medial gastrocnemius flap, should be preserved during surgical dissection. The myofascial flap is rotated transversely to cover the anteromedial tibia. The distal part of the flap is sutured to the anterior compartment fascia and the remnant of the patellar tendon (◘ Fig. 53.8a).

> This technique is reserved for patients who still have a patella and the adequate length of the remaining patella tendon to suture with the flap.

When the patient has a large defect and there is insufficient patellar tendon or patellar bone for reconstruction, the surgeon might choose to detach additional Achilles tendon by using an extended medial gastrocnemius flap by detaching a third to a half of the Achilles tendon (Jaureguito et al. 1997; Chiou et al. 1997) and rotate it with the medial gastrocnemius flap for additional coverage (◘ Fig. 53.8b).

The tension of the flap should be set when the patella is aligned at the top of the femoral flange and centered in the trochlear groove with the knee in full extension. Any soft tissue defect can be temporized with a negative pressure dressing or closed with a split-thickness skin graft.

Jaureguito et al. (1997) reported a mean residual extensor lag of 24° ± 19°. However, Busfield et al. (2004) reported more encouraging results with a mean residual extensor lag of 11°. Hence, this technique is commonly reserved for salvage procedures after multiple revision surgery (Jaureguito et al. 1997; Busfield et al. 2004) or failed allograft reconstruction (Burnett et al. 2006; Leopold et al. 1999).

53.5.4 Achilles Tendon Allograft

Allograft Achilles tendon reconstruction was originally introduced by Crossett et al. (2002). This method requires an intact patella or a smaller defect where the patella can be advanced (Jaureguito et al. 1997; Busfield et al. 2004).

> This technique is suitable for both intra- and postoperative patellar tendon ruptures.

The author's surgical technique (Jaureguito et al. 1997) begins with a medial parapatellar arthrotomy and the development of full-thickness medial and lateral flaps. The position and stability of the prosthesis are evaluated and revised, if necessary. Then, a rectangular keystone groove (2.5 cm in length, 1.5 cm in width, and 1 cm in thickness) is made with a round-tipped burr or small oscillating saw in the proximal tibial crest slightly distal and medial to the tibial tubercle. A fresh-frozen Achilles tendon allograft is then prepared. The calcaneal bone block of the Achilles tendon allograft is shaped to match the keystone groove in the tibia. One of many techniques may be selected to attach the calcaneal bone block to the tibial groove, including 4.5 mm malleolar or 6.5 mm cancellous screws or 18 g wires (Pawar et al. 2009; Browne and Hanssen 2011; Cadambi and Engh 1992; Lim et al. 2017; Fukuta et al. 2003; Chiou et al. 1997). The arthrotomy is closed, and the Achilles tendon is sutured over to the patella tendon with non-absorbent #5 Fiberwire suture with simple or running Krakow technique (◘ Fig. 53.9). The tension of the allograft should be reconstructed with the patella aligned at the top of the femoral flange and centered in the trochlear groove with the knee in full extension.

Crossett et al. (2002) reported the mean knee range of motion increased from 80° to 107° with Achilles tendon allograft patellar tendon reconstruction. Six of nine patients were able to fully extend the knee, and the mean residual extensor lag decreased from 44° to 3°.

Ares et al. (2014) reported a modified double-bundle Achilles allograft reconstruction technique in five patients diagnosed with a chronic postoperative patellar tendon rupture. The Achilles tendon allograft was divided into two bundles and crossed over at the patellar insertion of the quadriceps tendon. The calcaneal bone block was beveled at 45° (from anterior to posterior) to prevent superior displacement of the bone

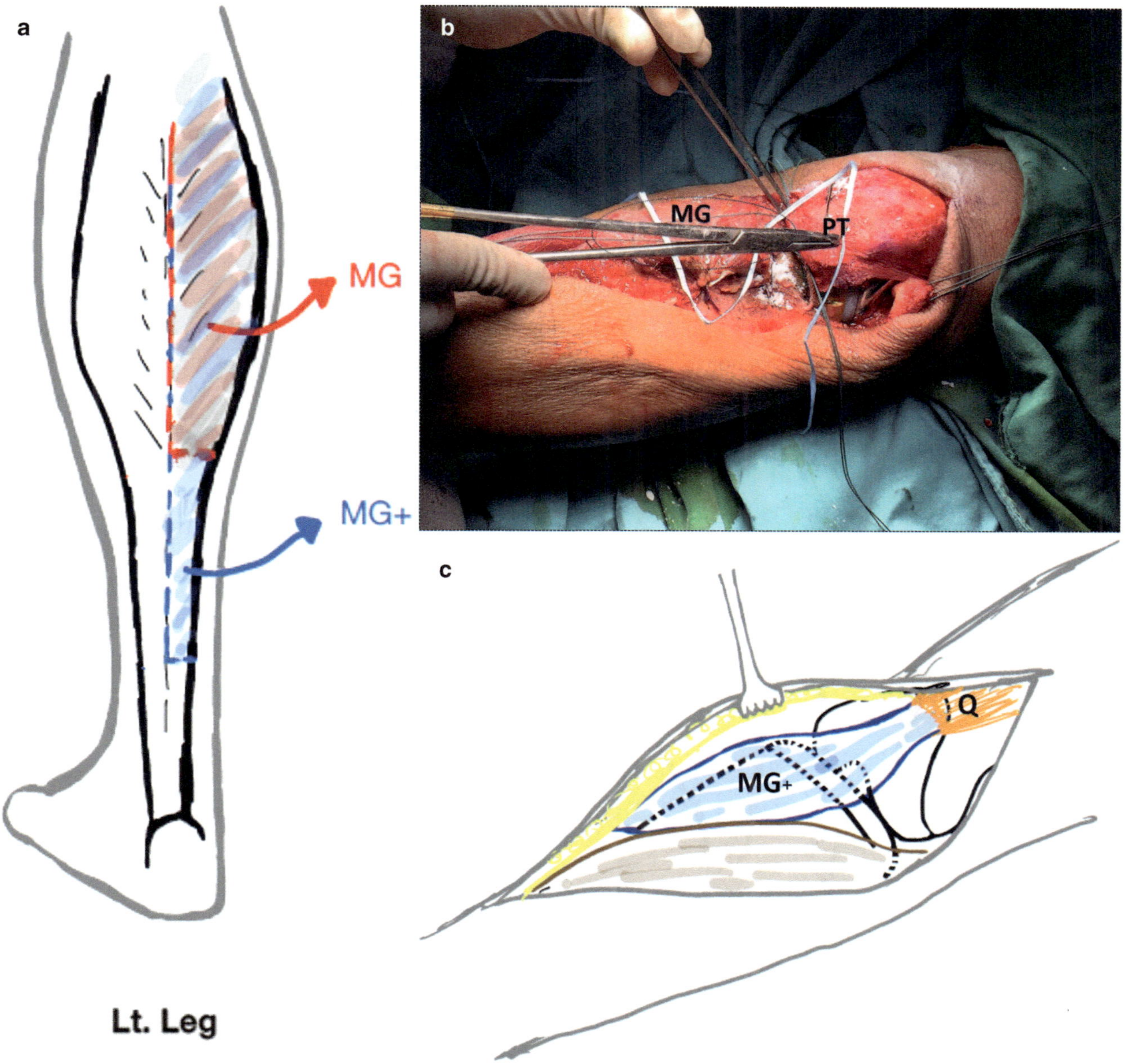

Fig. 53.8 **a–c** Illustration of the posterior aspect of left leg and the anterolateral aspect of left knee. **a, b** The medial gastrocnemius flap (*MG*) (at the musculotendinous junction) is rotated transversely to cover the anteromedial tibia, and the distal part of the flap is sutured to the anterior compartment fascia and the remnant of patellar tendon (*PT*). **c** An extended medial gastrocnemius flap (*MG+* = MG with half of the Achilles tendon) is rotated transversely to cover the anteromedial knee, and the distal part of the flap is sutured to the remnant of quadriceps muscle or tendon (*Q*)

block. Ares et al. (2014) reported that all patients discontinued using an ambulatory assistive gait aid. The mean knee flexion was 102°, and the residual extensor lag was just over 1° at 1 year.

Diaz-Ledezma et al. (2014) reported a large case series of ten Achilles tendon allograft reconstructions of chronic postoperative patellar tendon rupture with a short immobilization program (reduced to 3 weeks). The success rate was unsatisfactory (50%—three repeat mechanical failures and two infections).

> The authors advise immobilizing the knee in full extension until allograft incorporation with host bone and close monitoring for late infection.

53.5.5 Extensor Mechanism Allograft

Whole extensor mechanism allograft is used in chronic postoperative patellar tendon ruptures with a damaged patella or a large soft tissue defect where the patella cannot be manipulated to within 3–4 cm of the joint line (Springer and Della Valle 2008).

The author's surgical technique (Lim et al. 2017) for preparation of tibial bone block and postoperative rehabilitation protocol are similar to Achilles tendon allograft reconstruction (▶ Sect. 53.5.4).

> Fresh-frozen allograft is recommended because it has higher mechanical strength and lower antigenicity (Emerson et al. 1994). Freeze-dried allograft is to be avoided.

For proximal soft tissue reconstruction, nonabsorbable #5 Fiberwire suture is recommended to suture the allograft below the host quadriceps in a pants-over-vest fashion (e.g., the medial and lateral retinaculum are sutured to cover the allograft) (Nazarian and Booth 1999; Lim et al. 2017). Patellar resurfacing should be avoided in conjunction with extensor mechanism allograft (◘ Fig. 53.10).

Emerson et al. (1994) first reported using the whole extensor mechanism allograft technique to treat a gap in the patellar tendon or an unfixable patellar fracture. They originally suggested setting the tension for allograft in 60° of knee flexion. Nazarian and Booth (1999) suggested setting the allograft tension in full extension with a locked hinge knee brace or a well-padded long leg cast, including foot. At a mean 4-year follow-up, whole extensor mechanism allograft patellar tendon reconstruction had a mean knee flexion of 98°, and 21 of 36 patients could fully extend their knees, and the 15 patients who could not had a mean residual extension lag of 13°.

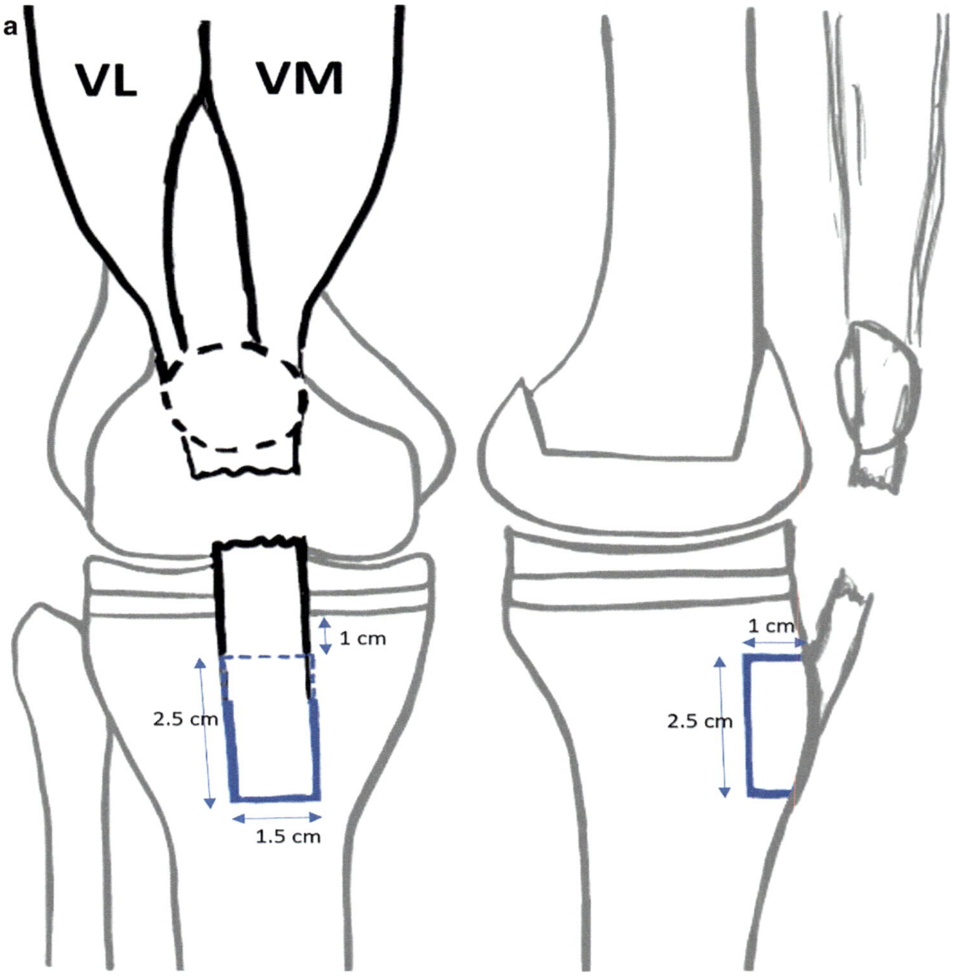

◘ **Fig. 53.9** **a, b** Achilles tendon allograft reconstruction. **a** A rectangular keystone groove (approx. Length 2.5 cm, approx. Width 1.5 cm, approx. Depth 1 cm) is burred to accept the Achilles tendon bone block. Preservation of proximal tibial bone stock (approx. 1 cm) above the keystone will help prevent proximal migration of bone block. **b** The Achilles tendon bone block is secured into the keystone with a bicortical lag screw and/or tensioned 18 g wires. The soft tissue portion of the Achilles tendon allograft (*AT*) is sewn to the residual host patellar tendon, quadriceps tendon, and vastus lateralis (*VL*) with nonabsorbable suture. The vastus medialis (*VM*) is advanced over the top of the Achilles tendon allograft (*AT*), creating a soft tissue casing around allograft (a.k.a., pants-over-vest)

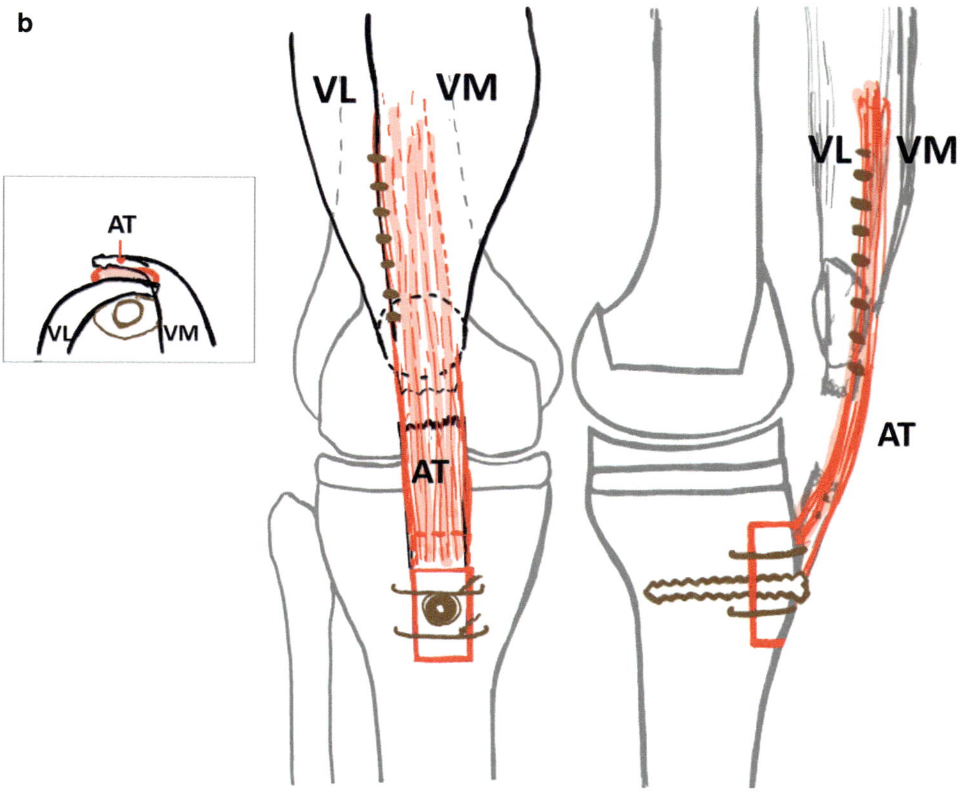

Fig. 53.9 (continued)

Brown et al. (2015) reported a large case series of 50 patients who underwent whole extensor mechanism allograft reconstruction for chronic extensor mechanism failure. They found a 38% failure rate—four for allograft failure (three for recurrent instability from graft stretching, one for an extensor mechanism rupture), five for deep infection, and ten for an extensor lag over 30°or a Knee Society score <60. Whole extensor mechanism allograft survival was 56% at 10 years.

53.5.6 Synthetic Mesh

Recently, the synthetic mesh has been used for extensor mechanism reconstruction carrying no concerning issues of donor soft tissue insufficiency, graft resorption, or disease transmission. Browne and Hanssen (2011) proposed the classical technique of extensor mechanism reconstruction using knitted monofilament polypropylene heavy-weight mesh (Marlex mesh™, C.R. Bard, Murray Hill, New Jersey, USA). The surgical technique begins with a medial parapatellar arthrotomy and the development of full thickness of medial and lateral subcutaneous flaps. The synthetic mesh (25 cm wide and 35.5 cm long) is rolled into an 8- to 10-layer tube about 2 cm in wide.

> Care must be taken to roll the mesh with the less stretchable side forming the long axis of the tube.

The synthetic mesh is sutured together with a running #5 Fiberwire. Next, a 2.5-cm trough is cut about 5–7 cm deep into the tibia just proximal to the tibial tubercle with a pencil-tipped burr. The distal part of the synthetic mesh is laminated with wet polymethylmethacrylate cement. Polymethylmethacrylate cement is then inserted into the tibial trough. The cement-laminated synthetic mesh is inserted into the trough, and the cement is allowed to cure.

After cementation, the synthetic mesh is transfixed with a 6.5 mm cortical screw placed through the tibia, cement, and synthetic mesh but avoiding the implant. A fibrous tissue flap or retinaculum is interposed between the synthetic mesh and the tibial component to prevent deterioration of the polyethylene insert or rupture of the synthetic mesh with a range of motion. A tunnel is created in the lateral retinaculum, and the proximal end of the synthetic mesh is then passed under the patellar tendon remnant through a tunnel from deep to superficial before being fixed to the host extensor mechanism in a pants-over-vest fashion. Patellar height is restored by placing traction on the synthetic mesh cranially while simultaneously pulling the residual patellar tendon,

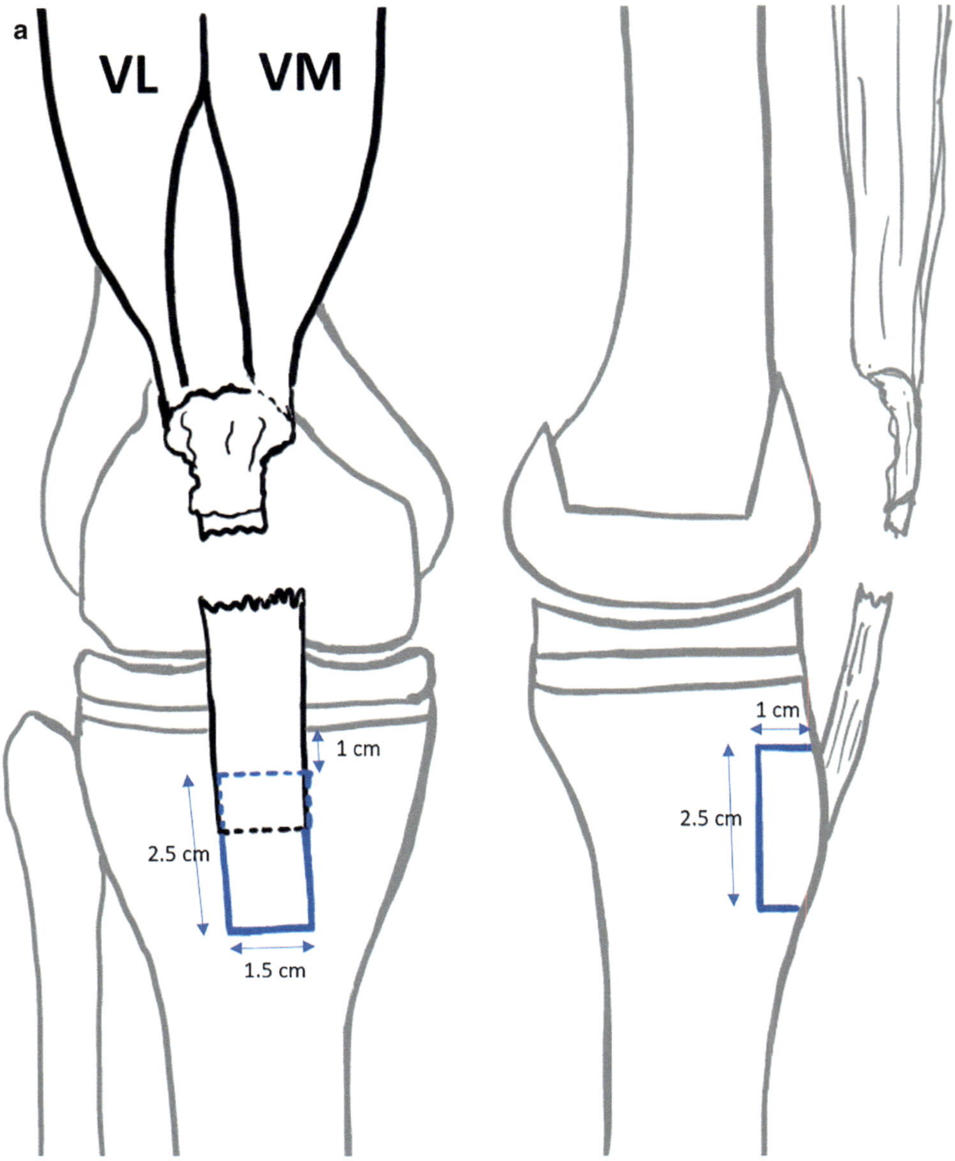

Fig. 53.10 **a, b** Whole extensor mechanism reconstruction. **a** A rectangular keystone groove (approx. Length 2.5 cm, approx. Width 1.5 cm, approx. Depth 1 cm) is burred to accept the tibial bone block. Preservation of proximal tibial bone stock (approx. 1 cm) above the keystone will help prevent proximal migration of bone block. **b** The tibial bone block is secured into the keystone with a bicortical lag screw and/or tensioned 18 g wires. The soft tissue portion of the extensor mechanism allograft (*EM*) is sewn to the residual quadriceps tendon and vastus lateralis (*VL*) with nonabsorbable suture. The vastus medialis (*VM*) is advanced over the top of the extensor mechanism allograft (*EM*), creating a soft tissue casing around allograft (a.k.a., pants-over-vest)

patella, and quadriceps distally. The proximal end of the synthetic mesh is sutured to the remaining quadriceps tendon and vastus lateralis fascia with the knee in full extension with nonabsorbable #5 Fiberwire that traverses the mesh and endogenous extensor mechanism with each interrupted suture. Once the synthetic mesh has been secured to the quadriceps tendon and vastus lateralis muscle, the vastus medialis muscle is sutured over the synthetic mesh with nonabsorbable #5 Fiberwire that traverses the mesh and vastus medialis fascia with each interrupted suture. Hence, the synthetic mesh is interposed between the vastus lateralis and medialis muscles (Fig. 53.11).

Browne and Hanssen (2011) reported outcomes of synthetic mesh graft reconstruction of patellar tendon rupture with a mean follow-up of 4 years, the mean knee flexion increased from 103° to 107°, and the mean extension lag was reduced from 36° to 10°. The successful cases comprised 9 out of 13 cases who had significant improvement of functional scores and had no progressive extension lag at final follow-up. Recently, a multicenter cohort study reported outcomes of synthetic reconstruction of

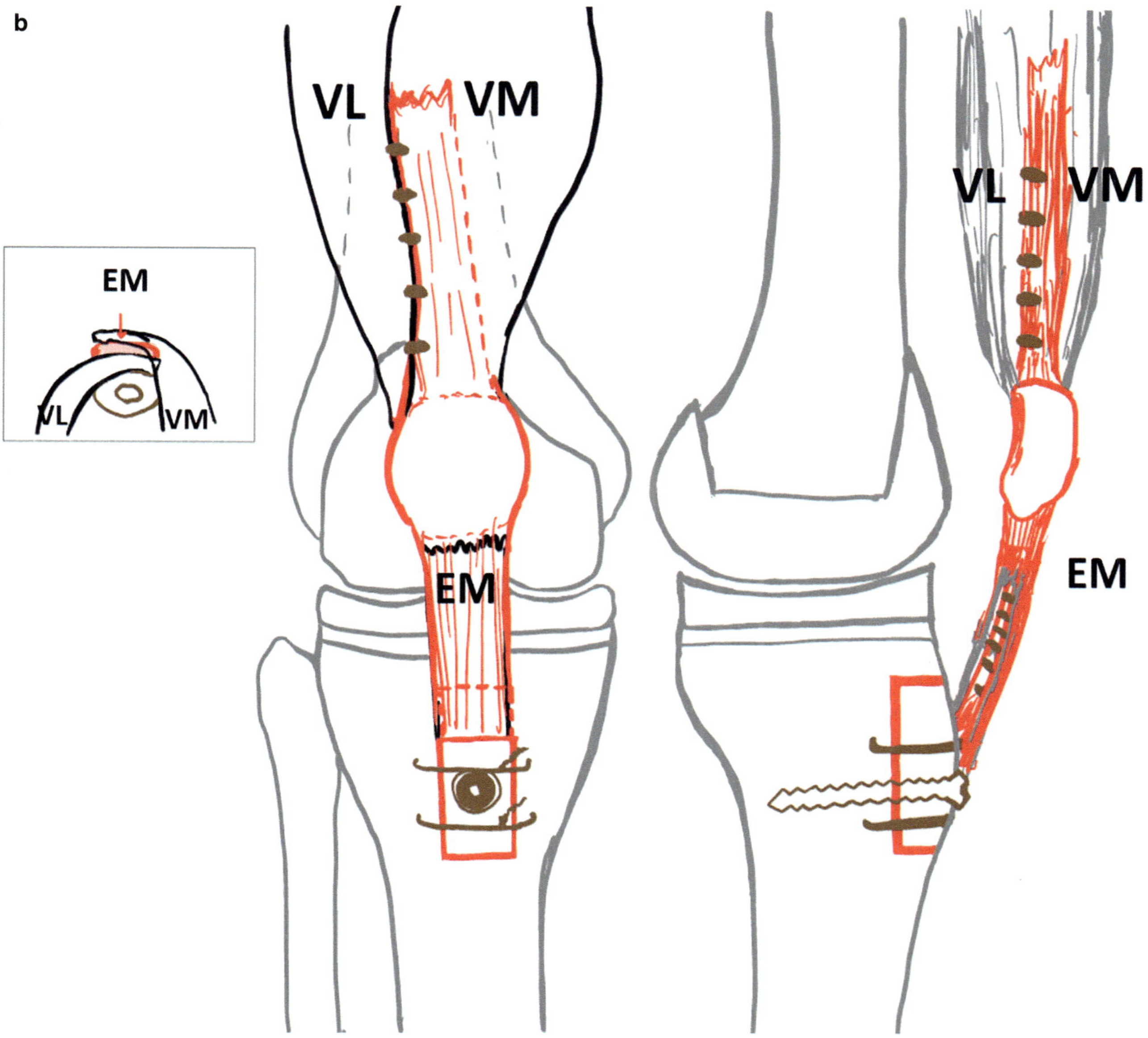

Fig. 53.10 (continued)

13 knees following TKA (Wood et al. 2019). After the mean follow-up of 3 years, the mean extension lag was improved from 45° to 14°, and the mean postoperative knee flexion was 95°. No graft failures were reported, and 62% of patients were able to ambulate without ambulatory aids at final follow-up. However, the infection rate after synthetic reconstruction was 15% (2 of 13 cases) and subsequently required revision surgery in this study.

53.6 Patella Fracture

Patella fractures occur from direct trauma after an accident or from contraction of the quadriceps during hyperflexion (e.g., manipulation under anesthesia). Direct repair of the patella fracture with screws and/or wires will not provide enough strength in the setting of a prior patellar prosthetic resurfacing. Fixation without augmentation will result in extension lag and a high nonunion rate (Schoderbek et al. 2006; Rand et al. 1989; Browne and Hanssen 2011). There are many augmentation techniques, including auto- and allograft tendon as well as synthetic mesh.

> The management of patella fractures can be categorized into conservative and surgical treatment.

There are three main factors to evaluate with regard to guiding treatment options:
- The stability of patellar component
- The function of the extensor mechanism
- The quality of the remaining bone stock

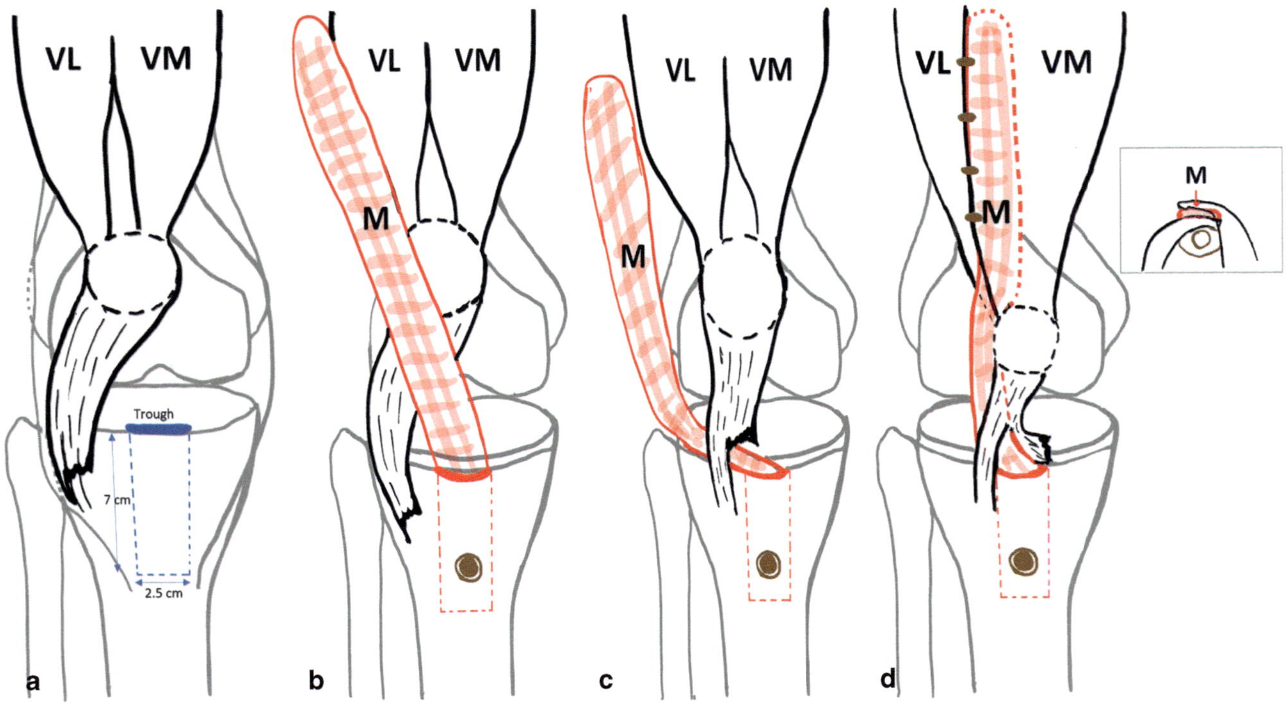

Fig. 53.11 **a–d** Synthetic mesh reconstruction. **a** A groove or trough (approx. Length 2.5 cm, approx. Depth 7 cm) is burred into the proximal tibia just above the tibial tubercle. **b** The synthetic mesh is cemented into that trough and transfixed with a screw once the cement has hardened. **c** The proximal end of the synthetic mesh is passed through a tunnel in the lateral retinaculum or patellar tendon from deep to superficial layer to place soft tissue between the mesh and the tibial component and polyethylene insert to avoid abrading the mesh when motion begins. **d** The reconstruction of the proximal end of the synthetic mesh is sewn to the residual patellar tendon, quadriceps tendon, and vastus lateralis (*VL*) with nonabsorbable suture. The vastus medialis (*VM*) is advanced over the top of the synthetic mesh creating a soft tissue casing around the synthetic mesh (a.k.a., pants-over-vest)

Ortiguera and Berry (2002) proposed a classification for guideline of patellar fractures in the setting of prior patellar resurfacing:

- Type 1: implant stable and extensor mechanism intact
- Type 2: implant stable and extensor mechanism disrupted
- Type 3A: implant loose with good bone stock
- Type 3B: implant loose with poor bone stock

Nonoperative management is restricted to *type 1* patella fractures and consists of 6–12 weeks of immobilization in extension with a locked hinged knee brace or a well-padded long leg cast including foot prior to a progressive range of motion. Weight bearing is permittable for type 1 fractures in patients who are able to perform a straight leg raise. Ortiguera and Berry reported 97% of bone union rate and satisfactory clinical outcome with conservative treatment in type 1 fracture.

Type 2 patella fractures leave the patient unable to fully extend the knee with an extension lag of more than 20°. Conservative treatment will fail, and surgical treatment is recommended for type 2 patella fractures. The remaining patellar bone is too thin and avascular for open reduction and internal fixation with screw or wiring. Hence, fixation is impractical. One option is removal of small boney fragments and attachment of the quadriceps or patellar tendon to the remaining bone by using a pull-through suture technique. The strength of attachment should be tested; if the suture is unstable after knee flexion less than 75°, tendon auto- or allograft reinforcement should be considered (Engh and Ammeen 1998). The complication rates of *type 2* patella fracture after open reduction and fixation is 50%, and the reoperation rate is 42%. Complications include nonunion, infection, and ipsilateral patella tendon rupture (Meding et al. 2008; Ortiguera and Berry 2002; Parker et al. 2003), which suggests the quality of remaining host bone and insufficiency of peripatellar blood supply as etiologies; hence, the authors would advise against any attempts to repair *type 2* patella fractures and instead proceed to extensor mechanism reconstruction with allograft or synthetic mesh (see reconstruction techniques in chronic patellar tendon rupture, ▶ Sect. 53.5).

Treatment of *type 3* patella fractures depends on the remaining bone stock. In cases with sufficient bone stock >10 mm, the patella can be resurfaced. However, in cases with insufficient bone stock <10 mm, there are various resurfacing options including biconvex patellar components, porous tantalum patellar augmentation, gullwing patelloplasty, or patellar bone grafting. However, resurfacing the patellar component may increase the risk of nonunion as a result of cement-induced thermal necrosis or cement penetration into the fracture site. In the case of comminution, a partial or complete patellectomy and suturing the remaining tendon with allograft or synthetic mesh augmentation are preferred (Chang et al. 2005). The complication rate for type 3 patellar fractures is 45%, including a 20% chance of reoperation (Ortiguera and Berry 2002).

53.7 Quadriceps Tendon Rupture

The incidence of quadriceps tendon rupture is less than that of patellar tendon rupture. Previous history of V–Y turndown, quadriceps snip, and over-resection of the patella are reported to be specific risk factors (Lynch et al. 1987; Parker et al. 2003). Quadriceps tendon rupture is often associated with post-traumatic injury and may be difficult to diagnose because the low alignment level of the patella is not usually found in radiographs. In some cases, patellar tilt could be found in skyline view, which represents a partial quadriceps tendon rupture.

Physical examination should concentrate on finding irregular soft tissue gaps, abnormal patellar tilting, and the strength of extensor mechanism when patients perform active knee extension against gravity. If patients cannot fully extend the knee, ultrasound or MRI should be requested to confirm the rupture.

> The treatment of quadriceps tendon rupture can be categorized according to the function of the remaining tendon.

For patients who are still able to perform active knee extension with an extension lag of <20° (partial rupture), nonoperative management with immobilization of the knee in full extension for 6–8 weeks can be considered (Dobbs et al. 2005; Bonnin et al. 2016), followed by gradual rehabilitation. For patients who have an extension lag of >20° (complete rupture), surgical treatment should be considered (Rosenberg 2012) because quadriceps weakness adversely affects the efficiency of the knee extensor mechanism and increases the chance of knee instability leading to falls.

Dobbs et al. (2005) reported treatment outcomes in patients who had quadriceps tendon rupture postoperatively. Seven patients with partial rupture (extension lag <20°) who received conservative treatment had all successful outcomes. With patients who had a complete rupture (extension lag >20°) and received surgical treatment with direct tendon repair, only four out of ten cases had satisfactory outcomes. As a result of isolated direct repair, the construction was not strong enough due to the 33–36% rate of re-rupture (Dobbs et al. 2005; Lynch et al. 1987). Therefore, additional augmentation techniques should be considered.

However, a recent study (Chhapan et al. 2018) reported 10 quadriceps tendon ruptures (7 complete ruptures vs. 3 partial ruptures) in 7 patients who sustained rupture within 90 days of primary TKA; early primary repair was performed in all cases. All patients achieved their preoperative range of motion without extension lag or restriction in range of movement within 6 months of repair of the quadriceps tendon.

Quadriceps tendon reconstruction can be performed by debridement of the fraying tissues. Then, the quadriceps tendon is detached and pulled down to an anatomical position and sutured to the patella with nonabsorbable suture in the extended knee position. Additional augmentation could be done by various techniques, including semitendinosus tendon and gracilis autograft (Pagnano 2003), Achilles or whole extensor mechanism allograft (Nazarian and Booth 1999; Diaz-Ledezma et al. 2014), and synthetic mesh (Abdel et al. 2018) (see reconstruction techniques in patellar tendon rupture, ► Sect. 53.5).

53.8 Rehabilitation Protocol Following Extensor Mechanism Reconstruction

The knee should be immobilized in full extension with a well-padded long leg cast, including the foot (Nazarian and Booth 1999). The patient should be nonweight bearing for at least 6 weeks with isometric quadriceps exercise. After 6 weeks, the cast can be removed and the patient can begin active motion from 0° to 30° in a hinged knee brace, but weight bearing is restricted for 6 more weeks. The range of motion can be increased within the knee brace in 30° increments every 2 weeks until motion exceeds 90°. Once beyond 90°, the hinged knee brace can be discarded and weight bearing and passive flexion can be resumed.

53.9 Outcome of Extensor Mechanism Disruption After TKA

> For the treatment of patellar tendon rupture after TKA, isolated direct repair should be avoided because of the high rate of complications.

Courtney et al. (2018) reported the largest case series comparing direct repair (58 patients) and allograft reconstruction (68 patients) for treatment of extensor mechanism rupture. The results showed that patellar tendon repair had the highest rate of poor outcomes compared to quadriceps repair and patellar fixation (63% vs. 22% vs 8%, $P = 0.002$). The most recent systemic review showed the complication rate after repair of patellar tendon (63%) was higher than the complication rate after repair of the quadriceps tendon (25%) (Vajapey et al. 2019). The complication rates for patellar and quadriceps tendon tears after autograft, allograft, or synthetic mesh reconstruction were similar (18% vs. 19%, respectively) (Courtney et al. 2018). The most common complication after extensor mechanism repair or reconstruction was an extension lag of 30° or greater (45%) (Courtney et al. 2018).

> For the treatment of quadriceps tendon rupture after TKA, partial tear or an extension lag of <20° could be treated with conservative treatment with a satisfactory outcome (Dobbs et al. 2005). Conversely, in the case of complete rupture (extension lag >20°), direct repair has shown a success rate of only 33–36% (Dobbs et al. 2005; Lynch et al. 1987).

Quadriceps tendon reconstruction with various techniques is recommended to reduce complications, especially re-rupture. However, from a recent published study, early identification (within 90 days) of quadriceps tendon rupture and direct repair followed by controlled postoperative rehabilitation could be another satisfactory option and showed excellent short-term and mid-term outcomes (Chhapan et al. 2018).

53.10 Authors' Preferred Approach

In the authors' opinion, *allograft* use for extensor mechanism reconstruction remains an option. There is no consensus in the literature as to the type of extensor mechanism reconstruction that yields the best results. Achilles tendon allograft reconstruction has been the gold standard for late patellar and quadriceps tendon reconstruction. Numerous studies in the past have shown acceptable results (Vajapey et al. 2019). Lim et al. reported 16 patients who underwent allograft extensor mechanism reconstruction at a mean 3-year follow-up (Lim et al. 2017), and 12 patients received Achilles tendon allograft and 4 patients received whole extensor tendon reconstruction. Patients had statistically significant improvements in the Knee Society score (both pain and function) and reduction in mean extensor lag from 35° preoperatively to 14° at final follow-up. However, 5 cases (31%) developed a recurrent extensor lag greater than 30° or had revision surgery. Hence, allograft using for extensor mechanism reconstruction remains a reasonable choice with moderate outcomes for a devastating injury. The *autograft* technique is suitable when the host tissue is competent, particularly when dealing with younger patients or postinfection. A full extensor mechanism allograft may represent a reliable solution when the defect involves the patella bone or the quadriceps tendon (Lamberti et al. 2018).

Synthetic mesh use for extensor mechanism reconstruction also reported satisfactory results especially from the largest case series of mesh graft reconstruction in 77 patients. After the mean follow-up of 4 years, 84% of the mesh reconstructions remained intact and the functional outcomes were excellent. The average extension lag was improved from 35° to 9° (Abdel et al. 2018).

> A recent systemic review comparing outcomes between synthetic mesh and allograft extensor mechanism reconstruction showed the equivalent success of allograft and synthetic mesh with approximately 25% failure rate in both groups (Shau et al. 2018).

Infection was the major cause of failure in both groups. However, synthetic mesh may have an advantage in terms of cost-effectiveness, disease transmission, and graft laxity.

Because *patella fractures* are more technically demanding due to the compromise of the bone stock and high risk for a loose component, we recommend against the fixation of patella fractures after TKA and would opt for excision of small fragments with poor vascularity and extensor mechanism reconstruction instead.

Conservative or postsurgical care should consist of immobilization with a long leg cast to include the foot with the knee in extension for at least 3 months followed by slowly increasing knee flexion over 6 weeks up to 90° or more.

53.11 Prevention

In high-risk patients with osteoporosis, rheumatoid arthritis, diabetes, or patella baja, excessive traction of the knee extensor mechanism should be avoided when exposing the knee. The surgeon should aggressively release the medial and lateral gutters, suprapatellar pouch, and posterior capsule as adequate surgical exposure is crucial to avoid excessive tension on the knee extensor mechanism. A posteromedial capsular peel can facilitate surgical exposure and reduce the risk of intraoperative patellar tendon rupture. Patellar tendon eversion should be avoided because it increases the traction force of patellar tendon. A lateral retinacular release should be avoided because it may damage the remaining blood supply to the patella. A quadriceps snip is very useful to aid exposure when needed. Patellar resurfacing should be avoided in patients with a residual patellar thickness of <12 mm.

Conclusion

Extensor mechanism compromise after TKA is a devastating complication. The results of direct repair after postoperative extensor mechanism disruption are historically poor; therefore, using soft tissue (e.g., allograft, autograft, and medial gastrocnemius rotational flap) or synthetic mesh reconstruction should be considered the gold standard in this setting. Reconstruction with synthetic mesh has demonstrated comparable outcomes with allograft in terms of success rate, postoperative extensor lag, knee range of motion, complication rate, and functional score. Periprosthetic joint infection was still the crucial cause for failure in both groups. However, synthetic materials may have favorable outcomes in terms of lower cost, graft stretch-out, and lack of disease transmission. Managing patient and surgical factors remain critical in preventing an extensor mechanism disruption. Patients should be informed of the varied surgical options, clinical outcomes, and failure rates since both soft tissue and synthetic mesh reconstructions have high complication rates. The ideal procedure that restores ambulation while avoiding re-rupture, infection, and residual extensor lag continues to remain elusive.

Take-Home Messages

- Extensor mechanism compromise after TKA is a devastating complication.
- Direct repair of extensor mechanism disruption after TKA will likely yield a poor result.
- Soft tissue (e.g., allograft, autograft) or synthetic mesh reconstruction is the current standard of care.
- There are several technical variations for treating an extensor mechanism disruption of the quadriceps or patellar tendons as well as a patella fracture.
- Complication rates are high for both soft tissue and synthetic mesh reconstructions, despite improved outcomes when compared to a direct repair.

References

Abdel MP, Salib CG, Mara KC, Pagnano MW, Perry KI, Hanssen AD (2018) Extensor mechanism reconstruction with use of Marlex mesh: a series study of 77 total knee arthroplasties. J Bone Joint Surg Am 100(15):1309–1318

Aracil J, Salom M, Aroca JE, Torro V, Lopez-Quiles D (1999) Extensor apparatus reconstruction with Leeds-Keio ligament in total knee arthroplasty. J Arthroplast 14(2):204–208

Ares O, Lozano LM, Medrano-Najera C, Popescu D, Martinez-Pastor JC, Segur JM et al (2014) New modified Achilles tendon allograft for treatment of chronic patellar tendon ruptures following total knee arthroplasty. Arch Orthop Trauma Surg 134(5):713–717

Barrack RL (1999) Specialized surgical exposure for revision total knee: quadriceps snip and patellar turndown. Instr Course Lect 48:149–152

Barrack RL, Stanley T, Allen BR (2003) Treating extensor mechanism disruption after total knee arthroplasty. Clin Orthop Relat Res 416:98–104

Bates MD, Springer BD (2015) Extensor mechanism disruption after total knee arthroplasty. J Am Acad Orthop Surg 23(2):95–106

Berger RA, Crossett LS, Jacobs JJ, Rubash HE (1998) Malrotation causing patellofemoral complications after total knee arthroplasty. Clin Orthop Relat Res 356:144–153

Berry DJ (1999) Epidemiology: hip and knee. Orthop Clin North Am 30(2):183–190

Bonnin M, Lustig S, Huten D (2016) Extensor tendon ruptures after total knee arthroplasty. Orthop Traumatol Surg Res 102(1 Suppl):S21–S31

Brown NM, Murray T, Sporer SM, Wetters N, Berger RA, Della Valle CJ (2015) Extensor mechanism allograft reconstruction for extensor mechanism failure following total knee arthroplasty. J Bone Joint Surg Am 97(4):279–283

Browne JA, Hanssen AD (2011) Reconstruction of patellar tendon disruption after total knee arthroplasty: results of a new technique utilizing synthetic mesh. J Bone Joint Surg Am 93(12):1137–1143

Burnett RS, Butler RA, Barrack RL (2006) Extensor mechanism allograft reconstruction in TKA at a mean of 56 months. Clin Orthop Relat Res 452:159–165

Busfield BT, Huffman GR, Nahai F, Hoffman W, Ries MD (2004) Gastrocnemius flap for extensor mechanism deficiency with and without total knee arthroplasty. Clin Orthop Relat Res 428:190–197

Cadambi A, Engh GA (1992) Use of a semitendinosus tendon autogenous graft for rupture of the patellar ligament after total knee arthroplasty. A report of seven cases. J Bone Joint Surg Am 74(7):974–979

Chang MA, Rand JA, Trousdale RT (2005) Patellectomy after total knee arthroplasty. Clin Orthop Relat Res 440:175–177

Chhapan J, Sankineani SR, Chiranjeevi T, Reddy MV, Reddy D, Gurava Reddy AV (2018) Early quadriceps tendon rupture after primary total knee arthroplasty. Knee 25(1):192–194

Chiou H-M, Chang M-C, Lo W-H (1997) One-stage reconstruction of skin defect and patellar tendon rupture after total knee arthroplasty: a new technique. J Arthroplast 12(5):575–579

Courtney PM, Edmiston TA, Pflederer CT, Levine BR, Gerlinger TL (2018) Is there any role for direct repair of extensor mechanism disruption following total knee arthroplasty? J Arthroplast 33(7s):S244–S2s8

Crossett LS, Sinha RK, Sechriest VF, Rubash HE (2002) Reconstruction of a ruptured patellar tendon with achilles tendon allograft following total knee arthroplasty. J Bone Joint Surg Am 84(8):1354–1361

Dalury DF, Dennis DA (2003) Extensor mechanism problems following total knee replacement. J Knee Surg 16(2):118–122

Diaz-Ledezma C, Orozco FR, Delasotta LA, Lichstein PM, Post ZD, Ong AC (2014) Extensor mechanism reconstruction with achilles tendon allograft in TKA: results of an abbreviate rehabilitation protocol. J Arthroplast 29(6):1211–1215

53

Dobbs RE, Hanssen AD, Lewallen DG, Pagnano MW (2005) Quadriceps tendon rupture after total knee arthroplasty. Prevalence, complications, and outcomes. J Bone Joint Surg Am 87(1):37–45

Emerson RH Jr, Head WC, Malinin TI (1990) Reconstruction of patellar tendon rupture after total knee arthroplasty with an extensor mechanism allograft. Clin Orthop Relat Res 260:154–161

Emerson RH Jr, Head WC, Malinin TI (1994) Extensor mechanism reconstruction with an allograft after total knee arthroplasty. Clin Orthop Relat Res 303:79–85. https://pubmed.ncbi.nlm.nih.gov/8194257/

Engh GA, Ammeen DJ (1998) Periprosthetic fractures adjacent to total knee implants: treatment and clinical results. Instr Course Lect 47:437–448

Fernandez-Baillo N, Garay EG, Ordoñez JM (1993) Rupture of the quadriceps tendon after total knee arthroplasty: a case report. J Arthroplast 8(3):331–333

Figgie HE 3rd, Goldberg VM, Figgie MP, Inglis AE, Kelly M, Sobel M (1989) The effect of alignment of the implant on fractures of the patella after condylar total knee arthroplasty. J Bone Joint Surg Am 71(7):1031–1039

Fujikawa K, Ohtani T, Matsumoto H, Seedhom BB (1994) Reconstruction of the extensor apparatus of the knee with the Leeds-Keio ligament. J Bone Joint Surg Br 76(2):200–203

Fukuta S, Kuge A, Nakamura M (2003) Use of the Leeds–Keio prosthetic ligament for repair of patellar tendon rupture after total knee arthroplasty. Knee 10(2):127–130

Järvelä T, Halonen P, Järvelä K, Moilanen T (2005) Reconstruction of ruptured patellar tendon after total knee arthroplasty: a case report and a description of an alternative fixation method. Knee 12(2):139–143

Jarvela T, Halonen P, Jarvela K, Moilanen T (2005) Reconstruction of ruptured patellar tendon after total knee arthroplasty: a case report and a description of an alternative fixation method. Knee 12(2):139–143

Jaureguito JW, Dubois CM, Smith SR, Gottlieb LJ, Finn HA (1997) Medial gastrocnemius transposition flap for the treatment of disruption of the extensor mechanism after total knee arthroplasty. J Bone Joint Surg Ser A 79(6):866–873

Lamberti A, Balato G, Summa PP, Rajgopal A, Vasdev A, Baldini A (2018) Surgical options for chronic patellar tendon rupture in total knee arthroplasty. Knee Surg Sports Traumatol Arthrosc 26(5):1429–1435

Leopold SS, Greidanus N, Paprosky WG, Berger RA, Rosenberg AG (1999) High rate of failure of allograft reconstruction of the extensor mechanism after total knee arthroplasty. J Bone Joint Surg Am 81(11):1574–1579

Lie DT, Gloria N, Amis AA, Lee BP, Yeo SJ, Chou SM (2005) Patellar resection during total knee arthroplasty: effect on bone strain and fracture risk. Knee Surg Sports Traumatol Arthrosc 13(3):203–208

Lim CT, Amanatullah DF, Huddleston JI 3rd, Harris AHS, Hwang KL, Maloney WJ et al (2017) Reconstruction of disrupted extensor mechanism after total knee arthroplasty. J Arthroplast 32(10):3134–3140

Lynch AF, Rorabeck CH, Bourne RB (1987) Extensor mechanism complications following total knee arthroplasty. J Arthroplast 2(2):135–140

Meding JB, Fish MD, Berend ME, Ritter MA, Keating EM (2008) Predicting patellar failure after total knee arthroplasty. Clin Orthop Relat Res 466(11):2769–2774

Nam D, Abdel MP, Cross MB, LaMont LE, Reinhardt KR, McArthur BA et al (2014) The management of extensor mechanism complications in total knee arthroplasty: AAOS exhibit selection. J Bone Joint Surg Ser A 96(6):e47(1)

Nazarian DG, Booth RE Jr (1999) Extensor mechanism allografts in total knee arthroplasty. Clin Orthop Relat Res 367:123–129

Ortiguera CJ, Berry DJ (2002) Patellar fracture after total knee arthroplasty. J Bone Joint Surg Am 84(4):532–540

Pagnano MW (2003) Patellar tendon and quadriceps tendon tears after total knee arthroplasty. J Knee Surg 16(4):242–247

Papalia R, Vasta S, D'Adamio S, Albo E, Maffulli N, Denaro V (2015) Complications involving the extensor mechanism after total knee arthroplasty. Knee Surg Sports Traumatol Arthrosc 23(12):3501–3515

Parker DA, Dunbar MJ, Rorabeck CH (2003) Extensor mechanism failure associated with total knee arthroplasty: prevention and management. J Am Acad Orthop Surg 11(4):238–247

Pawar U, Rao KN, Sundaram PS, Thilak J, Varghese J (2009) Scintigraphic assessment of patellar viability in total knee arthroplasty after lateral release. J Arthroplast 24(4):636–640

Rand JA, Morrey BF, Bryan RS (1989) Patellar tendon rupture after total knee arthroplasty. Clin Orthop Relat Res 244:233–238

Rorabeck CH, Angliss RD, Lewis PL (1998) Fractures of the femur, tibia, and patella after total knee arthroplasty: decision making and principles of management. Instr Course Lect 47:449–458

Rosenberg AG (2012) Management of extensor mechanism rupture after TKA. J Bone Joint Surg Br 94(11 Suppl A):116–119

Schoderbek RJ Jr, Brown TE, Mulhall KJ, Mounasamy V, Iorio R, Krackow KA et al (2006) Extensor mechanism disruption after total knee arthroplasty. Clin Orthop Relat Res 446:176–185

Seo JG, Moon YW, Park SH, Lee JH, Kang HM, Kim SM (2012) A case-control study of spontaneous patellar fractures following primary total knee replacement. J Bone Joint Surg Br 94(7):908–913

Shau D, Patton R, Patel S, Ward L, Guild G 3rd. (2018) Synthetic mesh vs. allograft extensor mechanism reconstruction in total knee arthroplasty – a systematic review of the literature and meta-analysis. Knee 25(1):2–7

Sheth NP, Pedowitz DI, Lonner JH (2007) Periprosthetic patellar fractures. J Bone Joint Surg Am 89(10):2285–2296

Springer BD, Della Valle CJ (2008) Extensor mechanism allograft reconstruction after total knee arthroplasty. J Arthroplast 23(7 Suppl):35–38

Vajapey SP, Blackwell RE, Maki AJ, Miller TL (2019) Treatment of extensor tendon disruption after total knee arthroplasty: a systematic review. J Arthroplast 34(6):1279–1286

Wood TJ, Leighton J, Backstein DJ, Marsh JD, Howard JL, McCalden RW et al (2019) Synthetic graft compared with allograft reconstruction for extensor mechanism disruption in total knee arthroplasty: a multicenter cohort study. J Am Acad Orthop Surg 27(12):451–457

Periprosthetic Fractures

Daniel O. Johansen and Adam A. Sassoon

Contents

E. Hansen, K.-D. Kühn (eds.), *Essentials of Cemented Knee Arthroplasty*,
https://doi.org/10.1007/978-3-662-63113-3_54

54

54.1 Introduction

Cases such as the one presented below are becoming more and more common, given the increase in the number of total knee arthroplasties (TKA) that are being performed each year (Inacio et al. 2017). The incidence of periprosthetic fractures around primary TKAs is estimated to be between 0.3% and 2.5% (Meek et al. 2011). As these types of injuries become more commonplace, orthopedic surgeons should be aware of the various challenges that these fractures pose. Knowledge of the risk factors, common fracture patterns, management options, and potential complications should be well understood.

54.2 Case Study

54.2.1 History of Present Illness

The patient is a 91-year-old female with multiple medical comorbidities who presents to the emergency department with left knee pain and inability to bear weight after suffering a ground-level fall while at home. She is found to have a closed deformity around the distal femur. She is neurovascularly intact on examination. Her past medical history is significant for atrial fibrillation for which she is treated with apixaban, past myocardial infarction, congestive heart failure, osteoporosis, and reports of several falls in the past. Her surgical history is significant for bilateral total hip arthroplasties and bilateral knee arthroplasties performed outside hospitals years ago. She has a history of a contralateral interprosthetic femur fracture 1 year prior to this fall, which required revision to distal femoral replacement. Her X-rays in the emergency department revealed a left-sided interprosthetic femur fracture (Fig. 54.1). The fracture is displaced, with a suspected loose femoral component (i.e., Lewis and Rorabeck type III fracture) and located distal to the proximal flange of the femoral component (i.e., Su et al. type III femur fracture).

54.2.2 Preoperative Planning

In cases such as these, involving a frail geriatric patient with multiple medical comorbidities, one of the first steps before proceeding with orthopedic management is to undergo a thorough medical evaluation to assess her overall medical condition. Optimization prior to surgery

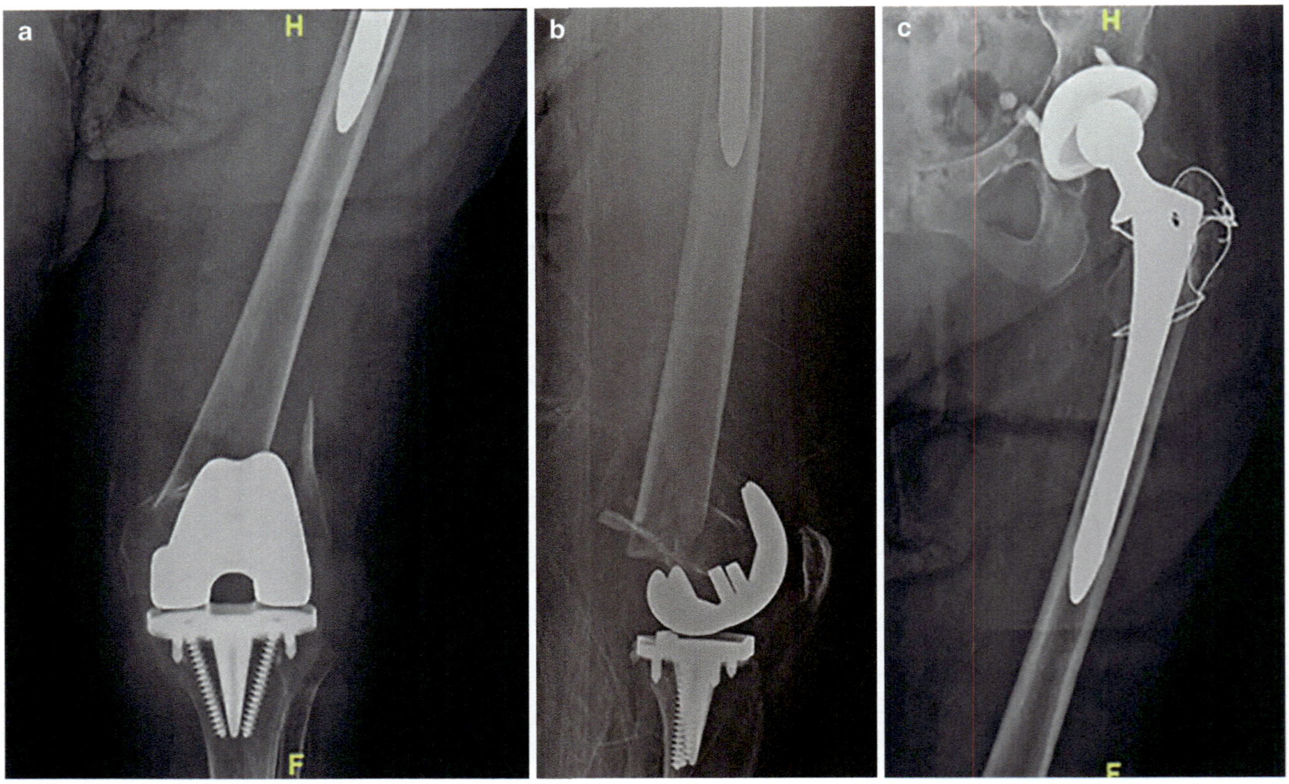

Fig. 54.1 Anteroposterior **a** and lateral **b** radiographs of a 91-year-old patient with a Lewis and Rorabeck type III periprosthetic distal femur fracture after a ground level fall. The patient was also found to have an ipsilateral total hip arthroplasty, which appeared stable on imaging **c**

should include cardiopulmonary workup by an internal medicine physician. Ideally, apixaban should be held 48 h prior to any planned orthopedic intervention (Sunkara et al. 2016). An assessment of the patient's preoperative functional status is also important to obtain as this could change surgical management.

Based on the location of the fracture in the presence of loose components, a revision is required. In this frail, geriatric patient, a distal femoral replacement (DFR) is chosen as the best option given her preoperative functional status, the fracture pattern, and the available bone stock. Preoperative templating with a DFR system is performed. Estimation of stem length is calculated based on measurements to the tip of the hip arthroplasty stem. In cases of ipsilateral hip arthroplasty, the stress riser between the tip of the hip stem and the DFR stem is cause for concern of fracture between the two implants. In order to bridge this zone of increased stress, an allograft strut is planned.

54.2.3 Surgical Procedure and Tips and Tricks

The previous anterior midline knee incision is extended proximally and laterally in a curvilinear fashion using a subvastus approach at the level of the planned strut graft (◘ Fig. 54.2). A medial parapatellar arthrotomy is performed with a quad snip to enhance our exposure. There is severe comminution of the osteoporotic distal femur with a loosened femoral component. The hematoma and fragments are extracted. The distal femur cut is then planned after measurement of the excised portion of the distal femur. A cerclage wire is placed around the diaphysis just proximal to the fracture in order to prevent the propagation of the fracture during the osteotomy (◘ Fig. 54.3). The cerclage wire also functions to control the proximal segment during the remainder of the procedure. A malleable retractor is bent and placed under the posterior femur, thereby preventing undue pressure on the underlying vascular structures (◘ Fig. 54.3). The tibial component is then revised to a stemmed prosthesis to mate the hinged bearing couple of the DFR system. Trial components are then placed. In this specific case, the stem of the femoral component of the prior THA is impeding the DFR stem. This potential issue was anticipated preoperatively, and a diamond cutting burr is available to cut the precise amount of stem tip. The rotation of the femoral component is noted during the trialing process to prevent patellar dislocation. The relative external rotation of the femoral component is marked. The final components are then cemented into place. Soft tissue tensioning is fine-tuned by selection of the thickness of the polyethylene liner. A subvastus approach is then undertaken to gain access to the interprosthetic region. A femoral strut graft is then measured to bypass the stress riser and is secured with cerclage cables. The edges of the strut allograft are beveled to prevent traumatic irritation of the vastus lateralis. The allograft strut is supplemented with morselized autograft taken from the distal femur resection. Additionally, the lateral cortex of the native femur is gently touched with a burr to stimulate bleeding and further aid in incorporation of the morselized autograft.

Infection prevention and wound management are crucial in these revision arthroplasty cases. Calcium sulfate beads impregnated with vancomycin and tobramycin are placed around the joint space. A meticulous layered wound closure is performed followed by application of a negative pressure wound dressing to optimize wound healing and prevent wound drainage. Postoperatively, the patient is made weight bearing as

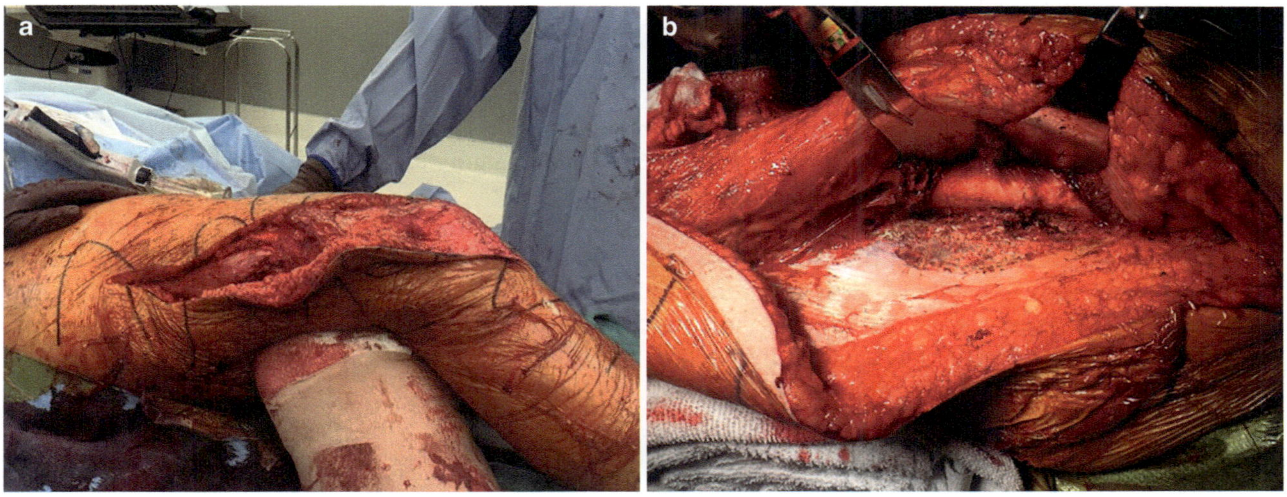

◘ **Fig. 54.2** **a** Intraoperative photo showing an example of a curvilinear shaped incision that can be utilized for accessing the knee. **b** Exposure of the femoral diaphysis using a subvastus approach

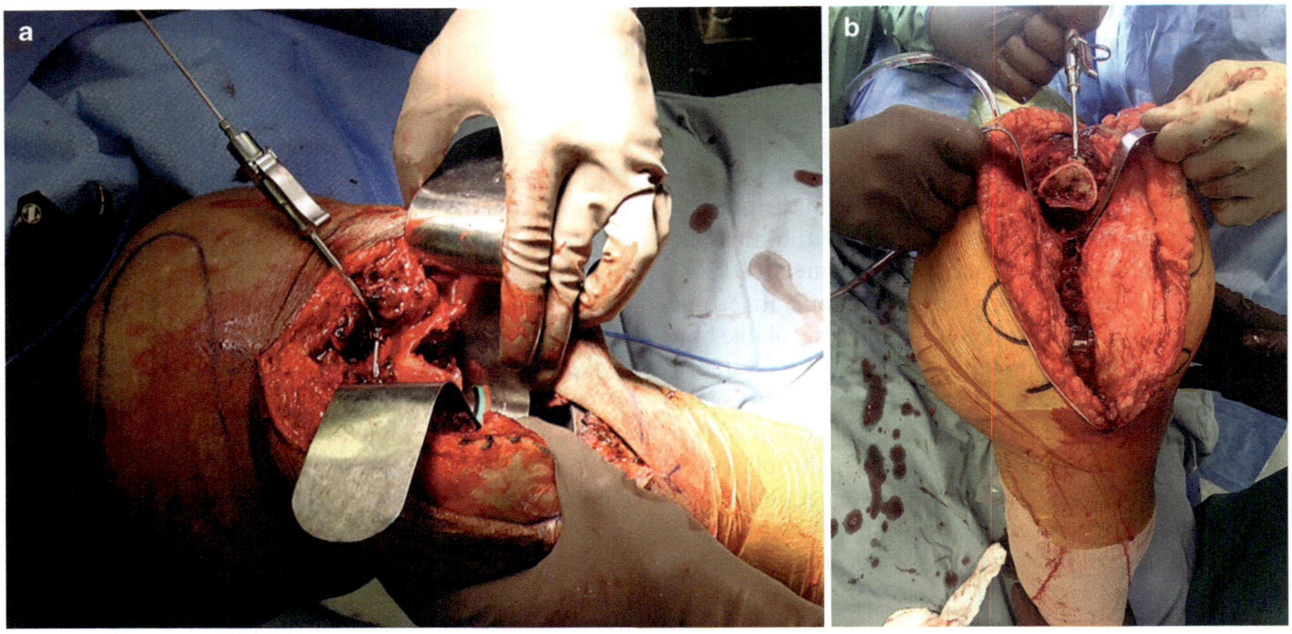

Fig. 54.3 **a**, **b** Intraoperative photos showing cerclage placement just proximal to the fracture in order to prevent fracture propagation proximally during the osteotomy. The cerclage can then be used as a leash during the remainder of the procedure to gain control of this segment of the femur. A malleable retractor is bent and placed posterior to the femur in order to protect the posterior neurovascular structures during the osteotomy and duration of the case as needed

tolerated. Postoperative X-rays demonstrate a well-aligned DFR with a well-fixed allograft strut bypassing the interprosthetic stress riser (Fig. 54.4).

54.3 Risk Factors

> Periprosthetic fractures around the knee can occur intraoperatively or postoperatively (Sunkara et al. 2016).

In one large retrospective study, intraoperative fractures during primary cemented TKAs were shown to occur at an incidence of 0.39% (Alden et al. 2010). In this series, most fractures occurred during exposure or bone preparation (40%) and during trialing components (33%) though 19% of their fractures occurred during the cementing process. In the revision arthroplasty setting, intraoperative fractures occur at an approximate 6-fold increase compared to primary TKA (Sassoon et al. 2014a, b). In the aseptic revision setting, fractures most commonly occur at the femur during exposure (Sassoon et al. 2014a). During two-staged revision for infected TKAs, fractures occur most commonly at the femur during component reimplantation rather than during component explant (Sassoon et al. 2014b).

Risk factors for *intraoperative* fractures include the following:

- Female sex
- Use of posterior stabilized femoral components
- Chronic steroid use
- Advanced age
- Rheumatoid arthritis
- Neurologic disorders (Alden et al. 2010)

Similarly, *postoperative* fractures share many of the same risk factors as intraoperative fractures, which tend to revolve around patient characteristics predisposing to poor bone quality. Some risk factors include the following:

- Patient age >70
- Female sex
- Chronic use of steroids
- Inflammatory arthropathy (Sunkara et al. 2016)

Additional factors are at higher risk for fracture postoperatively (Sunkara et al. 2016; Lim et al. 2017; Born et al. 2018), such as

- Anterior femoral notching
- Component malalignment
- Revised TKAs
- Patients with lower preoperative patient-reported outcome scores

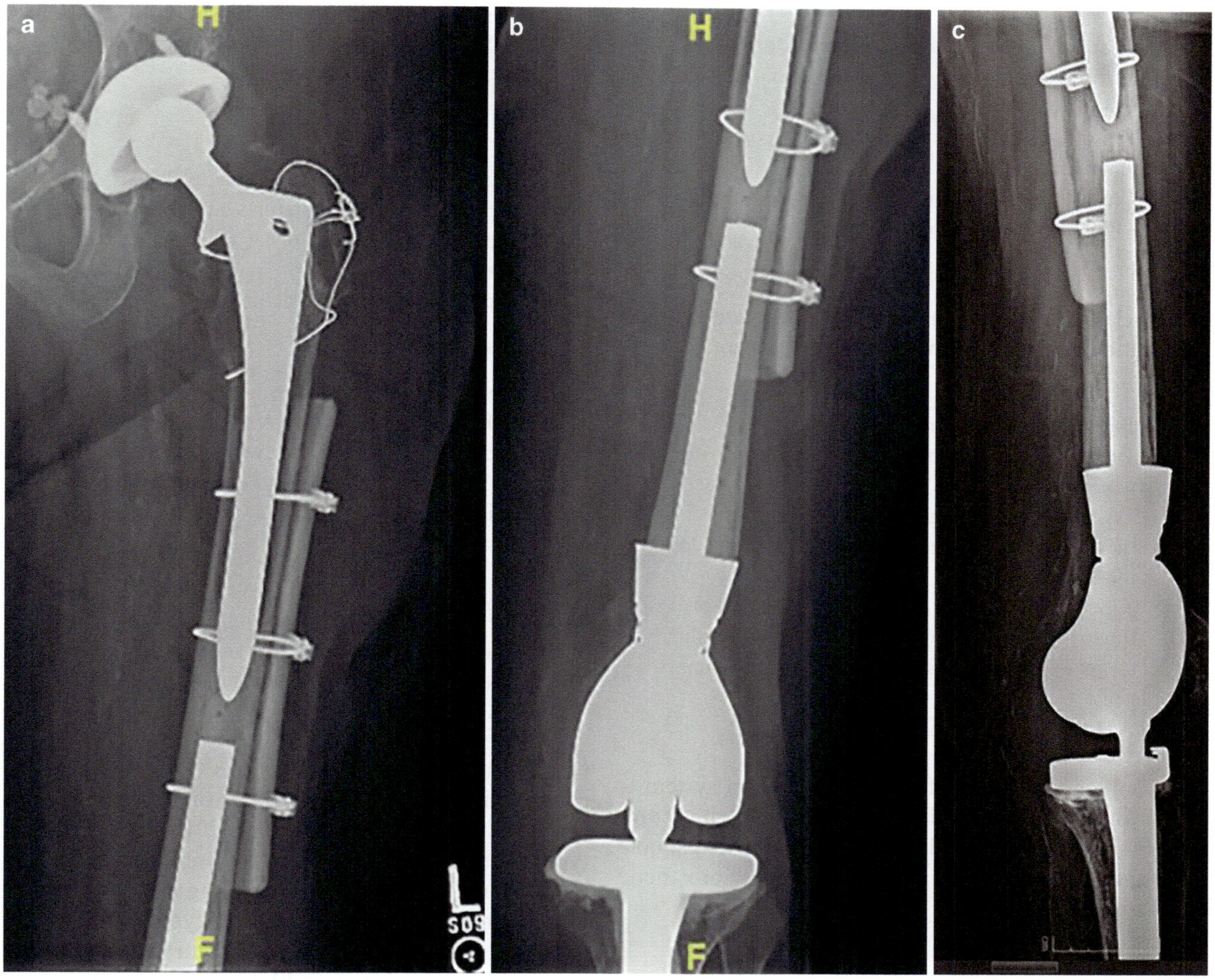

Fig. 54.4 **a–c** Due to the significant comminution and available bone stock in this low-demand 91-year-old patient, the decision is made to revise her knee to a distal femoral replacement (DFR). Due to the ipsilateral hip arthroplasty stem impeding the DFR stem, a measured cut of the most proximal aspect of the DFR stem is performed intraoperatively with a diamond-tipped burr. The interprosthetic region is now a stress riser for future fracture. Prophylactic placement of an allograft strut is cerclaged in place to bridge the interprosthetic region

54.4 Classification of Periprosthetic TKA Fractures

> Periprosthetic fractures around TKAs can occur at the femur, tibia, or patella. The most common fractures are located at the femur.

There are several classification systems that have been developed, which attempt to describe the location, fracture displacement, component fixation, and available bone stock. These classification systems are meant to provide an algorithm to help guide the surgeon in selecting the most appropriate management.

54.4.1 Periprosthetic Femur Fracture Classification Systems

There are several classification systems that have been created to describe periprosthetic femur fractures. To our knowledge, the most common classification systems that are used to describe periprosthetic fractures of the femur were developed and presented by Lewis and Rorabeck (1997) and Su et al. (2004).

The Lewis and Rorabeck classification system categorizes the supracondylar femur fracture into three types based on fracture displacement and component stability.

Lewis and Rorabeck Classification System

- Type I fractures are nondisplaced with a well-fixed femoral component.
- Type II fractures are displaced with components remaining well-fixed.
- Type III fractures are nondisplaced or displaced with loose or failing components.

The Su classification system describes the fracture based on the location in relation to the femoral component.

Su Classification System

- Type I fractures are proximal to the femoral component.
- Type II fractures begin at the proximal aspect of the femoral component and travel proximally along the femur.
- Type III fractures are ones in which any part of the fracture line extends distally to the most proximal aspect of the anterior flange of the femoral component.

The chapter authors' preferred classification system is the Lewis and Rorabeck classification because it accomplishes the goals of providing the surgeon with a simple algorithm for surgical management of periprosthetic fractures of the femur.

> The keys to this classification system are understanding if the fracture is displaced or nondisplaced, but more importantly, it addresses whether or not the implants will need to be revised based on the fixation of the implants.

Type I and II fractures can generally be fixed rather than revised as the components remain well fixed. Surgical fixation of type I and II fractures most commonly involves intramedullary fixation and/or plate fixation. Type III fractures will require revision and often will require the addition of plate fixation. The decision for revision to a long-stemmed prosthesis or to a distal femoral replacement is guided by the available bone stock and various patient characteristics.

54.4.2 Periprosthetic Tibia Fracture Classification

Periprosthetic fractures of the tibia are less common than those involving the femur. The incidence of periprosthetic tibial fractures is between 0.4% and 1.7% (Morwood et al. 2019). The most commonly used classification system to describe these types of fractures was first presented by Felix et al. (1997):

Felix Classification System

- Type I fractures involve the tibial plateau.
- Type II fractures are fractures near the tibial stem.
- Type III fractures are distal to the tibial component.
- Type IV fractures are fractures of the tibial tubercle.

Each type can also be subclassified based on the stability of the tibial implant: Type A fractures are well fixed, and type B fractures are those with a loose tibial component; Felix et al. (1997) also describe a subtype C, which is any tibial fracture occurring intraoperatively.

> The utility of the Felix classification system is that this simple descriptive system can be applied to guiding management based on fracture location and implant stability.

Certain type I and II fractures can be managed conservatively if the fracture is nondisplaced with a well-fixed component (Born et al. 2018). For displaced type IA and IIA fractures, the treatment generally involves internal fixation with plating (Morwood et al. 2019; Kim et al. 2017). For displaced type IIIA fractures, treatment can involve plating and/or intramedullary fixation (Morwood et al. 2019; Haller et al. 2014). Type IVA fractures can be treated with lag screws or plate fixation (Ruchholtz et al. 2013). For any Felix subtype B fractures, revision arthroplasty is required with conversion to long-stemmed tibial components or consideration of megaprosthesis in certain cases (Born et al. 2018).

54.5 Surgical Techniques

54.5.1 Periprosthetic Femur Fractures

54.5.1.1 Intramedullary Fixation

> Operative management of periprosthetic femur fractures with an intramedullary nail is a useful treatment option for Lewis and Rorabeck type I or II fractures that are proximal to the femoral component.

Intramedullary nails offer several advantages for fixation of these difficult-to-treat fractures. In the setting of periprosthetic femur fractures, nails function as a loadsharing device and stimulate secondary bone healing with callus formation. The ability to lock the nail proximally and distally provides an advantage of axial and rotational stability. The use of the previous midline TKA incision and less soft tissue stripping compared to the dissection needed for plate fixation offers an advantage of less soft tissue morbidity.

Preoperative imaging and planning are crucial for success with this method of fixation because the implant must be well fixed, the fracture needs to be proximal enough to allow for placement of distal locking screws, and the femoral component design must be able to accept a retrograde nail. The surgeon should obtain the operative reports for identifying the components in order to determine whether the intercondylar notch is open and to calculate the size of the opening for compatibility with the chosen retrograde nail (Ruchholtz et al. 2013; Thompson et al. 2014). Closed-box designs and femoral stems will preclude the use of a retrograde nail. If the operative report is not available and the femoral component design is unknown, an intraoperative notch view can be performed prior to incision, which can confirm the presence of an open notch for nail passage (Ricci 2015).

A potential disadvantage for intramedullary nailing is the difficult starting point with certain component designs. Some cruciate-retaining components with deep trochlear groves can displace the nail starting point posterior to Blumensaat's line, resulting in a recurvatum deformity (Service et al. 2015). Additionally, one should ensure the distal fracture fragment has at least 2–3 cm of bone to allow for at a minimum of two interlocking screws within the distal femur fracture fragment. Ideally, three to four interlocks should be used in the distal fragment to allow for improved construct stiffness and fatigue strength (Pekmezci et al. 2014). Finally, ipsilateral hip arthroplasty stems can prevent the planned use of a retrograde nail. This challenge with an ipsilateral hip arthroplasty can also be seen in cases of revision or distal femur replacement. In order to reduce the risk of creating a stress riser between the two stemmed implants, the use of a strut allograft can be employed (◘ Fig. 54.4).

When performing intramedullary fixation, the authors' preferred approach is via an open arthrotomy with direct visualization of the starting point and the components to ensure that they are not damaged during reaming. It is advisable to have back up articular inserts available in the event of damage to the insert during reaming.

Postoperative weight-bearing status after intramedullary fixation is determined by the initial fracture pattern. Most supracondylar periprosthetic fractures are displaced with some comminution. In these cases, it is recommended to protect weight bearing for 4–6 weeks (Ricci 2015). Weight bearing can be advanced as soon as there is radiographic evidence of healing at subsequent follow-up visits (Ricci 2015).

54.5.1.2 Plate Fixation

Historically, plate fixation for periprosthetic femur fractures was initially performed with nonlocked plates, blade plates, or dynamic condylar screws. Early studies using these fixation techniques tended to have high rates of varus collapse, nonunion, and required a large soft tissue dissection (Rorabeck and Taylor 1999; Bae et al. 2014). With the advent of periarticular locking plates, some of these disadvantages were mitigated and outcomes improved (Ricci et al. 2006).

> Fixation with modern locked plates provides a load-bearing construct that can achieve primary or secondary bone healing with the use of nonlocking and locking holes.

The multiple locked fixed-angle holes located at the distal end of the plate have reduced the rates of varus collapse (Ricci et al. 2006; Kim et al. 2015). Additionally, periarticular plates are able to be inserted in a biologically friendly, submuscular approach and then can be fixed utilizing minimally invasive techniques with percutaneous screw placement and with use of an outrigger. The addition of a second medial plate has also been described to enhance the fixation when there is limited distal bone stock (Kim et al. 2015). Plate fixation is used for fixation of fractures with well-fixed femoral components (i.e., Lewis and Rorabeck type I or II) and fractures that are at or above the femoral component (i.e., Su type I or II) (◘ Fig. 54.5). There are reports of successful plate fixation of Su type III fractures, but these cases can be particularly challenging given the limited amount of bone stock in the distal fragment for screw fixation (Kim et al. 2015).

Given the plate construct is load bearing, postoperative weight-bearing status generally must be restricted for a longer period of time than intramedullary fixation. Recommendations for some form of restricted weight bearing are between 8 and 12 weeks, depending on the level of fracture fixation and comminution (Ricci 2015; Wallace et al. 2017). Weight bearing can be advanced after this period with radiographic evidence of healing at subsequent visits. Immediate postoperative rehabilitation should be focused on knee range of motion.

54.5.1.3 Results of Intramedullary Nailing Versus Plate Fixation

In several early studies providing a comparison between intramedullary and locking plate fixation, plate fixation appeared to be superior in several outcome measures,

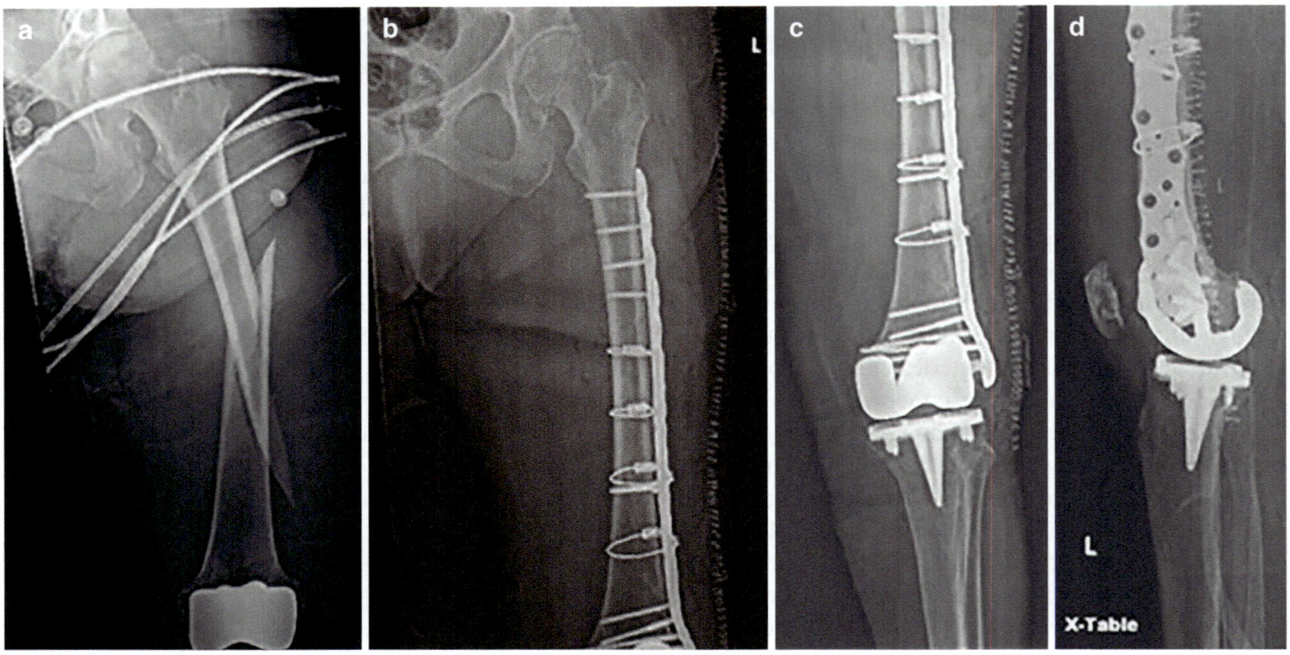

Fig. 54.5 **a** Anteroposterior radiograph of a 92-year-old patient with a Lewis and Rorabeck type II, Su type I periprosthetic fracture after a ground-level fall. Open reduction and internal fixation of the midshaft femur fracture were performed. The fracture was reduced, and initial fixation was performed with a lag screw and cerclage cables. A long, distal femur locking plate was then placed. **b–d** Final postoperative radiographs

including a lower rate of complications, reoperation, malunion, and nonunion (Horneff et al. 2013; Large et al. 2008). However, in more recent meta-analyses, there were found to be no significant differences in these outcome measures (Shin et al. 2017; Matlovich et al. 2017). Additionally, a recent biomechanical study testing various constructs to cyclical axial loading has not suggested superiority for either the locking plate or intramedullary nail (Mäkinen et al. 2015).

In the most recently published systematic review that included published studies from 2008 to 2018, there was found to be no significant differences in time to union or union rates between the two methods of fixation (Shah et al. 2020). However, they did find a significant decrease in the overall complication rate and reoperation rate of locked plating compared to intramedullary nailing (Shah et al. 2020). The most common complications reported in this study for locked plating were hardware failure (5%), malunion (2.5%), and deep infection (2.2%). In contrast, the most common complications reported for intramedullary nailing were malunion (11.5%), hardware failure (6.3%), and painful hardware (1.9%) (Shah et al. 2020).

The differences seen in all of these studies are likely related to the heterogeneity of these level III and IV studies included in their respective analyses. Unfortunately, there are no level I, randomized studies to compare the two treatment methods to help elucidate answers to these questions.

> It is clear, however, that both methods of fixation offer certain advantages and disadvantages. It is the role of the surgeon to choose the best implant based on patient characteristics, bone quality, fracture location, and fracture pattern.

54.5.2 Periprosthetic Tibia Fractures

54.5.2.1 Plate Fixation

> Internal fixation with plating is the most common method of treatment for periprosthetic tibia fractures not requiring revision (i.e., Felix subtype A fractures) (Morwood et al. 2019; Felix et al. 1997).

Locking plates are generally used due to the osteoporotic bone that is typically present in this older patient population. In the largest study of periprosthetic tibia fractures, Felix et al. (1997) note that they treated IIA and IIIA fractures with plate and screw fixation when surgical treatment was used. Type IA fractures were rare in their series as they classified most type I fractures as type IB due to loose or failing components.

When performing plate fixation for type IA, IIA, or IIIA fractures, a lateral-based approach is typically utilized (Kim et al. 2017; Schreiner et al. 2018). A minimally invasive plate osteosynthesis (MIPO) approach, when possible, is recommended for the theoretical benefit of lowering rates of wound complication, infection,

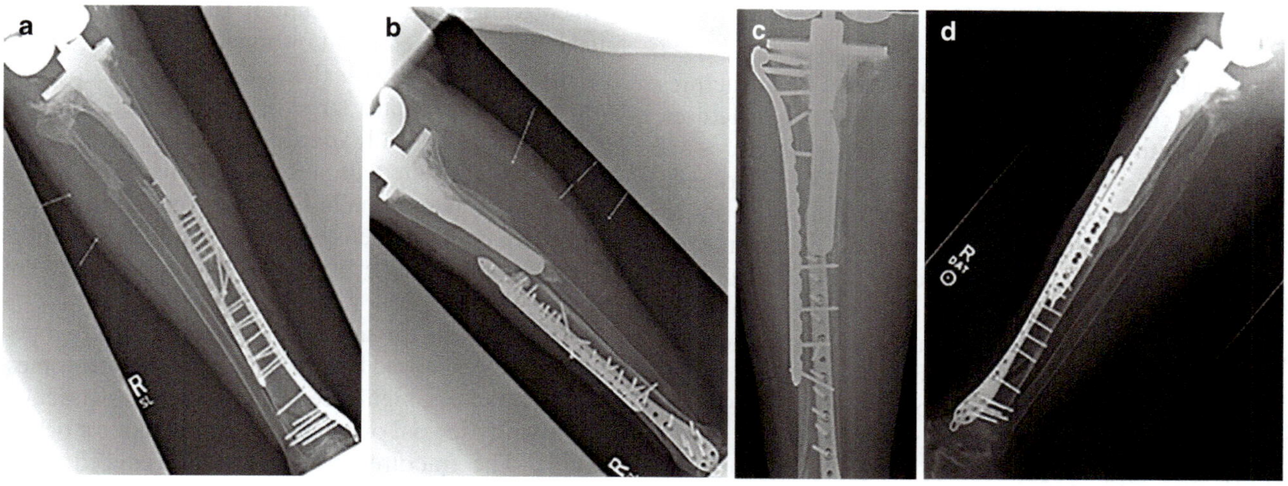

■ **Fig. 54.6** **a–d** A 75-year-old female patient with a history of a TKA and previous distal tibia fracture treated with internal fixation at an outside hospital now presents with a new fracture at the junction of the tip of the tibial stem and the most proximal plate after a ground-level fall. Anteroposterior **a** and lateral **b** radiographs reveal a Felix type IIA periprosthetic tibia fracture. Final radiographs **c, d** show that the previously placed lateral tibial plate was removed and exchanged for a longer proximal tibial locking plate to span the fracture and provide adequate fixation around the tibial component. Arthroplasty components were retained in this stable construct

and nonunion (Kim et al. 2017). Ideal fixation should be balanced within the proximal and distal segment of the fracture, but this can be difficult with the presence of the tibial implant and relative bone stock remaining (Kim et al. 2017) (■ Fig. 54.6).

Typically, the authors' preference is to include eight cortices of fixation above and below the fracture, but this can vary depending on the quality of bone in which the hardware is being placed. Dual plating for these fractures has also been described in cases where extra fixation was felt to be needed (Morwood et al. 2019). There were found to be no significant differences, however, in union rates when dual plating was used in one small study (Morwood et al. 2019).

54.5.2.2 Intramedullary Fixation

Historically, treatment of diaphyseal periprosthetic tibia fractures has been accomplished with nonoperative management or plate fixation (Morwood et al. 2019; Felix et al. 1997; Kim et al. 2017). Although not the first to perform intramedullary nailing, Haller et al. (Morwood et al. 2019) described their technique for performing intramedullary nailing of a type IIIA periprosthetic tibia fracture (Haller et al. 2014; Tabutin et al. 2007). The challenge of performing intramedullary fixation with a tibial implant in place is related to the lack of surrounding bone stock in and around the proximal tibia. Prior to attempting intramedullary fixation, the surgeon must be aware of the difficulty obtaining the proper start point, avoiding damage to the tibial component, and avoiding cortical blowout during the reaming process.

> An anterior starting point places the tibial tubercle at risk for fracture with the potential disruption of the extensor mechanism, a complication that must be avoided at all costs.

In their described technique, Haller et al. (2014) make several key points:

- Using a more distal transpatellar tendinous incision to obtain a distal starting point that will not disrupt the cement fixation of the tibial component
- Hand reaming the proximal tibia to avoid anterior cortical blowout or damage to the TKA components
- Use of a suction tip to help guide the ball tip guidewire past the posterior cortex
- Use of a nail size 9 mm or less
- Bending the tip of the nail to allow passage past the proximal tibia (Haller et al. 2014)

All four patients treated with an intramedullary nail using this technique went onto clinical and radiographic union.

More recently, a suprapatellar approach to intramedullary nailing has been described (Woyski and Emerson 2016). The potential benefit of this approach is that the nail should not have to be bent during the operation. In theory, this technique may have a higher chance of damage to the indwelling components.

54.5.2.3 Intramedullary Nailing Versus Plate Fixation

The available literature on periprosthetic tibia fractures is sparse compared to periprosthetic femur fractures, which is consistent with the fact that tibia fractures are less common around TKAs (Felix et al. 1997; Ebraheim et al. 2015). Overall, we see that treatment of periprosthetic tibia fractures with plate fixation or intramedullary fixation is a difficult task due to the difficulty of navigating the TKA implants, the poor soft tissue coverage around the tibia, and the general osteoporotic bone that is seen in patients with these fractures.

In the recent literature, the overall union rates after plate and screw fixation fall between 76.3% and 87.5% (Morwood et al. 2019; Kim et al. 2017; Triplet et al. 2020). Complication rates ranged from 18.75% to 31.6%, while reoperation rates ranged from 12.5% to 31.6% (Morwood et al. 2019; Kim et al. 2017; Triplet et al. 2020). The literature on periprosthetic tibia fractures treated with intramedullary nails is even more sparse. In the largest case series, which included only six patients, all type IIIA fractures treated with nailing had successful union (Tabutin et al. 2007). In the case series by Haller et al. (2014), all four patients healed their fractures by 6 months and there were no complications reported.

> Drawing direct comparisons between intramedullary and plate fixation is difficult because of the paucity of literature on periprosthetic tibia fractures.

Additionally, any comparison of the two treatment methods can only be made between type III fractures, which were found to be present in only 17% of the cases reported by Felix et al. (1997). Additional research is needed on the outcomes and results of treatment for these uncommon fractures.

54.5.3 Revision Arthroplasty

54.5.3.1 Periprosthetic Femur Fractures

> Periprosthetic femur fractures not amenable to internal fixation and Lewis and Rorabeck type III fractures of the femur require revision arthroplasty to address the loose or failing femoral component.

A treatment algorithm for these fractures first involves consideration of the metadiaphyseal bone stock (Kuzyk et al. 2017). For patients with good metaphyseal bone stock, the decision to use an unconstrained or constrained revision system is based on the integrity of the collateral ligaments. On the other hand, for patients with poor bone stock and defects larger than 2 cm, management can be more difficult. If the defects are contained, metal augments and/or bone graft will need to be used in conjunction with the constrained revision system. When defects are large or uncontained and the patient is physiologically younger and active, an allograft prosthetic composite will need to be considered with a constrained system. Finally, in cases where bone stock is poor, there are large defects present, and the patient is low functioning or elderly, a distal femoral replacement should be considered.

Similar to any revision TKA, the cemented components must be removed by a combination of osteotomes, cement extractors, high-speed burr, and other extraction devices with the goal of removing as little bone stock as possible. The fracture should then be reduced using standard fracture reduction techniques with supplementary fixation added as necessary. After reaming and canal preparation, any distal femur defects can be assessed for and treated with metal cones or bone graft (Fink and Mittelstädt 2018). Trialing and implantation of components can then be undertaken. Although there is no consensus on the specific components used, nearly all will require a conversion to a stemmed femoral component in order to bypass any deficient bone stock and distal fractures by at least two cortical femoral diameters. The tibial component is revised as needed to match the femoral component based on the selected level of constraint for the patient. Once components have been selected, we recommend using the modern cementing techniques that have been described in this book for fixation. Although fraught with many challenges in this patient population, one of the benefits of performing a revision arthroplasty is the ability to more quickly mobilize patients. Most patients will be able to fully weight bear after surgery, barring any additional injuries or extensor mechanism disruptions (Fink and Mittelstädt 2018; Saidi et al. 2014).

> Distal femoral replacement (DFR) is another potential option for the treatment of periprosthetic femur fractures.

DFR is best suited for the subset of patients with osteoporotic bone, large bony defects, and those who are low demand. The ability to get this group of patients, which oftentimes are frail and have many medical comorbidities, mobilizing after surgery with no to minimal weight-bearing restrictions makes DFR an attractive option (Khan and Schmidt 2019; Haidukewych 2019).

- **Results of Revision Arthroplasty and DFR**

The data for revision arthroplasty using standard revision components is limited, with most studies being small retrospective case series. In one early retrospective case series, all six patients went onto union, but there was a 33% complication rate (one for superficial infection and one for acute knee dislocation) (Srinivasan et al. 2005). In a more recent retrospective case series of 16 patients undergoing revision arthroplasty using standard revision components for Su type III fractures, all patients went onto union, and only two complications were reported (malunion in one case and instability requiring revision in another) (Fink and Mittelstädt 2018).

The results from studies on DFR for the treatment of periprosthetic femur fractures are overall promising for the treatment of complex periprosthetic femur fractures. A small retrospective case series of 11 patients treated with DFRs found none required revision at an average of 33 months and only 1 patient had died during their follow-up period (Jassim et al. 2014). More recent studies on outcomes following DFR for periprosthetic femur fractures have found revision rates between 10% and 14% and a mortality rate within their respective follow-up periods of 5.8–38.8% (Mortazavi et al. 2010; Darrith et al. 2019; Rahman et al. 2016). However, in a recent comparison of internal fixation to DFR, there was no significant difference between revision rates, 2-year mortality, or Knee Society scores (Darrith et al. 2019). In this study, revisions in the internal fixation group were more likely due to infection compared to patellar maltracking in the DFR group (Darrith et al. 2019).

54.5.3.2 Periprosthetic Tibia Fractures

> Although the treatment for periprosthetic fractures of the tibia with well-fixed tibial components generally requires some form of internal fixation, it is recommended that all Felix subtype B fractures undergo revision arthroplasty.

As described in the case series by Felix et al., the majority of type I and II fractures were found to be subtype B requiring revision surgery (Felix et al. 1997). It is not surprising that type 1 fractures were most commonly found to have loose components given the fracture line enters into the plateau at the bone–cement interface.

In type IB fractures, the fracture generally involves the medial plateau. The loosening around the tibial component is usually associated with a cavitary and segmental defect (Hanssen and Stuart 2000). Type IIB fractures tend to occur in the setting of osteolysis with severe segmental deficiencies in the metaphyseal–diaphyseal region (Hanssen and Stuart 2000). The difference in presentation in type I and IIB fractures generally requires different revision options.

Type IB fractures can generally be revised to a long-stemmed tibial component with management of the bony defects using a combination of cement fill (Fig. 54.7), bone graft, metal augments, or a custom prosthesis (Born et al. 2018; Kuzyk et al. 2017; Hanssen and Stuart 2000). Type IIB fractures can present a more

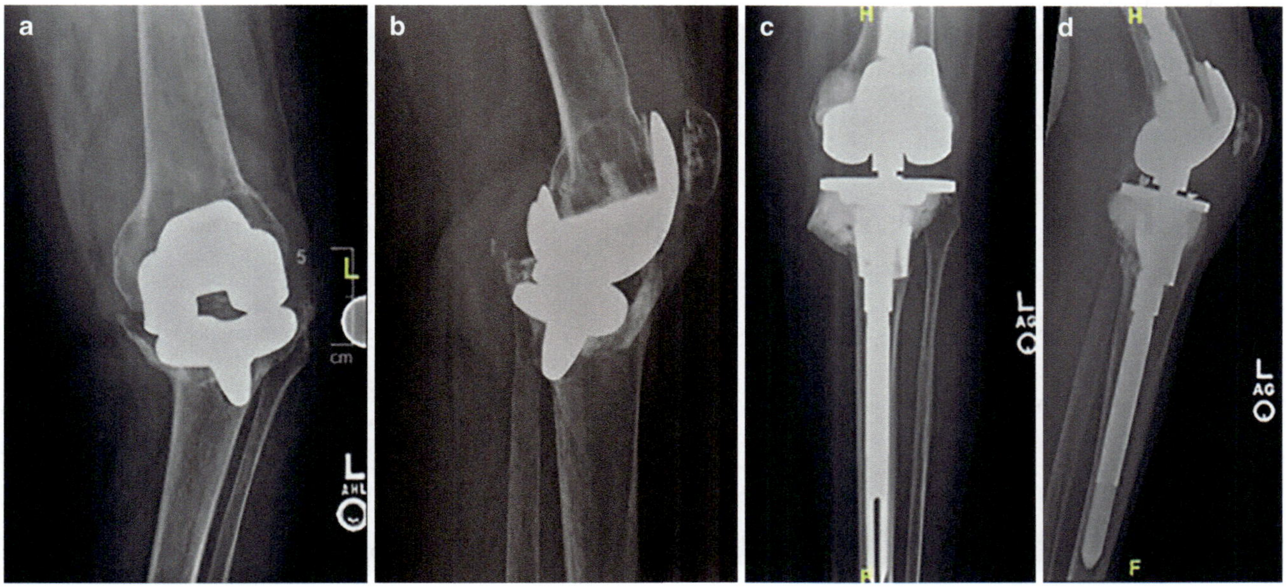

Fig. 54.7 Anteroposterior **a** and lateral **b** radiographs of a 70-year-old female with Charcot arthropathy associated catastrophic failure of a TKA with a type IB periprosthetic tibia fracture. Intraoperatively, she was found to have significant bone stock deficiencies of the tibia requiring trabecular metal metaphyseal cone augments. The final postoperative images **c**, **d** show conversion to a hinged implant with a long press-fit tibial stem with metaphyseal cement fill

difficult challenge due to the large cavitary and segmental deficiencies. In addition to a long-stemmed tibial component that bypasses the defects, structural bone graft may be necessary (Kuzyk et al. 2017; Hanssen and Stuart 2000). Additionally, consideration of the use of thicker polyethylene inserts may also be needed to reconstitute the joint line (Kuzyk et al. 2017).

Type IIIB fractures are rarely encountered (Felix et al. 1997). Management of these fractures will require early revision with a long stem, possibly being able to bypass the fracture based on the fracture location. It is recommended that additional fixation with plating is also used as most revision stems are not long enough to bypass these diaphyseal fractures. Another potential option is to stage the treatment with management of the fracture first, followed by revision of the tibial component once the fracture is healed (Hanssen and Stuart 2000).

> In cases when a proximal tibia fracture cannot be salvaged with internal fixation or standard revision implants, an endoprosthesis can be considered. In these cases, maintenance of the extensor mechanism is of utmost importance (Kuzyk et al. 2017; Windhager et al. 2016).

If the fracture involves the tibial tubercle, it must be repaired and allowed to heal to the tibia or direct healing to the prosthesis. Soft tissue coverage is another important factor for success with tibial endoprostheses. The soft tissue of the proximal tibia should be preserved with minimal local trauma, if possible. The surgeon will need to be ready to perform a rotational flap, if necessary (Kuzyk et al. 2017). Overall revision rates for endoprostheses in TKA revisions are as high as 55% (Windhager et al. 2016).

Take-Home Messages

- Success of treatment depends on accurate assessment of component stability.
- In the setting of stable implants, fracture location guides fixation methods.
- In the setting of loose components, revision to long-stemmed, constrained implants, or endoprostheses is favored.
- Surgeons should choose a treatment strategy that will allow for weight bearing and mobilization as early possible.
- In the setting of interprosthetic fractures, supplementation with cortical strut allograft or a plate is favored to mitigate the increased zone of stress between implants.

References

Alden KJ et al (2010) Intraoperative fracture during primary total knee arthroplasty. Clin Orthop Relat Res 468(1):90–95

Bae DK, Song SJ, Yoon KH, Kim TY (2014) Periprosthetic supracondylar femoral fractures above total knee arthroplasty: comparison of the locking and non-locking plating methods. Knee Surg Sports Traumatol Arthrosc 22(11):2690–2697. https://doi.org/10.1007/s00167-013-2572-2. Epub 2013 Jun 22. PubMed PMID: 23794003

Born CT, Gil JA, Johnson JP (2018) Periprosthetic tibial fractures. J Am Acad Orthop Surg 26(8):e167–e172. https://doi.org/10.5435/JAAOS-D-16-00387. Review. PubMed PMID: 29528870

Darrith B, Bohl DD, Karadsheh MS, Sporer SM, Berger RA, Levine BR (2019) Periprosthetic fractures of the distal femur: is open reduction and internal fixation or distal femoral replacement superior? J Arthroplast. https://doi.org/10.1016/j.arth.2019.12.033. pii: S0883-5403(19)31182-9. [Epub ahead of print] PubMed PMID: 31924488

Ebraheim NA, Ray JR, Wandtke ME, Buchanan GS, Sanford CG, Liu J (2015) Systematic review of periprosthetic tibia fracture after total knee arthroplasties. World J Orthop 6(8):649–654. https://doi.org/10.5312/wjo.v6.i8.649. eCollection 2015 Sep 18. PubMed PMID: 26396942; PubMed Central PMCID: PMC4573510

Felix NA, Stuart MJ, Hanssen AD (1997) Periprosthetic fractures of the tibia associated with total knee arthroplasty. Clin Orthop Relat Res 345:113–124. PubMed PMID: 9418628

Fink B, Mittelstädt A (2018) Treatment of periprosthetic fractures of the knee using trabecular metal cones for stabilization. Arthroplast Today 5(2):159–163. https://doi.org/10.1016/j.artd.2018.10.007. eCollection 2019 Jun. PubMed PMID: 31286037; PubMed Central PMCID: PMC6588680

Haidukewych GJ (2019) Role of distal femoral replacement for periprosthetic fractures above a total knee arthroplasty: when and how? J Orthop Trauma 33(Suppl 6):S33–S35. https://doi.org/10.1097/BOT.0000000000001566. PubMed PMID: 31404044

Haller JM, Kubiak EN, Spiguel A, Gardner MJ, Horwitz DS (2014) Intramedullary nailing of tibial shaft fractures distal to total knee arthroplasty. J Orthop Trauma 28(12):e296–e300. https://doi.org/10.1097/BOT.0000000000000096. PubMed PMID:24675750

Hanssen AD, Stuart MJ (2000) Treatment of periprosthetic tibial fractures. Clin Orthop Relat Res 380:91–98. PubMed PMID: 11064978

Horneff JG et al (2013) Intramedullary nailing versus locked plate for treating supracondylar periprosthetic femur fractures. Orthopedics 36(5):e561–e566

Inacio MCS, Paxton EW, Graves SE, Namba RS, Nemes S (2017) Projected increase in total knee arthroplasty in the United States – an alternative projection model. Osteoarthr Cartil 25(11):1797–1803. https://doi.org/10.1016/j.joca.2017.07.022. Epub 2017 Aug 8. PubMed PMID: 28801208

Jassim SS, McNamara I, Hopgood P (2014) Distal femoral replacement in periprosthetic fracture around total knee arthroplasty. Injury 45(3):550–553. https://doi.org/10.1016/j.injury.2013.10.032. Epub 2013 Nov 1. PubMed PMID: 24268192

Khan S, Schmidt AH (2019) Distal femoral replacement for periprosthetic fractures around total knee arthroplasty: when and how? J Knee Surg 32(5):388–391. https://doi.org/10.1055/s--0039-1683978. Epub 2019 Apr 8. Review. PubMed PMID: 30959548

Kim W, Song JH, Kim JJ (2015) Periprosthetic fractures of the distal femur following total knee arthroplasty: even very distal fractures can be successfully treated using internal fixation. Int

Orthop 39(10):1951–1957. https://doi.org/10.1007/s00264-015-2970-9. Epub 2015 Aug 25. PubMed PMID: 26300375

Kim HJ, Park KC, Kim JW, Oh CW, Kyung HS, Oh JK, Park KH, Yoon SD (2017) Successful outcome with minimally invasive plate osteosynthesis for periprosthetic tibial fracture after total knee arthroplasty. Orthop Traumatol Surg Res 103(2):263–268. https://doi.org/10.1016/j.otsr.2016.10.007. Epub 2016 Nov 25. PubMed PMID: 27890690

Kuzyk PRT, Watts E, Backstein D (2017) Revision total knee arthroplasty for the management of periprosthetic fractures. J Am Acad Orthop Surg 25(9):624–633. https://doi.org/10.5435/JAAOS-D-15-00680. Review. PubMed PMID: 28837455

Large TM et al (2008) Locked plating of supracondylar periprosthetic femur fractures. J Arthroplast 23(6 Suppl 1):115–120

Lewis PL, Rorabeck CH. Periprosthetic fractures. bz Engh GA, Rorabeck CH (eds): Revision total knee arthroplasty. Baltimore, Williams & Wilkins, 1997

Lim JBT, Bin Abd Razak HR, Zainul-Abidin S, Allen JC, JSB K, Howe TS (2017) What are the preoperative outcome measures that predispose to periprosthetic fractures after primary total knee arthroplasty? J Arthroplast 32(8):2531–2534. https://doi.org/10.1016/j.arth.2017.03.013. Epub 2017 Mar 16. PubMed PMID: 28390885

Mäkinen TJ, Dhotar HS, Fichman SG, Gunton MJ, Woodside M, Safir O, Backstein D, Willett TL, Kuzyk PR (2015) Periprosthetic supracondylar femoral fractures following knee arthroplasty: a biomechanical comparison of four methods of fixation. Int Orthop 39(9):1737–1742. https://doi.org/10.1007/s00264-015-2764-0. Epub 2015 Apr 16. PubMed PMID: 25877161

Matlovich NF, Lanting BA, Vasarhelyi EM, Naudie DD, McCalden RW, Howard JL (2017) Outcomes of surgical management of supracondylar periprosthetic femur fractures. J Arthroplast 32(1):189–192. https://doi.org/10.1016/j.arth.2016.06.056. Epub 2016 Aug 3. PubMed PMID: 27639307

Meek RM, Norwood T, Smith R, Brenkel IJ, Howie CR (2011) The risk of peri-prosthetic fracture after primary and revision total hip and knee replacement. J Bone Joint Surg Br 93(1):96–101. https://doi.org/10.1302/0301-620X.93B1.25087. PubMed PMID: 21196551

Mortazavi SM, Kurd MF, Bender B, Post Z, Parvizi J, Purtill JJ (2010) Distal femoral arthroplasty for the treatment of periprosthetic fractures after total knee arthroplasty. J Arthroplast 25(5):775–780. https://doi.org/10.1016/j.arth.2009.05.024. Epub 2010 Feb 19. PubMed PMID: 20171053

Morwood MP, Gebhart SS, Zamith N, Mir HR (2019) Outcomes of fixation for periprosthetic tibia fractures around and below total knee arthroplasty. Injury 50(4):978–982. https://doi.org/10.1016/j.injury.2019.03.014. Epub 2019 Mar 15. PubMed PMID: 30929804

Pekmezci M et al (2014) Retrograde intramedullary nails with distal screws locked to the nail have higher fatigue strength than locking plates in the treatment of supracondylar femoral fractures: a cadaver-based laboratory investigation. Bone Joint J 96-B(1):114–121

Rahman WA, Vial TA, Backstein DJ (2016) Distal femoral arthroplasty for management of periprosthetic supracondylar fractures of the femur. J Arthroplast 31(3):676–679. https://doi.org/10.1016/j.arth.2015.09.042. Epub 2015 Dec 3. PubMed PMID: 26657996

Ricci WM (2015) Periprosthetic femur fractures. J Orthop Trauma 29(3):130–137. https://doi.org/10.1097/BOT.0000000000000282. Review. PubMed PMID: 25699540

Ricci WM, Loftus T, Cox C, Borrelli J (2006) Locked plates combined with minimally invasive insertion technique for the treatment of periprosthetic supracondylar femur fractures above a total knee arthroplasty. J Orthop Trauma 20(3):190–196. PubMed PMID: 16648700

Rorabeck CH, Taylor JW (1999) Classification of periprosthetic fractures complicating total knee arthroplasty. Orthop Clin North Am 30(2):209–214. Review. PubMed PMID: 10196422

Ruchholtz S, Tomas J, Gebhard F, Larsen MS (2013) Periprosthetic fractures around the knee-the best way of treatment. Eur Orthop Traumatol 4:93–102. PubMed PMID: 24929282

Saidi K, Ben-Lulu O, Tsuji M, Safir O, Gross AE, Backstein D (2014) Supracondylar periprosthetic fractures of the knee in the elderly patients: a comparison of treatment using allograft-implant composites, standard revision components, distal femoral replacement prosthesis. J Arthroplast 29(1):110–114. https://doi.org/10.1016/j.arth.2013.04.012. Epub 2013 May 13. PubMed PMID: 23680503

Sassoon AA, Wyles CC, Norambuena Morales GA, Houdek MT, Trousdale RT (2014a) Intraoperative fracture during aseptic revision total knee arthroplasty. J Arthroplast 29(11):2187–2191. https://doi.org/10.1016/j.arth.2014.05.009. Epub 2014 May 22. PubMed PMID: 25189672

Sassoon AA, Nelms NJ, Trousdale RT (2014b) Intraoperative fracture during staged total knee reimplantation in the treatment of periprosthetic infection. J Arthroplast 29(7):1435–1438. https://doi.org/10.1016/j.arth.2014.01.021. Epub 2014 Jan 25. PubMed PMID: 24560463

Schreiner AJ, Schmidutz F, Ateschrang A, Ihle C, Stöckle U, Ochs BG, Gonser C (2018) Periprosthetic tibial fractures in total knee arthroplasty – an outcome analysis of a challenging and underreported surgical issue. BMC Musculoskelet Disord 19(1):323. https://doi.org/10.1186/s12891-018-2250-0. PubMed PMID: 30200931; PubMed Central PMCID: PMC6131855

Service BC, Kang W, Turnbull N, Langford J, Haidukewych G, Koval KJ (2015) Influenceof femoral component design on retrograde femoral nail starting point. J Orthop Trauma 29(10):e380–e384. https://doi.org/10.1097/BOT.0000000000000350. PubMed PMID: 25932527

Shah JK, Szukics P, Gianakos AL, Liporace FA, Yoon RS (2020) Equivalent union rates between intramedullary nail and locked plate fixation for distal femur periprosthetic fractures – a systematic review. Injury. https://doi.org/10.1016/j.injury.2020.02.043. pii: S0020-1383(20)30118-2. [Epub ahead of print]. PubMed PMID: 32115204

Shin YS, Kim HJ, Lee DH (2017) Similar outcomes of locking compression plating and retrograde intramedullary nailing for periprosthetic supracondylar femoral fractures following total knee arthroplasty: a meta-analysis. Knee Surg Sports Traumatol Arthrosc 25(9):2921–2928. https://doi.org/10.1007/s00167-016-4050-0. Epub 2016 Feb 20. Review. PubMed PMID: 26897137

Srinivasan K, Macdonald DA, Tzioupis CC, Giannoudis PV (2005) Role of long stem revision knee prosthesis in periprosthetic and complex distal femoral fractures: a review of eight patients. Injury 36(9):1094–1102. PubMed PMID:16054147

Su ET, DeWal H, Di Cesare PE (2004) Periprosthetic femoral fractures above total knee replacements. J Am Acad Orthop Surg 12(1):12–20. Review. PubMed PMID: 14753793

Sunkara T, Ofori E, Zarubin V, Caughey ME, Gaduputi V, Reddy M (2016) Perioperative management of Direct Oral Anticoagulants (DOACs): a systemic review. Health Serv Insights 9(Suppl

1):25–36. https://doi.org/10.4137/HSI.S40701. eCollection 2016. Review. PubMed PMID: 28008269

Tabutin J, Cambas PM, Vogt F (2007) Tibial diaphysis fractures below a total knee prosthesis. Rev Chir Orthop Reparatrice Appar Mot 93(4):389–394. French. PubMed PMID: 17646822

Thompson SM, Lindisfarne EA, Bradley N, Solan M (2014) Periprosthetic supracondylar femoral fractures above a total knee replacement: compatibility guide for fixation with a retrograde intramedullary nail. J Arthroplast 29(8):1639–1641. https://doi.org/10.1016/j.arth.2013.07.027. Epub 2014 Jun 11. Review

Triplet JJ, Taylor BC, Brewster J (2020) Outcomes and review of periprosthetic tibial fractures. Orthopedics 20:1–5. https://doi.org/10.3928/01477447-20200213-02. [Epub ahead of print]. PubMed PMID: 32077969

Wallace SS, Bechtold D, Sassoon A (2017) Periprosthetic fractures of the distal femur after total knee arthroplasty: plate versus nail fixation. Orthop Traumatol Surg Res 103(2):257–262. https://doi.org/10.1016/j.otsr.2016.11.018. Epub 2017 Jan 13. Review. PubMed PMID: 28089667

Windhager R, Schreiner M, Staats K, Apprich S (2016) Megaprostheses in the treatment of periprosthetic fractures of the knee joint: indication, technique, results and review of literature. Int Orthop 40(5):935–943. https://doi.org/10.1007/s00264-015-2991-4. Epub 2015 Sep 25. Review. PubMed PMID: 26404093

Woyski D, Emerson J (2016) Suprapatellar nailing of tibial shaft fractures in total knee arthroplasty. J Orthop Trauma 30(12):e409–e413. PubMed PMID: 27437612

Infection

Kyle H. Cichos and Elie S. Ghanem

Contents

E. Hansen, K.-D. Kühn (eds.), *Essentials of Cemented Knee Arthroplasty*,
https://doi.org/10.1007/978-3-662-63113-3_55

55.1 Introduction

Infection remains a serious and devastating complication after total knee arthroplasty (TKA).

> The risk of periprosthetic joint infection (PJI) after primary TKA is estimated at 1–2%. Additionally, revision TKA carries a higher 3–5% risk of PJI. Consequently, PJI accounts for 20–27% of all revision TKA procedures in the United States (Bozic et al. 2010; Delanois et al. 2017).

The highest risk of PJI occurs within the first year after surgery, but the lifetime risk is estimated at 2% (Garvin et al. 2018). Risk factors associated with increased infection rates include the following:

- Rheumatoid arthritis
- Peripheral vascular disease
- Heart failure
- COPD
- Anemia
- Diabetes
- Depression
- Renal disease
- Pulmonary circulation disorders
- Malignancy
- Obesity
- Malnutrition
- Male sex
- Tobacco use
- *Staphylococcus aureus* colonization
- Prior infection of another joint (Bozic et al. 2012; Crowe et al. 2015)

The organism profile for PJI varies geographically, by both country and institution. That said, some general trends have become apparent over the last 10–20 years.

> Coagulase-negative *S. aureus* was once considered the most common causative organism; however, this is shifting in recent years toward increasing rates of *S. aureus* and gram-negative infections.

> Recent trends further suggest increasing rates of antibiotic-resistant infections, including methicillin-resistant *S. aureus* (MRSA) (Bjerke-Kroll et al. 2014).

A biogram representing the distribution of PJI-causative organisms in the United States, based on averages from several large cohort studies (Bjerke-Kroll et al. 2014; Kheir et al. 2018), is shown in Fig. 55.1.

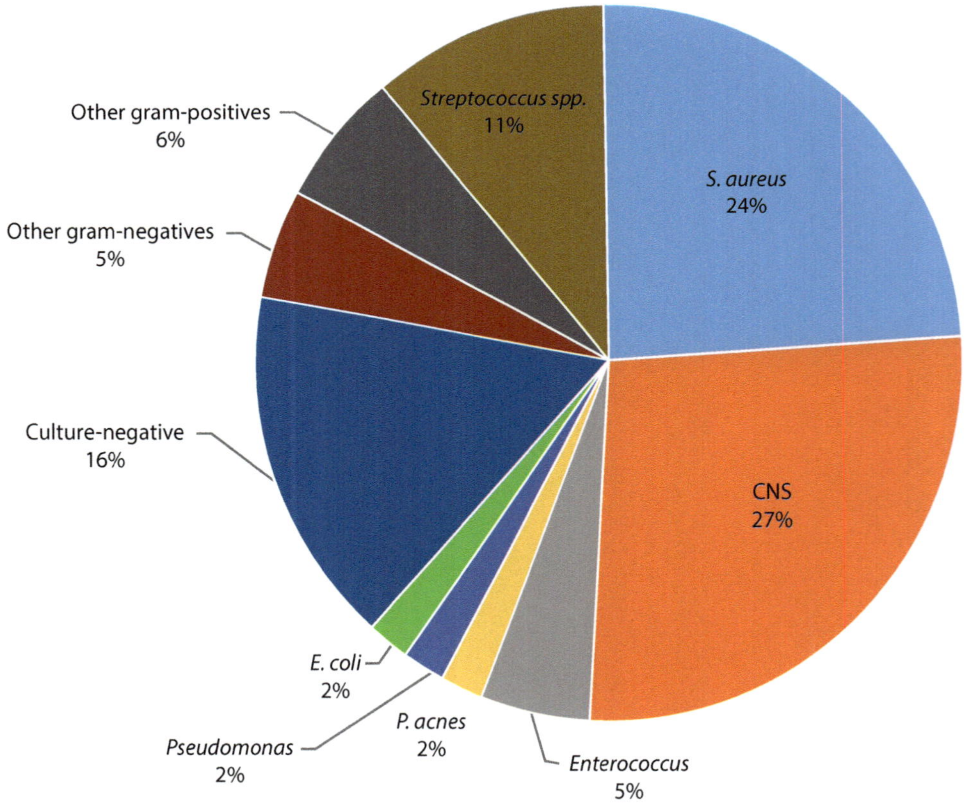

Fig. 55.1 Distribution of PJI-causative organisms in the United States. *CNS* coagulase-negative Staphylococci

55.2 Prevention

> The first step in preventing PJI is addressing modifiable patient risk factors preoperatively.

Smoking cessation at least 4 weeks prior to surgery reduces infection risk in patients using tobacco (Mills et al. 2011). Working with the patient's primary care provider to achieve glycemic control prior to surgery decreases infection risk in diabetic patients with a goal of HbA1c less than 8% or serum glucose levels less than 180 mg/dL (Iorio and Osmani 2017). Perioperative glycemic control in conjunction with a medical consult directly after surgery is an important factor in preventing infection in diabetic patients. Weight reduction should be recommended for all obese patients to achieve a BMI <40 kg/m^2 (Cizmic et al. 2019). Nutritional optimization focusing on achieving serum albumin levels ≥3.5 g/dL and prealbumin ≥15 mg/dL should be carried out in all patients presenting with malnutrition based on screening with albumin and prealbumin levels (Gu et al. 2019; Roche et al. 2018). One study found that malnutrition may play a more significant role in PJI compared to BMI (Nelson et al. 2015). Preoperative decolonization for *S. aureus* nasal colonization reduces the risk of postoperative infection (Stambough et al. 2017).

Perioperative protocols including minimizing traffic entering/exiting the operating room and timely administration (within an hour prior to incision) of intravenous preoperative antibiotics can help decrease the incidence of PJI (Panahi et al. 2012).

> A single dose of preoperative intravenous antibiotics has been shown to be as efficacious as administering multiple postoperative antibiotic doses in the prevention of PJI (Ryan et al. 2019; Tan et al. 2019a).

Dual-agent prophylaxis using a single preoperative dose of vancomycin effectively reduces PJI rates on the condition that the vancomycin is adequately weight-based dosed (Kheir et al. 2017; Burger et al. 2018). There is currently conflicting evidence supporting the use of laminar airflow in the operating room and the use of "space suits" (Aalirezaie et al. 2019a). Intraoperative prevention strategies include the use of solvents as components in the irrigation prior to closure. Current evidence suggests potential benefits utilizing dilute povidone-iodine (betadine) lavage in which the surgeon allows the solution to remain in the wound for 3 min prior to washing with normal saline irrigation (Brown et al. 2012). However, there are no level I reports on this strategy at this time. Additional options with even less evidence include chlorhexidine gluconate wash and the use of intrawound vancomycin powder dispersed into the surgical wound prior to closure (Frisch et al. 2017; Fleischman and Austin 2017). The use of ultraviolet light for decontamination of the operating room after the terminal case of the day allows for reduction of bacterial contamination and load (Aalirezaie et al. 2019a). Postoperative silver-impregnated incisional dressings have been shown to reduce the risk of PJI (Grosso et al. 2017).

55.3 Definition

The definition of PJI has varied over the years, with numerous arbitrary definitions utilized in research endeavors, especially when comparing outcomes of different treatments. The main driver for introducing specific time frames for PJI and to subdivide cases into acute and chronic infections was primarily based on clinical grounds to identify those patients with a high and low success rate when treated, specifically with debridement, antibiotics, and implant retention (DAIR) (Elkins et al. 2019).

> The recent International Consensus Meeting 2 (ICM2) for infection proposed not to include a time interval in the definition of acute and chronic PJI.

This is because the natural history of an infection is a continuum from initiation to chronicity linked to confounding variables, including host immune status and virulence of the organism.

The definition proposed by the general assembly at ICM2 was broad and encompassing to include acute PJI that was defined as a sudden onset of severe joint pain and/or swelling in a prior symptom-free prosthetic joint, and in the case of chronicity as the presence of mild or moderate pain in which its exact onset is hard to establish (Elkins et al. 2019). That being said, acute PJI presents in two different forms: early and late.

> Late acute (hematogenous) PJI is routinely defined as the appearance of sudden acute symptoms of infection occurring more than 3 months after the index arthroplasty in a previously asymptomatic prosthetic joint.

> Early acute PJI on the other hand appears in patients as less than 3 weeks of symptoms of infection and who are within 3 months of surgery (Wouthuyzen-Bakker et al. 2019, 2020).

55.4 Diagnosis

Diagnosing PJI begins with taking a careful history and physical examination. A history of native septic joint predisposes to increased risk of PJI after TKA with rates up to 15% (Aalirezaie et al. 2019b). Prolonged heavy wound drainage for more than 5 days after TKA is a red flag for potential PJI and warrants further workup (Jaberi et al. 2008).

> Serum white blood cell count (WBC) has not demonstrated consistent results as a diagnostic criterion for PJI (Toossi et al. 2012). Serological markers including C-reactive protein (CRP) and erythrocyte sedimentation rate (ESR) can be used to screen for PJI (Della Valle et al. 2011).

Other serum markers include interleukin-6 (IL-6), which correlates with PJI but is less commonly utilized in clinical practice (Patel et al. 2016). Serum D-dimer was introduced recently as a potential serum marker for diagnosing PJI that may replace traditional testing including ESR and CRP (Shahi et al. 2017). Soon after, D-dimer was found to have limited value as a screening tool for PJI, while plasma fibrinogen with a threshold value of 4.01 g/L was discovered to have similar diagnostic accuracy as the classical serological markers (Li et al. 2019; Wang et al. 2020). However, a recent study has called into question the utility and diagnostic accuracy of both plasma fibrinogen and D-dimer in comparison to the traditional markers, including ESR, CRP, and IL-6 (Xu et al. 2019).

> Aspiration of the knee remains the gold standard for diagnosing PJI after TKA.

Cell count (synovial white blood cells) >3000 cells/μL and differential (neutrophils) >80% of the fluid aspirate are suggestive of chronic infection, while a synovial white count >27,800 cells/μL and neutrophil differential >89% are suggestive of acute PJI within 6 weeks postoperatively (Parvizi and Gehrke 2014).

> α-Defensin immunoassay test has demonstrated excellent potential for diagnosis of PJI, with sensitivity and specificity ranging from 90% to 98% (Bonanzinga et al. 2017; Deirmengian et al. 2015).

Perhaps the best attribute of the α-defensin immunoassay is that its sensitivity does not appear to be impacted by prior administration of antibiotics (Shahi et al. 2016). Synovial fluid can also be applied to leukocyte esterase colorimetric strips that has shown promising results with high specificity (95–100%) for PJI (Parvizi et al. 2011).

Intraoperatively, frozen sections can be sent utilizing a cut-off for infection (>5 polymorphonuclear cells [PMN] per high-power field [hpf] in five or more fields), although its accuracy is dependent on the pathologist performing the analysis (Spangehl et al. 1999; Lonner et al. 1996). It is recommended to send at least 3–5 intraoperative tissue and/or fluid samples for culture to maximize yield for bacterial growth. Sonication of retrieved implants has also been shown to improve the diagnostic accuracy of culture results for PJI (Rothenberg et al. 2017).

The Musculoskeletal Infection Society (MSIS) guidelines of diagnostic criteria for PJI after TKA are presented in the following overview:

Musculoskeletal Infection Society (MSIS) Diagnostic Criteria for PJI

- *Major criteria* (PJI present if ≥1 exists):
  - Sinus tract communicating with the joint
  - 2 positive periprosthetic cultures of phenotypically identical organisms
- *Minor criteria* (PJI present if ≥3 of 5 exist):
  - Elevated CRP (acute: >100 mg/L, chronic: >10 mg/L) *and* ESR (acute: NA, chronic: >30 mm/h)
  - Elevated synovial fluid WBC count (acute: >10,000 cells/μL, chronic: >3000 cells/μL) *or* ++ change on leukocyte esterase test strip
  - Elevated synovial fluid PMN percentage (acute: >90%, chronic: >80%)
  - Positive histological analysis of periprosthetic tissue (>5 PMN per hpf at 400× magnification)
  - Single positive culture

Abbreviations see text; adapted from the 2014 MSIS criteria (Parvizi and Gehrke 2014).

A recent diagnostic algorithm was presented at the International Consensus Meeting II that weighted each test based on accuracy for diagnosing PJI (Parvizi et al. 2018). Diagnosis can be made if at least 1 major criterion is present, or when adding points for minor criteria in the absence of major criteria: ≥6 infected, 2–5 inconclusive, 0–1 not infected (Table 55.1).

55.5 Treatment

Multiple management strategies are currently utilized for the treatment of PJI.

> Nonoperative management with chronic suppressive antibiotic therapy is typically indicated for patients

Table 55.1 Weight-based diagnostic algorithm for PJI

Major criteria	
Sinus tract communicating to prosthesis	
Pathogen isolated by culture from two separate tissue/fluid samples from the affected joint	
Minor criteria (preoperative)	Points
Serum	
Elevated CRP (>10 mg/L) or D-dimer (>860 ng/mL)	2
Elevated ESR (>30 mm/h)	1
Synovial	
Elevated WBC (>3000 cells/μL) or ++ leukocyte esterase	3
Positive alpha-defensin	3
Elevated PMN (>80%)	2
Elevated CRP (>6.9 mg/L)	1
Inconclusive (preop score or dry aspiration)	
Positive histology (>5 PMN per hpf at 400× magnification)	3
Purulence in affected joint	3
Single positive intraoperative culture	2

Adapted from the International Consensus Meeting II (ICM2), weighted algorithm (Parvizi et al. 2018)
CRP C-reactive protein, *ESR* erythrocyte sedimentation rate, *WBC* white blood cell count, *PMN* polymorphonuclear cells

who are medically unfit for surgery. Chronic antibiotic suppressive therapy by itself has historically low success rates of eradication of PJI (25–67%) (Wouthuyzen-Bakker et al. 2017).

Operative strategies include the following:
- Irrigation and debridement with polyethylene exchange and component retention
- Single-stage revision arthroplasty
- Two-stage revision arthroplasty
- Salvage procedures—fusion or amputation

55.5.1 Irrigation and Debridement with Polyethylene Exchange (DAIR)

Indications for irrigation and debridement with polyethylene exchange and retention of components are acute infections. The polyethylene or modular components are exchanged, while the non-modular components are left in place. The key technical aspects of this treatment involve thorough tissue debridement and large-volume irrigation. Different additive antibacterial solvents can be added to the saline solution, although there is little data to support their efficacy in improving outcomes. This technique has a historically high failure rate that remains elevated up to 15–40% (Urish et al. 2018; Koyonos et al. 2011; Barros et al. 2019).

> Patients who are <2 weeks from their index TKA do significantly better than those >2 weeks from surgery (Narayanan et al. 2018).

A recent multicenter international study that utilized random forest machine learning algorithms determined the ten most significant variables that are associated with failure in order of importance:
- Elevated serum CRP values
- Positive blood cultures
- Indication for arthroplasty other than OA
- Not exchanging the modular components
- Use of immunosuppressive medication
- Late acute (hematogenous) infection
- MRSA infection
- Skin infection
- Polymicrobial infection
- Older age (Shohat et al. 2020)

Similarly, late acute (hematogenous) PJI was found to have a higher recurrence of infection with DAIR, especially when the inciting organism was *Staphylococcus* sp. compared to patients with early acute PJI (Wouthuyzen-Bakker et al. 2020).

> When compared to single-stage or two-stage exchange procedures in patients with late acute PJI, DAIR had significantly higher failure rates and recurrence of infection, especially in patients with high morbidity and *Staphylococcus* sp. as the inciting organism (Wouthuyzen-Bakker et al. 2019).

55.5.2 Single-Stage Revision TKA

This procedure involves performing revision TKA by removing all implants, thorough debridement of tissue and bone with irrigation, and then replacing them with new implant components.

> The International Consensus Meeting suggested that the best indications for this procedure are chronic PJI in an immunocompetent host, with a preoperatively known nonvirulent or resistant pathogen, with an

adequate soft tissue envelope, and without a sinus tract (Lichstein et al. 2014).

From a microorganism standpoint, low-virulence organisms with favorable antibiotic susceptibility profiles are more amenable to improved outcomes with single-stage revision TKA (Bialecki et al. 2019). However, a recent study concluded that only 19% of their patients treated for PJI would meet ICM criteria for single-stage procedure, so the applicability of this procedure may be limited to a selected group of patients (Dombrowski et al. 2020).

Potential advantages of single-stage revision compared to two-stage revision include lower medical cost, less morbidity, and improved mobility, but it also carries a higher risk of reinfection resulting from residual organisms not completely eradicated during the single revision surgery (Bialecki et al. 2019). Single-stage revision TKA has a variable failure rate of 5–18% (Bialecki et al. 2019).

Systematic reviews of the literature found no difference in outcomes between patients treated with single- and two-stage exchange for PJI.

It was concluded that it is a viable option, provided there are no contraindications, producing similar results in terms of eradication rates and functional outcomes, lower morbidity, and reduced costs (Pangaud et al. 2019; Nagra et al. 2016).

55.5.3 Two-Stage Revision TKA

The staged revision TKA is considered the gold standard for treating chronic PJI and involves removal of all prostheses with irrigation and debridement and insertion of an antibiotic spacer that allows for delivery of high local doses of antibiotics (stage 1).

Patients are given IV antibiotics for 4–6 weeks while they have the spacer in place. Delayed reconstruction then occurs by removal of antibiotic spacer and prosthesis implantation (stage 2). Choice of spacer includes static and articulating spacers. A prospective multisite study comparing spacer types revealed that articulating spacers have greater range of motion and higher Knee Society scores after reimplantation, while static spacers afforded no advantage but were associated with a longer hospital stay following removal of the infected implant (Nahhas et al. 2020). This is on the condition that the soft tissue envelope and osseous support are adequate to maintain and hold an articulating spacer.

While there is still debate regarding optimal timing to reimplantation, multiple studies have demonstrated no clear association between time to reimplantation and treatment failure when performing two-stage exchange arthroplasty for infection (Winkler et al. 2019; Aali Rezaie et al. 2018).

Challenges with two-stage revision TKA include confirming eradication of infection prior to performing the reimplantation procedure.

Having the antibiotic spacer in place makes this problematic, as typical serological tests (ESR and CRP) and knee fluid analysis are less reliable in diagnosing persistent infection than in a TKA.

Treatment with two-stage revision TKA results in reinfection rates of 5–20% at 2 years and 17% at 15 years (Petis et al. 2019), and failure rates vary significantly depending on how failure is defined (Tan et al. 2018).

Mortality rates in these patients are reported up to 11% at 1 year and up to 25% at 5 years (Lum et al. 2018). The success and reinfection rates may be overestimated since not all patients undergo the second-stage procedure due to numerous reasons.

In a large retrospective review of 504 stage-1 procedures, reimplantation occurred in 82.7%, and 11.9% required interim spacer exchange while the remaining required amputation, underwent arthrodesis, and the majority retained their spacer (Gomez et al. 2015). Patients who undergo spacer exchanges demonstrate lower survivorship and an increased risk of failure due to increased body mass index and higher rates of rheumatoid arthritis and were more likely to have PJI caused by resistant and polymicrobial organisms (Tan et al. 2019b). Another option in these high-risk patients is to retain their spacer for an extended period of time, up to 6 years, with less than 20% requiring revision of their spacer due to reinfection (Choi et al. 2014).

One plausible means of increasing treatment success rates after two-stage procedures is to administer extended oral antibiotics to the patients after reimplantation.

A multicenter randomized trial revealed that an additional 3 months of oral antibiotics can decrease the risk of reinfection from 19% to 5% after the two-stage reimplantation procedure with less than 1-year follow-up.

The authors did caution that long-term follow-up is needed for elucidation of the antibiotic safety profile and possible recurrence of PJI (Frank et al. 2017).

> A longer duration follow-up of more than 2 years to this study population revealed persistent results that conformed to the preliminary findings with lower reinfection rates in the group that received 3 months of oral antibiotics (Yang et al. 2020).

Given the tangible reinfection rates after reimplantation, some patients may require a second or third planned two-stage exchange procedure. Patients with a compromised or substantially compromised immune and extremity status based on MSIS criteria have decreased infection-free survivorship compared to their counterparts who undergo one two-stage procedure; thus, alternative salvage procedures should be considered for such patients (Fehring et al. 2017).

55.5.4 Salvage Options: Arthrodesis and Amputation

When the previously mentioned management strategies fail to eradicate infection, salvage options include arthrodesis (fusion) and amputation.

Arthrodesis allows for a generally painless stiff limb with some limb length discrepancy expected. Multiple techniques have been successfully used for arthrodesis, including external fixation, plating, and intramedullary nailing. Treatment success for arthrodesis, defined as infection eradication with bony fusion, ranges from 71% to 95% (Ghazavi et al. 2019).

When all treatment options have failed and the patient remains infected with a significant bone loss not amenable to fusion or in the case of life-threatening infection, the last treatment option is an above-knee amputation.

Conclusion

The risk of infection after primary TKA remains persistent at 1–2%, especially as the population ages with PJI constituting 20–27% of all revision TKA cases. Preoperative modification and optimization of modifiable risk patient factors described above are essential for prevention of PJI. Following good sterile technique perioperatively and proper administration of intravenous antibiotics is also key in the prevention of PJI. The diagnosis of PJI hinges upon utilizing a battery of tests readily available to the surgeon and is confirmed via the MSIS and ICM 2 criteria described above, with preoperative knee aspiration playing a pivotal diagnostic role. Treatment options include DAIR, 1-stage revision, 2-stage revision, and salvage options (arthrodesis and amputation). The optimal treatment method remains a topic of debate, and research continues into both the indications and contraindications for each strategy. Periprosthetic infection remains a devastating complication of TKA, significantly burdening both patients and the healthcare system but renders an opportunity for improved outcomes in the near future.

Take-Home Messages

- A total of 20–27% of all revision TKAs are performed for PJI, with *Staphylococcus* spp. being the most common causative bacteria.
- Modifying comorbid risk factors, nasal decolonization of *S. aureus* preoperatively, adhering to perioperative sterile protocols, and administering proper intravenous antibiotics in a timely fashion are optimal methods to prevent PJI.
- The diagnosis of PJI is a culmination of a battery of tests including a thorough clinical exam/history, serological markers, and knee aspirate analysis in conjunction with intraoperative findings and results that can be summarized in the MSIS criteria and ICM 2 scoring system.
- Accepted treatment modalities (excluding salvage options) include DAIR, 1-stage revision, and 2-stage revision. The optimal treatment is still debated, but DAIR has high failure rates in late acute PJI, while there is no difference in outcomes between 1-stage and 2-stage revision TKA in patients without contraindications for 1-stage revision.
- There is still significant room for improvement in all areas related to PJI, including prevention, diagnosis, and treatment. With infection coming to the front of the arthroplasty research focus, major improvements in each of these areas are anticipated in the coming years.

References

Aali Rezaie A, Goswami K, Shohat N, Tokarski AT, White AE, Parvizi J (2018) Time to reimplantation: waiting longer confers no added benefit. J Arthroplast 33(6):1850–1854. Epub 2018/04/02. J Arthroplasty. eng

Aalirezaie A, Akkaya M, Barnes CL, Bengoa F, Bozkurt M, Cichos KH et al (2019a) General assembly, prevention, operating room environment: proceedings of international consensus on orthopedic infections. J Arthroplast 34(2s):S105–Ss15. Epub 2018/10/24. J Arthroplasty. eng

Aalirezaie A, Arumugam SS, Austin M, Bozinovski Z, Cichos KH, Fillingham Y et al (2019b) Hip and knee section, prevention, risk mitigation: proceedings of international consensus on orthopedic infections. J Arthroplast 34(2s):S271–S2s8. Epub 2018/10/24. J Arthroplasty. eng

Barros LH, Barbosa TA, Esteves J, Abreu M, Soares D, Sousa R (2019) Early debridement, antibiotics and implant retention (DAIR) in patients with suspected acute infection after hip or knee arthroplasty – safe, effective and without negative func-

tional impact. J Bone Jt Infect 4(6):300–305. PMCID: PMC6960028. Epub 2020/01/23. J Bone Jt Infect. eng
Bialecki J, Bucsi L, Fernando N, Foguet P, Guo S, Haddad F et al (2019) Hip and knee section, treatment, one stage exchange: proceedings of international consensus on orthopedic infections. J Arthroplast 34(2s):S421–S4s6. Epub 2018/10/24. J Arthroplasty. eng
Bjerke-Kroll BT, Christ AB, McLawhorn AS, Sculco PK, Jules-Elysee KM, Sculco TP (2014) Periprosthetic joint infections treated with two-stage revision over 14 years: an evolving microbiology profile. J Arthroplast 29(5):877–882. Epub 2013/11/10. J Arthroplasty. eng
Bonanzinga T, Zahar A, Dutsch M, Lausmann C, Kendoff D, Gehrke T (2017) How reliable is the alpha-defensin immunoassay test for diagnosing periprosthetic joint infection? A prospective study. Clin Orthop Relat Res 475(2):408–415. PubMed PMID: 27343056. PMCID: PMC5213924. Epub 2016/06/28. eng
Bozic KJ, Kurtz SM, Lau E, Ong K, Chiu V, Vail TP et al (2010) The epidemiology of revision total knee arthroplasty in the United States. Clin Orthop Relat Res 468(1):45–51. PMCID: PMC2795838. Epub 2009/06/26. Clin Orthop Relat Res. eng
Bozic KJ, Lau E, Kurtz S, Ong K, Berry DJ (2012) Patient-related risk factors for postoperative mortality and periprosthetic joint infection in medicare patients undergoing TKA. Clin Orthop Relat Res 470(1):130–137. PMCID: PMC3237966. Epub 2011/08/30. Clin Orthop Relat Res. eng
Brown NM, Cipriano CA, Moric M, Sporer SM, Della Valle CJ (2012) Dilute betadine lavage before closure for the prevention of acute postoperative deep periprosthetic joint infection. J Arthroplast 27(1):27–30. Epub 2011/05/10. J Arthroplasty. eng
Burger JR, Hansen BJ, Leary EV, Aggarwal A, Keeney JA (2018) Dual-agent antibiotic prophylaxis using a single preoperative vancomycin dose effectively reduces prosthetic joint infection rates with minimal renal toxicity risk. J Arthroplast 33(7s):S213–S2s8. Epub 2018/04/17. J Arthroplasty. eng
Choi HR, Freiberg AA, Malchau H, Rubash HE, Kwon YM (2014) The fate of unplanned retention of prosthetic articulating spacers for infected total hip and total knee arthroplasty. J Arthroplast 29(4):690–693. Epub 2013/08/13. J Arthroplasty. eng
Cizmic Z, Feng JE, Huang R, Iorio R, Komnos G, Kunutsor SK et al (2019) Hip and knee section, prevention, host related: proceedings of international consensus on orthopedic infections. J Arthroplast 34(2s):S255–Ss70. Epub 2018/10/24. J Arthroplasty. eng
Crowe B, Payne A, Evangelista PJ, Stachel A, Phillips MS, Slover JD et al (2015) Risk factors for infection following total knee arthroplasty: a series of 3836 cases from one institution. J Arthroplast 30(12):2275–2278. Epub 2015/07/19. J Arthroplasty. eng
Deirmengian C, Kardos K, Kilmartin P, Cameron A, Schiller K, Booth RE Jr et al (2015) The alpha-defensin test for periprosthetic joint infection outperforms the leukocyte esterase test strip. Clin Orthop Relat Res 473(1):198–203. PMCID: PMC4390923. Epub 2014/06/20. Clin Orthop Relat Res. eng
Delanois RE, Mistry JB, Gwam CU, Mohamed NS, Choksi US, Mont MA (2017) Current epidemiology of revision total knee arthroplasty in the United States. J Arthroplast 32(9):2663–2668. Epub 2017/05/01. J Arthroplasty. eng
Della Valle C, Parvizi J, Bauer TW, DiCesare PE, Evans RP, Segreti J et al (2011) American Academy of Orthopaedic Surgeons clinical practice guideline on: the diagnosis of periprosthetic joint infections of the hip and knee. J Bone Joint Surg Am 93(14):1355–1357. Epub 2011/07/28. J Bone Joint Surg Am. eng
Dombrowski ME, Wilson AE, Wawrose RA, O'Malley MJ, Urish KL, Klatt BA (2020) A low percentage of patients satisfy typical indications for single-stage exchange arthroplasty for chronic periprosthetic joint infection. Clin Orthop Relat Res 478(8):1780–1786. Epub 2020/04/14. Clin Orthop Relat Res. eng
Elkins JM, Kates S, Lange J, Lichstein P, Otero J, Soriano A et al (2019) General assembly, diagnosis, definitions: proceedings of international consensus on orthopedic infections. J Arthroplast 34(2s):S181–S1s5. Epub 2018/10/24. J Arthroplasty. eng
Fehring KA, Abdel MP, Ollivier M, Mabry TM, Hanssen AD (2017) Repeat two-stage exchange arthroplasty for periprosthetic knee infection is dependent on host grade. J Bone Joint Surg Am 99(1):19–24. Epub 2017/01/07. J Bone Joint Surg Am. eng
Fleischman AN, Austin MS (2017) Local intra-wound administration of powdered antibiotics in orthopaedic surgery. J Bone Jt Infect 2(1):23–28. PMCID: PMC5423570. Epub 2017/05/23. J Bone Jt Infect. eng
Frank JM, Kayupov E, Moric M, Segreti J, Hansen E, Hartman C et al (2017) The Mark Coventry, MD, Award: oral antibiotics reduce reinfection after two-stage exchange: a multicenter, randomized controlled trial. Clin Orthop Relat Res 475(1):56–61. PMCID: PMC5174034. Epub 2016/07/09. Clin Orthop Relat Res. eng
Frisch NB, Kadri OM, Tenbrunsel T, Abdul-Hak A, Qatu M, Davis JJ (2017) Intraoperative chlorhexidine irrigation to prevent infection in total hip and knee arthroplasty. Arthroplast Today 3:294–297. Arthroplasty Today
Garvin KL, Miller RE, Gilbert TM, White AM, Lyden ER (2018) Late reinfection may recur more than 5 years after reimplantation of THA and TKA: analysis of pathogen factors. Clin Orthop Relat Res 476(2):345–352. Epub 2018/03/13. Clin Orthop Relat Res. eng
Ghazavi M, Mortazavi J, Patzakis M, Sheehan E, Tan TL, Yazdi H (2019) Hip and knee section, treatment, salvage: proceedings of international consensus on orthopedic infections. J Arthroplast 34(2s):S459–Ss62. Epub 2018/10/24. J Arthroplasty. eng
Gomez MM, Tan TL, Manrique J, Deirmengian GK, Parvizi J (2015) The fate of spacers in the treatment of periprosthetic joint infection. J Bone Joint Surg Am 97(18):1495–1502. Epub 2015/09/18. J Bone Joint Surg Am. eng
Grosso MJ, Berg A, LaRussa S, Murtaugh T, Trofa DP, Geller JA (2017) Silver-impregnated occlusive dressing reduces rates of acute periprosthetic joint infection after total joint arthroplasty. J Arthroplast 32(3):929–932. Epub 2016/10/26. J Arthroplasty. eng
Gu A, Malahias MA, Strigelli V, Nocon AA, Sculco TP, Sculco PK (2019) Preoperative malnutrition negatively correlates with postoperative wound complications and infection after total joint arthroplasty: a systematic review and meta-analysis. J Arthroplast 34(5):1013–1024. Epub 2019/02/13. J Arthroplasty. eng
Iorio R, Osmani FA (2017) Strategies to prevent periprosthetic joint infection after total knee arthroplasty and lessen the risk of readmission for the patient. J Am Acad Orthop Surg 25(Suppl 1):S13–Ss6. Epub 2016/12/17. J Am Acad Orthop Surg. eng
Jaberi FM, Parvizi J, Haytmanek CT, Joshi A, Purtill J (2008) Procrastination of wound drainage and malnutrition affect the outcome of joint arthroplasty. Clin Orthop Relat Res 466(6):1368–1371. PMCID: PMC2384013. Epub 2008/04/12. Clin Orthop Relat Res. eng
Kheir MM, Tan TL, Azboy I, Tan DD, Parvizi J (2017) Vancomycin prophylaxis for total joint arthroplasty: incorrectly dosed and has a higher rate of periprosthetic infection than cefazolin. Clin Orthop Relat Res 475(7):1767–1774. PMCID: PMC5449331. Epub 2017/04/13. Clin Orthop Relat Res. eng
Kheir MM, Tan TL, Ackerman CT, Modi R, Foltz C, Parvizi J (2018) Culturing periprosthetic joint infection: number of sam-

ples, growth duration, and organisms. J Arthroplast 33(11):3531–6.e1. Epub 2018/08/11. J Arthroplasty. eng
Koyonos L, Zmistowski B, Della Valle CJ, Parvizi J (2011) Infection control rate of irrigation and debridement for periprosthetic joint infection. Clin Orthop Relat Res 469(11):3043–3048. PMCID: PMC3183205. Epub 2011/05/10. Clin Orthop Relat Res. eng
Li R, Shao HY, Hao LB, Yu BZ, Qu PF, Zhou YX et al (2019) Plasma fibrinogen exhibits better performance than plasma D-dimer in the diagnosis of periprosthetic joint infection: a multicenter retrospective study. J Bone Joint Surg Am 101(7):613–619. Epub 2019/04/05. J Bone Joint Surg Am. eng
Lichstein P, Gehrke T, Lombardi A, Romano C, Stockley I, Babis G et al (2014) One-stage vs two-stage exchange. J Arthroplast 29(2 Suppl):108–111. Epub 2013/12/24. J Arthroplasty. eng
Lonner JH, Desai P, Dicesare PE, Steiner G, Zuckerman JD (1996) The reliability of analysis of intraoperative frozen sections for identifying active infection during revision hip or knee arthroplasty. J Bone Joint Surg Am 78(10):1553–1558. PubMed PMID: 8876584. Epub 1996/10/01. eng
Lum ZC, Natsuhara KM, Shelton TJ, Giordani M, Pereira GC, Meehan JP (2018) Mortality during total knee periprosthetic joint infection. J Arthroplast 33(12):3783–3788. Epub 2018/09/19. J Arthroplasty. eng
Mills E, Eyawo O, Lockhart I, Kelly S, Wu P, Ebbert JO (2011) Smoking cessation reduces postoperative complications: a systematic review and meta-analysis. Am J Med 124(2):144–54.e8. Epub 2011/02/08. Am J Med. eng
Nagra NS, Hamilton TW, Ganatra S, Murray DW, Pandit H (2016) One-stage versus two-stage exchange arthroplasty for infected total knee arthroplasty: a systematic review. Knee Surg Sports Traumatol Arthrosc 24(10):3106–3114. Epub 2015/09/24. Knee Surg Sports Traumatol Arthrosc. eng
Nahhas CR, Chalmers PN, Parvizi J, Sporer SM, Berend KR, Moric M et al (2020) A randomized trial of static and articulating spacers for the treatment of infection following total knee arthroplasty. J Bone Joint Surg Am 102(9):778–787. Epub 2020/05/08. J Bone Joint Surg Am. eng
Narayanan R, Anoushiravani AA, Elbuluk AM, Chen KK, Adler EM, Schwarzkopf R (2018) Irrigation and debridement for early periprosthetic knee infection: is it effective? J Arthroplast 33(6):1872–1878. Epub 2018/02/13. J Arthroplasty. eng
Nelson CL, Elkassabany NM, Kamath AF, Liu J (2015) Low albumin levels, more than morbid obesity, are associated with complications after TKA. Clin Orthop Relat Res 473(10):3163–3172. PMCID: PMC4562915. Epub 2015/05/23. Clin Orthop Relat Res. eng
Panahi P, Stroh M, Casper DS, Parvizi J, Austin MS (2012) Operating room traffic is a major concern during total joint arthroplasty. Clin Orthop Relat Res 470(10):2690–2694. PMCID: PMC3441983. Epub 2012/02/04. Clin Orthop Relat Res. eng
Pangaud C, Ollivier M, Argenson JN (2019) Outcome of single-stage versus two-stage exchange for revision knee arthroplasty for chronic periprosthetic infection. EFORT Open Rev 4(8):495–502. PMCID: PMC6719605. Epub 2019/09/21. EFORT Open Rev. eng
Parvizi J, Gehrke T (2014) Definition of periprosthetic joint infection. J Arthroplast 29(7):1331. Epub 2014/04/29. J Arthroplasty. eng
Parvizi J, Jacovides C, Antoci V, Ghanem E (2011) Diagnosis of periprosthetic joint infection: the utility of a simple yet unappreciated enzyme. J Bone Joint Surg Am 93(24):2242–2248. Epub 2012/01/20. J Bone Joint Surg Am. eng
Parvizi J, Tan TL, Goswami K, Higuera C, Della Valle C, Chen AF et al (2018) The 2018 definition of periprosthetic hip and knee infection: an evidence-based and validated criteria. J Arthroplast 33(5):1309–14.e2. The Journal of Arthroplasty
Patel R, Alijanipour P, Parvizi J (2016) Advancements in diagnosing periprosthetic joint infections after total hip and knee arthroplasty. Open Orthop J 10:654–661. PMCID: PMC5220175. Epub 2017/02/02. Open Orthop J. eng
Petis SM, Perry KI, Mabry TM, Hanssen AD, Berry DJ, Abdel MP (2019) Two-stage exchange protocol for periprosthetic joint infection following total knee arthroplasty in 245 knees without prior treatment for infection. J Bone Joint Surg Am 101(3):239–249. Epub 2019/02/08. J Bone Joint Surg Am. eng
Roche M, Law TY, Kurowicki J, Sodhi N, Rosas S, Elson L et al (2018) Albumin, prealbumin, and transferrin may be predictive of wound complications following total knee arthroplasty. J Knee Surg 31(10):946–951. Epub 2018/10/04. J Knee Surg. eng
Rothenberg AC, Wilson AE, Hayes JP, O'Malley MJ, Klatt BA (2017) Sonication of arthroplasty implants improves accuracy of periprosthetic joint infection cultures. Clin Orthop Relat Res 475(7):1827–1836. PMCID: PMC5449333. Epub 2017/03/16. Clin Orthop Relat Res. eng
Ryan SP, Kildow BJ, Tan TL, Parvizi J, Bolognesi MP, Seyler TM (2019) Is there a difference in infection risk between single and multiple doses of prophylactic antibiotics? A meta-analysis. Clin Orthop Relat Res 477(7):1577–1590. PMCID: PMC6999965 Related Research® editors and board members are on file with the publication and can be viewed on request. Epub 2019/02/28. Clin Orthop Relat Res. eng
Shahi A, Parvizi J, Kazarian GS, Higuera C, Frangiamore S, Bingham J et al (2016) The alpha-defensin test for periprosthetic joint infections is not affected by prior antibiotic administration. Clin Orthop Relat Res 474(7):1610–1615. PMCID: PMC4887359. Epub 2016/02/13. Clin Orthop Relat Res. eng
Shahi A, Kheir MM, Tarabichi M, Hosseinzadeh HRS, Tan TL, Parvizi J (2017) Serum D-dimer test is promising for the diagnosis of periprosthetic joint infection and timing of reimplantation. J Bone Joint Surg Am 99(17):1419–1427. Epub 2017/09/06. J Bone Joint Surg Am. eng
Shohat N, Goswami K, Tan TL, Yayac M, Soriano A, Sousa R et al (2020) Frank Stinchfield Award: identifying who will fail following irrigation and debridement for prosthetic joint infection. Bone Joint J 102-b(7_Supple_B):11–19. Epub 2020/07/01. Bone Joint J. eng
Spangehl MJ, Masri BA, O'Connell JX, Duncan CP (1999) Prospective analysis of preoperative and intraoperative investigations for the diagnosis of infection at the sites of two hundred and two revision total hip arthroplasties. J Bone Joint Surg Am 81(5):672–683. PubMed PMID: 10360695. Epub 1999/06/09. eng
Stambough JB, Nam D, Warren DK, Keeney JA, Clohisy JC, Barrack RL et al (2017) Decreased hospital costs and surgical site infection incidence with a universal decolonization protocol in primary total joint arthroplasty. J Arthroplast 32(3):728–34.e1. Epub 2016/11/09. J Arthroplasty. eng
Tan TL, Goswami K, Fillingham YA, Shohat N, Rondon AJ, Parvizi J (2018) Defining treatment success after 2-stage exchange arthroplasty for periprosthetic joint infection. J Arthroplast 33(11):3541–3546. Epub 2018/08/14. J Arthroplasty. eng
Tan TL, Shohat N, Rondon AJ, Foltz C, Goswami K, Ryan SP et al (2019a) Perioperative antibiotic prophylaxis in total joint arthroplasty: a single dose is as effective as multiple doses. J Bone Joint Surg Am 101(5):429–437. Epub 2019/03/08. J Bone Joint Surg Am. eng
Tan TL, Goswami K, Kheir MM, Xu C, Wang Q, Parvizi J (2019b) Surgical treatment of chronic periprosthetic joint infection: fate of spacer exchanges. J Arthroplast 34(9):2085-90.e1. Epub 2019/06/12. J Arthroplasty. eng

Toossi N, Adeli B, Rasouli MR, Huang R, Parvizi J (2012) Serum white blood cell count and differential do not have a role in the diagnosis of periprosthetic joint infection. J Arthroplast 27(8 Suppl):51–4.e1. Epub 2012/05/23. J Arthroplasty. eng
Urish KL, Bullock AG, Kreger AM, Shah NB, Jeong K, Rothenberger SD (2018) A multicenter study of irrigation and debridement in total knee arthroplasty periprosthetic joint infection: treatment failure is high. J Arthroplast 33(4):1154–1159. PMCID: PMC5858958. Epub 2017/12/10. J Arthroplasty. eng
Wang Y, Li Y, Qiao L, Sun S (2020) Comparison of a comprehensive set of fibrinolytic markers with C-reactive protein and erythrocyte sedimentation rate for the diagnosis of periprosthetic joint infection. J Arthroplast 35(9):2613–2618. Epub 2020/05/29. J Arthroplasty. eng
Winkler T, Stuhlert MGW, Lieb E, Muller M, von Roth P, Preininger B et al (2019) Outcome of short versus long interval in two-stage exchange for periprosthetic joint infection: a prospective cohort study. Arch Orthop Trauma Surg 139(3):295–303. Epub 2018/11/18. Arch Orthop Trauma Surg. eng
Wouthuyzen-Bakker M, Nijman JM, Kampinga GA, van Assen S, Jutte PC (2017) Efficacy of antibiotic suppressive therapy in patients with a prosthetic joint infection. J Bone Jt Infect 2(2):77–83. PMCID: PMC5423578. Epub 2017/05/23. J Bone Jt Infect. eng
Wouthuyzen-Bakker M, Sebillotte M, Lomas J, Kendrick B, Palomares EB, Murillo O et al (2019) Timing of implant-removal in late acute periprosthetic joint infection: a multicenter observational study. J Infect 79(3):199–205. Epub 2019/07/19. J Infect. eng
Wouthuyzen-Bakker M, Sebillotte M, Huotari K, Escudero Sánchez R, Benavent E, Parvizi J et al (2020) Lower success rate of débridement and implant retention in late acute versus early acute periprosthetic joint infection caused by Staphylococcus spp. results from a matched cohort study. Clin Orthop Relat Res 478(6):1348–1355. Epub 2020/02/28. Clin Orthop Relat Res. eng
Xu H, Xie J, Huang Q, Lei Y, Zhang S, Pei F (2019) Plasma fibrin degradation product and D-dimer are of limited value for diagnosing periprosthetic joint infection. J Arthroplast 34(10):2454–2460. Epub 2019/06/04. J Arthroplasty. eng
Yang J, Parvizi J, Hansen EN, Culvern CN, Segreti JC, Tan T et al (2020) 2020 Mark Coventry Award: microorganism-directed oral antibiotics reduce the rate of failure due to further infection after two-stage revision hip or knee arthroplasty for chronic infection: a multicentre randomized controlled trial at a minimum of two years. Bone Joint J 102-b(6_Supple_A):3–9. Epub 2020/06/02. Bone Joint J. eng

Management – Revision

Contents

Systematic Evaluation of Painful Total Knee Arthroplasty

Gwo-Chin Lee

Contents

E. Hansen, K.-D. Kühn (eds.), *Essentials of Cemented Knee Arthroplasty*,
https://doi.org/10.1007/978-3-662-63113-3_56

56.1 Introduction

Total knee arthroplasty (TKA) has been shown to be effective, reliable, and durable in relieving pain and improving function in patients with end-stage arthritis of the knee joint (Hopley and Dalury 2014). However, as the number of performed TKAs increases, there will be an expected corresponding increase in the number of failures and revisions (Bozic et al. 2010).

The reasons knees fail can be variable and sometimes multifactorial (Sharkey et al. 2014). While pain is nearly a universal complaint of patients with failing knee replacements, identifying and understanding the mechanism of failure and pain are critical for successful revision surgery.

> Mont et al. reported 59% poor results following exploration in patients with radiographically normal knees with unexplained pain (Mont et al. 1996).

Therefore, revision surgery should not be undertaken unless a definite and correctable cause can be identified preoperatively.

The evaluation of a painful TKA requires a systematic approach. Only the combination of the clinical history, physical examination, and radiographic and laboratory evaluations can provide the complete clinical picture that is critical to the understanding of why a particular knee has failed. This chapter will discuss the workup of the painful knee replacement.

56.2 Clinical History

A detailed clinical history is the starting point for the treatment of a painful TKA. Useful information includes the circumstances surrounding the initial arthroplasty including diagnosis, prior surgeries, and complications including wound healing complications and infection. Additionally, a review of preoperative radiographs prior to the initial TKA can provide important information with regard to the indications of surgery as well as information on whether the initial TKA relieved the preoperative knee pain.

Polkowski et al. showed that early-grade arthritis at the time of TKA was significantly associated with pain and dissatisfaction following TKA (Polkowski et al. 2013).

The type, characteristic, and duration of pain can also hint at the mechanism of failure. In general, symptoms such as pain with activities that is relieved at rest are associated with mechanical and aseptic failures, while rest pain and particularly pain at night should be suspicious for infection. Start-up pain, defined by initial worsening pain following rest (i.e., first few steps of the day or following periods of sitting), can be indicative of aseptic loosening. In addition, knee weakness, falls, and difficulty walking on uneven terrain is often associated with an unstable knee. Finally, recurrent hemarthrosis or sterile effusions with stair descent activities are characteristically seen in patients with flexion instability (Stambough et al. 2019).

56.3 Physical Examination

The clinical examination begins at the moment the patient walks through the exam room doors. Observing the patient's gait can provide significant information about the causes of dysfunction even before one lays hands on the knee joint. The presence of an abductor lurch (i.e., Trendelenburg gait) or ataxia points to the coexistence of hip or neural pathologies, respectively. The excursion of the knee joint through the gait cycle can demonstrate the presence of either fixed flexion contractures, knee recurvatum, or ligament instability (i.e., varus or valgus thrusts).

The systematic examination then progresses to the soft tissue envelope of the knee, where the incision and soft tissues are evaluated. The presence or absence of joint effusion or synovitis is noted. Draining wounds or nonhealing sinuses are seen in cases of infection while soft tissue defects with associated muscle dysfunction are present in cases with extensor mechanism disruptions. Both active and passive range of motion of the knee should be recorded, and the presence of any flexion contractures or extensor lags should be noted. The alignment of the knee joint is assessed in both the standing (weight-bearing) and supine (non-weight-bearing) positions. The presence of extra-articular deformities including excessive planovalgus foot deformity can significantly affect overall limb alignment (Meding et al. 2005). Patellar tracking is assessed throughout the entire arc of knee motion. The stability of the knee joint is then assessed in full extension, 30°, 60°, and 90° of knee flexion. Excessive differences in medial-lateral gapping represents medial-lateral gap imbalance, while excessive anterior-posterior translation and superior-inferior pistoning of the knee at 90° of flexion is seen in cases of flexion instability (◘ Fig. 56.1).

> It is important to note that since instability is poorly defined, a comparison to the contralateral knee and asking whether the patient is painful or uncomfortable during any of these maneuvers can distinguish physiologic vs. pathologic laxity.

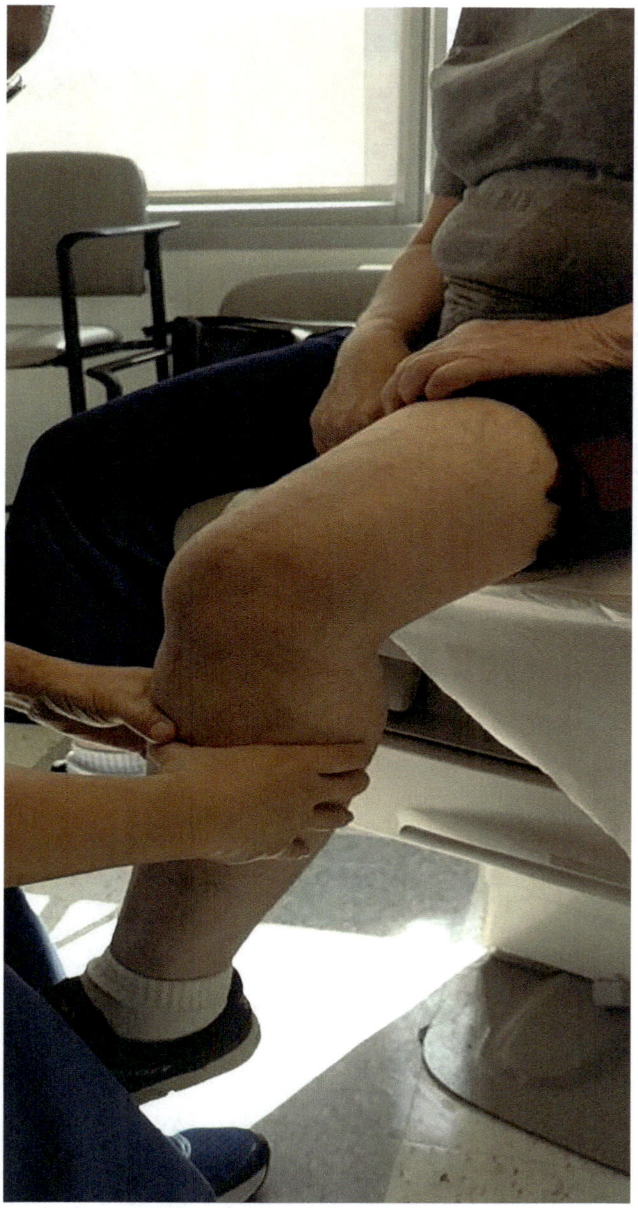

Fig. 56.1 Diagnosis of flexion instability. The patient is asked to sit at the edge of the exam table, and the examiner anchors the foot; this allows the patient to relax and allows the examiner to translate the knee anterior-posteriorly or "piston" the knee superior-inferiorly

Finally, an evaluation of the hip joint, spine, and a complete neurovascular exam is performed in order not to overlook coexisting pathologies and other potential sources of pain.

56.4 Radiographic Evaluation

A standard radiographic review includes standing anterior-posterior (AP), lateral, and Merchant or sunrise views of the knee. A long-standing hip-to-ankle radiograph can aid in the assessment of overall limb alignment, particularly in the setting of extra-articular deformities. Oblique radiographs have been shown to be more sensitive in the evaluation of osteolytic lesions (Nadaud et al. 2004). A critical evaluation of component fixation and position includes coronal and sagittal alignments, joint line position, posterior condylar offset, tibial slope, and the presence of radiolucent lines.

In general, the joint line should be positioned approximately 25–30 mm from the medial epicondyle of the femur, while the posterior condylar offset should measure approximately 25–30 mm from the posterior femoral cortex (Voleti et al. 2015). Failure to restore posterior condylar offset can result in flexion instability and loss of knee flexion. Comparing the prosthetic offset to the contralateral knee can also be helpful. In terms of tibial slope, depending on the type of prosthesis being used (PS vs. CR), it should be approximately 0–5°: 0–3° in PS knee implants and 3–5° in CR implants. Excessive posterior slope is associated with flexion instability, while anterior slope is associated with poor flexion (Song et al. 2019).

Fixation of the TKA components is determined by the presence or absence of signs of prosthetic loosening. A prosthesis is loose if there is

- Circumferential radiolucent lines around the entire implant greater than 2 mm
- Progressive radiolucent lines on serial radiographs
- Evidence of component migration on serial radiographs (Fig. 56.2)

In stemmed implants, a shift in stem position, subsidence, or pedestal formation are also signs of loosening (Fig. 56.3). While bone scans can show increased activity in loose TKA implants, their utility in the workup of a painful TKA has diminished over the past decade. Finally, it is also important to recognize that a positive bone scan up to 18 months following surgery can be normal and not indicative of component loosening (Niccoli et al. 2017).

Femoral and/or tibial component malrotation has been associated with extensor mechanism problems and persistent pain following TKA (Panni et al. 2018). While the sunrise or Merchant views can roughly assess femoral component rotation, in general, rotation is generally assessed using computed tomography (CT). On the femoral side, the femoral component should be parallel to the transepicondylar axis of the femur, while on the tibial side, the tibial component should not be internally rotated to the medial border of the tibial tubercle (Lee et al. 2004) (Fig. 56.4). While these rotational guidelines have been used over the past 30 years, recent studies in kinematically aligned knees have shown that small deviations from these landmarks can still be compatible with well-functioning TKAs (Nedopil et al. 2016).

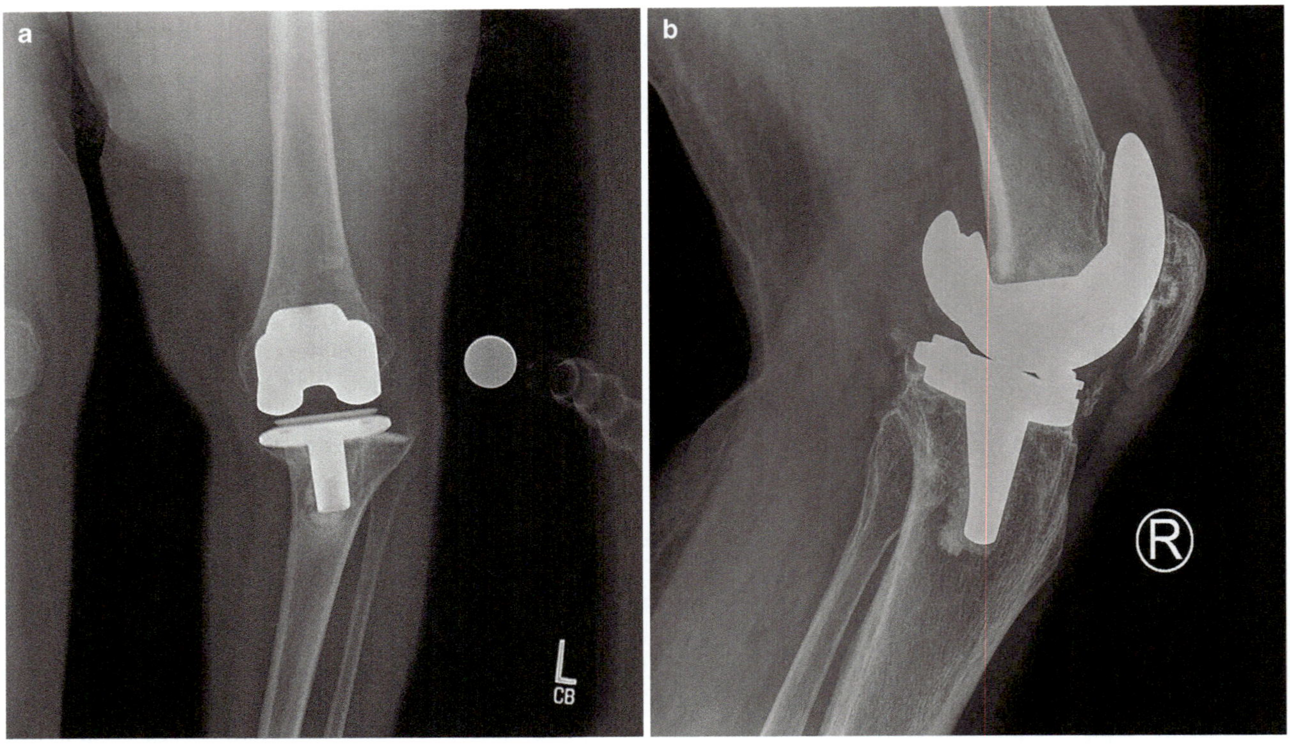

Fig. 56.2 **a** AP radiograph of the knee demonstrating a loose tibial component. Note the circumferential radiolucent lines and the collapse and migration of the prosthesis into varus. **b** Lateral radiograph of a loose femoral component. Radiolucencies are present around the entire implant, and the component has migrated proximally and into flexion

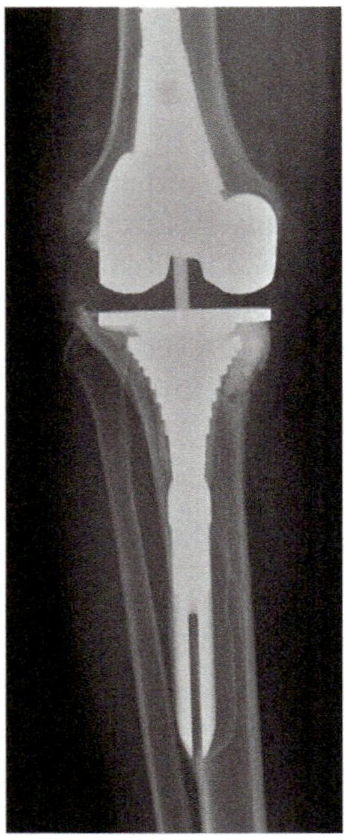

Fig. 56.3 AP radiograph of a loose stemmed tibial and femoral component. Notice again the lucent lines around the stem of the implant and migration of the stem into varus. In addition, notice the bony pedestal at the tip of the stem

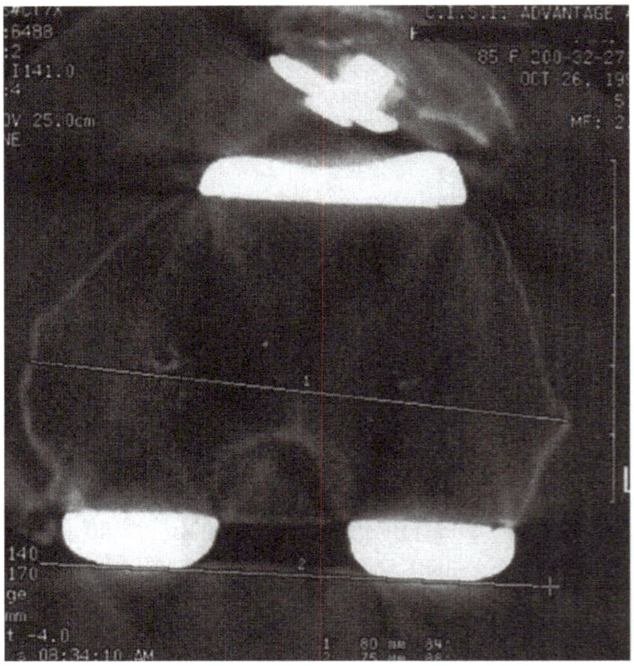

Fig. 56.4 CT scan of a knee with patellofemoral maltracking. The femoral component is internally rotated in relation to the transepicondylar axis of the knee (*line*)

> Consequently, one must consider the overall clinical picture and recommend revision only when the radiographic abnormality coincides with the patient's symptoms.

56.5 Laboratory Studies

There are three questions that need to be answered when evaluating a painful TKA:

1. Is the bone broken?
2. Is the implant well fixed, loose, or unstable?
3. Is the knee infected?

> Infection is the leading cause for early revision in some series following TKA today (Sharkey et al. 2014). Therefore, it is imperative that the workup of a painful knee replacement includes an evaluation for prosthetic joint infection (PJI).

The American Academy of Orthopaedic Surgery has published clinical practice guidelines for the diagnosis of prosthetic joint infections (Parvizi and Della Valle 2010). The first step in this algorithm is obtaining a serum erythrocyte sedimentation rate (ESR) and C-reactive protein (CRP) in all painful joint replacements. These markers are nonspecific inflammatory markers that have been shown to be highly sensitive when both are elevated to correlate with the presence of infection (Bingham et al. 2019). In rare instances, seronegative (negative ESR/CRP) prosthetic joint infections have also been reported (McArthur et al. 2015). The utility of other biomarkers including D-dimer and interleukin-6 remains undefined (Lee et al. 2017).

If the index of clinical suspicion for infection is high, joint aspiration of antibiotics is the most sensitive and specific way to diagnose prosthetic joint infections today. Synovial white blood cell count and differential have been shown to be correlated with infection. The thresholds can be variable, but the Musculoskeletal Infection Society (MSIS) currently recommends a synovial WBC threshold of 3000 cells and a PMN differential of 65% for chronic infections. For infections occurring within the first 6 weeks, a synovial WBC threshold of 10,000 cells and PMN differential greater than 90% is used (Aalirezaie et al. 2019). Leukocyte esterase and α-defensin have also been shown to be both sensitive and specific in the detection of PJI (Lee et al. 2017).

56.6 Preoperative Counseling

Finally, for the patient facing re-operation, a failed TKA can be the source of disappointment and anger. Questions such as why and how this condition did happen or whether anything done at the time of the initial operation prompted the current state of affairs can be uncomfortable. The surgeon should educate the patient and establish clear and realistic expectations in terms of the procedure, recovery, and likely successful outcome (i.e., motion, residual pain, stiffness, and activity levels) in order to assist the patient in the decision-making process.

> The physician's definition of successful revision must be aligned with the patient's definition of success in order to minimize patient dissatisfaction.

Conclusion

There are many reasons why a patient can present with a painful TKA. Accurate identification and understanding of the mode of failure (if any) is critical to successful management. A systematic approach including a detailed history, physical examination, and laboratory and radiographic studies is required to maximize success and minimize complications.

Take-Home Messages

- To successfully manage pain in TKA, accuracy in the identification and understanding of the mode of failure is key.
- A systematic approach including a detailed history, physical examination, and laboratory and radiographic studies is required to maximize success and minimize complications.
- All evaluations must include a workup for prosthetic joint infection. The presence or absence of infection must be established prior to revision.
- All causes of pain must be considered including referred sources such as the hip or spine and neurogenic pain.
- Setting realistic patient expectations prior to revision surgery in terms of recovery and ultimate function will assist the patient in the decision-making process of whether re-operation is necessary.

References

Aalirezaie A, Bauer TW, Fayaz H, Griffin W, Higuera CA, Krenn V, Krenn V, Molano M, Moojen DJ, Restrepo C, Shahi A, Shubnyakov I, Sporer S, Tanavalee A, Teloken M, Velázquez Moreno JD (2019) Hip and knee section, diagnosis, reimplantation: proceedings of international consensus on orthopedic infections. J Arthroplast 34(2S):S369–S379

Bingham JS, Hassebrock JD, Christensen AL, Beauchamp CP, Clarke HD, Spangehl MJ (2019) Screening for periprosthetic joint infections with ESR and CRP: the ideal cutoffs. J Arthroplast. https://doi.org/10.1016/j.arth.2019.11.040. pii:S0883-5403(19)31112-X. [Epub ahead of print]

Bozic KJ, Kurtz SM, Lau E, Ong K, Chiu V, Vail TP, Rubash HE, Berry DJ (2010) The epidemiology of revision total knee arthroplasty in the United States. Clin Orthop Relat Res 468(1):45–51

Hopley CD, Dalury DF (2014) A systematic review of clinical outcomes and survivorship after total knee arthroplasty with a contemporary modular knee system. J Arthroplast 29(7):1398–1411

Lee GC, Cushner FD, Scuderi GR, Insall JN (2004) Optimizing patellofemoral tracking during total knee arthroplasty. J Knee Surg 17(3):144–149; discussion 149–150

Lee YS, Koo KH, Kim HJ, Tian S, Kim TY, Maltenfort MG, Chen AF (2017) Synovial fluid biomarkers for the diagnosis of periprosthetic joint infection: a systematic review and meta-analysis. J Bone Joint Surg Am 99(24):2077–2084

McArthur BA, Abdel MP, Taunton MJ, Osmon DR, Hanssen AD (2015) Seronegative infections in hip and knee arthroplasty: periprosthetic infections with normal erythrocyte sedimentation rate and C-reactive protein level. Bone Joint J 97-B(7):939–944

Meding JB, Keating EM, Ritter MA, Faris PM, Berend ME, Malinzak RA (2005) The planovalgus foot: a harbinger of failure of posterior cruciate-retaining total knee replacement. J Bone Joint Surg Am 87(Suppl 2):59–62

Mont MA, Serna FK, Krackow KA, Hungerford DS (1996) Exploration of radiographically normal total knee replacements for unexplained pain. Clin Orthop Relat Res 331:216–220

Nadaud MC, Fehring TK, Fehring K (2004) Underestimation of osteolysis in posterior stabilized total knee arthroplasty. J Arthroplast 19(1):110–115

Nedopil AJ, Howell SM, Hull ML (2016) Does malrotation of the tibial and femoral components compromise function in kinematically aligned total knee arthroplasty? Orthop Clin North Am 47(1):41–50

Niccoli G, Mercurio D, Cortese F (2017) Bone scan in painful knee arthroplasty: obsolete or actual examination? Acta Biomed 88(2S):68–77

Panni AS, Ascione F, Rossini M, Braile A, Corona K, Vasso M, Hirschmann MT (2018) Tibial internal rotation negatively affects clinical outcomes in total knee arthroplasty: a systematic review. Knee Surg Sports Traumatol Arthrosc 26(6):1636–1644

Parvizi J, Della Valle CJ (2010) AAOS clinical practice guideline: diagnosis and treatment of periprosthetic joint infections of the hip and knee. J Am Acad Orthop Surg 18(12):771–772

Polkowski GG 2nd, Ruh EL, Barrack TN, Nunley RM, Barrack RL (2013) Is pain and dissatisfaction after TKA related to early-grade preoperative osteoarthritis? Clin Orthop Relat Res 471(1):162–168

Sharkey PF, Lichstein PM, Shen C, Tokarski AT, Parvizi J (2014) Why are total knee arthroplasties failing today--has anything changed after 10 years? J Arthroplast 29(9):1774–1778

Song SJ, Park CH, Bae DK (2019) What to know for selecting cruciate-retaining or posterior-stabilized total knee arthroplasty. Clin Orthop Surg 11(2):142–150

Stambough JB, Edwards PK, Mannen EM, Barnes CL, Mears SC (2019) Flexion instability after total knee arthroplasty. J Am Acad Orthop Surg 27(17):642–651

Voleti PB, Stephenson JW, Lotke PA, Lee GC (2015) No sex differences exist in posterior condylar offsets of the knee. Clin Orthop Relat Res 473(4):1425–1431

Periprosthetic Joint Infection: Consensus and Guidelines

Timothy L. Tan and Javad Parvizi

Contents

E. Hansen, K.-D. Kühn (eds.), *Essentials of Cemented Knee Arthroplasty*,
https://doi.org/10.1007/978-3-662-63113-3_57

57

57.1 Introduction

Infection is one of the major complications following total knee arthroplasty (TKA) (Gomez et al. 2015; Zmistowski et al. 2013; Berend et al. 2013) and is the most common reason for revision following modern TKA (Motififard et al. 2015; Bozic et al. 2010). In addition to the significant morbidity and mortality associated with this condition (Gomez et al. 2015; Zmistowski et al. 2013; Berend et al. 2013), periprosthetic joint infection (PJI) remains one of the most challenging conditions to diagnose and treat. In the last few years, there have been considerable efforts to better understand and treat PJI (◘ Fig. 57.1). However, there is often little evidence to guide surgeons regarding the proper prevention, diagnosis, and treatment of PJI.

Given the paucity of evidence in infection, consensus conferences are relied on to provide guidelines and establish a standard of care when limited evidence is available for clinically important questions. To answer these questions, the first International Consensus Meeting (ICM) on PJI was held in 2013, consisting of over 300 experts from 52 countries (Parvizi and Gehrke 2014). In addition to providing some guidelines regarding diagnosis, prevention, and treatment, the first ICM also established a definition for PJI that was adopted by the Center for Disease Control and has been widely adopted and used (Parvizi and Gehrke 2014). Due to its success, the Second International Consensus Meeting on PJI occurred in 2018, which included over 869 delegates from 92 countries (Parvizi et al. 2019).

The consensus utilized the Delphi method, which was originally developed by the RAND Corporation in the 1960s (Dalkey and Helmer 1963). This process sought to distribute questions to 2–3 delegates who would lend their expertise and perform a systematic review, followed by voting and feedback in a controlled-fashion 13-step process that occurred over 2 years. The level of evidence (LOE) (strong, moderate, low, or no evidence) was reported for each question in order to demonstrate the strength of recommendation for each question. Furthermore, the level of consensus was measured, which demonstrates the agreement among delegates.

Given the massive scale and amount of recommendations from the ICM, this chapter will highlight clinically important and relevant topics regarding cemented TKA.

57.2 Diagnosis

Within the last 5 years, a variety of novel tests have been introduced for the diagnosis of PJI, such as α-defensin and next-generation sequencing (Shahi et al. 2017; Li et al. 2019; Tarabichi et al. 2018; Deirmengian et al. 2015). One of the challenges for the orthopedic surgeon is incorporating these tests into clinical practice as these

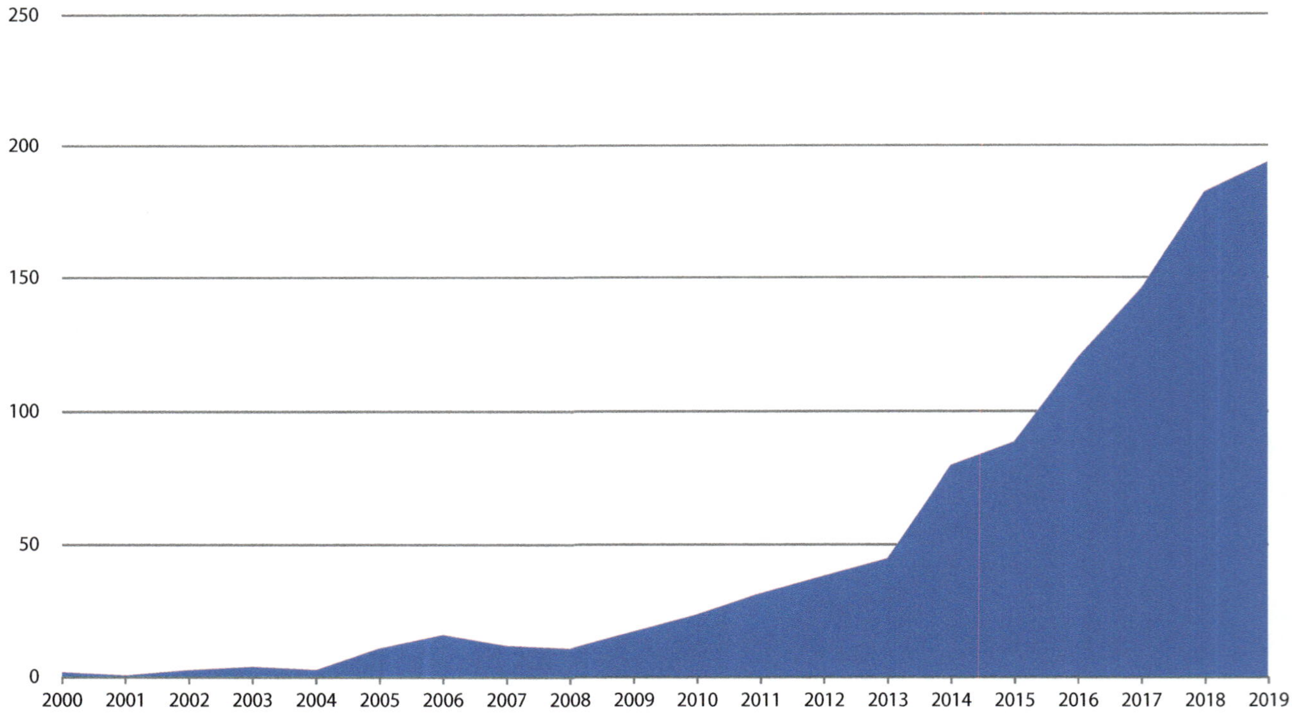

◘ **Fig. 57.1** Publications in PubMed for "Periprosthetic Joint Infection" and "Total Knee Arthroplasty" by year

tests were not accounted for in previous guidelines. Thus, one of the most important aspects of the ICM was the introduction of a new algorithm and definition for the diagnosis of PJI (Abdel Karim et al. 2019; Amanatullah et al. 2019).

> The introduction of the Musculoskeletal Infection Society definition of PJI has allowed for standardization and has greatly helped orthopedic surgeons diagnose PJI (Workgroup Convened by the Musculoskeletal Infection Society 2011).

However, this criterion is largely based on expert opinion and was not based on evidence or validated. One of the biggest issues with the previous definition is that culture-negative PJI was particularly hard to diagnose, as this relies on the minor criteria being ordered and positive.

> Thus, an evidence-based definition for PJI was developed through machine learning and a stepwise approach (Amanatullah et al. 2019; Parvizi et al. 2018).

In this new definition, the minor criteria are given differential weight, which recognizes the relative importance of various tests rather than considering all minor criteria equal. Furthermore, the new definition demonstrates higher sensitivity (97%) than the prior MSIS (79.3%) and ICM definition (86.9%). The new definition of PJI is depicted in Table 57.1 with a consensus of 68% and a level of evidence of moderate (Amanatullah et al. 2019).

In addition to the new definition, a new evidence-based algorithm was outlined to guide the orthopedic community on how to utilize the newer tests that were developed (Fig. 57.2).

> Similar to prior guidelines (Della Valle et al. 2011), a stepwise algorithm that first includes a physical examination followed by erythrocyte sedimentation rate and C-reactive protein was implemented with the introduction of D-dimer (Abdel Karim et al. 2019; Shohat et al. 2019).

> In patients with high clinical suspicion or elevated laboratory values, joint aspiration should be performed and sent for synovial white cell count, leukocyte esterase, neutrophil percentage, and culture.

While α-defensin has been introduced since the previous ICM and has gained popularity, the use of α-defensin did not reveal any improvement for the diagnosis of PJI.

Table 57.1 Definition of periprosthetic joint infection

Major criteria (at least one of the following)				Decision
Two positive growths of the same organism using standard culture methods				Infected
Sinus tract with evidence of communication to the joint or visualization of the prosthesis				
Minor criteria	**Threshold**		**Score**	**Decision**
	Acute	**Chronic**		
Serum CRP (mg/L) or D-dimer (μg/L)	100 Unknown	10 860	2	Combined preoperative and postoperative score: ≥6 Infection 3–5 Inconclusive <3 Not infected
Elevated serum ESR (mm/h)	–	30	1	
Elevated synovial WBC (cells/μL) or Leukocyte esterase or Positive α-defensin	10,000 ++ 1.0	3000 ++ 1.0	3	
Elevated synovial PMN (%)	90	70	2	
Single positive culture			2	
Positive histology			3	
Positive intraoperative purulence			3	

CRP C-reactive protein, *ESR* erythrocyte sedimentation rate, *WBC* white blood cell count, *PMN* polymorphonuclear cells

> Both the definition and the algorithm recognize that there will be cases in which the prior results are inconclusive, and thus purulence, histology, culture results, and next-generation sequencing should be considered.

The algorithm outlined above and in Fig. 57.2 received a level of evidence of strong and a consensus of 73%.

57.3 Prevention

57.3.1 Risk Factors

It is crucial to understand the risk factors for PJI in order to assess risk and implement strategies for modifiable risk factors with the aim of reducing the risk.

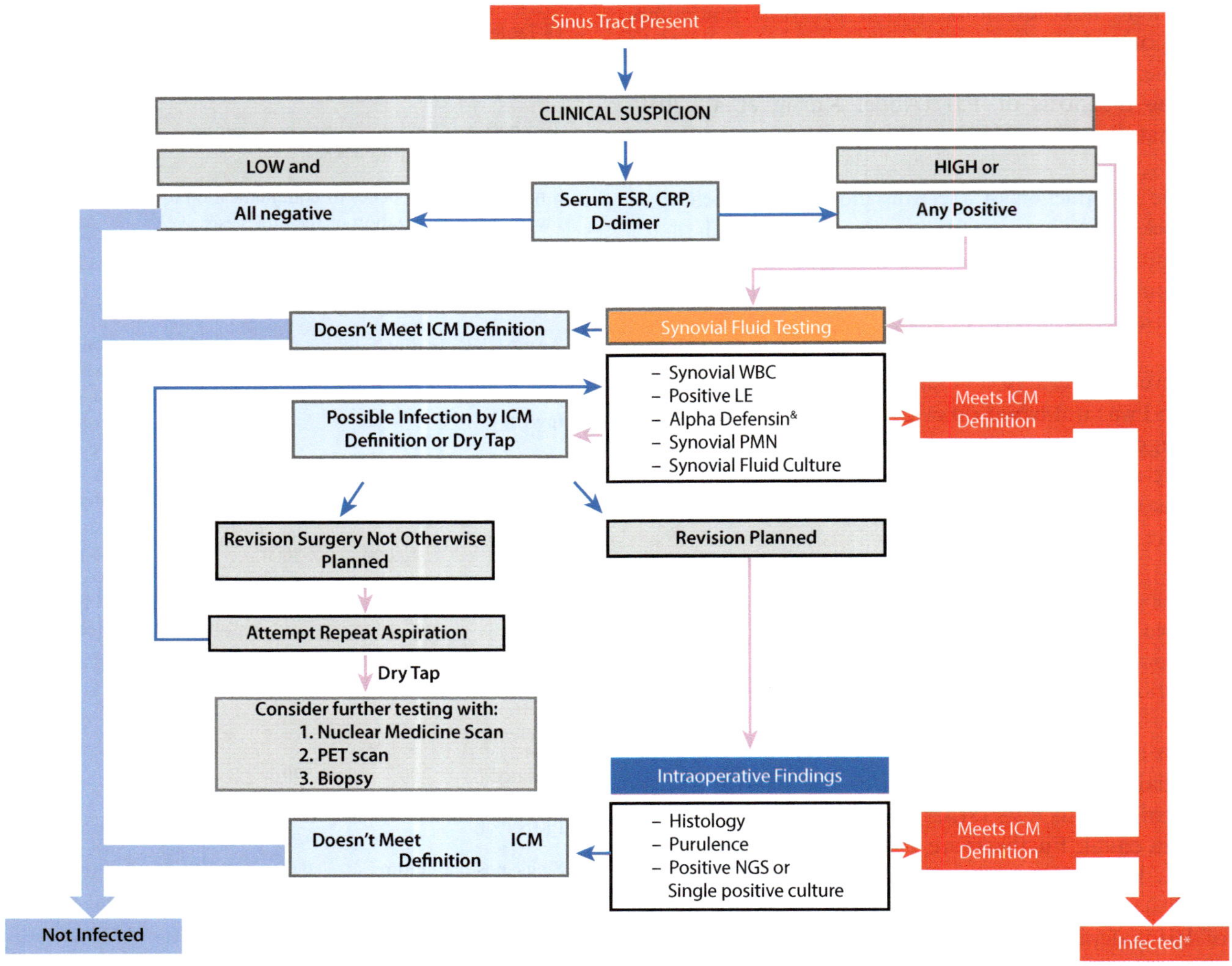

Fig. 57.2 Evidence-based algorithm for diagnosing periprosthetic joint infection. *At any time 2 positive cultures with the same organism or sinus tract are major criteria for infection. &Optional test; does not need to be performed routinely. ICM International Consensus Meeting, ESR erythrocyte sedimentation rate, CRP C-reactive protein, WBC white blood cell count, PMN polymorphonuclear cells, NGS next-generation sequencing

> The consensus identified several modifiable host-related factors, which included body mass index, smoking, alcohol consumption, diabetes, malnutrition, and other medical comorbidities.

> Nonmodifiable factors that were agreed upon were increasing age, male gender, and low socioeconomic status (98% consensus, strong LOE) (Cizmic et al. 2019).

Perioperative factors were also assessed and included the use of potent anticoagulation (80% consensus, moderate LOE), allogenic blood transfusion (Akonjom et al. 2019) (94% consensus, strong LOE), and general anesthesia as opposed to neuraxial anesthesia (Abdelaziz et al. 2019) (76% consensus, limited LOE). Laminar airflow was found to be not necessary for joint replacement surgery, as recent orthopedic literature has not demonstrated a reduction in infection (81% consensus, moderate LOE) (Aalirezaie et al. 2019).

57.3.2 Perioperative Antibiotics

Perioperative antibiotic prophylaxis has been a successful strategy to reduce infection in the setting of arthroplasty, and 24 hours of antibiotics has largely been used as this is the longest duration of antibiotics allowed by prior guidelines.

> However, with the introduction of new guidelines including the Center for Disease Control (CDC) Guidelines, the continuation of antibiotics in the postoperative period is no longer recommended (Surgical Site Infection | Guidelines | Infection Control | CDC 2019).

This is a highly controversial topic that prompted American Academy for Hip and Knee Surgeons (AAHKS) to release a position statement regarding the new CDC guideline.

> The recommendation from the ICM is that the current guidelines advocating for a single dose of perioperative antibiotics are primarily based on literature outside of orthopedics that is often underpowered and of limited evidence (Aboltins et al. 2019; Siddiqi et al. 2019; Ryan et al. 2019).

However, with the limited evidence available, it does appear that a single preoperative dose of antibiotics appears to be adequate, and there may not be a need for multiple doses (Tan et al. 2019). A large-scale randomized prospective study is certainly needed on this topic as there is a selection bias in the literature, with healthier patients often receiving a single dose compared to the multiple-dose counterparts.

57.3.3 Antibiotic Cement

The use of antibiotic cement was also a highly controversial topic in the ICM. The literature regarding antibiotic cement is highly conflicting.

> While a number of retrospective studies have correlated antibiotic cement with lower rates of wound infection and failure in TKA and THA, numerous studies could not find a difference (Fillingham et al. 2019; Namba et al. 2013; Bini et al. 2016; Tayton et al. 2016; Sanz-Ruiz et al. 2017; Jameson et al. 2019).

Furthermore, many of these studies were registry studies that make evaluating infection not ideal.

After an extensive discussion at the ICM, the recommendation is as follows:

> Antibiotic-impregnated cement may be used for patients at high risk of PJI undergoing primary total joint arthroplasty to reduce the risk of infection.

> The benefits vs. cost and other potential side effects such as the emergence of organisms resistant to antibiotics may be justified in patients at high risk of infection (93% consensus, limited LOE) (Fillingham et al. 2019).

57.3.4 Irrigation Solutions

While antibiotics can be used in cement, antibiotics such as polymyxin and bacitracin in the irrigation solution should not be routinely used.

> Guidelines from both the WHO and National Institute for Health and Care Excellence advise against the addition of topical antibiotics due to concerns for emergence of antimicrobial resistance, costs, and patient hypersensitivity (92% consensus, moderate LOE) (Blom et al. 2019).

Although a variety of irrigation solutions are available, the optimal irrigation solution is not known. However, the WHO and CDC support the use of dilute betadine as the irrigation solution of choice (75% consensus, strong LOE) (Blom et al. 2019).

57.4 Treatment

Once a diagnosis of PJI is made, prompt treatment includes a combination of both surgical and medical treatment. The indications and contraindications of the different surgical treatments were discussed extensively. Debridement, antibiotics, and implant retention (DAIR) was recommended for early postoperative PJI and acute hematogenous PJI, defined as symptoms existing for less than 4 weeks, in the setting of stable implants (80% consensus, moderate LOE) (Argenson et al. 2019). During a DAIR procedure, it is recommended that exchange of modular components be performed to reduce the rate of infection (94% consensus, moderate LOE) (Argenson et al. 2019) and that 6–8 L of saline or antiseptic solution be used (90% consensus, consensus LOE) (Argenson et al. 2019).

> For patients with a two-stage exchange arthroplasty, articulating spacers were found to provide a better range of motion and function, while nonarticulating spacers were indicated in patients with bone loss and deficient ligaments or abductor mechanism (91% consensus, strong LOE) (Abdel et al. 2019).

Furthermore, antibiotics in the cement spacer should be tailored to the infecting organism (94% consensus, moderate LOE) (Abdel et al. 2019). During re-implantation, it is recommended that antibiotics not exceed 5% weight per volume of cement in order to maintain the mechanical integrity of cement as fixation (Fillingham et al. 2019).

One-stage exchange arthroplasty is appealing for surgeons as there is decreased surgical morbidity and mortality, earlier functional return, and a decrease in healthcare costs. The ICM recognizes one-stage exchange as a viable option for chronic PJIs (Bialecki et al. 2019). However, a one-stage may not be an ideal option in patients with systemic sepsis, extensive comorbidities, resistant organisms, culture-negative infections, and poor soft tissue coverage (93% consensus, moderate LOE) (Bialecki et al. 2019).

Conclusion

Despite the abundance of research on PJI, there still remain many questions on how to diagnose, prevent, and treat this terrible complication. There are few guidelines to direct surgeons regarding PJI, and limited high-level studies on this topic are likely attributed to the relative rarity of this condition. Two of the biggest accomplishments from the ICM include the development of an evidence-based definition and the new algorithm for diagnosing PJI that incorporates recently developed tests. A wide arsenal of tests are available, and it can be very challenging for the treating surgeon on how to incorporate these new tests. The prevention of PJI may be the most effective way to limit its burden, and it is crucial to risk-stratify patients and optimize modifiable risk factors. Furthermore, the treatment of PJI remains far from perfect with high failure rates for all surgical modalities. It is crucial that we continue to elucidate the indications and contraindications for the different surgical options.

Take-Home Messages

- A new definition of PJI has been created with improved sensitivity and specificity.
- α-Defensin does not improve diagnostic accuracy in combination with other tests.
- Perioperative antibiotic guidelines have changed with antibiotics after skin closure no longer recommended but with minimal evidence in the arthroplasty literature.
- The literature regarding antibiotic cement is mixed but should be considered in patients at high risk for the development of periprosthetic joint infection.
- Local antibiotics should not be used in irrigation solutions.

References

Aalirezaie A, Akkaya M, Barnes CL et al (2019) General assembly, prevention, operating room environment: proceedings of international consensus on orthopedic infections. J Arthroplast 34(2S):S105–S115. https://doi.org/10.1016/j.arth.2018.09.060

Abdel Karim M, Andrawis J, Bengoa F et al (2019) Hip and knee section, diagnosis, algorithm: proceedings of international consensus on orthopedic infections. J Arthroplast 34(2S):S339–S350. https://doi.org/10.1016/j.arth.2018.09.018

Abdel MP, Barreira P, Battenberg A et al (2019) Hip and knee section, treatment, two-stage exchange spacer-related: proceedings of international consensus on orthopedic infections. J Arthroplast 34(2):S427–S438. https://doi.org/10.1016/j.arth.2018.09.027

Abdelaziz H, Citak M, Fleischman A et al (2019) General assembly, prevention, operating room – anesthesia matters: proceedings of international consensus on orthopedic infections. J Arthroplast 34(2S):S93–S95. https://doi.org/10.1016/j.arth.2018.09.058

Aboltins CA, Berdal JE, Casas F et al (2019) Hip and knee section, prevention, antimicrobials (systemic): proceedings of international consensus on orthopedic infections. J Arthroplast 34(2S):S279–S288. https://doi.org/10.1016/j.arth.2018.09.012

Akonjom M, Battenberg A, Beverland D et al (2019) General assembly, prevention, blood conservation: proceedings of international consensus on orthopedic infections. J Arthroplast 34(2S):S147–S155. https://doi.org/10.1016/j.arth.2018.09.065

Amanatullah D, Dennis D, Oltra EG et al (2019) Hip and knee section, diagnosis, definitions: proceedings of international consensus on orthopedic infections. J Arthroplast 34(2S):S329–S337. https://doi.org/10.1016/j.arth.2018.09.044

Argenson JN, Arndt M, Babis G et al (2019) Hip and knee section, treatment, debridement and retention of implant: proceedings of international consensus on orthopedic infections. J Arthroplast 34(2S):S399–S419. https://doi.org/10.1016/j.arth.2018.09.025

Berend KR, Lombardi AV, Morris MJ, Bergeson AG, Adams JB, Sneller MA (2013) Two-stage treatment of hip periprosthetic joint infection is associated with a high rate of infection control but high mortality. Clin Orthop 471(2):510–518. https://doi.org/10.1007/s11999-012-2595-x

Bialecki J, Bucsi L, Fernando N et al (2019) Hip and knee section, treatment, one stage exchange: proceedings of international consensus on orthopedic infections. J Arthroplast 34(2S):S421–S426. https://doi.org/10.1016/j.arth.2018.09.026

Bini SA, Chan PH, Inacio MCS, Paxton EW, Khatod M (2016) Antibiotic cement was associated with half the risk of re-revision in 1,154 aseptic revision total knee arthroplasties. Acta Orthop 87(1):55–59. https://doi.org/10.3109/17453674.2015.1103568

Blom A, Cho J, Fleischman A et al (2019) General assembly, prevention, antiseptic irrigation solution: proceedings of international consensus on orthopedic infections. J Arthroplast 34(2S):S131–S138. https://doi.org/10.1016/j.arth.2018.09.063

Bozic KJ, Kurtz SM, Lau E et al (2010) The epidemiology of revision total knee arthroplasty in the United States. Clin Orthop 468(1):45–51. https://doi.org/10.1007/s11999-009-0945-0

Cizmic Z, Feng JE, Huang R et al (2019) Hip and knee section, prevention, host related: proceedings of international consensus on orthopedic infections. J Arthroplast 34(2S):S255–S270. https://doi.org/10.1016/j.arth.2018.09.010

Dalkey N, Helmer O (1963) An experimental application of the DELPHI method to the use of experts. Manag Sci 9(3):458–467. https://doi.org/10.1287/mnsc.9.3.458

Deirmengian C, Kardos K, Kilmartin P, Gulati S, Citrano P, Booth RE (2015) The alpha-defensin test for periprosthetic joint infection responds to a wide spectrum of organisms. Clin Orthop 473(7):2229–2235. https://doi.org/10.1007/s11999-015-4152-x

Della Valle C, Parvizi J, Bauer TW et al (2011) American Academy of Orthopaedic Surgeons clinical practice guideline on: the diagnosis of periprosthetic joint infections of the hip and knee. J Bone Joint Surg Am 93(14):1355–1357. https://doi.org/10.2106/JBJS.9314ebo

Fillingham Y, Greenwald AS, Greiner J et al (2019) Hip and knee section, prevention, local antimicrobials: proceedings of international consensus on orthopedic infections. J Arthroplast 34(2S):S289–S292. https://doi.org/10.1016/j.arth.2018.09.013

Gomez MM, Tan TL, Manrique J, Deirmengian GK, Parvizi J (2015) The fate of spacers in the treatment of periprosthetic joint infection. J Bone Joint Surg Am 97(18):1495–1502. https://doi.org/10.2106/JBJS.N.00958

Jameson SS, Asaad A, Diament M et al (2019) Antibiotic-loaded bone cement is associated with a lower risk of revision following primary cemented total knee arthroplasty: an analysis of 731,214 cases using National Joint Registry data. Bone Joint J 101-B(11):1331–1347. https://doi.org/10.1302/0301-620X.101B11.BJJ-2019-0196.R1

Li R, Shao H-Y, Hao L-B et al (2019) Plasma fibrinogen exhibits better performance than plasma D-dimer in the diagnosis of periprosthetic joint infection: a multicenter retrospective study. J Bone Joint Surg Am 101(7):613–619. https://doi.org/10.2106/JBJS.18.00624

Motififard M, Pesteh M, Etemadifar MR, Shirazinejad S (2015) Causes and rates of revision total knee arthroplasty: local results from Isfahan, Iran. Adv Biomed Res 4. https://doi.org/10.4103/2277-9175.157829

Namba RS, Inacio MCS, Paxton EW (2013) Risk factors associated with deep surgical site infections after primary total knee arthroplasty: an analysis of 56,216 knees. J Bone Joint Surg Am 95(9):775–782. https://doi.org/10.2106/JBJS.L.00211

Parvizi J, Gehrke T (2014) Definition of periprosthetic joint infection. J Arthroplast 29(7):1331. https://doi.org/10.1016/j.arth.2014.03.009

Parvizi J, Tan TL, Goswami K et al (2018) The 2018 definition of periprosthetic hip and knee infection: an evidence-based and validated criteria. J Arthroplasty 33(5):1309–14.e2. https://doi.org/10.1016/j.arth.2018.02.078

Parvizi J, Gehrke T, Mont MA, Callaghan JJ (2019) Introduction: proceedings of international consensus on orthopedic infections. J Arthroplast 34(2):S1–S2. https://doi.org/10.1016/j.arth.2018.09.038

Ryan SP, Kildow BJ, Tan TL et al (2019) Is there a difference in infection risk between single and multiple doses of prophylactic antibiotics? A meta-analysis. Clin Orthop 477(7):1577–1590. https://doi.org/10.1097/CORR.0000000000000619

Sanz-Ruiz P, Matas-Diez JA, Sanchez-Somolinos M, Villanueva-Martinez M, Vaquero-Martín J (2017) Is the commercial antibiotic-loaded bone cement useful in prophylaxis and cost saving after knee and hip joint arthroplasty? The transatlantic paradox. J Arthroplasty 32(4):1095–1099. https://doi.org/10.1016/j.arth.2016.11.012

Shahi A, Kheir MM, Tarabichi M, Hosseinzadeh HRS, Tan TL, Parvizi J (2017) Serum D-dimer test is promising for the diagnosis of periprosthetic joint infection and timing of reimplantation. J Bone Joint Surg Am 99(17):1419–1427. https://doi.org/10.2106/JBJS.16.01395

Shohat N, Tan TL, Della Valle CJ et al (2019) Development and validation of an evidence-based algorithm for diagnosing periprosthetic joint infection. J Arthroplasty 34(11):2730–36.e1. https://doi.org/10.1016/j.arth.2019.06.016

Siddiqi A, Forte SA, Docter S, Bryant D, Sheth NP, Chen AF (2019) Perioperative antibiotic prophylaxis in total joint arthroplasty: a systematic review and meta-analysis. J Bone Joint Surg Am 101(9):828–842. https://doi.org/10.2106/JBJS.18.00990

Surgical Site Infection | Guidelines | Infection Control | CDC. https://www.cdc.gov/infectioncontrol/guidelines/ssi/index.html. Published March 25, 2019. Accessed 30 Jan 2020.

Tan TL, Shohat N, Rondon AJ et al (2019) Perioperative antibiotic prophylaxis in total joint arthroplasty: a single dose is as effective as multiple doses. J Bone Joint Surg Am 101(5):429–437. https://doi.org/10.2106/JBJS.18.00336

Tarabichi M, Shohat N, Goswami K et al (2018) Diagnosis of periprosthetic joint infection: the potential of next-generation sequencing. J Bone Joint Surg Am 100(2):147–154. https://doi.org/10.2106/JBJS.17.00434

Tayton ER, Frampton C, Hooper GJ, Young SW (2016) The impact of patient and surgical factors on the rate of infection after primary total knee arthroplasty: an analysis of 64,566 joints from the New Zealand Joint Registry. Bone Joint J 98-B(3):334–340. https://doi.org/10.1302/0301-620X.98B3.36775

Workgroup Convened by the Musculoskeletal Infection Society (2011) New definition for periprosthetic joint infection. J Arthroplast 26(8):1136–1138. https://doi.org/10.1016/j.arth.2011.09.026

Zmistowski B, Karam JA, Durinka JB, Casper DS, Parvizi J (2013) Periprosthetic joint infection increases the risk of one-year mortality. J Bone Joint Surg Am 95(24):2177–2184. https://doi.org/10.2106/JBJS.L.00789

Local Delivery of Antibiotics

Sherina Holland and Simon W. Young

Contents

E. Hansen, K.-D. Kühn (eds.), *Essentials of Cemented Knee Arthroplasty*,
https://doi.org/10.1007/978-3-662-63113-3_58

58.1 Introduction

Periprosthetic joint infection (PJI) is the most feared complication for both patient and surgeon following total knee arthroplasty (TKA). On average, a patient with a deep infection following a knee replacement spends an extra 21 days in hospital, undergoes an additional five operations, receives prolonged (>6 weeks) intravenous antibiotic therapy, and may eventually require removal of the prosthesis in order to eradicate the infection (Kapadia et al. 2014; Sculco 1993). Despite concerted efforts, infection rates following primary TKA continue to be reported at a rate of 0.86–2.5% (Bengtson and Knutson 1991; Blom et al. 2004; Nickinson et al. 2010; Phillips et al. 2006). Furthermore, there is evidence that the incidence of infection after TKA and total hip replacement has been increasing in recent decades (Dale et al. 2012; Kurtz et al. 2012).

The majority of early infections after TKA are believed to be due to bacterial contamination at the time of surgery (Fletcher et al. 2007). As a result, the use of prophylactic antibiotics is important in reducing the risk of infection (Davis et al. 1999; Fletcher et al. 2007).

> The aim of prophylactic antibiotics is not to sterilize already contaminated tissues but to act as an adjunct to host innate immune defenses and prevent any bacterial contamination proceeding to overt infection (Prokuski 2008).

> To be effective, the concentration of antibiotics in the tissues must exceed the minimum inhibitory concentration (MIC) for the organism responsible for the infection.

The tissue concentration should be maintained for the duration of the procedure, from the time of incision until the time of closure (Burke 1961).

58.2 Local Delivery of Prophylactic Antibiotics

> Prophylactic antibiotics are typically provided systemically via the intravenous route; the antibiotic distributes throughout the systemic circulation, including the tissues around the surgical site.

While systemic antibiotic prophylaxis has been shown to reduce infections in arthroplasty procedures (Espehaug et al. 1997), the tissue antibiotic concentrations that can be achieved via this route are limited by dose-dependent toxicity to major organs. Moreover, due to increased resistance, certain antibiotics such as cephalosporins may no longer provide adequate prophylaxis (Yamada et al. 2011). This has implications for both the choice of prophylactic agent and the clinical outcome, particularly as PJI in TKA caused by resistant organisms is associated with higher rates of treatment failure and reinfection (Parvizi et al. 2009; Salgado et al. 2007).

58.2.1 Intravenous Regional Administration

Prophylactic antibiotics can also be administered locally or regionally. "Regional" delivery of intravenous antibiotics (IVRA) involves the injection of antibiotics into a foot vein below an inflated tourniquet. The tourniquet interrupts circulation to the limb, so the distribution of antibiotics injected below the tourniquet is restricted to that limb. In the past, some authors have used a foot vein cannula for administering prophylactic antibiotics in TKA; this approach achieved substantially higher tissue concentrations at the surgical site without systemic side effects (de Lalla et al. 1993, 2000; Hoddinott et al. 1990; Lazzarini et al. 2003). However, cannulation of a foot vein is difficult, time-consuming, and often unsuccessful, particularly in obese patients. The skin of the foot is also known to have higher bacterial skin counts than other parts of the body (Belkin 1997) and is normally covered in sterile drapes during TKA. Therefore, cannulation of a foot vein may compromise sterility. These problems have limited the uptake of IVRA in clinical practice (Lazzarini et al. 2003).

58.2.2 Intraosseous Regional Administration (IORA)

An alternative means of regional administration is offered by intraosseous cannulation. The metaphysis of a long bone contains "venous sinusoids" that form a honeycomb-like structure containing a dense network of blood vessels. The contents of an injection into this area of bone travel directly to the circulation, as would those of an injection into a vein. Fluids or medications can be given using this method, and the pharmacokinetics of drugs administered this way are similar to those achieved by peripheral or central intravenous administration (Tobias and Ross 2010). Intraosseous administration of fluids and medications is well known in pediatric practice but works equally well in adults. Until recently, intraosseous regional administration (IORA) of prophylactic antibiotics in TKA had not been reported; our group has since described this method in

Table 58.1 Randomized controlled trials undertaken by our group investigating IORA of prophylactic antibiotics in TKA

Reference	Study design	Outcome
Young et al. (2013)	22 patients were randomized to receive either 1 g of cefazolin by IORA or 1 g of cefazolin by systemic administration	Overall mean cefazolin concentration in subcutaneous fat was 186 μg/g in the IORA group and 10.6 μg/g in the systemic group ($p < 0.01$) Overall mean concentration in bone was 130 μg/g in the IORA group compared to 11.4 μg/g in the systemic group ($p < 0.01$)
Young et al. (2014)	30 patients were randomized to receive either 250 mg or 500 mg of vancomycin by IORA or 1 g of vancomycin by systemic administration	Overall mean concentration of vancomycin in subcutaneous fat was 14 μg/g in the 250-mg IORA group, 44 μg/g in the 500-mg IORA group, and 3.2 μg/g in the systemic group Overall mean concentration in bone was 16 μg/g in the 250-mg IORA group, 38 μg/g in the 500-mg IORA group, and 4.0 μg/g in the systemic group
Young et al. (2018)	20 patients undergoing aseptic revision TKA were randomized to receive either 500 mg of vancomycin by IORA or 1 g of vancomycin by systemic administration	Overall mean tissue concentration of vancomycin in subcutaneous fat was 49.3 μg/g in the IORA group and 3.7 μg/g in the systemic group ($p < 0.001$) Overall mean concentration in the bone was 77.1 μg/g in the IORA group compared to 6.4 μg/g in the systemic group ($p < 0.001$)
Chin et al. (2018)	22 patients with a BMI >35 were randomized to receive either 500 mg of vancomycin by IORA or 15 mg/kg (maximum of 2 g) of vancomycin by systemic administration. The mean BMI was 41.1 in the IORA group and 40.1 in the IV systemic group	Overall mean concentration in subcutaneous fat was 39.3 μg/g in the IORA group and 4.4 μg/g in the IV systemic group ($p < .01$) Overall mean concentration in bone was 34.4 μg/g in the IORA group and 6.1 μg/g in the systemic group ($p < .01$)

several randomized control trials (Table 58.1) (Chin et al. 2018; Young et al. 2013, 2014, 2018).

> In our first study (Young et al. 2013), we demonstrated that IORA can achieve tissue concentrations of cefazolin 10–15 times higher than systemic administration.

Patients undergoing primary TKA ($n = 22$) were randomized to receive either 1 g of cefazolin systemically through a forearm vein or 1 g of cefazolin through an intraosseous cannula. The overall mean concentration of cefazolin in subcutaneous fat was 186 μg/g in the intraosseous group compared to 10.6 μg/g in the systemic group ($p < 0.01$) and in bone was 130 μg/g in the intraosseous group compared to 11.4 μg/g in the systemic group ($p < 0.01$).

> In order for prophylactic antibiotics to be effective in reducing the risk of PJI, their spectrum of activity must cover the organisms likely to cause intraoperative contamination.

Within our locality (Auckland, New Zealand), the majority of bacteria responsible for an early PJI are resistant to cefazolin (Ravi et al. 2016). Vancomycin is effective against cefazolin-resistant organisms; however, when provided systemically, vancomycin requires a prolonged administration time, risks promoting further antibiotic resistance, and may result in systemic toxicity.

Subsequently, in our second study, we assessed whether low doses of IORA vancomycin could result in equal or superior tissue concentrations to those achieved by systemic administration (Young et al. 2014). Patients undergoing primary TKA ($n = 30$) were randomized to receive 250 mg or 500 mg of vancomycin by IORA or 1 g of vancomycin by systemic administration. The overall mean tissue concentration of vancomycin in subcutaneous fat was14 μg/g in the 250-mg IORA group, 44 μg/g in the 500-mg IORA group, and 3.2 μg/g in the systemic group; mean concentrations in bone were 16 μg/g in the 250-mg IORA group, 38 μg/g in the 500-mg IORA group, and 4.0 μg/g in the systemic group. One patient in the systemic group developed “red man syndrome” during infusion.

> This suggests that IORA may allow a lower vancomycin dose (thereby reducing systemic toxicity) and avoids the difficulties associated with prolonged preoperative infusion times, while providing equal or enhanced prophylaxis in TKA.

In two further clinical trials, we demonstrated that low-dose IORA vancomycin could also result in equal or superior tissue concentrations to those achieved by systemic administration in high BMI patients (Chin et al. 2018) and in revision TKA (Young et al. 2018). As no cases of "red man syndrome" were seen with IORA, we recommend the use of the higher 500-mg vancomycin dose. The efficacy of antibiotic prophylaxis delivered by IORA was also demonstrated in a mouse model of methicillin-resistant *S. aureus* (MRSA) infected TKA (Young et al. 2015); IORA cefazolin and vancomycin were shown to be more effective at reducing the bacterial load than the same dose of antibiotic given systemically. Vancomycin in particular was enhanced by IORA even when provided at a low dose, suggesting that vancomycin may be more effective against MRSA when high tissue concentrations are achieved, such as with IORA.

Potential negatives of IORA include the cost of intraosseous needles and additional tourniquet time (inserting the intraosseous needle and performing the injection adds 3–5 minutes). Complications from intraosseous infusion are extremely rare; however, fluid extravasation with compartment syndrome due to incorrect needle placement has been reported when intraosseous (IO) injections are used in an emergency department setting (Tobias and Ross 2010), and there have been isolated reports of bone fracture following IO placement (Bowley et al. 2003; Tobias and Ross 2010), although this is thought to be related to the use of excessive force with manual needle placement in pediatric patients. There is also a risk of fat embolism. Although this seems more of a theoretical concern, subclinical lung microemboli have been observed following intraosseous infusion in animal models; however, this has not been shown to affect ventilation-perfusion performance in the clinical setting (Orlowski et al. 1989).

58.2.3 Other Methods of Delivering Local Antibiotics for Prophylaxis

Other methods of delivering local antibiotics have been used to enhance prophylaxis. Whiteside (Whiteside 2016) reported a single-surgeon series of 2293 arthroplasty cases with antibiotics added to the intraoperative irrigation solution. He used a solution of normal saline with vancomycin 1000 mg/l and polymyxin 250,000 units/L, administered regularly throughout the case via a hand-operated spray bottle. While there was no comparative group in the study, Whiteside reported no infections at a mean follow-up of 73 months (Whiteside 2016).

Local (intrawound) application of vancomycin powder (VP) during orthopedic surgery was first popularized by spinal surgeons, who demonstrated evidence that it may reduce the risk of surgical site infections (Chiang et al. 2014). More recently, a meta-analysis of primary and revision arthroplasty patients (Heckmann et al. 2019) calculated a decreased rate of PJI (OR 0.25, $p < .0001$) for patients that had received intrawound vancomycin. However, only six low-quality retrospective studies ($n = 3298$) were included in the meta-analysis, two of which utilized a betadine lavage protocol in addition to VP, which may have influenced the results. The authors subsequently cautioned against the use of intrawound VP during TKA and THA due to the lack of high-quality data regarding the safety of VP in this setting (Heckmann et al. 2019). To date, reported adverse events associated with intrawound VP include acute kidney injury (AKI) and (when the VP is placed in an extracapsular location) wound complications (Heckmann et al. 2019).

> As the goal of prophylaxis is to achieve adequate tissue levels from the time of skin incision until the time of closure, it is worth noting that neither intraoperative irrigation nor adding vancomycin powder at the end of the cases will achieve this.

> Furthermore, the adequacy of distribution through the tissues with these methods is uncertain.

58.3 Technique of Intraosseous Regional Administration

58.3.1 Indications and Contraindications

Intraosseous regional administration of antibiotics (IORA) can be used in primary and revision TKA performed under tourniquet. If intending to use IORA only in high-risk PJI patients, indications could include obesity (BMI >40), diabetes, previous ligamentous surgery or osteotomy, current or recent smokers, or patients who are immunocompromised for any reason. In settings where vancomycin is required, such as β-lactam allergy, known colonization with MRSA, or patients coming from high institutional MRSA prevalence, IORA allows the vancomycin to be administered with optimal timing and avoids the need for a prolonged IV infusion. Due to the relative ease of using cefazolin intravenously, we typically reserve the use of IORA for vancomycin infusion, although cefazolin can also be administered intraosseously. We have not mixed the two antibiotics together in the same syringe.

> Concurrent IV systemic administration of cefazolin may also be required to ensure compliance with local

hospital guidelines on prophylactic antibiotics; in this setting, the IORA vancomycin serves as an adjunct to the standard IV cefazolin prophylaxis.

Contraindications apply to patients with large cortical perforations or massive proximal tibial osteolysis. In the setting of revision TKA with a large stemmed tibial component and significant metaphyseal bone loss, intraosseous injection into the medial malleolus or distal femur can be used as an alternative IO injection site.

58.3.2 Procedure

To perform IORA, an intraosseous (IO) needle is required. At our hospital, we prefer the use of manual needles (Cook Medical, Bloomington, IN) (▪ Fig. 58.1). Powered options are available (EZ-IO, Teleflex Corp, San Antonio, TX); however, these are typically more expensive and require the sterilization of a battery-powered needle driver. Longer needles are available for obese patients.

IORA of antibiotics for TKA is administered in the proximal tibia distal to an inflated tourniquet. With the patient supine, we prep and drape the operative leg in the usual sterile fashion. Exsanguination is performed by leg elevation (alternatively, an Esmarch can be used), and the tourniquet is inflated to 250–300 mmHg. A small hole is made in the adhesive bandage (e.g., iodine-impregnated incision drapes) overlying the medial aspect of the proximal tibia (▪ Fig. 58.2). This allows the insertion of an IO needle without binding the adhesive dressing or advancing the adhesive drape below the skin. The IO needle is inserted into the proximal medial face of the tibia, just medial and slightly proximal to the tibial tubercle. We have found more proximal insertion (2–3 cm below the joint line) to be easier to penetrate with a manual needle (as the cortex is thinner) and results in faster flow rates (▪ Fig. 58.3). In revision knee replacements, the needle may be further distal to avoid the implant and cement—as long as the tip of the needle is in the cancellous bone, then flow will occur.

> In each instance, the needle should be inserted perpendicular to the cortical surface of the anteromedial tibia.

After inserting the IO needle, a large syringe containing the desired antibiotic is connected to the IO needle and the solution is administered over the course of 1–2 minutes (▪ Fig. 58.4). Once the antibiotic has been deliv-

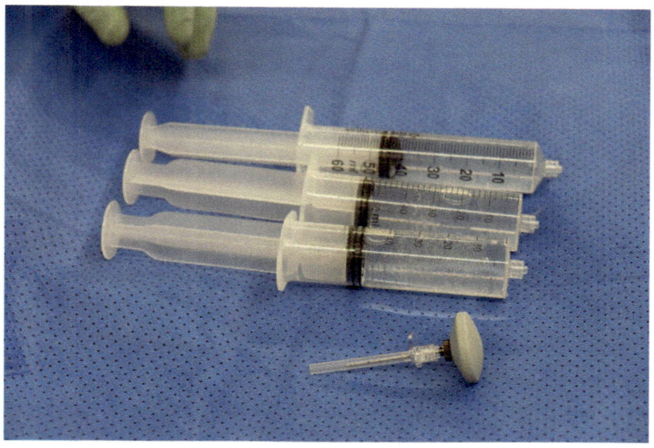

▪ **Fig. 58.1** Manual intraosseous (IO) needle and large syringes containing the injection solution

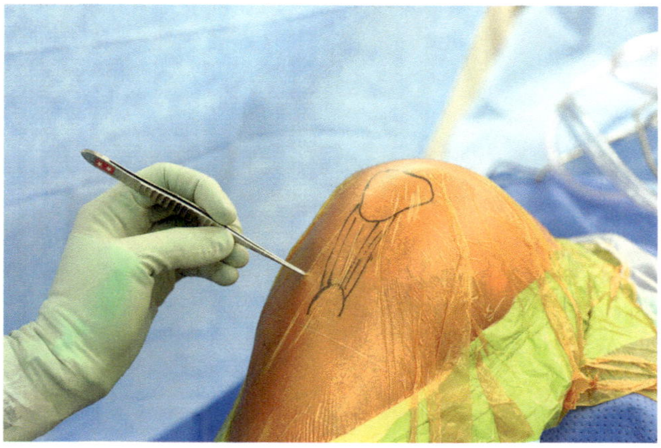

▪ **Fig. 58.2** A small hole is made in the adhesive bandage

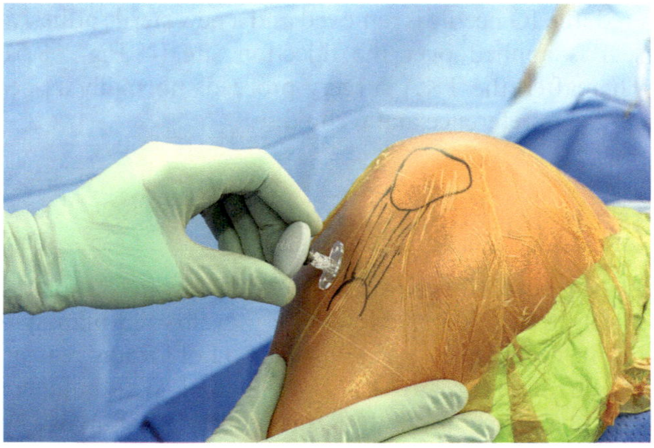

▪ **Fig. 58.3** The intraosseous needle is inserted into the proximal medial face of the tibia, just medial and slightly proximal to the tibial tubercle

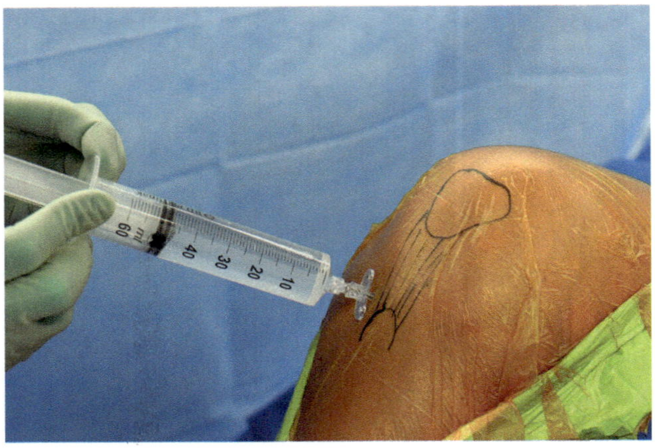

Fig. 58.4 Syringe containing the desired antibiotic is connected to the IO needle

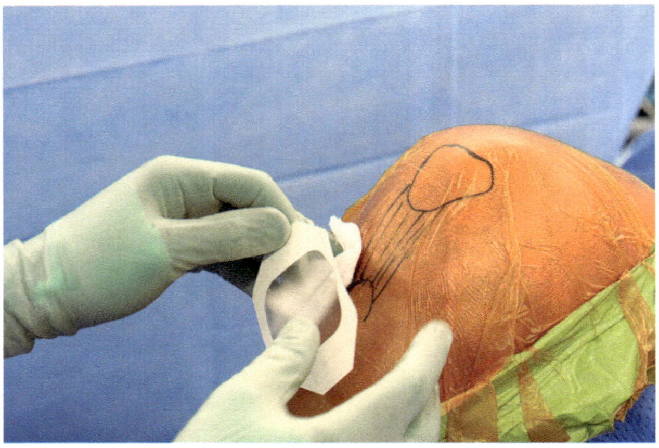

Fig. 58.5 The IO needle is removed and a sterile adhesive seal is applied over the injection site

ered, the IO needle is removed and a new sterile adhesive seal is applied over the injection site (Fig. 58.5). Thereafter, the TKA surgery proceeds normally as per surgeon preference and technique.

58.3.3 Injection Solution

At our hospital, we use 500 mg of vancomycin for the injection solution; the low dose prevents red man syndrome even if the tourniquet was to fail for any reason. If cefazolin is preferred, 1 g can be used. We administer 500 mg of vancomycin IORA in addition to standard IV prophylaxis, with an appropriate weight base dose of cefazolin, prior to incision. In our center, we mix the injection solution in the operating room. The 500 mg vial of vancomycin is mixed with 10 ml of saline then placed into a bowl on the sterile field. Saline is added to make a volume up to 120–140 ml, as this volume ensures the antibiotic will distribute throughout the limb. This is then drawn up into 2–3 50-ml syringes for injection (Fig. 58.1).

58.3.4 Keys to a Good Technique

> The optimal injection site is the proximal tibia; the cortex is thinner in this region, making needle insertion easier. Furthermore, the metaphyseal bone allows faster flow rates for the infusion.

We have found slightly more proximal insertions to be easier and have faster flow rates. Flow rates can be variable and typically take 1–2 minutes to complete. If the flow rate is slow, twisting and withdrawing the needle slightly (5 mm) may increase the rate; slower infusions may take 3–4 minutes. Revision cases usually require powered needle insertion (due to the thicker cortex distal to the implant); in complex revision cases with compromised proximal tibial bone, the medial malleolus can be used as an alternative IO injection site.

58.4 Local Antibiotic Delivery When Treating Established PJI to Supplement Debridement and Implant Retention

Local antibiotics for prophylaxis should be distinguished from their use in the treatment of an established infection. Prophylactic antibiotics support the body's innate (non-specific) immune system to *prevent* bacterial colonization, i.e., before bacterial adhesion, and other virulence factors can overcome these initial immune defenses and cause infection (Prokuski 2008).

> In contrast to prophylaxis, once an infection is established, antibiotics act instead to assist the body's adaptive (antigen-specific) immune response to *eradicate* the infection.

> The effectiveness of this treatment is dependent upon the concentration of antibiotic provided and the length of time it remains at that concentration.

Therefore, IORA has limited utility in this setting, as higher antibiotic concentrations are achieved only for a short period, whereas treatment of PJI typically requires many weeks of antibiotic therapy. Other methods may give more prolonged high local concentrations of antibiotics, such as the following:

- Application of local antibiotics via polymethylmethacrylate (PMMA)

- Calcium sulfate
- Intra-articular infusion or VP

However, their safety and ability to eradicate infection remain debated.

58.4.1 Antibiotic-Loaded PMMA Beads

Polymethylmethacrylate (PMMA) bone cement is used as a carrier material for antibiotics in the treatment of orthopedic joint infections and chronic osteomyelitis. The cement is prepared by mixing a PMMA polymer with a powdered antibiotic, followed by a liquid monomer. The resultant exothermic polymerization reaction produces a solid material that can be molded into beads, blocks, or a temporary spacer.

> Not all antibiotics can be used within bone cement.

Among other factors, the antibiotic must be heat-stable and water-soluble (van Vugt et al. 2019). Antibiotic-loaded bone cement (ALBC) is usually implanted (in the form of a spacer) during a two-stage revision procedure; however, several studies have described the use of antibiotic-loaded PMMA beads during DAIR. All have used a repeat (serial) debridement procedure, which may in itself have improved infection control by repeatedly disturbing any biofilm present.

Estes et al. (2010) retrospectively reviewed 20 acute PJIs treated with a two-stage DAIR procedure. Patients underwent an initial debridement with prosthesis retention and placement of antibiotic-loaded PMMA beads (comprising gentamicin or tobramycin, vancomycin, and cefazolin), the beads were removed within 7 days during a second debridement procedure, and new modular parts were inserted; 18 (90%) of the patients remained infection-free at a mean follow-up of 3.5 years. In a follow-up study, undertaken to determine the success rate of the same two-stage procedure in a larger group (48 primary TKA/THA, 35 revision TKA/THA), Chung et al. (2019) reported an infection control rate of 93.8% in the primary joints and 77.1% in the revision joints (Chung et al. 2019) at a mean follow-up of 3.5 years, although 55% of patients remained on suppressive antibiotics. Similarly, Tintle et al. (2009) reported a 100% infection control rate in a small case series ($n = 9$) of arthroplasty patients treated with a serial DAIR procedure and antibiotic-loaded PMMA beads (comprising vancomycin and tobramycin). However, less favorably, a retrospective review of acute–late-onset PJIs by Kuiper et al. (2013) reported a 66.6% failure rate in a subgroup analysis of 12 patients treated with DAIR and gentamicin-loaded PMMA beads.

> The principal downside of antibiotic-loaded PMMA beads is the need for an additional surgery to remove them; this may significantly increase the cost, length of stay, and potentially perioperative complications as compared to a single-stage procedure (Chung et al. 2019; Estes et al. 2010).

Furthermore, there is evidence that bacteria can colonize and form biofilm on the surface of PMMA (Anagnostakos et al. 2008; Neut et al. 2001). While high levels of antibiotics are eluted from bone cement immediately after placement, this is followed by a much lower concentration that may eventually fall below the MIC.

Systemic complications associated with ALBC are limited; however, there are reports of allergic reactions, acute renal failure, temporary hepatic enzyme elevation, and temporary bone marrow suppression in patients treated with antibiotic-loaded cement spacers for PJI (Luu et al. 2013). A meta-analysis of ten observational studies ($n = 544$) by Luu et al. (2013) calculated a 4.8% incidence of AKI in two-stage hip and knee revision patients, which was attributed to the nephrotoxicity of aminoglycosides loaded into the cement spacers.

> Due to the low number of published studies, it is difficult to determine whether antibiotic-loaded PMMA beads are associated with complications during DAIR.

However, Chung et al. (2019) reported three cases (3.6%) of renal failure with their two-stage DAIR approach, all of which required temporary dialysis.

58.4.2 Calcium Sulfate Beads

Calcium sulfate is an inorganic bioabsorbable bone substitute. Traditionally used as void filler, it can also act as a carrier material for antibiotics and other substances when impregnated into grafts or beads (Beuerlein and McKee 2010).

> Unlike PMMA beads, antibiotic-impregnated calcium sulfate (AICS) beads gradually absorb and do not require removal.

Moreover, AICS beads can accommodate a wider range of antibiotics as their formation does not result in an exothermic reaction and elute a higher, sustained, concentration of antibiotics as compared to PMMA beads (McConoughey et al. 2015) and have been shown to reduce biofilm formation (Howlin et al. 2015). To date, several studies have evaluated the use of AICS beads during DAIR, with varying success.

A retrospective review of 42 patients with chronic recurrent PJIs in the hip or knee joint (a group usually considered DAIR inappropriate) reported a 73.8% remission rate at a mean follow-up of 23 months (Gramlich et al. 2019) for patients treated with single-stage DAIR and antibiotic-impregnated calcium sulfate beads. Of those that failed, implant retention was achieved in five cases (11.9%) after performing a second DAIR procedure or long-term antibiotic suppression (Gramlich et al. 2019). However, a review by Flierl et al. (2017), in which 32 patients with an acute PJI were treated with DAIR and AICS beads, reported a 48% failure rate at a mean of 13 months; of the 16 patients who failed, 7 went onto a two-stage revision and 9 were treated with chronic antibiotic suppression. Complications associated with AICS beads include wound drainage, heterotopic bone formation, and hypercalcemia (Kallala and Haddad 2015; Kallala et al. 2018; McPherson et al. 2013).

A prospective study (Kallala et al. 2018) of 755 revision arthroplasty procedures treated with AICS beads reported 32 cases (4.2%) of wound drainage, 13 cases (1.7%) of heterotopic calcification, and 41 cases (5.4%) of transient hypercalcemia; bead volume (p = 0.0014) and patient grade (p = 0.0021) were shown to have a significant effect on the presence or absence of complications. The authors suggested, due to the risk of hypercalcemia, that patients undergoing treatment with AICS beads should be screened for contraindications, and calcium levels should be monitored pre- and postoperatively (Kallala et al. 2018). Moreover, it was recommended that the volume of calcium sulfate should be limited to a maximum of 40 cc per operation, increasing to 80 cc if it is placed within the medulla of the bone.

58

To date, there is limited data regarding AICS beads and the risk of nephrotoxicity. However, a case of acute tubular necrosis (Ma et al. 2019) has been reported in a patient treated with vancomycin and tobramycin AICS beads, presumed to be caused by acute tobramycin toxicity.

58.4.3 Intra-articular Infusion

Intra-articular (IA) delivery of antibiotics involves the injection of antibiotics into a Hickman catheter implanted into the joint cavity. The delivery technique is advocated by Whiteside et al. (2011, 2012, 2016) and requires two Hickman catheters to be implanted during revision surgery to provide an external portal for antibiotic injection. IA antibiotics are initiated the day after surgery and are continued for 6 weeks, after which point the catheters are removed under local anesthesia. Whiteside et al. have reported a 95% infection control rate for patients administered with IA antibiotics in two clinical studies: the first (n = 18) was composed of patients with MRSA (Whiteside et al. 2011) and the second group (n = 18) contained patients with a reinfected TKA (Whiteside et al. 2012). To date, only one study appears to have applied this technique following DAIR (Fukagawa et al. 2010). In a retrospective review of six infected primary TKAs, one revision TKA, and five tumor mega-prosthesis treated with IA antibiotics, Fukagawa et al. (2010) reported four failures, all of which occurred in the mega-prosthesis group.

> The principal disadvantage of IA is catheter management postoperatively and the need for additional surgery for removal; complications reported by Whiteside et al. (2012) include the occlusion and leakage of catheters.

58.4.4 Topical Vancomycin

As previously described, there is evidence to suggest that local administration of VP may reduce the risk of surgical site infections and PJIs during spinal (Chiang et al. 2014) and arthroplasty surgery (Heckmann et al. 2019), respectively. However, its effectiveness as an adjuvant therapy during the treatment of an acute PJI is unclear. A single study (Riesgo et al. 2018) has reviewed the use of topical vancomycin, in conjunction with dilute povidone-iodine lavage (VIP), during DAIR (with modular component and liner exchange). A total of 36 patients with acute TKA or THA PJI treated with DAIR and VIP were matched to a control cohort of patients who underwent DAIR for acute PJI in the 2 years prior to initiating VIP. With a primary outcome of failure (defined as a return to the operating room for an infection related problem) in the VIP group, 16.7% (6/36) failed at a mean follow-up of 27.1 months, compared to 37% (14/38) at a mean follow-up of 42.5 months in the control group ($p < .05$). Three patients (8.3%) in the VIP group were on chronic antibiotic suppression at final follow-up.

- **Conclusion**

Despite determined efforts, the incidence of PJI following TKA continues to rise. While systemic administration of prophylactic antibiotics has been shown to reduce the risk of infection following TKA, the tissue concentration of antibiotics achieved via this route is limited by dose-dependent toxicity. An alternative solution is to administer the antibiotics directly into the metaphysis of the long bone (via an intraosseous cannula) below an inflated tourniquet. This technique

(IORA) has been shown to achieve markedly higher tissue concentrations of antibiotics than systemic administration and may allow for a lower antibiotic dose, thereby reducing the risk of toxicity. We have found this method to be safe and effective in cohorts of primary, revision, and high-BMI patients.

There is growing interest in the use of local antibiotics for the treatment of an established PJI by enhancing the effectiveness of DAIR. In this review, we considered the application of antibiotic-impregnated PMMA or calcium sulfate beads (AICS), intra-articular infusion, and antibiotic powder as a supplement to DAIR. Two-stage DAIR with use of antibiotic PMMA beads appears to have promising results at the expense of requiring a second DAIR procedure for bead removal. The results of single-stage DAIR with dissolvable AICS beads are more mixed, and the potential increase in wound drainage remains a concern. Due to a paucity of published research, there is insufficient evidence to support the routine use of either intra-articular infusion or VP during DAIR.

Take-Home Messages

- Prophylactic antibiotics support the body's innate immune system to prevent bacteria colonization and infection.
- For effective prophylaxis, adequate concentrations of antibiotics must be present in the tissue from the time of incision to the time of closure.
- Intraosseous regional administration (IORA) of prophylactic antibiotics achieves approximately 10× higher tissue concentrations of antibiotics as compared to systemic administration.
- When provided as a *treatment* for infection, antibiotics support the body's adaptive immune response to eradicate the infection.
- Local antibiotics, when provided as a treatment for an established PJI, may help to achieve a high concentration of antibiotics in the tissue for a prolonged period of time.
- The safety and effectiveness of local antibiotic delivery techniques when used as a supplement to DAIR remain unclear.

References

Anagnostakos K, Hitzler P, Pape D, Kohn D, Kelm J (2008) Persistence of bacterial growth on antibiotic-loaded beads: is it actually a problem? Acta Orthop 79(2):302–307. https://doi.org/10.1080/17453670710015120

Belkin NL (1997) Use of scrubs and related apparel in health care facilities. Am J Infect Control 25(5):401–404. https://doi.org/10.1016/S01966553(97)90086-9

Bengtson S, Knutson K (1991) The infected knee arthroplasty. A 6-year followup of 357 cases. Acta Orthop Scand 62(4):301–311. https://doi.org/10.3109/17453679108994458

Beuerlein MJ, McKee MD (2010) Calcium sulfates: what is the evidence? J Orthop Trauma 24(Suppl 1):S46–S51. https://doi.org/10.1097/BOT.0b013e3181cec48e

Blom AW, Brown J, Taylor AH, Pattison G, Whitehouse S, Bannister GC (2004) Infection after total knee arthroplasty. J Bone Joint Surg Br 86(5):688–691. https://doi.org/10.1302/0301-620x.86b5.14887

Bowley DM, Loveland J, Pitcher GJ (2003) Tibial fracture as a complication of intraosseous infusion during pediatric resuscitation. J Trauma 55(4):786–787. https://doi.org/10.1097/01.TA.0000100170.61381.63

Burke JF (1961) The effective period of preventive antibiotic action in experimental incisions and dermal lesions. Surgery 50:161–168

Chiang HY, Herwaldt LA, Blevins AE, Cho E, Schweizer ML (2014) Effectiveness of local vancomycin powder to decrease surgical site infections: a meta-analysis. Spine J 14(3):397–407. https://doi.org/10.1016/j.spinee.2013.10.012

Chin SJ, Moore GA, Zhang M, Clarke HD, Spangehl MJ, Young SW (2018) The AAHKS clinical research award: intraosseous regional prophylaxis provides higher tissue concentrations in high BMI patients in total knee arthroplasty: a randomized trial. J Arthroplast 33(7):S13–S18. https://doi.org/10.1016/j.arth.2018.03.013

Chung AS, Niesen MC, Graber TJ, Schwartz AJ, Beauchamp CP, Clarke HD, Spangehl MJ (2019) Two-stage debridement with prosthesis retention for acute periprosthetic joint infections. J Arthroplast 34(6):1207–1213. https://doi.org/10.1016/j.arth.2019.02.013

Dale H, Fenstad AM, Hallan G, Havelin LI, Furnes O, Overgaard S, Pedersen AB, Kärrholm J, Garellick G, Pulkkinen P, Eskelinen A, Mäkelä K, Engesæter LB (2012) Increasing risk of prosthetic joint infection after total hip arthroplasty. Acta Orthop 83(5):449–458. https://doi.org/10.3109/17453674.2012.733918

Davis N, Curry A, Gambhir AK, Panigrahi H, Walker CR, Wilkins EG, Worsley MA, Kay PR (1999) Intraoperative bacterial contamination in operations for joint replacement. J Bone Joint Surg Br 81(5):886–889. https://doi.org/10.1302/0301-620x.81b5.9545

de Lalla F, Novelli A, Pellizzer G, Milocchi F, Viola R, Rigon A, Stecca C, Dal Pizzol V, Fallani S, Periti P (1993) Regional and systemic prophylaxis with teicoplanin in monolateral and bilateral total knee replacement procedures: study of pharmacokinetics and tissue penetration. Antimicrob Agents Chemother 37:2693–2698. https://doi.org/10.1128/AAC.37.12.2693

de Lalla F, Viola R, Pellizzer G, Lazzarini L, Tramarin A, Fabris P (2000) Regional prophylaxis with teicoplanin in monolateral or bilateral total knee replacement: an open study. Antimicrob Agents Chemother 44:316–319. https://doi.org/10.1128/AAC.44.2.316-319.2000

Espehaug B, Engesaeter LB, Vollset SE, Havelin LI, Langeland N (1997) Antibiotic prophylaxis in total hip arthroplasty. Review of 10,905 primary cemented total hip replacements reported to the Norwegian arthroplasty register, 1987 to 1995. J Bone Joint Surg Br 79:590–595. https://doi.org/10.1302/0301-620X.79B4.7420

Estes CS, Beauchamp CP, Clarke HD, Spangehl MJ (2010) A two-stage retention débridement protocol for acute periprosthetic joint infections. Clin Orthop Relat Res 468(8):2029–2038. https://doi.org/10.1007/s11999-010-1293-9

Fletcher N, Sofianos D, Berkes MB, Obremskey WT (2007) Prevention of perioperative infection. J Bone Joint Surg Am 89(7):1605–1618. https://doi.org/10.2106/JBJS.F.00901

Flierl MA, Culp BM, Okroj KT, Springer BD, Levine BR, Della Valle CJ (2017) Poor outcomes of irrigation and debridement in acute periprosthetic joint infection with antibiotic-impregnated calcium sulfate beads. J Arthroplast 32(8):2505–2507. https://doi.org/10.1016/j.arth.2017.03.051

Fukagawa S, Matsuda S, Miura H, Okazaki K, Tashiro Y, Iwamoto Y (2010) High-dose antibiotic infusion for infected knee prosthesis without implant removal. J Orthop Sci 15(4):470–476. https://doi.org/10.1007/s00776-010-1487-8

Gramlich Y, Walter G, Klug A, Harbering J, Kemmerer M, Hoffmann R (2019) Procedure for single-stage implant retention for chronic periprosthetic infection using topical degradable calcium-based antibiotics. Int Orthop 43(7):1559–1566. https://doi.org/10.1007/s00264-018-4066-9

Heckmann ND, Mayfield CK, Culvern CN, Oakes DA, Lieberman JR, Della Valle CJ (2019) Systematic review and meta-analysis of intrawound vancomycin in total hip and total knee arthroplasty: a call for a prospective randomized trial. J Arthroplast 34(8):1815–1822. https://doi.org/10.1016/j.arth.2019.03.071

Hoddinott C, Lovering AM, Fernando HC, Dixon JH, Reeves DS (1990) Determination of bone and fat concentrations following systemic cefamandole and regional cefuroxime administration in patients undergoing knee arthroplasty. J Antimicrob Chemother 26:823–829. https://doi.org/10.1093/jac/26.6.823

Howlin RP, Brayford MJ, Webb JS, Cooper JJ, Aiken SS, Stoodley P (2015) Antibiotic-loaded synthetic calcium sulfate beads for prevention of bacterial colonization and biofilm formation in periprosthetic infections. Antimicrob Agents Chemother 59(1):111–120. https://doi.org/10.1128/AAC.03676-14

Kallala R, Haddad FS (2015) Hypercalcaemia following the use of antibiotic-eluting absorbable calcium sulphate beads in revision arthroplasty for infection. Bone Joint J 97-B:1237–1241. https://doi.org/10.1302/0301-620X.97B9.34532

Kallala R, Harris WE, Ibrahim M, Dipane M, McPherson E (2018) Use of Stimulan absorbable calcium sulphate beads in revision lower limb arthroplasty: safety profile and complication rates. Bone Joint Res 7(10):570–579. https://doi.org/10.1302/2046-3758.710.BJR-2017-0319.R1

Kapadia BH, McElroy MJ, Issa K, Johnson AJ, Bozic KJ, Mont MA (2014) The economic impact of Periprosthetic infections following total knee arthroplasty at a specialized tertiary-care center. J Arthroplast 29(5):929–932. https://doi.org/10.1016/j.arth.2013.09.017

Kuiper JW, Vos SJ, Saouti R, Vergroesen DA, Graat HC, Debets-Ossenkopp YJ, Peters EJ, Nolte PA (2013) Prosthetic joint-associated infections treated with DAIR (debridement, antibiotics, irrigation, and retention): analysis of risk factors and local antibiotic carriers in 91 patients. Acta Orthop 84(4):380–386. https://doi.org/10.3109/17453674.2013.823589

Kurtz SM, Lau E, Watson H, Schmier JK, Parvizi J (2012) Economic burden of periprosthetic joint infection in the United States. J Arthroplasty 27(8 Suppl):61–65.e6. https://doi.org/10.1016/j.arth.2012.02.022

Lazzarini L, Novelli A, Marzano N, Timillero L, Fallani S, Viola R, de Lalla F (2003) Regional and systemic prophylaxis with teicoplanin in total knee arthroplasty: a tissue penetration study. J Arthroplast 18(3):342–346. https://doi.org/10.1054/arth.2003.50053

Luu A, Syed F, Raman G, Bhalla A, Muldoon E, Hadley S, Smith E, Rao M (2013) Two-stage arthroplasty for prosthetic joint infection: a systematic review of acute kidney injury, systemic toxicity and infection control. J Arthroplasty 28(9):1490–1498.e1. https://doi.org/10.1016/j.arth.2013.02.035

Ma AH, Hoffman C, McNeil JI (2019) Acute tubular necrosis associated with high serum vancomycin and tobramycin levels after revision of total knee arthroplasty with antibiotic-containing calcium sulphate beads. Open Forum Infect Dis 6(4):ofz141. https://doi.org/10.1093/ofid/ofz141

McConoughey SJ, Howlin RP, Wiseman J, Stoodley P, Calhoun JH (2015) Comparing PMMA and calcium sulfate as carriers for the local delivery of antibiotics to infected surgical sites. J Biomed Mater Res B Appl Biomater 103(4):870–877. https://doi.org/10.1002/jbm.b.33247

McPherson MD, Dipane BA, Sherif, MD (2013) Dissolvable antibiotic beads in treatment of periprosthetic joint infection and revision arthroplasty – the use of synthetic pure calcium sulfate (Stimulan®) impregnated with vancomycin & tobramycin. Reconstr Rev 3(1). https://doi.org/10.15438/rr.v3i1.27

Neut D, Van de Belt H, Stokroos I, Van Horn JR, Van der Mei HC, Busscher HJ (2001) Biomaterial-associated infection of getnamicin-loaded PMMA beads in orthopedic revision surgery. J Antimicrob Chemother 47(6):885–891. https://doi.org/10.1093/jac/47.6.885

Nickinson RSJ, Board TN, Gambhir AK, Porter ML, Kay PR (2010) The microbiology of the infected knee arthroplasty. Int Orthop 34(4):505–510

Orlowski JP, Julius CJ, Petras RE, Porembka DT, Gallagher JM (1989) The safety of intraosseous infusions: risks of fat and bone marrow emboli to the lungs. Ann Emerg Med 18(10):1062–1067. https://doi.org/10.1007/s00264-009-0797-y

Parvizi J, Azzam K, Ghanem E, Austin MS, Rothman RH (2009) Periprosthetic infection due to resistant staphylococci: serious problems on the horizon. Clin Orthop Relat Res 467(7):1732–1739. https://doi.org/10.1007/s11999-009-0857-z

Phillips JE, Crane TP, Noy M, Elliott TSJ, Grimer RJ (2006) The incidence of deep prosthetic infections in a specialist orthopaedic hospital: a 15-year prospective survey. J Bone Joint Surg Br 88-B(7):943–948. https://doi.org/10.1302/0301-620X.88B7.17150

Prokuski L (2008) Prophylactic antibiotics in orthopaedic surgery. J Am Acad Orthop Surg 16(5):283–293. https://doi.org/10.4103/0019-5413.159556

Ravi S, Zhu M, Luey C, Young SW (2016) Antibiotic resistance in early periprosthetic joint infection. ANZ J Surg 86(12):1014–1018. https://doi.org/10.1111/ans.13720

Riesgo AM, Park BK, Herrero CP, Yu S, Schwarzkopf R, Iorio R (2018) Vancomycin povidone-iodine protocol improves survivorship of periprosthetic joint infection treated with irrigation and debridement. J Arthroplast 33(3):847–850. https://doi.org/10.1016/j.arth.2017.10.044

Salgado CD, Dash S, Cantey JR, Marculescu CE (2007) Higher risk of failure of methicillin-resistant Staphylococcus aureus prosthetic joint infections. Clin Orthop Relat Res 461:48–53. https://doi.org/10.1097/BLO.0b013e3181123d4e

Sculco TP (1993) The economic impact of infected total joint arthroplasty. Instr Course Lect 42:349–351

Tintle SM, Forsberg JA, Potter BK, Islinger RB, Andersen RC (2009) Prosthesis retention, serial debridement, and antibiotic bead use for the treatment of infection following total joint arthroplasty. Orthopedics 32(2):87

Tobias JD, Ross AK (2010) Intraosseous infusions: a review for the anesthesiologist with a focus on pediatric use. Anesth Analg 110(2):391–401. https://doi.org/10.1213/ANE.0b013e3181c03c7f

van Vugt TAG, Arts JJ, Geurts JAP (2019) Antibiotic-loaded polymethylmethacrylate beads and spacers in treatment of orthopedic infections and the role of biofilm formation. Front Microbiol 10:1626. https://doi.org/10.3389/fmicb.2019.01626

Whiteside LA (2016) Prophylactic peri-operative local antibiotic irrigation. Bone Joint J 98-B(1 Suppl A):23–26. https://doi.org/10.1302/0301-620X.98B1.36357

Whiteside LA, Peppers M, Nayfeh TA, Roy ME (2011) Methicillin-resistant Staphylococcusaureus in TKA treated with revision and direct intra-articular antibiotic infusion. Clin Orthop Relat Res 469:26–33. https://doi.org/10.1007/s11999-010-1313-9

Whiteside LA, Nayfeh TA, LaZear R, Roy ME (2012) Reinfected revised TKA resolves with an aggressive protocol and antibiotic infusion. Clin Orthop Relat Res 470:236–243. https://doi.org/10.1007/s11999-011-2087-4

Whiteside LA, Roy ME, Nayfeh TA (2016) Intra-articular infusion: a direct approach to treatment of infected total knee arthroplasty. Bone Joint J 98-B(1 Suppl A):31–36. https://doi.org/10.1302/0301-620X.98B.36276

Yamada K, Matsumoto K, Tokimura F, Okazaki H, Tanaka S (2011) Are bone and serum cefazolin concentrations adequate for antimicrobial prophylaxis? Clin Orthop Relat Res 469(12):3486–3494. https://doi.org/10.1007/s11999-011-2111-8

Young SW, Zhang M, Freeman JT, Vince KG, Coleman B (2013) Higher cefazolin concentrations with intraosseous regional prophylaxis in TKA. Clin Orthop Relat Res 471(1):244–249. https://doi.org/10.1007/s11999-012-2469-2

Young SW, Zhang M, Freeman JT, Mutu-Grigg J, Pavlou P, Moore GA (2014) The Mark Coventry Award: higher tissue concentrations of vancomycin with low-dose intraosseous regional versus systemic prophylaxis in TKA: a randomized trial. Clin Orthop Relat Res 472(1):57–65. https://doi.org/10.1007/s11999-013-3038-z

Young SW, Roberts T, Johnson S, Dalton JP, Coleman B, Wiles S (2015) Regional intraosseous administration of prophylactic antibiotics is more effective than systemic administration in a mouse model of TKA. Clin Orthop Relat Res 473(11):3573–3584. https://doi.org/10.1007/s11999-015-4464-x

Young SW, Zhang M, Moore GA, Pitto RP, Clarke HD, Spangehl MJ (2018) The John N. Insall Award: higher tissue concentrations of vancomycin achieved with intraosseous regional prophylaxis in revision TKA: a randomized controlled trial. Clin Orthop Relat Res 476(1):9

Antibiotic-Loaded Bone Cement in Total Knee Arthroplasty

Hernan A. Prieto and Emmanuel Gibon

Contents

E. Hansen, K.-D. Kühn (eds.), *Essentials of Cemented Knee Arthroplasty*,
https://doi.org/10.1007/978-3-662-63113-3_59

59.1 Introduction

Total knee arthroplasty (TKA) is one of the most successful surgical procedures. A condylar design with good cementing technique has been considered the gold standard in TKA, due to the outstanding long-term results of cemented TKA in all age groups. Without stratifying for age, multiple published articles consistently cite a greater than 95% survivorship rate at 20 years (Scuderi et al. 1989; Ranawat et al. 1994; Font-Rodriguez et al. 1997; Milligan et al. 2019; Vessely et al. 2006). The practice of using polymethylmethacrylate (PMMA) in fixation of total joint arthroplasties has been present since its introduction by Sir John Charnley in the 1960s. The utility of PMMA in fixation of components and load distribution is not refuted. Addition of antibiotics to PMMA has been performed for the last 30 years in an effort to reduce the likelihood of infections, as well as part of the treatment of periprosthetic joint infections (PJIs).

> Buchholz and Engelbrecht (1970) incorporated antibiotics in PMMA bone cements to reduce the infection rates in orthopedic surgery, assuming that the antibiotic will gradually be released to give higher local concentrations than can be achieved by systemic therapy.

The concept of using bone cement as a depot for antibiotics is attractive, particularly in high-risk patients or complex reconstructions (Fig. 59.1) as it allows for delivery of antibiotics directly to the site of potential infection.

> The elution profile of antibiotic-loaded bone cement (ALBC) has been evaluated: the elution kinetics of vancomycin, tobramycin, gentamicin, moxifloxacin, and clindamycin are better than cefazolin, daptomycin, meropenem, ertapenem, cefotaxime, ampicillin, amoxicillin-clavulanate, and cefepime (Gálvez-López et al. 2014; Anagnostakos et al. 2009; Chang et al. 2013).

Thus, the two most common antibiotics mixed with bone cement are vancomycin and aminoglycosides such as tobramycin and gentamicin. Recent annual arthroplasty registries have shown that 96.3% of cemented TKAs and 93.7% of total hip arthroplasties (THAs) used ALBC (Australian National Joint Replacement Registry 2018). Plain cement has a slightly higher rate of revision than ALBC when used in TKA (Australian National Joint Replacement Registry 2018). However, the role of ALBC in the prevention of infection still remains a controversial topic (Jiranek et al. 2006; Hendriks et al. 2004; Blomgren and Lindgren 1981).

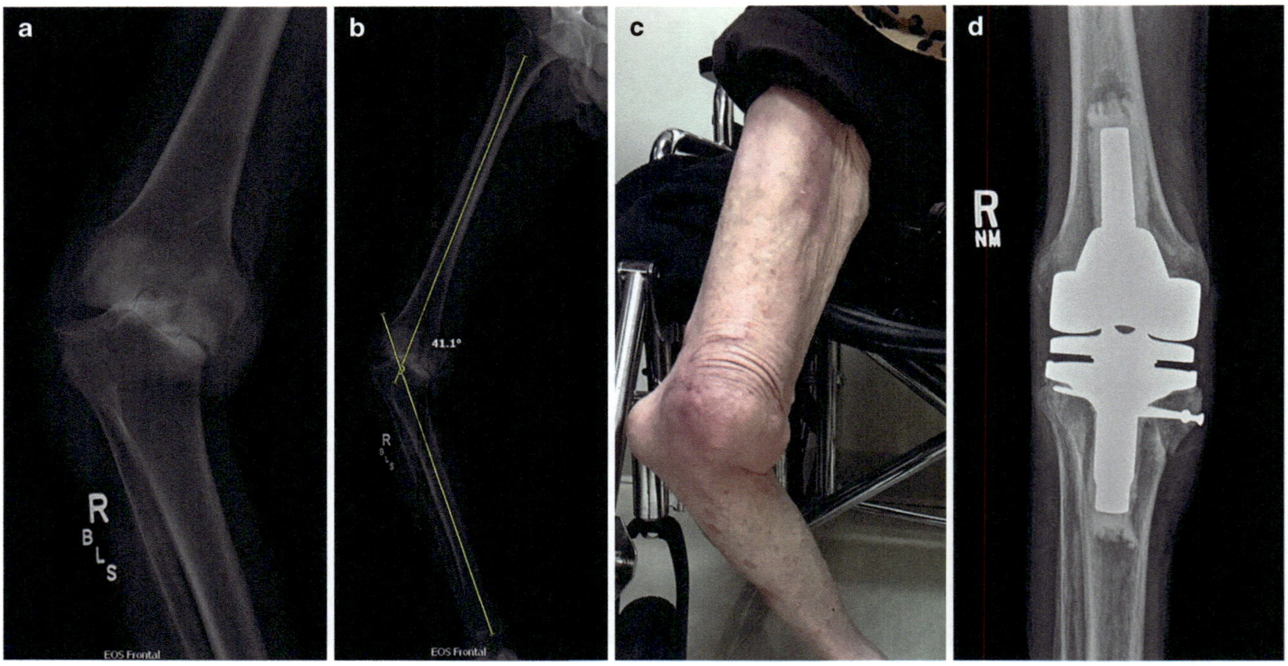

Fig. 59.1 **a–d** Complex primary TKA in a high-risk patient for PJI. A 67-year-old female patient with severe right knee OA **a**, severe varus deformity **b**, ligament instability **c**, and significant bone loss. She also has a long-standing history of rheumatoid arthritis in immunosuppressive therapy (leflunomide and prednisone) and is considered in the high-risk category for PJI/SSI. She underwent a complex primary constrained cemented TKA using bone autograft augmentation. ALBC was used at a prophylactic dose (1.2 g of tobramycin and 1 g of vancomycin mixed per batch of cement). At 3-year follow-up, her right TKA was functioning well, and there was no evidence of PJI **d**

59.2 Evidence

Previous evidence has shown that ALBC together with systemic antibiotic prophylaxis was effective in reducing PJI in TKA compared with plain cement and systemic antibiotic prophylaxis (Chiu et al. 2002; Eveillard et al. 2003; Randelli et al. 2010); however, more recent evidence suggests that this question is still debatable. Two recent prospective studies showed that ALBC did not reduce the rate of deep infection following primary TKA compared with plain cement (Wilairatana et al. 2017; Wang et al. 2015). More recently, a systematic review on the use of ALBC in total joint arthroplasty evaluated six articles encompassing 6318 arthroplasties. Among the study population, 3217 of these arthroplasties received ALBC and 3101 arthroplasties using plain cement served as the control. Only two studies showed a significant effect of ALBC in preventing deep infection in primary TKA. Contradictory results were reported in the remaining four prospective and randomized clinical trial studies that showed no statistical difference between the two groups in terms of the incidence of deep or superficial SSIs (Schiavone Panni et al. 2016). In another meta-analysis, Kleppel et al. reported 4092 patients following TKA (3903 primary TKAs and 189 revision TKAs). At an average follow-up time of 47.2 months for primary TKA, the use of ALBC demonstrates a nonsignificant reduction in PJI/SSI; however, there was a significant reduction in revision TKA infection rates in the ALBC group (Kleppel et al. 2017). Additionally, a recent analysis of 731,214 joints from the National Joint Registry (NJR) of England and Wales after adjusting for other variables demonstrated that the use of ALBC had a significantly lower risk of revision for any cause (HR 0.85, 95% CI 0.77–0.93; $p < 0.001$), as well as reduction of revisions for infection (HR 0.84, 95% CI 0.67–1.01; $p = 0.06$) (Jameson et al. 2019).

The 2018 Second International Consensus Meeting (ICM) on Musculoskeletal Infection, based on moderate evidence and with super majority-strong consensus, recommended:

» Antibiotic-impregnated cement may be used during primary TJA to reduce the risk of surgical site infections/periprosthetic joint infections. The benefits of antibiotic-impregnated cement vs. its cost and other potential adverse effects may be most justified in patients at high risk of infection (Parvizi 2019).

59.3 Indications for Antibiotic-Loaded Bone Cement

The prophylactic use of ALBC for the primary fixation of implants (▣ Fig. 59.1) must be clearly distinguished from its therapeutic use in the staged revision setting.

> Considerable variation exists in the use of ALBC in primary TKA; however, given the available evidence we feel that selective use in high-risk patients is warranted.

> In contrast, the routine use of ALBC in revision total joint arthroplasty is well accepted, with good supporting evidence in both aseptic and first-stage revision procedures utilizing articulating (▣ Fig. 59.2) or static spacers (▣ Fig. 59.3).

Although limited clinical evidence exists on the use of ALBC at the time of definitive component reimplantation after septic revision, the rationale for its use is strong.

Prophylactic and Therapeutic Use of ALBC

- *Prophylactic—low-dose antibiotic* (<1.2 g of antibiotic per 40 g pack of cement):
  - Primary TKA in high-risk groups for PJI*.
  - Revision TKA (aseptic revision and reimplantation).
- *Therapeutic—high-dose antibiotic* (>3 g of antibiotic per 40 g pack of cement):
  - First stage of a two-stage revision procedure in the antibiotic spacer.
  - Per 40 g pack of cement: 3 g of vancomycin and 3.6 g of tobramycin; if fungal infection is present or suspected, 150–200 mg of amphotericin B is added.

*Host risk factors for SSI/PJI in TJA: chronic kidney disease, diabetes mellitus, malnutrition, immunosuppression, rheumatoid arthritis, HIV/AIDS, peripheral vascular disease, obesity, smoking, clotting disorders, chronic obstructive pulmonary disease, untreated hepatitis C, MRSA colonization, chronic anticoagulation, previous joint surgery, previous joint infection, transplant, osteonecrosis, posttraumatic osteoarthritis, bariatric surgery (Parvizi 2019).

Although there is no consensus about the definition of high-dose ALBC, it is generally accepted that a dose

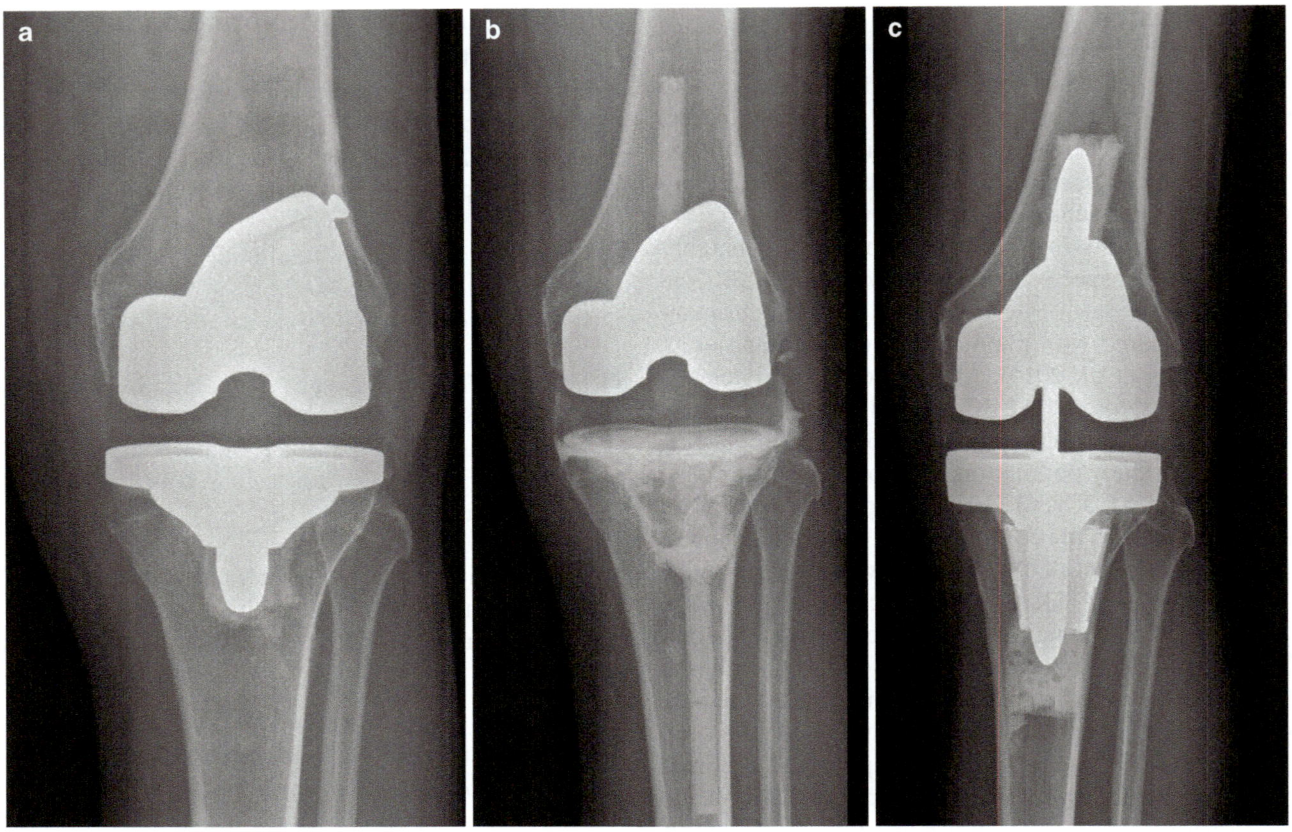

Fig. 59.2 **a–c** Two-stage revision for chronic PJI with articulating spacer. A 60-year-old male patient with a history of posttraumatic left knee OA who underwent left TKA after smoking cessation optimization **a**. The postoperative course was complicated with an acute PJI secondary to CoNS failing DAIR and 6 weeks of specific antibiotic therapy, subsequently he presented with infection recurrence, this time with *Candida albicans* and underwent two-stage revision surgery **b** with articulating spacer (high-dose antibiotics: 3 g of vancomycin, 3.6 g of tobramycin, 200 mg of amphotericin B per batch of cement, No.3 batch × 40 g of cement in total). The patient received 6 weeks of IV vancomycin and ertapenem, and oral fluconazole (12 weeks). He underwent left TKA re-implantation **c** using metaphyseal cones, short cemented stems, and ALBC was used at prophylactic dose. He received long-term oral suppressive antibiotic therapy (trimethoprim-sulfamethoxazole and fluconazole) for 6 months postoperatively. At 1-year follow-up after re-implantation, there is no clinical evidence of infection recurrence

higher than 2 g of antibiotic per 40 g of cement represents a high-dose ALBC (Hanssen and Spangehl 2004).

59.4 Industrially Manufactured Versus "Homemade" Preparations of ALBC

Commercially available ALBCs offer different options of viscosity (low, medium, and high viscosity) and antibiotics for the surgeon. The most common brands are included in Table 59.1; however, several concerns remain about having readily available ALBCs. Typically, aminoglycosides are included in the commercially ALBC, providing coverage against Gram-negative bacteria including *Pseudomonas*, *Proteus*, *Escherichia coli*, *Klebsiella pneumoniae*, Enterobacteriaceae, *Serratia*, and the Gram-positive *Staphylococcus*. However, tobramycin has the added benefit of superior activity against *Pseudomonas*. Additionally, vancomycin potentially has a higher antimicrobial activity when compared with gentamicin for methicillin-resistant *Staphylococcus aureus* (MRSA) while remaining heat-stable with adequate elution (Tunney et al. 1998; Kuechle et al. 1991; Adams et al. 1992). Studies have raised concerns regarding the following:

- Increasing microbial resistance
- Insufficient dose of antibiotic
- Additional unnecessary cost
- Reduced mechanical properties of the commercial preparations (Frew et al. 2017)

We must also consider the cost associated with the use of the ALBC. In the United States, the average cost of 1 pack (40 g) of industrially manufactured ALBC is somewhere between $215 and $325, compared to homemade preparations using pain cement that could be around $100. In a recent systematic review about cost implications of ALBC, King et al. conclude that hospital systems performing 1000 TKAs per year could save

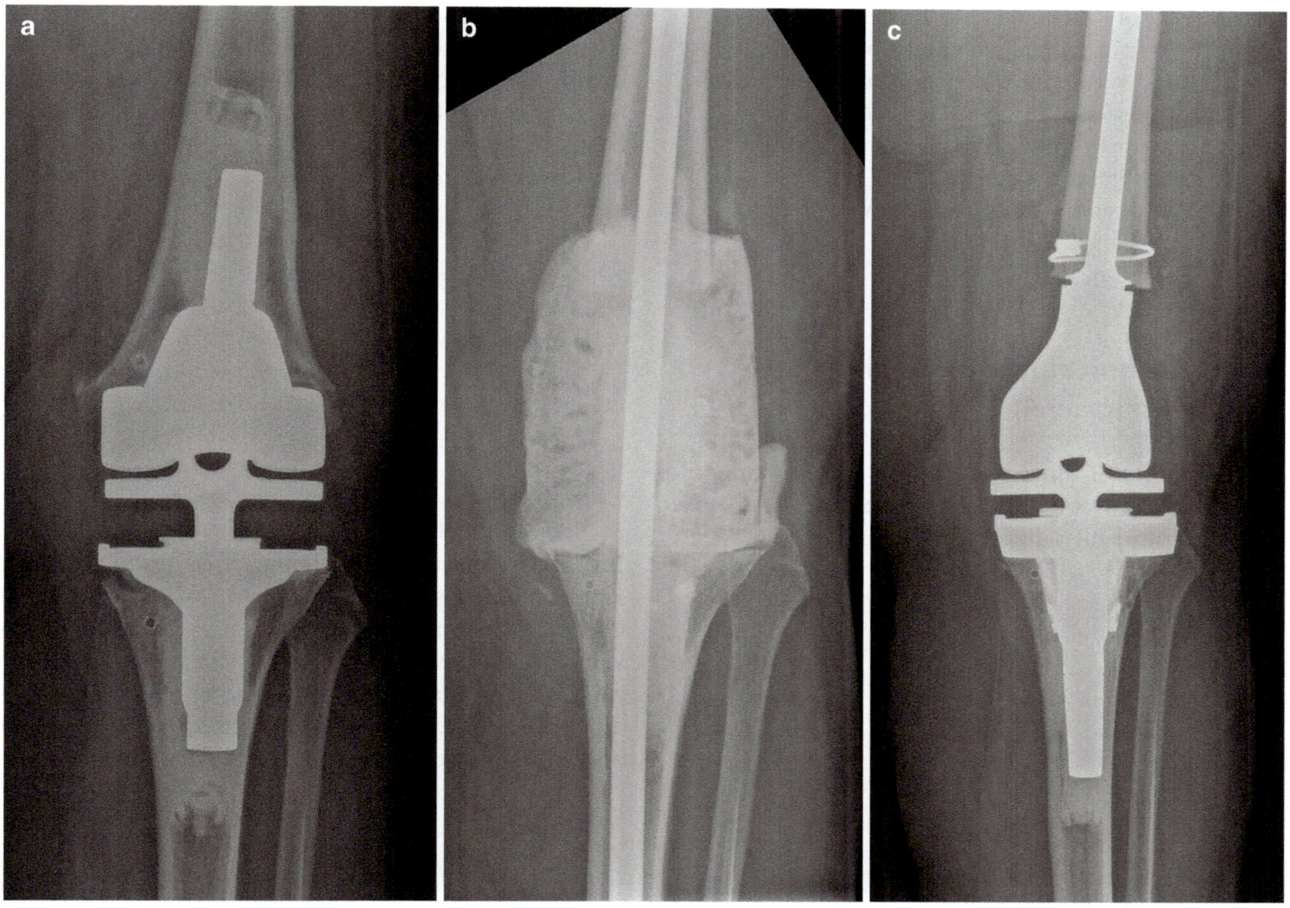

Fig. 59.3 **a–c** Two-stage revision for chronic PJI with static ALBC spacer. A 73-year-old male patient with a history of index left TKA and two aseptic revisions for aseptic loosening, and 1 year after the last revision, he was diagnosed with coagulase-negative *Staphylococcus* chronic PJI **a** and underwent two-stage revision surgery with static ALBC spacer **b** due to the massive bone loss and instability (high-dose antibiotics: 3 g of vancomycin and 3.6 g of tobramycin, per 40 g batch of cement, No.3 batch × 40 g of cement in total). He completed 6 weeks of IV vancomycin. He underwent left TKA reimplantation **c** using a distal femoral replacement and metaphyseal cones, cemented stems, and ALBC was used at a prophylactic dose (1.2 g of tobramycin, 1 g of vancomycin mixed per batch of cement). He received long-term oral suppressive antibiotic therapy (doxycycline) for 6 months postoperatively. At 1.5-year follow-up after reimplantation, there is no clinical evidence of infection recurrence

between $155,000 and $310,000 per year by switching to plain-cement homemade preparations (King et al. 2018). Industrially manufactured ALBC may be preferred due to the ease of access and time saving. However, biomechanical and elution testing has demonstrated that 1 g of vancomycin in homemade ALBC can reduce cost without compromising the mechanical strength or elution of the drug (Lee et al. 2016). Furthermore, a recent study comparing the elution properties of commercially available ALBC with homemade preparations using high-performance liquid chromatography mass spectrometry observed the highest peak concentrations of antibiotics from the homemade cements containing vancomycin added in the operating theater. The overall elution of antibiotics was fivefold (vancomycin) and twofold (gentamicin) greater from the homemade mix compared with commercially mixed cement (Frew et al. 2017).

> Considering the excellent elution properties and lower costs associated with the preparation of homemade ALBC in the operating theater by hand, it seems there is no significant advantage of using expensive commercially available ALBC.

59.4.1 Relevant Tips/Tricks of "Homemade" ALBC Articulating Spacers: Authors' Preferred Technique

Implants/Materials Needed

- Cruciate-retaining (CR) or posterior stabilized (PS) femoral component
- All-polyethylene CR or PS tibial component
- Bone Cement × 40 g pack (usually 3–4 batches are needed):

- 3 g of vancomycin powder per batch
- 3.6 g of tobramycin powder per batch
- 150 mg of amphotericin B powder per batch (if concerns for fungal infection)
- Methylene blue 1 mL per batch
- Mineral oil
- Two cement guns to make dowels
- Disposable cement spatula
- Hand-mixed

59.4.2 Technical Tips for Mixing ALBC (▫ Fig. 59.4)

High volumes of antibiotic powder make mixing difficult if the antibiotic and cement powders are mixed together before introducing the liquid monomer.

> It is rather recommended to first mix together the PMMA monomer and powder to form the liquid cement, followed by adding 1 mL/batch of methylene blue to obtain a homogeneously blue and fluid cement. Subsequently, the antibiotic powder is slowly added.

Vancomycin powder and some generic brands of tobramycin are crystalline in nature, which can make mixing difficult. It is preferable to leave many of the large crystals intact when preparing ALBC for use as beads or spacers because this makes a more porous mixture, which facilitates a higher volume of antibiotic elution.

> In contrast, when mixing crystalline antibiotics into cement to be used for prosthesis fixation, the crystals should be pulverized with a mortar and pestle before being added to the liquid cement because the crystalline defects significantly weaken the cement.

Step 1: Prepare Intramedullary Dowels and Augments of ALBC

Medullary dowels were popularized by Dr. Arlen Hanssen (Hanssen and Spangehl 2004) from Mayo Clinic, Rochester, MN, and have the advantages to provide a local-delivery antibiotic system in the medullary canal and facilitate its removal during re-implantation. To optimize time, this can be performed prior to incision at the back table working area using one batch 40 g of

▫ **Table 59.1** Available manufactured antibiotic-loaded bone cement

Brand	Manufacturer	Viscosity	Antibiotic dose (in 40 g pack of cement)	Setting time
Cemex® Genta ISO	Tecres SpA	High	Gentamicin 1 g	Regular
Cemex® Genta RX	Tecres SpA	Medium	Gentamicin 1 g	Medium
Cemex® Fast Genta	Tecres SpA	High	Gentamicin 1 g	Fast
CMW™ 1G	DePuy Synthes	High	Gentamicin 1 g	Medium
CMW™ 2G	DePuy Synthes	High	Gentamicin 1 g	Fast
Cobalt® G-HV	DJO Global	High	Gentamicin 1 g	Medium
Cobalt® G-MV	DJO Global	Medium	Gentamicin 1 g	Fast
Palacos® R+G	Heraeus Medical	High	Gentamicin 0.5 g	Regular
Palacos® LV+G	Heraeus Medical	Low	Gentamicin 1 g	Regular
Palacos® MV+G	Heraeus Medical	Medium	Gentamicin 0.5 g	Regular
Smartset™ GHV	DePuy Synthes	High	Gentamicin 1 g	Regular
Smartset™ GMV	DePuy Synthes	Medium	Gentamicin 1 g	Regular
Simplex™ HV Genta	Stryker	High	Gentamicin 0.5 g	Regular
Simplex™ P	Stryker	Medium	Tobramycin 1 g	Medium
Simplex™ P Speedset	Stryker	Medium	Tobramycin 1 g	Fast
VersaBond® AB	Smith & Nephew	Medium	Gentamicin 1 g	Regular

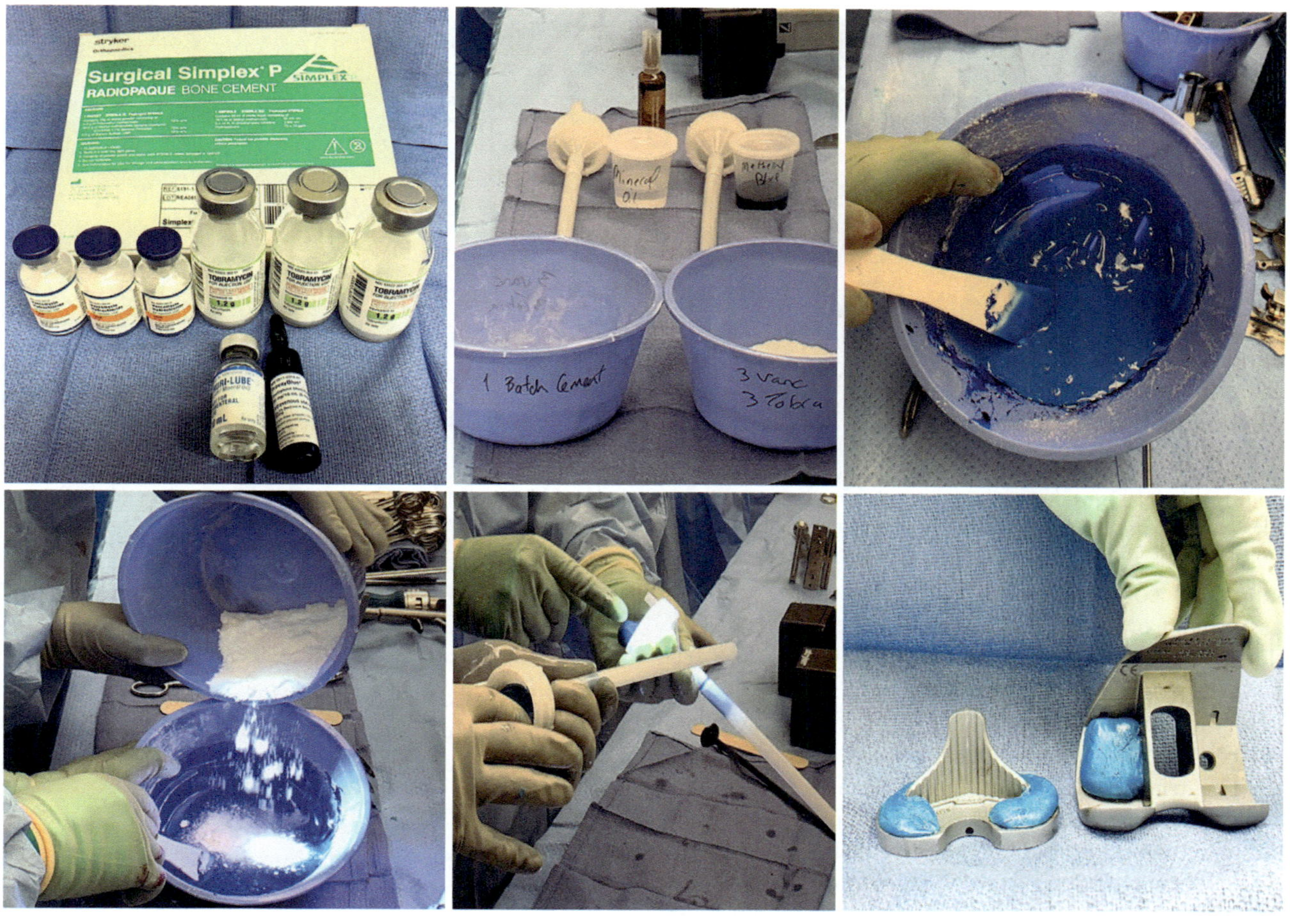

Fig. 59.4 ALBC Preparation—work on the back table. The cement powder and the liquid monomer are mixed together first until a fluid and homogeneous mixture is obtained. Then, 1 mL/batch of methylene blue is added, and antibiotics (powder) are added finally. The mixture is gently mixed with a spatula. The cement syringe nozzle tubes are generously covered with mineral oil inside in order to prevent adherence of the cement. Tibial augments can also be made and are useful in the case of a gap mismatch

cement, and 2 dowels of cement (10–15 cm long) are prepared by introducing high-dose ALBC into the cement gun nozzle tube, providing an excellent size and shape for a spacer to be inserted into the medullary canal (Fig. 59.5). The cement gun nozzle has been previously spread in the interior surface with sterile mineral oil to facilitate the extraction.

> It is important to create a small bulb at the end of the dowel to prevent migration into the femoral or tibial canal.

In roughly 1/3 of infected knee replacements without stems, there is extension of the infectious process into the medullary femoral or tibial canals (Hanssen and Spangehl 2004), and antibiotic beads in the medullary canals can be extremely difficult to remove at reimplantation. Also, 5-mm augments for the tibial and femur (distal and posterior) augments could be made using trial components, previously spread with mineral oil (Fig. 59.4).

- **Step 2: Refreshing the Cuts, Femur and Tibia Preparation (Fig. 59.5)**

After the infected implants are removed, a thorough synovectomy is performed. The tibia is prepared perpendicular to its mechanical axis. The intramedullary canal is reamed (usually up to 12–13 cm) and a minimal refreshing proximal cut is performed. Then, we proceed with the femoral preparation. The femoral component should be sized to fit the remaining distal femur in the sagittal plane. An intramedullary guide is placed. The distal femur cut is refreshed using a cutting guide with the proper rotation. The remaining cuts of the femur are refreshed (by either free-hand or using the 4-in-1 cutting block). This helps with the debridement of the remaining bone cement as well. A box for a PS implant is prepared if this is needed. Subsequently, assessment of the extension and flexion gaps is performed with the use of a laminar spreader in both extension and flexion, obtaining the respective gap measurement with a ruler (Fig. 59.5b, c). If a gap mismatch is anticipated (as usually happens), some ALBC femoral and/or tibial

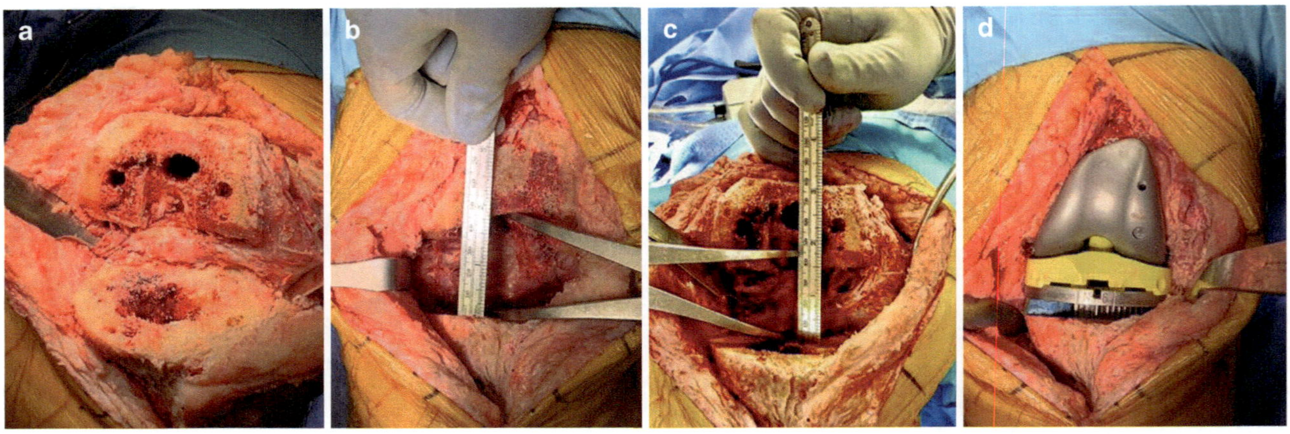

Fig. 59.5 **a–d** Bone preparation and trialing. After a thorough synovectomy, the proximal tibia and distal femur are refreshed **a**. Flexion **b** and extension **c** gaps are assessed, which helps anticipate any flexion/extension mismatch and, therefore, the use of previously made ALBC augments. Then multiple liner options (**d**) are put in place in order to obtain a balanced knee

augments could be made according to the previous assessment or at the beginning with the residual ALBC during the preparation of the medullary dowels. A trial is then placed. Multiple liner options are trialed to achieve appropriate stability in flexion/extension (Fig. 59.5d).

The trial implants are removed, and irrigation is performed. We use a total of 0.35% povidone-iodine solution for 3 minutes followed by pulse lavage, then disinfection with 1 L of 0.05% chlorhexidine gluconate (IrriSept) for another 3 minutes, and finally high-pressure pulse lavage irrigation with 6 L of sterile saline. We change the drapes for clean drapes. The tourniquet is released, and hemostasis is obtained. We change gloves and then proceed with cementation of the implants.

- **Step 3: Femoral and Tibial Implant Preparation and Cementation (Fig. 59.6)**

The tip of the all-polyethylene tibial component is removed with an oscillating saw in order to accommodate for the tibial dowel. Both medullary ALBC dowels are placed into the respective medullary canal, followed by gentle cementation of the bony surfaces of the femur and the tibia. While the cement is curing, small holes should be made for future cement interdigitations (this can be achieved with a freer). The all-polyethylene tibial implant and femoral components are precoated with cement (if ALBC augments are used, they must be included at this point) and impacted gently until fully seated, starting with the tibia and then applying the femoral component in deep knee flexion. Once the femur is seated, the knee is compressed in extension until the cement is dry. Any gaps between the femoral component and host bone can be filled with cement (Fig. 59.6).

59.4.3 Antibiotic Elution from "Homemade" High-Dose ALBC Spacers

Antibiotics used in "homemade" cement spacers must be water-soluble, thermostable, and available in powder form. Therefore, not all antibiotics can be mixed into bone cement.

> During polymerization, the exothermic reaction produces heat, ranging from 70 to 120 °C in vitro (Monzón et al. 2019), which warrants the use of heat-stable antibiotics.

Thus, the most commonly used antibiotics are gentamicin, tobramycin, vancomycin, and cefazolin. Elution of antibiotics from high-dose ALBC spacers depends on the concentration of antibiotics used, the brand of cement from which the mixing is made, the mixing methods, and porosity.

Lee et al. (2016) added 4 g of vancomycin (from three different manufacturers) into four different types of surgical-grade bone cements. Their elution study showed a constant burst release during the first hour, and then a plateau was reached at 72 hours. The authors also showed that regardless of the vancomycin manufacturer, Palacos cement resulted in the highest cumulative elution.

> Mixing two antibiotics has been shown to increase elution.

Paz et al. (2015) investigated the effect of adding cefazolin to vancomycin in high-dose ALBC. Their results showed that elution was significantly increased when cefazolin was added. Moreover, Hanssen et al. (2004) showed that mixing high-dose antibiotics creates

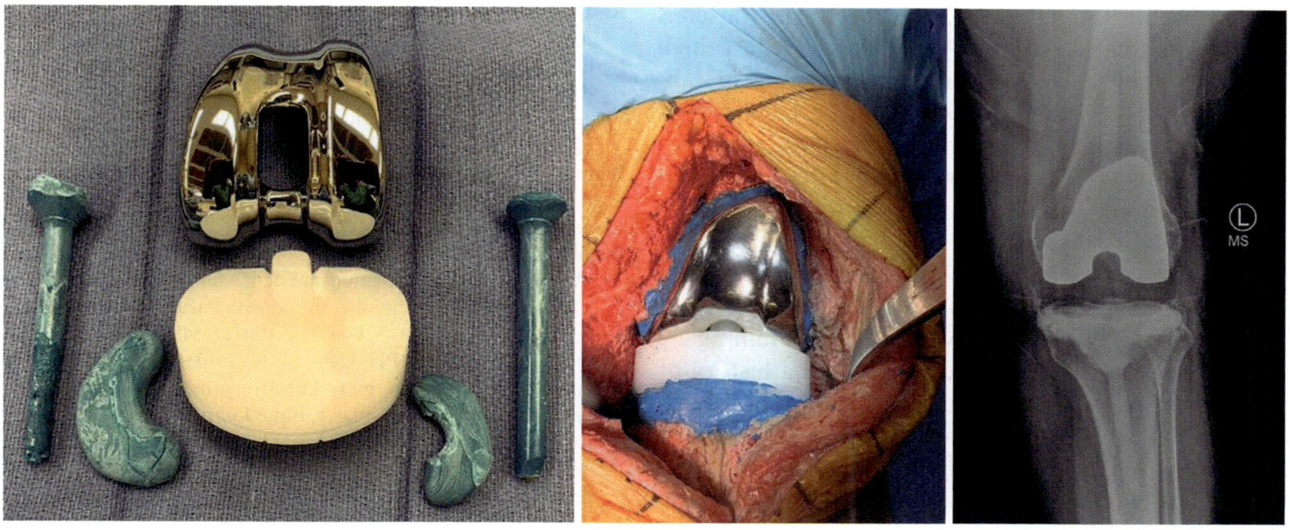

Fig. 59.6 Intraoperative and radiographic view of the ALBC articulating spacer. An excess of cement is left on purpose around the implants to enhance local delivery of antibiotics as well as to prevent further adhesion of the soft tissues and facilitate extraction at the time of re-implantation

considerable cement porosity facilitating elution for at least 4 weeks.

Interestingly, Martinez-Moreno et al. (2014) investigated the elution properties of 11 different antibiotics used in high-dose ALBC spherical beads for 30 days. Throughout the course of the investigation, the authors showed a triphasic pattern of elution with a progressive increase in the first 24 hours, then a rapid decrease, and a final phase of low and steady decline. Among the tested antibiotics, three were shown to be poor candidates (ampicillin, amoxicillin clavulanate, and cefepime) with undetectable concentrations at day 4.

Miller et al. (2012) compared three different mixing methods:

- Hand-stirred with bowl and spatula
- Bowl-mixed using a mechanical mixing bowl
- Dough-phase mixing with vancomycin left in chunks (1–5 mm)

Their elution analysis showed that dough-phase mixing leads to greater release. Several studies have investigated antibiotic levels at longer time points. Hsieh et al. (2006) mixed 4 g of vancomycin and 4 g of aztreonam with 40 g of cement. Their results showed that at a mean of 107 days after surgery, the concentration of antibiotics in the joint fluid was well above the minimal inhibitory concentration (MIC). Masri et al. (1998) blended high-dose tobramycin (between 1.2 and 4.8 g) and vancomycin (1–2 g) to 40 g of bone cement and implanted a knee Prostalac in 15 patients. The re-implantation was performed at a mean of 118 days. At that time, the authors showed that the use of at least 3.6 g of tobramycin and 1 g of vancomycin per cement batch was necessary to maintain intra-articular concentrations above the MIC.

59.4.4 Potential Complications of High-Dose ALBC Spacers

Considering the potential adverse effects of ALBC, it is important to distinguish between its prophylactic use (low-dose) and its high-dose use during the first stage of a two-stage revision procedure.

> For routine use of low-dose ALBC, Hansen et al. (2014) have shown no notable increase in bacteria resistance or changes in infecting pathogen profile. Otherwise, to date, no medical systemic complications have been reported with the use of low-dose ALBC (Gandhi et al. 2018).

Potential complications are associated with the use of high-dose ALBC. Thus, there are several case reports of nephrotoxicity (acute renal injury/failure) associated with the addition of aminoglycosides or other antibiotics in ALBC knee spacers (Geller et al. 2017; Menge et al. 2012; Aeng et al. 2015; James and Larson 2015; van Raaij et al. 2002; Curtis et al. 2005; Patrick et al. 2006; Roman and Slama 2015; Salim et al. 2018; Song et al. 2010; Berliner et al. 2018).

> Monitoring the renal function is recommended during and in the case of ongoing renal dysfunction; removal of the spacer as soon as possible should be considered.

Song et al. (2010) reported a case of a 69-year-old woman who developed pain, fever, generalized skin rash, and abnormal laboratory findings around 2 weeks after the placement of a spacer with high-dose piperacillin/tazobactam. Aeng et al. (2015) investigated a series of patients treated with an ALBC spacer with a high dose of tobramycin (3.6 g) and a moderate dose of vancomycin (1.5 g). The authors showed an incidence of acute kidney injury (AKI) of 20%. Interestingly, they also found two risk factors associated with AKI: intraoperative blood transfusion and postoperative treatment with NSAIDs.

Williams et al. (2014) described a case of a patient developing a painful blistering rash during the week following a TKA cemented with ALBC containing 2 g of vancomycin. However, the patient had a history of Stevens–Johnson syndrome to IV vancomycin 6 years prior. Such a history of life-threatening allergy reaction would represent the only contraindication to the addition of a specific antibiotic. Otherwise, there is no published contraindication to the use of high-dose ALBC.

Take-Home Messages

- ALBC in TKA could be used as a method of prophylaxis as compared with the treatment of an established PJI.
- Prophylactic ALBC (low dose): use in high-risk group patients in the setting of primary or revisions, therapeutic use (high dose): during the first-stage revision TKA for spacers (articulating or static).
- Homemade ALBC is cost-effective, providing excellent elution and mechanical properties with lower costs compared to commercial preparations.
- Antibiotic powder is preferred over liquid to improve elution and mechanical properties.
- The authors recommended the following sequence of mixing:
  1. Mix liquid monomer and powder to create a liquid cement.
  2. Add 1 cc of methylene blue/batch of cement for visualization purposes.
  3. Add antibiotic powder.

References

Adams K, Couch L, Cierny G, Calhoun J, Mader JT (1992) In vitro and in vivo evaluation of antibiotic diffusion from antibiotic-impregnated polymethylmethacrylate beads. Clin Orthop Relat Res 278:244–252

Aeng ESY, Shalansky KF, Lau TTY, Zalunardo N, Li G, Bowie WR, Duncan CP (2015) Acute kidney injury with tobramycin-impregnated bone cement spacers in prosthetic joint infections. Ann Pharmacother 49(11):1207–1213

Anagnostakos K, Wilmes P, Schmitt E, Kelm J (2009) Elution of gentamicin and vancomycin from polymethylmethacrylate beads and hip spacers in vivo. Acta Orthop 80(2):193–197

Australian National Joint Replacement Registry, Annual Report 2018. https://aoanjrr.sahmri.com/annual-reports-2018

Berliner ZP, Mo AZ, Porter DA, Grossman JM, Hepinstall MS, Cooper HJ, Scuderi GR (2018) In-hospital acute kidney injury after TKA revision with placement of an antibiotic cement spacer. J Arthroplast 33(7S):S209–S212

Blomgren G, Lindgren U (1981) Late hematogenous infection in total joint replacement: studies of gentamicin and bone cement in the rabbit. Clin Orthop Relat Res 155:244–248

Buchholz HW, Engelbrecht H. Uber die Depotwirkung einiger Antibiotica bei Vermischung mit dem Kunstharz Palacos [Depot effects of various antibiotics mixed with Palacos resins]. Chirurg. 1970 Nov;41(11):511–5. German. PMID: 5487941.

Chang Y, Tai CL, Hsieh PH, Ueng SWN (2013) Gentamicin in bone cement: a potentially more effective prophylactic measure of infection in joint arthroplasty. Bone Joint Res 2(10):220–226

Chiu F-Y, Chen C-M, Lin C-FJ, Lo W-H (2002) Cefuroxime-impregnated cement in primary total knee arthroplasty: a prospective, randomized study of three hundred and forty knees. J Bone Joint Surg Br Vol 84(5):759–762

Curtis JM, Sternhagen V, Batts D (2005) Acute renal failure after placement of tobramycin-impregnated bone cement in an infected total knee arthroplasty. Pharmacotherapy 25(6):876–880

Eveillard M, Mertl P, Tramier B, Eb F (2003) Effectiveness of gentamicin-impregnated cement in the prevention of deep wound infection after primary total knee arthroplasty. Infect Control Hosp Epidemiol 24(10):778–780

Font-Rodriguez DE, Scuderi GR, Insall JN (1997) Survivorship of cemented total knee arthroplasty. Clin Orthop Relat Res 345:79–86

Frew NM, Cannon T, Nichol T, Smith TJ, Stockley I (2017) Comparison of the elution properties of commercially available gentamicin and bone cement containing vancomycin with 'home-made' preparations. Bone Joint J 99(B-1):73–77

Gálvez-López R, Peña-Monje A, Antelo-Lorenzo R, Guardia-Olmedo J, Moliz J, Hernández-Quero J, Parra-Ruiz J (2014) Elution kinetics, antimicrobial activity, and mechanical properties of 11 different antibiotic loaded acrylic bone cement. Diagn Microbiol Infect Dis 78(1):70–74

Gandhi R, Backstein D, Zywiel MG (2018) Antibiotic-laden bone cement in primary and revision hip and knee arthroplasty. J Am Acad Orthop Surg 26(20):727–734

Geller JA, Cunn G, Herschmiller T, Murtaugh T, Chen A (2017) Acute kidney injury after first-stage joint revision for infection: risk factors and the impact of antibiotic dosing. J Arthroplast 32(10):3120–3125

Hansen EN, Adeli B, Kenyon R, Parvizi J (2014) Routine use of antibiotic laden bone cement for primary total knee arthroplasty: impact on infecting microbial patterns and resistance profiles. J Arthroplast 29(6):1123–1127

Hanssen AD, Spangehl MJ (2004) Practical applications of antibiotic-loaded bone cement for treatment of infected joint replacements. Clin Orthop Relat Res 427:79–85

Hendriks JGE, van Horn JR, van der Mei HC, Busscher HJ (2004) Backgrounds of antibiotic-loaded bone cement and prosthesis-related infection. Biomaterials 25(3):545–556

Hsieh P-H, Chang Y-H, Chen S-H, Ueng SWN, Shih C-H (2006) High concentration and bioactivity of vancomycin and aztreonam eluted from simplex cement spacers in two-stage revision of infected hip implants: a study of 46 patients at an average follow-up of 107 days. J Orthop Res 24(8):1615–1621

James A, Larson T (2015) Acute renal failure after high-dose antibiotic bone cement: case report and review of the literature. Ren Fail 37(6):1061–1066

Jameson SS, Asaad A, Diament M, Kasim A, Bigirumurame T, Baker P, Mason J, Partington P, Reed M (2019) Antibiotic-loaded bone cement is associated with a lower risk of revision following primary cemented total knee arthroplasty: an analysis of 731,214 cases using National Joint Registry data. Bone Joint J 101(B-11):1331–134
Jiranek WA, Hanssen AD, Greenwald AS (2006) Antibiotic-loaded bone cement for infection prophylaxis in total joint replacement. J Bone Joint Surg Br Vol 88(11):2487–2500
King JD, Hamilton DH, Jacobs CA, Duncan ST (2018) The hidden cost of commercial antibiotic-loaded bone cement: a systematic review of clinical results and cost implications following Total knee arthroplasty. J Arthroplast 33(12):3789–3792
Kleppel D, Stirton J, Liu J, Ebraheim NA (2017) Antibiotic bone cement's effect on infection rates in primary and revision total knee arthroplasties. World J Orthop 8(12):946–955
Kuechle DK, Landon GC, Musher DM, Noble PC (1991) Elution of vancomycin, daptomycin, and amikacin from acrylic bone cement. Clin Orthop Relat Res 264:302–308
Lee S-H, Tai C-L, Chen S-Y, Chang C-H, Chang Y-H, Hsieh P-H (2016) Elution and mechanical strength of vancomycin-loaded bone cement: in vitro study of the influence of brand combination. PLoS One 11(11):e0166545
Masri BA, Duncan CP, Beauchamp CP (1998) Long-term elution of antibiotics from bone-cement: an in vivo study using the prosthesis of antibiotic-loaded acrylic cement (PROSTALAC) system. J Arthroplast 13(3):331–338
Menge TJ, Koethe JR, Jenkins CA, Wright PW, Shinar AA, Miller GG, Holt GE (2012) Acute kidney injury after placement of an antibiotic-impregnated cement spacer during revision total knee arthroplasty. J Arthroplasty 27(6):1221–1227.e1221–1222
Miller R, McLaren A, Leon C, McLemore R (2012) Mixing method affects elution and strength of high-dose ALBC: a pilot study. Clin Orthop Relat Res 470(10):2677–2683
Milligan DJ, O'Brien S, Doran E, Gallagher NE, Beverland DE (2019) Twenty-year survivorship of a cemented mobile bearing total knee arthroplasty. Knee 26(4):933–940
Monzón RA, Coury JG, Disse GD, Lum ZC (2019) Bone cement in total hip and knee arthroplasty. JBJS Rev 7(12):e6
Parvizi J, Gehrke T. Part IX: biofilm. In: Parvizi J, Gehrke T, eds. Proceedings of the second international consensus meeting on musculoskeletal infection: data trace. 2019:959–982
Patrick BN, Rivey MP, Allington DR (2006) Acute renal failure associated with vancomycin- and tobramycin-laden cement in total hip arthroplasty. Ann Pharmacother 40(11):2037–2042
Paz E, Sanz-Ruiz P, Abenojar J, Vaquero-Martín J, Forriol F, Del Real JC (2015) Evaluation of elution and mechanical properties of high-dose antibiotic-loaded bone cement: comparative "in vitro" study of the influence of vancomycin and cefazolin. J Arthroplast 30(8):1423–1429
Ranawat CS, Flynn WF, Deshmukh RG (1994) Impact of modern technique on long-term results of total condylar knee arthroplasty. Clin Orthop Relat Res 309:131–135
Randelli P, Evola FR, Cabitza P, Polli L, Denti M, Vaienti L (2010) Prophylactic use of antibiotic-loaded bone cement in primary total knee replacement. Knee Surg Sports Traumatol Arthrosc 18(2):181–186
Roman C, Slama TG (2015) Acute renal failure related to implanted antibiotic-impregnated cement joint spacer. Infect Dis Clin Pract 23(3):e15–e16
Salim SA, Everitt J, Schwartz A, Agarwal M, Castenada J, Fülöp T, Juncos LA (2018) Aminoglycoside impregnated cement spacer precipitating acute kidney injury requiring hemodialysis. Semin Dial 31(1):88–93
Schiavone Panni A, Corona K, Giulianelli M, Mazzitelli G, Del Regno C, Vasso M (2016) Antibiotic-loaded bone cement reduces risk of infections in primary total knee arthroplasty? A systematic review. Knee Surg Sports Traumatol Arthrosc 24(10):3168–3174
Scuderi GR, Insall JN, Windsor RE, Moran MC (1989) Survivorship of cemented knee replacements. J Bone Joint Surg Br Vol 71(5):798–803
Song EK, Seon JK, Jeong MS (2010) Delayed-type hypersensitivity reaction to piperacillin/tazobactam in a patient with an infected total knee replacement. J Bone Joint Surg Br Vol 92(11):1596–1599
Tunney MM, Ramage G, Patrick S, Nixon JR, Murphy PG, Gorman SP (1998) Antimicrobial susceptibility of bacteria isolated from orthopedic implants following revision hip surgery. Antimicrob Agents Chemother 42(11):3002–3005
van Raaij TM, Visser LE, Vulto AG, Verhaar JAN (2002) Acute renal failure after local gentamicin treatment in an infected total knee arthroplasty. J Arthroplast 17(7):948–950
Vessely MB, Whaley AL, Harmsen WS, Schleck CD, Berry DJ (2006) The Chitranjan Ranawat Award: long-term survivorship and failure modes of 1000 cemented condylar total knee arthroplasties. Clin Orthop Relat Res 452:28–34
Wang H, Qiu G-X, Lin J, Jin J, Qian W-W, Weng X-S (2015) Antibiotic bone cement cannot reduce deep infection after primary total knee arthroplasty. Orthopedics 38(6):e462–e466
Wilairatana V, Sinlapavilawan P, Honsawek S, Limpaphayom N (2017) Alteration of inflammatory cytokine production in primary total knee arthroplasty using antibiotic-loaded bone cement. J Orthop Traumatol 18(1):51–57
Williams B, Hanson A, Sha B (2014) Diffuse desquamating rash following exposure to vancomycin-impregnated bone cement. Ann Pharmacother 48(8):1061–1065

Antibiotic Spacers for Prosthetic Joint Infections Following Total Knee Arthroplasty

Samik Banerjee, Scot Brown, and P. Maxwell Courtney

Contents

E. Hansen, K.-D. Kühn (eds.), *Essentials of Cemented Knee Arthroplasty*,
https://doi.org/10.1007/978-3-662-63113-3_60

60.1 Introduction

Periprosthetic joint infection (PJI) remains an infrequent, yet disastrous, complication after elective primary and revision total knee arthroplasty (TKA). Although the incidence of PJI is generally considered to be higher after revision TKA, with reported incidences up to 22%, the overall prevalence largely varies between 1% and 2% (Zhan et al. 2007). Most studies report a slightly higher incidence after total knee arthroplasties compared to total hip arthroplasties.

Eradication of chronic PJI and subsequent reconstruction is challenging for various reasons and is related to host factors, microbial characteristics, and the extent of local soft tissue and bone destruction (◘ Fig. 60.1). It was Bucholz and Engelbrecht who first introduced the concept of eradication of osteomyelitis with the use of local delivery of antibiotics through antibiotic-loaded acrylic bone cement in the 1970s. Marks in 1976 and Shurman in 1978 further demonstrated the role of antibiotic-loaded bone cement (ALBC) in eradication of orthopedic infections (Marks et al. 1976; Schurman et al. 1978).

> However, it was not until 1983 when Insall described two-stage surgery with the need for removing all components coupled with extensive debridement followed by systemic antibiotic therapy prior to reimplantation for prosthetic joint infections.

60

> Subsequently, this "two stage procedure" has emerged as the "gold standard" for the treatment of chronic PJIs in the United States.

Garvin and Hanssen found after evaluating 29 studies in a systematic review that the success of two-stage procedures with antibiotic-loaded cement spacers was better than one-stage exchange arthroplasties (82% of 158 TJAs vs. 58% of 60 TJAs) despite the use of systemic antibiotic therapy in both procedures (Garvin and Hanssen 1995).

Although two-stage surgery without the use of antibiotic-impregnated spacers allows complete removal of all foreign materials with later reimplantation following eradication of infection, the procedure leads to joint instability, soft tissue contractures, bone destruction, and substantial functional limitations. Moreover, from a technical viewpoint, reimplantation is exceedingly difficult due to arthrofibrosis and loss of tissue planes.

> This has led to the use of polymethylmethacrylate (PMMA) as a spacer for maintenance of soft tissue pliability, length, and tension, while promoting local delivery of high concentration of antibiotics.

Garvin and Hansen found that addition of antibiotic-containing PMMA bone cement in one- and two-stage techniques led to substantial improvements in eradication of PJIs for two-stage and one-stage reimplantation to 91% (385 out of 423 TJAs) and 82% (976 out of 1189 TJAs) (Garvin and Hanssen 1995).

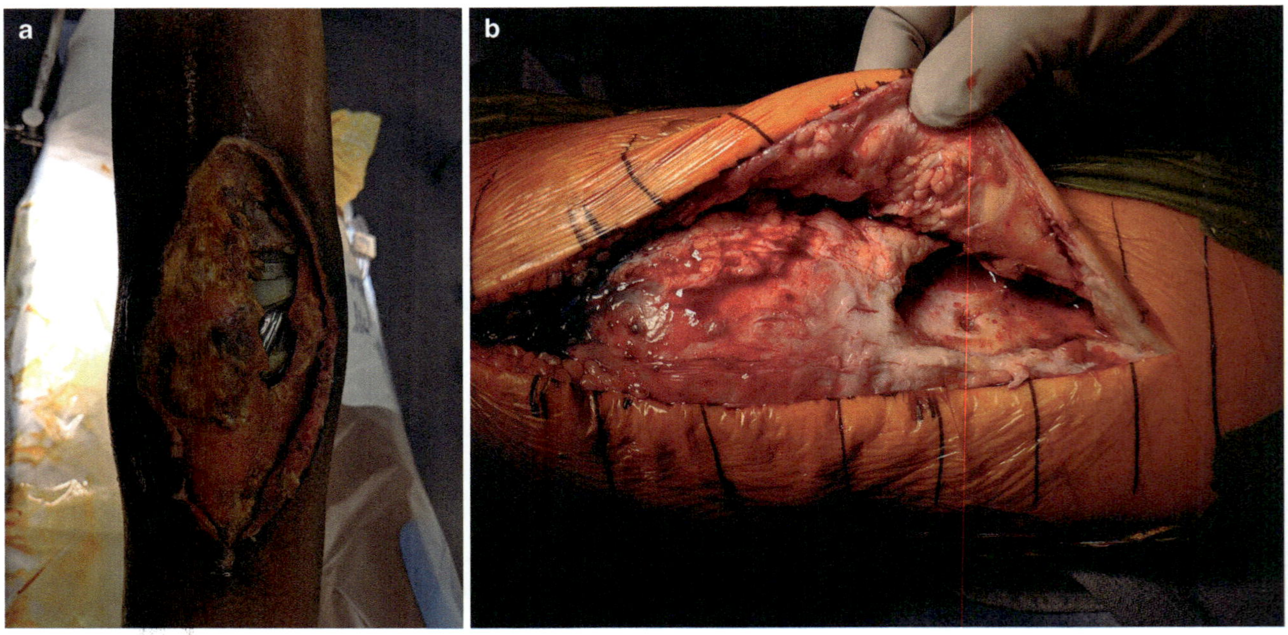

◘ **Fig. 60.1** **a** Chronic prosthetic joint infection with soft tissue loss. **b** Intraoperative photo of an infected knee with soft tissue loss on the medial proximal tibia secondary to infection

This chapter will focus on antibiotic cement spacers in prosthetic joint infection following TKA. Specifically, we will discuss on the following:

- Time-based classification of PJIs
- Antibiotics, elution characteristics, and systemic toxicity
- Types of spacers—articulating, nonarticulating, and functional spacers—duration of spacer use
- Fate of spacer implantation and options after failed spacers for recurrence of infection

60.2 Time-Based Classification of Prosthetic Joint Infections

This section has been covered in greater detail in a separate chapter of the book (▶ Chap. 55). However, as no discussion on antibiotic spacers is complete without an understanding of the time of presentation of PJIs, we briefly describe the time-based classification below. Typically, PJIs present at four different time intervals following any total joint arthroplasty procedure and are described as follows:

Time-Based Classification of PJIs (Cui et al. 2007)

- *Type 1:* Early postoperative infection within the first 3–4 weeks after prosthetic joint implantation
- *Type 2:* Late chronic infection presenting any time after the first 3–4 weeks following prosthetic joint implantation
- *Type 3:* Acute hematogenous infection in a seemingly well-functioning TJA following a bloodstream infection, typically from a distant source of infection
- *Type 4:* Unexpected ≥2 positive intraoperative cultures during an apparently aseptic revision arthroplasty or after reimplantation

For the most part, the currently accepted practice for the treatment of *Type 1* infection includes irrigation, synovectomy, bone and soft tissue debridement, and exchange of the tibial modular bearing surface. For early infection with cementless components, which are loose, and not osseointegrated, some authors would consider removal of all components with synovectomy, bone and soft tissue debridement, and reimplantation.

For *Type 2* infections, there is controversy in the optimal method of treatment, with some authors recommending a two-stage procedure with initial removal of all implants followed by delayed reimplantation and protracted course of antibiotic treatment, while others recommend one-stage reimplantation followed by prolonged postoperative antibiotic therapy. Still others believe that "functional spacers" with high-dose cemented implants may be considered a reasonable alternative in addition to systemic and prolonged antibiotic oral therapy in patients who are poor surgical candidates with multiple comorbidities. In select situations, with poor host conditions, a trial of debridement with retention of stable components and exchange of modular bearings may be considered.

In *Type 3* infections, most authors consider irrigation, synovectomy, bone and soft tissue debridement, and exchange of mobile and modular bearing surfaces as the initial treatment, unless loose components are found intraoperatively.

Most *Type 4* infections are treated postoperatively with appropriate systemic and oral antibiotics.

60.3 Antibiotics, Elution Characteristics, and Systemic Toxicity

> Various types of thermostable, water-soluble antibiotics, including glycopeptides, aminoglycosides, antifungals including amphotericin B and fluconazole, and, more recently, carbapenems and some "heat-sensitive" cephalosporins, have typically been combined for use with ALBC spacers (◘ Table 60.1) (Carli et al. 2018).

In addition to providing a synergistic effect and broad-spectrum coverage, combining antibiotics is essential for the treatment of polymicrobial infections. Spacers eluting these antibiotics achieve incrementally higher local concentrations in the joint and periarticular tissues compared to that which could be achieved with systemic therapy only.

> High antibiotic concentrations are deemed necessary, as the minimum bactericidal concentration for bacteria in biofilms is believed to be several-fold higher than planktonic bacteria (Nishimura et al. 2006).

> Moreover, high local concentration may prevent the development of resistant pathogens as prolonged exposure to antibiotic concentrations below the minimal inhibitory concentration (MIC) can contribute to the development of bacterial resistance.

> Elution of antibiotics from spacers is biphasic, with maximum diffusion in the first 3 days, followed by a steady constant release over the next 6–8 weeks.

The elution kinetics depends on several factors, including type, dosages of antibiotics, formulations, and their porosities, PMMA surface areas, and surface modifications such as indentations.

Table 60.1 Antibiotics commonly used with PMMA cement spacers

Antibiotic	Group	Suitability	Spectrum	Monitoring
Gentamicin	Aminoglycosides	Heat-stable; available in premixed formulations	Gram-negative aerobic bacteria; *Klebsiella, E. coli, Pseudomonas*	Needs postoperative serum concentration and BUN/Cr measurements Keep postoperative serum concentrations below 1.5 mg/L to reduce nephrotoxicity
Tobramycin	Aminoglycosides	Heat-stable; available in premixed formulations	Gram-negative bacteria; *Klebsiella, E. coli, Pseudomonas*	Needs postoperative serum concentration and BUN/Cr measurements Keep postoperative serum concentrations below 1.5 mg/L to reduce nephrotoxicity
Vancomycin	Glycopeptides	Heat-stable; enhanced elution with aminoglycosides—"passive opportunism," synergistic effect with aminoglycosides	Gram-positive bacteria—*Staphylococcus, Streptococcus*; MRSA and MRSE; Enterococci	Needs postoperative serum concentration and BUN/Cr measurements Keep postoperative serum concentrations below 15 μg/L to reduce nephrotoxicity
Clindamycin	Lincosamides	Heat-stable; enhanced elution with aminoglycosides	Gram-positive bacteria; MRSA; anaerobic infections	Usually no recommended drug monitoring necessary with ALBC use
Cefotaxime/ cefuroxime	Cephalosporins	Not heat stable; short acting due to hydrolysis	Depending on the generation; 1st and 2nd generation act against Gram-positive bacteria; 3rd and 4th generation against Gram-negative infections	Usually no recommended drug monitoring necessary with ALBC use
Rifampin	Ansamycin group	Not heat-stable; deleterious effect on mechanical properties; alginate microencapsulation may preserve compression properties and setting times	Gram-positive infections; *Staphylococcus* infections	Usually no recommended drug monitoring necessary with ALBC use
Meropenem	Carbapenems	Heat-stable	Effective against multiresistant Gram-negative infections; effective against *Enterobacter* sp.	Due to potential nephrotoxicity, will likely need postoperative serum concentration and BUN/Cr measurements
Colistin	Polymyxin E	Heat-stable, favorable elution characteristics; often combined with erythromycin for desirable antimicrobial effect	Effective against carbapenems and multidrug-resistant organisms	Due to potential nephrotoxicity, will likely need postoperative serum concentration and BUN/Cr measurements
Erythromycin	Macrolide	Heat-stable, favorable elution characteristics	Gram-positive organisms	No monitoring usually necessary
Amphotericin B	Subgroup of macrolides	Elution is variable; addition of poragen improves diffusion	Effective against fungi by binding to ergosterol in fungal membranes	Due to potential nephrotoxicity, will likely need postoperative serum concentration and BUN/Cr measurements

Table 60.1 (continued)

Antibiotic	Group	Suitability	Spectrum	Monitoring
Daptomycin	Cyclic lipopeptides	Heat-stable; favorable elution characteristics; effective against biofilms	Effective against Gram-positive organisms	Daptomycin dose in ALBC should be 3.3-times the original dose to double its release

PMMA polymethylmethacrylate, *BUN* blood urea nitrogen, *Cr* creatinine, *MRSA* methicillin-resistant *Staphylococcus aureus*, *MRSE* methicillin-resistant *Staphylococcus epidermidis*, *ALBC* antibiotic-loaded bone cement

> The type of cement used determines the diffusion of antibiotics.

Palacos® (Heraeus Medical, Yardley, PA) may be considered a more effective vehicle for drug delivery compared to other alternatives commercially available (Greene et al. 1998). It has been demonstrated that Palacos® has better diffusion characteristics with higher elution levels of vancomycin and tobramycin above MICs for organisms and were maintained for longer duration than Simplex® (Stryker Corp, Mahwah, NJ) PMMA cement. The elution profiles of Cobalt® HV and Bone Cement® R (DJO Global Carlsbad, CA) are intermediate between Simplex® and Palacos® LV for the most commonly tested antibiotics including vancomycin, tobramycin, and daptomycin (Meeker et al. 2019).

Combination of powdered vancomycin and tobramycin, in addition to the synergistic effect on microorganisms, can play a role in their individual elution characteristics from improvements in PMMA porosity, a phenomenon defined as "passive opportunism." One study on the long-term elution of antibiotics found a significant increase in the joint fluid concentration of tobramycin and vancomycin at 4 months when the dose was increased from 2.4 to 3.6 g per 40 g batch of PMMA cement (Masri et al. 1998). However, a similar increase in vancomycin dose from 1 to 1.5–2 g had no significant influence of vancomycin or tobramycin concentrations at long-term follow-up.

> Current data suggests that antibiotic levels usually remain above the MIC at approximately 3-month follow-up, although there is a trend toward declining levels over time partly related to the decrease in the diffusion gradient from tissue and joint fluid saturation (Klinder et al. 2019).

However, whether these lower levels are above bactericidal concentrations for biofilm bacteria is conjectural. Liquid gentamicin has similarly shown to improve the elution of vancomycin from PMMA cement by 1.5 times during the first 5 weeks, albeit with a 50% reduction in compressive mechanical properties of PMMA (Hsieh et al. 2009). Up to 6 g of antibiotics (for, e.g., 3 g vancomycin and 3 g flucloxacillin) per 40 g bag of cement can be incorporated without reducing the mechanical compressive strength below 70 MPa, which is considered the industry standard to prevent premature bone cement breakdown (Brock et al. 2010).

> Cement porosity, and thereby its elution, is increased by hand-mixing and curing the cement at 37 °C compared to room temperatures, with one study showing an up to 5-times increase in the elution concentrations of vancomycin and tobramycin (Sundblad et al. 2018).

In addition, delaying the addition of antibiotics until after 30 seconds of polymerization increased vancomycin elution for up to 6 weeks, while additional monomer use decreased the release of vancomycin from high-dose ALBC and can be potentially detrimental to the mechanical properties of PMMA (Masri et al. 1998; Amin et al. 2012). It is also noteworthy that use of closed suction drains in combination with ALBC does not affect the local antibiotic concentration released from the spacer at the initial 5 days after spacer insertion (Xu et al. 2019).

There is currently little agreement and no accepted guidelines on the optimum dosing of antibiotics for use in cement spacers. As explained above, there may be substantial inconsistency in the elution characteristics of the antibiotics used in cement spacers. Naturally, their systemic absorptions and concentrations can also vary. Although low-dose antibiotics (<2 g of antibiotic in 40 g of bone cement) in spacers are generally considered to be safe, due to lowered systemic exposures, there have been increasing concerns raised by authors about the systemic safety of high-dose antibiotics in spacers (Hanssen 2004; van Raaij et al. 2002; Patel et al. 2018; Kalil et al. 2012; Aeng et al. 2015; Berliner et al. 2018). Typically, antibiotic trough concentrations determine their renal toxic effects, with systemic levels of aminoglycosides above 2 mg/L and 15–20 μ/L for vancomycin considered to be associated with higher risks of nephrotoxicity (Aeng et al. 2015; Soto-Hall et al. 1983). One study demonstrated that the risks of renal toxicity are increased with the use of >4.8 g of tobramycin and >4.0 g of vancomycin in spacers with the serum creatinine levels peaking at 30 days and remaining elevated up to 3 months after insertion (Menge et al. 2012).

In conclusion, the elution kinetics of antibiotic PMMA spacers may be improved by the following factors:

Improvement of Elution Kinetics of Antibiotic PMMA Spacers

- Use of high-dose (for, e.g., vancomycin 2–4 g and tobramycin 2.4–3.6 g per 40 g bag of cement), 2 or 3 broad-spectrum antibiotics in Palacos® cement
- Hand-mixing at 37 °C
- Delaying antibiotic addition until initial polymerization
- Use of a power burr to form surface indentations
- Avoiding additional monomers during cement

Antibiotic-induced systemic toxicity commonly occurs within a week after surgery, although it can potentially manifest several days to weeks after ALBC spacer insertion. Careful and continuous monitoring of patients in the early postoperative period and at long-term follow-up is needed, especially those treated with concurrent nephrotoxic medications (for, e.g., nonsteroidal anti-inflammatory medications) and comorbidities predisposing them to enhanced side effects of these medications (for, e.g., increased age, elevated BMI, diabetes, preoperative anemia, elevated preoperative BUN and creatinine).

60.4 Types of Spacers

Several advantages have been reported with the use of various types of antibiotic spacers for eradication of infection. Maintaining soft tissue stability and allowing local elution of high-dose antibiotics in the joint act synergistically with systemically administered antibiotics for eradication of PJI. Broadly, there are two main types of knee spacers:

- Static spacers
- Articulating spacers

Articulating spacers can be prefabricated molds, which are commercially available, or custom-made intraoperatively. Another type of articulating spacer involves the use of autoclaved or new femoral components with polyethylene inserts implanted with ALBC. These will be discussed in further detail in the sections to follow.

60.4.1 Static Spacers

Static spacers are defined by designs that prevent ROM at the knee. The knee joint is kept in extension until the 2nd stage reimplantation. These static spacers were developed to avoid some of the issues associated with instability resulting from a knee resection arthroplasty after removal of TKA components. Multiple static spacers have been used, varying from the non-reinforced "hockey puck" type spacer to reinforced spacers with intramedullary spanning techniques (for, e.g., intramedullary rods, threaded Steinman pins). Static spacers aim to maintain soft tissue tension, elute antibiotics safely, avoid instability, and minimize bone loss during the interim stages of two-stage treatment for PJI. Instability can impede the eradication of PJI, and in the presence of massive bone (Nickinson et al. 2012) loss, soft tissue damage, extensor mechanism disruption, and collateral ligament disruption, maintenance of length and knee stability may only be reliably possible with the use of static reinforced endoskeleton type spacers (◘ Fig. 60.2). Additionally, keeping the knee stable and the wound at rest enables skin and soft tissue healing. Invagination of the "hockey puck" style spacer block is a definite concern, with one study reporting causing femoral and tibial bone loss up to 6 and 13 mm, respectively (Fehring et al. 2000).

Many techniques have been described for reinforcement of static antibiotic spacers to reduce bone loss and provide improved stability. These include threaded Steinman pins and humeral, tibial, or femoral intramedullary rods acting as an "endoskeleton" in the static spacers (Nickinson et al. 2012). Often, these intramedullary rods have to be custom-made on the table with a metal cutting burr so that a straight segment of the rod can be used, which is inserted easily. These reinforcements are also coated throughout their length with high-dose antibiotic cement to act as dowels to improve local elution of antibiotics in the intramedullary canals.

However, static spacers are not without drawbacks. When compared to functional antibiotic spacers, the authors also restrict weight bearing in static spacers. They may result in lower functional outcomes due to the restrictions in ROM and weight-bearing limitations they invariably impart. This can also lead to significant difficulty with exposure during reimplantation and subsequent ROM postoperatively due to quadriceps

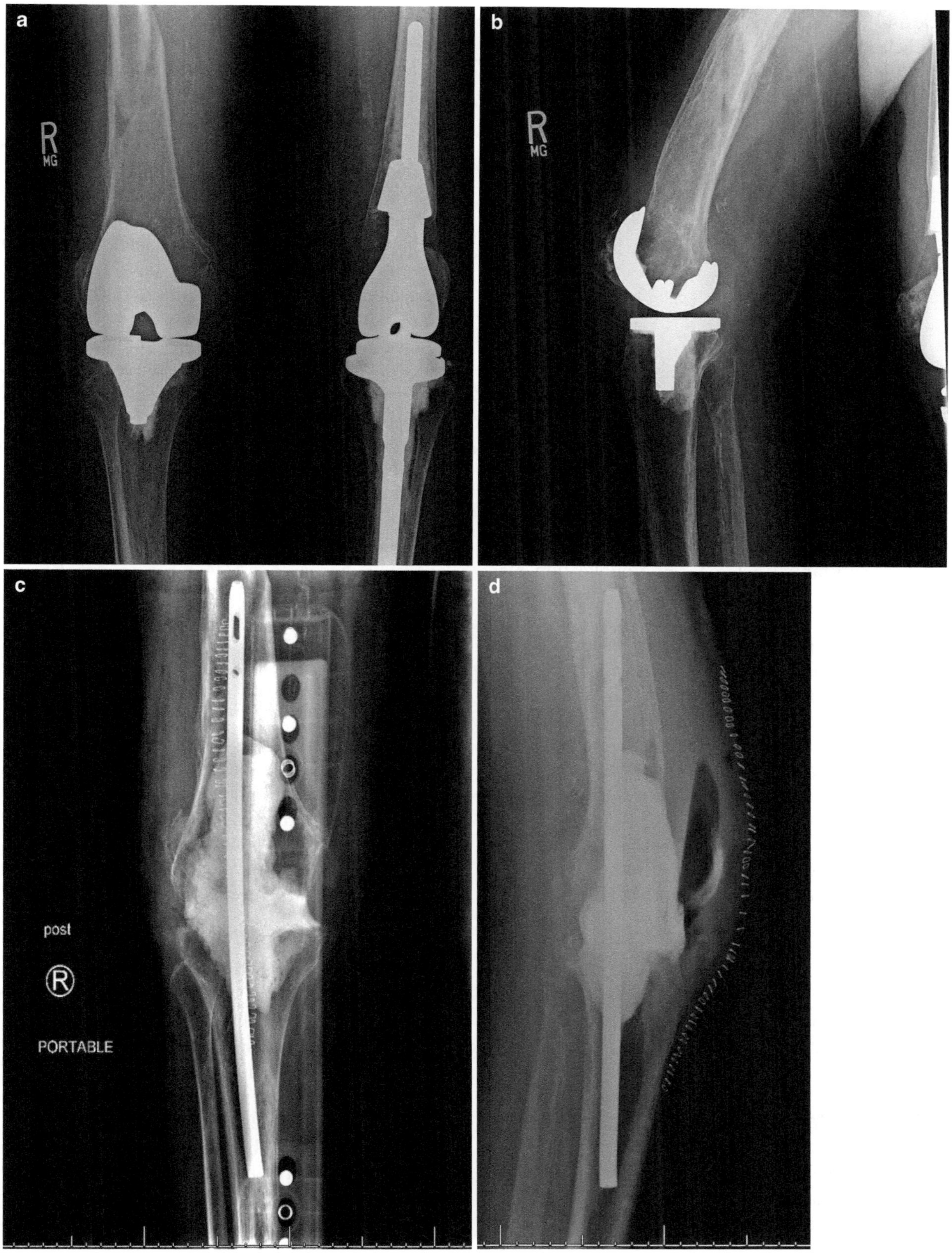

▣ **Fig. 60.2** **a** Preoperative radiographs of chronic right knee infection in an 85-year-old male. **b** Osteolysis under the femoral component—pre-op. **c** Postoperative AP view of static spacer placement due to significant bone loss found intraoperatively. **d** Postoperative lateral view of static spacer placement due to significant bone loss found intraoperatively muscle and collateral ligament scarring and shortening. Nevertheless, cumulative evidence suggests that there are no differences in the reinfection rates between static and articulating spacers.

In a systematic review, static spacers were compared with articulating spacers in 341 patients.

> The authors found that apart from a mean 10° improvement in ROM in favor of the articulating spacer cohort, there were no differences in reinfection rates (mean, 7% vs. 112%), functional outcome scores, and wound- and spacer-related complications (Voleti et al. 2013).

Use of static spacers should be based on multiple factors including assessment of bone and soft tissue defects, extensor mechanism integrity, collateral ligament stability, and surgeon familiarity. Similarly, other authors have reported no difference in the infection control rates, functional outcomes, complications, or reoperation rates with marginal improvements in ROM (mean 100° vs. 92°) in favor of articulating spacers (Pivec et al. 2014). But substantial heterogeneity, publication bias, and difference in treatment protocols exist among the studies evaluated. In a recent prospective randomized trial, involving 68 patients comparing static vs. articulating spacers, the authors found that articulating spacers had shorter lengths of hospital stay (mean 5 vs. 6 days), better ROM (mean arc of motion, 113° vs. 100°) and functional scores (mean Knee Society scores, 79 vs. 70 points), and less extensile exposures (4% vs. 17%) and reoperations (8% vs. 25%) than static spacers (Nahhas et al. 2020).

60

There is early but limited evidence in the literature currently to support the use of articulating spacers in the presence of adequate osseous and soft tissue support for improved ROM, easier exposure and reimplantations during 2nd stage procedures, and potentially better functional outcomes. Static may be used for extensor mechanism deficiencies, extensive bone loss, and lack of collateral ligament support predisposing to instability (Guild 3rd et al. 2014).

60.4.2 Articulating Cement Spacers

A variety of cements on cement articulating spacers have been described that facilitate maintenance of joint space, ROM, and protected weight bearing, to some extent, in the interval phases of two-stage treatment for PJIs (◘ Table 60.2). In theory, these articulating spacers prevent quadriceps shortening and contracture with improvements in ROM and function postoperatively; they preserve joint space and improve exposure during reimplantation by creating a pliable soft tissue envelope. Many authors have reported that 2nd stage reimplantation after previous articulating spacers requires less extensile exposures, such as tibial tubercle osteotomies and V–Y quadricepsplasties (Nahhas et al. 2020; Hsu et al. 2007).

Articulating spacers are either made intraoperatively on the back table by adding ALBC into commercially available silicone molds or are available off the shelf as prefabricated cement molds containing antibiotics, which are then stabilized to the host bone using surface cementation techniques. Prefabricated spacers compared to intraoperatively molded spacers may have better mechanical implant strength due to the more rigorous manufacturing regulatory processes and often can be extracted en bloc during reimplantation without chipping or fracturing requiring piecemeal removal. Furthermore, in one study of 58 patients who underwent two-stage reimplantations at a mean follow-up of 3.5 years, the authors reported that premolded spacers led to high patient satisfaction and improvements in functional scores (Meek et al. 2003).

> However, they usually have lower impregnated doses of antibiotics due to FDA regulations, and many authors prefer adding much higher doses of antibiotics and combinations of antibiotics in the cement used for fixation. Additionally, antibiotics cannot be customized to the infecting organism if the need arises.

For these reasons, the authors prefer manufacturing their own spacers with the appropriate high-dose antibiotic cement regimen. Either type of articulating spacer may need distal and/or posterior cement augmentation on the femur to improve flexion and extension stability. Additionally, both types of spacers can be reinforced with antibiotic PMMA coated Steinman pins serving as dowels for intramedullary antibiotic elution.

Several problems have been reported with the use of articulating spacers. Often these spacers may cause ratcheting or cause uncomfortable crepitus during ROM. Availability of a limited number of sizes of these cement components may additionally affect the soft tissue balance and stability of the knee, causing most patients to use some form of external stabilizing braces during the interval stages. Spacer fractures, dislocations, and posterior joint subluxations are not infrequently reported in most series on articulating spacers with one study on 154 patients reporting 57% incidence of spacer-related problems. These authors reported that spacer tilting in 24% and medial-lateral translations in 21% of patients to be the most common complications of articulating spacers (Struelens et al. 2013). Sagittal but not coronal subluxation spacers have been reported to lower the early and midterm functional outcomes following reimplantation (Lanting et al. 2017).

Table 60.2 Articulating spacer outcomes

Author	Year	Follow-up	Number of knees	Functional spacer type	Outcomes
Vasso et al.	2016	12 years (6–16 years)	46	Articulating cement on cement molds	ROM at follow-up mean, 115° (range 100°–128°) Recurrent infection 8.7% IKS knee and function scores 76 (range 52–94) points and 70 (range 55–90) points
Castelli et al.	2014	7 years (2–13 years)	50	Articulating preformed cement on cement spacer	Recurrent infection 8% ROM mean, 94° (0°–120°) KSS score mean 75 (clinical) and 81 (function)
Van Thiel et al.	2011	3 years (2–4.6 years)	60	Articulating cement on cement molds	Recurrent infection 12% ROM mean (103°) KSS mean 79
Ocguder et al.	2010	1.7 years (1.1–3.2 years)	17	Articulating preformed cement on cement spacer	Recurrent infection 12% ROM mean 95° (10°–120°)
Durbhakula et al.	2004	2.8 years (2.3–4.2 years)	24	Articulating cement on cement molds	HSS score mean 82 points (63–96 points) Recurrent infection 8% ROM 104°(range, 89°–122°)

ROM range of motion

In a gait study on patients with preformed articulating spacers, the authors reported a mean gait velocity reduction of 70% and substantial decrease in the ROM to 59% compared to controls. However, the ground reaction forces were only slightly reduced with minimal frontal and sagittal moments, thereby suggesting that useful postural modifications occur even in the absence of prosthetic components (Logoluso et al. 2012). Lastly, formation of particulate cement debris remains a concern with cement-on-cement articulation.

> In conclusion, articulating spacers may provide improvements in quality of life and independence, although the clinical decision on the type of spacer to be used should be made on an individual basis.

It is recommended that the spacer type is selected based on the type of infecting organism, planned duration of spacer implantation, type of host, ambulatory capacity, extent of host bone and soft tissue loss, stability of the collateral ligaments, and extensor mechanism integrity.

60.4.3 Functional Prosthetic Spacers

Despite improvement in outcomes of eradication of PJI with the use of articulating and nonarticulating cement spacers, complications including wound issues from spacer migration, instability, limb shortening, stiffness, pain, functional loss from prolonged nonweight bearing, poor residual bone quality from disuse osteoporosis, patient dissatisfaction, and unexpected bone loss are not uncommon. In addition, during revision surgery, surgical exposure is frequently difficult due to abundant scar tissue, necessitating extensile approaches such as quadriceps snip, tibial tubercle osteotomy, or V–Y quadricepsplasty for exposure (Windsor et al. 1990; Booth Jr. and Lotke 1989; Rosenberg et al. 1988). This led to the use of "functional articulating spacers" in the 1990s by Hofmann and colleagues providing patients with a "functional joint" for improved rehabilitation in the interim period, maintenance of extensor mechanism length and function, low-friction mobility, and easier revision during 2nd stage reimplantation (Table 60.3) (Hofmann et al. 1995; Hofmann et al. 2005).

In their original description, during the 1st stage procedure, after thorough irrigation and debridement, the femoral component was removed, cleaned, autoclaved, and reinserted with antibiotic cement. A tibial polyethylene insert, with or without an all-polyethylene patellar implant with the pegs removed, was inserted with antibiotic cement (Fig. 60.3). The tibial insert was implanted perpendicular to the mechanical axis of the tibia with 8° posterior slope using a tibial alignment jig. A standard tibial insert was chosen instead of an all-polyethylene tibial implant to provide a large amount of antibiotic cement in contact with the native bone surface. The cement was applied to the components only when it had

Table 60.3 Functional prosthetic spacer outcomes

Author	Year	Follow-up	Number of knees	Functional spacer type	Outcomes
Hofmann et al.	1995	2.6 years (1–5.8 years)	26	Autoclaved femoral w/polyethylene insert	Mean HSS Knee score 88 points; ROM at follow-up 5°–106°
Emerson et al.	2002	7.5 vs. 3.8 years	Static (n = 26) vs. mobile functional spacer (n = 22)	Static (block cement spacer) vs. Mobile (autoclaved femoral w/ polyethylene insert)	ROM at follow-up (mean, 108° vs. 94°; p = 0.01) Block spacer subluxation (n = 1) Recurrent infection (static vs. mobile; 7.6% vs. 9%; p > 0.05) Late recurrent infection with static spacer 23%
Hofmann et al.	2005	6 years (2–12.5 years)	50	Autoclaved femoral w/polyethylene insert	ROM at follow-up (mean, 100°) Improvement HSS knee score (mean, 64–89 points) Recurrent infection 12%
Cuckler et al.	2005	5.4 years (2–10 years)	44	Autoclaved femoral w/autoclaved polyethylene insert	Interval ROM (mean 110°); ROM at follow-up (mean 112°) Improvement Knee Society score (mean, 36–84 points) Recurrent infection 2.2% Delayed reimplantation in 9% due to patient comfort
Huang et al.	2006	4.3 years (2–9 years)	21	Autoclaved femoral w/autoclaved polyethylene insert	ROM mean, 98° Mean KSS 81 points Recurrent infection 5%
Trezies et al.	2006	6.7 years (0.1–12 years)	11	New femoral and new all-polyethylene tibial component	Recurrent infection 9%
Jamsen et al.	2006	2.1 years (0.2–5.7 years)	24	Autoclaved femoral w/all-polyethylene tibial insert new or sterilized	ROM mean 104° (range, 80°–120°) KSS score 82 (range, 56–99)
Anderson et al.	2009	4.5 years (2–9 years)	25	Autoclaved femoral w/all-polyethylene tibial insert	ROM at follow-up (mean, 2°–115°) Improvement HSS knee score (mean, 60–91 points) Recurrent infection 4%
Pietsch et al.	2009	4 years (2.6–5.6 years)	33	Autoclaved femoral w/autoclaved polyethylene insert	ROM at follow-up (mean, 0°–100°) Improvement HSS knee score (mean, 67–85 points) Reinfection 9%
Choi et al.	2012	4.8 years (1.2–9.8 years)	Static (n = 33) vs. mobile functional spacer (n = 14)	Static (block cement spacer) vs. Mobile (new [n = 6] or autoclaved [n = 8] femoral w/new [n = 7] or autoclaved polyethylene insert [n = 3] or block tibia cement [n = 4])	ROM at follow-up (static vs. mobile; 97° vs. 100°) Extensile approaches in 2nd stage (static vs. mobile; 29% vs. 76%) Recurrent infection (static vs. mobile; 67% vs. 71%; p > 0.05) 29% patients in the mobile spacer group did not undergo reimplantation due to patient comfort

Table 60.3 (continued)

Author	Year	Follow-up	Number of knees	Functional spacer type	Outcomes
Kalore et al.	2012	1 year (1–8.8 years)	53	Mobile (autoclaved; $n = 15$ vs. New femoral ($n = 16$) vs. Silicon-molded components ($n = 22$)	ROM (mean, flexion; autoclaved vs. new femoral vs. silicon-molded; 96° vs. 98° vs. 93°) Recurrent infection (autoclaved vs. new femoral vs. silicon-molded; 13% vs. 6% vs. 9%) Least cost with autoclaved femoral components
Kim et al.	2013	2 years	20	Autoclaved femoral w/all-polyethylene tibial cement spacer	Interval ROM (mean, 98° range 70°–115°) ROM at follow-up (mean, 103°; range 80°–130°) Reinfection 10%
Classen et al.	2014	4 years (1.6–8.6 years)	23	Autoclaved femoral w/block tibial cement spacer	Interval ROM (mean, 68° ± 28°) ROM at follow-up (mean, 105° ± 11°) Recurrent infection 13%
Juul et al.	2016	3.1 years (2–4.4 years)	22	New femoral component and all-polyethylene tibia	One AKA for persistent infection
Lyons et al.	2019	1.8 years (0.2–8.4 years)	55	New femoral component and all-polyethylene tibia	Postoperatively, KSS mean, 82 points (37–103 points) Recurrent infection rates 9.1%

ROM range of motion, *AKA* above-knee amputation

cured to a doughy state to avoid bone interdigitation and easy removal during reimplantation.

> In addition to the functional advantages, the prosthetic functional spacers can potentially prevent the need for a 2nd stage reimplantation, which is not a viable option for cement-on-cement molded articulating or static spacers.

Initial adoption of this technique was marked with skepticism due to concerns about reusing an implant designated for single-use and placing metal and polyethylene implants in an infected milieu, which may impede eradication of infection due to apprehensions about bacteria harboring on foreign devices. Recent evidence suggests that autoclaved Co-Cr femoral implants using standard gravity displacement cycle significantly reduce biofilm burden and can be considered sterile from commonly found bacterial species (Lyons et al. 2016).

> Furthermore, many hospitals do not allow for autoclave sterilization of previously infected implants.

> As a result, prosthetic spacers with new femoral, all-polyethylene tibial, and patellar components, instead of reusing a sterilized component, are becoming increasingly popular in two-stage treatment for PJI.

Multiple authors have reported equivalent reinfection rates with the benefits of preserved function and potentially improved patient comfort in the interim period, albeit at a higher cost compared to using autoclaved implants (Kalore et al. 2012). Cuckler and colleagues found that 9% (4 out of 44) patients in their series deferred their 2nd stage reimplantation for over a year as they were comfortable with their functional spacers (Cuckler 2005). Similarly, Choi et al. found that 4 out of 14 patients (28%) who had a functional spacer did not undergo any further procedures at a mean follow-up of 2 years as they were performing well with no recurrence of infection (Choi et al. 2012).

In a recent study by Goltz and others involving 59 patients who had undergone two-stage revision TKA with autoclaved femoral components and all-polyethylene tibia, the authors found that 15% (9

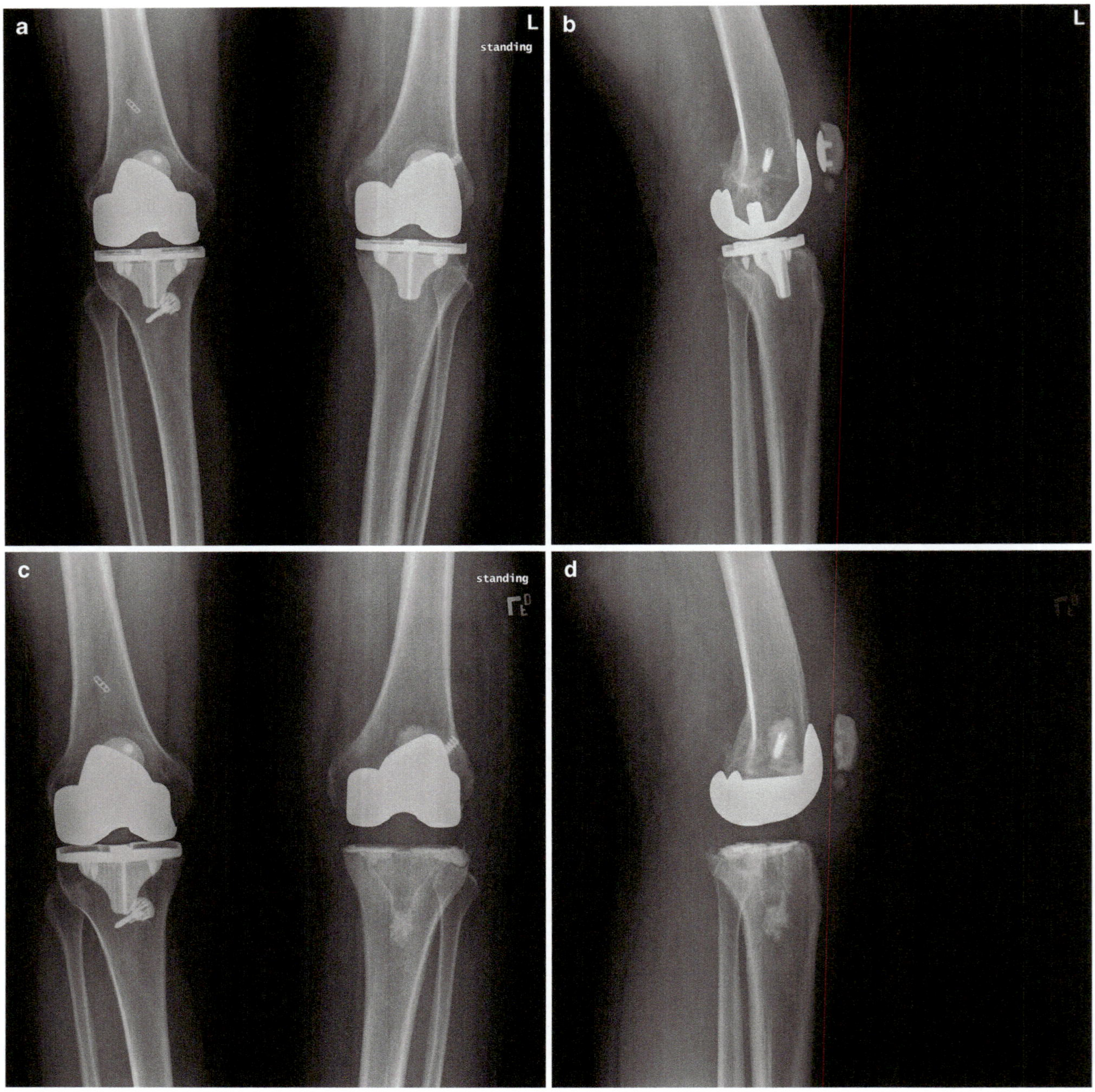

◘ **Fig. 60.3** **a** AP view showing tibial osteolysis pre-op. **b** Lateral view with tibial osteolysis with chronic infection. **c** Post-op after functional spacer placement. **d** Lateral view post-op after functional spacer

patients) had a recurrence with the same organism while 22% (13 patients) had reinfection with a different organism (Goltz et al. 2018). Diabetes was found to be significantly higher in patients who had a reinfection (55% vs. 19%; $p < 0.005$), suggesting that host factors play a substantial role in patients with PJIs. Nozdo and colleagues compared the outcomes of prefabricated spacers, spacer molds, and autoclaved femoral components in a study of 140 patients who had undergone two-stage revision TKA for PJIs. The authors reported no difference in the infection rates (Prefab cohort 89.7% vs. Mold cohort, 95.3%, vs. Autoclaved cohort, 87.2%), although the authors found that the on-table spacer molds had the lowest costs (mean, $1341) compared to the autoclaved (mean $3764) and prefabricated spacer cohorts (mean, $5439) (Nodzo et al. 2017).

A number of commercially prefabricated articulating "functional" spacers, initially developed for the hip and later for the knee, have been manufactured for ease of operating room workflow and avoid the need for autoclaving components (Haddad et al. 2000). These spacers are made predominantly of antibiotic-loaded

Table 60.4 Prefabricated metal-on-polyethylene spacers

Author	Year	Follow-up	Number of knees	Functional spacer type	Outcomes
Haddad et al.	2000	4 years (1.7–12.4 years)	45	PROSTALAC	Recurrence 9%
Gooding et al.	2011	9 years (5–12 years)	115	PROSTALAC	ROM (pre- vs. postoperative; mean, 86°–93°; $p = 0.11$) Spacer fracture 2.6% Dislocation 1.7% Recurrence 12%

ROM range of motion

cement with a small area of bicondylar metal shell on the femoral component and a corresponding area of ultrahigh molecular weight polyethylene on the tibial PMMA implant forming a low friction-bearing surface (Table 60.4). The femoral metal polycentric condyles are connected with a bar to form the cam that articulates with the spine of the tibial component forming a replica of a TKA implant. However, these preassembled implants are costly, require time for intraoperative fabrication, are less readily available, and often have a limited number of choices of sizes, precluding their universal use.

> As elaborated above, the advantages of antibiotic-loaded cement spacers, whether static or articulating, outweigh certain problems associated with their use.

These include antibiotic toxicity, cement fracture, dislocation, and persistence of foreign material in the presence of infection, femoral and tibial fractures, and bone loss either from instability or during spacer removal at the time of reimplantation. Many of these complications are related to young age and the presence of chronic infection (Yang et al. 2019). Nonetheless, patients who have these spacer complications have lower functional scores compared to those without complications.

60.5 Fate of Spacers and Options for Failed Spacers

The clinical course of patients who undergo the first of the two stages of treatment for PJI is variable. A substantial proportion of patients do not undergo reimplantation for a multitude of reasons.

> Nearly 20% of patients encounter reinfection with the same organism or recurrence of infection with a different organism (Gomez et al. 2015).

Additionally, many patients undergo multiple debridements due to wound-related issues, spacer exchanges, and plastic surgical procedures. Patients who do not have the 2nd stage reimplantation either undergo arthrodesis, resection arthroplasty, and amputation or live with the implanted spacer. Results of debridement with retention of components for failed two-stage procedure carries a high failure rate of more than 50%, and a further intended two-stage procedure was possible in about 60% reported in one study (Kheir et al. 2017). Many of these patients have multiple comorbidities, and some of them have readmissions with systemic sepsis.

> Sadly, death accounts for a substantial proportion of these patients who never undergo reimplantation with one study reporting 7% death (36 out of 504 patients) among patients in the interstage period (Gomez et al. 2015).

> In a study of 504 hip and knee PJIs planned for a two-stage procedure, the authors reported that reimplantation occurred in 82.7% of the patients (417 out of 504 cases) (Gomez et al. 2015).

A total of 83% (Gomez et al. 2015) of patients who did not have the 2nd stage procedure had a retained spacer, 7% needed an amputation, while 5% underwent an arthrodesis at minimum 1-year follow-up. Similar outcomes were reported in another large Medicare database study, with only 62% of patients undergoing the 2nd stage reimplantation. The authors reported that the risk of death increases in the presence of increasing age (OR

>3 for age >85 years), diabetes, congestive heart failure, chronic liver disease (OR 1.2), chronic lung disease (OR 1.2), alcohol abuse (OR 1.4), and hemodialysis (OR 3.4) (Cancienne et al. 2017).

Options for failed two-stage procedure for reinfection include a repeat two-stage exchange, amputation, or arthrodesis. Knee arthrodesis as a one-stage or delayed two-stage procedure is a reasonable option for failed two-stage reimplantation with recurrence of infection. Frequently, these patients have large bony deficiencies and unreconstructible extensor mechanism disruptions. Despite many authors reporting successful outcomes with union rates varying between 75% and 100% after knee arthrodesis for failed spacers, a substantial amount of limb length discrepancy (LLD) results from the repeat debridements, excision of infected and necrotic bone, and need to achieve bony contact for successful arthrodesis (Makhdom et al. 2019). In a study of 22 patients who had undergone knee arthrodesis for persistent infection after TKA, union was achieved with eradication of infection in 87% of patients, although the mean LLD was 4.9 cm in this series (Robinson et al. 2018). Several authors have reported similar results, with most reporting better union rates with intramedullary nails than external fixation.

In the past few years, intercalary fusion nails have been introduced as a potential viable option to preserve leg length by not relying on bone-to-bone fusion in patients with recurrent infections and salvage situations. Sacrponi et al., in a series of 38 patients at a mean follow-up of 5 years, found no recurrence of infection in 89% (34 patients) of patients, with only 53% reporting mild to moderate handicap (Scarponi et al. 2014).

60

> The decision-making for failed two-stage exchange is challenging as high complication rates up to 35% have been reported with both knee arthrodesis and above-knee amputations (AKAs).

Although the functional outcomes are similar in both of these groups as reported in one study, patients who were fitted with a modern-generation microprocessor-controlled prosthesis demonstrated better functional outcome scores than knee arthrodesis (Hungerer et al. 2017).

Conclusion

Antibiotic-loaded spacers with high-dose antibiotics remain an integral part of two-stage treatment for prosthetic joint infections. PMMA with its mechanical and elution characteristics is currently the most commonly employed method for delivering high concentration of antibiotics locally. There is no consensus on the superiority of static endoskeleton-type spacers compared to articulating spacers regarding wound complications, functional outcomes, and reinfection rates, although some studies report a small improvement in the ultimate ROM and potentially easier reimplantation with articulating spacers. Nevertheless, the treatment needs to be individualized based on a variety of host factors, microbial characteristics, ambulatory and functional capacity, and surgeon expertise. There has been an increasing interest and popularity in the use of prosthetic components as functional spacers to provide a low-friction-articulating surface and the functional benefits of these devices, especially in situations where a 2nd stage procedure may not be possible. Despite the best efforts, a substantial proportion of patients have reinfection or have recurrence from a different organism than the initial infecting organisms and need further procedures, including resection, arthrodesis, or amputation.

Take-Home Messages

- Use of vancomycin with tobramycin in bone cement can improve their individual elution characteristics from increased PMMA porosity—a phenomenon defined as "passive opportunism."
- Articulating spacers may provide improved ROM and potentially easier reimplantation with less need for extensile exposures compared to static spacers.
- Static spacers are typically used in conditions associated with poor soft tissue envelope, substantial bone loss, extensor mechanism disruptions, and intraoperative instability with deficient collateral ligaments.
- Implantation of new femoral components and polyethylene inserts with antibiotic-loaded PMMA cement is becoming increasingly popular as a functionally viable alternative to prefabricated or custom-molded spacers.
- Close monitoring of patients for early detection of mechanical and systemic complications of antibiotic-loaded cement spacers is critical during follow-up.

References

Aeng ES, Shalansky KF, Lau TT et al (2015) Acute kidney injury with tobramycin-impregnated bone cement spacers in prosthetic joint infections. Ann Pharmacother 49(11):1207–1213

Amin TJ, Lamping JW, Hendricks KJ, McIff TE (2012) Increasing the elution of vancomycin from high-dose antibiotic-loaded bone cement: a novel preparation technique. J Bone Joint Surg Am 94(21):1946–1951

Berliner ZP, Mo AZ, Porter DA et al (2018) In-hospital acute kidney injury after TKA revision with placement of an antibiotic cement spacer. J Arthroplast 33(7S):S209–S212

Booth RE Jr, Lotke PA (1989) The results of spacer block technique in revision of infected total knee arthroplasty. Clin Orthop Relat Res 248:57–60

Brock HS, Moodie PG, Hendricks KJ, McIff TE (2010) Compression strength and porosity of single-antibiotic cement vacuum-mixed with vancomycin. J Arthroplast 25(6):990–997

Cancienne JM, Werner BC, Bolarinwa SA, Browne JA (2017) Removal of an infected total hip arthroplasty: risk factors for repeat debridement, long-term spacer retention, and mortality. J Arthroplast 32(8):2519–2522

Carli AV, Sethuraman AS, Bhimani SJ, Ross FP, Bostrom MPG (2018) Selected heat-sensitive antibiotics are not inactivated during polymethylmethacrylate curing and can be used in cement spacers for periprosthetic joint infection. J Arthroplast 33(6):1930–1935

Choi HR, Malchau H, Bedair H (2012) Are prosthetic spacers safe to use in 2-stage treatment for infected total knee arthroplasty? J Arthroplast 27(8):1474–1479 e1471

Cuckler JM (2005) The infected total knee: management options. J Arthroplast 20(4 Suppl 2):33–36

Cui Q, Mihalko WM, Shields JS, Ries M, Saleh KJ (2007) Antibiotic-impregnated cement spacers for the treatment of infection associated with total hip or knee arthroplasty. J Bone Joint Surg Am 89(4):871–882

Fehring TK, Odum S, Calton TF, Mason JB (2000) Articulating versus static spacers in revision total knee arthroplasty for sepsis. The Ranawat Award. Clin Orthop Relat Res 380:9–16

Garvin KL, Hanssen AD (1995) Infection after total hip arthroplasty. Past, present, and future. J Bone Joint Surg Am 77(10):1576–1588

Goltz DE, Sutter EG, Bolognesi MP, Wellman SS (2018) Outcomes of articulating spacers with autoclaved femoral components in total knee arthroplasty infection. J Arthroplast 33(8):2595–2604

Gomez MM, Tan TL, Manrique J, Deirmengian GK, Parvizi J (2015) The fate of spacers in the treatment of periprosthetic joint infection. J Bone Joint Surg Am 97(18):1495–1502

Greene N, Holtom PD, Warren CA et al (1998) In vitro elution of tobramycin and vancomycin polymethylmethacrylate beads and spacers from Simplex and Palacos. Am J Orthop (Belle Mead NJ) 27(3):201–205

Guild GN 3rd, Wu B, Scuderi GR (2014) Articulating vs. static antibiotic impregnated spacers in revision total knee arthroplasty for sepsis. A systematic review. J Arthroplast 29(3):558–563

Haddad FS, Masri BA, Campbell D, McGraw RW, Beauchamp CP, Duncan CP (2000) The PROSTALAC functional spacer in two-stage revision for infected knee replacements. Prosthesis of antibiotic-loaded acrylic cement. J Bone Joint Surg Br 82(6):807–812

Hanssen AD (2004) Prophylactic use of antibiotic bone cement: an emerging standard--in opposition. J Arthroplast 19(4 Suppl 1):73–77

Hofmann AA, Kane KR, Tkach TK, Plaster RL, Camargo MP (1995) Treatment of infected total knee arthroplasty using an articulating spacer. Clin Orthop Relat Res 321:45–54

Hofmann AA, Goldberg T, Tanner AM, Kurtin SM (2005) Treatment of infected total knee arthroplasty using an articulating spacer: 2- to 12-year experience. Clin Orthop Relat Res 430:125–131

Hsieh PH, Tai CL, Lee PC, Chang YH (2009) Liquid gentamicin and vancomycin in bone cement: a potentially more cost-effective regimen. J Arthroplast 24(1):125–130

Hsu YC, Cheng HC, Ng TP, Chiu KY (2007) Antibiotic-loaded cement articulating spacer for 2-stage reimplantation in infected total knee arthroplasty: a simple and economic method. J Arthroplast 22(7):1060–1066

Hungerer S, Kiechle M, von Ruden C, Militz M, Beitzel K, Morgenstern M (2017) Knee arthrodesis versus above-the-knee amputation after septic failure of revision total knee arthroplasty: comparison of functional outcome and complication rates. BMC Musculoskelet Disord 18(1):443

Kalil GZ, Ernst EJ, Johnson SJ et al (2012) Systemic exposure to aminoglycosides following knee and hip arthroplasty with aminoglycoside-loaded bone cement implants. Ann Pharmacother 46(7–8):929–934

Kalore NV, Maheshwari A, Sharma A, Cheng E, Gioe TJ (2012) Is there a preferred articulating spacer technique for infected knee arthroplasty? A preliminary study. Clin Orthop Relat Res 470(1):228–235

Kheir MM, Tan TL, Gomez MM, Chen AF, Parvizi J (2017) Patients with failed prior two-stage exchange have poor outcomes after further surgical intervention. J Arthroplast 32(4):1262–1265

Klinder A, Zaatreh S, Ellenrieder M et al (2019) Antibiotics release from cement spacers used for two-stage treatment of implant-associated infections after total joint arthroplasty. J Biomed Mater Res B Appl Biomater 107(5):1587–1597

Lanting BA, Lau A, Teeter MG, Howard JL (2017) Outcome following subluxation of mobile articulating spacers in two-stage revision total knee arthroplasty. Arch Orthop Trauma Surg 137(3):375–380

Logoluso N, Champlon C, Melegati G, Dell'Oro F, Romano CL (2012) Gait analysis in patients with a preformed articulated knee spacer. Knee 19(4):370–372

Lyons ST, Wright CA, Krute CN, Rivera FE, Carroll RK, Shaw LN (2016) Confirming sterility of an autoclaved infected femoral component for use in an articulated antibiotic knee spacer: a pilot study. J Arthroplast 31(1):245–249

Makhdom AM, Fragomen A, Rozbruch SR (2019) Knee arthrodesis after failed total knee arthroplasty. J Bone Joint Surg Am 101(7):650–660

Marks KE, Nelson CL, Lautenschlager EP (1976) Antibiotic-impregnated acrylic bone cement. J Bone Joint Surg Am 58(3):358–364

Masri BA, Duncan CP, Beauchamp CP (1998) Long-term elution of antibiotics from bone-cement: an in vivo study using the prosthesis of antibiotic-loaded acrylic cement (PROSTALAC) system. J Arthroplast 13(3):331–338

Meek RM, Masri BA, Dunlop D et al (2003) Patient satisfaction and functional status after treatment of infection at the site of a total knee arthroplasty with use of the PROSTALAC articulating spacer. J Bone Joint Surg Am 85(10):1888–1892

Meeker DG, Cooper KB, Renard RL, Mears SC, Smeltzer MS, Barnes CL (2019) Comparative study of antibiotic elution profiles from alternative formulations of polymethylmethacrylate bone cement. J Arthroplast 34(7):1458–1461

Menge TJ, Koethe JR, Jenkins CA et al (2012) Acute kidney injury after placement of an antibiotic-impregnated cement spacer during revision total knee arthroplasty. J Arthroplasty 27(6):1221–1227 e1221–1222

Nahhas CR, Chalmers PN, Parvizi J et al (2020) A randomized trial of static and articulating spacers for the treatment of infection following total knee arthroplasty. J Bone Joint Surg Am 102(9):778–787

Nickinson RS, Board TN, Gambhir AK, Porter ML, Kay PR (2012) Two stage revision knee arthroplasty for infection with massive bone loss. A technique to achieve spacer stability. Knee 19(1):24–27

Nishimura S, Tsurumoto T, Yonekura A, Adachi K, Shindo H (2006) Antimicrobial susceptibility of Staphylococcus aureus and Staphylococcus epidermidis biofilms isolated from infected total hip arthroplasty cases. J Orthop Sci 11(1):46–50

Nodzo SR, Boyle KK, Spiro S, Nocon AA, Miller AO, Westrich GH (2017) Success rates, characteristics, and costs of articulating antibiotic spacers for total knee periprosthetic joint infection. Knee 24(5):1175–1181

Patel RA, Baker HP, Smith SB (2018) Acute renal failure due to a tobramycin and vancomycin spacer in revision two-staged knee arthroplasty. Case Rep Nephrol 2018:6579894

Pivec R, Naziri Q, Issa K, Banerjee S, Mont MA (2014) Systematic review comparing static and articulating spacers used for revision of infected total knee arthroplasty. J Arthroplast 29(3):553–557 e551

Robinson M, Piponov HI, Ormseth A, Helder CW, Schwartz B, Gonzalez MH (2018) Knee arthrodesis outcomes after infected total knee arthroplasty and failure of two-stage revision with an antibiotic cement spacer. J Am Acad Orthop Surg Glob Res Rev 2(1):e077

Rosenberg AG, Haas B, Barden R, Marquez D, Landon GC, Galante JO (1988) Salvage of infected total knee arthroplasty. Clin Orthop Relat Res 226:29–33

Scarponi S, Drago L, Romano D et al (2014) Cementless modular intramedullary nail without bone-on-bone fusion as a salvage procedure in chronically infected total knee prosthesis: long-term results. Int Orthop 38(2):413–418

Schurman DJ, Trindade C, Hirshman HP, Moser K, Kajiyama G, Stevens P (1978) Antibiotic-acrylic bone cement composites. Studies of gentamicin and Palacos. J Bone Joint Surg Am 60(7):978–984

Soto-Hall R, Saenz L, Tavernetti R, Cabaud HE, Cochran TP (1983) Tobramycin in bone cement. An in-depth analysis of wound, serum, and urine concentrations in patients undergoing total hip revision arthroplasty. Clin Orthop Relat Res 175:60–64

Struelens B, Claes S, Bellemans J (2013) Spacer-related problems in two-stage revision knee arthroplasty. Acta Orthop Belg 79(4):422–426

Sundblad J, Nixon M, Jackson N, Vaidya R, Markel D (2018) Altering polymerization temperature of antibiotic-laden cement can increase porosity and subsequent antibiotic elution. Int Orthop 42(11):2627–2632

van Raaij TM, Visser LE, Vulto AG, Verhaar JA (2002) Acute renal failure after local gentamicin treatment in an infected total knee arthroplasty. J Arthroplast 17(7):948–950

Voleti PB, Baldwin KD, Lee GC (2013) Use of static or articulating spacers for infection following total knee arthroplasty: a systematic literature review. J Bone Joint Surg Am 95(17):1594–1599

Windsor RE, Insall JN, Urs WK, Miller DV, Brause BD (1990) Two-stage reimplantation for the salvage of total knee arthroplasty complicated by infection. Further follow-up and refinement of indications. J Bone Joint Surg Am 72(2):272–278

Xu C, Jia CQ, Kuo FC, Chai W, Zhang MH, Chen JY (2019) Does the use of a closed-suction drain reduce the effectiveness of an antibiotic-loaded spacer in two-stage exchange arthroplasty for periprosthetic hip infection? A prospective, randomized, controlled study. BMC Musculoskelet Disord 20(1):583

Yang FS, Lu YD, Wu CT, Blevins K, Lee MS, Kuo FC (2019) Mechanical failure of articulating polymethylmethacrylate (PMMA) spacers in two-stage revision hip arthroplasty: the risk factors and the impact on interim function. BMC Musculoskelet Disord 20(1):372

Zhan C, Kaczmarek R, Loyo-Berrios N, Sangl J, Bright RA (2007) Incidence and short-term outcomes of primary and revision hip replacement in the United States. J Bone Joint Surg Am 89(3):526–533

Does Antibiotic-Loaded Bone Cement Trigger Widespread Antibiotic Resistance Affecting Prosthetic Joint Infection Treatment?

Christof Berberich

Contents

E. Hansen, K.-D. Kühn (eds.), *Essentials of Cemented Knee Arthroplasty*,
https://doi.org/10.1007/978-3-662-63113-3_61

61.1 Introduction

Since the description of the strong depot effect of local antibiotics mixed with Palacos resin by Buchholz and Engelbrecht in 1970, antibiotic-loaded bone cement (ALBC) has been widely used in the prevention and treatment of orthopedic infections (Buchholz and Engelbrecht 1970). The selection of the antibiotics added to bone cement powder either during the commercial production of ALBC or during manual admixture in the operating theatre should be based on the expected bacterial spectrum present in surgical-site contaminations (empiric use in prophylaxis) or on the prior identification of the pathogen following culture of aspiration fluid or tissue biopsies in septic cases (targeted use, e.g., in bone cement spacers). The advantage of this in situ delivery method of antibiotics directly to where the implant is most vulnerable to infections is the high initial peak concentration followed by a gradual antibiotic release over time. Several in vitro and in vivo studies have demonstrated that far higher concentrations are achieved by this local application mode than with systemic antibiotic administration without causing notable systemic side effects (Wahlig et al. 1978, 1984; Wahlig and Dingeldein 1980).

Because of its wide antimicrobial spectrum and the strict concentration-dependent bactericidal effects, gentamicin is a preferred antimicrobial drug in bone cements. Combinations of gentamicin with an additional antibiotic partner, such as clindamycin, vancomycin, or others, have been proven to be even more potent against biofilm formation due to synergistic release effects, broader antimicrobial efficacy, and simultaneous inhibitory effects on different targets in the bacterial cells (Kühn 2014; Della Valle et al. 2001; Ensing et al. 2009; Mohamed et al. 2020).

61

Several registry- or clinical study-based publications have reported a protective effect of ALBC against prosthetic joint infections (PJIs) in cemented primary or revision arthroplasty (Engesaeter et al. 2003; Jämsen et al. 2009; Parvizi et al. 2008; Jameson et al. 2019). However, in times of increasing awareness of antibiotic stewardship programs, concerns are growing whether the widespread empiric use of ALBC in arthroplasty may trigger antibiotic resistance and counterbalance the benefit of a possibly lower PJI risk (Fig. 61.1).

61.2 Differences in Classification of "Susceptible" or "Resistant" Bacteria After Systemic or Local Administration of Antibiotics

> Predictions of antibiotic success or failure are clinically based on the antibiogram that determines whether the bacteria are susceptible or resistant to the antibiotics tested in different concentrations in vitro.

For systemic antibiotic therapy, information on the typical tissue concentrations achieved with standard antibiotic doses is integrated with the minimal inhibitory concentrations (MICs) of a pathogen in order to determine the MIC breakpoints (MICBPs). Both values determine whether the pathogen can be considered sus-

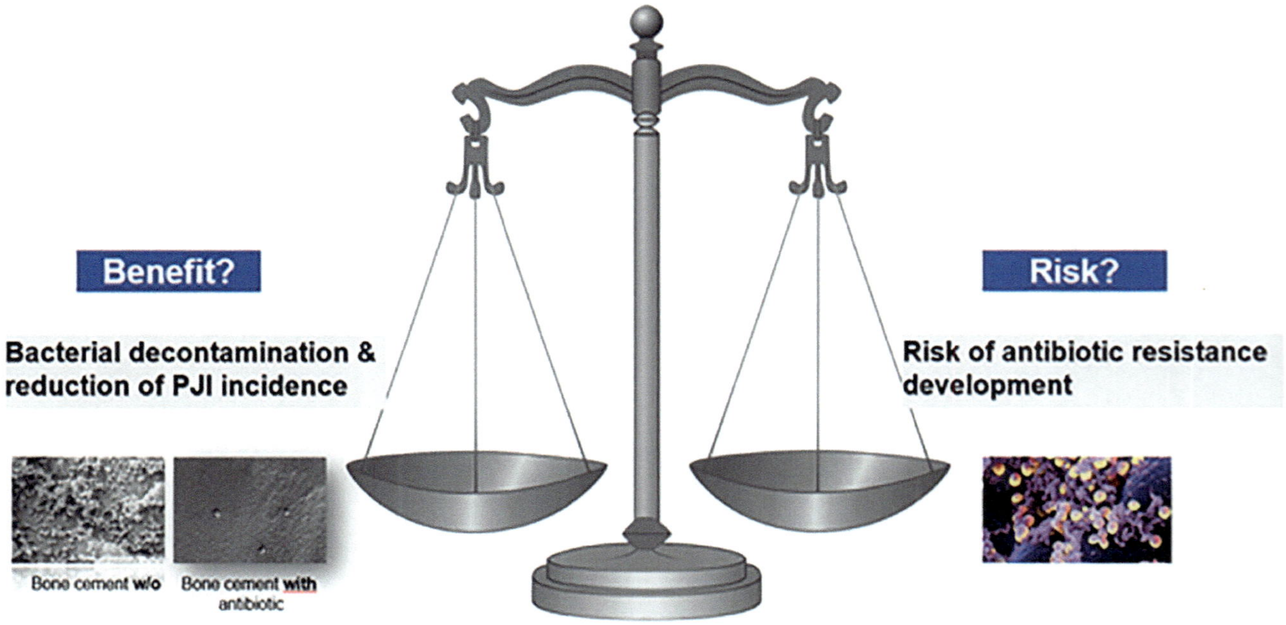

Fig. 61.1 Benefit vs. risk consideration of ALBC use

ceptible, intermediate, or resistant to the chosen antibiotic therapy in a patient. They also provide a minimal dosage recommendation in order to prevent exposure to sub-therapeutic antibiotic concentrations.

While the pharmacokinetic parameters and the therapeutic framework are relatively well established for systemic antibiotics, no such equivalent guidance is available for antibiotics administered locally into the surgical wound bed or used to coat cement or implants. The antibiotic concentrations achieved locally are often much higher than those that typically result from systemic administration (see schematic illustration in ◘ Fig. 61.2).

Thus, in this situation, standard susceptibility reporting criteria and MICBP often do not apply. The pharmacokinetics (change of drug concentrations over time) of the local antibiotic delivery mode is also very different from the systemic antibiotic application with a high initial peak concentration, which may exceed that achieved via the systemic route by a factor of 100 and more, followed by gradually decreasing elution from bone cement over time (Hendriks et al. 2003; Neut et al. 2010).

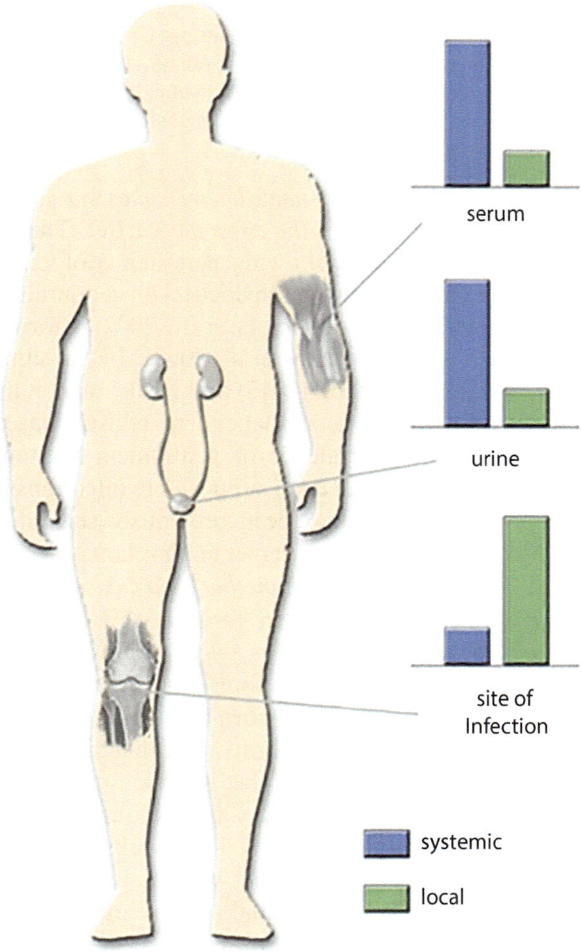

◘ **Fig. 61.2** Comparison of antibiotic concentrations in serum, urine, and site of infection after systemic treatment with 1 × 80 g of gentamicin given i.m. i.m. and local treatment with 1.25% gentamicin mixed into Palacos® R bone cement

> This means in clinical practice that some of the bacterial strains that are classified as intermediate or resistant in "normal" antibiograms may still be susceptible at the locally high concentrations after peak elution from bone cement.

This is particularly true for those antibiotics that show a bactericidal and strict concentration-dependent action, such as the aminoglycosides.

As an experimental proof of concept, Hendriks et al. (2005) demonstrated the following in their interfacial gap model simulating the physiological conditions at the cement–prosthesis interface:

- All susceptible coagulase-positive and -negative *Staphylococcus* strains (MIC = 0.25–4 mg/L) were killed in the presence of the eluted gentamicin.
- The intermediate resistant strains of *Pseudomonas* (strain 5148; MIC = 2 mg/L) and *S. epidermidis* (strain 5234; MIC = 24 mg/L) did also not survive.
- Only the high-level gentamicin-resistant *S. epidermidis* strain 5115 (MIC values ≥256 mg/L) withstood the antibiotic action (◘ Fig. 61.3).

61.3 Only Bacterial Strains with a Priorly Acquired High-Level Antibiotic Resistance May Survive and Get Selected in the Presence of ALBC

The above-mentioned observations confirm the efficacy of ALBC to form an antimicrobial colonization barrier around the prothesis against all susceptible and intermediate resistant bacterial intruders. However, bacteria that have previously acquired a high-level antibiotic-resistant genotype by random mutational changes are able to survive. At the end, such mutants will replace the former mixed bacterial population, and only resistant bacteria will dominate.

When discussing the reasons for antibiotic resistance development, it is important to differentiate between induction and selection of resistance (Araos et al. 2015). The first requires the existence of antimicrobial resistance determinants in the bacterial cell, the expression of which is modulated by the presence or absence of the antibiotic drug (e.g., regulation of β-lactamase expression in *S. aureus*). The latter simply confers a preexisting, antibiotic-resistant genotype a survival advantage against other competitors under the selection pressure of the antibiotic. At the end, all surviving bacteria would then be of the high-level gentamicin-resistant form (◘ Fig. 61.3).

Bacterial strain	MIC (mg/l)	Inoculum	CMW™ 1 ⊕	CMW™ 1 •	Palacos® ⊕	Palacos® •	Palamed® ⊕	Palamed® •
CNS 7334	0.25	4.8	•	6.7	-	5.3	-	6.3
Staph. aureus 7323	1.0	5.7	-	7.0	-	6.7	-	6.8
Pseudomonas aeruginosa 5148	2.0	6.3	-	6.8	-	7.3	-	7.3
CNS 7353	3.0 to 4.0 (32)†	5.7	-	5.2	-	6.3	-	5.5
CNS 5234	24.0	6.7		6.5		6.3		6.2

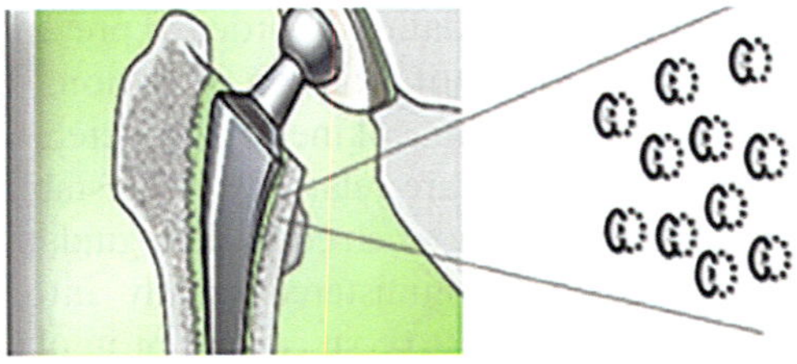

Bacterial strain	MIC (mg/l)	Inoculum	CMW™ 1 ⊕	CMW™ 1 •	Palacos® ⊕	Palacos® •	Palamed® ⊕	Palamed® •
CNS 7334	0.25	4.8	•	6.7	-	5.3	-	6.3
Staph. aureus 7323	1.0	5.7	-	7.0	-	6.7	-	6.8
Pseudomonas aeruginosa 5148	2.0	6.3	-	6.8	-	7.3	-	7.3
CNS 7353	3.0 to 4.0 (32)†	5.7	-	5.2	-	6.3	-	5.5
CNS 5234	24.0	6.7		6.5		6.3		6.2
CNS 5115	>256.0	5.9	6.0‡	7.0‡	6.1‡	6.8‡	5.4	6.9

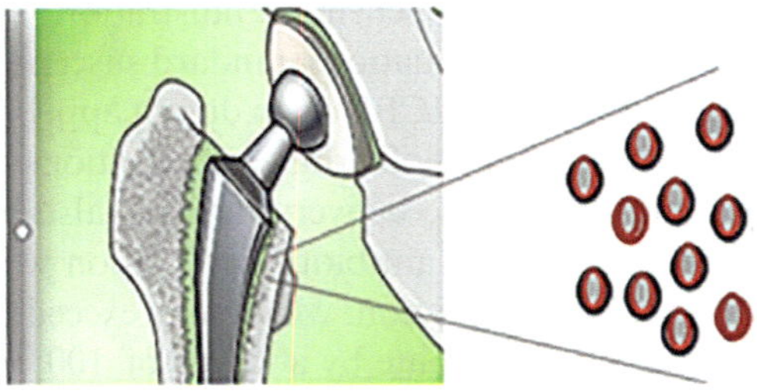

Fig. 61.3 **a** Five clinically isolated bacterial strains: three gentamicin-susceptible *Staphylococcus* strains (CNS 7334, *S. aureus* 7323, and CNS 7353) and two gentamicin intermediate resistant strains (*Pseudomonas aeruginosa* 5148 and CNS 5234) are killed in gaps in the presence of gentamicin (+) eluted from the tested bone cements CMW™ 1, Palacos®, and Palamed®. All bacterial strains in the row (−) were all able to grow on the same bone cements without antibiotic loading (numbers given as ^{10}log CFU/cm^2). **b** The clinically isolated bacterial CNS strain 5115 survives in the gap even in the presence of gentamicin (+) eluted from the tested bone cements CMW™ 1, Palacos®, and Palamed®. The same bacterial strain in the row (−) grew at even higher CFU numbers (numbers given as ^{10}log CFU/cm^2) on cement without antibiotic loading. MIC minimal inhibitory concentration, CFU colony-forming unit

> From a clinical point of view, it is important to point out that the antibiotic-mediated selection of previously resistant bacteria is typically not broad and only directed against one particular antibiotic class.

61.4 Clinical Implications if Using (Single or Dual) ALBC

Experimental data and clinical observations, mainly derived from experiences with gentamicin-loaded bone cement, suggest the following hypotheses:

1. *Prophylactic use of gentamicin-loaded bone cement may protect against infections if gentamicin-sensitive germs have been inoculated during or immediately after surgery.* This is supported by direct comparisons of early revision and PJI rates after the use of ALBC vs. plain cement (Pellegrini and Suardi 2020). The higher the gentamicin elution from the bone cement matrix in the first days, the better is its protective effect. It should be noted that not all ALBC elute antibiotics equally depending on parameters such as cement polymer composition, micro- and macroporosity of the cement matrix, and nature of the admixed antibiotic (Kühn et al. 2005; Kühn 2014; Meyer et al. 2011; Meeker et al. 2019).
2. Although less common as a consequence of the initially high drug concentrations in the joint compartment, *previous high-resistance bacteria may survive by selection and subsequently grow on ALBC.* This is supported by reports showing persistence of resistant coagulase-negative staphylococci on gentamicin-impregnated PMMA (Arciola et al. 2002; Thornes et al. 2002, Anagnostakos et al. 2008). In the same way, Stefánsdóttir et al. (2013) and Holleyman et al. (2019) observed in two independent registry-based studies that the prevalence of gentamicin-resistant bacteria was higher in deep surgical-site infections if primary prostheses had been previously cemented with ALBC instead of uncemented implants.
3. *Even if selection of resistant bacteria has occurred upon exposure to ALBC, the resistance is limited to the antibiotic that exerted the selection pressure.* For clinical practice, it is, therefore, important to note that gentamicin resistance normally does not influence the possible susceptibility to other antibiotic classes. When comparing the infection rates and antibiotic resistance profiles of germs found in deep surgical-site infections among 1941 necks of femur fracture patients treated either with a single ALBC (control group) or with a dual ALBC (intervention group), Tyas et al. (2018) observed a significantly lower PJI rate in the intervention group (1.2% vs. 3.4%). Although the bacteria in the fewer PJI cases of the intervention group showed almost logically a higher percentage of resistance to gentamicin and

clindamycin, there were proportionally fewer infections resistant to clindamycin, gentamicin, and to both antibiotics in this group. Of highest clinical impact was the finding that the levels of resistance to those antibiotics used for the treatment of PJI remained largely unchanged. It was, therefore, reassuring to know that these antimicrobial options remain effective and do not lower the probability for a successful eradication of the infection.

4. *Dual ALBCs (e.g., impregnated with gentamicin and clindamycin or with gentamicin and vancomycin) should be used in and after local treatment of PJI cases* (in spacers in two-stage treatment protocols and in the fixation cement in one-stage or two-stage treatment protocols if cementation of the revision implants is preferred). Because of the simultaneous action on different bacterial targets, parallel resistances against both antibiotics at the same time are much rarer. Even if a gentamicin resistance due to ALBC use in primary arthroplasty has occurred via selection, the other antibiotic should still remain active.

Take-Home Messages

- Use of ALBC in arthroplasty appears justified for prophylactic purposes and for the support of the treatment of septic cases due to its strong in situ antimicrobial effect on susceptible and even intermediate resistant bacteria.
- As with any other antibiotic exposure, resistance development is possible. This occurs, however, mainly by selection of previously high-level resistant mutants and is limited to the antibiotic that has exerted the selection pressure.
- The use of antibiotic combinations in bone cement may lead to lower treatment failure and lowers the risk of concomitant resistance development.
- There is no hard clinical evidence that the routine use of bone cement impregnated with appropriate bactericidal antibiotics promotes the development of broad antibiotic resistance and would negatively affect antibiotic treatment options in PJI cases.

References

Anagnostakos K, Hitzler P, Pape D et al (2008) Persistence of bacterial growth on antibiotic-loaded beads: is it actually a problem? Acta Orthop 79:302–307

Araos R, Munita JM, Arias CA (2015) Antimicrobial resistance: selection vs. induction. In: LaPlante K et al (eds) Antimicrobial stewardship: principles and practice. CABI, Wallingford

Arciola CR, Campoccia D, Montanaro L (2002) Effects on antibiotic resistance of *Staphylococcus epidermidis* following adhesion to polymethylmethacrylate and to ailicone surfaces. Biomaterials 23(6):1495–1502. https://doi.org/10.1016/s0142-9612(01)00275-7

Buchholz HW, Engelbrecht H (1970) Depot effects of various antibiotics mixed with Palacos resins. Chirurg 41(11):51

Della Valle AG, Bostrom M, Brause B et al (2001) Effective bactericidal activity of tobramycin and vancomycin eluted from acrylic bone cement. Acta Orthop Scand 72(3):237–240. https://doi.org/10.1080/000164701528465 47

Engesaeter LB, Lie SA, Espehaug B et al (2003) Antibiotic prophylaxis in total hip arthroplasty: effects of antibiotic prophylaxis systemically and in bone cement on the revision rate of 22,170 primary hip replacements followed 0–14 years in the Norwegian Arthroplasty Register. Acta Orthop Scand 74(6):644–651. https://doi.org/10.1080/00016470310018135

Ensing GT, van Horn JR, van der Mei HC et al (2009) Copal bone cement is more effective in preventing biofilm formation than Palacos R-G. Clin Orthop Relat Res 466(6):1492–1498. https://doi.org/10.1007/s11999-008-0203-x

Hendriks JG, Neut D, van Horn JR et al (2003) The release of gentamicin from acrylic bone cements in a simulated prosthesis-related interfacial gap. J Biomed Mater Res B Appl Biomater 64(1):1–5. https://doi.org/10.1002/jbm.b.10391

Hendriks JG, Neut D, van Horn JR et al (2005) Bacterial survival in the interfacial gap in gentamicin-loaded acrylic bone cements. J Bone Joint Surg Br 87(2):272–276. https://doi.org/10.1302/0301-620x.87b2

Holleyman RJ, Deehan DJ, Walker L et al (2019) Staphylococcal resistance profiles in deep infection following primary hip and knee arthroplasty: a study using the NJR dataset. Arch Orthop Trauma Surg 139(9):1209–1215. https://doi.org/10.1007/s00402-019-03155-1

Jämsen E, Huhtala H, Puolakka T, Moilanen T (2009) Risk factors for infection after knee arthroplasty. A register-based analysis of 43,149 cases. J Bone Joint Surg Am 91:38–47

Jameson SS, Asaad A, Diament M et al (2019) Antibiotic-loaded bone cement is associated with a lower risk of revision following primary cemented total knee arthroplasty: an analysis of 731,214 cases using National Joint Registry data. Bone Joint J 101-B(11):1331–1347

Kühn KD (2014) PMMA cements, 2013th edn. Springer, Berlin Heidelberg/New York

Kühn KD, Ege W, Gopp U (2005) Acrylic bone cements: composition and properties. Orthop Clin North Am 36(1):17–28, v. https://doi.org/10.1016/j.ocl.2004.06.010

Meyer J, Piller G, Spiegel CA et al (2011) Vacuum-mixing significantly changes antibiotic elution characteristics of ommercially available antibiotic-impregnated bone cements. J Bone Joint Surg Am 93(22):2049–2056

Meeker DG, Cooper KB, Renard RL et al (2019) Comparative study of antibiotic elution profiles from alternative formulations of polymethylmethacrylate bone cement. J Arthroplast 34(7):1458–1461. https://doi.org/10.1016/j.arth.2019.03.008

Mohamed NS, Wilkie WA, Remily EA et al (2020) Antibiotic choice: the synergistic effect of single vs dual antibiotics. J Arthroplast 35(3S):S19–S23. https://doi.org/10.1016/j.arth.2019.11.002

Neut D, Kluin OS, Thompson J et al (2010) Gentamicin release from commercially-available gentamicin-loaded PMMA bone cements in a prosthesis-related interfacial gap model and their antibacterial efficacy. BMC Musculoskelet Disord 11:258. https://doi.org/10.1186/1471-2474-11-258

Parvizi J, Saleh KJ, Ragland PS et al (2008) Efficacy of antibiotic-impregnated cement in total hip replacement. Acta Orthop 79:335

Pellegrini AV, Suardi V (2020) Antibiotics and cement: what I need to know? Hip Int 30(1_suppl):48–53. https://doi.org/10.1177/1120700020915463

Stefánsdóttir A, Johansson A, Lidgren L et al (2013) Bacterial colonization and resistance patterns in 133 patients undergoing a primary hip- or knee replacement in Southern Sweden. Acta Orthop 84(1):87–91. https://doi.org/10.3109/17453674.2013.773120

Thornes B, Murray P, Bouchier-Hayes D (2002) Development of resistant strains of *Staphylococcus epidermidis* on gentamicin-loaded bone cement in vivo. J Bone Joint Surg Br 84:758–760

Tyas B, Marsh M, Oswald T et al (2018) Antibiotic resistance profiles of deep surgical site infections in hip hemiarthroplasty. Comparing low dose single antibiotic versus high dose dual antibiotic impregnated cement. J Bone Joint Infect 3(3):123–129. https://doi.org/10.7150/jbji.22192. eCollection 2018

Wahlig H, Dingeldein E (1980) Antibiotics and bone cements. Experimental and clinical long-term observations. Acta Orthop Scand 51(1):49–56

Wahlig H, Dingeldein E, Bergmann R, Reuss K (1978) The release of gentamicin from polymethylmethacrylate beads. An experimental and pharmacokinetic study. J Bone Joint Surg Br 60-B(2):270–275

Wahlig H, Dingeldein E, Buchholz HW et al (1984) Pharmacokinetic study of gentamicin-loaded cement in total hip replacements. Comparative effects of varying dosage. J Bone Joint Surg Br 66(2):175–179

Infection Risk-Adjusted Antibiotic Prophylaxis Strategies in Arthroplasty: Low-Dose Single vs. High-Dose Dual Antibiotic-Loaded Bone Cement

Pablo Sanz-Ruiz and Christof Berberich

Contents

E. Hansen, K.-D. Kühn (eds.), *Essentials of Cemented Knee Arthroplasty*,
https://doi.org/10.1007/978-3-662-63113-3_62

62.1 Introduction

Periprosthetic joint infection (PJI) is a rare, but devastating complication following joint replacement. The overall PJI incidence is in the range of 1–3% in primary arthroplasty, but it is higher in some high-risk situations such as revision procedures (Zimmerli et al. 2004; Ong et al. 2009; Kasch et al. 2017; Bosco et al. 2015). PJI treatment is complex and often requires multiple surgeries resulting in a high burden for the patient and in high costs for the health care system (Kasch et al. 2016). The number of PJI cases is expected to further increase as a consequence of the growing numbers of primary and revision arthroplasty procedures worldwide. Despite higher awareness of this complication, infection rates have not changed much over the last two decades. This observation may be explained by the trend to operate more on older patients with many comorbidities together with the spread of more resistant pathogens (Fernandez-Fairen et al. 2013).

Many surgeons in Europe use local antibiotics in cemented arthroplasty procedures in the form of antibiotic-loaded bone cement (ALBC) as a complementary strategy to perioperative antibiotic prophylaxis (PAP). The rationale behind this strategy is the formation of an additional antimicrobial "frontline" in the joint cavity itself (Kühn et al. 2014).

> One of the major advantages of this strategy is that high-peak concentrations of bactericidal antibiotics are achieved where contaminations may have occurred without exposing the patient to a major risk of side effects.

62

In fact, several clinical studies and arthroplasty registry results have provided evidence for lower revision rates when systemic and local antibiotic prophylaxis are combined (Engesaeter et al. 2003; Jämsen et al. 2009; Jiranek et al. 2006; Wu et al. 2016). In line with these registry observations, a meta-analysis of the available clinical data has concluded that the systematic use of ALBC may reduce PJI incidence by up to 50% in primary procedures and up to 40% in revision operations (Parvizi et al. 2008).

We have recently reported on our own experiences made since the implementation of routine use of the ALBC PALACOS R+G for all cemented primary hip and knee procedures in our institution leading to a reduction of PJI cases by 60–70% compared to the period when non-ALBC was used (Sanz-Ruiz et al. 2017). The introduction of ALBC was further found to be highly cost-efficient with cost savings of 2672 € per patient in hip arthroplasty as a consequence of considerably lower PJI treatment costs (Sanz-Ruiz et al. 2017).

62.2 Risk Factors for Infection and the Idea of a Risk-Tailored Antibiotic Prophylaxis

It is now widely accepted that arthroplasty patients may have a different PJI risk profile, which can be quantified using validated risk calculators (Tan et al. 2018). A recent prospective observational cohort study analyzing 623,253 primary hip procedures performed between 2003 and 2013 in England and Wales has determined to which extent each of these factors may contribute to a higher infection risk (Lenguerrand et al. 2018). BMI ≥40 kg/m^2, malnutrition, wound dehiscence, surgical-site infections, and previous surgeries were found to be associated with a much higher PJI incidence than "normal" (3- to 9-fold higher PJI rate). However, it should be noted that the exact hazard ratio of each potential risk factor is still a matter of debate.

> Given the fact that the majority of arthroplasty patients suffer from several risk factors, the practical conclusions for surgeries from such risk factor tables are also not yet clear and must be further discussed.

However, assuming that the prior identification of individuals at higher PJI risk (in particular if several risk factors are combined) may, indeed, help to further optimize prophylactic strategies during surgery, the extra effort may appear justified. So far, the implementation of a risk-adjusted antibiotic prophylactic regimen is still rather an idea than an evidence-proven concept. If taken further, two possible complementary modifications to standard protocols exist:

- Modification of the routine perioperative antibiotic prophylaxis scheme by either extending the postoperative duration (e.g., beyond 24 hours [Inabathula et al. 2018]) and/or by adding a second antibiotic to the standard regimen (e.g., vancomycin or teicoplanin to a cephalosporin [Tornero et al. 2015]).
- Use of high-dose ALBC with antibiotic combinations for implant fixation in the joint cavity.

Proof of concept that the latter strategy may have a positive impact on the incidence of surgical-site and deep-implant infections has been recently demonstrated in a quasi-randomized clinical trial on 848 patients with an intracapsular neck-of-femur fracture (NOF) treated with cemented hemiarthroplasty in the Northumbria Hospital Trust in the UK (Sprowson et al. 2016). Treatment in the clinical study was performed either with a low-dose single antibiotic cement (PALACOS® R+G; G = gentamicin) in the group representing the current standard of care or with a high-dose dual antibiotic cement (COPAL® G+C;

gentamicin + clindamycin) in the intervention group. It was found that the rate of deep infections was significantly reduced from 3.5% (PALACOS® group) to 1.1% (COPAL® group). The rate of complications was similar in both groups.

62.3 Results

62.3.1 PJI Risk Classification at the University Hospital Gregorio Maranon, Madrid

Based on our own experiences as a large tertiary hospital and taking into account the practicality and clinical relevance of some literature-supported risk factors, in 2012 some surgeons in our hospital developed their own risk algorithm, which they then followed. Its calculation is based on the following general health-specific and orthopedic/trauma-specific risk factors (Table 62.1).

In the case of TKA, a patient at high risk for PJI was defined if he/she has at least two or more of these comorbidities or risk factors, and in the case of THA, at least three or more (Fig. 62.1). In addition, some isolated risk factors were identified, which justify a direct classification as a high-risk patient:

High Risk!
- Severe kidney or cardiac disease
- Immunodeficiency
- Previous infection or colonization (hips)
- Previous surgery at the same joint
- Revision surgery

62.3.2 Outcome Analysis with High-Dose Antibiotic Cement in High-Risk Patients to Reduce PJI

Based on this risk algorithm, all our cemented primary arthroplasty operations performed in the time period 2015–2018 on a total of 2551 patients (primary arthroplasties included TKA, THA, and hemiarthroplasties) were grouped into those who received single antibiotic-loaded low-dose cement PALACOS® R+G (92.8% = 2368 patients with a mixed low and high-risk profile) vs. a high-risk patient group receiving double antibiotic-loaded high dose cement COPAL® G+C (183 patients = 7.2%). The post-analysis of PJI cases that occurred in this time period was 3.7% for all patients, but only 2.45% in the more homogeneous high-risk patient COPAL® cohort ($p = 0.65$) (Fig. 62.2). This trend toward a reduction of PJI cases in the COPAL® group, albeit not statistically significant because of the heterogeneous patient profile in the comparator group, was contradictory to what we expected in this high-risk patient group (Sanz-Ruiz and Berberich 2020).

Table 62.1 Differentiation of general and specific risk factors that to our experience in combination justify the classification of patients as PJI risk patients

General risk factors	Specific risk factors
Age >80 years	Previous infection/steroid injection <6 months
Nutritional status and weight (BMI >30 >19)	Pernicious anemia
Diabetes mellitus	Inflammatory disease
Tobacco consumption	Organic disease: kidney, cardiac
Rectal or urinary tract bacterial colonization	Revision surgery
Immunodeficiency	Hip fracture surgery
Previous hospital stay or institutionalized patient	Previous orthopedic or trauma surgery with implantation of hardware

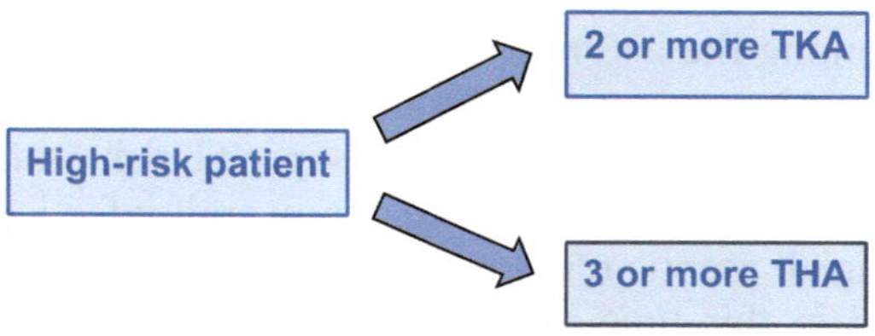

Fig. 62.1 Classification of risk patients based on the risk factors described in Table 62.1

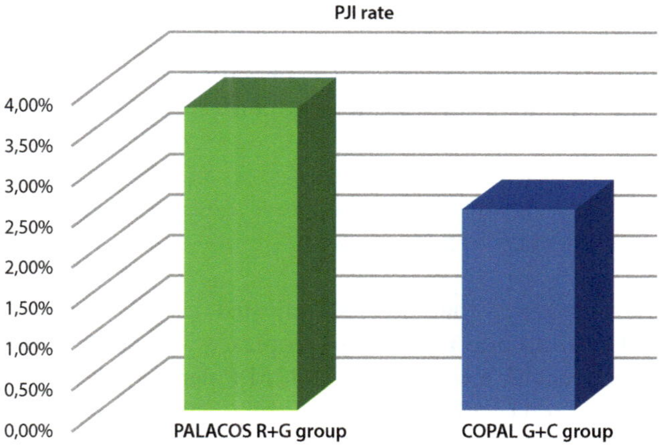

Fig. 62.2 PJI rate within 1 year between 2015 and 2018 in the group "PALACOS® R+G" with mixed PJI risk profiles (92.8%) and in the group "COPAL® G+C" (7.2%) with exclusive high-risk profile according to our recent risk stratification algorithm

Table 62.2 Comparison of PJI rate in aseptic revision cases occurring 2015–2018 in patients receiving PALACOS® R+G vs. patients receiving COPAL® G+C[a]

Cases	PALACOS® R+G	COPAL® G+C	All
No. of aseptic revision cases	143	103	246
PJI cases	6	0	6
% PJI	**4.1%**	**0%**	**2.44%**

[a]Septic revisions, oncologic cases, or periprosthetic fractures excluded; comparable patient profile in both groups

In order to determine the "true effect" of the bone cement COPAL® G+C for fixation and infection prophylaxis, it was necessary to compare strictly homogeneous groups. Therefore, we focused our analysis on solely aseptic cemented revision knee arthroplasty cases, which were performed between 2015 and 2018.

Among the 246 retrospectively analyzed TKA revisions, 143 were cemented with PALACOS® R+G and 103 with COPAL® G+C. Patient-specific risk profiles in each group were comparable. An overall infection rate among all aseptic revision patients of 2.44% was determined in this time period. However, when comparing the infection rate between the individual cement groups, a statistically significant reduction ($p = 0.035$) of PJI cases was found in the COPAL® G+C group (no infection case in 103 patients = 0% infection rate) compared to the number of infections in the PALACOS® R+G group (6 infection cases in 143 patients = 4.1% infection rate – Table 62.2) (Sanz-Ruiz et al. 2020).

> It should be noted that the surgical practice and the choice of perioperative antibiotic prophylaxis did not differ between both groups.

It was shown that the risk-adjusted use of COPAL® G+C in aseptic revision arthroplasty was highly cost-effective with a cost saving of 1261 € per patient treated with COPAL® G+C (Sanz-Ruiz et al. 2020).

Conclusion

Our data appear to confirm the hypothesis that a prior PJI risk classification of arthroplasty patients may be beneficial if combined with special risk-adjusted prophylactic measures. For the first time, we show here that the rationale of using either PALACOS® R+G as low-dose cement for relatively healthy patients in primary procedures or COPAL® G+C as high-dose double antibiotic-loaded cement for patients with multiple comorbidities and in revision situations leads to less PJI cases in the orthopedic ward and is highly cost-effective. These data extend the observations from a randomized clinical trial with neck-of-femur fracture patients in the UK that COPAL® G+C can, indeed, substantially lower the superficial and deep infection risk in patients at high infection risks. The principle of a more effective in situ protection appears to hold true also in a more general perspective and deserves further investigations.

Take-Home Messages

- The risk for PJI is significantly higher in patients with multiple comorbidities and in revision arthroplasties.
- Among the prophylactic measures taken to prevent PJI, use of ALBC can be an important tool. Its effect may be stronger in patients at higher infection risk.
- Prior risk classification can be helpful to determine whether an infection risk-adjusted prophylactic regimen should be considered.
- Several factors exposing a patient to an increased infection risk in joint replacement procedures have been defined, but the exact hazard ratios of each risk factor are still debated. A simple risk algorithm and scoring system as the one developed in our hospital may overcome this complexity.
- Our risk scoring model on the basis of two or three risk factors, respectively, has proven easy, practical, and effective to differentiate patients with lower and higher risk profiles for PJI. Some single risk factors were even weighted as sufficient in our clinical practice to classify a patient as a high-risk patient.
- Our retrospective analysis of patient groups treated with either the low-dose cement PALACOS® R+G or with the high-dose dual antibiotic-loaded cement COPAL® G+C has provided evidence that the latter can be even more useful in reducing the number of PJI cases in high-risk patients, especially after hip fracture and aseptic knee revision surgery.
- The prophylactic use of the dual ALBC COPAL® C+G in aseptic revision was found to be cost-effective.

References

Bosco JA, Bookman J, Slover J et al (2015) Principles of antibiotic prophylaxis in total joint arthroplasty: current concepts. J Am Acad Orthop Surg 23(8):e27–e35. https://doi.org/10.5435/JAAOS-D-15-00017

Engesaeter LB, Lie SA, Espehaug B et al (2003) Antibiotic prophylaxis in total hip arthroplasty: effects of antibiotic prophylaxis systemically and in bone cement on the revision rate of 22,170 primary hip replacements followed 0–14 years in the Norwegian Arthroplasty Register. Acta Orthop Scand 74(6):644–651. https://doi.org/10.1080/00016470310018135

Fernandez-Fairen M, Torres A, Menzie A et al (2013) Economical analysis on prophylaxis, diagnosis, and treatment of periprosthetic infections. Open Orthop J 7:227–242. https://doi.org/10.2174/1874325001307010227

Inabathula A, Dilley JE, Ziemba-Davis M et al (2018) Extended oral antibiotic prophylaxis in high-risk patients substantially reduces primary total hip and knee arthroplasty 90-day infection rate. J Bone Joint Surg Am 100(24):2103–2109

Jämsen E, Huhtala H, Puolakka T, Moilanen T (2009) Risk factors for infection after knee arthroplasty. A register-based analysis of 43,149 cases. J Bone Joint Surg Am 91(1):38–47. https://doi.org/10.2106/JBJS.G.01686

Jiranek WA, Hanssen AD, Greenwald AS (2006) Antibiotic-loaded bone cement for infection prophylaxis in total joint replacement. J Bone Joint Surg Am 88:2487–2500

Kasch R, Assmann G, Merk S et al (2016) Economic analysis of two-stage septic revision after total hip arthroplasty: what are the relevant costs for the hospital's orthopedic department? BMC Musculoskelet Disord 17:112. https://doi.org/10.1186/s12891-016-0962-6

Kasch R, Merk S, Assmann G et al (2017) Comparative analysis of direct hospital care costs between aseptic and two-stage septic knee revision. PLoS One 12(1):e0169558. https://doi.org/10.1371/journal.pone.0169558

Kühn KD, Lieb E, Berberich C (2014) PMMA bone cements – what is the role of local antibiotics. Maitrise Orthop Proc N 243:1–15

Lenguerrand E, Whitehouse MR, Beswick AD et al (2018) Risk factors associated with revision for prosthetic joint infection after hip replacement: a prospective observational cohort study. Lancet Infect Dis 18(9):1004–1014

Ong KL, Kurtz SM, Lau E et al (2009) Prosthetic joint infection risk after total hip arthroplasty in the Medicare population. J Arthroplast 24:105–109

Parvizi J, Saleh KJ, Ragland PS et al (2008) Efficacy of antibiotic-impregnated cement in total hip replacement. Acta Orthop 79(3):335–341. https://doi.org/10.1080/17453670710015229

Sanz-Ruiz P, Berberich C (2020) Infection risk-adjusted antibiotic prophylaxis strategies in arthroplasty: ahort review of evidence and experiences of a tertiary center in Spain. Orthop Res Rev 12:89–96

Sanz-Ruiz P, Matas-Diez JA, Sanchez-Somolinos M et al (2017) Is the commercial antibiotic-loaded bone cement useful in prophylaxis and cost saving after knee and hip joint arthroplasty? The transatlantic paradox. J Arthroplast 32(4):1095–1099. https://doi.org/10.1016/j.arth.2016.11.012

Sanz-Ruiz P, Matas-Diez JA, Villanueva-Martínez M et al (2020) Is dual antibiotic-loaded bone cement more effective and cost-efficient than a single antibiotic-loaded bone cement to reduce the risk of prosthetic joint infection in aseptic revision knee arthroplasty? J Arthroplast 35(12):3724–3729. https://doi.org/10.1016/j.arth.2020.06.045

Sprowson AP, Jensen C, Chambers S et al (2016) The use of high-dose dual-impregnated antibiotic-laden cement with hemiarthroplasty for the treatment of a fracture of the hip: the fractured hip infection trial. Bone Joint J 98-B(11):1534–1541. https://doi.org/10.1302/0301-620X.98B11.34693

Tan TL, Maltenfort MG, Chen AF et al (2018) Development and evaluation of a preoperative risk calculator for periprosthetic joint infection following total joint arthroplasty. J Bone Joint Surg Am 100(9):777–785

Tornero E, García-Ramiro S, Martínez-Pastor JC et al (2015) Prophylaxis with teicoplanin and cefuroxime reduces the rate of prosthetic joint infection after primary arthroplasty. Antimicrob Agents Chemother 59(2):831–837

Wu CT, Chen IL, Wang JW et al (2016) Surgical site infection after total knee arthroplasty: risk factors in patients with timely administration of systemic prophylactic antibiotics. J Arthroplast 31(7):1568–1573. https://doi.org/10.1016/j.arth.2016.01.017

Zimmerli W, Trampuz A, Ochsner PE (2004) Prosthetic-joint infections. N Engl J Med 351:1645–1654

Revision Total Knee Arthroplasty Stems: Cemented Versus Cementless

Daniel A. Oakes and Thomas M. Steck

Contents

E. Hansen, K.-D. Kühn (eds.), *Essentials of Cemented Knee Arthroplasty*,
https://doi.org/10.1007/978-3-662-63113-3_63

63.1 Introduction

With nearly 600,000 primary cases performed annually, total knee arthroplasty (TKA) is arguably among the most common and most successful surgical procedures performed in the United States (Kurtz et al. 2005). Given the increasing frequency of this procedure and the changing patient demographics to include younger patients who are undergoing TKA, the revision burden will subsequently increase.

> Currently, approximately 55,000 revision TKAs are performed annually in the United States (Bhandari et al. 2012). According to a recent retrospective review, the most common reasons for revision TKA are mechanical loosening (39.9%), infection (27.4%), instability (7.5%), periprosthetic fracture (4.7%), and arthrofibrosis (4.5%) (Sharkey et al. 2014).

63.2 Case Example

A 66-year-old male presents with a history of right TKA complicated by periprosthetic infection requiring explantation and articulating antibiotic cement spacer placement at an outside facility approximately 1 year prior to presentation (Fig. 63.1). After demonstrating that the infection resolved, the patient undergoes revision right TKA with re-implantation. Both medial and lateral femoral and tibial trabecular metal augments are used to address bone loss, a constrained liner is used given lateral laxity, and fully cemented tibial and femoral stems are used, with antibiotic-loaded cement (ALBC) (Fig. 63.2).

Postoperatively the patient has an unremarkable course, and the knee is functioning well at the last follow-up.

63.3 The Challenge of the Revision Knee

Osteolysis resulting in compromised metaphyseal bone stock complicates the ability to achieve durable fixation in revision TKA. One must balance often compromised ligaments or substitute for them with increasing levels of constraint. A successful revision is predicated on stable implant fixation. To enhance fixation, the role of modular stems in revision TKA is well accepted.

> Stems increase the relative length of the femoral and tibial components and allow for transfer of loads from compromised, osteolytic bone at the prior prosthesis–bone interface to previously unviolated metadiaphyseal and diaphyseal bone.

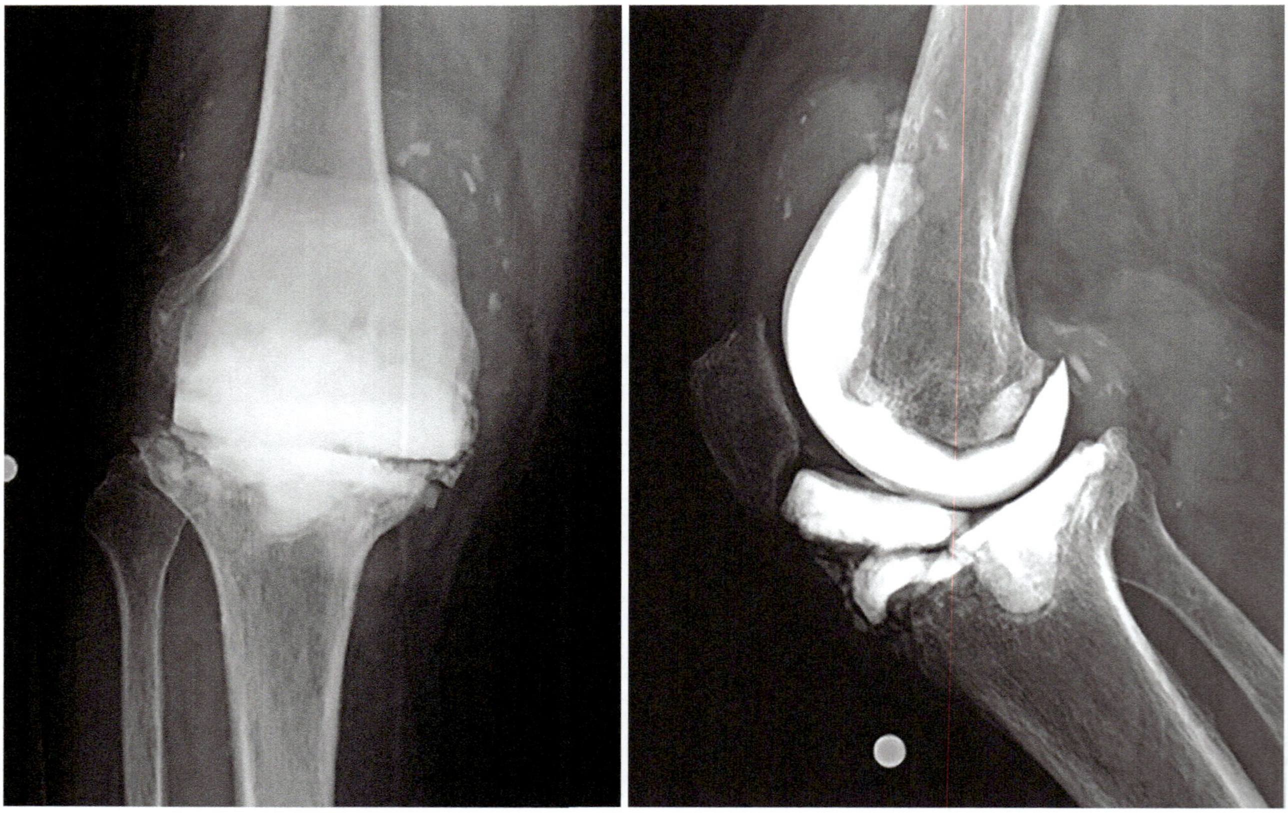

Fig. 63.1 Preoperative radiographs

63

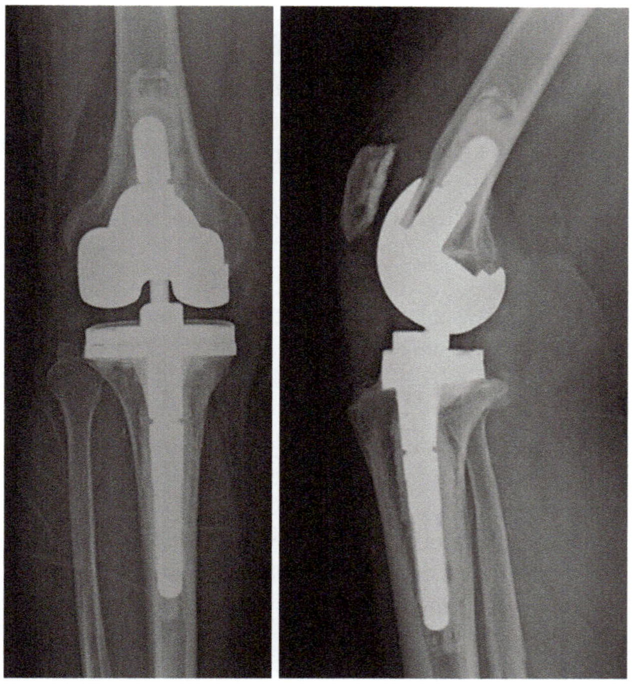

Fig. 63.2 Postoperative radiographs

By more evenly distributing the forces and providing a more mechanically stable construct, stems allow for decreased strain at the bone–prosthesis interface. Stemmed implants have been associated with a decreased likelihood of implant loosening (Bugbee et al. 2001).

63.4 Optimal Stem Fixation

Despite general agreement regarding the benefit of stemmed implants in revision TKA, there remains considerable controversy regarding the optimal length, diameter, and fixation method. Stems (short or long) may be fully cemented with or without the use of cement restrictors. Longer stems can be placed using an "uncemented" technique, which is better described as a hybrid surface cementing technique and utilizes a press-fit technique in the diaphysis and more proximally cements the interface. This technique relies on cortical contact in diaphyseal bone for both alignment and stabilization distally, while support closer to the joint is achieved by the cement in the metaphyseal region and the joint interfaces.

> Use of small-diameter cementless stems that do not engage the cortex or so-called "dangle stems" should be avoided, as this limits fixation and may lead to increased loosening.

63.4.1 Cementless Stems

The use of a cementless stem requires preoperative templating to ensure that the patient's specific anatomy is amenable to the use of a press-fit stem. Tibias noted on long-standing films to have excessive tibia vara, or tibia valga may increase the difficulty of achieving a distal press-fit fixation and the desired alignment. Offset stems and offset couples can aid in navigating these bony geometries. Press-fit stems are designed to engage the diaphysis, as opposed to fully cemented stems, which are designed to engage either the metaphysis, metadiaphysis, or the diaphysis.

To achieve an optimal diaphyseal fit, the majority of press-fit stem systems include reaming the medullary canal to a diameter at which chatter is felt or heard so as to improve the cortical contact with the prosthesis. Reaming also allows for debridement of a potentially sclerotic false inner cortex, which reduces the probability of referencing from a false cortex. Reaming is typically performed approximately 1 cm past the templated stem tip to reduce the risk of tip impingement.

After reaming a trial implant may be used to ensure that the stem can be fully seated and to ensure that a deformity is not induced by the diaphyseal fit.

> If there is difficulty with seating the stem or if a deformity is induced, offset stems or couples can be used to adjust the position of the implant relative to the diaphysis.

While the end of the stem provides diaphyseal stability, the metaphyseal region of the femoral stem or the tibial keel is often in need of cement to enhance metaphyseal stability. Additionally, cement can manually be impacted into the metaphyseal cancellous bone at the prosthesis–bone interface to create interdigitation and improve the interface stability of the implant.

Proponents of cementless stems offer several advantages relative to cemented stems, including decreased operative time and ease of removal in subsequent revisions (Table 63.1). Additionally, cementless stems have been associated with decreased proximal stress shielding in biomechanical studies (Completo et al. 2008). Haas et al. reported 84% good to excellent results at 42 months post-op following revision TKA with uncemented stemmed implants, with a reported 83% survivorship rate at 8 years post-op (Haas et al. 1995). Vince and Long (1995) followed 44 patients who underwent revision TKA with uncemented press-fit stems for 2–6 years and found that 3 of the 13 patients who were revised to a constrained condylar articulation

Table 63.1 Relative advantages and disadvantages of cemented stems vs. press-fit stems

Advantages/disadvantages	Cemented stem	Press-fit stem
Advantages	Immediate stability Helpful in cases of aberrant anatomy Able to elute antibiotics	Less stress shielding Allows for diaphyseal referencing during insertion Potentially easier to remove
Disadvantages	Difficult to remove Unable to reference diaphysis during insertion	End of stem pain Alignment may be altered by stem fit in cases of aberrant anatomy Risk of periprosthetic fracture with canal preparation and insertion

implant showed evidence of loosening, whereas none of the 31 patients who were reconstructed with a posterior stabilized implant demonstrated. The authors noted that all 3 of the patients who showed loosening had re-implantations after a two-stage protocol for infection and concluded that use of a cementless stem may not provide adequate fixation in the setting of poor bone quality. This study also highlights that uncemented stems may be useful in assisting with alignment, but these stems in the current forms (the absence of an ingrowth surface) may not actually be a significant contributor to implant fixation.

63

There are several additional disadvantages to cementless stems (Table 63.1). Use of cementless stems may induce displacement of the femoral or tibial component, requiring the use of offset stems. Similarly, in the case of aberrant metadiaphyseal anatomy such as an excessive femoral bow, obtaining a press-fit with a stem of sufficient length may not be possible. The need to prepare the canal prior to stem insertion also raises the potential for periprosthetic fracture during stem insertion or canal preparation. Finally, end-of-stem pain is a theoretical disadvantage of cementless stems; however, this may be diminished using slotted stems (Barrack et al. 2004).

63.4.2 Cemented Stems

The cemented stem allows for uniform and consistent fixation along the length of the construct. Similar to placing a femoral stem in a total hip arthroplasty, proper cement technique is essential to achieving durable fixation. The canal and bone interface needs to be cleared of fibrous tissue. A cement restrictor should be placed to allow at least a 1-cm cement plug at the tip of the stem. The canal should be irrigated and dried. Cementation is typically performed using a cement gun to ensure adequate delivery of cement into the canal and allow for pressurization that will enhance the cement interdigitation.

> Care must be taken when inserting the stem, as alignment is determined by the surgeon at the time of insertion, not as a result of a diaphyseal press-fit.

A cemented stem is more easily paired with a metaphyseal engaging porous metal cone, which can further enhance metaphyseal fixation.

The cemented stem offers several advantages (Table 63.1). Cemented stems may allow for flexibility in component placement and may be beneficial in cases of excessive diaphyseal bowing or other anatomic variants. For example, generally when using a fully cemented stem, offset stems or couplers are rarely necessary.

> In the setting of re-implantation for a prior periprosthetic infection, use of cement allows for the selection of organism-specific local antibiotic delivery as it elutes from the bone cement.

There are also several disadvantages to cemented stems (Table 63.1). Primarily, by not obtaining a diaphyseal fit, there is decreased ability to reference the anatomic axis, providing challenges when attempting to optimize mechanical alignment. This is a theoretical limitation as the surgeon can always prepare the distal femur and proximal tibia based on diaphyseal referencing and then cement a shorter stem in place. One distinct disadvantage of cemented stems is that removing a well-placed and fully cemented stem can pose significant technical challenges at future surgeries. That said, it behooves the revision surgeon to provide the patient with the most stable implant fixation at the time of the revision procedure. While concerns about future surgeries are prudent, it is best to provide the best outcome for the current procedure.

63.5 Clinical Outcomes

Edwards et al. compared two cohorts of patients from two centers treated with cementless and cemented stems in a second-stage re-plantation for infection. The revision rate for both groups was similar. The radiographic loosening was more prevalent in the cemented vs. uncemented group. However, loosening was also associated with poor bone quality. While this study proposes a difference between the two groups, a careful review of this retrospective data does not seem to support this claim (Edwards et al. 2014).

Relatively few high-quality studies exist comparing the two fixation strategies. A recent meta-analysis (Wang et al. 2016) was performed to compare survivorship of revised implants with regard to cemented or cementless stems and found no significant difference in failure for any reason, re-operation, aseptic, and infection between the two fixation methods.

To the authors' best knowledge, only two randomized control trials comparing cemented vs. uncemented stems have been performed. In a study by Heesterbeek et al. (2016) 32 patients with AORI Type-I or Type-II bone loss undergoing revision TKA were randomly allocated to undergo revision TKA with either a fully cemented stem or a hybrid implantation technique (cemented femoral component or tibial base plate with a press-fit stem). Patients were followed for a total of 2 years post-op, and both clinical and radiographic outcomes were assessed. At 2 years post-op, there was no difference in clinical outcome scores or in rates of radiographic micromotion as captured using radiostereometric analysis, and none of the 32 patients displayed radiographic or clinical signs of loosening. In the other randomized control trial by Kosse et al. (2017) 23 patients who underwent revision TKA were randomized to cemented or cementless stems, and the authors demonstrated no difference in median micromotion or clinical outcomes at 6.5 years post-op. The short follow-up on both of these studies further emphasizes that this question of superiority has not been clearly answered.

Several retrospective studies have also compared the two fixation techniques. Lachiewicz and O'Dell (2020) retrospectively compared patients who underwent revision TKA with either a cemented (34 patients) or an uncemented stem (50 patients) and found no difference in clinical or radiographic outcomes at a mean of 6 years post-op between the two groups, though they estimated that the study was underpowered by a factor of 4 to assess for differences between the two groups. Gililland et al. (2014) performed a multicenter retrospective cohort study comparing 82 patients who underwent revision TKA with either a cemented or an uncemented stem for aseptic loosening and found no differences in Knee Society scores or in radiographic loosening at a mean of 8 years follow-up.

Several biomechanical studies have also investigated the difference between the two fixation methods. In a cadaveric study Jazrawi et al. (2001), compared micromotion of the tibial tray and strain of the component between cemented and cementless stems of varying lengths and diameters. Longer and larger diameter stems were found to have less micromotion of the tibial tray as compared to shorter and smaller diameter stems; however, the short (75 mm) cementless stems did demonstrate a 33–85% increase in tibial tray motion as compared to short (75 mm) cemented stems, which was statistically significant.

The concept that short cementless stems that do not engage the diaphysis are more susceptible to loosening has been corroborated in clinical studies. Fehring et al. (2003) performed a retrospective clinical and radiographic review of revision TKAs performed with either cemented or cementless stems. In this series, all cementless stems engaged the metaphysis. Also, 93% of the cemented stems were considered stable at the last follow-up; however, only 71% of the cementless stems were considered stable at the last follow-up, which was a statistically significant difference.

Whether a cemented or cementless stem is chosen, the length and diameter of the stem must be accounted for in preoperative templating. The current body of literature has failed to identify an ideal length or diameter for revision stems, though some data do exist to guide implant selection.

› In particular, a higher canal filling ratio (CFR), i.e., the percentage of the intramedullary canal taken up by the stem, has been shown to correlate with improvement in survivorship.

Parsley et al. (2003) retrospectively reviewed revision TKAs with both cemented and cementless tibial stems with variable length and diameter.

› They determined that a CFR of >85% in cementless stems correlated with improved coronal plane alignment relative to stems with a CFR of <85%, and varus malalignment of the tibia occurred more frequently with fully cemented stems.

Additionally, Fleischman et al. (2017) performed a retrospective review of 223 patients with revision TKAs with a mean follow-up of 61.6 months and found that for hybrid stems in which cement is placed on the undersurface and metaphyseal portions of the articular components but not around the diaphyseal portion of stems, risk of failure was reduced by 41.2% for each additional 10% of canal fill regardless of length or diameter.

› In conclusion, both cemented and uncemented stems in the setting of revision TKA have been associated with good midterm results. Yet, this debate is still lacking clear evidence of a technique with overwhelming clinical superiority.

63.6 Author's Preferred Technique

The senior author's revision practice has evolved over a 16-year period from using a press-fit diaphyseal technique with or without metaphyseal cone augmentation to one that utilizes fully cemented short to midlength stems. Long-term follow-up showing loosening of what would have been identified radiographically as well-positioned press-fit stems led to this practice change. Currently, the senior author utilizes diaphyseal referencing of the canals to identify the alignment of the distal femur and proximal tibia. Metaphyseal augmentation is utilized with porous metal cones more often on the tibia than the femur. Cement restrictors are utilized. Fully cemented short to midlength stems are utilized. This construct can safely allow the use of all levels of articular constraint.

Take-Home Messages

- The use of stems in revision TKA is associated with a decreased risk of loosening.
- Fully cemented stems provide immediately durable fixation and are useful in situations with aberrant metadiaphyseal anatomy; however, they may be more difficult to revise if future revisions are warranted.
- Uncemented stems may be easier to revise and are potentially associated with less stress shielding and may facilitate marginally shorter operative times, however, They may potentially result in tip of stem pain, malalignment, and periprosthetic fracture.
- Uncemented stems should be of sufficient length and diameter to fill the diaphysis and to engage the diaphyseal cortex.
- Successful stem augmentation in a revision TKA should provide stable enough fixation to allow the use of all levels of articular constraint.
- There is no conclusive evidence to date that clinical or radiographic outcomes differ when either a cemented or an uncemented stem is used in revision TKA.

References

Barrack RL, Stanley T, Burt M, Hopkins S (2004) The effect of stem design on end-of- stem pain in revision total knee arthroplasty. J Arthroplast 19(7 Suppl 2):119–124

Bhandari M, Smith J, Miller LE, Block JE (2012) Clinical and economic burden of revision knee arthroplasty. Clin Med Insights Arthritis Musculoskelet Disord 5:89–94

Bugbee WD, Ammeen DJ, Engh GA (2001) Does implant selection affect outcome of revision knee arthroplasty? J Arthroplast 16(5):581–585

Completo A, Fonseca F, Simões JA (2008) Strain shielding in proximal tibia of stemmed knee prosthesis: experimental study. J Biomech 41:560–566

Edwards PK, Fehring TK, Hamilton WG, Perricelli B, Beaver WB, Odum SM (2014) Are cementless stems more durable than cemented stems in two-stage revisions of infected total knee arthroplasties? Clin Orthop Relat Res 472:206–211

Fehring TK, Odum S, Olekson C, Griffin WL, Mason JB, McCoy TH (2003) Stem fixation in revision total knee arthroplasty: a comparative analysis. Clin Orthop Relat Res 416:217–224

Fleischman AN, Azboy I, Fuery M, Restrepo C, Shao H, Parvizi J (2017) Effect of stem size and fixation method on mechanical failure after revision total knee arthroplasty. J Arthroplast 32(9 Supp):S202–S208

Gililland JM, Gaffney CJ, Odum SM, Fehring TK, Peters CL, Beaver WB (2014) Clinical & radiographic outcomes of cemented vs. diaphyseal engaging cementless stems in aseptic revision TKA. J Arthroplast 29(Suppl 2):224–228

Haas SB, Insall JN, Montgomery W III, Windsor RE (1995) Revision total knee arthroplasty with use of modular components with stems inserted without cement. J Bone Joint Surg Am 77A:1700–1707

Heesterbeek PJC, Wymenga AB, van Hellemondt GG (2016) Difference in implant micromotion between hybrid fixation and fully cemented revision total knee arthroplasty. J Bone Joint Surg Am 98(16):1359–1369

Jazrawi LM, Bai B, Kummer FJ, Hiebert R, Stuchin SA (2001) The effect of stem modularity and mode of fixation on tibial component stability in revision total knee arthroplasty. J Arthroplast 16(6):759–767

Kosse NM, van Hellemondt GG, Wymenga AB, Heesterbeek PJC (2017) Comparable stability of cemented vs press-fit placed stems in revision total knee arthroplasty with mild to moderate bone loss: 6.5 year results from a randomized control trial with radiostereometric analysis. J Arthroplast 32(1):197–201

Kurtz S, Mowat F, Ong K, Chan N, Lau E, Halpern M (2005) Prevalence of primary and revision total hip and knee arthroplasty in the United States from 1990 through 2002. J Bone Joint Surg Am 87(7):1487–1497

Lachiewicz PF, O'Dell JA (2020) Is there a difference between cemented and uncemented femoral stem extensions in revision knee arthroplasty? J Knee Surg 33(1):84–88

Parsley BS, Sugano N, Bertolusso R, Conditt MA (2003) Mechanical alignment of tibial stems in revision total knee arthroplasty. J Arthroplast 18(7 Suppl 1):33–36

Sharkey PF, Lichstein PM, Shen C, Tokarski AT, Parvizi J (2014) Why are total knee arthroplasties failing today has anything changed after 10 years? J Arthroplast 29:1774e8

Vince KG, Long W (1995) Revision knee arthroplasty: the limits of press fit medullary fixation. Clin Orthop Relat Res 317:172–177

Wang C, Pfitzner T, von Roth P, Mayr HO, Sostheim M, Hube R (2016) Fixation of stem in revision of total knee arthroplasty: cemented versus cementless – a meta-analysis. Knee Surg Sports Traumatol Arthrosc 24:3200–3211

Metaphyseal Fixation: Sleeves and Cones

Robert Pivec and Matthew S. Austin

Contents

E. Hansen, K.-D. Kühn (eds.), *Essentials of Cemented Knee Arthroplasty*,
https://doi.org/10.1007/978-3-662-63113-3_64

64.1 Introduction

Revision total knee arthroplasty (TKA) is generally synonymous with varying degrees of bone loss, and finding solutions for rigid and durable fixation in the face of an often poor biomechanic and biologic foundation has been the impetus leading to the development of modern revision knee systems. The iterative and generational advances in improving total knee revision (TKR) longevity has gone hand-in-hand with the transition away from structural allograft and long diaphyseal engaging stems toward metaphyseal sleeves and cones.

Although beyond the scope of this chapter, the use of bulk structural allografts has several distinct disadvantages including available supply, poor osseointegration, limited revascularization (leading to diminished mechanical properties), postoperative weight-bearing restrictions, and the potential for disease transmission (Dennis and Little 2005; Panegrossi et al. 2014). Similarly, the use of long diaphyseal engaging stems (both cemented and press-fit) has fallen out of favor due to stress shielding, modulus mismatch concerns causing end-of-stem pain and periprosthetic fracture, and difficulty with subsequent implant removal (Completo et al. 2008; Murray et al. 1994). The rates of progressive radiolucencies and aseptic revisions at midterm follow-up with these systems have been variably reported as high as 35% and 20%, respectively (Murray et al. 1994; Panegrossi et al. 2014).

Cones and sleeves have gained increasing popularity to address large bone defects as classified by the Anderson Orthopaedic Research Institute (AORI) classification system:

Anderson Orthopaedic Research Institute (AORI) Classification of Bone Defects

- *Type 1*: Minor femoral or tibial defects with intact metaphyseal bone, not compromising the stability of a revision component.
- *Type 2*:
  - *2A*: Damaged metaphyseal bone. Loss of cancellous metaphyseal bone requiring reconstruction to provide stability of the revision component. Defects in one femoral or tibial condyle.
  - *2B*: Damaged metaphyseal bone. Loss of cancellous metaphyseal bone requiring reconstruction to provide stability of the revision component. Defects in both femoral or both tibial condyles.
- *Type 3*: Deficient metaphyseal segment compromising a major portion of either femoral condyles or tibial plateau.

> The transition from structural allografts, which act more in a buttress fashion, and long stems, which provide diaphyseal fixation, toward sleeves or cones has allowed surgeons to create stable metaphyseal fixation that preferentially loads proximally in the tibia and vice versa in the femur.

A recent systematic review comparing outcomes of 476 structural allografts compared to 223 cones demonstrated a combined failure rate of 6.5% for allograft and 0.9% for cones (Beckmann et al. 2015). While another systematic review by Kim et al. comparing cones to sleeves demonstrated no difference between the two fixation strategies and overall aseptic failure rates less than 1%, which is consistent with previously reported failure rates for these more modern devices (Kim et al. 2018).

Cones

Cone types differ from manufacturers, but all have the same consistent rationale of achieving biologic fixation along the outer diameter with cementation of the tibial tray and stem into the inner diameter of the cone. Cone tribology may consist completely of highly porous metal such as tantalum (e.g., Zimmer Trabecular Metal; Zimmer, Warsaw, IN) or more rigid designs with a highly porous titanium surface coating, which can either be symmetric (e.g., Legion RK, Smith and Nephew, Nashville, TN) or asymmetric (Stryker TS; Stryker, Kalamazoo, MI).

> In general, the rationale for cone choice rests primarily on being able to accommodate the defect through intimate bone contact on its outer diameter and accommodate the stem of the implant through its inner diameter.

In certain situations, the cone (or host bone) may need to be further shaped to accommodate a precise fit. If reamers are used for preparation, particularly with asymmetric style cones, care must be used to avoid excessive bone loss. The clinical and radiographic outcomes of cones are elaborated on further in the discussion.

Sleeves

> Metaphyseal sleeves offer the potential option of purely cementless fixation as the tibial tray and stem engage the sleeve via a taper (DePuy MBT; DePuy-Synthes, Warsaw, IN).

Sleeve–bone fixation occurs at the peripheral rim with bony ingrowth into a highly porous titanium matrix, but this can be supplemented with a hybrid technique where the under-surface of the tibial tray (but not the stem) is cemented to give further initial stability. Similar to cones, distal stem cement is an option. However, this has consequences for end-of-stem pain as well as greater difficulty with any future implant removal. The clinical and radiographic outcomes of cones are elaborated on further in the discussion. Technical tips and an overview of the surgical technique are further discussed in the respective section (▶ Sect. 64.3).

64.2 Case Example

A 74-year-old male patient with a past medical history of chronic kidney disease presents to the office with left knee pain for the past several months, which is not associated with a fall and is exacerbated by activity (particularly getting out of a chair and when taking his first steps). He had undergone a primary bilateral total knee arthroplasty with a cemented posterior-cruciate retaining knee system approximately 15 years prior at an outside institution (◘ Fig. 64.1). Prior to this, the patient had developed similar pain in his contralateral knee and required revision TKA for aseptic loosening.

▪ **Physical Exam**

- Height: 5 feet, 9 inches; weight: 240 pounds; BMI: 35
- Well healed midline incision
- Knee range of motion 0–110°
- Varus knee alignment
- Normal distal lower extremity motor and sensory exam
- Palpable pedal pulses

▪ **Laboratory Tests**

- Serum WBC: 9.5
- ESR: 6 mm/h
- CRP: 6 mg/L
- Preoperative culture: negative
- Intraoperative culture: negative

▪ **Imaging**

Routine preoperative anteroposterior and lateral radiographs (◘ Fig. 64.1a, b) demonstrate a TKA in varus position with loosening and subsidence of the tibial baseplate and findings suggestive of femoral loosening as well. Long-leg standing films, which had been

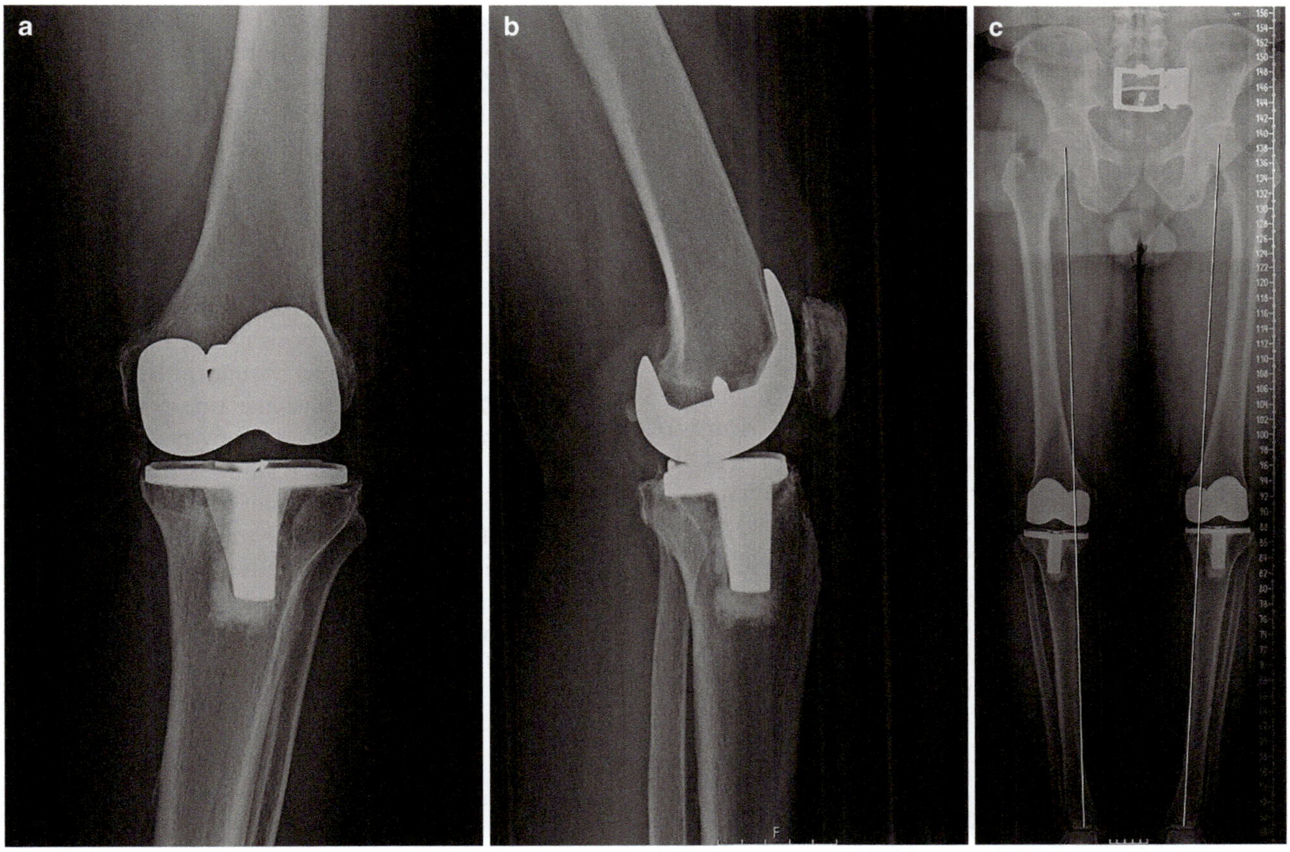

◘ **Fig. 64.1** Preoperative anteroposterior **a** and lateral **b** radiographs demonstrate varus positioning of the tibial component with associated loosening and subsidence. Review of prior long-leg standing radiograph **c** demonstrates initial placement of both tibial components in approximately 6–8° of varus with medial deviation of the mechanical axis bilaterally

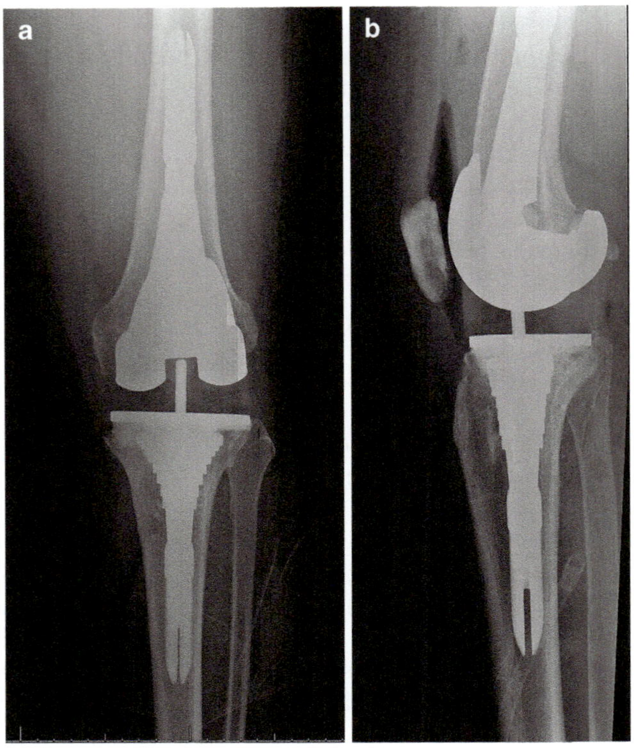

Fig. 64.2 Postoperative anteroposterior **a** and lateral **b** radiograph following revision TKA utilizing a press-fit metaphyseal sleeve with a fluted stem (Depuy Sigma and Depuy MBT, Warsaw, IN) and cement directly under the tibial baseplate without any distal cement

obtained during a prior visit, demonstrate medial deviation of the mechanical axis.

- **Diagnosis**

Aseptic loosening of the tibial and femoral component.

- **Treatment**

64

Planned revision TKA with removal of both components and placement of metaphyseal sleeves for reconstruction of any boney defects. Surgical goals are to achieve implant stability while also restoring the native joint line (Fig. 64.2). Intraoperatively, the tibial component is noted to be grossly loose and removed manually with minimal effort; the femoral component is also noted to be loose and removed without difficulty and with minimal iatrogenic bone loss. Postoperatively, the patient is allowed to fully weight bear without restrictions and at early follow-up has a stable, painless knee with no radiolucencies.

64.3 Surgical Technique

The patient is placed in a routine supine position with a tourniquet, and the prior skin incision is utilized and extended as necessary. The workflow (Fig. 64.3) proceeds in a systematic and sequential manner from initial implant removal, thorough debridement, and lavage followed by canal reaming to establish stem diameter (Fig. 64.4). After each canal is reamed, attention is turned then to the femur followed by the tibia.

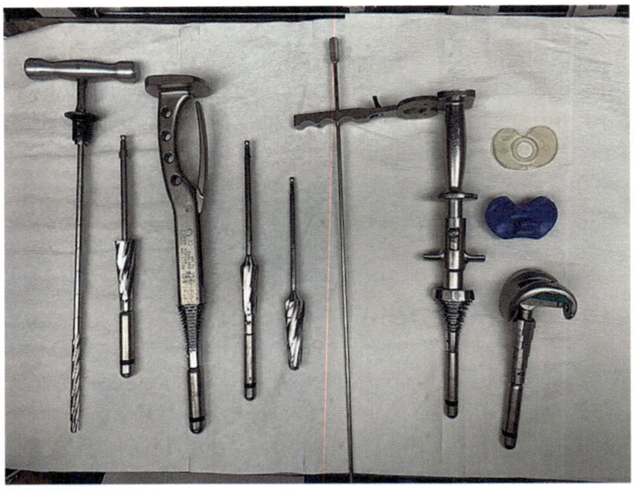

Fig. 64.3 Summary view of the instrumentation and associated usage and workflow moving from left to right

Femoral preparation begins with assessing for any bone loss and identifying anatomic landmarks to establish the native joint line. Initial distal reaming prior to broaching (Fig. 64.5a) is critical to avoid iatrogenic fracture (Fig. 64.5b). After broaching, the femoral trials are placed and checked relative to the prior identified landmarks for alignment and joint line position (Fig. 64.5c, d).

Following femoral preparation, attention is turned to the tibia (Fig. 64.6). Similarly, a proximal reamer is used prior to broaching to avoid iatrogenic fracture. After seating of the final broach, the upper flat surface of the broach is used as an uncaptured tibial cutting guide (Fig. 64.6c) to make a perpendicular and flat cut of the proximal tibia, thereby maximizing contact area (Fig. 64.6d, e). Trialing is then performed (Fig. 64.6f), and the final joint line position, range-of-motion, stability, and patellar tracking are assessed.

With satisfactory trialing, attention is then turned to implantation. The surgical team changes gloves, and the final components are assembled on the back table (Fig. 64.7a). The femur is implanted first, followed by the tibia.

> In order to maximize initial stability and also facilitate implant removal in the event of a re-revision, cement is only placed under the tibial baseplate (Fig. 64.7b, c).

In this situation, the amount of anteromedial bone loss was filled in completely with cement (Fig. 64.2a).

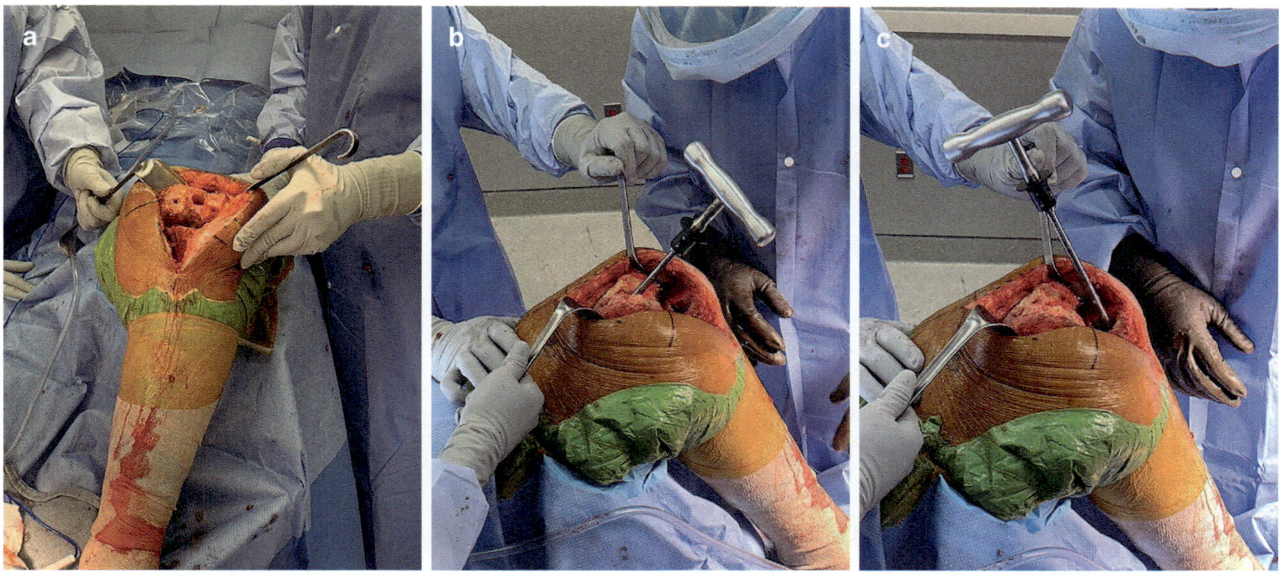

Fig. 64.4 Femoral and tibial bone loss following implant removal, thorough debridement, and lavage **a**, which was followed by initial manual reaming to establish the femoral **b** and tibial **c** canals

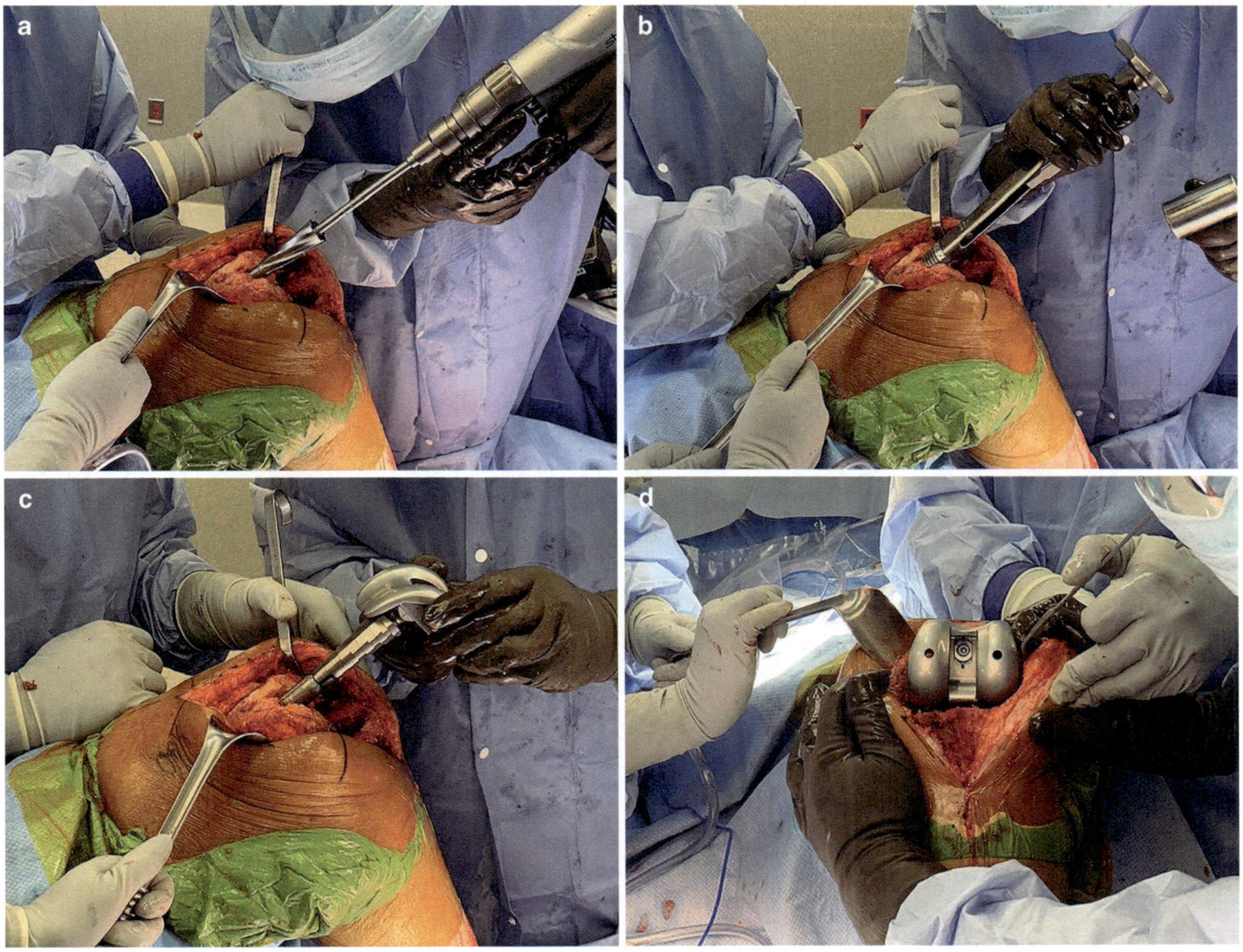

Fig. 64.5 **a–d** Preparation of the femur after reaming to establish canal diameter. The distal portion of the femoral metadiaphysis is reamed **a** to accommodate the broach **b** after which sizing is sequentially increased until a stable interference fit is obtained. The trial femur is then placed **c** and checked for proper position and rotation **d**

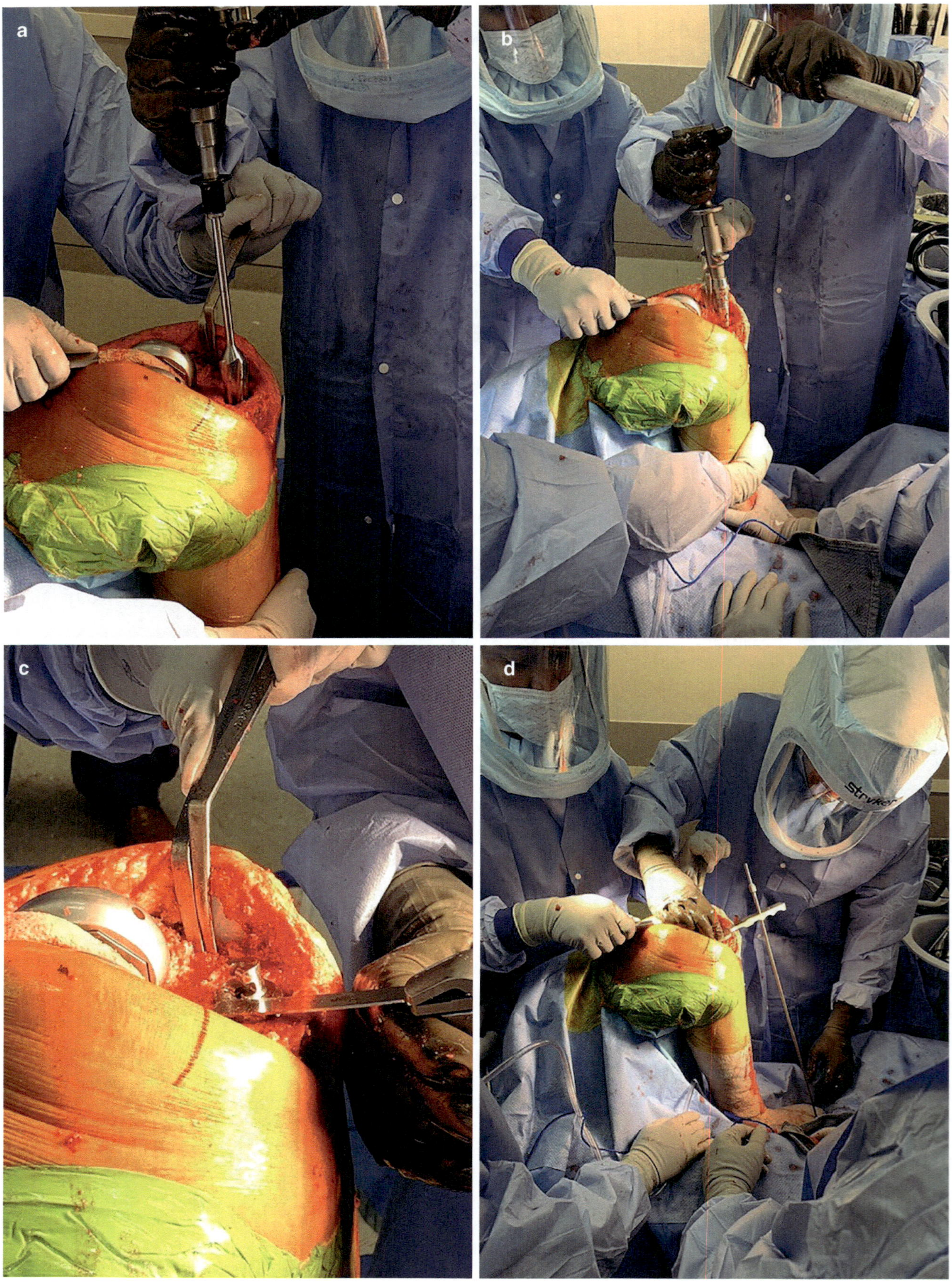

64

■ **Fig. 64.6** Tibia preparation begins with proximal tibia reaming **a** followed by sequential broaching **b**. The final broach is used as an uncaptured tibial guide to remove any remaining bone **c** in order to achieve a tibial cut that is neutral to the mechanical axis **d**. A flat cut maximizes contact area **e** for implant stability (note bone loss isolated to the antero-medial tibia). Trialing **f** is then performed using the last sized broach

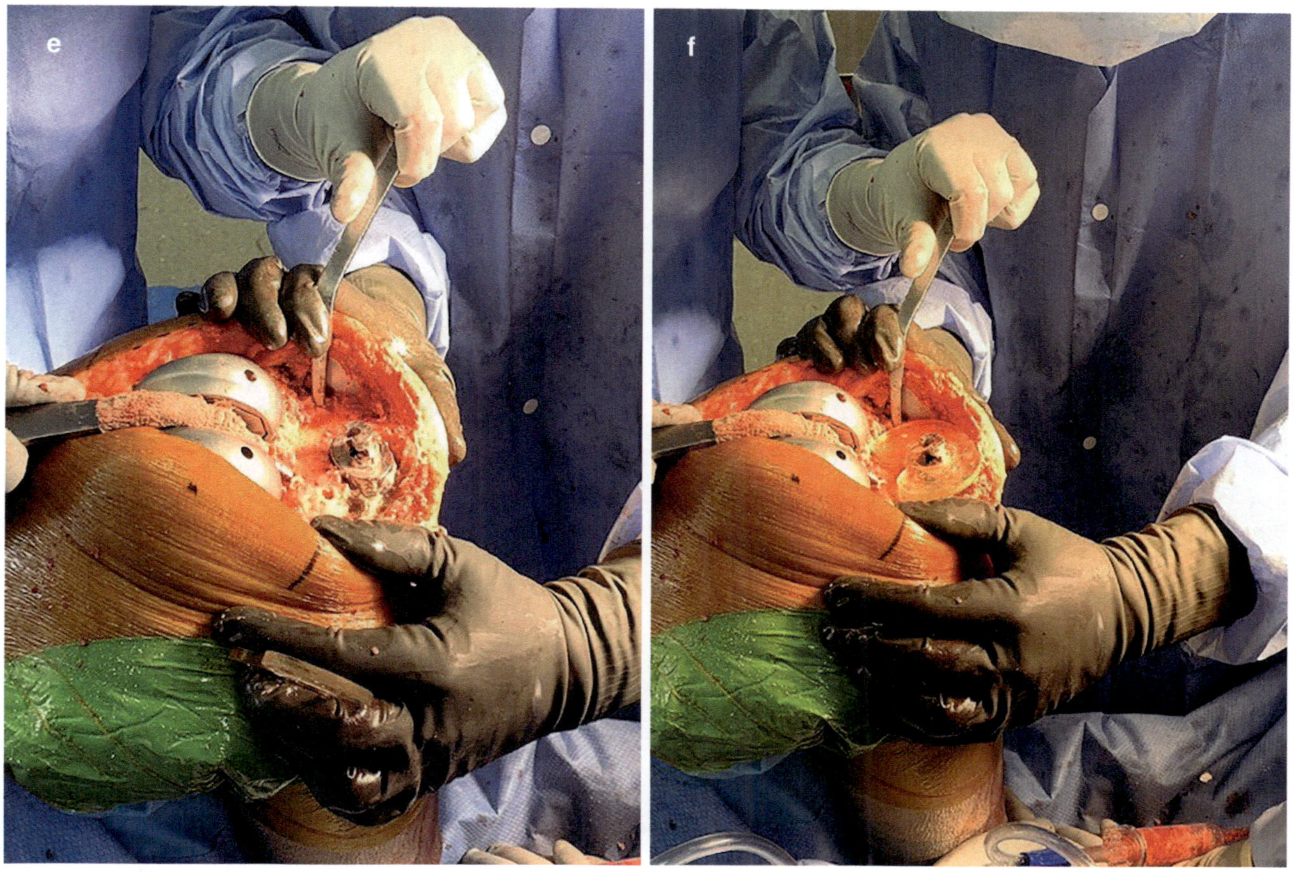

Fig. 64.6 (continued)

Final reduction is then performed, and the surgical arthrotomy and incision are closed in a routine fashion.

64.4 Discussion and Literature Review

The recent literature for metaphyseal cones and sleeves has been encouraging with both cones (Table 64.1) and sleeves (Table 64.2) demonstrating excellent osseointegration and low aseptic loosening rates at early to mid-term follow-up. Although promising when compared to results with allograft or long cemented stems, which were observed to have loosening rates of 6.5% at similar time points, further long-term surveillance is warranted.

Sleeves were recently reviewed by Martin-Hernandez and colleagues (Martin-Hernandez et al. 2017) who in a retrospective study of 134 patients at mean 6-year follow-up (range, 3–9 years) observed no cases of aseptic loosening and ingrowth in >99% of stems. When septic failures were excluded, osseointegration was seen in 100% of the cases. No progressive radiolucencies or implant migration was seen; however, the authors did report three cases of end-of-stem pain.

Outcomes of metaphyseal cones with a similar follow-up period were reported by Kamath et al. (2015) who reviewed 66 porous tantalum cones at a mean 6-year follow-up (range, 5–9 years). Osseous ingrowth was observed in 65 of 66 cones, and progressive radiolucencies were observed in two of the cones; however, only one cone needed to be revised.

> The choice between a cone or a sleeve is primarily surgeon preference as both options have thus far demonstrated successful outcomes. While cones require cement at the cone–implant interface, the use of sleeves gives the surgeon flexibility to use both hybrid cemented and fully cementless options.

Although there are theoretical concerns with the durability of the cone cement–implant interface since it experiences more sheer stress, this has not been manifest in the literature as greater rates of aseptic loosening.

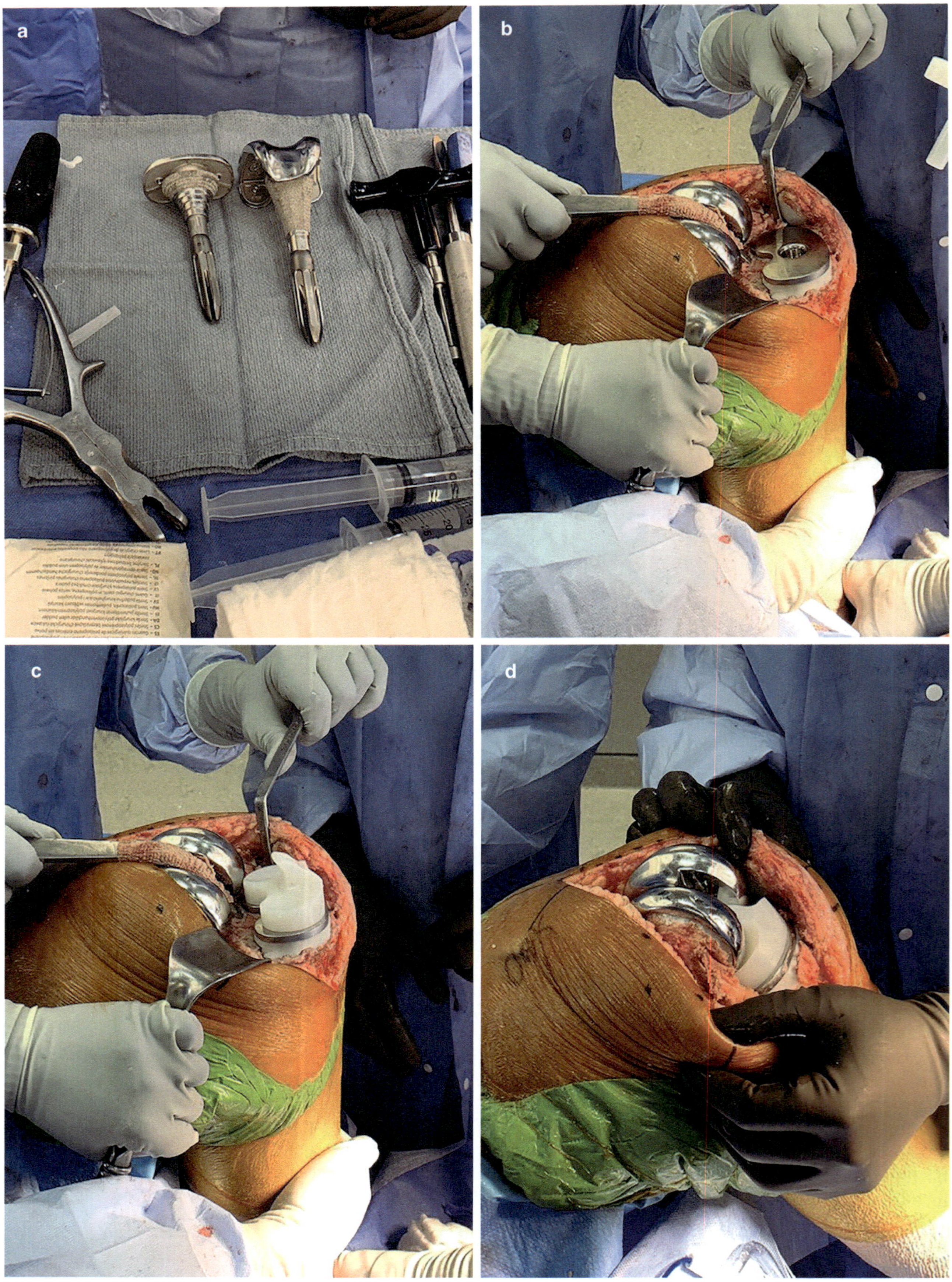

64

Fig. 64.7 Femoral and tibial components are assembled **a**; a hybrid fixation method is used where cement is only placed under the tibial baseplate **b** and **c** with satisfactory final reduction **d**

Table 64.1 Outcomes of sleeve in revision TKA

Study	Patients (*n*)	Follow-up (years)	Ingrowth	Aseptic revisions
Alexander et al. (2013)	30	2	100%	0%
Agarwal et al. (2013)	103	3.5	98%	2%
Huang et al. (2014)	83	2	97%	2.7%
Barnett et al. (2014)	36	3	96%	0%
Bugler et al. (2015)	34	2	100%	0%
Dalury and Barrett (2016)	45	4	99%	1%
Martin-Hernandez et al. (2017)	134	6	99%	0%
Zanirato et al. (2018)	46	2	91%	0%
Watters et al. (2017)	104	5	99%	0%
Fedorka et al. (2018)	50	5	93%	2.7%

Table 64.2 Outcomes of cones in revision TKA

Study	Patients (*n*)	Follow-up (years)	Ingrowth	Aseptic revisions
Rao et al. (2013)	72	3	100%	0%
Jensen et al. (2012)	36	3.5	97.3%	2.7%
De Martino et al. (2015)	73	7	100%	0%
Brown et al. (2015)	83	4	99%	1.2%
Kamath et al. (2015)	63	6	96.8%	1.5%
You et al. (2019)	15	2	100%	0%

Similarly, the concern for iatrogenic fracture with broaching for sleeves can be avoided with a careful broaching technique.

It is the recommendation of the authors that surgeons choose the approach with which they are most familiar in order to maximize patient outcomes (Kim et al. 2018).

Take-Home Messages

- Identify patients with significant bone loss preoperatively and be equipped with the proper implants and instrumentation to reconstruct the defects.
- Use anatomic landmarks (epicondyles, distance from inferior patellar pole, medial meniscus remnant) to identify the native joint line.
- Take care when broaching, particularly with sclerotic bone, as there is a risk for intraoperative fracture.
- A hybrid cement technique where cement is placed under the tibia baseplate will enhance initial implant stability.
- Stems, if oversized or too distal, may cause end-of-stem pain. Using a slotted or "clothespin" design may help prevent this occurrence.
- Full, immediate, weight bearing is allowed postoperatively.

References

Agarwal S, Azam A, Morgan-Jones R (2013) Metal metaphyseal sleeves in revision total knee replacement. Bone Joint J 95-B(12):1640–1644. https://doi.org/10.1302/0301--620X.95B12.31190

Alexander GE, Bernasek TL, Crank RL, Haidukewych GJ (2013) Cementless metaphyseal sleeves used for large tibial defects in revision total knee arthroplasty. J Arthroplast 28(4):604–607. https://doi.org/10.1016/j.arth.2012.08.006

Barnett SL, Mayer RR, Gondusky JS, Choi L, Patel JJ, Gorab RS (2014) Use of stepped porous titanium metaphyseal sleeves for tibial defects in revision total knee arthroplasty: short term results. J Arthroplast 29(6):1219–1224. https://doi.org/10.1016/j.arth.2013.12.026

Beckmann NA, Mueller S, Gondan M, Jaeger S, Reiner T, Bitsch RG (2015) Treatment of severe bone defects during revision total knee arthroplasty with structural allografts and porous metal cones-a systematic review. J Arthroplast 30(2):249–253. https://doi.org/10.1016/j.arth.2014.09.016

Brown NM, Bell JA, Jung EK, Sporer SM, Paprosky WG, Levine BR (2015) The use of trabecular metal cones in complex primary and revision total knee arthroplasty. J Arthroplast 30(9 Suppl):90–93. https://doi.org/10.1016/j.arth.2015.02.048

Bugler KE, Maheshwari R, Ahmed I, Brenkel IJ, Walmsley PJ (2015) Metaphyseal sleeves for revision total knee arthroplasty: good

short-term outcomes. J Arthroplast 30(11):1990–1994. https://doi.org/10.1016/j.arth.2015.05.015
Completo A, Fonseca F, Simões JA (2008) Strain shielding in proximal tibia of stemmed knee prosthesis: experimental study. J Biomech 41(3):560–566. https://doi.org/10.1016/j.jbiomech.2007.10.006
Dalury DF, Barrett WP (2016) The use of metaphyseal sleeves in revision total knee arthroplasty. Knee 23(3):545–548. https://doi.org/10.1016/j.knee.2016.02.005
De Martino I, De Santis V, Sculco PK, D'Apolito R, Assini JB, Gasparini G (2015) Tantalum cones provide durable mid-term fixation in revision TKA. Clin Orthop Relat Res 473(10):3176–3182. https://doi.org/10.1007/s11999-015-4338-2
Dennis DA, Little LR (2005) The structural allograft composite in revision total knee arthroplasty. Orthopedics 28(9):1005–1007. http://www.ncbi.nlm.nih.gov/pubmed/16190088
Fedorka CJ, Chen AF, Pagnotto MR, Crossett LS, Klatt BA (2018) Revision total knee arthroplasty with porous-coated metaphyseal sleeves provides radiographic ingrowth and stable fixation. Knee Surg Sports Traumatol Arthrosc 26(5):1500–1505. https://doi.org/10.1007/s00167-017-4493-y
Huang R, Barrazueta G, Ong A et al (2014) Revision total knee arthroplasty using metaphyseal sleeves at short-term follow-up. Orthopedics 37(9):e804–e809. https://doi.org/10.3928/01477447--20140825-57
Jensen CL, Petersen MM, Schrøder HM, Flivik G, Lund B (2012) Revision total knee arthroplasty with the use of trabecular metal cones: a randomized radiostereometric analysis with 2 years of follow-up. J Arthroplast 27(10):1820–1826, e2. https://doi.org/10.1016/j.arth.2012.04.036
Kamath AF, Lewallen DG, Hanssen AD (2015) Porous tantalum metaphyseal cones for severe tibial bone loss in revision knee arthroplasty: a five to nine-year follow-up. J Bone Joint Surg Am 97(3):216–223. https://doi.org/10.2106/JBJS.N.00540
Kim HJ, Lee O-S, Lee SH, Lee YS (2018) Comparative analysis between cone and sleeve in managing severe bone defect during revision total knee arthroplasty: a systematic review and meta-analysis. J Knee Surg 31(7):677–685. https://doi.org/10.1055/s--0037-1606564
Martin-Hernandez C, Floria-Arnal LJ, Muniesa-Herrero MP et al (2017) Mid-term results for metaphyseal sleeves in revision knee surgery. Knee Surg Sports Traumatol Arthrosc 25(12):3779–3785. https://doi.org/10.1007/s00167-016-4298-4
Murray PB, Rand JA, Hanssen AD (1994) Cemented long-stem revision total knee arthroplasty. Clin Orthop Relat Res 309:116–123. http://www.ncbi.nlm.nih.gov/pubmed/7994949
Panegrossi G, Ceretti M, Papalia M, Casella F, Favetti F, Falez F (2014) Bone loss management in total knee revision surgery. Int Orthop 38(2):419–427. https://doi.org/10.1007/s00264-013-2262-1
Rao BM, Kamal TT, Vafaye J, Moss M (2013) Tantalum cones for major osteolysis in revision knee replacement. Bone Joint J 95-B(8):1069–1074. https://doi.org/10.1302/0301-620X.95B8.29194
Watters TS, Martin JR, Levy DL, Yang CC, Kim RH, Dennis DA (2017) Porous-coated metaphyseal sleeves for severe femoral and tibial bone loss in revision TKA. J Arthroplast 32(11):3468–3473. https://doi.org/10.1016/j.arth.2017.06.025
You JS, Wright AR, Hasegawa I et al (2019) Addressing large tibial osseous defects in primary total knee arthroplasty using porous tantalum cones. Knee 26(1):228–239. https://doi.org/10.1016/j.knee.2018.11.001
Zanirato A, Cavagnaro L, Basso M, Divano S, Felli L, Formica M (2018) Metaphyseal sleeves in total knee arthroplasty revision: complications, clinical and radiological results. A systematic review of the literature. Arch Orthop Trauma Surg 138(7):993–1001. https://doi.org/10.1007/s00402-018-2967-0

Technology

Contents

Custom Cutting Blocks

Ankit Bansal, David Craig Loucks, Robert Greenhow, and Russell Presley Swann

Contents

E. Hansen, K.-D. Kühn (eds.), *Essentials of Cemented Knee Arthroplasty*,
https://doi.org/10.1007/978-3-662-63113-3_65

65.1 Introduction

Patient-specific instrumentation (PSI), or custom cutting blocks, can be an effective tool in performing total knee arthroplasty (TKA). Modern applications of PSI can yield precise restoration of alignment. It is a cost-effective means of reproducibly achieving targeted resections in TKA. The authors of this chapter prefer kinematic balancing as opposed to conventional mechanical techniques. This chapter outlines the history of PSI, modern design rationale, authors' preferred technique, and the results of custom cutting blocks.

65.2 History of Custom Cutting Blocks

Custom cutting blocks have been used over the past two decades for TKA, often leading to mixed results (Kosse et al. 2018; Laende et al. 2019; Li et al. 2019; Nunley et al. 2012; Zhu et al. 2017). Many early versions of this technology relied on alternative imaging sources for modeling the distal femur and proximal tibia.

> Although debate exists regarding ideal axial imaging source (An et al. 2017; Li et al. 2019; Wu et al. 2017), early failures may have been associated with the use of MRI, yielding inexact delineation between subchondral bone and cartilage.

The less reproducible positioning of the guide on cartilage could potentially lead to surgeon uncertainty and limit intra- and inter-observer reliability (Cucchi et al. 2018; Yamamura et al. 2019). Other manufacturers have used axial imaging with standing full-length X-rays to properly align the hip-knee-ankle axis. Severe flexion deformities or just position changes of the limb can alter these axes, also limiting the precision of implant position.

Newer designs use 3D CT technology, and they can manufacture 3D-printed models of the distal femur and proximal tibia with etchings to denote resection levels (Qiu et al. 2017). They retain the ability to attach extramedullary alignment rods to verify intended resections.

> Nonetheless, the ultimate goals of using custom cutting blocks in TKA remain the same: facilitate preoperative planning, optimize efficient surgical workflow, and achieve reproducible implant positions.

65.3 Modern PSI Design Rationale

The underlying quality of any patient-specific instrumentation (PSI) system is dependent on its ability to yield reproducible results (Huijbregts et al. 2016). Many of the previous failures of PSI have largely been associated with inaccuracies of the underlying system itself (Sassoon et al. 2015; Zhang et al. 2015). In fact, several authors have discouraged their routine use in TKA altogether (Kosse et al. 2018; Teeter et al. 2019). However, not all custom cutting blocks are created equally, and each has its own set of limitations (Cucchi et al. 2018; Randelli et al. 2019). Based on our extensive experience, we have identified a few qualities that an ideal PSI system should offer.

First, as mentioned previously, CT-based cutting blocks tend to be more precise than MRI-based ones (Li et al. 2019). MRI scans occasionally have difficulty differentiating subchondral bone with surrounding cartilage or ligamentous structures. They are also more expensive, necessitate longer scan times, and are more susceptible to patient artifacts. Periarticular implants about the knee could yield significant imaging scatter, limiting its ability to generate precise cutting blocks. Instead, CT-based technology yields a better tactile confirmation for the surgeon when placing the cutting block on bone once cartilage is removed using electrobovie cautery. Large osteophytes and prominent bony landmarks can serve as contact points with minimal surgical variability.

Second, the PSI system preferred by the authors provides 3D printed bone models. Distal femur and proximal tibia replicas are provided sterile intraoperatively (◘ Fig. 65.1). Intended resection thickness and angulation can be confirmed via direct comparison to the replica, which includes etchings for contact points and intended cuts (◘ Fig. 65.2).

> In addition, an ideal system should offer the ability for the surgeon to confirm alignment prior to actually making the cut.

Extramedullary alignment rod for the tibia, e.g., should pair with the cutting block for yet another visual confirmation (◘ Fig. 65.3). Therefore, the registration of the patient-specific guide to the patient's anatomy should be seamless.

65.4 Authors' Preferred Surgical Technique

The authors' preferred TKA technique employs kinematic balancing principles. The primary objective is to restore the native pre-arthritic femoral and tibial articular surfaces, with respect to angulation and slope (Howell et al. 2013a, b) (◘ Fig. 65.4). This begins with "anatomic resurfacing" of the distal and posterior femur, thereby restoring the flexion–extension axis and the patellofemoral axis of the knee (Eckhoff et al. 2005; Lee et al. 2017). The PSI plan generally calls for a 7-mm

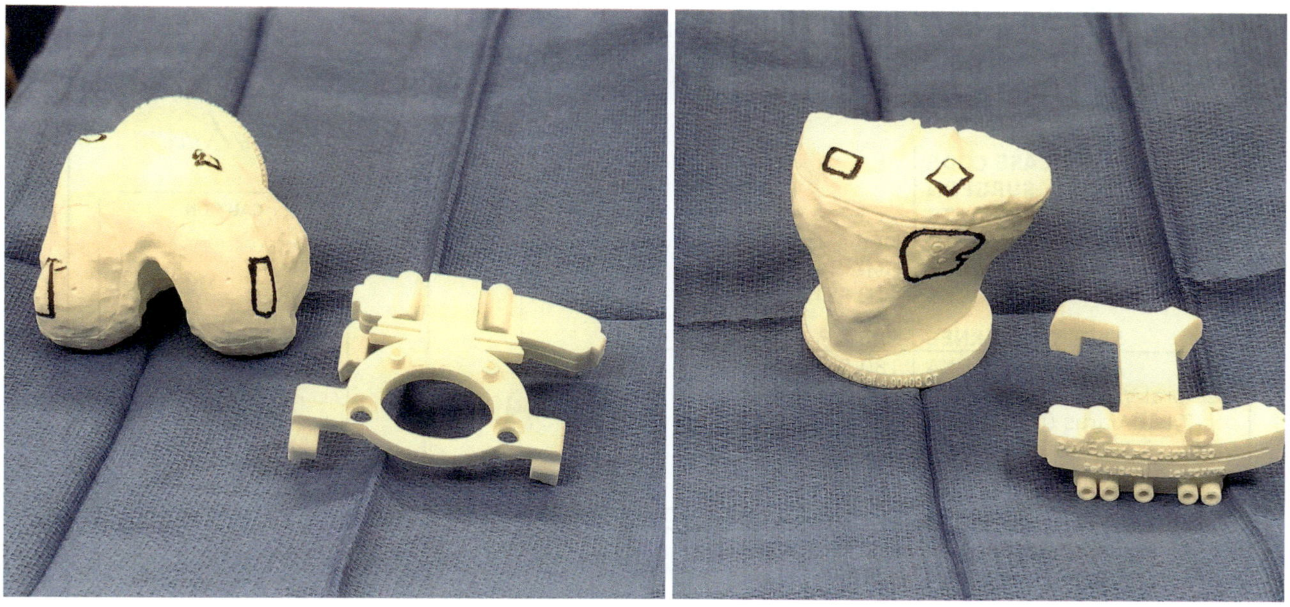

Fig. 65.1 Patient-specific 3D bone models of the distal femur and proximal tibia, with their respective cutting blocks

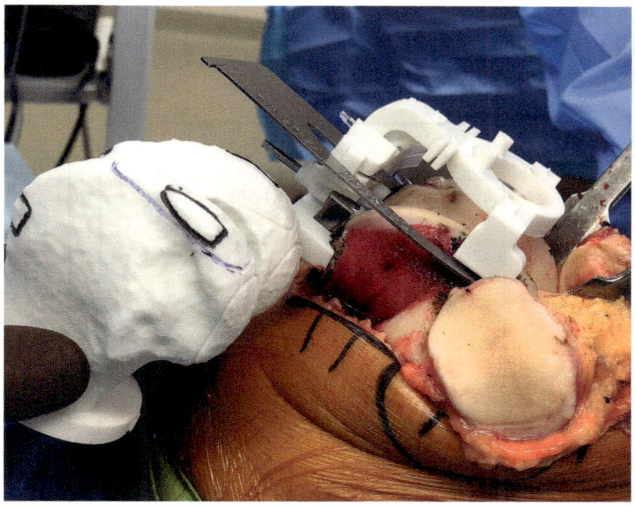

Fig. 65.2 Femoral bone model (with purple marker highlight showing distal femoral resection) beside exposed femur

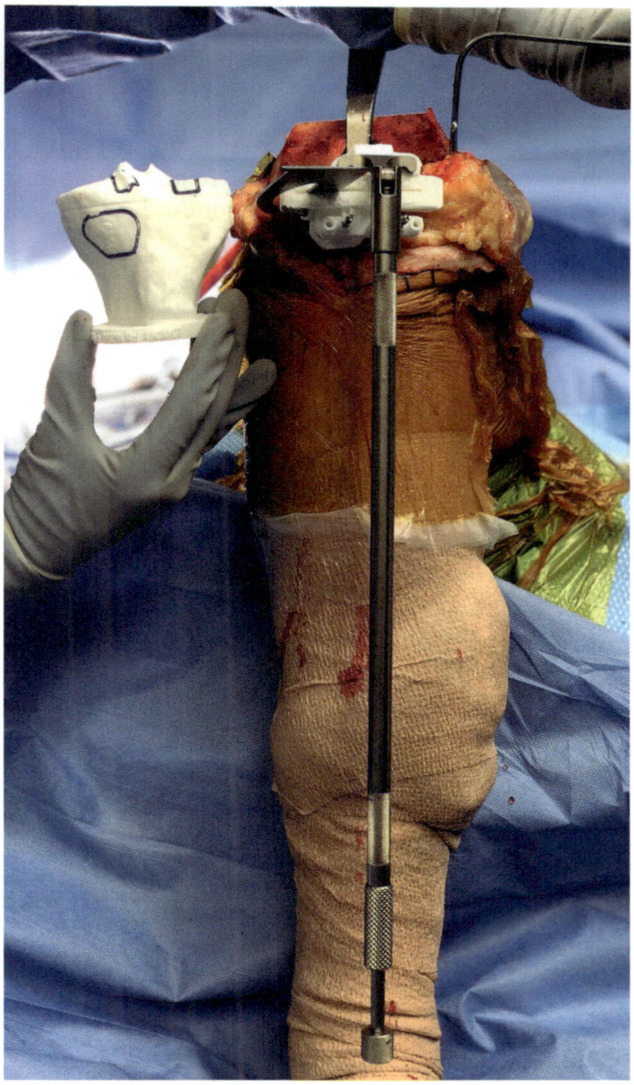

Fig. 65.3 Pinned tibial block with a drop rod and angel wing while holding a bone model

distal femoral and 6-mm posterior femoral bony resection. If we assume 2 mm cartilage thickness throughout, this corresponds to 9 mm and 8 mm, respectively, which are the exact dimensions of the femoral implant. Caliper measurements of each cut should facilitate immediate feedback to the surgeon. Patient-specific instrumentation can not only create this preoperative plan but can also help guide the surgeon's progress through the case, via these calipered cuts. Small adjustments can be made along the way to ensure intended alignment and eventual balancing.

As many have alluded previously, the flexion–extension placement of the distal femoral component is critical to the overall balancing of the knee. It determines

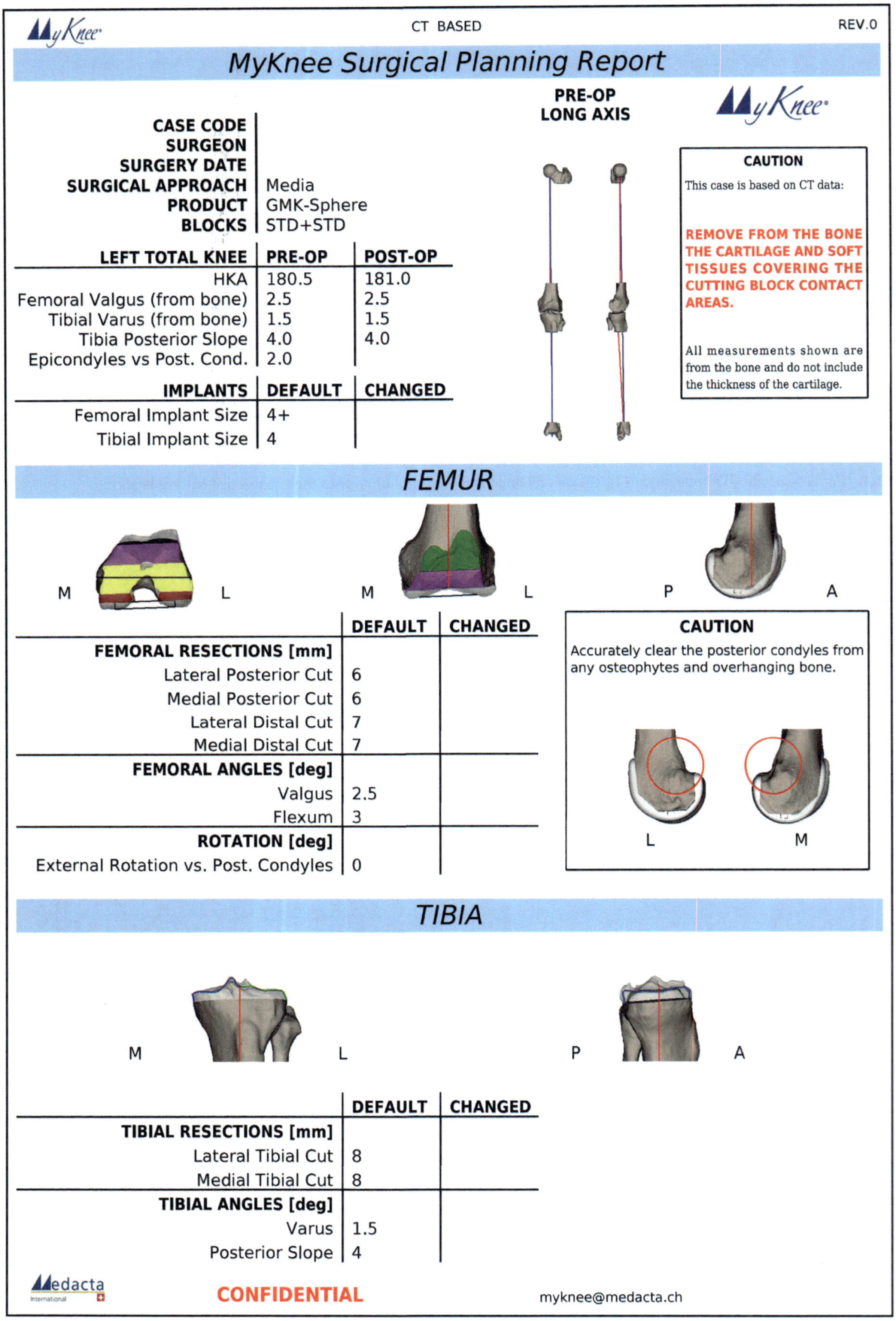

MyKnee CT BASED REV.0

MyKnee Surgical Planning Report

CASE CODE	
SURGEON	
SURGERY DATE	
SURGICAL APPROACH	Media
PRODUCT	GMK-Sphere
BLOCKS	STD+STD

LEFT TOTAL KNEE	PRE-OP	POST-OP
HKA	180.5	181.0
Femoral Valgus (from bone)	2.5	2.5
Tibial Varus (from bone)	1.5	1.5
Tibia Posterior Slope	4.0	4.0
Epicondyles vs Post. Cond.	2.0	

IMPLANTS	DEFAULT	CHANGED
Femoral Implant Size	4+	
Tibial Implant Size	4	

PRE-OP LONG AXIS

CAUTION

This case is based on CT data:

REMOVE FROM THE BONE THE CARTILAGE AND SOFT TISSUES COVERING THE CUTTING BLOCK CONTACT AREAS.

All measurements shown are from the bone and do not include the thickness of the cartilage.

FEMUR

	DEFAULT	CHANGED
FEMORAL RESECTIONS [mm]		
Lateral Posterior Cut	6	
Medial Posterior Cut	6	
Lateral Distal Cut	7	
Medial Distal Cut	7	
FEMORAL ANGLES [deg]		
Valgus	2.5	
Flexum	3	
ROTATION [deg]		
External Rotation vs. Post. Condyles	0	

CAUTION

Accurately clear the posterior condyles from any osteophytes and overhanging bone.

TIBIA

	DEFAULT	CHANGED
TIBIAL RESECTIONS [mm]		
Lateral Tibial Cut	8	
Medial Tibial Cut	8	
TIBIAL ANGLES [deg]		
Varus	1.5	
Posterior Slope	4	

Medacta International

CONFIDENTIAL

myknee@medacta.ch

Fig. 65.4 Resting knee alignment and planned resections in patient-specific kinematically balanced knee arthroplasty. MyKnee preoperative planning prepared by Medacta International MySolutions department. (Courtesy of Medacta International SA) the native arc of flexion and extension of the tibia on the femur (Howell et al. 2013a; Roth et al. 2015). In conventional TKA instruments, variability exists for the distal femoral starting drill, through which an intramedullary guide determines sagittal alignment. Instead, PSI guides allow very little variability in this plane of motion and can restore the neutral sagittal plane quite reproducibly (Li et al. 2019; Yamamura et al. 2019).

Once the distal femoral cut is made, the 4-in-1 cutting block can be placed using the planned pinholes. Check for anterior notching should be performed at this time. Posterior femoral condyle cuts are addressed first. Similar to the distal cuts, the posterior cuts should be merely a resurfacing of the femur, accounting for cartilage loss. Planned resections are generally 6 mm of bone on each side. Calipered measurements should equal 5 mm in worn and 7 mm in unworn situations. Upon confirmation of these, the remaining chamfer cuts can be completed.

The proximal tibial resection is made using similar principles. If no bony wear is noted, an even resurfacing cut is made on the tibia. Kinematic balancing can be achieved by accounting for constitutional varus or valgus alignment into the preoperative plan. We most commonly set the proximal tibial resection at 6–8 mm. Native tibial slope is preserved up to 5°. Special consideration should be given to the sagittal alignment when planning for cruciate-retaining (CR), posterior stabilized (PS), ultracongruent (UC), or UC-medial sphere designs. In the implant advocated by the lead authors, asymmetric tibial trays lower the likelihood of malrotation and also gain better plateau coverage on cortical bone. Overall, PSI guides provide secondary checks for planned cuts when compared to the 3D model. Caliper measurements are used to confirm the depths of resection as tertiary confirmation (◘ Fig. 65.5).

Spacer blocks or trial components can provide an assessment of overall stability and motion. A variety of options exist to achieve a fine-tuned balancing of TKA. Commonly, 2° varus or valgus tibial recutting guides are used (◘ Fig. 65.6).

> The multistep quality assurance checks for femoral and tibial component positioning should be followed (Roth et al. 2015).

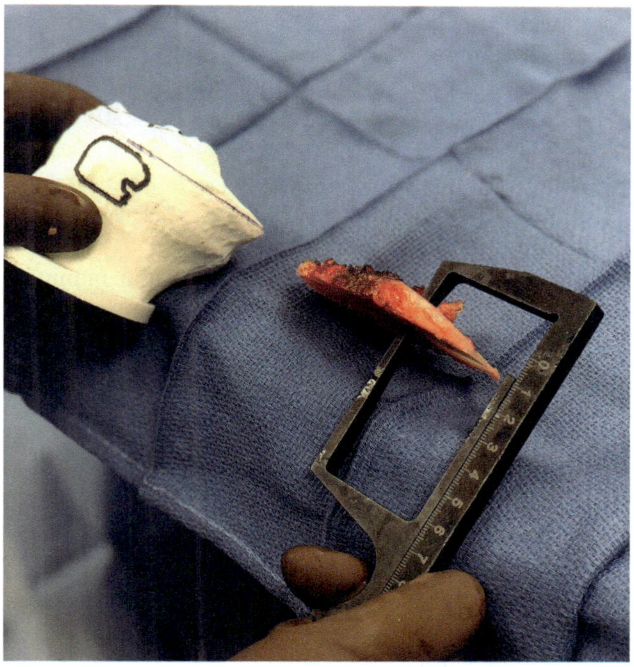

◘ **Fig. 65.5** C-caliper measuring tibial resection in comparison to the tibial bone model

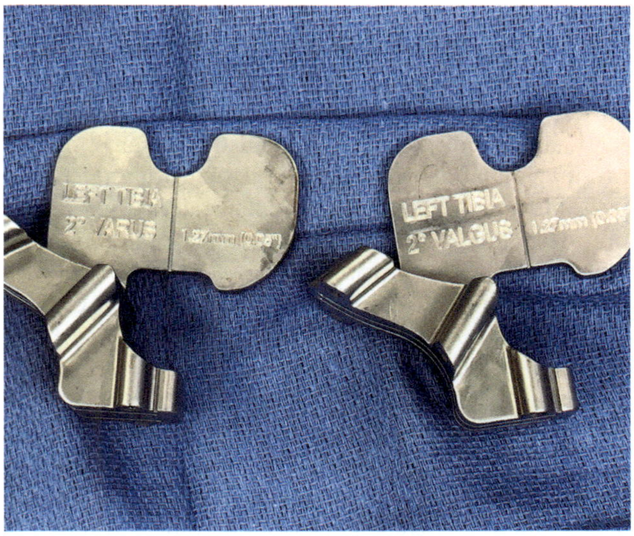

◘ **Fig. 65.6** Varus/valgus 2° recut guides

65.5 Results of Patient-Specific Instrumentation

The quality of any PSI system is directly linked to its ability to reproducibly achieve the intended target. Our published retrospective series of 132 patients showed that the average hip–knee–ankle (HKA) axis was restored within 1° of intended alignment. In a radiographic analysis of 1257 patients, PSI prevented severe limb malalignment and component position outliers better than conventional instruments (Pauzenberger et al. 2019). The mean deviation from the intended target was also significantly less. In a meta-analysis of 23 randomized trials Gong et al. (2019), reported a mean improved rotational alignment of the femoral component by 0.4°, a faster operative time by 7 min, and a lower perioperative blood loss by 90 cc relative standard instrumentation. No differences were found in the alignment of remaining components or the number of outliers. Recent advances in 3D CT technology have yielded an even closer restoration of implant position to their intended targets (Nabavi et al. 2017; Vide et al. 2017; Yamamura et al. 2019).

> Historically though, the translation from PSI's surgical precision to better clinical outcomes has lagged.

A randomized trial evaluating one particular manufacturer's PSI not only showed a lack of improvement in implant position but also found no significant improvement in blood loss or operative time (Randelli et al. 2019). Their PSI required a greater number of tibial recuts than conventional instruments. Kizaki et al. (2019) published a meta-analysis of 38 studies, 24 of which were randomized trials, totaling 3487 patients. They concluded that PSI did not improve patient-reported outcome scores any greater than conventional techniques. Although there was a small effect size improvement in blood loss, no difference was found in transfusion rates, as well as operative time and complication rates.

To comprehend this lack of clinical improvement, one must consider the concept of precision vs. accuracy. Although most modern PSI designs add precision in achieving certain target resections or alignment, it is possible that surgeons have been aiming for the wrong target. Trying to reach neutral mechanical alignment in all patients may be a mistake. The transition to kinematic alignment, keeping in mind the patients' constitutional alignment and their pre-arthritic state, may yield more reproducible results. This, added with PSI's improved precision, may improve total knee replacement outcomes in the future.

Several studies have supported this theory. Calliess et al. (2017) compared PSI kinematically aligned (KA) knees with non-PSI mechanically aligned (MA) ones in a prospective randomized study of 200 patients. PSI-KA knees showed greater mean Knee Society score (KSS) and WOMAC score improvements than MA. However, the authors noted some outliers in the KA group with worse outcomes, which correlated with deviations from the PSI plan. Laende et al. (2019) evaluated KA-PSI knees vs. mechanically aligned computer-assisted knees. No difference in longitudinal migration of the tibial component was found at 2-year follow-up in a study of 47 patients. Both groups showed mean migrations below acceptable thresholds. In addition, the degree of migration did not correlate with varus or valgus "malalignment" of the tibial component, relative to those placed neutral to the tibial axis, indicating stable fixation in both groups.

Aside from added surgical precision, using custom cutting blocks has some inherent advantages. PSI allows for proper preoperative planning, accommodating even the smallest extra-articular deformities.

> It averts the need to remove periarticular hardware unless directly impinging with the eventual components.

In fact, it can predict whether certain pins or resections will directly interfere with indwelling implants such as a femoral nail or screws.

> It obviates the need to enter the femoral intramedullary canal altogether, which itself has been correlated with decreased risk of fat embolus syndrome and overall blood loss (Cucchi et al. 2019; Leon et al. 2017).

PSI can also facilitate the commonly performed conversion from unicompartmental knee arthroplasty (UKA) to TKA. Its CT mapping accounts for the UKA prosthesis, and kinematic or mechanical alignment can be achieved thereafter. In addition, the overall efficient PSI workflow can translate to a single-use disposable system (Attard et al. 2019).

> Since component sizes are already planned, most cases can be optimized with minimal trays and trials, especially relevant to those operating at freestanding ambulatory surgery centers (ASCs) with limited sterilization capacity.

Modern advancements in computer navigation and robotic surgery have become increasingly popular in TKA. However, surgeons and health systems must consider the added costs associated with this, relative to the gain in surgical precision. Many require a similar preoperative CT scan as PSI but necessitate intraoperative registration and additional pinholes in the femoral and tibial shafts, which themselves can lead to complications (Blue et al. 2018; Wysocki et al. 2008). Furthermore, the significant capital costs in acquisition of these robots are not trivial. When comparing custom cutting blocks with robotically assisted surgery, PSI clearly has a distinct advantage in cost and intraoperative efficiency (Attard et al. 2019; DeHaan et al. 2014). Nonetheless, one could still argue against the routine use of any enhancing technology in certain healthcare environments. A recently published study from the Canadian healthcare system found that patient-specific instrumentation contributed very little to the overall perioperative efficiency, which did not justify the added cost per case (Teeter et al. 2019).

> Routine use of PSI is not without limitations. First, a limited CT scan is still required, which means added radiation and cost to the patient. Second, a 3-week planning period exists, where the guides and 3D bone replicas are engineered and manufactured, which in turn has a 6-month expiration.

This exists to retain the precision of the guides to the patients' anatomy, as progression of arthritis or changes in bony morphology can occur with time.

Conclusion

Use of custom cutting blocks, or patient-specific instrumentation (PSI), is a growing technology in TKA. It holds advantages in operating efficiency, surgical precision, and thorough preoperative planning. Although the translation to improved clinical outcomes relative to mechanical instrumentation lags behind, principles in kinematic balancing are showing a promising future. The combination of PSI in kinematically placed TKA may be a viable option for years to come.

Take-Home Messages

- Success after use of custom cutting blocks in TKA is dependent on imaging technique, surgical precision toward intended target, and its application to the patient with respect to alignment.
- Intraoperative secondary checks should be present to confirm intended resection and alignment prior to and after resections are made. Thereby, corrections can be made with each step.
- Use of patient-specific instrumentation has not yet translated to improved clinical outcomes when aiming for mechanical alignment in TKA. Combining PSI with kinematic alignment may yield improved outcomes.
- PSI allows proper preoperative planning, accommodates extra-articular deformities, and permits added OR efficiency.
- PSI is cost-effective when compared to navigated or robotically assisted TKA.

References

An VV, Sivakumar BS, Phan K, Levy YD, Bruce WJ (2017) Accuracy of MRI-based vs. CT-based patient-specific instrumentation in total knee arthroplasty: a meta-analysis. J Orthop Sci 22(1): 116–120

Attard A, Tawy GF, Simons M, Riches P, Rowe P, Biant LC (2019) Health costs and efficiencies of patient-specific and single-use instrumentation in total knee arthroplasty: a randomised controlled trial. BMJ Open Qual 8(2):e000493

Blue M, Douthit C, Dennison J, Caroom C, Jenkins M (2018) Periprosthetic fracture through a unicortical tracking pin site after computer navigated total knee replacement. Case Rep Orthop 2018:2381406

Calliess T, Bauer K, Stukenborg-Colsman C, Windhagen H, Budde S, Ettinger M (2017) PSI kinematic versus non-PSI mechanical alignment in total knee arthroplasty: a prospective, randomized study. Knee Surg Sports Traumatol Arthrosc 25(6):1743–1748

Cucchi D, Menon A, Compagnoni R, Ferrua P, Fossati C, Randelli P (2018) Significant differences between manufacturer and surgeon in the accuracy of final component size prediction with CT-based patient-specific instrumentation for total knee arthroplasty. Knee Surg Sports Traumatol Arthrosc 26(11):3317–3324

Cucchi D, Menon A, Zanini B, Compagnoni R, Ferrua P, Randelli P (2019) Patient-specific instrumentation affects perioperative blood loss in total knee arthroplasty. J Knee Surg 32(6):483–489

DeHaan AM, Adams JR, DeHart ML, Huff TW (2014) Patient-specific versus conventional instrumentation for total knee arthroplasty: peri-operative and cost differences. J Arthroplast 29(11):2065–2069

Eckhoff DG, Bach JM, Spitzer VM et al (2005) Three-dimensional mechanics, kinematics, and morphology of the knee viewed in virtual reality. J Bone Joint Surg Am 87(Suppl 2):71–80

Gong S, Xu W, Wang R et al (2019) Patient-specific instrumentation improved axial alignment of the femoral component, operative time and perioperative blood loss after total knee arthroplasty. Knee Surg Sports Traumatol Arthrosc 27(4):1083–1095

Howell SM, Papadopoulos S, Kuznik KT, Hull ML (2013a) Accurate alignment and high function after kinematically aligned TKA performed with generic instruments. Knee Surg Sports Traumatol Arthrosc 21(10):2271–2280

Howell SM, Howell SJ, Kuznik KT, Cohen J, Hull ML (2013b) Does a kinematically aligned total knee arthroplasty restore function without failure regardless of alignment category? Clin Orthop Relat Res 471(3):1000–1007

Huijbregts HJ, Khan RJ, Fick DP et al (2016) Component alignment and clinical outcome following total knee arthroplasty: a randomised controlled trial comparing an intramedullary alignment system with patient-specific instrumentation. Bone Joint J 98-B(8):1043–1049

Kizaki K, Shanmugaraj A, Yamashita F et al (2019) Total knee arthroplasty using patient-specific instrumentation for osteoarthritis of the knee: a meta-analysis. BMC Musculoskelet Disord 20(1):561

Kosse NM, Heesterbeek PJC, Schimmel JJP, van Hellemondt GG, Wymenga AB, Defoort KC (2018) Stability and alignment do not improve by using patient-specific instrumentation in total knee arthroplasty: a randomized controlled trial. Knee Surg Sports Traumatol Arthrosc 26(6):1792–1799

Laende EK, Richardson CG, Dunbar MJ (2019) A randomized controlled trial of tibial component migration with kinematic alignment using patient-specific instrumentation versus mechanical alignment using computer-assisted surgery in total knee arthroplasty. Bone Joint J 101-B(8):929–940

Lee YS, Howell SM, Won YY et al (2017) Kinematic alignment is a possible alternative to mechanical alignment in total knee arthroplasty. Knee Surg Sports Traumatol Arthrosc 25(11): 3467–3479

Leon VJ, Lengua MA, Calvo V, Lison AJ (2017) Use of patient-specific cutting blocks reduces blood loss after total knee arthroplasty. Eur J Orthop Surg Traumatol 27(2):273–277

Li Z, Yang Z, Liao W et al (2019) Fewer femoral rotational outliers produced with CT- than with MRI-based patient-specific instrumentation in total knee arthroplasty. Knee Surg Sports Traumatol Arthrosc 28(9):2930–2941

Nabavi A, Olwill CM, Do M, Wanasawage T, Harris IA (2017) Patient-specific instrumentation for total knee arthroplasty. J Orthop Surg (Hong Kong) 25(1):2309499016684754

Nunley RM, Ellison BS, Zhu J, Ruh EL, Howell SM, Barrack RL (2012) Do patient-specific guides improve coronal alignment in total knee arthroplasty? Clin Orthop Relat Res 470(3):895–902

Pauzenberger L, Munz M, Brandl G et al (2019) Patient-specific instrumentation improved three-dimensional accuracy in total knee arthroplasty: a comparative radiographic analysis of 1257 total knee arthroplasties. J Orthop Surg Res 14(1):437

Qiu B, Liu F, Tang B et al (2017) Clinical study of 3D imaging and 3D printing technique for patient-specific instrumentation in total knee arthroplasty. J Knee Surg 30(8):822–828
Randelli PS, Menon A, Pasqualotto S, Zanini B, Compagnoni R, Cucchi D (2019) Patient-specific instrumentation does not affect rotational alignment of the femoral component and perioperative blood loss in total knee arthroplasty: a prospective, randomized, controlled trial. J Arthroplasty 34(7):1374–1381. e1371
Roth JD, Howell SM, Hull ML (2015) Native knee laxities at 0 degrees, 45 degrees, and 90 degrees of flexion and their relationship to the goal of the gap-balancing alignment method of total knee arthroplasty. J Bone Joint Surg Am 97(20):1678–1684
Sassoon A, Nam D, Nunley R, Barrack R (2015) Systematic review of patient-specific instrumentation in total knee arthroplasty: new but not improved. Clin Orthop Relat Res 473(1):151–158
Teeter MG, Marsh JD, Howard JL et al (2019) A randomized controlled trial investigating the value of patient-specific instrumentation for total knee arthroplasty in the Canadian healthcare system. Bone Joint J 101-B(5):565–572
Vide J, Freitas TP, Ramos A, Cruz H, Sousa JP (2017) Patient-specific instrumentation in total knee arthroplasty: simpler, faster and more accurate than standard instrumentation-a randomized controlled trial. Knee Surg Sports Traumatol Arthrosc 25(8):2616–2621
Wu XD, Xiang BY, Schotanus MGM, Liu ZH, Chen Y, Huang W (2017) CT- versus MRI-based patient-specific instrumentation for total knee arthroplasty: a systematic review and meta-analysis. Surgeon 15(6):336–348
Wysocki RW, Sheinkop MB, Virkus WW, Della Valle CJ (2008) Femoral fracture through a previous pin site after computer-assisted total knee arthroplasty. J Arthroplast 23(3):462–465
Yamamura K, Minoda Y, Sugama R et al (2019) Design improvement in patient-specific instrumentation for total knee arthroplasty improved the accuracy of the tibial prosthetic alignment in the coronal and axial planes. Knee Surg Sports Traumatol Arthrosc 28(5):1560–1567
Zhang QM, Chen JY, Li H et al (2015) No evidence of superiority in reducing outliers of component alignment for patient-specific instrumentation for total knee arthroplasty: a systematic review. Orthop Surg 7(1):19–25
Zhu M, Chen JY, Chong HC et al (2017) Outcomes following total knee arthroplasty with CT-based patient-specific instrumentation. Knee Surg Sports Traumatol Arthrosc 25(8):2567–2572

Navigation in Total Knee Arthroplasty

Robert P. Runner, Travis Scudday, and Nader A. Nassif

Contents

E. Hansen, K.-D. Kühn (eds.), *Essentials of Cemented Knee Arthroplasty*,
https://doi.org/10.1007/978-3-662-63113-3_66

66.1 Introduction and History

Many factors contribute to the long-term success of total knee arthroplasty (TKA):

- Patient selection
- Prosthesis design
- Soft tissue balancing
- Overall alignment of the limb

> Surgical factors for proper translational and rotational placement of the prosthetic components are key as incorrect positioning can lead to accelerated wear, component loosening, or poor functional performance (Delp et al. 1998).

With the goal of an overall neutral mechanical axis, studies sought to identify the average normal anatomic angles during functional motion to help determine appropriate knee arthroplasty component position. In most patients, the native tibia is in slight varus and the native distal femur in valgus with 75% of the knee joint load passing through the medial tibial plateau during single-limb stance (Hsu et al. 1990). Even early on in long-term follow-up of knee replacements, coronal alignment has been key for long-term success of implants. One early retrospective review of a single implant design from patients from 1971 to 1975 published in 1983 found higher failure rates, as high as 88% (8 of 9 knees), in implants placed where the overall coronal alignment of the limb was greater than 6° of varus (Bargren et al. 1983). Different guide systems have been developed for intramedullary and extramedullary techniques for cutting the tibia with reasonable success (Evans et al. 1995). However, using conventional tools in early arthroplasty cases, 26% failed to achieve the satisfactory alignment of the limb of 4–10° valgus (Petersen and Engh 1988). In another study, up to a quarter of proximal tibial cuts were improper when using conventional-technique guides (Cates et al. 1993).

Accurate component placement is essential for long-term success in knee replacement (Lotke and Ecker 1977). Studies of early knee replacement designs show postoperative alignment and its effect on radiolucent lines (Hvid and Nielsen 1984). In one study, when the mechanical axis of the limb (Maquet's line) drawn from the center of the femoral head to the center of the talus passes through the middle third of the prosthesis, there was significantly less loosening (3%) vs. when the line passed medial or lateral to the middle third of the prosthesis (24% loosening) (Jeffery et al. 1991). Another longer-term follow-up of early TKA patients showed overall varus alignment leading to higher failure rates. It recommended neutral to slight valgus alignment for the best chance at long-term survival (Ritter et al. 1994).

> Given that malalignment of the femoral and tibial components can lead to early failure, navigation systems have been developed to assist in component placement with the idea that better component alignment will result in improved implant survival and outcomes.

Some of the first computer-assisted knee replacements were performed over 2 decades ago, in 1997 (Delp et al. 1998). The initial focus was on coronal plane alignment of the mechanical axis. Nonimage-based (Krackow et al. 1999) and image-based systems have been around for decades dating back to the 1980s. Active robotic devices were also developed in this same timeframe, with many companies from across the world emerging to innovate on this new technology. Further technology for sensors for component rotation and intraoperative measurement of forces across the knee with a range of motion are currently available as well and are the focus of another chapter (▶ Chap. 68). Within orthopedics, new devices or technology are frequently developed with proposed theoretical benefits but do not guarantee better patient outcomes, and adaptation in the market can take time (Bhattacharyya et al. 2006). Navigation within knee arthroplasty is one emerging technology, and these tools are becoming more mainstream but still are not used in a majority of TKA cases (Antonios et al. 2019; Delp et al. 1998).

There are several definitions that need to be clarified when discussing navigation systems:

Definitions Concerning Navigation Systems

- *Calibration* is the process performed on the surgical tools to allow them to be identified with great accuracy within the 3D anatomical model.
- *Registration* is the process of collecting the data using tracked instruments of relevant positions of anatomic landmarks in space for the computer to build the frame of reference of the leg/knee.
- The *frame of reference* is the 3D anatomical model of the knee that is created in the digital space. In navigation systems that use preoperative imaging (often CT scans), matching is performed to overlay the frame of reference onto the patient's anatomy.
- The *working volume* is the volume in three-dimensional space where the tracking system can accurately reproducibly trace a calibrated object with trackers (Picard et al. 2016).

In orthopedics, three types of computer-assisted systems exist:

- Active systems use robotic tools to perform the surgical tasks of cutting or drilling with no intervention of the surgeon.

- Semi-active systems utilize controlled robotic tools that only allow a surgeon to perform a task within a specific predetermined frame of reference.
- Passive systems guide the position of standard templates/cutting blocks, but the surgeon uses traditional instruments (i.e., saws) to perform the task under surgeon control.

> Knee navigation systems are an example of a passive system as the surgeon uses the technology to assist the orientation of guides but performs the cuts him-/herself (Picard et al. 2016).

> Computer navigation is increasing worldwide over time, with a documented use across the United States (Gholson et al. 2017) of up to 7% of computer navigation or robotic-assisted TKA in 2014 (Antonios et al. 2019), and up to 22.8% in 2012 in Australia (de Steiger et al. 2015) steadily increasing to 33.2% in the Australian registry in 2018 (Australian Orthopaedic Association National Joint Replacement Registry (AOANJRR) 2019).

> There are marked regional differences in the adaptation of this technology, and they are associated with increased hospital charges (Antonios et al. 2019).

This chapter explores indications and contraindications for the technology, type of devices, registration techniques, complications, current evidence on results of navigation, and pearls and pitfalls in current practice.

66.2 Uses/Indications

Some surgeons are routinely using navigation in all cases with the hope to decrease the incidence of malposition of components, especially the tibia, outside the acceptable range of 90 ± 3° (Berend et al. 2004; D'Lima et al. 2001; Ritter et al. 2011; Werner et al. 2005).

Even in nondeformed anatomy, when using conventional femoral intramedullary guides, the starting point for entry into the femoral canal can drastically affect the varus/valgus and flexion/extension of the cut relative to the diaphysis of the femur. Anterior translation of the entry point leads to extension; posterior translation leads to flexion (Gangadharan et al. 2010; Mihalko et al. 2005).

The advantage of navigation, however, is to help execute total knee replacements in clinical settings where it would be difficult to perform with standard instrumentation. Patients with extra-articular deformities (especially on the femoral side) can benefit from navigation (Fehring et al. 2006; Hazratwala et al. 2016; Lee et al. 2014; Matassi et al. 2019; Shah et al. 2013; Takasaki et al. 2010).

> Navigation allows the surgeon to establish the overall mechanical axis of the limb irrespective of the deformity for appropriate component positioning to restore a neutral mechanical axis (Fig. 66.1).

Additionally, the accuracy of the cuts when using navigation is validated in cadavers and intraoperative measurements—thus, the navigation works when there is

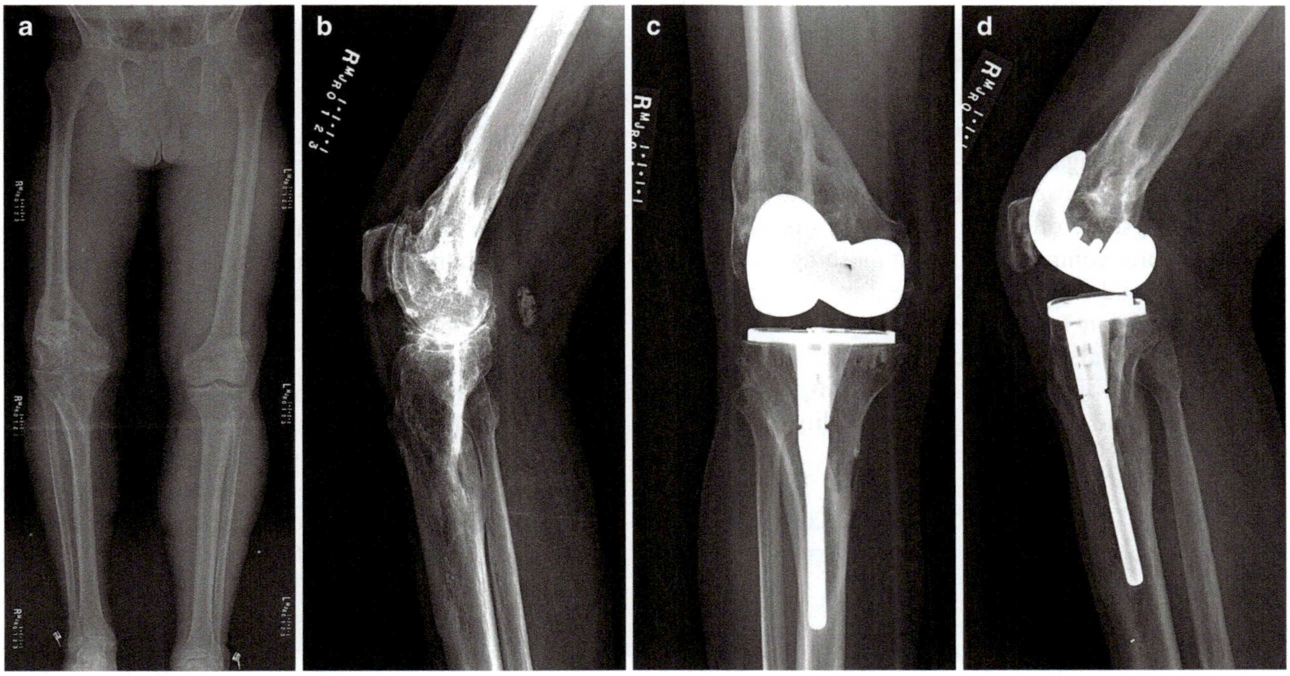

Fig. 66.1 Scanogram of bilateral lower extremity **a** and a lateral of the right knee **b** of a patient with a distal femur fracture malunion where standard intramedullary instrumentation cannot be used on the femoral side. AP **c** and lateral **d** radiographs showing a TKA using navigation to avoid femoral instrumentation. The tibia was navigated using an intramedullary guide for stem placement to bypass the defect in the tibial shaft

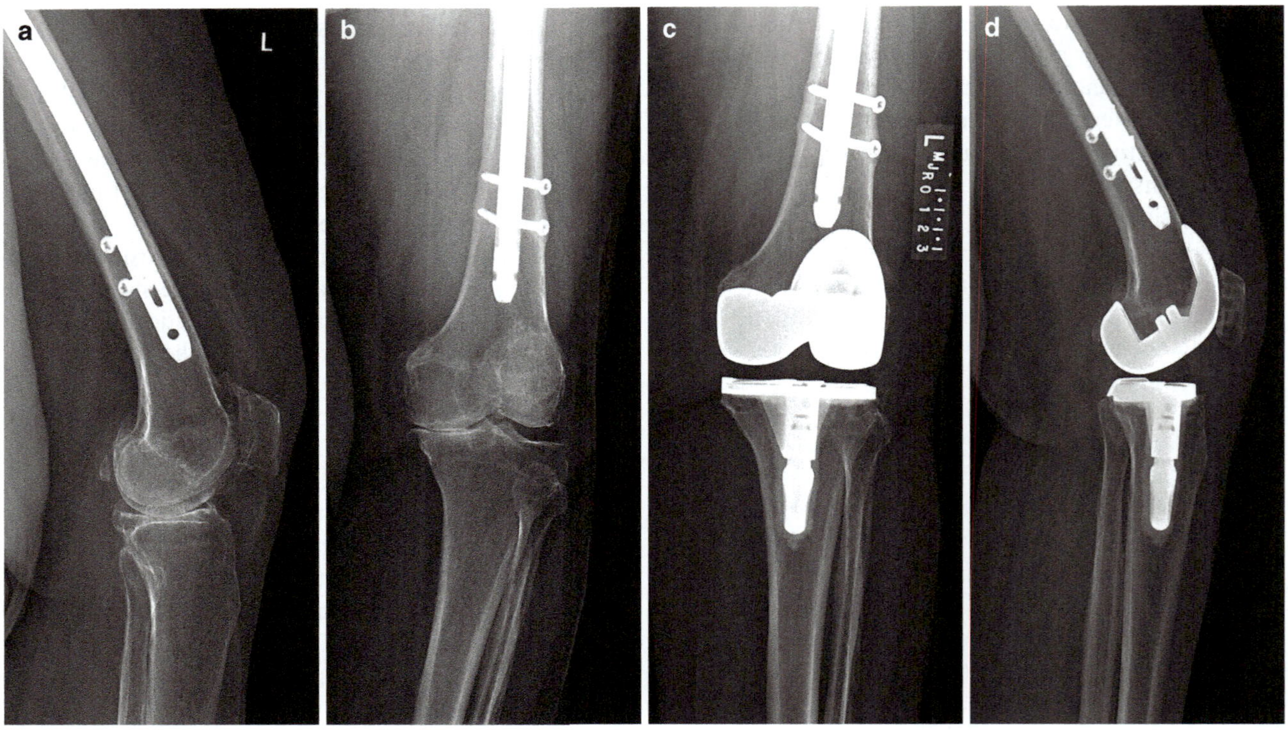

■ **Fig. 66.2** AP **a** and lateral **b** radiographs showing an arthritic knee distal to a cephalomedullary nail. A TKA was performed **c**, **d**; using navigation; standard intramedullary femoral instrumentation could not be used given the presence of previous femoral hardware

accurate registration, no movement of the pins, and good surgical technique (Biant et al. 2008).

Patients with prior fractures and hardware in place may also benefit from the use of navigation (Fehring et al. 2006; Lin et al. 2014). On the tibial side, the proximal tibial cut can usually be made with standard extramedullary instrumentation; however, femoral hardware can interfere with the placement of the intramedullary cutting jig. Again, navigation in this circumstance would be an advantage to the surgeon (■ Fig. 66.2).

Although navigation has been traditionally utilized for establishing an overall neutral mechanical axis, some navigation systems offer features to aid with placement of the femoral component and establishing its rotation as well as to aid with the assessment of the flexion and extension tension to help reproduce a more balanced knee (Siston et al. 2005; Stiehl and Heck 2015; Stockl et al. 2004) (■ Fig. 66.3). These functions, however, are less accurate and result in higher variability that is both surgeon- and system-dependent.

> Understanding the abilities of the particular system that a surgeon uses is essential to understanding its limitations.

Other less common indications for navigation use include patients with a prior history of osteomyelitis as well as patients who have intramedullary enchondroma. In both instances, surgeons should avoid instrumenting the medullary canal to avoid possible sequelae. Patients with poor pulmonary status may also realize some theoretical benefit from navigation as the medullary canal is not violated, resulting in a decreased risk of fat embolism, although this has not been demonstrated in the literature thus far (Kim et al. 2008).

66.3 Contraindications

Surgeons must also be aware of cases where navigation can lead them down the wrong path. The most common reason for inability to use a particular system is an inability to properly register the anatomy. Whether accelerometer-based or imaging-based systems are utilized, there is the potential at the time of surgery that the anatomic registration may not be accurate. Following registration, surgeons should confirm its accuracy before proceeding further. Surgeons must also be diligent in evaluating the quality and angles of the cuts recommended by the navigation system on the patient in order to avoid a poor outcome (Hasegawa et al. 2013; Laskin 2003; Plaskos et al. 2002; Robinson et al. 2006).

> Some factors that can lead to improper registration include obesity (Fehring et al. 2006) and improperly placed tracking pins.

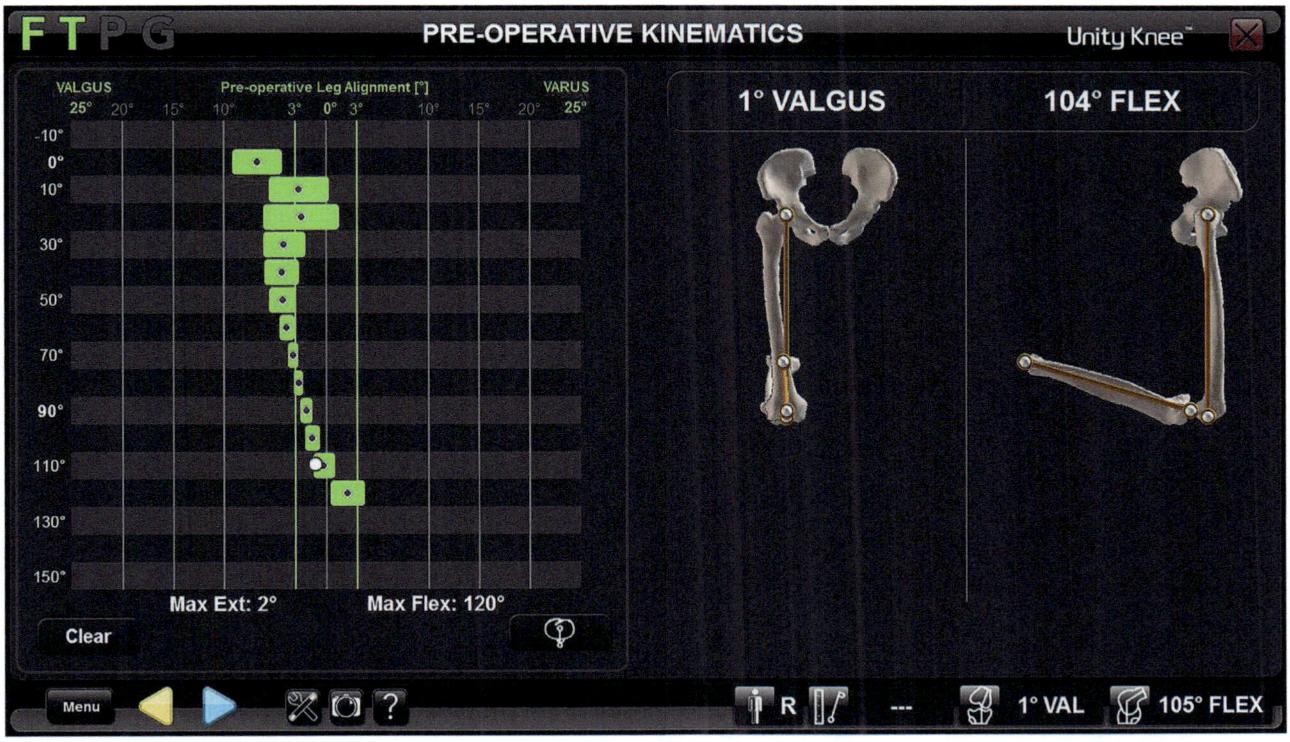

Fig. 66.3 Navigation screen showing alignment/ligament tension throughout the arc of motion prior to any bony resections. Following the reconstruction, surgeons can perform the same measurements to assess changes in the knee kinematics following the TKA

Placement of the additional pins for fixation of the optical tracking arrays results in additional stress risers around the knee. *Periprosthetic fractures* through pin sites are a rare but a known complication, which is addressed in ▶ Sect. 66.6 (Hernandez-Vaquero and Suarez-Vazquez 2007; Hoke et al. 2011; Kim et al. 2010; Wysocki et al. 2008). Navigation should be avoided in patients with osteoporotic bone as the pins increase the risk of fractures or can shift during the case in the soft bone and lead to inaccurate cuts.

> Although not a clinical contraindication, the added cost of the navigation (both in cost of the technology itself and the possible extra time in the operating room) should also be considered when deciding on the use of navigation (Antonios et al. 2019).

The additional cost incurred to the health care system should be justified by the advantage of the use of navigation on a case-by-case basis.

66.4 Types of Devices/Preoperative Planning

Modern knee arthroplasty navigation systems continue to multiply. Despite the myriad of options currently available, they can be categorized into three groups:

Types of Knee Arthroplasty Navigation Systems

- Preoperative three-dimensional image-guided systems
- Imageless systems
- Accelerometer-based systems

Both image-guided and imageless systems are based on earlier large console navigation systems. As such, both techniques rely on line-of-sight infrared arrays, which are rigidly fixed to the tibia and femur (Fig. 66.4). Once secure fixation of the reference optical arrays is

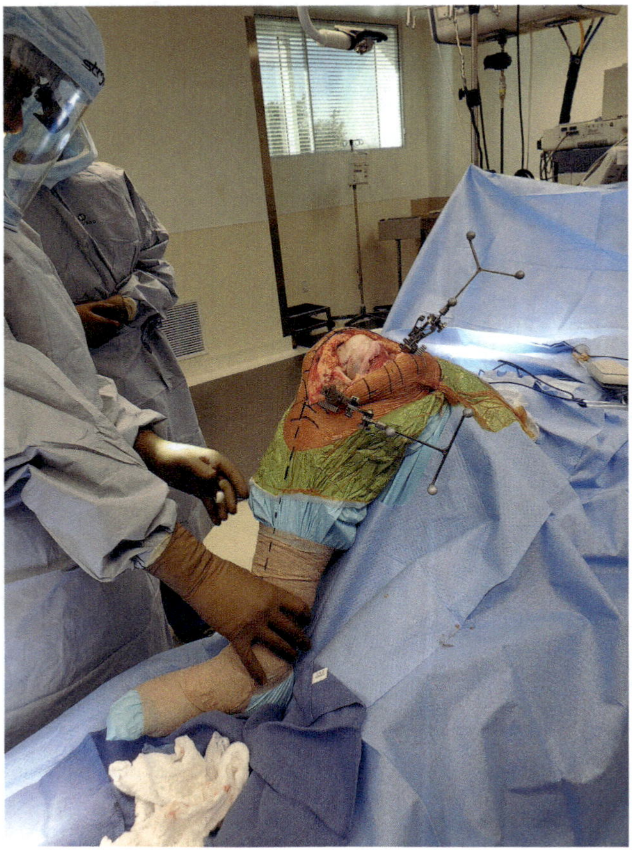

Fig. 66.4 Rigid fixation of the optical array is required in the distal femur and proximal tibia for accurate registration

established, the knee is exposed and mapped with an infrared stylus on systematic sequential anatomic points specific to each system. The center of rotation of the hip as well as the mechanical axis of the femur is established. The anatomic or mechanical axis of the tibia is also determined. The computer model created allows both systems to guide the bony cuts accurately and reproducibly (Perlick et al. 2004).

The biggest difference between the two methods lies in the preoperative workup.

- Image-based navigation relies on preoperative CT or MRI evaluation of the knee. These three-dimensional models are used to create a preoperative template. The intraoperative mapping allows the preoperative model to be synced to the operative knee.
- Imageless systems require no preoperative three-dimensional imaging instead relying solely on the intraoperative registering without a cross reference.

Once mapped, both imageless and image-guided systems work similarly. Line of sight is needed throughout the surgery, and any loss of array fixation results in delay of the workflow. Often large sensor towers are used intraoperatively to maintain the line of sight to the arrays.

> Image-based systems do add cost due to the need for preoperative imaging and added administrative burden; however, having a preoperative reference anatomy can reduce the risk of malregistration (Nam et al. 2013; Tabatabaee et al. 2018).

In an effort to reduce the reliance on the sometimes-cumbersome line of sight arrays and to decrease the initial cost of some large console units, handheld accelerometer systems have been developed (Fig. 66.5) (Fujimoto et al. 2017). With limited intraoperative mapping, these systems fit well with a conventional alignment workflow. The mechanical axis of the tibia is mapped in a similar fashion as the large console systems except the accelerometers attached to the cutting jigs remove the need for line of sight arrays. With the tibia registered, the center of the hip is identified with short arc motions, and the distal femur can then be navigated.

> Currently, these systems are unable to aid in femoral or tibial rotation.

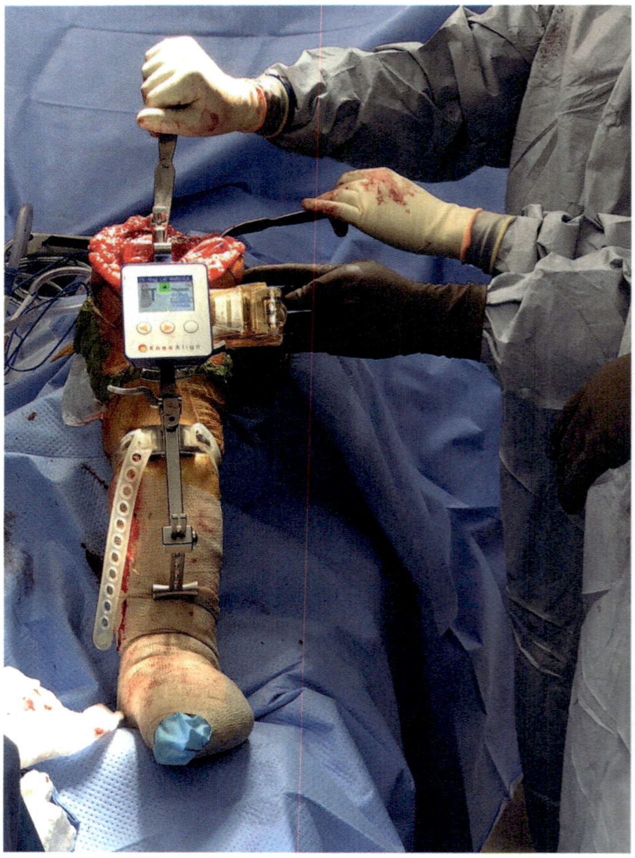

Fig. 66.5 Accelerometer-based systems do not require a large footprint in the operating room and rely on the small accelerometers on the cutting jigs themselves that are then used for registration and calibration

Preoperative workup for imageless and accelerometer-based systems is minimal.

66.5 Surgical Technique and Intraoperative Calibration

Adequate exposure of the knee is needed for any and all navigation systems. Once exposure of the knee has been established, the navigation setup can begin. Image-guided systems often rely on bony osteophytes as part of the preoperative map, and as such, these are not removed prior to beginning the navigation workflow. Most imageless systems recommend osteophyte removal before navigation. Stable rigid pin fixation for infrared arrays is the starting point of both image-guided and imageless systems. This can be achieved either intra-incisional or outside of the incision, depending on the specific system used.

Once pin arrays have been attached to the femur and the tibia and line of site are established, intraoperative registration can begin. Systematic and sequential anatomic registration can differ slightly between systems. Often the tibial surface is mapped including the center near the ACL footprint or tibial spines and then both the medial and lateral plateaus. The malleoli are then identified for the mechanical axis of the tibia (◘ Fig. 66.6). With the tibia completed, the center of rotation of the hip is identified using wide arcs of motion of the hip while keeping the arrays visible. The femoral surface is then mapped with the infrared stylus. Femoral registration typically requires registration of the medial and lateral femoral condylar surfaces along with the medial and lateral epicondyles, anterior cortex, and Whiteside's line to evaluate rotation of the femoral component (◘ Fig. 66.7).

With the computer model built, the bony resection can then be completed in the order desired by the surgeon. Both femoral and tibial rotation can be checked with these detailed maps (◘ Fig. 66.8). Newer systems are allowing soft tissue tension to be applied as well while setting the surgical plan. Most systems currently fall into a measured resection workflow giving the surgeon read back in the form of millimeter gaps before and after a planned resection. The surgeon can virtually plan the resection prior to making any bony cuts. Once the plan is established, the cutting guides are applied. Often these are identical to the conventional guides but are placed and secured using arrays to verify that the surgical plan can be executed.

The accelerometer-based systems work well into the workflow of traditional cutting jigs. Often these systems are implant agnostic; the surgery is carried out identically to a conventional surgery. Once exposure is completed, the extramedullary cutting guide is applied to the tibia. The center of the proximal tibia at the ACL footprint is identified, and then the malleoli are registered. With this, the coronal and sagittal alignment for the tibial resection can be set. The depth of resection is often still caliper-based (via an external 2 mm/10 mm stylus) or set by the height resection on the navigation.

The femur is then independently registered. A rigid pin is placed in the center of the distal femur. The hip center of rotation is identified with short arc movements of the hip. The distal femoral resection can then be completed to the coronal and sagittal alignment set by the surgeon. With both tibia and distal femoral resections completed, the surgery proceeds with conventional jigs. Currently, accelerometer-based systems cannot set femoral rotation.

66.6 Complications

> Several potential complications exist that are unique to TKA performed with navigation, including pin site infection (0.47%) (Brown et al. 2017), neurologic or vascular injury from pin placement, fracture through the pin site on the tibial or femoral side (Kamara et al. 2017), and inaccurate registration.

Surgeon technique for achieving accurate bone cuts based on navigated guide placement is also key to ensure that the final component positioning matches the planned template.

For many navigation devices, reference pins are required to be placed in the femur and/or tibia to accurately record their position in space during the procedure. These pins can be placed either within the surgical wound in the bones or may require a separate small incision away from the surgical wound. They can be inserted unicortically, transcortically, or bicortically. One retrospective cohort study showed pin site complications in 839 patients to be low with 3 infections, 1 neurapraxia, and 1 suture abscess that were all able to be treated non-operatively (Kamara et al. 2017).

Postoperatively, these pinholes can become a location of stress and lead to fracture in as low as 0.065–0.16% (Brown et al. 2017) and up to 1.38% of cases (Blue et al. 2018). Several case reports exist for fracture through a pin site. Femoral pin site fractures were first reported in the United States in two cases in 2008 (Wysocki et al. 2008). These fractures most commonly occur in the first 3 months post-op, and supracondylar femur fractures or diaphyseal fractures may require intramedullary nailing if the component is stable (Blue et al. 2018; Li et al. 2008).

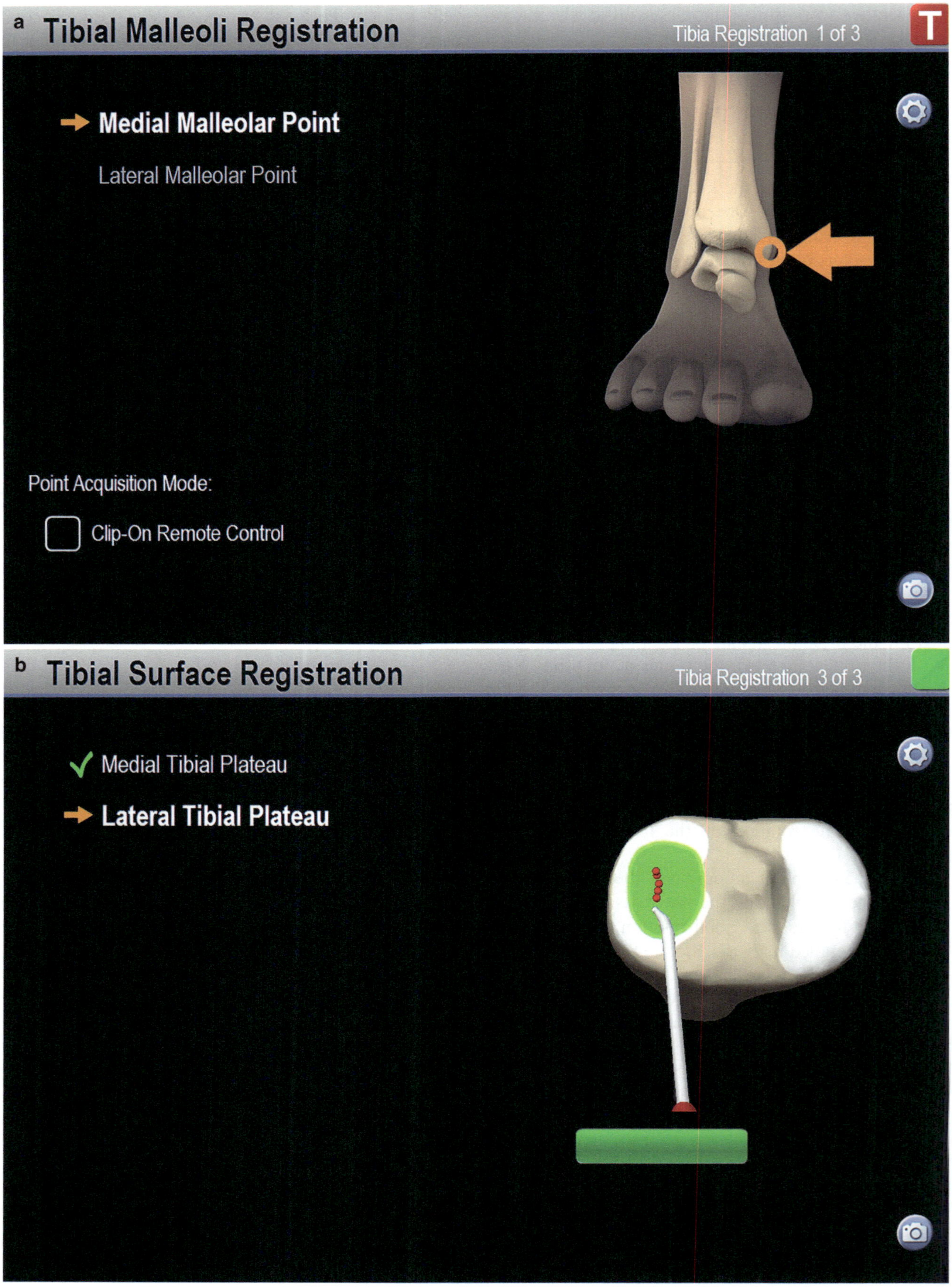

Fig. 66.6 **a** Along with the footprint of the ACL, the medial and lateral malleoli are used to establish the mechanical axis of the tibia. Inaccurate registration of the mechanic axis will result in an error in the tibial cut. **b** Identifying the medial and lateral plateau and borders of the proximal tibia aids with determining the appropriate sizing

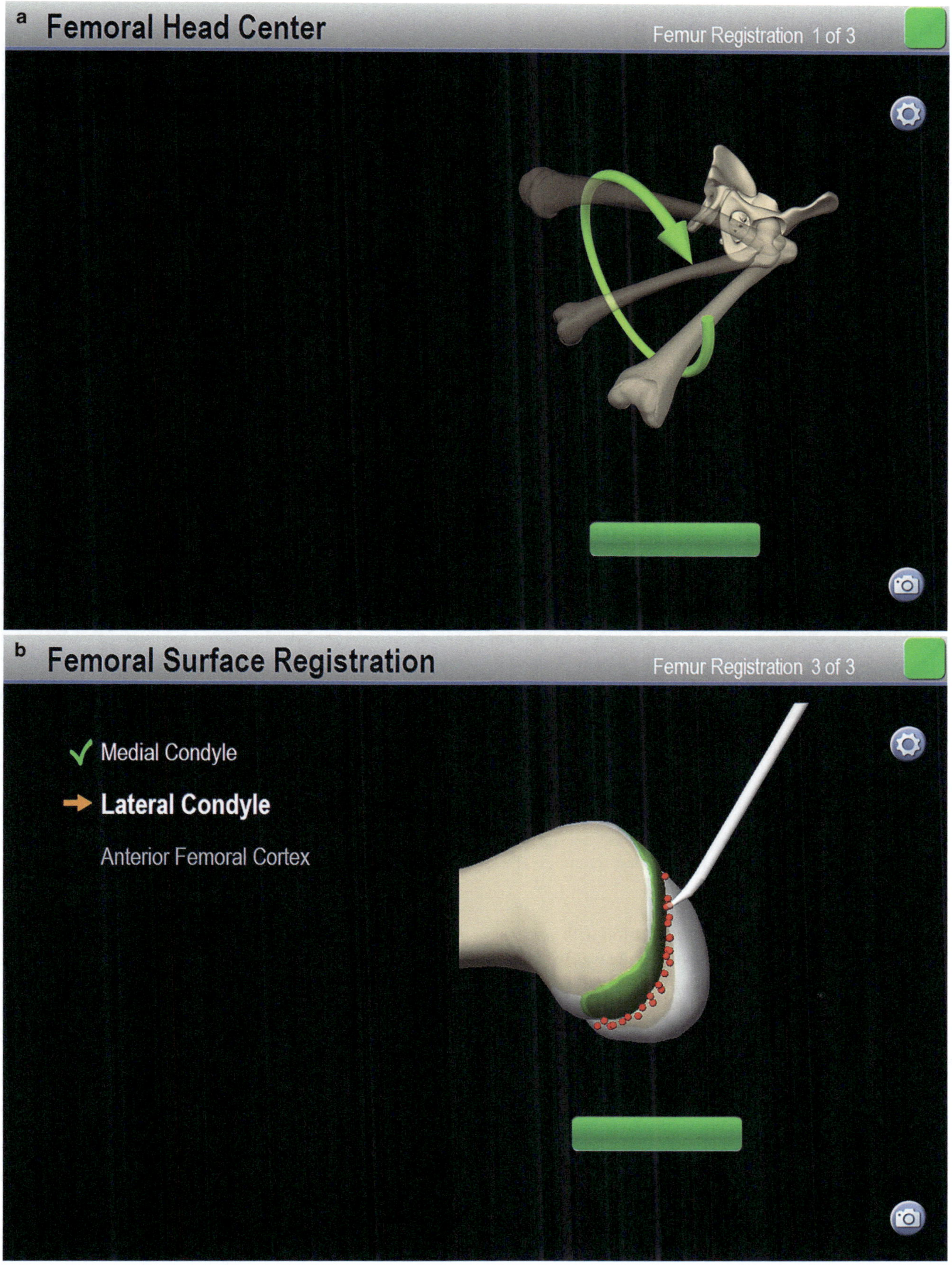

Fig. 66.7 **a** Determining the center of rotation of the hip using small arcs of motion of the femur. **b** Registration of the bony anatomy of the femoral condyles allow for appropriate evaluation of resection level and sizing

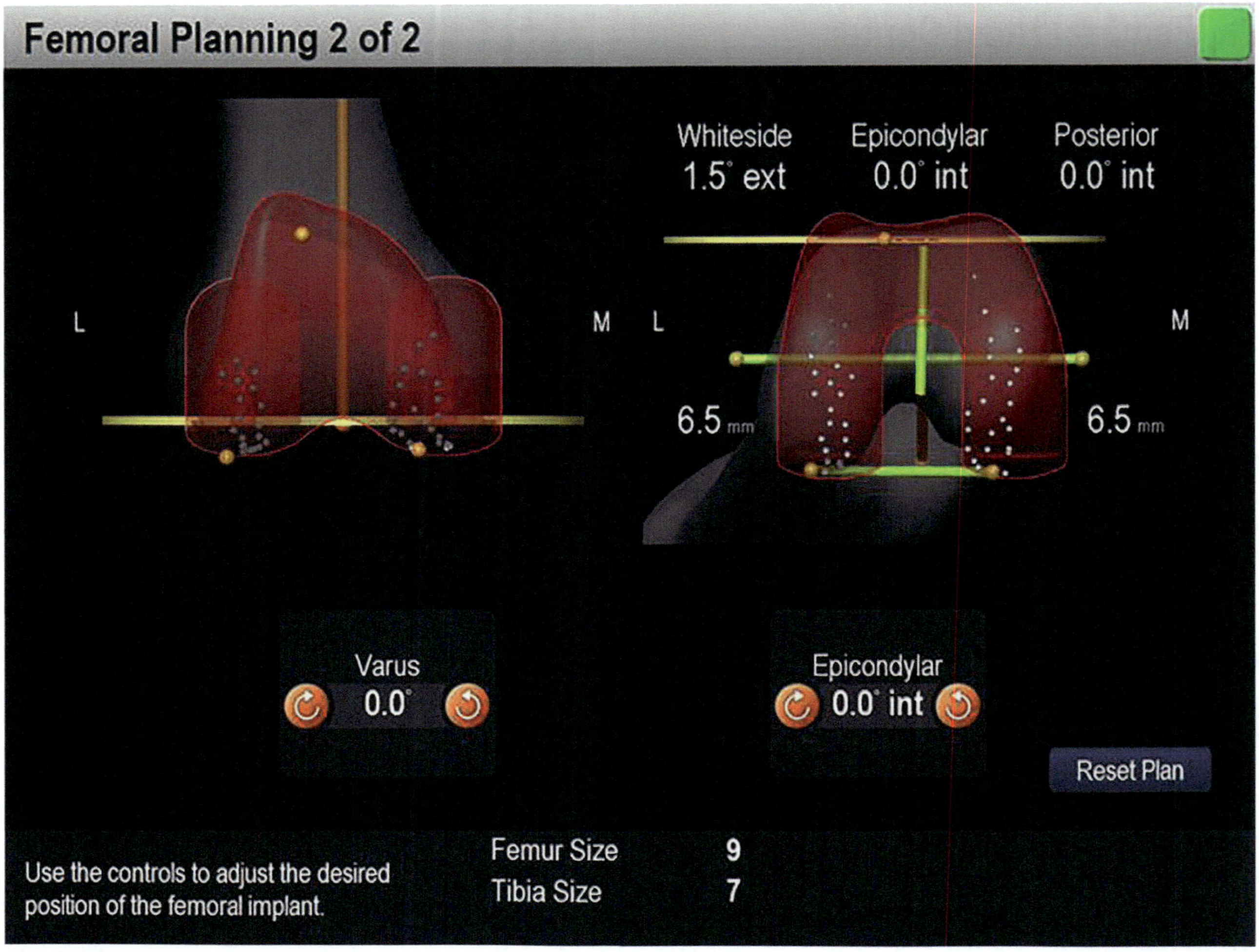

Fig. 66.8 The computer model built from the registration process allows for sizing and appropriate rotation and translation of the femoral and tibial components

> Surgeons must be aware of post-op patients with disproportionally high thigh pain as it could be a sign of a stress fracture or impending fracture (Jung et al. 2011).

Fractures may have a delayed presentation with one fracture reported at 12 months post-op, which was thought to be associated with transcortical pin placement (Jung et al. 2011); however, femoral fractures have been reported even with unicortical pin placement (Blue et al. 2018).

Fractures through pinholes can also occur following tibial pin placement and can even occur intraoperatively (Manzotti et al. 2008). One retrospective cohort found diaphyseal tibial stress fractures in 3 out of 220 cases and recommended using smaller-diameter self-drilling, self-tapping pins in different planes in the metaphysis to reduce this complication (Hoke et al. 2011). Finite element analysis showed increases in pin diameter and poor bone strength from osteoporosis intensified the stress around the pinhole, especially with transcortical pins (Kim et al. 2010).

Vascular injury is rare but can occur. One reported case of vascular injury related to two 3.0 mm threaded bicortical femoral pin insertion from an anterior start point with the knee in flexion. A large quadriceps hematoma was found 6 days postoperatively with active bleeding from a branch of the superficial femoral artery as it entered the linea aspera at the pin site and was treated with evacuation placement of unicortical screws (Gulhane et al. 2013).

Additionally, intraoperative landmark identification can be difficult and can affect registration and building the frame of reference. This source of error can lead to inaccurate placement of the cutting guides and final components (Robinson et al. 2006). In a cadaveric study, the error range of the mechanical axis was 5.2° of valgus to 2.9° of varus while the transepicondylar axis error range was even larger at 11.1° of external rotation to 6.3° of internal rotation (Davis et al. 2014). These registration errors can drastically affect the final alignment and cause surgeons to think they are doing the correct intraoperative steps only to have the final product with components malpositioned (Davis et al. 2014).

Even with better guide positioning through navigation, bone-cutting errors that affect final alignment can still occur in TKA (Laskin 2003). In one cadaveric study, the variability from the cutting jig guide was 0.4–0.8° different in the varus–valgus plane and 1.3° different in the sagittal plane (Plaskos et al. 2002). Slotted cutting guides did reduce the variability of the bone cuts, and guide movement contributed to 10–40% of the total cutting error (Plaskos et al. 2002).

> Diligent surgical technique is required in navigated cases as well to avoid these errors.

66.7 Results

In theory, navigated knee replacement improves the accuracy of bone cuts and subsequent implant positioning and postoperative limb alignment. Several studies corroborate this intuitive finding with improved alignment in the coronal and sagittal plane as well as rotational alignment on the femur (Ballas et al. 2013; Bathis et al. 2004a; Bolognesi and Hofmann 2005; Brin et al. 2011; Burnett and Barrack 2013; Carter et al. 2008; Chauhan et al. 2004; Chen et al. 2014; Chin et al. 2005; Clayton et al. 2014; Decking et al. 2005; Fehring et al. 2006; Hankemeier et al. 2005; Huang et al. 2011; Johnson et al. 2013; Jones and Jerabek 1989; Kim et al. 2005; Lee et al. 2014; Matziolis et al. 2007; Moskal et al. 2014; Nam et al. 2014; Novak et al. 2007; Perlick et al. 2004; Picard et al. 2007; Rebal et al. 2014; Rhee et al. 2019; Selvanayagam et al. 2019; Sparmann et al. 2003; Spencer et al. 2007; Stockl et al. 2004; Stulberg 2003; Venkatesan et al. 2013; Victor and Hoste 2004). A 2019 meta-analysis of nine randomized controlled trials found navigation-improved sagittal alignment of the femoral component and coronal alignment of the tibial component compared to conventional techniques, though the mechanical axis, coronal alignment of the femoral, and sagittal alignment of the tibial components were not significantly different (Rhee et al. 2019). A similar 2014 meta-analysis of 47 studies with 22 randomized trials found similar results with improved component alignment (Moskal et al. 2014). One meta-analysis comparing imageless navigation systems to conventional methods found navigation to be within 3° of the ideal mechanical axis significantly more frequently (87.1% vs. 73.7%, $p < 0.01$) (Rebal et al. 2014). An earlier 2011 Bayesian meta-analysis found navigation-reduced outliers in the mechanical axis by 80% (Brin et al. 2011). There are other studies, however, showing no difference in alignment when navigation is compared to conventional tools (Bauwens et al. 2007; Cip et al. 2018; Jawhar et al. 2013; Kuzyk et al. 2012; Mihalko et al. 2005; Shin et al. 2016; Siston et al. 2005; Yau et al. 2008). One 2007 meta-analysis of 33 studies with 11 randomized trials found the mechanical axis alignment was not different for conventional or navigated methods with a weighted mean difference of 0.2°, but navigation had a lower risk of critical threshold outliers >3° and >2° (Bauwens et al. 2007). A 2012 meta-analysis of ten studies evaluating sagittal plane alignment of tibial components in navigation vs. conventional methods found no reduction in outliers (Kuzyk et al. 2012).

> Overall, given the large body of evidence supporting improved precision and accuracy of alignment using computer navigation, this is one generally agreed upon the advantage of navigation.

With improved alignment achieved via navigation and the reduction of outliers, patient-reported outcomes should theoretically be superior in patients with navigated components. However, many studies in both short-, medium-, and longer-term follow-up are inconsistent with regard to results. Several show no differences in patient-reported outcomes between the groups (Burnett and Barrack 2013; Chin et al. 2019; Czurda et al. 2010; Johnson et al. 2013; Kim et al. 2018; Rhee et al. 2019; Roberts et al. 2015; Selvanayagam et al. 2019; Spencer et al. 2007; Victor and Hoste 2004). The 2017 Chitranjan S. Ranawat Award-winning randomized study out of CORR found no difference in minimum 14-year follow-up for pain function or survivorship in young patients (age 48–64 years) and did not recommend widespread use of navigation due to its risks and cost (Kim et al. 2018). A few show improved clinical outcomes with the use of navigation (Chin et al. 2019; Moskal et al. 2014; Petursson et al. 2018; Rebal et al. 2014), and even some show improved outcomes with conventional alignment tools (Chin et al. 2019). One 2018 multicenter parallel-group randomized controlled trial found computer navigation improved KOOS subscales for symptoms and sport/recreation and WOMAC subscale for stiffness, showing improved function at 2 years post-op (Petursson et al. 2018). One of the main benefits of improved alignment would be reduced revision rates in the navigated patients; however, in several studies, no significant differences in revision rates were found (Cip et al. 2018; Kim et al. 2018; Rhee et al. 2019; Roberts et al. 2015). A 2018 Austrian prospective randomized trial of 100 conventional and 100 navigated TKAs found no difference at 12 years post-op in long-term implant survival, outcome scores, or clinical exam (Cip et al. 2018).

> An earlier 2015 evaluation of the Australian National Joint Replacement Registry found navigation-improved revision rates for patients under age 65 (6.3% vs. 7.8% revision at 9 years) with a significant reduction in the revision rate from loosening/lysis (hazard ratio 1.38, $p = 0.001$).

> Thus, there may be a benefit for younger patients in regard to revision risk, and further studies are warranted in this group (de Steiger et al. 2015).

Further study in the 2019 annual report found similar findings with patients under age 65 having a lower rate of revision when navigation is used at all time points (Australian Orthopaedic Association National Joint Replacement Registry (AOANJRR) 2019). In patients over age 65, use of navigation was associated with a higher rate of revision in the first 6 months but a lower rate of revision at all time points afterward (Australian Orthopaedic Association National Joint Replacement Registry (AOANJRR) 2019).

Another theoretical benefit of navigation is avoiding intramedullary instrumentation of the femoral and/or tibial canals. This could lead to reduced blood loss and reduced transfusion rate. Several studies have found reduced blood loss in navigated cases (Chauhan et al. 2004; Licini and Meneghini 2015; Millar et al. 2011; Moskal et al. 2014; Venkatesan et al. 2013) and even one that found reduced transfusions (Liodakis et al. 2016). Yet, others showed that transfusion rates were not affected by navigation (Gholson et al. 2017; Millar et al. 2011) even though blood loss may be reduced. Given the current advantages of tranexamic acid and perioperative blood pressure control, transfusion rates have been significantly reduced in recent years; thus, this theoretical advantage of navigated systems may not be as clinically relevant in practice today.

As fat embolism and pulmonary complications from fat embolism are risks with intramedullary instrumentation to set bony alignment, navigation could theoretically reduce or avoid this risk. One study was able to clinically show lower rates of fat emboli with navigation (Venkatesan et al. 2013); however, several others showed no difference between the embolism risks (Kim et al. 2008; O'Connor et al. 2010) as measured via the Mini Mental State Exam (Haytmanek et al. 2010). Multiple studies have also shown no difference in respiratory complications between navigation and conventional techniques (Browne et al. 2010; Liodakis et al. 2016).

> The additional steps required to set up the navigation and implement the technique do appear to increase operative time in several studies, especially as providers are learning the techniques (Bauwens et al. 2007; Bolognesi and Hofmann 2005; Burnett and Barrack 2013; Carter et al. 2008; Chauhan et al. 2004; Moskal et al. 2014; Watters et al. 2011).

The added time is found to be between 11 and 39 minutes and up to 23% of additional time for the case, which can add up when performing multiple TKA procedures per day (Bauwens et al. 2007; Bolognesi and Hofmann 2005; Watters et al. 2011). Other studies show no difference in operative time between the two techniques; thus, the literature is mixed (Chen et al. 2014; Gholson et al. 2017; Shin et al. 2016). In terms of the accuracy of providers who perform the navigated TKA, studies show that seven new trainees, such as residents or providers inexperienced with navigation, are equally as accurate in alignment when using navigation (Ballas et al. 2013; Schnurr et al. 2011). Just as with any new technology, the more a provider uses it, the faster and more efficient they will become with the steps.

When comparing image-based navigation to non-image-based navigation, there does not appear to be a difference in postoperative leg alignment (Bathis et al. 2004b); thus, both types of modalities can be utilized for navigation. For conventional alignment techniques, intramedullary femoral guides appear to have an advantage over extramedullary devices for femoral alignment (Cates et al. 1993), but there are minimal differences for intramedullary and extramedullary tibial alignment guides (Dennis et al. 1993; Ishii et al. 1995).

66.8 Economic Value

> In the current era of value-based healthcare of quality/cost, the monetary cost of new technology like computer navigation must be considered before its widespread implementation.

One decision-analysis model found that computer-assisted surgery was at higher cost but more effective than conventional alignment systems. Based on their assumption, the additional cost of $1500 per case with a possible 14% improvement in coronal alignment to within 3° of neutral mechanical axis and an 11-fold reduction in revision rates at 15 years (4.7% vs. 54% in coronal malalignment), the computer navigation would add $45,554 per quality-adjusted life-year and result in cost savings if the added cost is $629 or less (Novak et al. 2007).

Interestingly, a Markov decision model evaluating the cost-effectiveness of computer-assisted surgery based on high- and low-volume TKA centers found that the lower volume centers would require a larger reduction in annual revision rate (13%) if only 25 navigated TKAs were performed per year, compared to centers of 250 TKAs that only require a 2% reduction in annual revision (Slover et al. 2008). The benefit of buying the high initial cost computer navigation for lower volume surgeons or centers requires significant reductions in 20-year revision rates (Clayton et al. 2014; Gothesen et al. 2013; Slover et al. 2008; Venkatesan et al. 2013).

A systematic review from 2013 found a few short- and medium- with no long-term studies showing improved clinical outcomes with navigated TKA and recommended longer-term follow-up to show improved function, reduced long-term revision, and appropriate cost prior is ubiquitous adoption (Burnett and Barrack 2013). Data shows that navigation can be cost-effective for reducing outlines and improving precision for mechanical alignment, but further study on the effect on patient satisfaction or functional outcomes will be required before true cost-effectiveness can be determined (Beal et al. 2016; Jones and Jerabek 1989).

Conclusion

Many fields within orthopedics are incorporating the use of computers and navigation (Karkenny et al. 2019). The use of navigation in TKA appears to be increasing across the United States with many devices on the market (Antonios et al. 2019; Boylan et al. 2018). The Nationwide Inpatient Sample Data from 2014 shows 6.3% utilization of navigation (Antonios et al. 2019), while National Surgical Quality Improvement Program (NSQIP) data found 3.06% utilization (Gholson et al. 2017), and those percentages are rapidly rising in recent years. Many studies show improved accuracy in alignment with navigation, but the definitive effect on improving patient-reported outcomes or reducing revisions is yet to be determined (Carter et al. 2008; Jones and Jerabek 1989). The cost-effectiveness of computer-assisted navigation in TKA is yet to be determined and will depend on the direct cost of the devices and the effect of improved accuracy on improving revision rate and longevity of the implants associated with malalignment (Novak et al. 2007).

As An Author's Note

We currently use navigation in cases of severe deformity or retained hardware where intramedullary alignment of the femur would be difficult.

Take-Home Messages

- The use of navigation has not shown substantial improvement in outcomes but does appear to improve alignment.
- Selective use of the technology appears to be the most common use at this time.
- Beware of pin placement as it can result in additional stress risers and an increased risk of periprosthetic fracture.
- Verification of appropriate registration is critical for the success of a navigated knee.
- Cost and the possible added time required will be important factors before widespread use is adopted.

References

Antonios JK, Korber S, Sivasundaram L, Mayfield C, Kang HP, Oakes DA, Heckmann ND (2019) Trends in computer navigation and robotic assistance for total knee arthroplasty in the United States: an analysis of patient and hospital factors. Arthroplast Today 5(1):88

Australian Orthopaedic Association National Joint Replacement Registry (AOANJRR) (2019) Hip, knee & shoulder arthroplasty: 2019 annual report. AOA, Adelaide

Ballas R, Philippot R, Cartier JL, Boyer B, Farizon F (2013) Computer-assisted total knee arthroplasty: impact of the surgeon's experience on the component placement. Arch Orthop Trauma Surg 133(3):397

Bargren JH, Blaha JD, Freeman MA (1983) Alignment in total knee arthroplasty. Correlated biomechanical and clinical observations. Clin Orthop Relat Res 173:178

Bathis H, Perlick L, Tingart M, Luring C, Zurakowski D, Grifka J (2004a) Alignment in total knee arthroplasty. A comparison of computer-assisted surgery with the conventional technique. J Bone Joint Surg Br 86(5):682

Bathis H, Perlick L, Tingart M, Luring C, Perlick C, Grifka J (2004b) Radiological results of image-based and non-image-based computer-assisted total knee arthroplasty. Int Orthop 28(2):87

Bauwens K, Matthes G, Wich M, Gebhard F, Hanson B, Ekkernkamp A, Stengel D (2007) Navigated total knee replacement. A meta-analysis. J Bone Joint Surg Am 89(2):261

Beal MD, Delagramaticas D, Fitz D (2016) Improving outcomes in total knee arthroplasty-do navigation or customized implants have a role? J Orthop Surg Res 11(1):60

Berend ME, Ritter MA, Meding JB, Faris PM, Keating EM, Redelman R, Faris GW, Davis KE (2004) Tibial component failure mechanisms in total knee arthroplasty. Clin Orthop Relat Res 428:26

Bhattacharyya T, Blyler C, Shenaq D (2006) The natural history of new orthopaedic devices. Clin Orthop Relat Res 451:263

Biant LC, Yeoh K, Walker PM, Bruce WJ, Walsh WR (2008) The accuracy of bone resections made during computer navigated total knee replacement. Do we resect what the computer plans we resect? Knee 15(3):238

Blue M, Douthit C, Dennison J, Caroom C, Jenkins M (2018) Periprosthetic fracture through a unicortical tracking pin site

after computer navigated total knee replacement. Case Rep Orthop 2018:2381406
Bolognesi M, Hofmann A (2005) Computer navigation versus standard instrumentation for TKA: a single-surgeon experience. Clin Orthop Relat Res 440:162
Boylan M, Suchman K, Vigdorchik J, Slover J, Bosco J (2018) Technology-assisted hip and knee arthroplasties: an analysis of utilization trends. J Arthroplast 33(4):1019
Brin YS, Nikolaou VS, Joseph L, Zukor DJ, Antoniou J (2011) Imageless computer assisted versus conventional total knee replacement. A Bayesian meta-analysis of 23 comparative studies. Int Orthop 35(3):331
Brown MJ, Matthews JR, Bayers-Thering MT, Phillips MJ, Krackow KA (2017) Low incidence of postoperative complications with navigated total knee arthroplasty. J Arthroplast 32(7):2120
Browne JA, Cook C, Hofmann AA, Bolognesi MP (2010) Postoperative morbidity and mortality following total knee arthroplasty with computer navigation. Knee 17(2):152
Burnett RS, Barrack RL (2013) Computer-assisted total knee arthroplasty is currently of no proven clinical benefit: a systematic review. Clin Orthop Relat Res 471(1):264
Cartėr RE, Rush PF, Smid JA, Smith WL (2008) Experience with computer-assisted navigation for total knee arthroplasty in a community setting. J Arthroplast 23(5):707
Cates HE, Ritter MA, Keating EM, Faris PM (1993) Intramedullary versus extramedullary femoral alignment systems in total knee replacement. Clin Orthop Relat Res 286:32
Chauhan SK, Scott RG, Breidahl W, Beaver RJ (2004) Computer-assisted knee arthroplasty versus a conventional jig-based technique. A randomised, prospective trial. J Bone Joint Surg Br 86(3):372
Chen JY, Chin PL, Tay DK, Chia SL, Lo NN, Yeo SJ (2014) Less outliers in pinless navigation compared with conventional surgery in total knee arthroplasty. Knee Surg Sports Traumatol Arthrosc 22(8):1827
Chin PL, Yang KY, Yeo SJ, Lo NN (2005) Randomized control trial comparing radiographic total knee arthroplasty implant placement using computer navigation versus conventional technique. J Arthroplast 20(5):618
Chin BZ, Seck VMH, Syn NL, Wee IJY, Tan SSH, O'Neill GK (2019) Computer-navigated versus conventional total knee arthroplasty: a meta-analysis of functional outcomes from level I and II randomized controlled trials. J Knee Surg 34(6):648–658
Cip J, Obwegeser F, Benesch T, Bach C, Ruckenstuhl P, Martin A (2018) Twelve-year follow-up of navigated computer-assisted versus conventional total knee arthroplasty: a prospective randomized comparative trial. J Arthroplast 33(5):1404
Clayton AW, Cherian JJ, Banerjee S, Kapadia BH, Jauregui JJ, Harwin SF, Mont MA (2014) Does the use of navigation in total knee arthroplasty affect outcomes? J Knee Surg 27(3):171
Czurda T, Fennema P, Baumgartner M, Ritschl P (2010) The association between component malalignment and post-operative pain following navigation-assisted total knee arthroplasty: results of a cohort/nested case-control study. Knee Surg Sports Traumatol Arthrosc 18(7):863
D'Lima DD, Hermida JC, Chen PC, Colwell CW (2001) Polyethylene wear and variations in knee kinematics. Clin Orthop Relat Res 392:124
Davis ET, Pagkalos J, Gallie PA, Macgroarty K, Waddell JP, Schemitsch EH (2014) Defining the errors in the registration process during imageless computer navigation in total knee arthroplasty: a cadaveric study. J Arthroplast 29(4):698
de Steiger RN, Liu YL, Graves SE (2015) Computer navigation for total knee arthroplasty reduces revision rate for patients less than sixty-five years of age. J Bone Joint Surg Am 97(8):635
Decking R, Markmann Y, Fuchs J, Puhl W, Scharf HP (2005) Leg axis after computer-navigated total knee arthroplasty: a prospective randomized trial comparing computer-navigated and manual implantation. J Arthroplast 20(3):282
Delp SL, Stulberg SD, Davies B, Picard F, Leitner F (1998) Computer assisted knee replacement. Clin Orthop Relat Res 354:49
Dennis DA, Channer M, Susman MH, Stringer EA (1993) Intramedullary versus extramedullary tibial alignment systems in total knee arthroplasty. J Arthroplast 8(1):43
Evans PD, Marshall PD, McDonnell B, Richards J, Evans EJ (1995) Radiologic study of the accuracy of a tibial intramedullary cutting guide for knee arthroplasty. J Arthroplast 10(1):43
Fehring TK, Mason JB, Moskal J, Pollock DC, Mann J, Williams VJ (2006) When computer-assisted knee replacement is the best alternative. Clin Orthop Relat Res 452:132
Fujimoto E, Sasashige Y, Nakata K, Yokota G, Omoto T, Ochi M (2017) Technical considerations and accuracy improvement of accelerometer-based portable computer navigation for performing distal femoral resection in total knee arthroplasty. J Arthroplast 32(1):53
Gangadharan R, Deehan DJ, McCaskie AW (2010) Distal femoral resection at knee replacement - the effect of varying entry point and rotation on prosthesis position. Knee 17(5):345
Gholson JJ, Duchman KR, Otero JE, Pugely AJ, Gao Y, Callaghan JJ (2017) Computer navigated total knee arthroplasty: rates of adoption and early complications. J Arthroplast 32(7):2113
Gothesen O, Slover J, Havelin L, Askildsen JE, Malchau H, Furnes O (2013) An economic model to evaluate cost-effectiveness of computer assisted knee replacement surgery in Norway. BMC Musculoskelet Disord 14:202
Gulhane S, Holloway I, Bartlett M (2013) A vascular complication in computer navigated total knee arthroplasty. Indian J Orthop 47(1):98
Hankemeier S, Hufner T, Wang G, Kendoff D, Zheng G, Richter M, Gosling T, Nolte L, Krettek C (2005) Navigated intraoperative analysis of lower limb alignment. Arch Orthop Trauma Surg 125(8):531
Hasegawa M, Yoshida K, Wakabayashi H, Sudo A (2013) Cutting and implanting errors in minimally invasive total knee arthroplasty using a navigation system. Int Orthop 37(1):27
Haytmanek CT, Pour AE, Restrepo C, Nikhil J, Parvizi J, Hozack WJ (2010) Cognition following computer-assisted total knee arthroplasty: a prospective cohort study. J Bone Joint Surg Am 92(1):92
Hazratwala K, Matthews B, Wilkinson M, Barroso-Rosa S (2016) Total knee arthroplasty in patients with extra-articular deformity. Arthroplast Today 2(1):26
Hernandez-Vaquero D, Suarez-Vazquez A (2007) Complications of fixed infrared emitters in computer-assisted total knee arthroplasties. BMC Musculoskelet Disord 8:71
Hoke D, Jafari SM, Orozco F, Ong A (2011) Tibial shaft stress fractures resulting from placement of navigation tracker pins. J Arthroplast 26(3):504. e5
Hsu RW, Himeno S, Coventry MB, Chao EY (1990) Normal axial alignment of the lower extremity and load-bearing distribution at the knee. Clin Orthop Relat Res 255:215
Huang TW, Hsu WH, Peng KT, Hsu RW, Weng YJ, Shen WJ (2011) Total knee arthroplasty with use of computer-assisted navigation compared with conventional guiding systems in the same patient: radiographic results in Asian patients. J Bone Joint Surg Am 93(13):1197
Hvid I, Nielsen S (1984) Total condylar knee arthroplasty. Prosthetic component positioning and radiolucent lines. Acta Orthop Scand 55(2):160

Ishii Y, Ohmori G, Bechtold JE, Gustilo RB (1995) Extramedullary versus intramedullary alignment guides in total knee arthroplasty. Clin Orthop Relat Res 318:167

Jawhar A, Shah V, Sohoni S, Scharf HP (2013) Joint line changes after primary total knee arthroplasty: navigated versus non-navigated. Knee Surg Sports Traumatol Arthrosc 21(10):2355

Jeffery RS, Morris RW, Denham RA (1991) Coronal alignment after total knee replacement. J Bone Joint Surg Br 73(5):709

Johnson DR, Dennis DA, Kindsfater KA, Kim RH (2013) Evaluation of total knee arthroplasty performed with and without computer navigation: a bilateral total knee arthroplasty study. J Arthroplast 28(3):455

Jones CW, Jerabek SA (1989) Current role of computer navigation in total knee arthroplasty. J Arthroplast 33(7):2018

Jung KA, Lee SC, Ahn NK, Song MB, Nam CH, Shon OJ (2011) Delayed femoral fracture through a tracker pin site after navigated total knee arthroplasty. J Arthroplast 26(3):505. e9

Kamara E, Berliner ZP, Hepinstall MS, Cooper HJ (2017) Pin site complications associated with computer-assisted navigation in hip and knee arthroplasty. J Arthroplast 32(9):2842

Karkenny AJ, Mendelis JR, Geller DS, Gomez JA (2019) The role of intraoperative navigation in orthopaedic surgery. J Am Acad Orthop Surg 27(19):e849

Kim SJ, MacDonald M, Hernandez J, Wixson RL (2005) Computer assisted navigation in total knee arthroplasty: improved coronal alignment. J Arthroplast 20(7 Suppl 3):123

Kim YH, Kim JS, Hong KS, Kim YJ, Kim JH (2008) Prevalence of fat embolism after total knee arthroplasty performed with or without computer navigation. J Bone Joint Surg Am 90(1):123

Kim K, Kim YH, Park WM, Rhyu KH (2010) Stress concentration near pin holes associated with fracture risk after computer navigated total knee arthroplasty. Comput Aided Surg 15(4–6):98

Kim YH, Park JW, Kim JS (2018) 2017 Chitranjan S. Ranawat award: does computer navigation in knee arthroplasty improve functional outcomes in young patients? A randomized study. Clin Orthop Relat Res 476(1):6

Krackow KA, Bayers-Thering M, Phillips MJ, Bayers-Thering M, Mihalko WM (1999) A new technique for determining proper mechanical axis alignment during total knee arthroplasty: progress toward computer-assisted TKA. Orthopedics 22(7):698

Kuzyk PR, Higgins GA, Tunggal JA, Sellan ME, Waddell JP, Schemitsch EH (2012) Computer navigation vs extramedullary guide for sagittal alignment of tibial components: radiographic study and meta-analysis. J Arthroplast 27(4):630

Laskin RS (2003) Instrumentation pitfalls: you just can't go on autopilot! J Arthroplast 18(3 Suppl 1):18

Lee CY, Lin SJ, Kuo LT, Peng KT, Huang KC, Huang TW, Lee MS, Hsu RW, Shen WJ (2014) The benefits of computer-assisted total knee arthroplasty on coronal alignment with marked femoral bowing in Asian patients. J Orthop Surg Res 9:122

Li CH, Chen TH, Su YP, Shao PC, Lee KS, Chen WM (2008) Periprosthetic femoral supracondylar fracture after total knee arthroplasty with navigation system. J Arthroplast 23(2):304

Licini DJ, Meneghini RM (2015) Modern abbreviated computer navigation of the femur reduces blood loss in total knee arthroplasty. J Arthroplast 30(10):1729

Lin SY, Chen CH, Huang PJ, Fu YC, Huang HT (2014) Computer-navigated minimally invasive total knee arthroplasty for patients with retained implants in the femur. Kaohsiung J Med Sci 30(8):415

Liodakis E, Antoniou J, Zukor DJ, Huk OL, Epure LM, Bergeron SG (2016) Navigated vs conventional total knee arthroplasty: is there a difference in the rate of respiratory complications and transfusions? J Arthroplast 31(10):2273

Lotke PA, Ecker ML (1977) Influence of positioning of prosthesis in total knee replacement. J Bone Joint Surg Am 59(1):77

Manzotti A, Confalonieri N, Pullen C (2008) Intra-operative tibial fracture during computer assisted total knee replacement: a case report. Knee Surg Sports Traumatol Arthrosc 16(5):493

Matassi F, Cozzi Lepri A, Innocenti M, Zanna L, Civinini R, Innocenti M (2019) Total knee arthroplasty in patients with extra-articular deformity: restoration of mechanical alignment using accelerometer-based navigation system. J Arthroplast 34(4):676

Matziolis G, Krocker D, Weiss U, Tohtz S, Perka C (2007) A prospective, randomized study of computer-assisted and conventional total knee arthroplasty. Three-dimensional evaluation of implant alignment and rotation. J Bone Joint Surg Am 89(2):236

Mihalko WM, Boyle J, Clark LD, Krackow KA (2005) The variability of intramedullary alignment of the femoral component during total knee arthroplasty. J Arthroplast 20(1):25

Millar NL, Deakin AH, Millar LL, Kinnimonth AW, Picard F (2011) Blood loss following total knee replacement in the morbidly obese: effects of computer navigation. Knee 18(2):108

Moskal JT, Capps SG, Mann JW, Scanelli JA (2014) Navigated versus conventional total knee arthroplasty. J Knee Surg 27(3):235

Nam D, Weeks KD, Reinhardt KR, Nawabi DH, Cross MB, Mayman DJ (2013) Accelerometer-based, portable navigation vs imageless, large-console computer-assisted navigation in total knee arthroplasty: a comparison of radiographic results. J Arthroplast 28(2):255

Nam D, Cody EA, Nguyen JT, Figgie MP, Mayman DJ (2014) Extramedullary guides versus portable, accelerometer-based navigation for tibial alignment in total knee arthroplasty: a randomized, controlled trial: winner of the 2013 HAP PAUL award. J Arthroplast 29(2):288

Novak EJ, Silverstein MD, Bozic KJ (2007) The cost-effectiveness of computer-assisted navigation in total knee arthroplasty. J Bone Joint Surg Am 89(11):2389

O'Connor MI, Brodersen MP, Feinglass NG, Leone BJ, Crook JE, Switzer BE (2010) Fat emboli in total knee arthroplasty: a prospective randomized study of computer-assisted navigation vs standard surgical technique. J Arthroplast 25(7):1034

Perlick L, Bathis H, Tingart M, Perlick C, Grifka J (2004) Navigation in total-knee arthroplasty: CT-based implantation compared with the conventional technique. Acta Orthop Scand 75(4):464

Petersen TL, Engh GA (1988) Radiographic assessment of knee alignment after total knee arthroplasty. J Arthroplast 3(1):67

Petursson G, Fenstad AM, Gothesen O, Dyrhovden GS, Hallan G, Rohrl SM, Aamodt A, Furnes O (2018) Computer-assisted compared with conventional total knee replacement: a multicenter parallel-group randomized controlled trial. J Bone Joint Surg Am 100(15):1265

Picard F, Deakin AH, Clarke JV, Dillon JM, Gregori A (2007) Using navigation intraoperative measurements narrows range of outcomes in TKA. Clin Orthop Relat Res 463:50

Picard F, Deep K, Jenny JY (2016) Current state of the art in total knee arthroplasty computer navigation. Knee Surg Sports Traumatol Arthrosc 24(11):3565

Plaskos C, Hodgson AJ, Inkpen K, McGraw RW (2002) Bone cutting errors in total knee arthroplasty. J Arthroplast 17(6):698

Rebal BA, Babatunde OM, Lee JH, Geller JA, Patrick DA, Macaulay W (2014) Imageless computer navigation in total knee arthroplasty provides superior short term functional outcomes: a meta-analysis. J Arthroplast 29(5):938

Rhee SJ, Kim HJ, Lee CR, Kim CW, Gwak HC, Kim JH (2019) A comparison of long-term outcomes of computer-navigated and conventional total knee arthroplasty: a meta-analysis of randomized controlled trials. J Bone Joint Surg Am 101(20):1875

Ritter MA, Faris PM, Keating EM, Meding JB (1994) Postoperative alignment of total knee replacement. Its effect on survival. Clin Orthop Relat Res 299:153
Ritter MA, Davis KE, Meding JB, Pierson JL, Berend ME, Malinzak RA (2011) The effect of alignment and BMI on failure of total knee replacement. J Bone Joint Surg Am 93(17):1588
Roberts TD, Clatworthy MG, Frampton CM, Young SW (2015) Does computer assisted navigation improve functional outcomes and implant survivability after total knee arthroplasty? J Arthroplast 30(9 Suppl):59
Robinson M, Eckhoff DG, Reinig KD, Bagur MM, Bach JM (2006) Variability of landmark identification in total knee arthroplasty. Clin Orthop Relat Res 442:57
Schnurr C, Eysel P, Konig DP (2011) Do residents perform TKAs using computer navigation as accurately as consultants? Orthopedics 34(3):174
Selvanayagam R, Kumar V, Malhotra R, Srivastava DN, Digge VK (2019) A prospective randomized study comparing navigation versus conventional total knee arthroplasty. J Orthop Surg (Hong Kong) 27(2):2309499019848079
Shah RR, Patel RM, Puri L (2013) Computer-assisted total knee arthroplasty for significant tibial deformities. J Arthroplast 28(1):28
Shin YS, Kim HJ, Ko YR, Yoon JR (2016) Minimally invasive navigation-assisted versus conventional total knee arthroplasty: a meta-analysis. Knee Surg Sports Traumatol Arthrosc 24(11):3425
Siston RA, Patel JJ, Goodman SB, Delp SL, Giori NJ (2005) The variability of femoral rotational alignment in total knee arthroplasty. J Bone Joint Surg Am 87(10):2276
Slover JD, Tosteson AN, Bozic KJ, Rubash HE, Malchau H (2008) Impact of hospital volume on the economic value of computer navigation for total knee replacement. J Bone Joint Surg Am 90(7):1492
Sparmann M, Wolke B, Czupalla H, Banzer D, Zink A (2003) Positioning of total knee arthroplasty with and without navigation support. A prospective, randomised study. J Bone Joint Surg Br 85(6):830
Spencer JM, Chauhan SK, Sloan K, Taylor A, Beaver RJ (2007) Computer navigation versus conventional total knee replacement: no difference in functional results at two years. J Bone Joint Surg Br 89(4):477
Stiehl JB, Heck DA (2015) How precise is computer-navigated gap assessment in TKA? Clin Orthop Relat Res 473(1):115
Stockl B, Nogler M, Rosiek R, Fischer M, Krismer M, Kessler O (2004) Navigation improves accuracy of rotational alignment in total knee arthroplasty. Clin Orthop Relat Res 426:180
Stulberg SD (2003) How accurate is current TKR instrumentation? Clin Orthop Relat Res 416:177
Tabatabaee RM, Rasouli MR, Maltenfort MG, Fuino R, Restrepo C, Oliashirazi A (2018) Computer-assisted total knee arthroplasty: is there a difference between image-based and imageless techniques? J Arthroplast 33(4):1076
Takasaki M, Matsuda S, Fukagawa S, Mitsuyasu H, Miura H, Iwamoto Y (2010) Accuracy of image-free navigation for severely deformed knees. Knee Surg Sports Traumatol Arthrosc 18(6):763
Venkatesan M, Mahadevan D, Ashford RU (2013) Computer-assisted navigation in knee arthroplasty: a critical appraisal. J Knee Surg 26(5):357
Victor J, Hoste D (2004) Image-based computer-assisted total knee arthroplasty leads to lower variability in coronal alignment. Clin Orthop Relat Res 428:131
Watters TS, Mather RC 3rd, Browne JA, Berend KR, Lombardi AV, Bolognesi MP (2011) Analysis of procedure-related costs and proposed benefits of using patient-specific approach in total knee arthroplasty. J Surg Orthop Adv 20(2):112
Werner FW, Ayers DC, Maletsky LP, Rullkoetter PJ (2005) The effect of valgus/varus malalignment on load distribution in total knee replacements. J Biomech 38(2):349
Wysocki RW, Sheinkop MB, Virkus WW, Della Valle CJ (2008) Femoral fracture through a previous pin site after computer-assisted total knee arthroplasty. J Arthroplast 23(3):462
Yau WP, Chiu KY, Zuo JL, Tang WM, Ng TP (2008) Computer navigation did not improve alignment in a lower-volume total knee practice. Clin Orthop Relat Res 466(4):935

Robot-Assisted Total Knee Arthroplasty

Chad A. Krueger and Jess H. Lonner

Contents

E. Hansen, K.-D. Kühn (eds.), *Essentials of Cemented Knee Arthroplasty*,
https://doi.org/10.1007/978-3-662-63113-3_67

67.1 Introduction

Few procedures in all of medicine have demonstrated the impact on patient function and pain relief as total knee arthroplasty (TKA). Nonetheless, improper component positioning, limb malalignment, and soft tissue imbalance can negatively impact these beneficial results and may lead to patient dissatisfaction, suboptimal function, and premature failure (Antonios et al. 2020; Kazarian et al. 2019; Sharkey et al. 2014). While a variety of methods have been used in an attempt to perform an "ideal" TKA, outliers in a component position beyond the target goal and errors in soft tissue balance are commonplace (Abdel et al. 2018; Kazarian et al. 2019). Robotic technologies have been advanced to improve component alignment and soft tissue balance in TKA (rTKA), with the ultimate goal of impacting functional outcomes and implant durability (Boylan et al. 2018; de Steiger et al. 2015; Koenig et al. 2012; Liow et al. 2014; Lonner and Fillingham 2019). While the use of robotics in unicompartmental knee arthroplasty (UKA) has grown substantially since 2007, its application in TKA in the United States has been more recent.

> Early experience with robotics in UKA, which has shown improved alignment, safety, conservative bone resection, durability, and early function (Battenberg et al. 2019; Dunbar et al. 2012; Gilmour et al. 2018; Lonner and Kerr 2019; Lonner and Klement 2019; Sherman and Wu 2020; Ponzio and Lonner 2016), has been a catalyst for the currently growing interest in robotics in TKA.

In addition to the desire to improve outcomes and surgical efficiencies, economic pressures and regional competition may also be influencing adoption of robotic technology for TKA (Barbash et al. 2014; Lonner and Fillingham 2019). Despite the "promise" of robot assistance, there will naturally be surgeon adopters on the one hand and nonusers on the other hand (BenMessaoud et al. 2011; Yarbrough and Smith 2007). A surgeon's perceptions regarding the usefulness and ease of use of the technology, as well as extrinsic factors such as regional competition, patient requests, technology costs, and learning curves, may at once serve as either motivators or deterrents to using robots in surgery (Barbash et al. 2014; Barbash Glied 2010; BenMessaoud et al. 2011; Blute and Prestipino 2014; Sherman and Wu 2020; Lonner and Fillingham 2019). Indeed, in healthcare, the decision to acquire and implement a new technology is largely based on the perceived "value" of that technology, which is traditionally determined by considering the applicable costs and benefits (Barbash et al. 2014). Some surgeons remain concerned about the increased costs, longer operative times during the "learning curve," or the need for additional preoperative imaging associated with some rTKAs (Lonner and Fillingham 2018). Furthermore, many are hesitant to adopt rTKAs unless studies show improved functional or patient-related outcomes compared to conventional TKA. While additive costs of robotic surgery with the current existing systems are often high, increased competition from manufacturers and wider dissemination of alternative technologies should drive costs down, as we have observed with emerging orthopedic robotic systems (Buckingham and Buckingham 1995; Lonner and Fillingham 2019; Lonner and Moretti 2016).

> With these concepts in mind, at the current time, in some regions, roughly 12% of all TKA procedures are performed with robotic assistance (Boylan et al. 2018), but in some areas of the country, the rate of rTKAs has almost doubled since 2008 (Lonner and Fillingham 2018).

> A recent analysis of potential market penetration over the next decade projected that nearly 23% of TKAs will be performed with robotics in 5 years (MDDI 2015).

Analysts suggest that once robotic penetration in the joint arthroplasty market achieves a 35% level, orthopedic surgeons and hospitals will routinely demand access to the robotic technologies (Newswire 2016). That threshold may be just around the corner. In this chapter, we will review the basics of available robotic systems approved for TKA by the United States Food and Drug Administration (US FDA) and highlight some of the potential benefits, downsides, and other considerations of rTKA technology.

67.2 Robotic TKA Systems

There are three general categories of robotic systems:

Types of Robotic Systems for TKA (Jacofsky and Allen 2016)

- Autonomous systems
- Semiautonomous systems
- Passive systems

Autonomous systems perform bone resection independent of surgeon guidance after surgeon input of preoperative and intraoperative parameters such as

67

resection depth and orientation and implant sizing. Passive systems provide guidance to the surgeon during the procedure, but the surgeon actively places all cutting guides and performs all cuts.

Semiautonomous systems are those in which the surgeon performs the procedure while obtaining live feedback from, and collaborating with, the robotic system during the actual surgery. There is a preoperative and/or intraoperative plan that the surgeon determines and references and may actively change during the procedure. The semi-active systems provide protective mechanisms against inadvertent bone preparation, including haptically constraining the saw blade or burr, modulating the speed or exposure of the motorized burr, or by robotically constraining the cutting blocks (Jacofsky and Allen 2016; Lang et al. 2011).

Some robotic systems use a form of advanced imaging in order to create a preoperative plan for the surgical procedure. These images, typically obtained via a computer tomography (CT) scan, but occasionally from calibrated plain radiographs, allow the computer to create a three-dimensional model of the patient's anatomy from which the operation can be planned. A preoperative plan is then formulated in which the surgeon can preoperatively or intraoperatively determine the provisional implant sizes and position, and how intraoperative variations in those may affect the range of motion and soft tissue balance of the TKA. Other systems only rely on intraoperative referencing; these are generically referred to as "image-free" robotic systems (Jinnah et al. 2019). While these obviously preclude preoperative case simulation, they prevent the patient from being exposed to the radiation, expense, and inconvenience of CT scans (Ponzio and Lonner 2015) and still allow the surgeon to intraoperatively determine how component sizing, alignment, and position may affect the soft tissue tension through a joint range of motion without compromising radiographic or clinical outcomes (Lonner and Fillingham 2019; Lonner and Moretti 2016).

> There is no data to date showing that patient outcomes, implant positioning, or soft tissue balancing is improved with any specific type of robotic assistance compared to another, so it is important for surgeons to determine which system they prefer within their surgical practice.

A summary of the robotic systems discussed below and their features is provided in Table 67.1. All are approved for use in TKA by the US FDA.

67.2.1 TSolution-One® (ROBODOC) Surgical System (Think Surgical Inc., Fremont, CA)

The oldest robotic TKA system is the ROBODOC (now, TSolution One®) (Fig. 67.1).

> This is an "open," autonomous system that was first used in 1992 for femoral canal preparation in THA and has been shown to be successful in several published reports for improving alignment in both total hip and knee arthroplasty (Bargar 2007).

The system develops a surgical plan based on preoperative CT imaging and modeling, and after surgeon input of intraoperative bone parameters, the system autonomously mills away bone with no other surgeon input other than controlling the on–off switch. The system does not distinguish between bone or other surfaces, so careful soft tissue retraction is critical to avoid inadvertent damage to the surrounding soft tissues (Chun et al. 2011; Park and Lee 2007; Schulz et al. 2007). While only recently FDA-

Table 67.1 Overview of common robotic systems for TKA and their particular features

Feature	TSOlution-One® (ROBODOC)	MAKO	NAVIO/CORI	ROSA Knee®	Omnibot
Pre-op CT requirement?	Yes	Yes	No	No	No
Control	Autonomous	Semiautonomous	Semiautonomous	Semiautonomous	Autonomous
Resection tool	Navigated Mill	Navigated burr Navigated saw	Navigated burr Navigated pins for blocks Manual saw	Navigated blocks Manual saw	Navigated blocks Manual saw
Soft tissue balancing algorithm	No	Yes	Yes	Yes	Yes
FDA Status for TKA	Approved	Approved	Approved	Approved	Approved

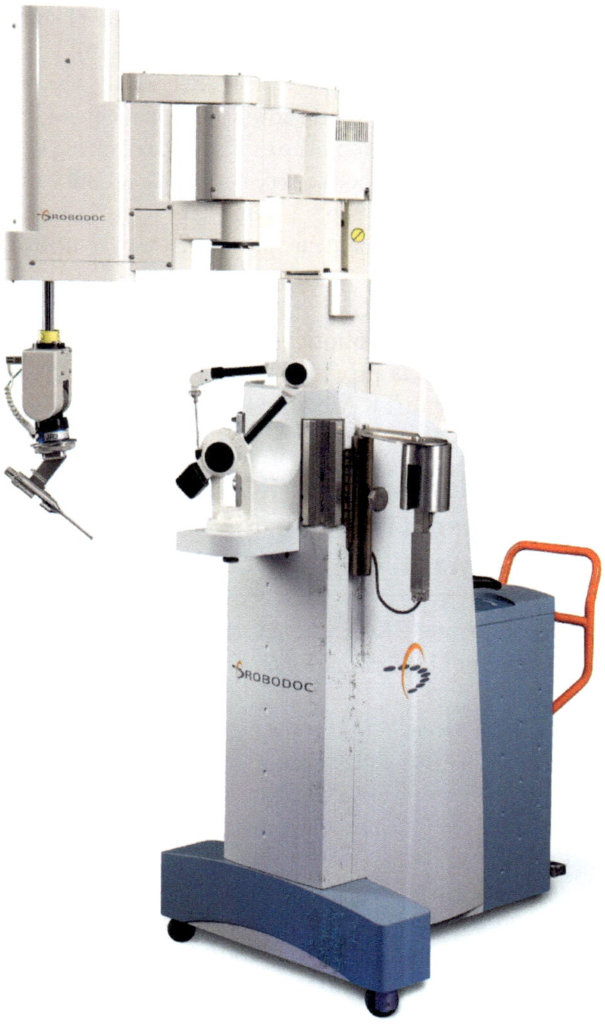

Fig. 67.1 TSolution-One® (ROBODOC) surgical system (Lonner and Fillingham 2019)

approved for TKA in the United States, this technology has been used for TKA in other countries for over a decade (Song et al. 2011). Unlike other available robotic systems, it does not include a soft tissue balancing algorithm.

67.2.2 MAKO (Stryker, Fort Lauderdale, FL)

67

The MAKO robotic system (Fig. 67.2) is a semiautonomous system that provides haptic feedback and allows the surgeon to make adjustments to the surgical plan preoperatively and intraoperatively. The surgical plan is based on a preoperative CT scan that is then executed through the use of stereotactic reference pins that are placed intraoperatively.

> The system provides real-time haptic feedback to the surgeon during surgical execution that helps prevent the surgeon from deviating from the plan. This system also allows for computer-based or manually guided soft-tissue balancing.

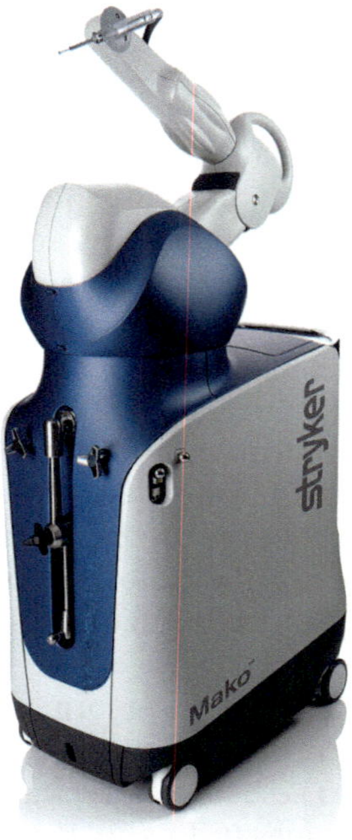

Fig. 67.2 MAKO robotic system (Lonner and Fillingham 2019)

The requirement of the preoperative CT scan adds increased radiation exposure, inconvenience, and cost to the patient (Liow et al. 2014).

67.2.3 NAVIO/CORI (Smith and Nephew, Memphis, TN)

The NAVIO/CORI system (Fig. 67.3) is a handheld semiautonomous platform. It is image-free in that it does not require additional preoperative imaging for planning or landmark mapping. It uses intraoperative referencing to create a virtual model of the patient's knee anatomy and limb alignment, coupled with a soft tissue balancing algorithm to determine the surgical plan and guide the procedure.

> NAVIO does not rely on haptic feedback. Instead, it provides protective control against inadvertent bone removal by modulating the exposure and speed of the motorized burr.

The safety of the burr retraction is limited to its sensitivity and retraction speed, but nonetheless, it has proven effective.

67.2.4 ROSA® Knee Robot (Zimmer Biomet, Warsaw, IN)

The ROSA® Knee System (Fig. 67.4) is a robotically assisted semiautonomous surgical system. It is unique in that it has two options for case planning.

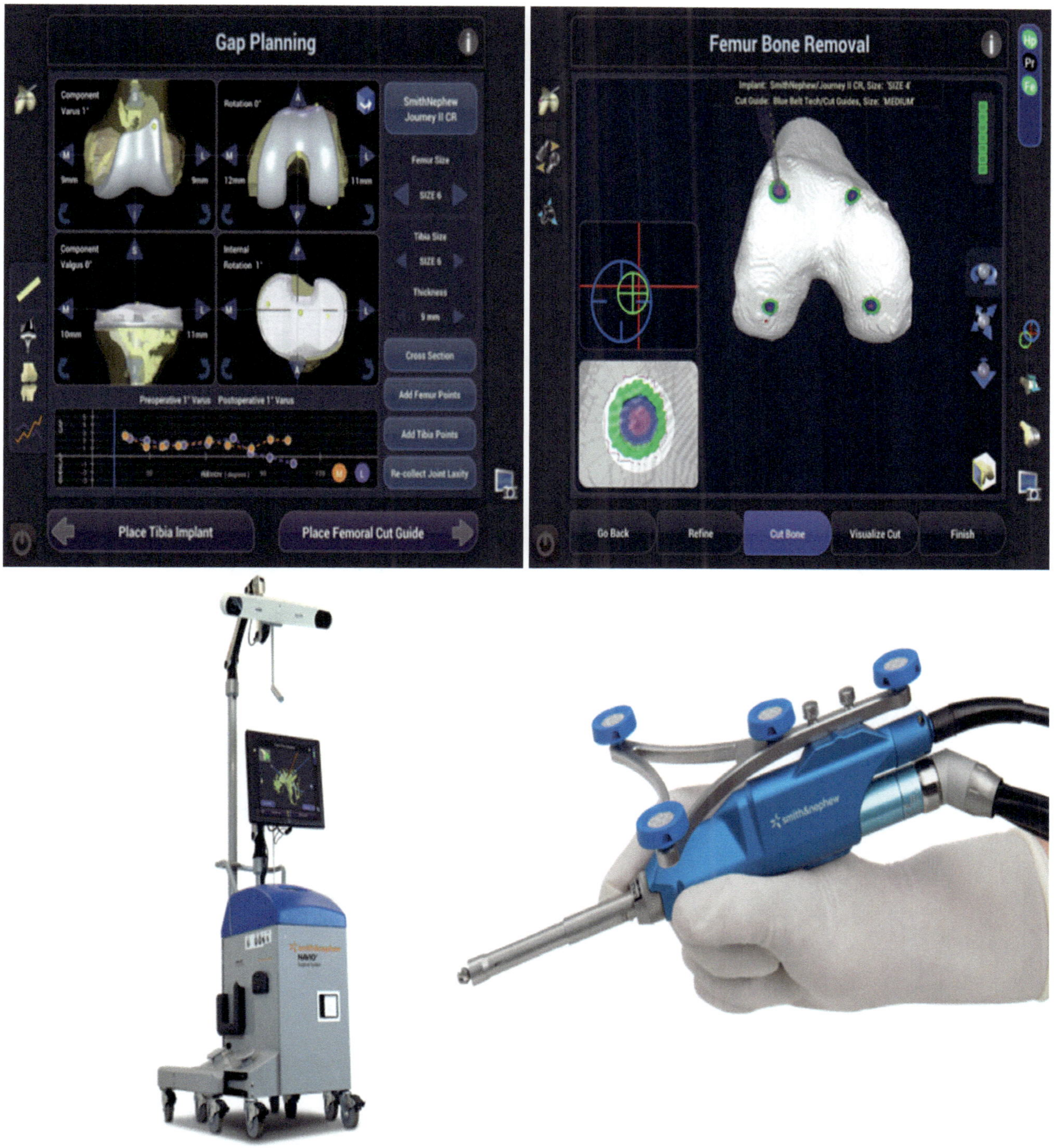

◘ **Fig. 67.3** NAVIO robotic system (Lonner and Fillingham 2019)

- One option for case planning merges information gained from calibrated preoperative radiographs with intraoperative anatomical landmark identification.

- Another option exclusively uses intraoperative condylar surface and limb landmark registration for three-dimensional virtual knee modeling, determination of component sizing and positioning, and soft tissue balancing.

Both options are equally effective and accurate and obviate the need for supplemental preoperative imaging with CT scanning. The robotic end effector positions and constrains cutting blocks in place based on the virtual planning algorithm, after which the surgeon uses a conventional saw blade to resect the degenerated bone surfaces. The saw is neither haptically nor otherwise constrained, which allows the surgeon to retain a comfortable, ergonomic, efficient,

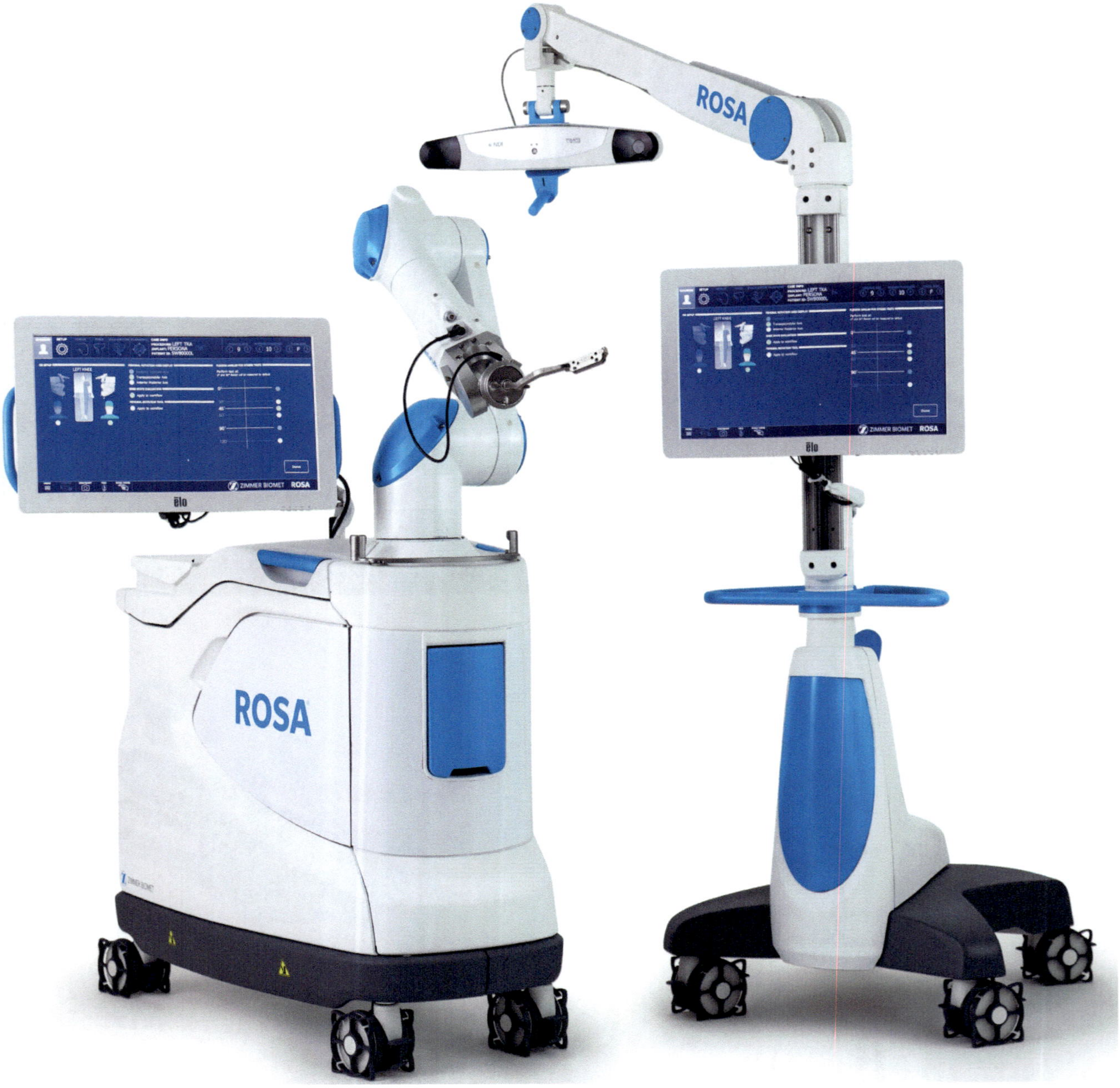

Fig. 67.4 ROSA® Knee Robot (Lonner and Fillingham 2019)

and tactile "feel" during bone resections. The system also prioritizes a soft tissue balancing algorithm.

67.2.5 Omnibot (Corin, Tampa, FL)

OMNIBbotics® (Fig. 67.5) is another image-free system that robotizes the positioning of the cutting guides for femoral (iBlock) and tibial (NanoBlock) cuts based entirely on intraoperative surgical planning, again including surface mapping, landmark registration, and soft tissue balancing.

> The surgeon then manually performs the resections using a standard saw, providing a vehicle for accurate and efficient surface resection coupled with kinematic balancing (Koenig and Plaskos 2019).

67.3 Outcomes of Robotic-Assisted TKA

67.3.1 Radiographic Outcomes

Several studies evaluating robotic TKA in comparison to conventional TKA have demonstrated improved accuracy of component position and alignment and fewer radiographic outliers with robotic assistance, even early in the learning curve (Table 67.2) (Hampp et al. 2019a; Ren et al. 2019; Yang et al. 2017).

> Furthermore, early experience with newer robotic technologies expanding in the TKA space is showing sub-degree precision and elimination of error compared to the preoperative plan (Table 67.3).

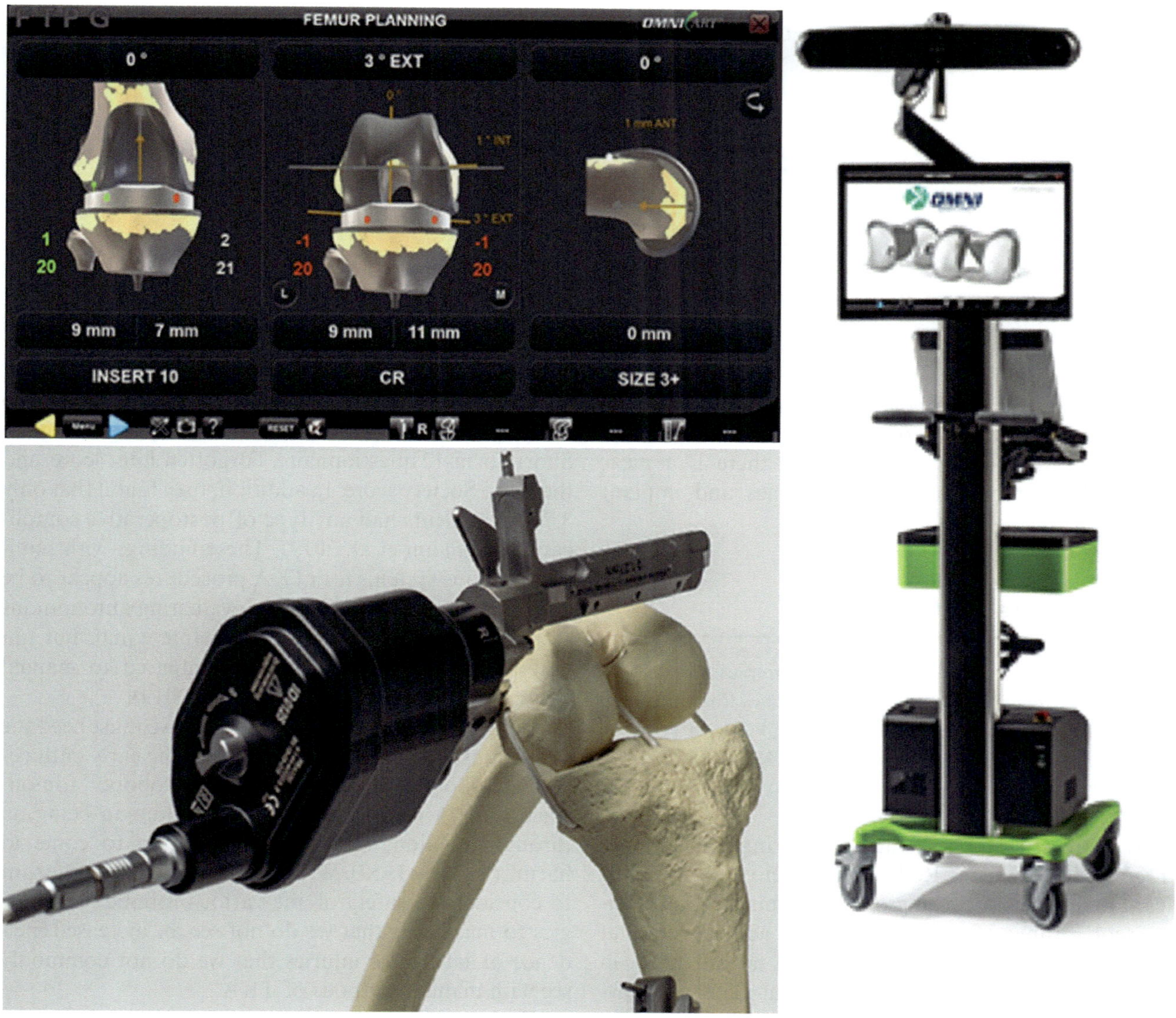

Fig. 67.5 Omnibot system (Lonner and Fillingham 2019)

Table 67.2 Studies comparing the accuracy of mechanical alignment for robotic and conventional TKAs

Study	Robotic		Conventional	
	Mean deviation (°)	SD	Mean deviation (°)	SD
Siebert et al. (2002)	0.8	1	2.6	2.2
Song et al. (2011)	0.2	1.6	1.2	2.1
Song et al. (2013)	0.5	1.4	1.2	2.9
Kim et al. (2019)	2	2	3	3
Liow et al. (2014)	1.3	0.9	1.8	1.2

Mean deviation: The mean number of degrees (°) between the preoperatively planned or neutral mechanical axis and the postoperative mechanical axis. *SD*: Standard deviation (°)

Table 67.3 Relative error in degrees of the final implant alignment compared to the planned implant alignment from the robotic devices

Study	Robot	Parameters relative to plan			
		Femur		Tibia	
		Coronal	Sagittal	Coronal	Sagittal
Parratte et al. (2019)	ROSA®	0.03 (0.51)	−0.95(0.88)	−0.06 (0.69)	0.2 (0.84)
Casper et al. (2018)	NAVIO	−0.1 (0.9)	−2 (2.2)	−0.2 (0.9)	−0.2 (1.3)

Standard deviation in parentheses

While these studies support the improved accuracy of component positioning obtained with robotic assistance, the question remains whether there is a measurable impact on functional outcomes and implant durability.

67.3.2 Clinical Outcomes

> Despite the improved accuracy of component positioning using rTKA, most studies have not found substantial clinical differences between rTKA with an autonomous robot and conventional TKA (Kim et al. 2019; Song et al. 2013; Yim et al. 2013).

In the largest long-term study comparing conventional TKA and rTKA using ROBODOC, there were no significant differences between groups in terms of Knee Society scores, range of motion, or UCLA activity scores at an average follow-up of 13 years and no difference in implant survivorship between groups at a mean follow-up of 15 years (Kim et al. 2019). Several other studies, including one prospective randomized controlled trial, and another large retrospective series, showed similar clinical outcomes at 4- and 10-year follow-up (Park and Lee 2007; Yang et al. 2017).

On the other hand, newer data, using semiautonomous robotic systems that combine quantified bone resection and soft tissue balancing algorithms, may be demonstrating some measurable improvements in clinical outcomes. Kayani et al. demonstrated increased function and shorter hospital lengths of stay for rTKA compared to conventional TKA, although it is not clear whether perioperative protocols were different between groups (Kayani et al. 2018a). In another study that evaluated the short-term (3 months) effects of rTKA compared to manual TKA, Khlopas et al. found that rTKA patients had greater or equal improvements in 9 out of 10 Knee Society scores compared to manual TKA patients (Khlopas et al. 2020). In a longer-term study by Malkani et al. that followed patients for at least 2 years postoperatively, the authors found that all patients who underwent rTKA had excellent outcomes regarding the Short Form-12 questionnaire, Forgotten Joint score, and the Knee Society score. In addition, they found that only 3.7% of patients had any type of postoperative complication (Malkani et al. 2019). These findings with semiautonomous systems for rTKA procedures appear to be even more favorable than those evaluating autonomous systems, which found them to generate equal, but not necessarily improved, outcomes compared to manual TKA procedures (Karunaratne et al. 2019).

Finally, when considering robotics, we must heed the sage counsel of Isaac Asimov, one of the early enthusiasts of robotics, whose First Law of Robotics admonished that "A robot may not injure a human being or, through inaction, allow a human being to come to harm" (Asimov 1950). With that in mind, it is important to consider the safety of the various robotic technologies to make sure that we do not see an increased incidence of iatrogenic injuries that we do not commonly see with manual methods of TKA.

In two early studies of one autonomous robotic system for TKA, inadvertent injuries of the patellar tendon occurred in 3% and 8%, respectively (Chun et al. 2011; Park and Lee 2007). This is considerably greater than the incidence of patellar tendon disruption following TKA with conventional methods, which has ranged from 0.17% to 1.4% (Lynch et al. 1987; Rand et al. 1989). Park et al. also experienced a supracondylar femur fracture and patella fracture in their initial cohort of rTKAs. However, the authors noted that with improved surgical exposure and soft tissue retraction, these major complications are mitigated (Park and Lee 2007). More recent experience with the system using appropriate extensile exposures and soft tissue retraction has led to a substantial reduction in soft tissue complications (Naziri et al. 2019). Furthermore, semiautonomous systems, by virtue of controlling the saw blade or motorized burr, have enjoyed few iatrogenic soft tissue injuries to date (Hampp et al. 2019b; Lonner and Kerr 2019).

67.4 Disadvantages of Robotic-Assisted TKA

The most obvious disadvantages of using robotics to assist with TKA are the additional costs and prolonged surgical times (Lonner and Fillingham 2018; Song et al. 2011; Song et al. 2013).

The initial capital required to purchase some systems is roughly 1 million dollars, with operating costs, disposables, and service agreements adding as much as $1000 per case (Davey 2011; Liow et al. 2014; Lonner and Klement 2019), in addition to preoperative CT imaging that may be required with some systems. Ongoing efforts should be taken to offset these increased expenses by reducing unnecessary inventory and instrumentation, decreasing surgical times, increasing surgical efficiency, avoiding expensive preoperative CT imaging when feasible, and hopefully decreasing the number of revision surgeries with robotics assistance. While there are some data suggesting that robotic TKA may decrease the 90-day episode of care costs for some patients by over $2000 (Cool et al. 2019), we must be clear to acknowledge when cost savings attributed to a robot actually result from reductions in postoperative rehabilitation, home health services, and length of stay that have more to do with protocol modifications rather than the use of the robot per se. Further cost–benefit analyses comparing robotic and conventional approaches, with standardized perioperative protocols, will be necessary to better define the value equation of these technologies.

There is also a predictable learning curve associated with the use of rTKA (Kayani et al. 2018a; Liow et al. 2014). Much of this learning curve appears to take place during the registering of patient anatomy and with learning the robotic system itself, although surgical precision occurs immediately (Chun et al. 2011). The learning curves associated with rTKA are also associated with increased surgical times.

It is widely published that performing rTKA adds an additional 15–25 minutes of operative time per case, which has its own inherent costs and potential risks of surgical infection.

While many of these time figures are based on older robotic systems and more modern systems have been found to not add significant operative time once surgeons are out of their learning curve (Kayani et al. 2018b), the added time of surgical planning, model adjustments, and increased use of disposable instrumentation need to be accounted for when considering a robotic system.

67.5 The Future

It is our expectation that the application of robotics for TKA will continue to evolve and expand as we learn further how to best use these powerful tools. In time, the robotic systems should be able to track planning parameters and soft tissue balancing and interface that information with clinical results to seamlessly determine the optimal positioning, sizing, and kinematics to optimize outcomes for future cases. As costs continue to diminish and surgical efficiencies improve, robotic surgery will likely become more normative. As of now, it seems that rTKA is a valuable tool for improving the accuracy of component positioning, especially for lower-volume surgeons. Whether contemporary robotic systems that include soft tissue balancing algorithms will accelerate recovery, reduce postoperative pain, and improve functional outcomes and implant durability remains to be seen. Nonetheless, as we embark on the next generation of arthroplasty technology, even equivalence may be a reasonable target, given the remarkable success of contemporary TKA, if we can use robotics to decrease inventory, streamline workflows, and improve efficiency for these common procedures.

Take-Home Messages

- Robotic-assisted TKA is a safe alternative to conventional TKA that allows for more precise placement of both the tibial and femoral components.
- There is limited data showing that robotic-assisted TKA yields improved outcomes compared to conventional TKA. However, the literature also clearly shows that patients do not do worse after robotic-assisted TKA.
- There are several different robotic-assisted TKA systems available. Each has its own unique benefits and shortcomings. Becoming familiar and facile with the robotic device you choose will assist in shortening the learning curve.
- Robotic-assisted TKA can be associated with substantial start-up costs. Working toward improving operating room efficiency, decreasing instrument volume, and other similar changes can help offset some of these costs.
- There are many companies heavily invested in robotic-assisted TKA. It is likely that this field will continue to expand, driving down the costs and improving the end-user experience with these devices.

References

Abdel MP, Ollivier M, Parratte S, Trousdale RT, Berry DJ, Pagnano MW (2018) Effect of postoperative mechanical axis alignment on survival and functional outcomes of modern total knee arthroplasties with cement: a concise follow-up at 20 years. J Bone Joint Surg Am 100(6):472–478

Antonios JK, Kang HP, Robertson D, Oakes DA, Lieberman JR, Heckmann ND (2020) Population-based survivorship of computer-navigated versus conventional total knee arthroplasty. J Am Acad Orthop Surg 28(20):857–864

Asimov I (1950) In: Robot I (ed) The Isaac Asimov collection. Doubleday, New York, p 40

Barbash Glied SA (2010) New technology and health care costs – the case of robotic-assisted surgery. N Engl J Med 363:701–704

Barbash GI, Friedman B, Glied SA, Steiner CA (2014) Factors associated with adoption of robotic surgical technology in US hospitals and relationship to radical prostatectomy procedure. Ann Surg 259:1–6

Bargar WL (2007) Robots in orthopaedic surgery. Clin Orthop Relat Res 463:31–36

Battenberg AK, Netravali NA, Lonner JH (2019) A novel handheld robotic-assisted system for unicompartmental knee arthroplasty: surgical technique and early survivorship. J Robot Surg 14(1):55–60

BenMessaoud C, Kharrazi H, MacDorman KF (2011) Facilitators and barriers to adopting robotic-assisted surgery: contextualizing the unified theory of acceptance and use of technology. PLoS One 6:e16395

Blute ML, Prestipino AL (2014) Factors associated with adoption of robotic surgical technology in US hospitals and relationship to radical prostatectomy procedure volume. Ann Surg 259:7–9

Sherman WF, Wu VJ. Robotic Surgery in Total Joint Arthroplasty: A Survey of the AAHKS Membership to Understand the Utilization, Motivations, and Perceptions of Total Joint Surgeons. J Arthroplasty 2020:S0883540320307373. https://doi.org/10.1016/j.arth.2020.06.072

Boylan M, Suchman K, Vigdorchik J, Slover J, Bosco J (2018) Technology-assisted hip and knee arthroplasties: an analysis of utilization trends. J Arthroplast 33(4):1019–1023

Buckingham RA, Buckingham RO (1995) Robots in operating theatres. BMJ 311(7018):1479–1482

Casper M, Mitra R, Khare R, Jaramaz B, Hamlin B, McGinley B, Mayman D, Headrick J, Urish K, Gittins M, Incavo S, Neginhal V (2018) Accuracy assessment of a novel image-free handheld robot for total knee arthroplasty in a cadaveric study. Comput Assist Surg (Abingdon) 23(1):14–20

Chun YS, Kim KL, Cho YJ, Kim YH, Yoo MC, Rhyu KH (2011) Causes and patterns of aborting a robot-assisted arthroplasty. J Arthroplast 26(4):621–625

Cool CL, Jacofsky DJ, Seeger KA, Sodhi N, Mont MA (2019) A 90-day episode-of-care cost analysis of robotic-arm assisted total knee arthroplasty. J Comp Eff Res 8(5):327–336

Davey SM (2011) Surgeon opinion on new technologies in orthopaedic surgery. J Med Eng Technol 35:139–148

de Steiger RN, Liu Y, Graves SE (2015) Computer navigation for total knee arthroplasty reduces revision rate for patients less than sixty-five years of age. J Bone Joint Surg Am 97(8):635–642

Dunbar NJ, Roche MW, Park BH, Branch SH, Conditt MA, Banks SA (2012) Accuracy of dynamic tactile-guided unicompartmental knee arthroplasty. J Arthroplast 27:803–808

Gilmour A, MacLean AD, Rowe PJ, Banger MS, Donnelly I, Jones BG, Blyth MJG (2018) Robotic-arm-assisted vs conventional unicompartmental knee arthroplasty. The 2-year clinical outcomes of a randomized controlled trial. J Arthroplast 33:S109–S115

Hampp EL, Chughtai M, Scholl LY, Sodhi N, Bhowmik-Stoker M, Jacofsky DJ, Mont MA (2019a) Robotic-arm assisted total knee arthroplasty demonstrated greater accuracy and precision to plan compared with manual techniques. J Knee Surg 32(3):239–250

Hampp EL, Sodhl N, Scholl L et al (2019b) Less iatrogenic soft-tissue damage utilizing robotic-assisted total knee arthroplasty when compared with a manual approach. Bone Joint Res 8:495–501

Jacofsky DJ, Allen M (2016) Robotics in arthroplasty: a comprehensive review. J Arthroplast 31(10):2353–2363

Jinnah AH, Luo TD, Plate JF, Jinnah RH (2019) General concepts in robotics in orthopedics. In: Lonner JH (ed) Robotics in knee and hip arthroplasty. Springer Nature, Cham

Karunaratne S, Duan M, Pappas E, Fritsch B, Boyle R, Gupta S, Stalley P, Horsley M, Steffens D (2019) The effectiveness of robotic hip and knee arthroplasty on patient-reported outcomes: a systematic review and meta-analysis. Int Orthop 43(6):1283–1295

Kayani B, Konan S, Tahmassebi J, Pietrzak JRT, Haddad FS (2018a) Robotic-arm assisted total knee arthroplasty is associated with improved early functional recovery and reduced time to hospital discharge compared with conventional jig-based total knee arthroplasty: a prospective cohort study. Bone Joint J 100-B(7):930–937

Kayani B, Konan S, Pietrzak JRT, Huq SS, Tahmassebi J, Haddad FS (2018b) The learning curve associated with robotic-arm assisted unicompartmental knee arthroplasty: a prospective cohort study. Bone Joint J 100-B(8):1033–1042

Kazarian GS, Lawrie CM, Barrack TN, Donaldson MJ, Miller GM, Haddad FS, Barrack RL (2019) The impact of surgeon volume and training status on implant alignment in total knee arthroplasty. J Bone Joint Surg Am 101(19):1713–1723

Khlopas A, Sodhi N, Hozack WJ, Chen AF, Mahoney OM, Kinsey T, Orozco F, Mont MA (2020) Patient-reported functional and satisfaction outcomes after robotic-arm-assisted total knee arthroplasty: early results of a prospective multicenter investigation. J Knee Surg 33(07):685–690

Kim YH, Yoon SH, Park JW (2019) Does robotic-assisted TKA result in better outcome scores or long-term survivorship than conventional TKA? A randomized, controlled trial. Clin Orthop Relat Res 478(2):266

Koenig JA, Plaskos C (2019) Total knee arthroplasty technique: OMNIbotics. In: Lonner JH (ed) Robotics in knee and hip arthroplasty. Springer Nature, Cham

Koenig JA, Suero EM, Plaskos C (2012) Surgical accuracy and efficiency of computer-navigated TKA with a robotic cutting guide–report on the first 100 cases. Orthopaedic Proc 94-B:103

Lang JE, Mannava S, Floyd AJ et al (2011) Robotic systems in orthopaedic surgery. J Bone Joint Surg Br 93(10):1296–1299

Liow MH, Xia Z, Wong MK, Tay KJ, Yeo SJ, Chin PL (2014) Robot-assisted total knee arthroplasty accurately restores the joint line and mechanical axis. A prospective randomised study. J Arthroplast 29(12):2373–2377

Lonner JH, Fillingham YA (2018) Pros and cons: a balanced view of robotics in knee arthroplasty. J Arthroplast 33(7):2007–2013

Lonner JH, Fillingham Y (2019) A brief history of robotics in surgery. In: Lonner JH (ed) Robotics in knee and hip arthroplasty. Springer Nature, Cham, pp 3–10

Lonner JH, Kerr G (2019) Low rate of iatrogenic complications during unicompartmental knee arthroplasty with two semiautonomous robotic systems. Knee 26(3):745–749

Lonner JH, Klement MR (2019) Robotic-assisted medial unicompartmental knee arthroplasty: options and outcomes. J Am Acad Orthop Surg 27(5):e207–e214

Lonner JH, Moretti VM (2016) The evolution of image-free robotic assistance in unicompartmental knee arthroplasty. Am J Orthop (Belle Mead NJ) 45:249–254

Lynch AF, Rorabeck CH, Bourne RB (1987) Extensor mechanism complications following total knee arthroplasty. J Arthroplast 9:135–140

Malkani AL, Roche MW, Kolisek FR, Gustke KA, Hozack WJ, Sodhi N, Acuña A, Vakharia R, Salem HS, Jaggard C, Smith L, Mont MA (2019) New technology for total knee arthroplasty provides excellent patient-reported outcomes: a minimum two-year analysis. Surg Technol Int 36:276–280

MDDI (2015) [cited 2015 March 5]. Available from: http://www.mddionline.com

Naziri Q, Cusson BC, Chaudhri M, Shah NV, Sastry A (2019) Making the transition from tradition to robotic-arm assited TKA: what to expect? A single-surgeon comparative-analysis of the first-40 consecutive cases. J Orthop 16(4):364–368

Newswire G (2016) Orthopedic surgical and surgical assist robots market – hip and knee orthopedic surgical robot device markets will reach $5 billion by 2022: ResearchMoz. [cited 2020 March 2]. Available from: https://www.globenewswire.com/newsrelease/2016/05/23/842396/0/en/Orthopedic-Surgical-and-Surgical-Assist-Robots-Market-Hip-and-Knee-Orthopedic-Surgical-Robot-Device-Markets-will-reach-5-billion-by-2022-ResearchMoz.html

Park SE, Lee CT (2007) Comparison of robotic-assisted and conventional manual implantation of a primary total knee arthroplasty. J Arthroplast 22(7):1054–1059

Parratte S, Price AJ, Jeys LM, Jackson WF, Clarke HD (2019) Accuracy of a new robotically assisted technique for total knee arthroplasty: a cadaveric study. J Arthroplast 34(11):2799–2803

Ponzio DY, Lonner JH (2015) Preoperative mapping in unicompartmental knee arthroplasty using computed tomography scans is associated with radiation exposure and carries high cost. J Arthroplast 30:964–967

Ponzio DY, Lonner J (2016) Robotic technology produces more conservative tibial resection than conventional techniques in UKA. Am J Orthop (Belle Mead NJ) 45:e465–e468

Rand JA, Morrey BF, Bryan RS (1989) Patellar tendon rupture after total knee arthroplasty. Clin Orthop Relat Res 244:233–238

Ren Y, Cao S, Wu J, Weng X, Feng B (2019) Efficacy and reliability of active robotic-assisted total knee arthroplasty compared with conventional total knee arthroplasty: a systematic review and meta-analysis. Postgrad Med J 95(1121):125–133

Schulz AP, Seide K, Queitsch C, von Haugwitz A, Meiners J, Kienast B, Tarabolsi M, Kammal M, Jürgens C (2007) Results of total hip replacement using the Robodoc surgical assistant system: clinical outcome and evaluation of complications for 97 procedures. Int J Med Robot 3:301–306

Sharkey PF, Lo P, Shen C, Tokarski AT, Parvizi J (2014) Why are total knee arthroplasties failing today-has anything changed after 10 years? J Arthroplast 29:1774–1778

Siebert W, Mai S, Kober R, Heeckt PF (2002) Technique and first clinical results of robot-assisted total knee replacement. Knee 9(3):173–180

Song EK, Seon JK, Park SJ, Jung WB, Park HW, Lee GW (2011) Simultaneous bilateral total knee arthroplasty with robotic and conventional techniques: a prospective, randomized study. Knee Surg Sports Traumatol Arthrosc 19(7):1069–1076

Song EK, Seon JK, Yim JH, Netravali NA, Bargar WL (2013) Robotic-assisted TKA reduces postoperative alignment outliers and improves gap balance compared to conventional TKA. Clin Orthop Relat Res 471(1):118–126

Yang HY, Seon YJ, Shim YJ, Lim HA, Song EK (2017) Robotic total knee arthroplasty with a cruciate-retaining implant: a 10-year follow-up study. Clin Orthop Surg 9(2):169–176

Yarbrough AK, Smith TB (2007) Technology acceptance among physicians: a new take on TAM. Med Care Res Rev 64:650–672

Yim JH, Song EK, Khan MS, Sun ZH, Seon JK (2013) A comparison of classical and anatomical total knee alignment methods in robotic total knee arthroplasty: classical and anatomical knee alignment methods in TKA. J Arthroplast 28(6):932–937

The Role of Tibial Force Sensors in Total Knee Arthroplasty

Jimmy Chow, Martin Roche, Jessica Lee, and Tsun-Yee Law

Contents

E. Hansen, K.-D. Kühn (eds.), *Essentials of Cemented Knee Arthroplasty*,
https://doi.org/10.1007/978-3-662-63113-3_68

68.1 Introduction

Despite the overall successes of total knee arthroplasty (TKA), the risk for all-cause failure requiring revision at 10 years postoperatively is nearly 5%, with patients reporting dissatisfaction 15–30% of the time (Mulhall et al. 2006; Sharkey et al. 2014). Infection, instability, and stiffness have been implicated as the leading causes for revision and dissatisfaction (Khan et al. 2016; Le et al. 2014; Lombardi et al. 2011; Mulhall et al. 2006). With the evolution of modern implant designs and improved polyethylene processing techniques, which have decreased the impact of aseptic loosening secondary to wear, instability, and stiffness, have been implicated in 26% and 18% of early and 18% and 14% of late failures, respectively (Le et al. 2014).

Surgical strategies aimed at preventing these complications and improving outcomes include judicious soft tissue balancing and appropriate alignment to achieve a successful TKA (Garvin and Wright 2017; Kappel et al. 2019; Lombardi et al. 2011). However, only recently have various alignment parameters on soft tissue balance and their clinical relevance (anatomic, kinematic) been investigated (Kappel et al. 2019; Peters et al. 2013).

- Historically, achieving proper soft tissue balance relied heavily upon the surgeon's subjectively perceived tactile feel of ligamentous tension, the use of distractors such as laminar spreaders, and block spacers combined with subjective personal experience (Kappel et al. 2019; Roth et al. 2017).

- Newly emerging intraoperative load bearing sensor technologies provide surgeons with a means to accurately measure soft tissue balance before and after component implantation to objectively achieve intercompartmental balance 3D (coronal, sagittal, and rotational) through a full range of motion.

Currently, two disposable intra-op devices that utilize load data technology during TKA are commercially available.

68.2 Verasense™

Verasense™ (Verasense™ Knee System, Orthosensor Inc, Dania Beach, FL) is a wireless, sensorized, implant agnostic device that is presently compatible with Stryker, Zimmer-Biomet, and Smith-Nephew implants. It consists of a disposable load sensing platform embedded in an implant-specific trial polyethylene insert with variable thickness augments. The surgeon inserts the Verasense™ trial, reduces the extensor mechanism, as this has been demonstrated to impact intercompartmental load difference (Schnaser et al. 2015), and captures data at any point through a full range of motion (Fig. 68.1).

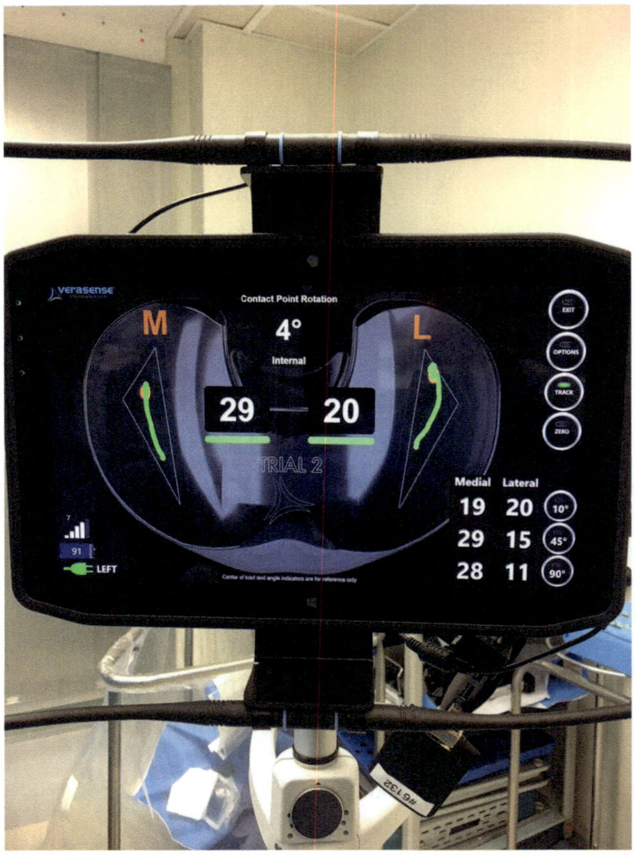

Fig. 68.1 Surgeon evaluates implant rollback and soft tissue pressures on computer screen through a full ROM

- The numeric pressure differentials and visualized femoral contact point cues, combined with knee position, give the surgeon objective information on mediolateral pressure symmetry, implant incongruency, kinematic rollback, and flexion stability.

- This is guiding him/her to make specific adjustments related to implant rotation, bony re-alignments, and selective soft tissue releases.

- The Verasense™ system requires all bony cuts to be made in order to trial; however, it is not preventative of additional subsequent bony adjustments should the need arise.

Of note, it is important to reference load pressures during cementation, as elements of imbalance were observed in 44% of patients during initial cementing techniques (Chow et al. 2017). This data can be saved and can be later referenced during the patient's postoperative course.

In terms of meaningful data, soft tissue tension is best defined at 10°, 45°, and 90° of flexion, with the hip and leg in a neutral position during ROM (Elmallah et al. 2016; Nodzo et al. 2017; Woon et al. 2019). A balanced knee is determined when mediolateral loading differential of ≤15 lbs through the ROM with absolute loading pressures falling between 10 and 40 lbs along with a stable endpoint (minimal translation <2 mm) on posterior drawer testing (Gustke et al. 2014a, b, c, 2017; Jarvelin et al. 2012; Su et al. 2010).

68.3 eLIBRA®

The other commercially available device is the eLIBRA® Dynamic Knee Balancing System (DKBS) (Synvasive Technology, Zimmer® Warsaw, IN) (Fig. 68.2).

> It is a force measurement system designed to allow the surgeon to assess the flexion gap with the intention of minimizing flexion instability by adjusting femoral component rotation relative to the existing collateral soft tissue envelope (Camarata 2014).

This knee system allows for measured balanced resection utilizing an electronic force measurement device along with an adjustable femoral component device to achieve a symmetrical flexion gap. This system was designed to address anatomic variants that could deter the use of typical landmarks guiding femoral component rotation (Olcott and Scott 2000). This device does not measure femoral component contact pressures geographically and is compatible only with the Zimmer Persona and Vanguard knee systems and instrumentation.

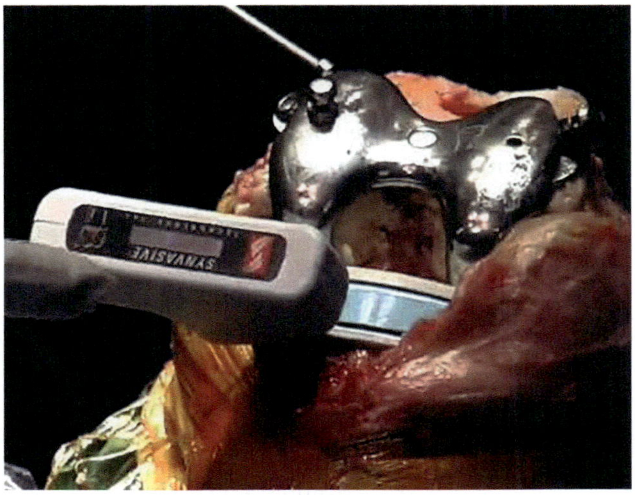

Fig. 68.2 eLIBRA® device

Following the distal femur and proximal tibia resections, the eLIBRA® is superimposed on the tibial cut with the knee exposed in flexion. The femoral posterolateral implant is then adjusted to obtain load pressures, which are received by an embedded force plate and represented on a graphical user interface. The values depicted can range from 1 through 20, with each unit representing approximately 15 Newtons (3.4 lbs of force). Following adequate symmetrical mediolateral balancing as dictated by symmetric load, femoral rotation is marked by creating the pin holes for the femoral cutting block and the femoral cutting block is secured. Once the flexion gap and rotation of the femur are determined, the TKA is completed as usual. The force plate may then be inserted under the trial insert following all bony cuts or underneath the gap spacer paddle for additional adjustments to soft tissue and the tibial component rotation.

68.4 Benefits of Sensor-Guided TKA

68.4.1 Improved Outcomes

Multiple studies have called into question whether surgeons are competent at achieving consistent soft tissue balance in TKA (D'Lima et al. 2007; Elmallah et al. 2016; Golladay et al. 2019), and further, if "balance" as measured by sensor acquired data is actually associated with superior clinical outcomes (Chow and Breslauer 2017; Golladay et al. 2019).

> At least three independent studies demonstrate that when blinded to sensor data, experienced surgeons only balanced knees 50% of the time (as measured by sensors) in situ (D'Lima et al. 2007; Golladay et al. 2019).

Additionally, Griffin et al. (2000) found that only 47–57% of flexion and extension gaps were matched utilizing manual soft tissue tensioning.

A recent multicenter study comparing both surgeon- and sensor-guided arthroplasties observed both improved balance (84% vs. 50%) and superior clinical results in the sensor-guided group (Golladay et al. 2019). A comparative cohort study of 114 patients (57 manual, 57 sensor-assisted) also yielded superior KSS and Oxford Knee Scores at 6 months in the sensor-guided group (Elmallah et al. 2016). In addition, studies have shown a significant reduction in the rate of postoperative arthrofibrosis/stiffness and subsequent manipulation under anesthesia when utilizing intraoperative sensor assistance during TKA (Chow and Breslauer 2017; Geller et al. 2017).

68.4.2 In Situ Adjustments

Data gathered from using sensor-based technologies can be applied to address tibiofemoral rotational incongruency, subtle mediolateral joint imbalance, sagittal plane imbalance, and component malalignment (Roche et al. 2014).

A single-center study observed that an average of 2–3 sensor-guided corrections were necessary to achieve ligament balance, as visualized by targeted loading parameters (Gustke et al. 2017). Similarly, MacDessi et al. associated use of sensor guidance with 46.5% additional surgical adjustments beyond manual assessment in their cohort, while Roche et al. (2014) found excessive medial/lateral load discrepancies necessitating soft tissue release to be present 92.6% of the time. The ability to make small soft tissue adjustments with immediate meaningful feedback can potentially lessen the implant constraint requirement per surgeon discretion at the time of primary TKA. Amundsen et al. (2017) utilized sensor guidance to implement an algorithmic pie crusting of the MCL technique and attributed guidance with a decreased number of varus deformity cases requiring constrained inserts.

Further studies on safe zones of bony alignment (±3° coronal plane) have found that soft tissue balance obtained with 1–2° of bone adjustments may reduce the risk of instability from overaggressive soft tissue release (Allen and Pagnano 2016; Verstraete et al. 2017).

Beyond soft tissue release, sensor-based technologies can be utilized to address rotational incongruencies in the tibiofemoral articulation and optimize patellofemoral tracking.

In a study of 75 ELibra® force measurement assisted TKA patients, postoperative cone beam computed tomography (CBCT) found that there was optimal orientation of the femoral component with a mean of 2.18° of external rotation as well as improvement in KSS clinical and functional scores (preoperative means of 48.35 and 47.53; postoperative means of 88.03 and 91.2 [$p < 0.001$]) (D'Angelo et al. 2015). Conversely, Roche et al. (2015) assessed referencing off of the tibial tubercle for tibial tray rotation prior to using sensor assistance and determined that 68% demonstrated excessive external rotation and the remaining 32% demonstrated excessive internal rotation. Also, 53% of knees exhibited asymmetric tibiofemoral congruency in extension, but all were subsequently corrected using sensor assistance with acceptable tibiofemoral tracking following component implantation.

68.4.3 Balancing Revision Cases

The sensor can be utilized during revision surgery as a means to determine the etiology of a painful knee when imaging, injection/aspiration, and laboratory workup are negative. This enables a potentially modified revision leading to less morbidity and economic resource expenditure. Specifically, planned both component and single component revisions have been downgraded to single component and polyethylene exchange in isolation, respectively, because of information provided by sensors and subsequent tissue adjustments.

68.4.4 Surgical Training

Sensor-based technology may have beneficial application in surgical training to achieve the "feel" of a balanced knee but needs to be reinforced.

A single center study demonstrated that after proficiency was achieved in sensor-guided TKA, reliable balance was achieved by the surgeon without the use of a sensor to a point. After this time point, however, skills attrition manifested in unacceptable force differences at 45°, 90°, and finally 10° of flexion in subsequent procedures (Woon et al. 2019). Additionally, a single center study defined the learning curve to achieve similar operative times between a sensor naïve and sensor competent state to be a mere 41 procedures (Lakra et al. 2019), whereas Gharaibeh et al. (2018) determined that after 30 cases, a surgeon's capacity to achieve balance was improved to significance.

Beyond achieving a "feel" for a balanced knee, sensor guidance can serve as a means of controlling balance as an achievable and quantifiable outcome, so that other techniques in arthroplasty might be evaluated. Nodzo et al. (2017) utilized sensor guidance to determine that setting femoral component rotation parallel to the transepicondylar axis (TEA) achieved adequate balance as defined by a <15 lb mediolateral compartment differential in 84% of their cohort and concluded that this was more meaningful than referencing the posterior condylar axis.

68.5 Robotic and Sensor-Assisted Surgery Synergy

The future integration of sensors that quantify the patient's soft tissue tension and knee stability through a full range of motion and robotic microadjustments enables the surgeon to make incremental implant and bone cuts to allow true customization of a patient's total knee soft tissue balance and alignment. Although there is no literature available that evaluates the relationship between a patient's preoperative, preresection ligamentous assessment captured by robot (regardless of make) and the post-cut tension with trial implants as measured by sensors, all robotic and sensor data can be collected for future use. In combination with PROs, this data has strong future implications for developing surgical algorithms to achieve an optimal balance for patient-specific deformities.

Conclusion

Intraoperative load-bearing sensors deliver real-time dynamic and objective data to the surgeon through a full range of motion. This assists the surgeon in accurately and consistently balancing the knee during TKA. Further, sensor technology can be employed simultaneously with multiple implant systems and exhibits synergy with robotic and navigated surgeries. The knowledge of the implant design and superior tibiofemoral tracking as guided by sensor technology enables the surgeon to minimize component malrotation as a potential cause of revision morbidity. Additionally, sequential soft tissue releases such as pie crusting or needling at the joint line can be assessed quantitatively with sensor-guided in situ tensioning, potentially mitigating eccentric load and subsequent asymmetric wear as etiologies for long-term failure (Amundsen et al. 2017; Clarke et al. 2005; Verdonk et al. 2009). As machine learning advances, surgeons will be provided consistent zones and outputs, with data-driven techniques to improve outcomes by establishing clinically relevant parameters for sensor metrics. Further study needs to address whether soft tissue balance is maintained at mid- and long-term intervals and whether the significance of measurable balance is borne out in PROs (MacDessi et al. 2019).

Take-Home Messages

- Puts a number on a concept—sensor-based technologies provide meaningful and measurable intraoperative data allowing surgeons to assess and adjust soft tissue tension during TKA.
- Numbers are more objective and reliable than surgeon's "feel(ing)" of balance.
- Patient-reported outcomes are significantly increased with the use of sensor-based compared to manual instrumentation.
- Compatible with multiple industry designs.
- The per-case savings are justifiable—the utilization cost of sensor-based technology is less than the projected savings extrapolated from downgraded procedure codes resultant from sensor use.
- Regular use leads to more consistent balancing and tibial component rotation during surgery; however, there is an attrition point after a period of disuse.

References

Allen M, Pagnano MW (2016) Neutral mechanical alignment: is it necessary? Bone Joint J 98-b(1 Suppl A):81

Amundsen S, Lee Y, González Della Valle A (2017) Algorithmic pie-crusting of the medial collateral ligament guided by sensing technology affects the use of constrained inserts during total knee arthroplasty. Int Orthop (SICOT) 41:1139–1145. https://doi.org/10.1007/s00264-017-3413-6

Camarata DA (2014) Soft tissue balance in total knee arthroplasty with a force sensor. Orthop Clin North Am 45(2):175

Chow JC, Breslauer L (2017) The use of intraoperative sensors significantly increases the patient-reported rate of improvement in primary total knee arthroplasty. Orthopedics 40(4):e648

Chow J, Wang K, Elson L et al (2017) Effects of cementing on ligament balance during total knee arthroplasty. Orthopedics 40(3):e455

Clarke HD, Fuchs R, Scuderi GR et al (2005) Clinical results in valgus total knee arthroplasty with the "pie crust" technique of lateral soft tissue releases. J Arthroplast 20(8):1010

D'Angelo F, Puricelli M, Binda T et al (2015) The use of an electronic system for soft tissue balancing in primary total knee arthroplasties: clinical and radiological evaluation. Surg Technol Int 26:261

D'Lima DD, Patil S, Steklov N et al (2007) An ABJS best paper: dynamic intraoperative ligament balancing for total knee arthroplasty. Clin Orthop Rel Res 463:208

Elmallah RK, Mistry JB, Cherian JJ et al (2016) Can we really "feel" a balanced total knee arthroplasty? J Arthroplast 31(9 Suppl):102

Garvin KL, Wright TM (2017) Strategies to improve total knee arthroplasty: a multidisciplinary research conference. J Am Acad Orthop Surg 25(Suppl 1):S1–S3. https://doi.org/10.5435/JAAOS-D-16-00633

Geller JA, Lakra A, Murtaugh T (2017) The use of electronic sensor device to augment ligament balancing leads to a lower rate of arthrofibrosis after total knee arthroplasty. J Arthroplast 32(5):1502

Gharaibeh MA, Chen DB, MacDessi SJ (2018) Soft tissue balancing in total knee arthroplasty using sensor-guided assessment: is there a learning curve? ANZ J Surg 88(5):497–501. https://doi.org/10.1111/ans.14437

Golladay GJ, Bradbury TL, Gordon AC et al (2019) Are patients more satisfied with a balanced total knee arthroplasty? J Arthroplast 34(7S):S195–S200

Griffin FM, Insall JN, Scuderi GR (2000) Accuracy of soft tissue balancing in total knee arthroplasty. J Arthroplast 15:970–973

Gustke KA, Golladay GJ, Roche MW et al (2014a) A new method for defining balance: promising short-term clinical outcomes of sensor-guided TKA. J Arthroplast 29(5):955

Gustke KA, Golladay GJ, Roche MW et al (2014b) Primary TKA patients with quantifiably balanced soft-tissue achieve significant clinical gains sooner than unbalanced patients. Adv Orthop 2014:628695. https://doi.org/10.1155/2014/628695

Gustke KA, Golladay GJ, Roche MW et al (2014c) Increased satisfaction after total knee replacement using sensor-guided technology. Bone Joint J 96-b(10):1333

Gustke KA, Golladay GJ, Roche MW et al (2017) A targeted approach to ligament balancing using kinetic sensors. J Arthroplast 32(7):2127

Jarvelin J, Hakkinen U, Rosenqvist G, Remes V (2012) Factors predisposing to claims and compensations for patient injuries following total hip and knee arthroplasty. Acta Orthop 83(2):190

Kappel A, Laursen M, Nielsen PT, Odgaard A (2019) Relationship between outcome scores and knee laxity following total knee

arthroplasty: a systematic review. Acta Orthop 90(1):46–52. https://doi.org/10.1080/17453674.2018.1554400
Khan M, Osman K, Green G, Haddad FS (2016) The epidemiology of failure in total knee arthroplasty: avoiding your next revision. Bone Joint J 98-b(1 Suppl A):105
Lakra A, Sarpong NO, Jennings EL et al (2019) The learning curve by operative time for soft tissue balancing in total knee arthroplasty using electronic sensor technology. J Arthroplast 34(3):483–487
Le DH, Goodman SB, Maloney WJ, Huddleston JI (2014) Current modes of failure in TKA: infection, instability, and stiffness predominate. Clin Orthop Rel Res 472(7):2197
Lombardi AV, Berend KR, Ng VY (2011) Neutral mechanical alignment: a requirement for successful TKA: affirms. Orthopedics 34(9):e504
MacDessi SJ, Bhimani A, Burns AWR et al (2019) Does soft tissue balancing using intraoperative pressure sensors improve clinical outcomes in total knee arthroplasty? A protocol of a multicentre randomised controlled trial. BMJ Open 9:e027812. https://doi.org/10.1136/bmjopen-2018-027812
Mulhall KJ, Ghomrawi HM, Scully S et al (2006) Current etiologies and modes of failure in total knee arthroplasty revision. Clin Orthop Rel Res 446:45
Nodzo S, Franceschini V, Della Valle AG (2017) Intraoperative load sensing variability during cemented, posterior stabilized total knee arthroplasty. J Arthroplast 32(1):66–70
Olcott CW, Scott RD (2000) A comparison of 4 intraoperative methods to determine femoral component rotation during total knee arthroplasty. J Arthroplast 15(1):22
Peters CL, Jimenez C, Erickson J et al (2013) Lessons learned from selective soft-tissue release for gap balancing in primary total knee arthroplasty: an analysis of 1216 consecutive total knee arthroplasties: AAOS exhibit selection. J Bone Joint Surg Am 95(20):e152
Roche M, Elson L, Anderson C (2014) Dynamic soft tissue balancing in total knee arthroplasty. Orthop Clin North Am 45(2):157
Roche M, Elson L, Anderson C (2015) A novel technique using sensor-based technology to evaluate tibial tray rotation. Orthopedics 38:e217–e222. https://doi.org/10.3928/01477447-20150305-60
Roth JD, Howell SM, Hull ML (2017) An improved tibial force sensor to compute contact forces and contact locations in vitro after total knee arthroplasty. J Biomech Eng 139(4). https://doi.org/10.1115/1.4035471
Schnaser E, Lee L, Della Valle AG (2015) Position affects intraoperative compartmental loads during TKA: a pilot study using a novel radiofrequency knee soft-tissue aalancer. J Arthroplast 30:1348–1353, e3
Sharkey PF, Lichstein PM, Shen C et al (2014) Why are total knee arthroplasties failing today – has anything changed after 10 years? J Arthroplast 29:1774–1778
Su EP, Su SL, Della Valle AG (2010) Stiffness after TKR: how to avoid repeat surgery. Orthopedics 33(9):658
Verdonk PC, Pernin J, Pinaroli A et al (2009) Soft tissue balancing in varus total knee arthroplasty: an algorithmic approach. Knee Surg Sports Traumatol Arthrosc 17(6):660–666. https://doi.org/10.1007/s00167-009-0755-7
Verstraete MA, Meere PA, Salvadore G et al (2017) Contact forces in the tibiofemoral joint from soft tissue tensions: implications to soft tissue balancing in total knee arthroplasty. J Biomech 58:195
Woon CY, Carroll KM, Lyman S, Mayman DJ (2019) Dynamic sensor-balanced knee arthroplasty: can the sensor "train" the surgeon? Arthroplast Today 5(2):202–210. https://doi.org/10.1016/j.artd.2019.03.001

Accelerometers

Cynthia A. Kahlenberg and Michael P. Ast

Contents

E. Hansen, K.-D. Kühn (eds.), *Essentials of Cemented Knee Arthroplasty*,
https://doi.org/10.1007/978-3-662-63113-3_69

69.1 Introduction

Component alignment has been shown to play a role in survivorship, functional outcome, and patient satisfaction after total knee arthroplasty (TKA) (Ritter et al. 1994, 2011; Matsuda et al. 2013). Multiple prior studies have demonstrated that using conventional instruments, optimal component positioning is achieved in less than 80% of cases (Mizu-uchi et al. 2008; Mason et al. 2007). Large-console robotic systems are available to assist in defining resection planes. However, these systems have several drawbacks including initial costs that may exceed $1 million (Jacofsky and Allen 2016). As an alternative, handheld accelerometers were introduced for navigation in TKA.

69.2 Case Examples

- Case 1

The following case demonstrates use of accelerometer-based navigation in a complex primary TKA. An 80-year-old female with prior history of spiral supracondylar femur fracture 1 year prior presents for evaluation of right knee pain (▫ Fig. 69.1). The patient complains of increasing pain with progressive deformity and difficulty walking. She has well-healed incisions from prior surgery and no signs or symptoms of infection. She is indicated for TKA.

The presence of hardware in the femoral canal does not allow for placement of an intramedullary femoral alignment guide. KneeAlign® navigation is used for accurate restoration of the mechanical axis without intramedullary guidance. Only the distal-most screws are removed in order to place the new femoral component. A constrained insert is used due to stretching of the medial collateral ligament from the valgus deformity. The surgeon is able to avoid the morbidity of plate removal by using the accelerometer-based handheld navigation (▫ Fig. 69.2).

- Case 2

Accelerometer-based navigation may also prove useful in cases of extra-articular deformity. The following is a case of a 62-year-old male who had sustained a mid-shaft femur fracture 30 years prior to presentation that was treated with traction. The patient has residual valgus and recurvatum deformity at the fracture site, as well as end-stage osteoarthritis affecting the lateral compartment (▫ Fig. 69.3). He complains of knee pain and walks with a walker. He has a valgus thrust with ambulation and range of motion from 10° of recurvatum to 80° of flexion.

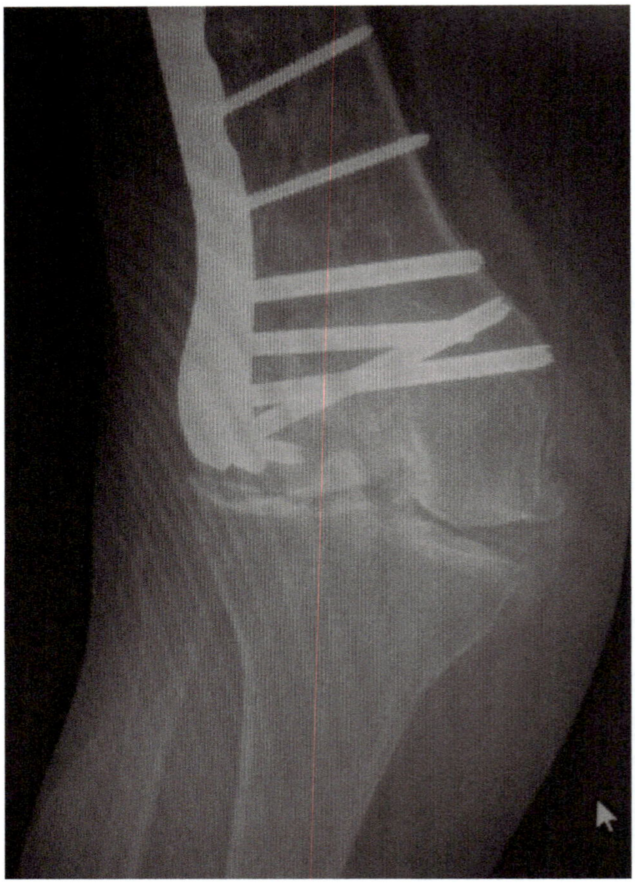

▫ **Fig. 69.1** 80-year-old female with prior hardware from distal femur open reduction and internal fixation. The patient is indicated for TKA

The diaphyseal femoral deformity precludes use of standard intramedullary femoral instrumentation, similar to the prior case. Handheld accelerometer-based navigation is used to make the distal femoral cut perpendicular to the mechanical axis in both the coronal and sagittal planes. A constrained liner is used in this case due to the laxity from the valgus deformity. Postoperative radiographs show accurate restoration of mechanical alignment in both the coronal and sagittal planes (▫ Fig. 69.4).

69.3 What Are Handheld Accelerometers?

Handheld accelerometers are sterile handheld devices used during TKA to more accurately define resection angles of the distal femur and proximal tibia.

> They consist of a handheld computer device with metal jigs that allow for navigated bony resections of the knee. Current commercially available accelerometer systems are single use and imageless; they do not

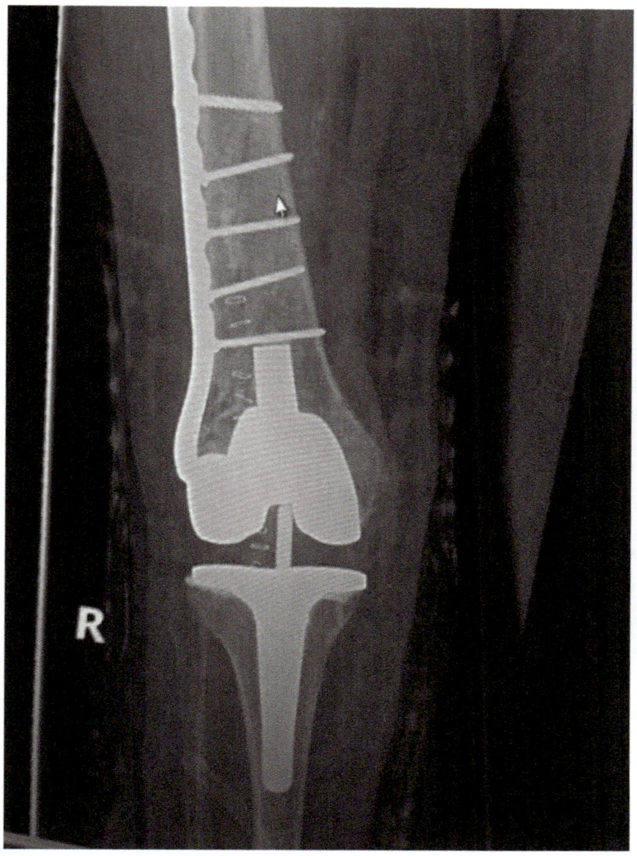

Fig. 69.2 Postoperative radiograph shows well-aligned TKA with maintenance of distal femoral plate

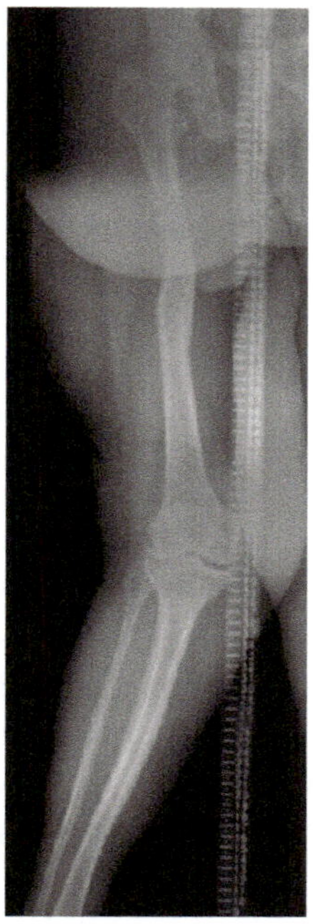

Fig. 69.3 Preoperative radiograph showing extra-articular femoral deformity and valgus angulation at the knee

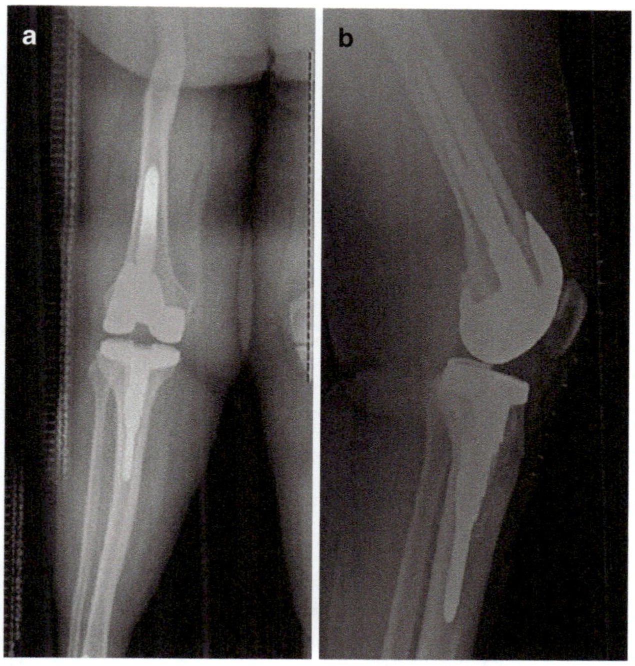

Fig. 69.4 Postoperative radiographs demonstrating accurate restoration of mechanical alignment in both the coronal **a** and sagittal **b** planes

require preoperative imaging, large consoles, or external connections to laptops.

These navigation devices may require the use of a specific implant (iAssist®, Zimmer, Inc., Warsaw, IN) or may allow for use with any implant (KneeAlign®, Orthalign Inc., Aliso Viejo, CA).

In general, handheld accelerometer navigation systems define the mechanical axis of the tibia and femur and give real-time feedback on both sagittal and coronal alignment for bony resection in reference to this mechanical axis (Lackey and Berend 2012).

Once alignment is obtained using accelerometer technology, a cutting slot is pinned into place, and the resection is performed.

69.4 How Are Handheld Accelerometer Systems Used?

For the KneeAlign® system, the tibial cut utilizes an extramedullary tibial jig. Attached to this jig is a triaxial accelerometer inside a reference sensor and a display console with another triaxial accelerometer attached to the mobile portion of the jig (Nam et al. 2012a). The

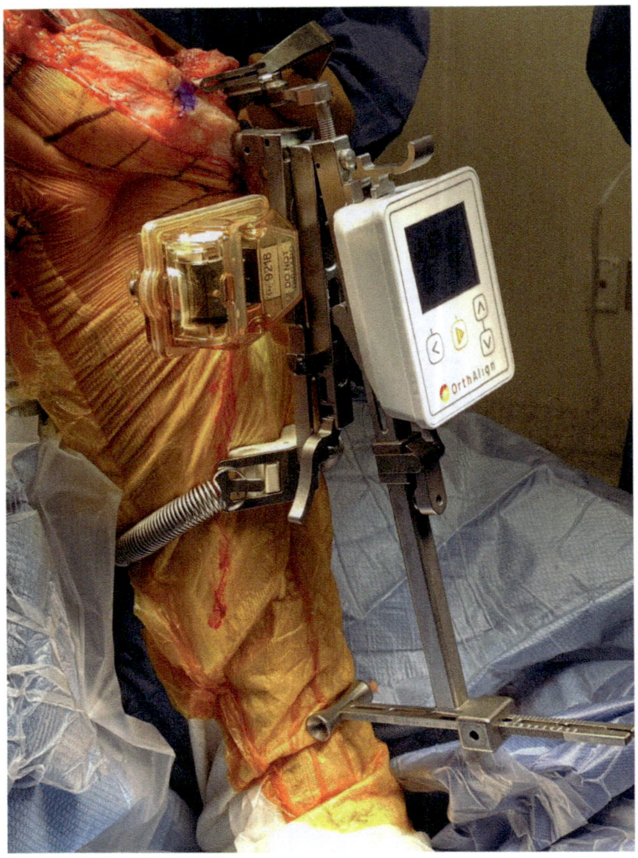

Fig. 69.5 Intraoperative view of the tibial KneeAlign® jig during the registration process

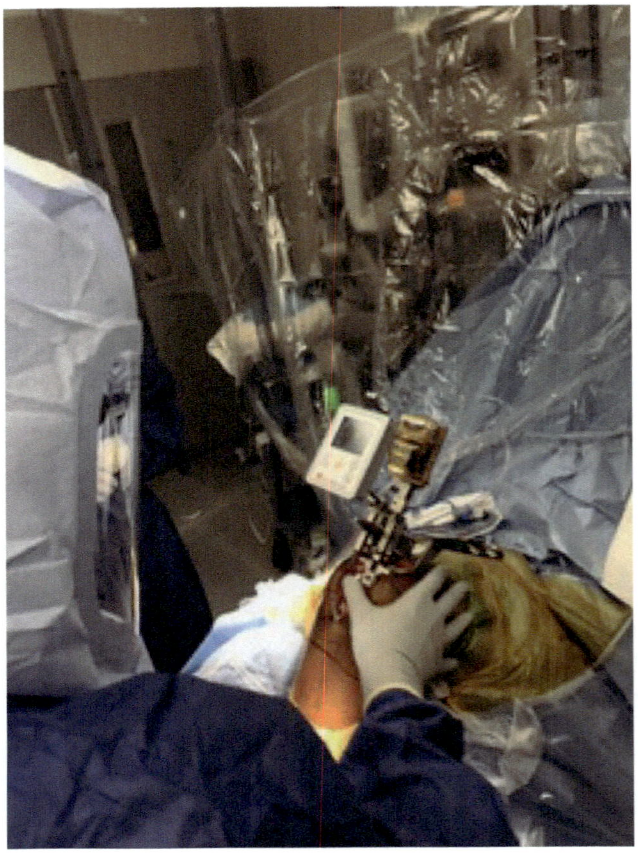

Fig. 69.6 Intraoperative view of the KneeAlign® distal femoral jig with sensors attached

two accelerometers communicate wirelessly. Registration is performed using the mobile portion of the jig (Fig. 69.5). The mechanical axis is defined proximally by the anterior cruciate ligament (ACL) footprint and distally using most prominent points of the medial and lateral malleoli to calculate the location of the middle of the tibial plafond. After registration is completed and the mechanical axis of the tibia is determined, the mobile portion of the jig is used to set the desired coronal resection angle and posterior slope in relation to the mechanical axis. These numbers are displayed on the console.

On the femoral side, a cutting jig without any intramedullary component is fixed to the distal femur (Fig. 69.6). A reference sensor, which contains a triaxial accelerometer and a triaxial angular rate sensor, is attached to the fixed jig. In addition, a display unit containing another triaxial accelerometer is attached to the mobile portion of the jig. A flexion and external rotation maneuver at the hip is performed to allow the accelerometers and angular rate sensor to calculate the location of the center of the femoral head and the location of the mechanical axis using a mathematical algorithm with data from sensors.

> Flexion/extension and varus/valgus angulation can then be adjusted on the mobile portion of the jig in relation to the mechanical axis of the femur, and the cutting slot is pinned into place with these parameters of resection for the distal femur (Nam et al. 2012b).

The iAssist® accelerometer-based handheld navigation system operates on similar principles (Scuderi et al. 2014). On the tibial side, an electronic digitizing pod containing a gyroscope is fixed to the tibia along with the tibial extramedullary guide. The guide is fixed proximally in the center of the tibia between the tibial spines and distally using a clamp around the malleoli to center the jig in the middle of the ankle. The tibia is registered using movements in an abduction, adduction, and neutral position. This creates a coordinate system to define the mechanical axis of the tibia, and the coronal and sagittal alignments of the resection plane can then be adjusted using the electronic pod.

On the femoral side, similar to KneeAlign®, the iAssist® system registers the mechanical axis of the femur using the center of the hip and the distal femoral sulcus. The center of the hip is determined using multiple movements performed by the surgeon. Alignment information is displayed on the electronic pod, and adjustments are made in both the coronal and sagittal plane to guide appropriate resection (Scuderi et al. 2014).

> Of note, both systems use standard manual guides to adjust the depth of resection on both the tibial and femoral sides.

69.5 Benefits of Accelerometers in TKA

As a handheld navigation device used in the surgical field, accelerometer-based systems hold unique advantages.

> First, in contrast to most large-console robotic computer navigation systems, accelerometer-based navigation does not require tibial or femoral pins to affix sensors or markers for registration (Ikawa et al. 2017).

In large-console navigation requiring femoral pins, the rate of periprosthetic fracture has been reported to be above 1% in some series (Beldame et al. 2010; Blue et al. 2018; Jung et al. 2011; Thomas et al. 2015). Accelerometer-based navigation may allow for some of the benefits of computer-assisted surgery without the risk of pin site fracture or associated pin complications.

> Another potential advantage of accelerometer-based navigated TKA over conventional TKA is that there is no instrumentation of the femoral canal, potentially leading to a lower incidence of fat emboli and blood loss from the femur.

Ikawa et al. showed statistically significantly lower blood loss (a difference of nearly 300 mL) after TKA using accelerometer-based navigation compared to a conventional system (Ikawa et al. 2017). Furthermore, avoidance of instrumenting the femoral canal with accelerometer-based navigation may be beneficial in complex cases of extra-articular femoral deformity (Sculco et al. 2019).

> Finally, accelerometer-based handheld navigation has been associated with a shorter learning curve (Kamenaga et al. 2019) and less increased operative time compared to large-console computer navigation.

Ikawa et al. showed an increased operating time of <3 minutes using accelerometer-based navigation compared to an additional 20 minutes for routine computer-assisted TKA (Ikawa et al. 2017). Similarly, Nam et al. showed in a direct comparison of accelerometer handheld navigation with an imageless large-console computer navigation system that these modalities produced similar accuracy but with significantly shorter operating time using the accelerometer navigation (Nam et al. 2013).

69.6 Clinical and Radiographic Outcomes of TKA Using Accelerometer Technology

Since it was released for widespread use, several studies have evaluated the clinical and radiographic outcomes of accelerometer-based technology in TKA.

> In a systematic review of 11 studies comparing conventional with accelerometer-based TKA, the authors noted small benefits in alignment of accelerometer-based TKA in some studies but no difference in functional outcomes, complications, or revisions (Budhiparama et al. 2019).

Goh et al. compared primary TKA using accelerometer-based navigation with conventional techniques as well as large-console computer assistance (Goh et al. 2018). They found fewer radiographic outliers in the navigated groups compared to conventional TKA. They found shorter operative times in the accelerometer and conventional groups compared to large-console navigation. However, there was no difference among any of the groups in the functional outcomes, quality of life measures, or patient satisfaction at 2 years postoperatively.

In one radiographic study of KneeAlign®, Nam et al. noted that among 80 patients who underwent TKA, 96.2% had a tibial cut within 2° of perpendicular to mechanical axis and 94.9% had a femoral cut within 2° perpendicular to mechanical axis (Nam et al. 2013). Similarly, Desseaux et al. showed a neutral mechanical axis and optimal coronal plane alignment in 95% of cases using iAssist® (Desseaux et al. 2016). However, in a prospective randomized controlled trial using KneeAlign®, Gharaibeh et al. found no statistically significant increase in accuracy of achieving a postoperative coronal limb alignment within 3° of neutral alignment in comparison to conventional techniques (Gharaibeh et al. 2016).

In a meta-analysis of 10 studies comparing handheld accelerometer-based navigation vs. conventional techniques for TKA, Shigemura et al. found significantly fewer outliers in the overall mechanical axis alignment and the femoral component coronal alignment when navigation was used. However, there was no difference in coronal alignment of the tibial component between the two groups (Shigemura et al. 2019). This finding is significant given that prior studies citing malalignment as a cause of early TKA failure have shown that the tibial component malalignment is the key mechanism of failure (Ritter et al. 2011; Berend et al. 2004). In a recent study by Shoji et al. using KneeAlign® 2 in 40 cases, there were 0 outliers (>3° from planned resection) in the tibial coronal component angle. However, outliers reached 19% for the sagittal femoral component angle and 9% for the sagittal tibial component angle (Shoji et al. 2018). Thus, these results demonstrated greater accuracy in the coronal than sagittal plane using accelerometer-based navigation.

In many studies using accelerometer-based navigation, tibial alignment has consistently been shown to be slightly more accurate than femoral alignment (Nam et al. 2013; Huang et al. 2015). Fujimoto et al. showed that errors can occur with locating the center of the hip during the registration maneuver, especially with large adduction movements, and thus recommended that surgeons make smaller movements during registration and be aware of the possibility of inaccuracy based on registration (Fujimoto et al. 2016).

Accelerometer-based navigation has also been compared with patient-specific instrumentation (PSI) in a retrospective study by Kawaguchi et al. (Kawaguchi et al. 2017) The authors found that the accelerometer-based navigation was more likely to result in optimal alignment in both the coronal and sagittal planes compared to PSI.

69.7 Future Directions for the Use of Accelerometers in TKA

Long-term outcomes are not yet available to demonstrate the effects of use of accelerometers in TKA.

> Future longitudinal outcome studies are needed to define whether accelerometer-based navigation is able to help decrease long-term complications and revision rates.

Given the potentially increased accuracy of mechanical alignment using this technology, there may be long-term benefits that will be shown on a large population scale. However, future studies are needed to define these potential benefits.

Additional work is needed to define the benefits of accelerometer-based navigation in complex primary and revision settings. With a projected increase in future demand for revision TKA, accelerometers may prove useful in improving revision outcomes. The available literature has demonstrated that accelerometer-based navigation adds minimal time to the operation, which may make it an excellent tool for achieving appropriate alignment in revision TKA.

> Long-term outcome data for TKA using accelerometer-based navigation will also help to define the cost-effectiveness of this technology.

Early studies have shown that computer assistance in knee arthroplasty is potentially cost-effective (Novak et al. 2007), but further work is needed to make this determination. The economics of single-use handheld accelerometer navigation compared to large-console robotic navigation, which may require significantly higher up-front costs, must be critically evaluated.

Finally, it is unknown to what extent alignment parameters influence outcomes in the increasingly popular cementless TKA. Future studies may demonstrate a benefit of accelerometer-based navigation in this setting.

Take-Home Messages

- Accelerometer-based handheld navigation aids in achieving more accurate bony cuts and mechanical alignment compared to conventional techniques.
- Accelerometers have been shown to add less operative time compared to large-console navigation systems.
- No proven difference in clinical outcomes is found between accelerometer-based handheld navigation and conventional techniques.
- Accelerometer-based navigation may prove particularly useful in cases of retained hardware or extra-articular deformity, which would be challenging with conventional TKA techniques.
- Future studies should evaluate this type of technology in complex primary, cementless primary, and revision settings, as well as its cost-effectiveness for TKA.

References

Beldame J, Boisrenoult P, Beaufils P (2010) Pin track induced fractures around computer-assisted TKA. Orthop Traumatol Surg Res 96(3):249–255. https://doi.org/10.1016/j.otsr.2009.12.005

Berend ME, Ritter MA, Meding JB et al (2004) Tibial component failure mechanisms in total knee arthroplasty. Clin Orthop Relat Res 428:26–34. https://doi.org/10.1097/01.blo.0000148578.22729.0e

Blue M, Douthit C, Dennison J, Caroom C, Jenkins M (2018) Periprosthetic fracture through a Unicortical tracking pin site after computer navigated total knee replacement. Case Rep Orthop 2018:2381406. https://doi.org/10.1155/2018/2381406

Budhiparama NC, Lumban-Gaol I, Ifran NN, Parratte S, Nelissen R (2019) Does accelerometer-based navigation have any clinical benefit compared with conventional TKA? A systematic review. Clin Orthop Relat Res 477(9):2017–2029. https://doi.org/10.1097/CORR.0000000000000660

Desseaux A, Graf P, Dubrana F, Marino R, Clavé A (2016) Radiographic outcomes in the coronal plane with iASSIST™ versus optical navigation for total knee arthroplasty: a preliminary case-control study. Orthop Traumatol Surg Res 102(3):363–368. https://doi.org/10.1016/j.otsr.2016.01.018

Fujimoto E, Sasashige Y, Nakata K, Yokota G, Omoto T, Ochi M (2016) Primary arthroplasty technical considerations and accuracy improvement of accelerometer-based portable computer navigation for performing distal femoral resection in total knee arthroplasty. J Arthroplast 32(1):53–60. https://doi.org/10.1016/j.arth.2016.05.067

Gharaibeh MA, Solayar GN, Harris IA, Chen DB, MacDessi SJ (2016) Primary arthroplasty accelerometer-based, portable navigation (KneeAlign) vs conventional instrumentation for total knee arthroplasty: a prospective randomized comparative trial. J Arthroplast. https://doi.org/10.1016/j.arth.2016.08.025

Goh GS-H, Liow MHL, Tay DK-J, Lo N-N, Yeo S-J, Tan M-H (2018) Accelerometer-based and computer-assisted navigation in total knee arthroplasty: a reduction in mechanical Axis outliers does not lead to improvement in functional outcomes or quality of life when compared to conventional total knee arthroplasty. J Arthroplast 33(2):379–385. https://doi.org/10.1016/j.arth.2017.09.005

Huang EH, Copp SN, Bugbee WD (2015) Accuracy of a handheld accelerometer-based navigation system for femoral and Tibial resection in total knee arthroplasty. J Arthroplast 30:1906–1910. https://doi.org/10.1016/j.arth.2015.05.055

Ikawa T, Takemura S, Kim M, Takaoka K, Minoda Y, Kadoya Y (2017) Usefulness of an accelerometer-based portable navigation system in total knee arthroplasty. Bone Joint J 99-B(8):1047–1052. https://doi.org/10.1302/0301-620X.99B8.BJJ-2016-0596.R3

Jacofsky DJ, Allen M (2016) Robotics in arthroplasty: a comprehensive review. J Arthroplast. https://doi.org/10.1016/j.arth.2016.05.026

Jung KA, Lee SC, Ahn NK, Song MB, Nam CH, Shon OJ (2011) Delayed femoral fracture through a tracker pin site after navigated total knee arthroplasty. J Arthroplast 26(3):505.e9–505.e11. https://doi.org/10.1016/j.arth.2010.01.006

Kamenaga T, Hayashi S, Hashimoto S et al (2019) Accuracy of cup orientation and learning curve of the accelerometer-based portable navigation system for total hip arthroplasty in the supine position. J Orthop Surg 27(2):230949901984887. https://doi.org/10.1177/2309499019848871

Kawaguchi K, Michishita K, Manabe T, Akasaka Y, Higuchi J (2017) Comparison of an accelerometer-based portable navigation system, patient-specific instrumentation, and conventional instrumentation for femoral alignment in total knee arthroplasty. Knee Surg Relat Res 29(4):269–275. https://doi.org/10.5792/ksrr.17.032

Lackey WG, Berend ME (2012) Hand-held navigation in total knee arthroplasty. J Bone Joint Surg Br 94(11 Suppl A):151–152. https://doi.org/10.1302/0301-620X.94B11.30831

Mason JB, Fehring TK, Estok R, Banel D, Fahrbach K (2007) Meta-analysis of alignment outcomes in computer-assisted total knee arthroplasty surgery. J Arthroplast 22(8):1097–1106. https://doi.org/10.1016/j.arth.2007.08.001

Matsuda S, Kawahara S, Okazaki K, Tashiro Y, Iwamoto Y (2013) Postoperative alignment and ROM affect patient satisfaction after TKA. Clin Orthop Relat Res 471(1):127–133. https://doi.org/10.1007/s11999-012-2533-y

Mizu-uchi H, Matsuda S, Miura H, Okazaki K, Akasaki Y, Iwamoto Y (2008) The evaluation of post-operative alignment in total knee replacement using a CT-based navigation system. J Bone Joint Surg Br 90-B(8):1025–1031. https://doi.org/10.1302/0301-620X.90B8.20265

Nam D, Dy CJ, Cross MB, Kang MN, Mayman DJ (2012a) Cadaveric results of an accelerometer based, extramedullary navigation system for the tibial resection in total knee arthroplasty. Knee 19(5):617–621. https://doi.org/10.1016/j.knee.2011.09.008

Nam D, Jerabek SA, Cross MB, Mayman DJ (2012b) Cadaveric analysis of an accelerometer-based portable navigation device for distal femoral cutting block alignment in total knee arthroplasty. Comput Aided Surg 17(4):205–210. https://doi.org/10.3109/10929088.2012.689335

Nam D, Weeks KD, Reinhardt KR, Nawabi DH, Cross MB, Mayman DJ (2013) Accelerometer-based, portable navigation vs imageless, large-console computer-assisted navigation in total knee arthroplasty. A comparison of radiographic results. J Arthroplast 28(2):255–261. https://doi.org/10.1016/j.arth.2012.04.023

Novak EJ, Silverstein MD, Bozic KJ (2007) The cost-effectiveness of computer-assisted navigation in total knee arthroplasty. J Bone Joint Surg Am 89(11):2389–2397. https://doi.org/10.2106/JBJS.F.01109

Ritter MA, Faris PM, Keating EM, Meding JB (1994) Postoperative alignment of total knee replacement. Its effect on survival. Clin Orthop Relat Res 299:153–156. http://www.ncbi.nlm.nih.gov/pubmed/8119010. Accessed September 9, 2019

Ritter MA, Davis KE, Meding JB, Pierson JL, Berend ME, Malinzak RA (2011) The effect of alignment and BMI on failure of total knee replacement. J Bone Joint Surg Am 93(17):1588–1596. https://doi.org/10.2106/JBJS.J.00772

Scuderi GR, Fallaha M, Masse V, Lavigne P, Amiot L-P, Berthiaume M-J (2014) Total knee arthroplasty with a novel navigation system within the surgical field. Orthop Clin North Am 45(2):167–173. https://doi.org/10.1016/j.ocl.2013.11.002

Sculco PK, Kahlenberg CA, Fragomen AT, Rozbruch SR (2019) Management of extra-articular deformity in the setting of total knee arthroplasty. J Am Acad Orthop Surg 27(18):1. https://doi.org/10.5435/JAAOS-D-18-00361

Shigemura T, Murata Y, Yamamoto Y, Mizuki N, Toki Y, Wada Y (2019) No definite advantage of a portable accelerometer-based navigation system over conventional technique in total knee arthroplasty: a systematic review and meta-analysis. Orthop Traumatol Surg Res 105:619–626. https://doi.org/10.1016/j.otsr.2019.03.006

Shoji H, Teramoto A, Suzuki T, Okada Y, Watanabe K, Yamashita T (2018) Radiographic assessment and clinical outcomes after total knee arthroplasty using an accelerometer-based portable navigation device. Arthroplast Today 4:319–322. https://doi.org/10.1016/j.artd.2017.11.012

Thomas A, Pemmaraju G, Nagra G, Bassett J, Deshpande S (2015) Complications resulting from tracker pin-sites in computer navigated knee replacement surgery. Acta Orthop Belg 81(4):708–712. http://www.ncbi.nlm.nih.gov/pubmed/26790794. Accessed September 12, 2019

Supplementary Information

E. Hansen, K.-D. Kühn (eds.), *Essentials of Cemented Knee Arthroplasty*,
https://doi.org/10.1007/978-3-662-63113-3

Index

A

B

C

D

E

F

G

H

N

O

P

Q

R

S

T

U

V

W

Y

Z

GPSR Compliance

The European Union's (EU) General Product Safety Regulation (GPSR) is a set of rules that requires consumer products to be safe and our obligations to ensure this.

If you have any concerns about our products, you can contact us on ProductSafety@springernature.com

In case Publisher is established outside the EU, the EU authorized representative is:

Springer Nature Customer Service Center GmbH
Europaplatz 3
69115 Heidelberg, Germany

Batch number: 10731657

Printed by Printforce, the Netherlands